Occupational Therapy *for*
Physical Dysfunction

FIFTH EDITION

Editors

Catherine A. Trombly, ScD, OTR, FAOTA

Professor Emerita Department of Occupational Therapy
Sargent College of Health and Rehabilitation Sciences
Boston University
Boston, Massachusetts

Mary Vining Radomski, MA, OTR, FAOTA

Coordinator, Rehabilitation Outcomes, Quality, and Clinical Research
Occupational Therapist, Brain Injury Program
Sister Kenny Rehabilitation Services
Minneapolis, Minnesota

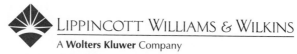

LIPPINCOTT WILLIAMS & WILKINS
A **Wolters Kluwer** Company
Philadelphia • Baltimore • New York • London
Buenos Aires • Hong Kong • Sydney • Tokyo

Editor: Timothy L. Julet
Managing Editor: Linda S. Napora
Marketing Manager: Debby Hartman
Production Editor: Paula C. Williams
Compositor: Graphic World, Inc.
Printer: Quebecor-World

351 West Camden Street
Baltimore, Maryland 21201-2436 USA

530 Walnut Street
Philadelphia, Pennsylvania 19106-3621 USA

The publisher is not responsible (as a matter of product liability, negligence, or otherwise) for any injury resulting from any material contained herein. This publication contains information relating to general principles of medical care which should not be construed as specific instructions for individual patients. Manufacturers' product information and package inserts should be reviewed for current information, including contraindications, dosages, and precautions.

Printed in the United States of America

Library of Congress Cataloging-in-Publication Data
Occupational therapy for physical dysfunction / editors, Catherine A. Trombly, Mary Vining Radomski.— 5th ed.
    p. cm.
  Includes bibliographical references and index.
  ISBN 0-7817-2461-9
    1. Occupational therapy. 2. Physically handicapped—Rehabilitation.   I. Trombly, Catherine Anne.   II. Radomski, Mary Vining.

RM735 .O33 2001
615.8′515—dc21

               2001029671

The publishers have made every effort to trace the copyright holders for borrowed material. If they have inadvertently overlooked any, they will be pleased to make the necessary arrangements at the first opportunity.

To purchase additional copies of this book call our customer service department at **(800) 638-3030** or fax orders to **(301) 824-7390**. International customers should call **(301) 714-2324.**

Visit Lippincott Williams & Wilkins on the Internet: **http://www.lww.com.** Lippincott Williams & Wilkins customer service representatives are available from 8:30 am to 6:00 pm, EST, Monday through Friday, for telephone access.

01 02 03
1 2 3 4 5 6 7 8 9 10

To the occupational therapists, persons with physical dysfunction, and students who taught me in the past and to the therapists of the future and the patients they will serve.

Catherine A. Trombly

To Virginia E. Vining, who embodies rich and robust occupational functioning and who is proud of her three daughters no matter what.

Mary Vining Radomski

Preface

*T*his textbook is written for the professional-level student and as a resource for experienced therapists. Although the *Fifth Edition* has undergone major revision, it continues to emphasize that practice should be based on a conceptual foundation. The premise is that the goal of occupational therapy is to enable patients and clients to recover occupational role performance to the greatest extent possible so they can be in control of their lives and enjoy the concomitant sense of self-efficacy. The *Fifth Edition* is organized around this premise, using the language of the Model of Occupational Functioning, that is, restoring competence in life roles and optimizing abilities, capacities, context, and environment to enable that competence. This model incorporates respect for the individuality of each person by promoting a collaborative approach to reestablishing role competency rather than an expert-driven, prescriptive emphasis on impairment.

Three aspects of the *Fifth Edition* immediately draw attention. First, Mary Vining Radomski joins me as coeditor for this edition. Mary brings a wealth of knowledge about occupational therapy for persons with acquired brain damage, experience in writing for the profession, and her vantage point as chairperson of AOTA's Physical Disabilities Special Interest Section. Second, the publisher is now Lippincott Williams & Wilkins, and it has been a pleasure to work with both the new Lippincott personnel and our familiar coworkers from Williams & Wilkins. Third, the look is new. A second color has been used to emphasize teaching points. Procedures and lengthy definitions have been boxed to facilitate learning.

The goals for writing this textbook more than 25 years ago are preserved in this edition. Those goals were the transmission of current information on the evaluation and treatment of adults with occupational dysfunction secondary to physical impairment and the presentation of the material within a conceptual frame-work. The scientific basis for practice, including evidence to support choice of assessments and intervention decisions, continues to be emphasized. In addition, the *Fifth Edition* has these two goals:

1. To place proper emphasis on therapy that acknowledges the context or environment as enabler or barrier to occupational functioning, in keeping with the greater emphasis on these in contemporary models of health.
2. To model task analysis, problem formulation, and treatment planning through expanded and more numerous case examples. Opportunities for practice of the reasoning processes that are essential to the practice of occupational therapy are offered throughout.

The *Fifth Edition* consists of six sections with 48 chapters. These sections are organized as follows:

Section I describes the historical and social influences on the current practice of occupational therapy for those with physical impairment. This section also lays the foundation for the rest of the textbook and the theoretical foundation for practice by introducing the Model of Occupational Functioning.

Section II presents the areas of assessment for which an occupational therapist working with adults with occupational dysfunction secondary to physical impairment is responsible. The chapters in this section begin with assessment of the person's occupational roles and competence of performance in those roles and follow with assessment of the person's abilities and capacities that support role performance and of the environmental and contextual constraints and enablers of performance.

Section III presents three mechanisms of therapeutic change: occupation, learning, and therapeutic rapport.

Section IV presents therapeutic technologies that enable and support occupational functioning: splinting, wheelchairs, adapted or assistive devices, and physical agent modalities.

Section V elucidates treatment principles and practices of therapy for persons with physical dysfunction, including documentation of practice, so important in current health care practice. As in earlier editions, this section does not provide recipes for the treatment of persons with particular diagnoses but rather descriptions of best practice. The professional occupational therapist can choose from these for a particular patient who has his or her own particular goals and manifestation of a diagnosis.

Section VI includes discussions of the practice of occupational therapy for particular major diagnostic categories written by specialists. These experts alert therapists who are beginning to practice with one of these populations to the various commonly encountered impairments that affect occupational functioning and to the specialized assessments and treatments developed for persons carrying the diagnosis.

This text is meant to be used by learners who have knowledge gained in previous courses. Before studying assessment and treatment of persons with neurological trauma or disease, the reader should understand neuroanatomy, neurophysiology, motor science, and clinical neurological disorders. Knowledge of anatomy, physiology, kinesiology, biomechanics, and clinical orthopaedic and general medical disorders is needed before studying assessment and treatment of persons with trauma or disease to their musculoskeletal, cardiopulmonary, or integumentary systems. Other prerequisites include construction skills needed for making splints and adaptations and ability to do the occupations that the therapist will need to use as occupation-as-means and occupation-as-end in the treatment of clients.

Fifty-four outstanding clinical and academic occupational therapists and experienced lay persons contributed to this edition. Each did so with the desire to contribute to the profession of occupational therapy by sharing their knowledge and skills with occupational therapists preparing to practice in this new century.

Catherine A. Trombly
Mary Vining Radomski

Acknowledgments

I am grateful to the Gracious Author of my story for plans, challenges, and opportunities that I alone could not have orchestrated or completed. Thanks also to Jim, Lauren, and Allison, who cheered me along and then loaded the dishwasher. I appreciate the tutelage of many of the textbook's authors and Linda Napora at Lippincott Williams & Wilkins, who patiently worked with this apprentice. Finally, thank you to Catherine A. Trombly for inviting me aboard.

M. V. R.

Contributors

Jennifer Angelo, PhD, OTR, FAOTA, ATP
Department of Rehabilitation Science and Technology
University of Pittsburgh
Pittsburgh, Pennsylvania

Michal S. Atkins, MA, OTR
Clinical Specialist
Spinal Cord Injury Service
Rancho Los Amigos National Rehabilitation Center
Downey, California

Wendy Avery-Smith, MS, OTR/L
Occupational Therapist
Whittier Rehabilitation Hospital
Haverhill, Massachusetts
Professional Associate
Department of Rehabilitation Medicine
New York Presbyterian Hospital
New York Weill Cornell Center
New York, New York

Julie Bass-Haugen, PhD, OTR
Associate Professor and Chair
Department of Occupational Therapy
College of St. Catherine
St. Paul, Minnesota

Jane Bear-Lehman, PhD, OTR, FAOTA
Assistant Professor of Clinical Occupational Therapy
Programs in Occupational Therapy
College of Physicians and Surgeons
Columbia University
New York, New York

Karen S. Bentzel, MS, OTR/L
Clinical Lecturer
Department of Occupational Therapy
Elizabethtown College
Elizabethtown, Pennsylvania

Bette R. Bonder, PhD, OTR/L, FAOTA
Professor
Department of Health Sciences and Psychology
Cleveland State University
Cleveland, Ohio

Alfred G. Bracciano, EdD, OTR
Director and Professor
Department of Occupational Therapy
Saginaw Valley State University
University Center, Michigan

Mary Ellen Buning, MS, OTR, ATP
Research Associate
Department of Rehabilitation Science and Technology
University of Pittsburgh
Pittsburgh, Pennsylvania

Nancy Callinan, MA, OTR, CHT
Supervisor, Hand Therapy
Park Nicollet Clinic
St. Louis Park, Minnesota

Felice Gadaleta Celikyol, MA, OTR, FAOTA
Formerly Director
Occupational Therapy Services
Kessler Institute for Rehabilitation, Inc.
West Orange, New Jersey

Barbara Acheson Cooper, MHSc, PhD, OT(C)
Professor
School of Rehabilitation Science
Institute of Applied Health Sciences
McMaster University
Hamilton, Ontario, Canada

Cynthia Cooper, MFA, MA, OTR/L, CHT
Hand Therapist and Out-Patient Team Lead
Mayo Clinic Hospital
Phoenix, Arizona
Assistant Professor
Department of Physical Medicine and Rehabilitation
Mayo Medical School
Rochester, Minnesota

Lois F. Copperman, PhD, OTR/L
Occupational Therapist
Department of Rehabilitation
Department of Neurology
Oregon Health Sciences University
Portland, Oregon

Elin Schold Davis, OTR/L, CDRS
Lead Therapist
Outpatient Brain Injury Clinic
Program in Advanced Rehabilitation Technologies
Sister Kenny Institute
Minneapolis, Minnesota

Jean C. Deitz, PhD, OTR, FAOTA
Professor and Coordinator of Graduate Programs
Division of Occupational Therapy
Department of Rehabilitation Medicine
University of Washington
Seattle, Washington

Lisa D. Deshaies, OTR, CHT
Clinical Specialist
Department of Occupational Therapy
Rancho Los Amigos National Rehabilitation Center
Downey, California

Brian J. Dudgeon, PhD, OTR/L
Lecturer, Division of Occupational Therapy
Department of Rehabilitation Medicine
University of Washington
Seattle, Washington

Donald W. Earley, MA, OTR
Assistant Professor
Occupational Therapy Program
Saginaw Valley State University
University Center, Michigan

Susan E. Fasoli, ScD, OTR/L
Post-Doctoral Fellow
Department of Mechanical Engineering
Massachusetts Institute of Technology
Cambridge, Massachusetts

Nancy A. Flinn, MA, OTR, BCN
Assistant Professor
College of St. Catherine
Staff Therapist
Allina Home Care and Hospice
St. Paul, Minnesota

Susan Jane Forwell, MA, OT(C)
Senior Instructor
Division of Occupational Therapy
School of Rehabilitation Sciences
University of British Columbia
Vancouver, British Columbia

Glenn Goodman, PhD, OTR
Associate Professor
Occupational Therapy Program
Cleveland State University
Cleveland, Ohio

Julie McLaughlin Gray, MA, OTR
Instructor of Clinical Occupational Therapy
Department of Occupational Science and Occupational Therapy
University of Southern California
Los Angeles, California

Carolyn Schmidt Hanson, PhD, OTR
Assistant Professor
Department of Occupational Therapy
University of Florida
Gainesville, Florida

Lucinda L. Hugos, MS, PT
Physical Therapist
Department of Rehabilitation
Department of Neurology
Oregon Health Sciences University
Portland, Oregon

Nancy E. Huntley, OTR, CES
Department of Rehabilitation Services
Fairview Southdale Hospital
Edina, Minnesota

Jeanne Jackson, PhD, OTR
Associate Professor
Department of Occupational Science and Occupational
    Therapy
University of Southern California
Los Angeles, California

Douglas D. Jones, JD, MEd
Director
Center for Student Leadership and Activities
Santa Fe Community College
Gainesville, Florida

Theodore I. King, II, PhD, OT, FAOTA
Associate Professor
Occupational Therapy Department
University of Wisconsin—Milwaukee
Milwaukee, Wisconsin

Mary Law, PhD, OT(C)
Professor
School of Rehabilitation Science
Department of Clinical Epidemiology and Biostatistics
McMaster University
Research Associate
Department of Occupational Therapy
Chedoke-McMaster Hospitals
Hamilton, Ontario, Canada

Lori Letts, PhD (ABD), OT(C)
Assistant Professor
School of Rehabilitation Science
McMaster University
Hamilton, Ontario, Canada

Kathryn Levit, MA, OTR
Making Progress
Alexandria, Virginia

Jaclyn Faglie Low, PhD, OTR, FAOTA
Associate Professor and Associate Dean
School of Occupational Therapy
Texas Women's University—Houston Center
Houston, Texas

Lieutenant Colonel Stephen Luster, MS, OTR/L, CHT
Chief, Occupational Therapy
Brooke Army Medical Center
Fort Sam Houston,
San Antonio, Texas

Virgil Mathiowetz, PhD, OTR, FAOTA
Associate Professor
Program in Occupational Therapy
Department of Physical Medicine and Rehabilitation
University of Minnesota
Minneapolis, Minnesota

Amy C. Orroth, OTR/L, CHT
Senior Burn Therapist
Massachusetts General Hospital
Boston, Massachusetts

Monica A. Pessina, MEd, OTR,
Doctoral student
Department of Anatomy and Neurobiology
Boston University
School of Medicine
Boston, Massachusetts

Susan L. Pierce, OTR, CDRS
President
Adaptive Mobility Services, Inc.
Orlando, Florida

Carolyn Robinson Podolski, MS, OTR/L
Clinical Assistant Professor
Department of Occupational Therapy
Sargent College of Health and Rehabilitation Sciences
Boston University
Boston, Massachusetts

Lee Ann Quintana, MS, OTR
Preferred Rehabilitation Services
Albuquerque Manor
Albuquerque, New Mexico

Mary Vining Radomski, MA, OTR, FAOTA
Coordinator, Rehabilitation Outcomes, Quality, and
    Clinical Research
Occupational Therapist, Brain Injury Program
Sister Kenny Rehabilitation Services
Minneapolis, Minnesota

Colonel Valerie J. Rice, PhD, CPE, OTR/L, FAOTA
Director, Operation Aegis—Injury Control
U.S. Army Medical Department Center and School
Fort Sam Houston
San Antonio, Texas

Patricia Rigby, MHSc, OT(C)
Assistant Professor
Department of Occupational Therapy
Faculty of Medicine
University of Toronto
Professional Advisor
Bloorview McMillan Children's Centre
Toronto, Ontario

Joyce Shapero Sabari, PhD, OTR, BCN
Associate Professor and Chair
Occupational Therapy Program
State University of New York
Downstate Medical Center
Brooklyn, New York

Shoshana Shamberg, OTR/L, MSEd
President
Abilities Occupational Therapy Services, Inc.
Accessibility and Independent Living Consultant
Baltimore, Maryland

Jo M. Solet, EdM, PhD, OTR/L
Clinical Instructor in Psychology
Department of Psychiatry
Harvard Medical School and
Behavioral Medicine Program
Cambridge Health Alliance
Cambridge, Massachusetts

Debra Stewart, MSc, OT(C)
Assistant Clinical Professor
School of Rehabilitation Science
McMaster University
Hamilton, Ontario, Canada

Susan Strong, MSc, OT(C)
Assistant Clinical Professor
Work Function Unit
School of Rehabilitation Science
McMaster University
Hamilton, Ontario, Canada

Linda Tickle-Degnen, PhD, OTR/L, FAOTA
Associate Professor
Department of Occupational Therapy
Sargent College of Health and Rehabilitation Sciences
Boston University
Boston, Massachusetts

Catherine A. Trombly, ScD, OTR/L, FAOTA
Professor Emerita
Department of Occupational Therapy
Sargent College of Health and Rehabilitation Sciences
Boston University
Boston, Massachusetts

Anne M. Woodson, OTR
Occupational Therapist III
Department of Occupational Therapy
University of Texas Medical Branch
Galveston, Texas

Y. Lynn Yasuda, MSEd, OTR, FAOTA
Education Specialist
Education and Staff Development
Rancho Los Amigos National Rehabilitation Center
Downey, California

Ruth Zemke, PhD, OTR, FAOTA
Professor and Post-Professional Programs Coordinator
Department of Occupational Science and Occupational
     Therapy
University of Southern California
Los Angeles, California

Contents

1

Conceptual Foundations for Practice

Catherine A. Trombly

LEARNING OBJECTIVES

After studying this chapter, the reader will be able to do the following:

1. Describe the Occupational Functioning Model.
2. State the similarities and differences in definitions among the Occupational Functioning Model, the American Occupational Therapy Association (AOTA) Uniform Terminology, and the World Health Organization's International Classification of Functioning, Disability and Health (ICIDH-2).
3. Define and give examples of the levels of the Occupational Functioning Model.
4. Organize assessment and treatment planning according to the Occupational Functioning Model.

*H*ow do occupational therapists know what to do when a person with **occupational dysfunction** secondary to a disease or injury that results in physical impairment is referred to them? First, they have *specific knowledge* about what the diagnosis means in terms of limitations of bodily structure or function and limitation of engagement in activities, and they know the outcome of research on the effectiveness of treatments available. Second, they have *specific skills* for assessing and treating persons with occupational dysfunction secondary to physical impairment. Third, they know *how therapy is organized*.

The organization of occupational therapy is found in various conceptual models of practice. A model of practice guides therapy to convert states of occupational dysfunction to states of occupational function. It guides data gathering, interpretation, and treatment planning. It specifies the types of intervention used to restore occupational performance and provides a scaffold for creative problem solving within the ongoing therapeutic situation (Kielhofner, 1997). There are several models from which the therapist may choose (Box 1-1). One model, the **Occupational Functioning Model**, is described here.

GLOSSARY

Ability—Competence in doing; ability to use knowledge effectively and readily in performance (Mish, 1989). A general trait an individual brings to learning a new task (Fleishman, 1972).

Activity, activities—In the OFM, activities are smaller units of behavior that make up tasks. The behavior accomplishes a functional goal. In the ICIDH-2, activity is defined as the nature and extent of functioning at the level of the person and includes everything a person does at any level of complexity from basic physical and mental functions of the person as a whole (e.g. acquisition of knowledge or grasp) to complex skills and behavior (e.g. driving a car or interacting with persons in formal settings) (World Health Organization, 2000). AOTA (1997) defines purposeful activity as goal-directed behaviors or tasks that the individual considers meaningful.

Activity analysis—A process used to identify the properties inherent in a given occupation, task, or activity, as well as the skills, abilities, and capacities required to complete it. Activity analysis is used to select an activity to remediate deficient capacities and abilities or, knowing the person's skills, abilities, and capacities, to ensure successful completion of the activity or to motivate engagement in activity.

Adaptive therapy—Therapy that promotes a balance among a person's goals, capabilities, and environmental demands by use of assistive technology, adaptation of the environment or methods of accomplishing an activity, and/or redefinition of goals.

Augmented maturation—Therapeutic techniques that use controlled sensory stimulation and activities that promote responses in developmental sequences to develop first-level capacities or developed capacities.

Capacities—Potential attributes that, once developed into abilities and skills, will contribute to occupational functioning. Capacities are the basis of performance.

Context—The interrelated conditions in which something exists or occurs (Mish, 1989). In health care, context refers to the whole situation, background, or environment that is relevant to a particular event or personality. In this sense, context has personal, social, cultural, and physical dimensions. In movement science, context is a more circumscribed concept that refers to the immediate physical and social constraints of action.

Environment—The complex of external factors, circumstances, objects, or conditions by which one is surrounded. The aggregate of social and cultural conditions that influence the life of an individual (Mish, 1989).

Impairment—Any loss or abnormality of body structure or of a physiological or psychological function (World Health Organization, 2000).

Occupation-as-end—Occupation is the functional goal (activity, task) to be learned. Its therapeutic impact comes from its characteristics of purpose and meaning (Trombly, 1995a). Example: learning to put on a blouse by a person who has had a stroke.

Occupation-as-means—Occupation that is "therapeutically constructed everyday activities" (Wood, 1998, p. 405) used as the therapeutic change agent to remediate impaired abilities or capacities. Its therapeutic effect derives from characteristics of purpose and meaning (Trombly, 1995a). Also termed therapeutic occupation (Fisher, 1998). Example: peeling a carrot to develop gross grasp by a person who likes to cook.

Occupational dysfunction—Inability to maintain one's self, that is, care for self, dependents, and home; to advance oneself through work, learning, and financial management; or to enhance the self by engaging in self-actualizing activities that add enjoyment to life.

Occupational Functioning Model—A conceptual model that guides occupational therapy evaluation and treatment of persons with physical dysfunction. The propositions of the model: (1) To engage satisfactorily in a life role, a person must be able to do the tasks that in his opinion make up that role. (2) Tasks are composed of activities, which are small units of behavior. (3) To be able to do a given activity, one must have certain sensorimotor, cognitive, perceptual, emotional, and social abilities. (4) Abilities are developed from capacities that the person has gained through learning or maturation. (5) These developed capacities depend on first-level capacities that derive from a person's genetic endowment or spared organic substrate (Trombly, 1993, 1995a).

Participation—The nature and extent of a person's involvement in life situations in relation to impairments, activities, health conditions, and contextual factors (World Health Organization, 2000). A fundamental property of participation is the complex interaction between a person with impairment and/or disability and the context (World Health Organization, 2000). Participation consists of all areas or aspects of human life, including full experience of being involved in a practice, custom or social behavior (World Health Organization, 2000).

Performance area—Broad category of human activities that are typically part of daily life (AOTA, 1994).

Performance components—Fundamental human abilities that are required, in varying degrees and in differing combinations, for successful engagement in performance areas (AOTA, 1994).

BOX 1-1
Occupational Therapy Conceptual and Practice Models Appropriate for Use With Persons With Physical Dysfunction

- ▶ Appraisal method of coping (Gage, 1992).
- ▶ Ecology of human performance (Dunn et al., 1994).
- ▶ Life Style Performance Model (Fidler, 1996).
- ▶ Model of human occupation (MOHO) (Kielhofner & Burke, 1980; Kielhofner, 1995).
- ▶ Occupational adaptation (Schkade & Schultz, 1992; Schultz & Schkade, 1992).
- ▶ Occupational Functioning Model (Trombly, 1993, 1995a).
- ▶ Occupational Performance Model (Baum & Law, 1997).
- ▶ Occupational Performance Process Model (Fearing et al., 1997).
- ▶ Occupational Therapy Intervention Process Model (Fisher, 1998).
- ▶ Person–Environment–Occupation Model (Law et al., 1996).
- ▶ Person–Environment Occupational Performance Model (Christiansen & Baum, 1997).

The Occupational Functioning Model

One assumption of the Occupational Functioning Model (OFM) is that people strive to achieve feelings of satisfaction, defined here as a sense of self-efficacy and self-esteem. Self-efficacy and self-esteem derive from being in charge of one's own life, being competent in one's life roles. Research partially supports the idea that competency is related to satisfaction. For example, of 30 persons with multiple sclerosis who were studied by Lundmark and Bränholm (1996), those who were satisfied with life were significantly more independent in self-care and housekeeping and engaged in more leisure activities than those who were not. Furthermore, actual performance has been found to strengthen efficacy beliefs in older adults (Resnik, 1998).

Another assumption of the OFM is that the ability to carry out one's roles and activities of life depends on basic abilities and capacities (e.g., strength, perception, ability to sequence information). This hierarchical organization assumes that lower-level capacities and abilities are related to a higher-level functioning. This organization has been preliminarily supported in a study of patients with spinal cord injury (Dijkers, 1999). It appears from that research that the relationship between two adjacent levels is stronger than between two nonadjacent levels. The relationship between levels is strong both at the low end of the model (Pendlebury et al., 1999) and at the high end (Dijkers, 1997, 1999), but there is a multivariate relationship between lower levels of the model and higher levels of functioning. The relationship is not as simple as depicted in Figure 1-1. No single

activity accounts for role performance. Many capacities contribute to development of one ability, and many abilities are needed to engage successfully in an activity. When one capacity or ability is impaired, occupational dysfunction does not automatically occur (Rogers & Holm, 1994; Rondinelli et al., 1997). Other capacities and abilities may adaptively adjust to allow accomplishment of the activity.

Research is needed to clarify the multivariate relationships among lower-level abilities and capacities and higher-level activities, tasks, and roles (Trombly, 1993, 1995a). Bivariate relationships between ability and function have been examined; however, as suggested earlier, only part of the variance associated with function is accounted for by one ability. For example, Lynch and Bridle (1989) found a moderately strong ($r = -0.65$, $p < .01$) relationship between the scores of the *Jebsen-Taylor Hand Function Test* (Jebsen et al., 1969) and the scores of the *Klein–Bell ADL* [activities of daily living] *Scale* (Klein & Bell, 1982). The negative correlation occurs because the lower the score (time) on the *Jebsen-Taylor*, the better the performance; while the

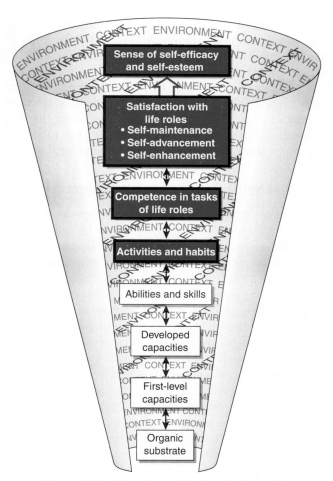

Figure 1-1 Paradigm of occupational functioning model.

higher the score on the *Klein–Bell*, the better the performance. Filiatrault et al. (1991) found a similar relationship ($r = 0.6$) between the *Fugl-Meyer Motor Function Test* (upper extremity subtest) (Fugl-Meyer et al., 1975) and the *Barthel Index* (ADL) (Mahoney & Barthel, 1965). These outcomes do indicate that sensorimotor control of the upper extremities is related to self-care. But because the r^2 value is only approximately 40%, other unidentified variables account for the remaining 60% variance associated with ADL. This makes sense because in addition to upper extremity function, ADL independence requires such skills as sitting and standing balance, perception of positions of objects in space, and ability to sequence steps of a procedure.

Researchers also must verify whether remediation of impaired capacities and abilities results in more complete and more versatile participation in the activities and tasks of importance to people's lives than learning specific routines of activities in an adapted way. This is a key question for the practice of occupational therapy with persons having physical dysfunction. Thorndike (1924) addressed the question for education and concluded, "The best way to develop knowledge or skill in any subject area is to study that subject" (Mayer et al., p. 219). Similar conclusions are emerging concerning motor skill learning (Marteniuk et al., 1987; Trombly & Wu, 1999). But the actual test of relative therapeutic effectiveness has not been done.

Another assumption of the OFM is that satisfactory occupational functioning occurs only within environmental and contextual constraints particular to the individual. The constructs of the occupational functioning model shown in Figure 1-1 are described next.

Sense of Self-Efficacy and Self-Esteem

The goal of occupational therapy is the development of competence, which promotes a sense of self-efficacy and self-esteem. Competence refers to effective interaction with the physical and social **environments** (Fig. 1-2). To be competent means to have the skills to be sufficient or adequate to meet the demands of a situation or task (White, 1959). It does not equate to excellence, normality, or the ability to do everything, and it recognizes that there are degrees of sufficiency and adequacy in people (Mocellin, 1992; White, 1971). The sense of competence allows people to believe in their own control rather than being controlled by the social or physical environments (Trombly, 1993). Competence develops by enabling a person to engage in graduated, goal-directed activity that is accomplishable by that person and produces a feeling of satisfaction (White, 1959). Occupational therapists help people achieve competence through occupation, developmental and instrumental learning, and therapeutic interaction with the therapist.

When people feel competent, they are likely to esteem themselves. Self-esteem is that aspect of self-concept that attributes a negative or positive value to the self. Self-esteem is created by individuals' analysis of their competency in socially relevant areas (Gage & Polatajko, 1994). People's level of self-esteem depends on their confidence, based on experience, that they can make desired things happen and that others will appreciatively recognize this competence (White, 1971).

Efficacy, as it is used in the OFM, refers both to Bandura's (1977) concepts of perceived self-efficacy and outcome expectancy and Rogers' (1983) concept of response efficacy. Perceived self-efficacy refers to people's beliefs in their performance capabilities with respect to a specific task (Bandura, 1977; Gage et al., 1994; Resnik, 1998). It is concerned not with the skills one possesses but with the judgments of what one can do with those skills. Perceived self-efficacy is influenced through an ongoing evaluation of success and failure with each task people participate in over the course of their lives (Gage & Polatajko, 1994). Response efficacy and outcome expectancy refer to a judgment of the consequences that certain behavior will produce

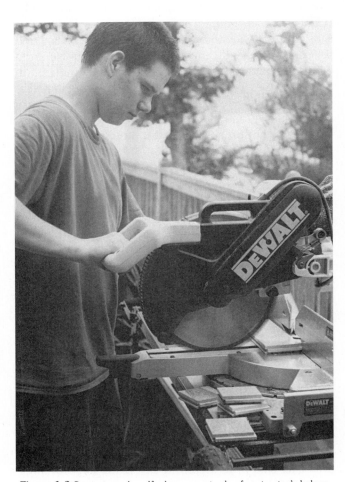

Figure 1-2 Competency in self-advancement role of contractor's helper.

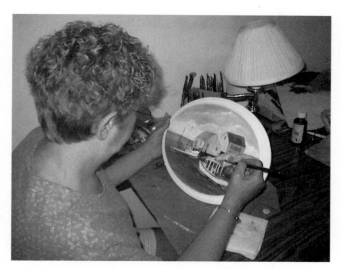

Figure 1-3 Accomplished artist painting a picture.

(Resnik, 1998). It is the individual's judgment of how effective his or her responses to cope with a given problem will be (Rogers, 1983). The most powerful source of efficacy expectations is past accomplishments in similar situations (Fig. 1-3).

Satisfaction With Life Roles

A sense of efficacy is derived from being in control of one's life. This means being able to engage satisfyingly in one's life roles or to voluntarily reassign a role to another. Roles are socially expected behavior patterns associated with an individual's status in a particular society (Mish, 1989). The role of independent person is highly prized by most people in North American

cultures, but is not in other cultures, for example, the Maori, and therapists must be sensitive to cultural differences (Hocking, 1998). Various thinkers have proposed taxonomies of roles. For example, Reilly (1962) categorized occupational roles according to gender and age, identifying four: preschooler, student, housewife or paid worker, and retiree. She saw play and work roles on a continuum. Kielhofner (1995) elaborated on Reilly's work and defined three roles: play, ADL, and work. Fidler (1996) defined four domains: self-care and self-maintenance, intrinsic gratification, social contribution, and interpersonal relatedness. The OFM sorts roles into three domains related to aspects of self-definition: self-maintenance, self-advancement, and self-enhancement (Trombly, 1993, 1995a).

Assignment of roles to a particular category is not absolute. Some roles may be classified in one domain by one person but in another domain by another person, depending on the motivation. For example, volunteering may be classified by one person as a self-advancement role because volunteering promotes skills that will be useful in a worker role. Another may classify volunteering as self-enhancement because it promotes a sense of satisfaction without expectation of gain. The individuality of motivation underscores the importance of assessing each person from his or her own point of view, letting each define his or her roles and their meaning.

Self-Maintenance Roles

Self-maintenance roles are associated with development and maintenance of the self, including family and home. This domain exceeds AOTA's (1994) **performance area** of ADL (Table 1-1) to include care of home and

---

> **TABLE 1-1**
> **Occupational Functioning Model Related to AOTA's Uniform Terminology, 3rd edition, 1994**

Occupational Functioning Model	AOTA Terminology
Self-efficacy and self-esteem	No corresponding term
Satisfaction with life roles	Performance areas
Self-maintenance	Activities of daily living
Self-advancement	Work and productive activities
Self-enhancement	Play and leisure activities
Competence in tasks of life roles	
Activities and habits	
Abilities and skills	**Performance Components**: the elements that make up or
Developed capacities	provide the ability to do activities (Moyers, 1999).
First-level capacities	
Organic substrate	No corresponding term
Environment and context: the milieu in which occupation occurs, including natural and built physical environments, tools and utensils, social relationships, cultural situations, and time.	Performance contexts: the situations or factors that may influence the client's ability to perform a task. May be temporal, physical, social, cultural, or environmental (AOTA, 1994; Moyers, 1999).

family. Examples of roles in this domain are independent person, grandparent, parent, son, daughter, homemaker (Fig. 1-4), home maintainer (Fig. 1-5), exerciser, and caregiver.

Self-Advancement Roles

Self-advancement roles are those that draw the person into productive community activities and add to the person's skills, possessions, or other betterment. This domain corresponds to the **participation** category of the ICIDH-2 (Table 1-2) and to the AOTA occupational performance area of work and productive activity (Table 1-1) but extends that to include the instrumental roles that enable work. Examples of roles in this domain include worker (Figs. 1-2 and 1-6), student, intern, commuter, shopper, investor, manager, and voter.

Self-Enhancement Roles

Self-enhancement roles contribute to the person's sense of accomplishment and enjoyment (Figs. 1-3 and 1-7). This domain loosely corresponds to AOTA's (1994) occupational performance area of play and leisure (Table 1-1) and fits within the ICIDH-2 category of participation (Table 1-2). Examples of roles in this domain include hobbyist, friend, club member, parishioner, vacationer, golfer, moviegoer, and violinist.

Competency in Tasks of Life Roles

Roles consist of constellations of tasks. For example, the role of homemaker may include the tasks of food preparation (Fig. 1-4) and service, housecleaning, laundry, and decorating (Fig. 1-5). The tasks identified for the same role by different people may be different (Nelson & Payton, 1991; Trombly, 1993, 1995a; Yerxa & Locker, 1990). The value ascribed to tasks varies among people of similar situations and may vary from what therapists consider important for patients. Because people have different values, each person must define his or her role by identifying the tasks that he or she believes are crucial to satisfactory engagement in that particular role. The therapist cannot assume that particular tasks are or are not important to a person's interpretation of a role.

Tasks consist of constellations of related activities and are therapeutically developed using **occupation-as-end**, that is, practicing the activities constituting the task in normal temporal order and environmental demand, with or without assistive technology as required.

Activities and Habits

Activities, in this context, are smaller units of behavior that comprise tasks (Figs. 1-2–1-7). Activities bring to-

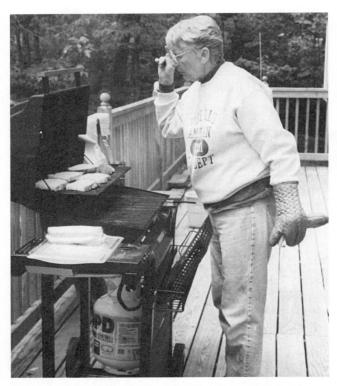

Figure 1-4 Self-maintenance role: homemaker; task: meal preparation; activity: grilling fish.

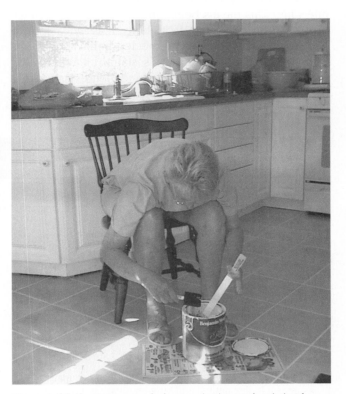

Figure 1-5 Self-maintenance role: home maintainer; task: painting the walls; activity: preparing the paint.

TABLE 1-2

Occupational Functioning Model Related to the World Health Organization ICIDH-2 Classification (World Health Organization, 2000)

Occupational Functioning Model	ICIDH-2
Self-efficacy and self-esteem	No corresponding term

Satisfaction with life roles
    Self-maintenance
    Self-advancement
    Self-enhancement
	Participation: the nature and extent of a person's involvement in life situations. The interaction between a person having a disability and/or impairment with contextual factors.

Competence in tasks of life roles Activities and habits Abilities and skills Developed capacities	**Activity**: nature and extent of functioning at the level of the person. All that a person does at any level of complexity.
First-level capacities Organic substrate	Bodily structure and psychological and physiological function
Environment and context: the milieu in which occupation occurs, including natural and built physical environments, tools and utensils, social relationships, cultural situations, and time.	Contextual factors: complete background to a person's life and living, including both external environmental factors [a] and internal personal factors.[b]

[a]Natural environment (weather or terrain), human-made environment (tools, furnishings, the built environment), social attitudes, customs, rules, practices and institutions, and other individuals.
[b]Age, race, gender, educational background, experiences, personality, and character style, aptitudes, fitness, lifestyle, habits, upbringing, coping styles, social background, profession, and experience.

gether abilities and skills within a functional context. For example, one task of the gardener is pest control. Activities that make up this task include hanging lures, spreading granular insect killer, mixing and spraying liquids, and picking insects off plants. Furthermore, each of these activities consists of smaller units of behavior, such as opening the package and pouring granular insect killer into a garden spreader. Some activities, such as picking insects off plants, require full attention. Others, called habits, do not. Habits are chains of subroutines that are so well learned that the person does not have to pay attention to do them under ordinary circumstances and in familiar contexts. Occupational therapy seeks to help the person sustain adaptive habits, let go of habits that are no longer adaptive, and develop new habits, given the person's changed abilities and capacities.

Activities and habits are learned using occupation-as-end. Functional and meaningful activities are practiced using assistive technology, adaptive methods, or adapted environment to enable performance.

Abilities and Skills

Activities depend on more basic abilities (Clark et al., 1990; Fleishman, 1972; Fleishman & Quaintance, 1984; Kielhofner, 1997). A person with a great number of highly developed abilities can become proficient at a

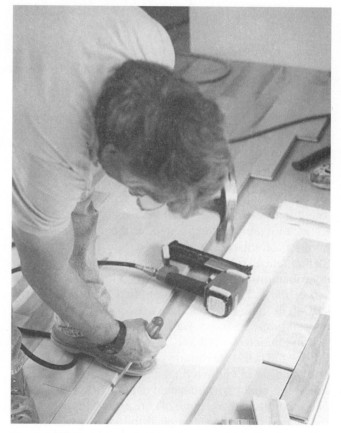

Figure 1-6 Self-advancement role: contractor; task: installing floor; activity: moving the wood into place.

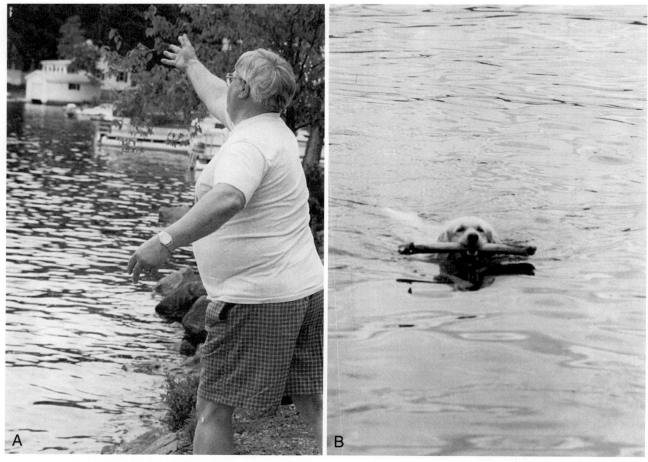

Figure 1-7 **A.** Self-enhancement role: pet owner; task: exercise dog; activity: throw the stick. **B.** Molly with stick.

greater variety of activities. An **ability** is a general trait, such as muscle strength or certain actions that individuals bring with them when they begin to learn a new task (Fleishman, 1972). Actions such as reaching, stooping, grasping, pinching, manipulating, pulling, and pushing are abilities that underlie many activities. Fleishman found in numerous studies of thousands of subjects that 52 general abilities explained proficiency in a large number of job-related activities. Some of those are mathematical reasoning, perceptual speed, multilimb coordination, and manual dexterity (Fleishman & Quaintance, 1984). Fisher (1997) identified abilities similarly; she labels them motor and process skills. Some of these are stabilizes, positions, walks, transports, chooses, gathers, and initiates.

In the OFM taxonomy, abilities are seen as a combination of endowed talents and acquired skills. A skill is the ability to achieve a goal under a wide variety of conditions with a degree of consistency and economy (Higgins, 1991). To accomplish the activity of hanging lures in the above example of the gardener, the person needs certain abilities, such as coordination, dexterity,

CLINICAL REASONING
in OT Practice

Occupational Self-Analysis

1. Make an occupational diary by listing awake hours along the left side of a piece of 11×8 inch paper and the days of the week across the top.
2. Fill in activities or tasks you do hour by hour in a typical week.
3. Classify these into role categories: self-maintenance, self-advancement, or self-enhancement.
4. Calculate what percentage of time you engaged in these role categories by using this formula: hours spent in one role category divided by total awake hours times 100%.
5. Make another chart. Choose your favorite role (e.g., student, mother). What tasks make up this role for you?
6. Choose the key task from your answer to question 5. What activities comprise this task?
7. Choose one activity from your answer to question 6. What abilities are needed to do this activity?
8. What type of impairments would prevent you from doing the activity as you usually do it?

and ability to follow directions. The person also needs to be able to translate these endowed talents into skilled actions required to hang the lures. Carefully analyzed **occupation-as-means** is used to develop deficient abilities and skills. In the process of repeatedly accomplishing occupations that demand greater levels of the deficient ability or skill, in varying contexts, the patient gains greater levels of that ability or skill (See Chapter 11 for a more complete discussion of the use of occupation-as-means). By varying the context, the therapist encourages more robust learning.

Developed Capacities

Developed **capacities** reflect the organization of first-level capacities into more mature, less reflexive, and more voluntary responses. For example, to support dexterity, which is an ability, the person needs independent use of fingers, graded release, and pinch, which are developed capacities that derive from reflexive grasp and automatic release (first-level capacities). This organization is normally acquired through maturation. In therapy, occupation-as-means is used to develop these capacities. Therapeutic demands for gradually more mature and varied responses are made through repeated opportunities to engage in selected occupations.

First-Level Capacities

First-level capacities are the functional foundation for movement, cognition, perception, and emotional life based on the integrity of the organic substrate. In the motor domain, first-level capacities are reflex-based motor responses that reflect the organization of primary visual, sensory, and motor systems. Examples include reflexive grasp, reflexive release, primitive reaching, kicking, and stepping. They are the subroutines that Bruner (1973) described as underlying development of all voluntary movement. Related to cognition and perception, the ability to recognize a connection between an instrumental, nonreflexive response given consistently within a particular perceptual situation is a first-level capacity. In relation to the socioemotional domain, an example is the fascination of babies with human faces.

Organic Substrate

Organic substrate is the structural foundation for movement, cognition, perception, and emotions, including the primordial central nervous system (CNS) organization in the neonate, the CNS organization that is spared or recovers spontaneously after injury or illness; and the integrity of the skeleton, muscles, sensory and motor

nerves, heart, lungs, and skin. If the organic substrate is not present, therapy cannot generate it. If it exists at all, therapy attempts to develop first level capacities through techniques classified as **augmented maturation** (see Chapter 26).

Environment and Context

The words *environment* and **context** are often used interchangeably. In current health care literature the term *context* is used to encompass all that surrounds and influences any aspect of human functioning—physical environment as well as social, personal, and cultural contexts. In the dictionary, context is defined as the interrelated conditions in which something exists or occurs (Mish, 1989). Environment is defined as the complex of external factors, circumstances, objects, and social and cultural beliefs and practices that influence the life of an individual (Mish, 1989). In the OFM model, context and environment surround and permeate all levels of the occupational functioning hierarchy but have greater influence at the higher levels of the hierarchy than the lower. At the lower levels, the immediate physical and personal contexts influence the actions. For example, organization of a reaching movement was shown to differ when actual, natural objects and utensils were used versus when simulated objects were used (Wu et al., 1998). Cultural and social contexts pertain less to this level. At the higher levels of activities, tasks, and roles, on the other hand, all aspects of context—personal, social, cultural, and physical—interact with the person's abilities to yield occupational functioning for the particular person. Figure 1-1 depicts these ideas within the limitations of two-dimensional representation. Chapter 9 discusses the influence of personal, social, and cultural contexts on occupational functioning, and Chapter 10 discusses the influence of physical context.

When a person cannot meet the challenges of the environment, that person is said to be disabled (Institute of Medicine, 1997). However, a person with impaired abilities and capacities may be able to accomplish activities and tasks of his or her roles if the environment is adapted to enable that. Therefore, treatment may focus on that goal rather than on remediation of the person's impaired abilities or capacities.

Assessment and Treatment

The hierarchical organization of the OFM indicates that higher-level occupational functioning is established on a foundation of abilities and capacities. Both assessment and treatment take this organization into account.

Case Example

RELATION BETWEEN ABILITIES AND TASK PERFORMANCE

History of Injury

Mr. J. got a fracture dislocation of C6-7 in a diving accident. A cervical fusion and laminectomy were performed on the day of the accident without medical complications. The spinal cord injury was incomplete, and he exhibited a C6 functional level after surgery. Once Mr. J. was medically stable, he was discharged from acute care to a rehabilitation center near his home.

On admission, the occupational therapist engaged Mr. J. in an interview about his social and occupational histories to determine what his roles were before the accident and what his expectations were for himself after rehabilitation. The therapist then determined whether he was capable of performing any of the tasks or activities Mr. J. associated with those roles. The therapist found that he was dependent in all self-care, and other more complicated activities were not evaluated at this time. To determine why Mr. J. was unable to do his ADL, the therapist evaluated Mr. J.'s strength. Mr. J.'s proximal upper extremity musculature rated 4 to 5, with the exception of the triceps, which graded 2 (see Table 4-2, which describes muscle strength grading). Wrist extensors graded 3+ on the left and 4– on the right; wrist flexors and finger and thumb muscles graded 2 bilaterally. He was paralyzed in both lower extremities.

Social History

The interview with Mr. J. revealed that he is 24 years old, a college graduate, and living with his parents in a second-floor apartment in a small city. He has many friends from college and work. He has four older siblings who are all married. The family is supportive and plans that Mr. J. will go to live with a brother and sister-in-law on discharge until the parents move to a more accessible house. It is important to the family that Mr. J. be independent in self-care at discharge.

Occupational History and Expectations

The interview further revealed that Mr. J. is a computer programmer with a thriving start-up software company. The company is holding his job for him. He identified keyboarding as one of the major physical tasks of his role as computer programmer. Another task he identified was troubleshooting programs on large, fan-folded sheets of computer paper. He expects to return to work, but to do so, Mr. J. needs to regain not only the essential tasks of his job but also his roles of independent person and commuter. Before the accident, he enjoyed swimming, basketball, and camping with his friends. He plans on resuming these activities after discharge.

Rehabilitation

During rehabilitation, Mr. J. engaged in occupation-as-means within the biomechanical approach to remediate the weakness of his wrists, fingers, and thumbs, and occupation-as-end within the rehabilitative approach to recover important tasks and activities.

Status at Discharge: Abilities and Residual Impairments

Mr. J. did not regain strength in his trunk or lower extremities, necessitating the use of a wheelchair for locomotion. He learned to use gravity, momentum, and leverage to move his body in the wheelchair and on the bed. The proximal upper extremity musculature recovered to normal strength, allowing shoulder movements that enabled use of momentum for postural adjustment. The triceps remained at less than functional strength, so he could not relieve ischial pressure on his buttocks by elevating himself off the wheelchair cushion. Mr. J.'s wrist strength improved to 4+ bilaterally, which allowed a functional tenodesis grasp (see Chapter 43 for a description of this condition, including special circumstances such as tenodesis grasp). Finger and thumb strength recovered to 3+, but that is not a functional strength.

Status at Discharge: Occupational Functioning

In spite of these residual impairments, Mr. J. was successfully rehabilitated. Mr. J. became proficient in use of his wheelchair, which was adapted to allow propulsion without grasp. He also learned how to relieve ischial pressure to maintain skin integrity. At present, Mr. J. requires 2 hours to bathe and dress. He showers using a shower bench and handheld shower head, which he holds using tenodesis grasp. He is able to manage his bowel and bladder programs and to dress, using adaptive methods and devices. While he is saving for an adapted van with a hydraulic lift to allow him to drive independently, he attends adaptive driving class at the rehabilitation center as an outpatient. In the meantime he uses the handicapped travel service of the public transportation system to get to and from work and appointments. He has resumed work part time (noon to 4 PM). He keyboards with increasing speed using universal cuffs with typing sticks tipped with rubber ends. His computer is adapted to allow one key depression for all operations. He also uses the typing sticks to turn pages of the computer printouts.

Mr. J. attends sports games with his friends. At a recent benefit game of the regional wheelchair basketball league, audience members were challenged by the local champion team to use wheelchairs and play against them. Mr. J. and one of his nondisabled friends took the challenge. As a result, Mr. J. was issued an invitation to join the team next season. Although Mr. J. is doing well socially with his group of old friends and although he is personable, he felt the need to learn to interact with acquaintances and strangers. Therefore Mr. J. attends outpatient group occupational therapy for social, emotional, and practical problem solving. Members of the group are other persons with similar activity limitations.

CLINICAL REASONING
in Occupational Therapy Practice

Treatment Planning for Mr. J.

Mr. J. has extensive impairments. What are the pros and cons of concentrating therapeutic intervention on enablement of activities, tasks, and roles versus remediation of capacities and abilities? From this deliberation, state a goal your treatment might be directed toward. Which treatment approach would you choose to achieve the goal? Which treatments would you use to achieve that goal?

Assessment

Assessment *always* follows a top-down approach. That is, the therapist determines what roles and tasks the person was responsible for in life before the accident or disease and what the person is expected to be and wants to be responsible for in postrehabilitation life, including the context in which the person typically engaged in these valued roles and tasks (Coster, 1998; Mathiowetz, 1993; Mayer et al., 1986; Trombly, 1993, 1995a). The *Role Checklist* (Barris et al., 1988) and the *Canadian Occupational Performance Measure* (*COPM*) (Law et al., 1998) are two of several assessments the therapist can use to gather this information. The therapist may also measure the patient's sense of self-efficacy concerning ability to fulfill particular roles by having the patient assign a number on a visual analogue scale that ranges from 0 (not at all confident) to 100 (absolutely certain) for each major task that defines a specific role. For example, "on this scale from 0 to 100, how confident are you that you can dress yourself without help?" (Gill et al., 1994).

When evaluating a patient's competence to accomplish the roles identified as important in the interview, the therapist observes the patient attempting to do the tasks and activities of those roles in the most familiar context. The *AMPS* (*Assessment of Motor and Process Skills*) (Fisher, 1997) and the *Klein–Bell ADL Scale* (Klein & Bell, 1982) are examples of assessments. Based on that observation and the probabilities established by the diagnosis and age of the person, the therapist hypothesizes which of the myriad abilities and capacities assumed to be related to accomplishment of these activities might be impaired (the process of **activity analysis** applied to assessment). For example, if one of the patient's goals is to shave with an electric razor but

he appears to lack the grasp strength and endurance to do so, those abilities and capacities are assessed according to the procedures described in Chapter 4. A person whose abilities and capacities are found deficient may be treated to optimize them, allowing not only shaving but other occupational performance.

Also to be considered as part of the assessment is whether the environment enables or hinders occupational functioning. There is no formal assessment of that construct yet, although researchers are working on it. In the meantime, the occupational therapist should ask about and observe performance in physical and social environments typical for the patient.

Treatment

Treatment may focus on changing the environment, changing the impaired skills and abilities of the person, or teaching compensatory ways to accomplish activities and tasks. Treatment to improve occupational functioning, then, may start toward the bottom of the OFM hierarchy, focusing on optimizing abilities and capacities, or may start higher, at the activity level of the hierarchy, focusing on restoring competence in doing the activities and tasks of valued roles that the patient has identified as concerns. The starting point should acknowledge the problem that the patient has identified as of immediate concern, although treatment may not actually start there. For example, if the patient identified resuming fishing as the goal, the therapist may choose to teach adaptive methods to enable that. However, if in the experience of the therapist it would be more effective to start treatment by regaining finger dexterity to enable baiting the hook and removing the fish from the line and doing other tasks of other roles, the therapist must help the patient understand how treatment of this lower-level ability addresses the stated concern at the task level. And the therapist must ensure carryover of any gained dexterity to the fishing task.

Optimizing impaired abilities and capacities is accomplished through remedial therapy in which a change in physiological structure, function, or organization is sought. If remediation of deficit abilities or capacities does not restore occupational functioning, if the political and economic constraints prevent such thorough treatment, or if the patient is not committed to the extensive work required to recover abilities and capacities, a degree of competence can be restored using **adaptive therapy**. Adaptive therapy seeks to find and promote a balance among the person's goals, capabilities, and environmental demands in daily occupations (Thorén-Jönsson et al., 1999). The method of doing an activity may be modified, assistive technology may be employed to enable completion of the activity, and/or the physical or social environments may be modified. The person may be counseled to reassess the need to accomplish a particularly difficult activity alone and opt to employ another to do it.

Optimizing Abilities and Capacities

It is believed that remediating impaired sensorimotor, cognitive, perceptual, and emotional capacities and abilities to as good a level as a person's organic substrate allows will enable versatile performance of activities. Versatile performance allows the person to adjust to changes in the social and physical environments, whereas if a person learns only one compensatory response, adaptation to new situations is unlikely. As in the typical development of these capacities and abilities, therapy engages the patient in circumscribed encounters with the environment, using occupation-as-means. Using the example of the man who wanted to shave, the therapist might provide a cuff to hold the razor (eliminating the need for grasp) and let the patient shave as much as he could. The occupational therapist would finish the activity. Day by day, the patient's endurance for shaving would increase and he would do more of the task on his own. Simultaneously, the therapist would engage the patient in activities that require increased grasp strength until the patient was able to pick up and hold the razor.

The cognitive-perceptual approach and two motor approaches to optimize abilities and capacities are described here. The two approaches for motor impairments were first identified by Trombly and Scott in 1977: the biomechanical approach and the neurodevelopmental approach. In more recent years, the title of the latter was amended to the motor learning–neurodevelopmental approach (Trombly, 1995b).

Cognitive-Perceptual Approach

The cognitive-perceptual approach is actually a loose amalgamation of several treatment models or interventions, including Warren's (1993) hierarchical model, Toglia's (1991) multicontext approach, and other interventions described in this textbook.

Performance in occupations requires the ability to perceive and evaluate sensory information from the environment; the ability to conceive of, plan, and execute a purposeful action on the environment; and the ability to remember and sequence information and solve problems. Secondary to disease or injury to the central nervous system, perceptual and/or cognitive abilities can be lost or diminished. The nervous system has plasticity, which implies that intervention can produce organic or behavioral change. Interventions, therefore, try to affect the organic organization through controlled sensory input and/or to affect the behavioral organization through a teaching–learning format, using occupation-as-means (Trombly, 1995a). The evaluation and treatment techniques for the cognitive-perceptual approach are described in Chapters 7, 8, 12, 28, and 29, and application is discussed in Chapters 38–40.

Biomechanical Approach

The biomechanical approach has been used in some manner since occupational therapists began treating persons with physical dysfunction (Spackman, 1968). The basic assumption is that occupation requires the ability to move the limbs (range of motion and muscle strength) and the endurance to persist in movement until the goal is accomplished (central and peripheral endurance). Problems such as edema, contractures, joint destruction (arthritis), cardiopulmonary disease, peripheral nerve injury, spinal cord injury, and cumulative trauma disorders are treated using the biomechanical approach. This approach would be chosen, therefore, to move a patient from the developed capacity level forward to the ability level in the OFM.

The primary mechanism that brings about therapeutic change within the biomechanical approach is occupation-as-means, that is, activities that provide stretch of soft tissues, active or passive movement to preserve and restore full range of motion, resistance and other stress to strengthen weak muscles, or graduated, increasing levels of aerobic exercise to improve endurance. The evaluation and intervention techniques are described in Chapters 4, 11, and 20; adjunctive therapies that support this approach are discussed in Chapters 14, 15, 18, and 25; and the application of the approach, in combination with complementary approaches, is illustrated in Chapters 41–47.

Motor Learning–Neurodevelopmental Approaches

According to the motor learning–neurodevelopmental approaches, dysfunction exists when impairment of the CNS results in the inability to move voluntarily to effect a desired change in the environment. Stroke, Parkinson's disease, traumatic brain injury, and brain tumors are examples of disorders that can be treated using this approach. A therapist following these approaches may use sensory input and developmental sequences (augmented maturation) to facilitate change in sensorimotor organization. Or the therapist may use motor learning principles to bring about change in voluntary movement behavior and thereby improve the overall functioning of the client.

These approaches are used to help the person move from first-level capacities through the ability level to the activity and task levels. The neurodevelopmental approaches may be most applicable to remediation of capacities, whereas the motor learning approaches are best for developing abilities and activity and task performance.

The motor learning-neurodevelopmental approach is actually composed of several minitheories relating to neurophysiological, developmental, and motor learning aspects of acquiring voluntary human movement.

Motor Learning Approaches to Recovery of Motor Behavior. Two approaches apply motor learning principles and methods to treatment of persons with CNS impairment. These are the Carr and Shepherd *Motor Relearning Programme for Stroke* (see Chapter 22) and the task-oriented approach described by Horak (1991) and Bass-Haugen and Mathiowetz (see Chapter 21). Both approaches emphasize motor performance using functional tasks; include remediation of performance components and modification of the environment to improve task performance; stress practice that fits the nature of the task; and reject assumptions of the reflex-hierarchical theories of motor control and traditional developmental theories. Both approaches heed the research findings on the effect of context on the organization of movement, which indicate that practicing a skill under simplified, non–context-specific conditions is different from practicing with an actual object in a context-specific situation (Mathiowetz & Wade, 1995; Trombly & Wu, 1999; Wu et al., 1998).

Neurodevelopmental Approaches to Recovery of Motor Behavior. Several approaches have been developed to remediate impairments of motor control in persons who have suffered CNS disease or trauma. They are based on a hierarchical representation of the CNS in which the lesion is thought to release reflex activity from higher control. To some extent, these approaches all use techniques such as controlled sensory input to affect motor output and ontogenetic or recovery-based developmental sequences for both assessment and treatment. The approaches share the idea of the importance of the need for repetition. All emphasize the development of basic movements and postures and assume that when movement is "normalized," skilled movement and occupational performance will occur automatically. The approaches of Bobath and Brunnstrom, representative of this group of treatments, are described in Chapters 23 and 24.

Restoring Competence

Restoration of occupational functioning depends on developing competence in the valued tasks and activities of the patient's life roles. Competence in tasks and activities is synthesized through successful engagement with the environment. Occupational therapists are skilled in developing graduated encounters with objects and the surrounding physical and social environments to promote successful performance. They are also expert in teaching compensatory methods to accomplish activities. Some therapists use this approach exclusively (Christiansen & Baum, 1997; Mayer et al., 1986). Others believe that first optimizing the impaired abilities and capacities requires less compensation and produces more versatility of performance. There is no research to support one point of view over the other. Methods to restore competence are embodied in the rehabilitative approach (Trombly & Scott, 1977).

Rehabilitative Approach

The rehabilitative approach is applicable to the activity, task, and role levels of the OFM. The rehabilitative approach aims at making people as independent as possible in spite of any residual impairment. If people must live with an impairment that decreases independent functioning, the occupational therapist will concentrate on helping them find ways to compensate by reorganizing activity patterns or adapting techniques, equipment, or the environment. The goal is independence. People are considered independent when they perform tasks for themselves, using assistive equipment, alternative methods, or adapted environments as required, or when they appropriately oversee completion of activities by others on their own behalf (Moyers, 1999).

Interventions under the rehabilitative approach are compensatory, and they focus on teaching physical and emotional adaptation. The therapist teaches the patient to recognize and use remaining abilities in adapted ways and teaches the principles and concepts of adapted methods so that the person can become an independent problem solver. Therapeutic mechanisms of change include occupation-as-end, teaching–learning, and therapeutic rapport. The assessment and treatment procedures are described in Chapters 3, 9–13, 16, 17, and 37.

Summary Review Questions

1. Describe the Occupational Functioning Model.
2. What is the overall goal of occupational therapy for persons with occupational dysfunction due to physical impairments?
3. Using the OFM as your conceptual model of practice, what would you assess first in a patient with stroke: level of spasticity of the upper extremity, ADL, or role history and expectations?
4. Define ability and developed capacity. Give an example of each. To what levels of AOTA's Uniform Terminology and ICIDH-2 do these correspond?
5. Define *task* and *activity*. Give an example of each. To what levels of AOTA's Uniform Terminology and ICIDH-2 do these correspond?
6. What distinguishes occupation-as-means from occupation-as-end?

References

American Occupational Therapy Association [AOTA]. (1994). Uniform terminology for occupational therapy (3rd ed.). *American Journal of Occupational Therapy, 48,* 1047–1054.

American Occupational Therapy Association [AOTA]. (1997). Statement: Fundamental concepts of occupational therapy: Occupation, purposeful activity, and function. *American Journal of Occupational Therapy, 51,* 864–866.

Bandura, A. (1977). Self-efficacy: Toward a unifying theory of behavior change. *Psychological Review, 84,* 191–215.

Barris, R., Oakley, F., & Kielhofner, G. (1988). The *Role Checklist.* In B. J. Hemphill (Ed.), *Mental health assessment in occupational therapy* (pp. 73–91). Thorofare, NJ: Slack.

Baum, C. M., & Law, M. (1997). Occupational therapy practice: Focusing on occupational performance. *American Journal of Occupational Therapy, 51,* 277–288.

Bruner, J. (1973). Organization of early skilled action. *Child Development, 44,* 1–11.

Christiansen, C. H., & Baum, C. M. (1997). *Occupational therapy: Enabling functional well-being* (2nd ed.). Thorofare, NJ: Slack.

Clark, M. C., Czaja, S. J., & Weber, R. A. (1990). Older adults and daily living task profiles. *Human Factors, 32,* 537–549.

Coster, W. (1998). Occupation-centered assessment of children. *American Journal of Occupational Therapy, 52,* 337–344.

Dijkers, M. (1997). Quality of life after spinal cord injury: A meta-analysis of the effects of disablement components. *Spinal Cord, 35,* 829–840.

Dijkers, M. P. J. M. (1999). Correlates of life satisfaction among persons with spinal cord injury. *Archives of Physical Medicine and Rehabilitation, 80,* 867–876.

Dunn, W., Brown, C., & McGuigan, A. (1994). The ecology of human performance: A framework for considering the effect of context. *American Journal of Occupational Therapy, 48,* 595–607.

Fearing, V. G., Law, M., & Clark, J. (1997). An Occupational Performance Process Model: Fostering client and therapist alliances. *Canadian Journal of Occupational Therapy, 64,* 7–15.

Fidler, G. S. (1996). Life-style performance: From profile to conceptual model. *American Journal of Occupational Therapy, 50,* 139–147.

Filiatrault, J., Arsenault, A. B., Dutil, E. M., & Bourbonnais, D. (1991). Motor function and activities of daily living assessments: A study of three tests for persons with hemiplegia. *American Journal of Occupational Therapy, 45,* 806–810.

Fisher, A. G. (1997). *Assessment of Motor and Process Skills* (2nd ed.). Fort Collins, CO: Three Star Press.

Fisher, A. G. (1998). Uniting practice and theory in an occupational framework. *American Journal of Occupational Therapy, 52,* 509–521.

Fleishman, E. A. (1972). On the relation between ability, learning, and human performance. *American Psychologist, 27,* 1017–1032.

Fleishman, E. A., & Quaintance, M. K. (1984). *Taxonomies of human performance.* New York: Academic Press.

Fugl-Meyer, A. R., Jääskö, L., Leyman, I., Olsson, S., & Steglind, S. (1975). The post stroke hemiplegic patient: 1. A method for evaluation of physical performance. *Scandinavian Journal of Rehabilitation Medicine, 7,* 13–31.

Gage, M. (1992). The Appraisal Model of Coping: An assessment and intervention model for occupational therapy. *American Journal of Occupational Therapy, 46,* 353–362.

Gage, M., Noh, S., Polatajko, H. J., & Kaspar, V. (1994). Measuring perceived self-efficacy in occupational therapy. *American Journal of Occupational Therapy, 48,* 783–790.

Gage, M., & Polatajko, H. (1994). Enhancing occupational performance through an understanding of perceived self-efficacy. *American Journal of Occupational Therapy, 48,* 452–461.

Gill, D. L., Kelley, B. C., Williams, K., & Martin, J. J. (1994). The relationship of self-efficacy and perceived well-being to physical activity and stair climbing in older adults. *Research Quarterly for Exercise and Sport, 65,* 367–371.

Higgins, S. (1991). Motor skill acquisition. *Physical Therapy, 71,* 123–139.

Hocking, C. (1998). Partnership and participation: The bicultural New Zealand context. *World Federation of Occupational Therapists (WFOT) Bulletin, 37,* 51–55.

Horak, F. B. (1991). Assumptions underlying motor control for neurologic rehabilitation. In M. Lister (Ed.), *Contemporary management of motor control problems. Proceedings of the II STEP Conference* (pp. 11–27). Alexandria, VA: The Foundation for Physical Therapy.

Institute of Medicine. (1997). *Enabling America: Assessing the role of rehabilitation science and engineering.* Washington: National Academy Press.

Jebsen, R. H., Taylor, N., Trieschmann, R., Trotter, M., Howard, L. (1969). An objective and standardized test of hand function. *Archives of Physical Medicine & Rehabilitation, 50,* 311–319.

Kielhofner, G. (Ed.). (1995). *A Model of Human Occupation: Theory and application* (2nd ed.). Baltimore: Williams & Wilkins.

Kielhofner, G. (1997). *Conceptual foundations of occupational therapy* (2nd ed.). Philadelphia: F. A. Davis.

Kielhofner, G., & Burke, J. (1980). A model of human occupation: Part 1. Conceptual framework and content. *American Journal of Occupational Therapy, 34,* 572–581.

Klein, R. M., & Bell, B. (1982). Self-care skills: behavioral measurement with *Klein–Bell ADL Scale. Archives of Physical Medicine & Rehabilitation, 63,* 335–338.

Law, M., Cooper, B., Strong, S., Stewart, S., Rigby, P., & Letts, L. (1996). The person-environment-occupational model: A transactive approach to occupational performance. *Canadian Journal of Occupational Therapy, 63,* 9–23.

Law, M., Baptiste, S., Carswell, A., McColl, M., Polatajko, H., & Pollack, N. (1998). *Canadian Occupational Performance Measure* (3rd ed.). Ottawa: CAOT.

Lundmark, P., & Bränholm, I-B. (1996). Relationship between occupation and life satisfaction in people with multiple sclerosis. *Disability and Rehabilitation, 18,* 449–453.

Lynch, K. B., & Bridle, M. J. (1989). Validity of the *Jebsen-Taylor Hand Function Test* in predicting activities of daily living. *Occupational Therapy Journal of Research, 9,* 316–318.

Mahoney, F. I., & Barthel, D. W. (1965). Functional evaluation: The *Barthel Index. Maryland State Medical Journal, 14,* 61–65.

Marteniuk, R. G., MacKenzie, C. L., Jeannerod, M., Athenes, S., & Dugas, C. (1987). Constraints on human arm movement trajectories. *Canadian Journal of Psychology, 41,* 356–378.

Mathiowetz, V. (1993). Role of physical performance component evaluations in occupational therapy functional assessment. *American Journal of Occupational Therapy, 47,* 225–230.

Mathiowetz, V., & Wade, M. G. (1995). Task constraints and functional motor performance of individuals with and without multiple sclerosis. *Ecological Psychology, 7,* 99–123.

Mayer, N. H., Keating, D. J., & Rapp, D. (1986). Skills, routines, and activity patterns of daily living: A functional nested approach. In B. Uzzell & Y. Gross (Eds.), *Clinical Neuropsychology of Intervention* (pp. 205–222). Boston: Martinus Nijhoff.

Mish, F. C. (Ed.). (1989). *Webster's ninth new collegiate dictionary.* Springfield, MA: Merriam-Webster.

Mocellin, G. (1992). An overview of occupational therapy in the context of the American influence on the profession: Part 2. *British Journal of Occupational Therapy, 55,* 55–60.

Moyers, P. (1999). The guide to occupational therapy practice. *American Journal of Occupational Therapy, 53,* 247–322.

Nelson, C. E., & Payton, O. D. (1991). The issue is: A system for involving patients in program planning. *American Journal of Occupational Therapy, 45,* 753–755.

Pendlebury, S. T., Blamire, A. M., Lee, M. A., Styles, P., & Matthews, P. M. (1999). Axonal injury in the internal capsule correlates with motor impairment after stroke. *Stroke, 30,* 956–962.

Reilly, M. (1962). Occupational therapy can be one of the great ideas of 20th century medicine. *American Journal of Occupational Therapy, 16,* 1–9.

Resnik, B. (1998). Efficacy beliefs in geriatric rehabilitation. *Journal of Gerontological Nursing, 24,* 34–44.

Rogers, R. W. (1983). Cognitive and psychological processes in fear appeals and attitude change: A revised theory of protection motivation. In J. T. Cacioppo, R. E. Petty, & D. Shapiro (Eds.), *Social psychophysiology* (pp. 153–176). New York: Guilford.

Rogers, J. C., & Holm, M. B. (1994). Accepting the challenge of outcome research: Examining the effectiveness of occupational therapy practice. *American Journal of Occupational Therapy, 48,* 871–876.

Rondinelli, R. D., Dunn, W., Hassanein, K. M., Keesling, C. A., Meredith, S. C., Schulz, T. L., & Lawrence, N. J. (1997). A simulation of hand impairments: Effects on upper extremity function and implications toward medical impairment rating and disability determination. *Archives of Physical Medicine and Rehabilitation, 78,* 1358–1363.

Schkade, J. K., & Schultz, S. (1992). Occupational adaptation: Toward a holistic approach for contemporary practice, Part 1. *American Journal of Occupational Therapy, 46,* 829–837.

Schultz, S., & Schkade, J. K. (1992). Occupational adaptation: Toward a holistic approach for contemporary practice, Part 2. *American Journal of Occupational Therapy, 46,* 917–925.

Spackman, C. S. (1968). A history of the practice of occupational therapy for the restoration of physical function: 1917–1967. *American Journal of Occupational Therapy, 22,* 67–71.

Thorén-Jönsson, A-L, Möller, A., & Grimby, G. (1999). Managing occupations in everyday life to achieve adaptation. *American Journal of Occupational Therapy, 53,* 353–362.

Thorndike, E. L. (1924). Mental discipline in high school studies. *Journal of Educational Psychology, 15,* 1–22.

Toglia, J. P. (1991). Generalization of treatment: A multicontext approach to cognitive perceptual impairment in adults with brain injury. *American Journal of Occupational Therapy, 45,* 505–516.

Trombly, C. (1993). Anticipating the future: Assessment of occupational function. *American Journal of Occupational Therapy, 47,* 253–257.

Trombly, C. A. (1995a). Occupation: Purposefulness and meaningfulness as therapeutic mechanisms. *American Journal of Occupational Therapy, 49,* 960–972.

Trombly, C. A. (Ed.). (1995b). *Occupational Therapy for Physical Dysfunction* (4th ed.) Baltimore: Williams & Wilkins.

Trombly, C. A., & Scott, A. D. (1977). *Occupational Therapy for Physical Dysfunction.* Baltimore: Williams & Wilkins.

Trombly, C. A., & Wu, C-Y. (1999). Effect of rehabilitation tasks on organization of movement after stroke. *American Journal of Occupational Therapy, 53,* 333–344.

Warren, M. (1993). A hierarchical model for evaluation and treatment of visual perceptual dysfunction in adult acquired brain injury, Parts 1 & 2. *American Journal of Occupational Therapy, 47,* 42–54; 55–66.

White, R. W. (1959). Motivation reconsidered: The concept of competence. *Psychological Reviews, 66,* 297–333.

White, R. W. (1971). The urge towards competence. *American Journal of Occupational Therapy, 25,* 271–274.

Wood, W. (1998). It is jump time for occupational therapy. *American Journal of Occupational Therapy, 52,* 403–411.

World Health Organization. (2000). *ICIDH-2: The international classification of Functioning, Disability and Health.* (pre-final version) [On-line], Available: www.who.int/icidh. Geneva: Author.

Wu, C.-Y., Trombly, C., Lin, K.-C., & Tickle-Degnen, L. (1998). Effects of object affordances on reaching performance in person with and without cerebrovascular accident. *American Journal of Occupational Therapy, 52,* 447–456.

Yerxa, E. J., & Locker, S. B. (1990). Quality of time use by adults with spinal cord injuries. *American Journal of Occupational Therapy, 44,* 318–326.

2

Historical and Social Foundations for Practice

Jaclyn Faglie Low

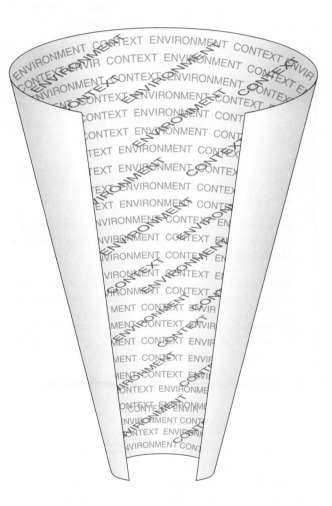

LEARNING OBJECTIVES

After studying this chapter, the reader will be able to do the following:

1. Describe the changes in hospital structure and function that fostered the development of occupational therapy.
2. Identify the factors that generated a concern for age-related expectations for occupational function.
3. Compare the provision of occupation as therapy for soldiers in World War I with that for World War II servicemen.
4. Describe the relationship between rehabilitation medicine and occupational therapy.
5. Describe the relationship between occupational therapy for persons with tuberculosis and work-hardening programs.
6. Identify early concerns about the adequacy of crafts as treatment modalities.
7. Describe the adjunctive equipment and modalities that occupational therapists use to augment traditional therapeutic modalities.
8. Explain the introduction of orthotic fabrication into occupational therapy practice.
9. Describe the introduction of neurodevelopmental theories to occupational therapy practice and literature.

*O*ccupational therapists today are concerned with their patients' abilities to resume life roles upon discharge from abbreviated hospital stays. Occupational therapists in earlier times questioned whether patients would assume vocational and other responsibilities after prolonged hospitalizations. Occupational therapists today debate the inclusion of physical agent modalities into their repertoire of techniques, whereas occupational therapists in earlier times questioned the adequacy of crafts and devel-

GLOSSARY

Adaptive equipment—Equipment designed to help persons with disabilities compensate for functional limitations; equipment ranges from simple, such as a long-handled reacher for those unable to bend over, to complex computerized environmental control systems.

Battle fatigue—See war neurosis.

Bleeding—Incision into a vein to allow blood loss to restore the proper balance of body humors.

Blistering—Application of irritants to the skin to raise blisters and draw putrid humors or infection from the body.

Habit training—A regimen wherein patients hospitalized with mental illness were expected to follow a rigid daily schedule that included responsibility for personal hygiene, making one's bed, and attending treatment sessions at prescribed times; regimens were designed to help patients develop good habits as an aid to restoration of good mental health and for the therapeutic value of work and routine.

Homeopathy—Medical practice based on treating disorders with minuscule doses of substances that produce the same symptoms as the illness.

Hydrotherapy—Use of water as a therapeutic agent; hydropathy incorporated both the prescription of drinking water and the use of bathing to treat illness.

Military medicine—Health care practiced within the military system; focus is on treatment of war-related injuries or illnesses.

Moral treatment—Treatment approach for mental illness that focused on work as a therapeutic agent rather than restraint and isolation.

Neurorehabilitation—Treatment approach for persons with central nervous system dysfunction; uses specific sensory input to influence motor responses.

Orthotics—External devices fitted to specific body parts to support the body part, immobilize the body part, or facilitate movement of the body part.

Physical agent modalities—Treatment methods that act on soft tissue and prepare the body part for improved functional movement patterns; includes heat and electrical stimulation.

Purging—Induction of severe vomiting to remove putrid substances from the body and restore the balance of body humors.

Purposeful activity—Activity used in treatment that is goal directed and that the patient perceives as meaningful or purposeful.

Rehabilitation—An approach to treatment for the person who has a permanent disability; focuses on training in the use of special equipment or techniques to facilitate independence rather than on remediation.

War neurosis, battle fatigue—Physical and emotional responses to combat experiences.

Work hardening—Treatment program aimed at returning the injured worker to productive activity through a structured, interdisciplinary program of increasing endurance, work tolerance, and improved body mechanics.

Work therapy—Work activity with primary purpose of therapeutic benefit rather than productivity.

---

oped therapeutic equipment when crafts were not sufficient to meet goals.

Although the specific details of the questions have changed over time, the fundamental character of questions about the practice of occupational therapy is the same: How can we best prepare our patients to return to appropriate life roles after a life-changing illness or injury? What are the appropriate tools of practice?

The roots of contemporary concerns are discernible in the experiences of forebears. This chapter explores the social and historical foundations of physical disability practice, beginning with the history of activity in the service of health and an introduction to the founders of the profession. It describes two facets of late 19th and early 20th century American life that were crucial to the development of occupational therapy: the evolution of the structure and role of the hospital and a burgeoning concern for age norms for life tasks. Historical foundations are disclosed in professional literature that documents early involvement of occupational therapists in **military medicine**, **rehabilitation** and **work hardening**, and the introduction of **physical agent modalities**, **adaptive equipment**, **orthotics**, and **neurorehabilitation** techniques into practice.

Activity As Therapy

Occupational therapy is based on the belief that **purposeful activity** (occupation) prevents or mediates dysfunction of physical or psychological origin. Fitness was considered necessary for optimal functioning in occupational roles determined by age, gender, and socioeconomic class. Writings attributed to Hippocrates, Galen, and Aesculapius proclaimed exercise, activity treatment, and employment as important therapeutic agents. Centuries later, physicians in European asylums for the insane instituted **work therapy** for inmates. They noted that lower-class patients who were required to perform tasks while incarcerated recovered more quickly than did idle upper-class patients. The value of physical activity and productive work was central to the **moral treatment** advanced by the French physician Phillipe Pinel in the 18th century and the Tuke family in 18th- and 19th-century England.

Ideas about the value of activity were transported to colonial America. The first hospital chartered in Great Britain's North American colonies included as part of its equipment and supplies spinning wheels, wool, and flax for use by patients. Dr. Benjamin Rush, a signer of the Declaration of Independence, wrote to the managers of the Pennsylvania Hospital in 1797 and again in 1813 in support of the therapeutic value of work for patients (Dunton, 1917).

Attitudes in the United States changed as immigrants with different values and habits swelled the population of the asylums. Mental illness was seen as a permanent condition for which little could be done except to lock the sufferer away. Thus the use of activity as therapy in institutions for the mentally ill lay dormant for decades. Dunton (1917) surmised that the decline in work as therapy from 1860 to 1890 was related to the demands of post–Civil War conditions.

Hospitals for the physically ill required work of their patients. However, jobs were done in the service of the institution rather than for therapeutic benefit. As recovery progressed, women patients cared for sicker patients. In New York City's Bellevue and Charity hospitals, women's jobs required sewing, and men's required maintenance skills such as carpentry, cleaning, and even rowing a boat to ferry passengers on a twice-daily schedule (Rosenberg, 1978).

The formal idea of occupation as therapy did not emerge until the late 19th and early 20th centuries. However, 19th-century Americans valued work and activity, especially outdoor activity, as vital to good health. Until the introduction of the germ theory of disease and asepsis, traditional medical care was frequently more harmful than helpful. Emphasis on curing disease through **bleeding**, **blistering**, and **purging** to restore the balance of the body's humors was challenged by sectarian or nontraditional approaches to health care. Health reformers advocated education, regular exercise, dress reform, and dietary restrictions in addition to specific curative practices such as **hydrotherapy** and **homeopathy**.

The Growth of a Profession

Professions are made up of practitioners with special skills, knowledge, attitudes, and shared beliefs. Professions are not created instantaneously but evolve over time and within social, cultural, and environmental contexts. Identifiable factors influenced the development of occupational therapy as a profession. These include the personalities and experiences of the individuals who recognized the idea of occupation as therapy and the world in which they lived. The late 19th and early 20th centuries were characterized by changes in the effectiveness and ways of provision of health care and influenced by burgeoning emphasis on the relation between chronological age and appropriate roles in life. These factors helped create the conditions in which the ideas and ideals of the founders could flourish.

The Founders and the Near-Founders

In the first decades of the 20th century, individuals in various fields of endeavor began almost simultaneously to practice and promote the use of occupation as therapy. George Barton, an architect with numerous health problems, was convinced that he could help others with similar problems. He opened Consolation House in Clifton Springs, New York, where he provided education, vocational assistance, and workshop activities for convalescents.

Barton assembled five like-minded individuals to meet with him in 1917 to establish the National Society for the Promotion of Occupational Therapy, which in 1923 was renamed the American Occupational Therapy Association. Joining Barton was psychiatrist William Rush Dunton Jr., a descendent and namesake of Benjamin Rush. Dunton directed the occupations program at the Sheppard and Pratt Institute in Maryland and wrote a number of books and articles on occupation as therapy and on training nurses to provide occupation. His major works included *Occupational Therapy* (1915), *Reconstruction Therapy* (1919), and *Prescribing Occupational Therapy* (1928). He also cowrote, with Dr. Sidney Licht, *Occupational Therapy: Principles and Practice* (1950, 1957).

Also present was Eleanor Clarke Slagle. She worked with Dunton at Johns Hopkins in Baltimore, where she developed a program called **habit training** for chronically schizophrenic patients. Slagle later went to Chicago, where she directed the Henry P. Favill School of Occupations until it closed in 1920 (History, 1940). Other founding members were Susan Cox Johnson and Thomas Kidner. Johnson, director of occupations for the New York State Department of Public Charities, wrote a textbook on textiles and spent 2 years as a teacher of arts and crafts in the Philippines (Licht, 1967; Johnson, 1917). Kidner, a London-born architect, was the vocational secretary of the Canadian Military Hospitals Commission and a special adviser to the U.S. government on problems of rehabilitation (Licht, 1967). Isabel Newton, Barton's secretary, was also present. She later married Barton and worked with him as a teacher of occupations to invalids.

Susan Tracy, born in 1864, graduated from nurse training at the Massachusetts Homeopathic Hospital in 1889. She studied manual arts at Teachers College at Columbia University while working as a private-duty nurse. Tracy taught courses in invalid occupations for nursing students. She incorporated her course material into her textbook *Studies in Invalid Occupations* (1910). In 1916, she introduced an occupational therapy program for general medicine patients at Michael Reese Hospital in Chicago (Occupational Therapy, 1917, p. 425).

Although she did not attend the organizational meeting, Tracy was one of the five directors of the society listed on the certificate of incorporation. Peloquin (1991) referred to Tracy and Herbert J. Hall as near-founders because of their influence on the profession. Hall was the director of Devereux Mansion in Marblehead, Massachusetts, where he established an experimental workshop.

Rationales for Occupation as Therapy

The early practitioners of occupational therapy validated the idea of occupation as therapy in various ways. Barton emphasized the scientific aspects of occupational therapy in a speech presented at the First Consolation House Conference (March 15–17, 1917). The speech, entitled "Inoculation of the Bacillus of Work," included numerous medical metaphors:

Preparation of the patient

The occupational diagnosis

Occupational "applications," "hypodermics," and "lumbar punctures"

The therapeutic value of drawing and modeling

Like water, a tonic and alterative (Barton, 1917, p. 399).

Barton (1917) compared occupational dysfunction with medical conditions and interventions. He referred to certain occupations as hypodermics, to be used, in his words, "where superficial stimulation is not sufficient, cases in which one has to get inside into the blood, or into the muscle itself" (p. 400). For even more severe problems, he termed the appropriate curative occupations "lumbar punctures" (p. 400).

Dunton acknowledged the lack of a scientific basis for occupation as therapy (Serrett, 1985) but proposed nine principles of occupational therapy to imbue the work with greater precision. His principles emphasized that the work be interesting, focused on cure, tailored to the patient's needs, and culminating in a useful product.

Elizabeth Upham, director of the art department at Milwaukee-Downer College, referred to "the modern science of therapeutic occupations for the handicapped" (Upham, 1917, p. 409). Other authors added their views to the debate. An unsigned history of occupational therapy credited Tracy's book *Studies in Invalid Occupation* as "the first attempt to place occupational therapy on a scientific basis" (History, 1940, p. 31). Hall defined occupational therapy as "the science of organized work for invalids" (Definitions of Occupational Therapy, 1940, p. 37). At an organizational level, the National Society for the Promotion of Occupational Therapy emphasized the scientific aspects of practice by selecting engineer and efficiency expert Frank Gilbreth as an honorary member in 1917 (American Occupational Therapy Association, 1967).

The Professional Literature

The directors of the National Society for the Promotion of Occupational Therapy selected the Maryland Psychiatric Quarterly as its official periodical. *The Modern Hospital* also carried information on occupational therapy. Articles focused equally on physical rehabilitation and mental illness, with authors emphasizing returning people to productive lives. In 1915, *The Modern Hospital* began featuring a monthly column, "Occupational Therapy, Vocational Re-Education and Industrial Rehabilitation."

A new journal, *Archives of Occupational Therapy*, appeared in 1922. Dunton owned and edited it and the *Maryland Psychiatric Quarterly*. *Archives of Occupational Therapy* was renamed *Occupational Therapy in Rehabilitation*. When he retired in 1947, Dunton attempted to transfer ownership of *Occupational Therapy in Rehabilitation* to the American Occupational Therapy Association, but the publisher, Williams & Wilkins, owned the copyrights to the journal name and its contents (Bone, 1971). The American Occupational Therapy Association began publication of the *American Journal of Occupational Therapy* in 1947.

The founders and the near-founders contributed to the developing body of knowledge by writing books, many of which became required textbooks. Among them were *Studies in Invalid Occupation: A Manual for Nurses and Attendants* and *Rake Knitting, and Its Special Adaptation to Invalid Workers* by Susan E. Tracy, Dunton's *Occupational Therapy: A Manual for Nurses*, and Barton's *Occupational Nursing: How the Installation of Invalid Occupation Work in Institutions Will Affect the Nursing Profession, and a Practical Example of Its Therapeutic Value* and *A View of Invalid Occupation: An Explanation of the New Idea of Providing Convalescents with Occupation* (Textbooks Required, 1920).

Occupational Therapy Finds Its Place

Social changes in the late 19th and early 20th centuries created an environment that fostered the development of occupational therapy. Among these were changes in the organizational structure and role of the hospital, the increasing effectiveness of traditional medical care, and the professionalization of health care providers.

The Development of Hospitals

Under earlier configurations, hospitals had no place for services of the type provided by occupational therapy. Although work was required of patients, it was for the benefit of the institution rather than the patient. For centuries, hospitals existed only as institutions of refuge for those without family members to care for them during illness. There was little emphasis on cure because there was often little that could cure.

From 1870 to 1910, two factors operated to change the role of the hospital. First, people moved to the cities in response to industrialization and thus were cut off from family support systems. Second, the introduction of aseptic techniques and anesthesia made surgery not only effective but survivable. According to Starr (1982), "The reconstitution of the hospital involved its redefinition as an institution of medical science rather than of social welfare, its reorganization on the lines of a business rather than a charity, and its reorientation to professionals and their patients rather than to patrons and the poor" (pp. 147–148).

Within the hospital, divisions of labor developed to increase efficiency. Hospitals "projected ideals of specialization and technical competence" (Starr, 1982, p. 146). Patients no longer provided their own care. The population of hospitalized patients shifted from the poor to the middle class.

Nursing as a profession emerged within the hospital setting. Nursing care was initially provided in the home, with women caring for family members. Nursing next was incorporated into a market economy as women began to nurse for hire in their patients' homes and then was concentrated in central plants where workers were subject to close supervision and new forms of control (Melosh, 1982, p. 8).

During the late 19th century, hospitals offered training programs for nursing students. Students did the ward work. Most nurses left the institution for private-duty work after graduation. Middle- and upper-class patients convalesced at home under the care of the hospital-trained professional nurse. By the end of the 1930s, however, the cost of private-duty nursing was prohibitive for most middle-class families (Melosh, 1984). These patients moved to hospitals for care.

The history of occupational therapy differs from that of nursing. When patients were cared for in their homes, activities to pass the time during convalescence and adaptations to activities for those with permanent impairments were provided according to the resources and imaginations of family and patient.

Patients in hospitals of the late 19th and early 20th centuries had to work to keep the hospital functioning, so there was no place or time for occupation as therapy. Professional nurses who provided convalescent care in the home may have offered, as did Susan Tracy, invalid occupations to clients, but that was a matter of individual circumstance. It was not until hospitals became curative centers for middle-class patients that there was a place for occupational therapy.

The Timeliness of Life Events

The ancients observed that there is a predetermined and established order to changes that occur in human beings as they grow up and grow old. Observations culminated in theories dividing human life into specific periods with associated actions or behaviors. Hippocrates was credited in a Latin translation of a Greek text with describing seven seasons, or ages, in human life. During the Middle Ages, medicine adopted a four-age theory: childhood, youth, maturity, and old age. Astrological theory included seven stages. Because astrology was considered a science, theories based on astrology were accepted on an equal basis with medicine (Burrow, 1986). Subsequent representations of the seven-age schemata were common. The best-known to the English-speaking world appeared in William Shakespeare's *As You Like It*. It begins thus:

> All the world's a stage,
> And all the men and women merely players:
> They have their exits and their entrances,
> And one man in his time plays many parts,
> His acts being seven ages. (act II, scene 7)

Kern (1983) identified the introduction of standard time, which occurred at the end of the 19th century, as the event that set the stage for the development of concepts about the timeliness of life events. Chudacoff (1989) placed the origin of age grading in "the education and medical care of children" (p. 50). He traced the former to the work of Pestalozzi, a Swiss educator, and the latter to the development of pediatrics as a medical specialty in the late 19th century. Chudacoff (1989) observed, "these [educational and medical] theories were refined and applied to older age groups as well as to youths. Moreover, spokespersons in popular and professional journals . . . began to delineate the ideal sequencing of a wide variety of experiences" (p. 50). He noted, "Such delineations not only implied norms but also often specified them. As a result, the concept of being on, ahead of, or behind schedules . . . meant matching the timing of one's personal experiences and achievements to cultural standards" (p. 50). Chudacoff (1989) noted that "the proliferation of intelligence testing in the 1910s and 1920s evidences a near obsession with age norms in American social science" (p. 81).

Emphasis on accuracy in the measurement of time created a framework in which all activities were categorized as being on time, ahead of time, or behind time. This set the stage for theories outlining appropriate times for important life events. Neugarden et al. (1968) characterized the powerful influence of ideas about age and stage related behaviors thus: "There exists what might be called a prescriptive time-table for the ordering of major life events: a time in the life span when men and women are expected to marry, a time to raise children, a time to retire" (p. 22).

Although the study of stage theories of human development was not a part of the preparation of the founders or the early occupational therapists, implicit in the belief systems of the founders of occupational therapy was the idea that role and activity have age and stage specificity. From the beginning, occupational therapists formulated goals that focused on occupational function and selected treatment activities based on "the relation of the age, sex, interests, physical and mental limitations of the patient to the occupation selected . . . " (Occupations for Invalids, 1916).

The World War I experience illustrates this focus. The acceptable roles of the young man were soldier and worker. The first reconstruction aides sent to France during World War I were stationed near the front lines and were charged with returning to duty as quickly as possible men suffering from **war neurosis** (Low, 1992). In the postwar years, the concern was for return to productive employment.

Subsequent writings in occupational therapy literature incorporated the works of such stage theorists as Gesell, Piaget, Erikson, and Havighurst as bases for understanding human behavior and occupational roles.

CLINICAL REASONING
in OT Practice

Influence of Historical and Social Foundations of Occupational Therapy Practice

The account of Ora Ruggles's career as a reconstruction aide working with injured servicemen after World War I (Carlova & Ruggles, 1946) included the story of Ben. Ben's war injuries resulted in the amputation of one leg and a spinal cord injury that caused some paralysis which interfered with his ability to sit up. Ben was described as "a grizzled Tennessee mountain man" (p. 80) who rebuffed the overtures of others until he became interested in Ruggles's work with patients. Acting on his interest, Ruggles taught Ben to make knotted belts. She noted both psychological and physical benefits from this activity. According to the authors, "In working the cords, which were tied to the rail at the foot of his bed, he exercised and strengthened his hands, arms and back. After a while, he could sit up straight, and, in time, even learned to say good morning" (Carlova & Ruggles, 1946, p. 81).

Consider how the choices of activity might have differed if the patient described had been a man with similar injuries in World War II. Think about the differences between the work of the reconstruction aides and the occupational therapist described in military hospitals during and after World War II. Think further about how a patient with such injuries would be treated today.

Treatment planning incorporates implications of the patient's age, gender, and life role expectations. Deviations from age-related life role expectations are often regarded as evidence of pathology.

Occupational Therapy Finds Its Place

Just as humans must adapt to various environments and challenges as they pass through the stages of life, so must professions adapt. Several significant periods in the history of occupational therapy practice influenced the profession and practitioners in significant ways. Among them are the two world wars and the period between them, a challenge to professional autonomy, and shifts in locations of service delivery and types of patients served.

Occupational Therapy and Military Medicine

The rapid growth of occupational therapy was credited in part to World War I (Gutman, 1995). The reconstruction aides were civilian women appointed to help in rehabilitation efforts for servicemen suffering from **battle fatigue**, war neurosis, or war-related injuries. The occupational therapy aides used craft activities that were carefully selected to meet each patient's physical and psychological needs. The work of one reconstruction aide, Ora Ruggles, is recounted in *The Healing Heart* (Carlova & Ruggles, 1946).

Women were selected for training and service as reconstruction aides on the basis of proficiency in a variety of crafts. Although training courses included psychology, specific handicapping conditions, the history of occupational therapy, and hospital etiquette, the use of crafts remained the focus (Emergency Course of Instruction). An Army medical department circular dated March 27, 1918, described the job and the qualifications for appointment: "trained women to furnish forms of occupation to convalescents in long illness . . . to give to patients the therapeutic benefit of activity. . . . She shall have a High School Education, or its equivalent." In addition to the educational requirement, applicants were required to be accomplished in at least three crafts, including basketry, weaving, wood carving, block printing, and needlework.

The seriousness of purpose of occupational therapy was subject to question because the providers of occupational therapy were women and their primary tools were craft activities and their own personalities. Colonel Frank Billings (1918) of the Office of the Surgeon General characterized the work of the reconstruction aides: "as diversional in character, in the form of knitting, in the form of basket weaving, etc." (p. 1925). He contrasted it with "more purposeful" activities that would serve "training of the soldier for employment after his discharge from the Army" (p. 1925).

This differentiation between women's work and men's work culminated in a distinction between bedside activities and vocational activities. Prolonged engagement in bedside activities provided by women reconstruction aides was criticized as promoting dependence and invalidism (Sexton, 1918). Vocational activities conducted by male vocational teachers prepared the men to return to economic productivity.

Following the armistice, many of the short training courses for reconstruction aides that had sprung up in response to the war emergency effort closed. Most of the reconstruction aides returned to civilian life and their former occupations of teacher, artist, or artisan. Some remained as occupational therapists employed in Veterans Bureau hospitals or public heath service facilities. Although the reconstruction aides did not have military status during their service time, they were allowed to apply for credit for service time toward civil service appointments (Low, 1992).

Opportunities for occupational therapists working with the civilian population grew with the passage of the 1923 Federal Industrial Rehabilitation Act, which mandated that hospitals providing care to persons with industrial injuries or illness include occupational therapy as "an integral part of its treatment" (American

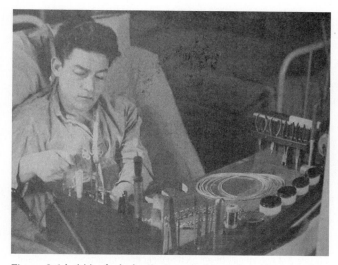

Figure 2-1 Activities for bed patients can be interesting and constructive; jewelry is an excellent project for long term bed patients. (Department of the Army. [1951]. *Occupational Therapy*. Department of the Army Technical Manual TM 8-291, p. 8. Washington: US Government Printing Office.)

Occupational Therapy Association, 1967, p. 10). This did not immediately result in a greater number of occupational therapists working with patients with physical disabilities. In 1937, nearly 80% of occupational therapists worked in mental health settings (Reed & Sanderson, 1983).

The outbreak of World War II increased the demand for occupational therapists to care for wounded servicemen. Occupational therapy literature is replete with descriptions of programs in military hospitals (Fig. 2.1). The activities and equipment described confirm emphasis on remediation of specific physical problems. Vetting (1945) described the equipment and activities of the occupational therapy clinic at the U.S. Naval Hospital at Bethesda: "A large carpentry shop . . . primarily for activities . . . to increase joint motion and muscle strength . . . will include workbenches designed specifically for patients who must work at shoulder height, adjustable workbenches to be used by patients who need to improve their posture . . . a height comfortable for the wheelchair patients" (p. 134). Other activities described were "Clay modeling . . . for increasing joint motions of the hands . . . floor looms adapted for shoulder and back exercise . . ."(Vetting, p. 135) (Fig. 2.2). A report on the Naval Hospital at Jacksonville, Florida, described the use of bicycle saws, bicycle lathes, and foot treadle looms to strengthen lower extremities (Egan, 1945).

Occupational Therapy and Rehabilitation

Rehabilitation became a recognized medical specialty in World War II. Although the idea of helping people

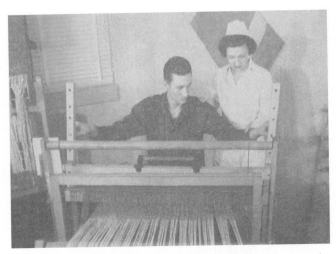

Figure 2-2 A loom may be adapted to meet many objectives of upper and lower extremity treatment. (Department of the Army. [1951]. *Occupational Therapy*. Department of the Army Technical Manual TM 8-291, p. 8. Washington: US Government Printing Office.)

with handicapping conditions to become productive and useful citizens was evidenced earlier by establishment of curative workshops, histories of rehabilitation link its development not to treatment through activity but to physical medicine. The latter approach developed during the years between the world wars and encompassed uses of "physical and other effective properties of light, heat, cold, water, electricity, massage, manipulation, exercise, and mechanical devices for physical and occupational therapy in the diagnosis or treatment of disease" (Berkowitz, 1981, p. 531).

The first department of physical medicine in an American medical school was established during the 1920s at Northwestern University (Berkowitz, 1981). In 1936 the establishment of a certifying board in physical medicine was proposed before the Advisory Board of Medical Specialties. It was not approved until 1947. By 1949, 234 physicians identified themselves as specialists in this area (Stevens, 1971). Although the two specialties were not identical, the overlapping domains of physical medicine and rehabilitation resulted in the creation in 1948 of a new medical specialty board, the American Board of Physical Medicine and Rehabilitation (Stevens, 1971).

As an Army Air Force physician, Howard Rusk "received orders to minimize his patients' hospital stays and to return as many people to combat as possible" (Berkowitz, 1981, p. 532), reminiscent of the orders under which the reconstruction aides acted. Rusk aimed to establish convalescent centers where the wounded would be sent when their conditions stabilized sufficiently for them to leave acute care and engage in programs of reconditioning and vocational guidance.

Rusk and his colleagues envisioned rehabilitation centers serving the special needs of military and civilian patients: "Unlike a general hospital, a rehabilitation clinic could contain the special facilities needed to train a paraplegic to go up and down a curb or to manipulate a wheelchair" (Berkowitz, 1981, p. 536). Occupational therapists were seen as "an important adjunct in the treatment and early recovery in injury and disease; and [occupational therapy] has an extremely important role in the modern concept of total rehabilitation" (Samberg, 1947, p. 290).

Poor relationships and communication between the physiatrists and vocational rehabilitation agencies slowed the initial growth of rehabilitation centers. In addition, territorial disputes with orthopaedic surgeons caused problems. To solidify their place in the health care arena, the physiatrists attempted to assume control of both the registration of occupational therapists and the standards and structure of occupational therapy education. From 1943 through the early 1950s the board of managers of the American Occupational Therapy Association resisted their efforts. Although successful in retaining professional autonomy, the board of managers and others in leadership positions within the association chose to avoid publicizing the actions of the physiatrists and their responses. They feared many of the rank and file occupational therapists might support the physiatrists' position because of positive interactions with physical medicine and rehabilitation doctors in military health care (Colman, 1992).

Friedland (1998) proposed that occupational therapists did in fact align themselves with rehabilitation medicine and abandoned commitment to the value of occupation in favor of reductionistic goals of increasing joint range of motion and muscle strength. However, this emphasis, along with concern for returning persons to economic productivity, was evidenced much earlier in writings that included description of equipment to accomplish such goals when crafts were not sufficient (Hickinson, 1934; Taylor, 1929).

In Hospital and at Home

Occupational therapists working in general hospitals dealt with a variety of diagnostic categories. Fay and March (1947) discussed grading downward for patients with neurosyphilis, a degenerative disorder, grading from large to fine movements to increase coordination for persons with hemiplegia and paraplegia, adapting activities for persons with Parkinson's disease, and focusing on muscle reeducation and avoidance of fatigue for persons with poliomyelitis. Their description of recommended management of patients with burns will be familiar to contemporary therapists: "the first object . . . is to help overcome the secondary stiffness resulting from immobilization" (p. 135). Therapists are advised to stretch contractures gently and gradually, "since the scar tissue and the new skin are sensitive and must not be torn or irritated" (p. 135). Rumsey's (1946) description of the occupational therapy principles for the treatment of peripheral nerve injuries mandated that the involved joint be kept flexible, that involved muscles be contracted and relaxed, and that the treatment plan incorporate both permanent and temporary compensatory techniques and equipment.

Home health was an arena of practice for occupational therapists from the early days of the profession. The aim of most home-based therapy was to help the person improve sufficiently to attend a curative workshop.

Work Hardening From Tuberculosis to Back Injury

Within the professional literature, occupational function was identified as the goal of therapy. Techniques varied with diagnostic categories. For many years, sanatoria for the treatment of tuberculosis were major employers of occupational therapists. Patients moved through a graduated regimen from bed rest to light activity to vocational training, a program easily recognizable as work hardening. The general superintendent of the Cook County (Illinois) Tuberculosis Hospital proclaimed the desired outcome of treatment for tuberculosis was that the patient be "cured and fitted for work" (Bailey, 1917, p. 378). A number of sanatorium-based programs included workshops where patients produced goods for sale.

Work programs for other injuries simulated actual job conditions as much as possible. Goodman (1922) described a work program for industrial injuries: "[the clients] would be in the atmosphere of work all the time" (p. 200). The director of occupational therapy at a curative workshop for orthopaedic conditions and industrial injuries reported on the program of physical and occupational therapy: "Our patients report for treatment at 8:00 in the morning, so that they will continue the habit of starting out early, thus making it easier for readjustment to work later on" (Taylor, 1929, p. 337).

Concerns about malingering by injured patients are longstanding. Spackman (1947) noted complications arising from industrial compensation programs: "The trouble occurs in instances when it is not financially profitable for the patient to return to work" (p. 227).

Many of the clients seen today in work-hardening programs are laborers or unskilled workers; back injury is the most common reason for referral (Hanson & Walker, 1992). In addition to addressing the reconditioning needed for return to work, occupational therapists are widely engaged in injury prevention programs.

Tools of Practice

The evolution of a profession requires practitioners to be open to new tools and approaches. However, transitions are rarely smooth. Professional identity may be threatened by methods perceived as radical departures from the early ideals. Incorporation of new techniques or technologies may generate territorial disputes with other professionals.

Use of Crafts and Exercise

Although expertise in activity analysis and selecting activities specific to treatment goals has been a hallmark of occupational therapy from the beginning, occupational therapists in many settings were concerned about the adequacy of handicrafts to prepare patients for occupational function. According to an editorial in a 1918 issue of *Maryland Psychiatric Quarterly*, activities used in therapy "may appear trivial" ("Occupational Aides," 1918, p. 27).

Hall (1917), several times president of the National Society for the Promotion of Occupational Therapy, commented, "The occupations that are employed therapeutically range all the way from work in the service of the institution to virtual play in the construction of rather useless articles of the so-called arts and crafts order" (p. 383).

Practicing therapists recognized the limitations of their traditional approaches. Decrying the scarcity of crafts that required finger extension, Taylor (1929) reported, "Mechanical means are often necessary because of the limitations in occupations" (p. 337). She was equally concerned about activities for lower extremity function: "The problem ahead of us in the use of occupational therapy for functional restoration is to readapt and make jig saws, looms, etc., so that all physical exercises may be obtained through occupations" (p. 337).

After describing adaptations of loom, bicycle saw, and treadle saw for lower extremity strengthening, one director of occupational therapy noted, "As ankle flexion is usually limited, I am going to mention two ways of getting it by mechanical appliances" (Hickinson, 1934, p. 34). The first was a cot with a pulley at one end. The patient lay on his or her side, and "a band around the patient's foot is fastened to the cord over the pulley, and a weight attached. Flexion of the foot uses the flexor muscles to pull up the weight, which may be gradually increased" (Hickinson, 1934, p. 34). The second was described thus: "The foot may be strapped in the ankle circumductor, and the circumductor turned entirely by pulling the foot away from the pedal. [The term circumductor suggests a device that moves the ankle through full circumduction.] The handle is not used except to start. This makes a heavy exercise" (Hickinson, 1934, p. 34). Subsequent attempts at developing equipment for specific muscle patterns included such inventions as the Extensorcisor, described as "an apparatus to provide progressive resistive exercises for the finger extensor muscles" (Heather et al., 1962, p. 10).

Mosey (1970) noted that following World War II, "Occupational therapists were uncomfortable with their operating principle that it was good for disabled people to keep active and busy doing the things they enjoyed" (p. 235). Emphasis on crafts gave way to exercise, and practice became specialized. One of the specialized areas was the treatment of patients with poliomyelitis. Treatment, which was based on the work of Sister Elizabeth Kenny, was directed toward maintaining or improving muscle strength and joint range of motion.

Exercises and activities aimed at restoring or increasing motion at specific joints required that occupational therapists be proficient in joint measurement. The first volume of the *American Journal of Occupational Therapy* included articles on joint measurement (Hurt, 1947a, b, c) and a printed paper goniometer with directions for cutting out and assembling it (Goniometer, 1947). Over time, information on specific exercise techniques and equipment appeared in the professional literature.

Physical Agent Modalities

By the late 1970s and early 1980s, occupational therapists working with patients with physical disabilities began to incorporate other less traditional modalities into their treatments. To facilitate joint and muscle function, they used paraffin baths, hot and cold packs, ultrasound, and electrical stimulation. These approaches and others selected to produce changes in soft tissue were known collectively as physical agent modalities.

In 1992, the American Occupational Therapy Association issued a position paper on the use of physical agent modalities. The techniques in question were labeled as adjunctive modalities (American Occupational Therapy Association, 1992a, p. 1075) to convey that use of these techniques was considered adjunctive or supplemental to purposeful activity in meeting patients' objectives. The position paper mandated that use be restricted to "a practitioner who has documented evidence of possessing the theoretical background and technical skills for safe and competent

integration of the modality" (American Occupational Therapy Association, 1992b, p. 1090).

However, as late as 1997, a survey of occupational therapists revealed that most users of physical agent modalities had no formal training in either theoretical basis for use or technique (Cornish-Painter et al., 1997). Occupational therapy education programs incorporate specific instruction in physical agent modalities into their curricula, and continuing education opportunities for clinicians are readily available.

Adaptive Equipment

Adaptive equipment for performing occupational tasks and activities of daily living was first described for a patient at Michael Reese Hospital in Chicago. The patient was paralyzed by a gunshot wound. Susan Tracy strapped a polishing pad to the man's right hand and taught him to polish articles placed in front of him by moving his arm. The benefit of this was realized when, as the author reported, "This man had not been able to put anything into his own mouth for 4 months, but, with the aid of a second leather palm which holds a fork or spoon, he can now feed himself" (Occupational Therapy in the General Hospital, 1917, p. 426).

Some 30 years later, Haas provided directions for making a knife-and-fork combination (Haas, 1946). Haas published a booklet, *Equipment Aids for Those Having One Hand* (Haas, 1947, p. 1). He recommended the use of clamps, vacuum cups, and clips for stabilizing projects and proposed attaching fine sandpaper to tools to increase friction and prevent slipping (Haas, 1947).

In the years following World War II, much adapted equipment addressed the needs of disabled veterans. An unsigned article in a 1945 *Occupational Therapy and Rehabilitation* issue was illustrated with photographs of aids designed to permit war veterans with amputations to drive. The adaptations were designed by the war engineering board of the Society of Automotive Engineers, and the information was provided to occupational therapists so they could advise their patients (Simple devices enable veterans to drive motor vehicles safely, 1945).

Patients with poliomyelitis had long convalescent periods in which activities were limited by poor endurance and disability. Occupational therapists developed activity programs to provide mental stimulation without overtaxing damaged neuromuscular systems. McFarland & Lukins (1946), respectively a physician and an occupational therapist, described a mouth stick page turner for patients in respirators and included instructions for fabrication. MacLean (1949) described the development and adaptation of arm slings, lapboards, adjustable tables, and built-up armrests to improve functional abilities. For the next several years, adaptations to meet the needs of patients who had had poliomyelitis were frequently featured in occupational therapy literature.

New products were regularly introduced to occupational therapists in the *American Journal of Occupational Therapy.* A 1952 column of products and techniques included a collapsible reacher for the bed or wheelchair patient (Have You Tried? 1952). Contemporary occupational therapists have access to extensive collections of adaptive equipment for almost every disabling condition. Today's challenges are found in selecting equipment that is reliable, affordable, and acceptable to the patient, both functionally and cosmetically.

Orthotics

An article by Slagle (1938) was illustrated with a photograph of a patient identified as having a brachial plexus injury wearing an airplane splint "to rest shoulder muscles" (p. 378). The patient is engaged in an activity identified as Egyptian card weaving with the stated purpose of providing "motion of grasp, wrist and elbow flexion" (p. 378). There is no indication that the splint is itself part of the occupational therapy program.

Writing on the management of patients with arthritis, Sammons (1945) reported, "Splints are frequently used to prevent flexion deformities of the hands or spinal rigidity in faulty position in rheumatoid spondylitis" (p. 18). The author referred to the use of a cock-up splint for wrist drop, but no information was provided as to whether the occupational therapist was involved in the fabrication or fitting. In a chapter on treating persons with physical injuries, Spackman (1947) referred to a cock-up splint but did not give information on construction, application, or management.

Hand surgeon Sterling Bunnell outlined a sequence of care for hand injuries, with occupational therapy initiated once the wound had healed and continuing until the patient was "ready for work" (Bunnell, 1950, p. 148). His article was illustrated with photographs of a variety of commercial splints with an address from which they could be ordered.

Fabrication of orthoses was addressed in 1952. The chief of occupational therapy at the Veterans Administration Hospital in Portland, Oregon, reported on the use of plastic to fabricate splints for patients with poliomyelitis. She included principles of a well-designed splint and directions for making several splints, including an opponens cuff and a foot-drop splint (Boyce, 1952).

Silverstein (1953) described clinic-made adaptations of several of Bunnell's hand splints. She noted, "It became possible . . . to adapt these splints to fit hands of unusual sizes or peculiar deformities . . . to supply these new splints quickly and at a much lower cost than previously. . . . Familiarity with the mechanics of the devices allowed alteration of the splints as the patient's condition improved" (Silverstein, 1953, p. 213).

Neurorehabilitation Techniques

As patients with head injury and stroke achieved higher rates of survival, interest in treating the sequelae of neurological insults developed. In 1948, Berta Bobath's "The Importance of the Reduction of Muscle Tone and the Control of Mass Reflex Action in the Treatment of Spasticity" was published in *Occupational Therapy and Rehabilitation.* Subsequent writings on the management of adult hemiplegia by the Bobaths appeared in physical therapy journals.

Herbert Kabat, a physician, was among the first to introduce ideas about neuromuscular mechanisms into treatment techniques. In 1950, Kabat and occupational therapist Dorothy Rosenberg described a program aimed at " . . . accelerating the development of voluntary motion in severely paralyzed muscles . . . [by] . . . using reinforcement techniques for guided resistive exercise utilizing primitive mass movement patterns, certain reflexes, synergistic motions, symmetrical bilateral motions, etc." (Kabat & Rosenberg, 1950, p. 6).

Patients with a variety of neurological disorders were admitted to the Kabat–Kaiser Institute for medical care, physical therapy, occupational therapy, and vocational counseling. Physical therapists helped patients establish individual motions before occupational therapists began working on movement combinations necessary for self-care.

Carroll studied the efficacy of Kabat's reinforcement techniques in treatment of hemiplegia. The techniques she used were "(1) the tonic neck reflexes, (2) the stimulation of synergists, (3) the use of resistance, and (4) rhythmic stabilization" (Carroll, 1950, p 212). Relating inconclusive results to a limited treatment time and interruptions because of medical complications, Carroll recommended that occupational therapists "devise a variety of techniques which are based on these principles and which may lead to better results in the total rehabilitation of the hemiplegic patient" (p. 213).

In the third of a three part series, "Proprioceptive Facilitation Elicited Through the Upper Extremities," Ayres described the selection and adaptation of "simple, normal, life-like activities" (Ayres, 1955, p. 121) using proprioceptive facilitatory mechanisms.

Margaret Rood, trained as both physical therapist and occupational therapist, based her work on use of sensory input to influence motor output. Although she was not a prolific writer, her work influenced occupational therapy education. Information on the muscle spindle and on proprioception was incorporated into anatomy and physiology courses (Cohen & Reed, 1996).

Signe Brunnstrom, also a physical therapist, presented her theory and techniques to occupational therapists in a 1961 article, "Motor Behavior of Adult Hemiplegic Patients: Hints for Training" (Brunnstrom, 1961). Subsequent publications by occupational therapists and professionals from other disciplines provided readers further explanations of neuromuscular mechanisms and applications of theoretical information to clinical practice. Street (1963) discussed the theories of Rood, Sherrington, and others and the clinical implications of techniques for inhibiting or facilitating antagonists.

In the abstract of her 1968 article "A New Look at the Nervous System in Relation to Rehabilitation Techniques," Moore said, "More recent concepts concerning learning, plasticity and facilitatory and inhibitory systems in the nervous system are covered" (Moore, 1968, p. 489). Rider (1971) studied Rood's techniques and reported a study, "Effects of Neuromuscular Facilitation on Cross Transfer."

Contemporary research indicates that neurological functions occur concurrently at many levels of the nervous system rather than in the rigidly hierarchical model of earlier theorists. While new information is increasing its influence on practice, occupational therapists have not discarded the works of these earlier theorists and practitioners. Techniques introduced by Kabat, the Bobaths, Brunnstrom, and Rood are still in evidence in many clinical settings.

Past, Present and Future: Will the Questions Be the Same?

Occupational therapists have met many challenges throughout the course of the profession. Today's occupational therapists are discovering that challenges once met reappear, sometimes in familiar form and sometimes in different guise. Treatment planning for short hospital stays and limited reimbursable visits are formidable tasks for occupational therapists trained in more traditional fee-for-service practices, as daunting as the challenges our predecessors faced in preparing patients to return to productive lives after long hospitalizations.

The types of diagnoses that occupational therapists see have changed with changes in health care. New technologies and treatment techniques become available and must be evaluated for effectiveness and appropriateness. Individuals today are less bound by economic and societal definitions of occupational roles appropriate for age and gender. In many ways, this makes treatment planning more difficult, because neither patient nor therapist can rely on prescribed occupational roles. Assumptions about life roles based on age, gender, and education may be inaccurate.

In 1929, Marjorie Taylor, director of the department of occupational therapy at Milwaukee-Downer College and advisory director of the Junior League Curative Workshop in Milwaukee, exhorted: "The therapists must bend all their energies to rapidity of functional gain with every patient. In no other field is the pressure of time felt so keenly, or the loss of money through inexact or unintelligent treatment so great" (Taylor, 1929, p. 335). Although the fees charged for her program were $2.50 per day for combined treatments in occupational therapy and physical therapy, her message is both familiar and vital to occupational therapists today.

Summary Review Questions

1. What changes in hospitals fostered development of occupational therapy?
2. What factors facilitated development of standards for the timeliness of life task accomplishment?
3. How do practices of the 19th-century health reformers relate to occupational therapy in the 20th century?
4. How did occupational therapy for World War I servicemen differ from occupational therapy in military hospitals during World War II?
5. Describe the relationship between rehabilitation medicine and the leaders of occupational therapy in the years following World War II.
6. How was treatment for persons with tuberculosis similar to work-hardening programs?
7. What were early concerns about crafts and adjunctive equipment modalities that occupational therapists have used to augment more traditional therapeutic modalities?

References

American Occupational Therapy Association. (1967). *Then—and now!* Bethesda, MD: author.

American Occupational Therapy Association. (1992a). Use of adjunctive modalities in occupational therapy. *American Journal of Occupational Therapy, 46,* 1075–1081.

American Occupational Therapy Association. (1992b). Position paper: Physical agent modalities. *American Journal of Occupational Therapy, 46,* 1090–1091.

Ayers, A. J. (1955). Proprioceptive facilitation elicited through the upper extremities. Part III: Specific application to occupational therapy. *American Journal of Occupational Therapy, 9,* 121–126, 143.

Bailey, H. L. (1917). The Cook County Tuberculosis Hospital, Oak Forest, Ill. *The Modern Hospital, 8,* 377–379.

Barton, G. E. (1917). Inoculation of the bacillus of work. *The Modern Hospital, 8,* 399–402.

Berkowitz, E. D. (1981). The federal government and the emergence of rehabilitation medicine. *The Historian, 43,* 530–545.

Billings, F. (1918). Chairman's address. The national program for the reconstruction and rehabilitation of disabled soldiers. *Journal of the American Medical Association, 70,* 1924–1925.

Bobath, B. (1948). The importance of the reduction of muscle tone and the control of mass reflex action in the treatment of spasticity. *Occupational Therapy and Rehabilitation, 27,* 371–373.

Bone, C. D. (1971). Origin of the *American Journal of Occupational Therapy. American Journal of Occupational Therapy, 25,* 48–52.

Boyce, M. H. (1952). Plastic splints. *American Journal of Occupational Therapy, 6,* 203–207.

Brunnstrom, S. (1961). Motor behavior of adult hemiplegic patients. *American Journal of Occupational Therapy, 15,* 6–12, 47.

Bunnell, S. (1950). Occupational therapy of hands. *American Journal of Occupational Therapy, 4,* 145–153, 177.

Burrow, J. A. (1986). *The Ages of Man: A Study in Medieval Writing and Thought.* Oxford UK: Clarendon.

Carlova, J., & Ruggles, O. (1946). *The Healing Heart.* New York: Messner.

Carroll, J. (1950). The utilization of reinforcement techniques in the program for the hemiplegic. *American Journal of Occupational Therapy, 4,* 211–213, 239.

Chudacoff, H. P. (1989). *How Old Are You? Age Consciousness in American Culture.* Princeton, NJ: Princeton University.

Cohen, H., & Reed, K. L. (1996). The historical development of neuroscience in physical rehabilitation. *American Journal of Occupational Therapy, 50,* 561–568.

Colman, W. (1992). Maintaining autonomy: The struggle between occupational therapy and physical medicine. *American Journal of Occupational Therapy, 46,* 63–70.

Cornish-Painter, C., Peterson, C. Q., & Lindstrom-Hazel, D. K. (1997). Skill acquisition and competency testing for physical agent modality use. *American Journal of Occupational Therapy, 51,* 681–685.

Definitions of Occupational Therapy. (1940). *Occupational Therapy and Rehabilitation, 19,* 35–38.

Dunton, W. R. (1915). *Occupational Therapy.* Philadelphia: Saunders.

Dunton, W. R. (1917). History of occupational therapy. *The Modern Hospital, 8,* 380–382.

Dunton, W. R. (1919). *Reconstruction Therapy.* Philadelphia: Saunders.

Dunton, W. R. (1928). *Prescribing Occupational Therapy.* Baltimore: Thomas.

Dunton, W. R., & Licht, S. (1950). *Occupational Therapy, Principles and Practices.* Springfield, IL: Charles C. Thomas.

Dunton, W. R., & Licht, S. (1957). *Occupational Therapy, Principles and Practices* (2nd ed.). Springfield, IL: Charles C. Thomas.

Egan, H. (1945). U.S. Naval Hospital, Jacksonville, Florida. *Occupational Therapy and Rehabilitation, 25,* 143–145.

Emergency Course of Instruction for Reconstruction Aides. *American Occupational Therapy Association Archives,* Series 1, Box 01, Folder 06. Rockville, MD.

Fay, E. V., & March, I. (1947). Occupational therapy in general and special hospitals. In H. S. Willard & C. S. Spackman (Eds.), *Principles of Occupational Therapy* (pp. 1118–1140). Philadelphia: Lippincott.

Friedland, J. (1998). Occupational therapy and rehabilitation: An awkward alliance. *American Journal of Occupational Therapy, 52,* 373–380.

Goniometer. (1947). *American Journal of Occupational Therapy, 1,* 268.

Goodman, H. B. (1922). The industrial case from the accident back to the job. *Archives of Occupational Therapy, 1,* 193–204.

Gutman, S. (1995). Influence of the U.S. military and occupational therapy reconstruction aides in World War I on the development of occupational therapy. *American Journal of Occupational Therapy, 49,* 256–262.

Haas, L. J. (1946). Eating with one hand. *Occupational Therapy and Rehabilitation, 25,* 233–234.

Haas, L. J. (1947). Equipment aids for the aging person. *Occupational Therapy and Rehabilitation, 25,* 1–4.

Hall, H. J. (1917). Remunerative occupations for the handicapped. *The Modern Hospital, 8,* 383–386.

Hanson, C. S., & Walker, K. W. (1992). The history of work in physical dysfunction. *American Journal of Occupational Therapy, 46,* 56-62.

Have you tried? (1952). *American Journal of Occupational Therapy, 6,* 281.

Heather, A. J., Smith, T. A., & Walsh, D. (1962). Extensorcisor. *American Journal of Occupational Therapy, 16,* 10–12.

Hickinson, L. M. (1934). Anatomical considerations and technique in using occupations as exercise for orthopedic disabilities. *Occupational Therapy and Rehabilitation, 13,* 30–34.

History. (1940). *Occupational Therapy and Rehabilitation, 19,* 27–34.

Hurt, S. (1947a). Considerations in muscle function and their application to disability evaluation and treatment. *American Journal of Occupational Therapy, 1,* 69–73.

Hurt, S. (1947b). Joint measurement. *American Journal of Occupational Therapy, 1,* 209–214.

Hurt, S. (1947c). Joint measurement Part II. *American Journal of Occupational Therapy, 1,* 218–285.

Johnson, S. (1917). Occupational therapy in New York City institutions. *The Modern Hospital, 8,* 414–415.

Kabat, H., & Rosenberg, D. (1950). Concepts and techniques of occupational therapy for neuromuscular disorders. *American Journal of Occupational Therapy, 4,* 6–11.

Kern, S. (1983). *The Culture of Time and Space.* Cambridge, MA: Harvard University.

Licht, S. (1967). The founding and founders of the American Occupational Therapy Association. *American Journal of Occupational Therapy, 21,* 269–277.

Low, J. F. (1992). The reconstruction aides. *American Journal of Occupational Therapy, 46,* 45–48.

MacLean, F. M. (1949). Occupational therapy in the management of poliomyelitis. *American Journal of Occupational Therapy, 3,* 20–27.

McFarland, J. W., & Lukins, N. M. (1946). A page turning device for respiratory patients. *Occupational Therapy and Rehabilitation, 25,* 42–44.

Melosh, B. (1982). *The physician's hand: Work, culture and conflict in American nursing.* Philadelphia: Temple University.

Melosh, B. (1984). More than "the physician's hand": Skill and authority in twentieth-century nursing. In J. W. Leavitt (Ed.), *Women and Health in America* (pp. 482-496). Madison: University of Wisconsin.

Moore, J. C. (1968). A new look at the nervous system in relation to rehabilitation techniques. *American Journal of Occupational Therapy, 22,* 489–501.

Mosey, A. C. (1970). *Three Frames of Reference for Mental Health.* Thorofare, NJ: Charles B. Slack.

Neugarten, B., Moore, J., & Lowe, J. (1968). Age norms, age constraints, and adult socialization. In B. L. Neugarten (Ed.), *Middle Age and Aging: A Reader in Social Psychology.* Chicago: University of Chicago.

Occupation aides. (1918). *Maryland Psychiatric Quarterly, 8,* 27.

Occupational therapy in the general hospital. (1917). *The Modern Hospital, 8,* 425–427.

Occupations for Invalids. (1916). School of Practical Arts, Teachers College, Columbia University. American Occupational Therapy Association Archives, Series 12, Box 101, File 733. Rockville, MD.

Peloquin, S. M. (1991). Occupational therapy service: Individual and collective understandings of the founders, part 1. *American Journal of Occupational Therapy, 45,* 352–360.

Reed, K. L., & Sanderson, S. R. (1983). *Concepts of Occupational Therapy* (2nd ed). Baltimore: Williams & Wilkins.

Rider, B. A. (1971). Effects of neuromuscular facilitation on cross transfer. *American Journal of Occupational Therapy, 25*, 84–89.

Rosenberg, C. E. (1978). The practice of medicine in New York a century ago. In J. W. Leavitt & R. L. Numbers (Eds.), *Sickness and Health in America* (pp. 55–74). Madison: University of Wisconsin.

Rumsey, R. (1946). Occupational therapy in the treatment of peripheral nerve injuries. *Occupational Therapy and Rehabilitation, 25*, 180–183.

Samberg, H. H. (1947). Occupational therapy in a general hospital. *American Journal of Occupational Therapy, 1*, 285–290.

Sammons, D. D. (1945). Arthritis (I). *Occupational Therapy and Rehabilitation, 24*, 13–22.

Serrett, K. D. (1985). Another look at occupational therapy's history: Paradigm or pair-of-hands? *Occupational Therapy in Mental Health, 3*, 1–31.

Sexton, F. H. (1918). Vocational rehabilitation of soldiers suffering from nervous diseases. *Mental Hygiene, 2*, 265–276.

Shakespeare, W. (1975). The Complete Works of William Shakespeare. New York: Avenel.

Simple devices enable veterans to drive motor vehicles safely. (1945). *Occupational Therapy and Rehabilitation, 45*, 263.

Silverstein, F. (1953). Occupational therapy and the hand splint. *American Journal of Occupational Therapy, 7*, 213–216, 222.

Slagle, E. C. (1938). Occupational therapy. *Trained Nurse and Hospital Review, 100*, 375–382.

Spackman, C. S. (1947). Occupational therapy for patients with physical injuries. In H. S. Willard & C. S. Spackman (Eds.), *Principles of Occupational Therapy* (pp. 175–273). Philadelphia: Lippincott.

Starr, P. (1982). *The Social Transformation of American Medicine*. New York: Basic Books.

Stevens, R. (1971). *American Medicine and the Public Interest*. New Haven: Yale University.

Street, D. R. (1963). Antagonistic activity in voluntary motion. *American Journal of Occupational Therapy, 17*, 10–15.

Taylor, M. (1929). Occupational therapy in industrial injuries. *Occupational Therapy and Rehabilitation, 8*, 335–338.

Textbooks required for the January 1920 term at the School of Diversional Occupation in Colorado Springs, Colorado. (1920). American Occupational Therapy Association Archives, Series 12, Box 101, File 731. Rockville, MD.

Tracy, S. (1910). *Studies in Invalid Occupations: A Manual for Nurses and Attendants*. Boston: Whitcomb & Barrows.

Upham, E. G. (1917). Some principles of occupational therapy. *The Modern Hospital, 8*, 409–413.

Vetting, M. L. (1945). U.S. Naval Hospital, N.N.M.C., Bethesda, Maryland. *Occupational Therapy and Rehabilitation, 25*, 131–135.

3

Assessing Roles and Competence

Mary Law

LEARNING OBJECTIVES

After studying this chapter, the reader will be able to do the following:

1. Understand the nature and importance of assessment in occupational therapy.
2. Evaluate roles, competence, and occupational function, beginning with clients' perception of their **occupational performance** issues.
3. Understand the measurement criteria necessary for reliable and valid assessments for use in occupational therapy practice.
4. Discuss and use current validated assessments of competence in occupational function (roles, tasks, and activities).

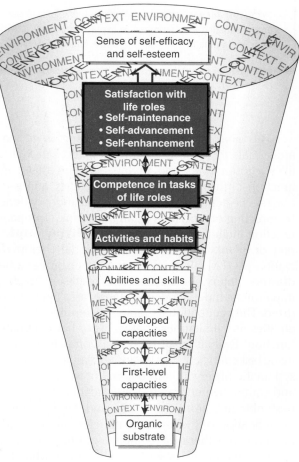

The determination of the status of the client in terms of the services that the professional provides is the basis for evidence-based practice in any health profession. Occupational therapists provide services relative to occupational function and offer services to persons who have or are at risk for developing occupational dysfunction. Occupational dysfunction is defined as the inability to engage in one or more of the roles that are important to the client in the manner in which he or she wants to engage in them. The occupational therapy assessment necessarily begins with the determination of the client's past roles, probable future roles, ability to accomplish the tasks and activities he or she associates with a given role, and satisfaction with performance. Later chapters discuss assessment of the component abilities and capacities (components of occupational function) required to carry out the tasks and activities of a given role.

GLOSSARY

Activities of daily living—Activities or tasks that a person does every day to maintain personal care.

Instrumental activities of daily living—Complex activities or tasks that a person does to maintain independence in the home and community.

Leisure—Activities or tasks that are not obligatory and that are done for enjoyment.

Occupational performance—Ability of individuals to perform and be satisfied with performance in purposeful daily activities in their environment, developmental stage, and societal roles.

Reliability—Consistency or reproducibility of an assessment under various conditions (Streiner & Norman, 1989).

Validity—Ability of an instrument to assess the intended characteristic (Law, 1987).

Work—Activities or tasks in the areas of home management, care of others, education, vocation, and avocation (AOTA, 1994).

The goal of occupational therapy is to enable individuals to achieve competency and satisfaction in life's chosen roles and in the activities that support function of these roles. Such competency and satisfaction can be achieved through personal independence or by directing others, such as an attendant. Occupational function includes **activities of daily living**, **work**, and play or **leisure** (American Occupational Therapy Association [AOTA], 1994). Whenever a person has a health disorder, injury, or disease that results in a physical impairment, independence in these tasks may be jeopardized. The occupational therapist determines the client's abilities and limitations, that is, his or her occupational function. Evaluation of roles and competence in daily living tasks and activities begins with an interview and/or systematic observation to determine what activities can and cannot be performed. This functional information is best obtained from the client and family. Following identification of the issues of difficulty in occupational function, the therapist completes further assessments (often impairment based) to determine what factors limit performance. If the limiting factors can be improved or eliminated by direct intervention, the therapist chooses an intervention approach that is appropriate to the problem. If, however, the limiting factors are not amenable to change, the therapist teaches the individual to compensate for these limitations by adapting the task or by changing the environment in which it is performed.

In the past, therapists have assessed roles and competence by administering standardized evaluations or checklists of activities of daily living (ADL), work, and leisure. However, occupational function, or the ability to carry out activities during daily life, depends on the individual's culture, gender, roles that he or she wishes to undertake, and environment (Law, 1991; Trombly, 1995a). Thus occupational function is a personal concept. The individuality of a person's roles and his or her day-to-day functioning make it both difficult and time-consuming for one standardized evaluation to assess all aspects of occupational function. As outlined by Trombly (see Chapter 1), assessment should be a top-down approach beginning with an evaluation of roles, tasks, and activities. Roles include self-maintenance (e.g. caregiver, home maintainer), self-enhancement (e.g. friend, movie-goer) and self-advancement (e.g. worker, student, shopper) (Trombly, 1995b).

This approach to assessment includes consideration of the environment in which a person lives. Assessment does not ignore components of occupational function, such as strength, endurance, problem solving, and depth perception. However, it begins with a function-based assessment of the tasks and activities that the client needs, wants, or is expected to accomplish and is having difficulty in performing (Law et al., 1998). Looking at this process from the perspective of the revised World Health Organization's Classification of Functioning, Disability and Health (ICIDH-2) (WHO, 2000), occupational therapists begin by assessing activities and participation and assess impairments only if necessary to explain difficulties in performance.

By beginning with a focus on the clients' needs and considering their roles and the environment in which they live, therapists recognize the values and goals that clients bring to occupational therapy. This approach reflects a change in philosophy to a client-centered approach, recognizing that it is the person who is engaged in therapy who should be articulating the goals of therapy and driving the process (Law, 1998).

Measurement Concepts

Several important concepts of measurement must be considered in assessing roles and competence in occupational therapy. The format of the evaluation instrument can be an interview or a standardized list of activities on which the therapist indicates whether each item can be performed. The use of nonstandardized checklists is not recommended because of their inherent lack of evidence of **reliability** and **validity**. The tasks listed in nonstandardized checklists are rarely even operationally defined, the initial step in establishing reliability and validity.

The level of measurement of most evaluations of roles, tasks, and activities is ordinal, that is, the score can range from "dependent, is unable" to "independent, is able." Space is usually available on forms for periodic reevaluation. It is important to record the level of performance at a minimum at admission and discharge, because these records may be used for program evaluation, to justify service to third-party payers, in legal actions, and in determining whether a patient will be discharged home or to an extended-care facility. It is also important to note whether an assessment is measuring a person's capacity to perform a task or actual performance.

The clinical utility of an assessment tool is an important consideration. Clinical utility refers to all of the practical factors of an instrument, such as cost, training required, availability of a manual, and ease of administration and interpretation. In most occupational therapy services, managers want to use assessments that are time efficient and provide information useful for planning and evaluating treatment.

Assessment of roles and competence by occupational therapists can take place in many different environments, such as a rehabilitation center, workplace, school, or community setting. The setting in which an assessment is done affects a person's performance. Research indicates that occupational therapists cannot take results of assessment at one location (e.g., rehabilitation center) and assume that these results apply to performance in another location (e.g., home) (Brown et al., 1996).

Evaluation instruments should be valid, reliable, and responsive enough to detect important changes (Law & Letts, 1989). A valid assessment is one that measures what it purports to measure. Most evaluations of functional performance have content validity. The items are samples of a universe of behavior, but some are more important than others (Hasselkus & Safrit, 1976). For example, in the universe of meal preparation, "can use the stove safely" is more important than "can stir batter."

A reliable assessment is one that measures the attribute under study consistently no matter who is scoring (interrater reliability) or when the assessment occurs (test–retest reliability). Responsiveness, the third characteristic of a good assessment, refers to the ability to detect the smallest clinically important increment of change. As an example, for a therapist working on a day-to-day basis with a patient to increase his or her ability to dress, the assessment should be sensitive enough to allow progress to be noted when different areas of the body can be dressed or different articles of clothing applied. Responsiveness is directly related to the number of items on an assessment and to the number of categories on the scoring scale. An assessment with 50 items is likely to be more responsive than one with 10 items. A scoring system using a 1–7 Likert scale is likely to be more responsive than one using a 1–3 scale.

After clients identify the activities that are important to them, observation of those activities is the most direct method of assessing functional ability and is preferred for accuracy, detection of inefficient or unsafe methods, and determination of the underlying reason that a particular task cannot be performed. It can, however, be time-consuming and costly (Law & Letts, 1989). Self-report of actual performance through interview is the easiest, fastest, and most inexpensive method of assessing functional abilities. There is a concern, however, that such reports may not accurately reflect what the person can do. If a person reports questionable data and does not permit observation, the therapist should verify the report with others who have knowledge of the client's actual performance. False information is not necessarily the result of a conscious intent to deceive but may reflect the fact that a patient is in a health care facility and does not have an accurate sense of his or her abilities. Studies comparing results of self-report with observation of functional performance have found high agreement between the two, especially for self-care tasks performed daily (Collin et al., 1988; Harris et al., 1986). Conversely, Edwards (1990) and Sagar et al. (1992) found that patients consistently overrated their ability. Sinoff & Ore (1997) found that persons older than 85 years of age had larger discrepancy scores between self-report and actual performance on the *Barthel Index*. In some instances, proxy reports from family or caregivers are used in assessment. However, the information given is the family member's perspective, not that of the client. Long et al. (1998) have found that caregivers with a large burden of care tend to rate their family members low on assessments.

Tasks and activities are not all evaluated at the same time. Ability to do self-care, personal mobility, and leisure activities within the limits of a disability are usually done early, and they form the basis for the therapy plan that includes restorative therapy and/or adaptation to enable occupational function. As recovery continues and discharge planning decisions are being considered, evaluations concerned with access to home and community, transportation, care of the home and children, hobbies, sports and family recreation, and job and educational abilities are done as applicable.

Evaluation Methods

A comprehensive assessment of occupational function begins with identification of occupational needs, is followed by evaluation of client's ability to carry out roles, and continues with evaluation of the person's ability to carry out specific tasks and activities.

Identification of Occupational Needs

A client-centered occupational therapy assessment begins with the evaluation of what tasks and activities the client needs, wants, or is expected to accomplish and is having difficulty in performing (Law et al., 1994). Such an assessment recognizes that performance of the occupations of one's choice is an individual issue and that a person's perception is the important force that drives the occupational therapy process. Information about an individual's occupations, roles, developmental stage, and the environment in which he or she lives is best obtained through an interview. This can be done through a narrative interview or through use of more structured interview-based assessments.

Informal Interview Methods

Neistadt (1994), using survey research, found that most occupational therapists establish goals through an informal client interview. Her research indicates that the difficulty with such an unstructured process is that therapy goals tend to be vague and not specifically related to occupation. Gitlin et al. (1995) discuss the use of narrative or ethnographic methods as a way to gain information from clients and their families.

Semistructured Interview Methods

A semistructured interview method that can be used to assess a person's perception of his occupational performance is the *Canadian Occupational Performance Measure (COPM)* (Law et al., 1998). The Resources section has information regarding purchase of this and other tests discussed in this chapter. *COPM* helps clients to identify occupational function issues, assists in goal setting, and measures changes in their perception of occupational performance over the course of occupational therapy intervention. *COPM* measures an individual's perception of occupational performance among

people with a variety of disabilities and across all developmental stages. It is client centered and incorporates roles and role expectations within the client's own environment.

During the *COPM* interview, clients or caregivers identify areas of ADL, work, and leisure that are important to them and are in need of occupational therapy intervention. *COPM* is administered in a four-step process that includes problem definition, priority setting, scoring, and reassessment. For each occupational performance area, the therapist gives several illustrations of the kinds of activities that fall in that area and determines from clients whether they need to, want to, or are expected to perform any of these activities. If clients do not feel that they have a problem with daily activities in a performance area, the next occupational performance area is explored. If clients must do an activity, current performance is explored. If clients are unable to perform the activity or are not satisfied with the way they do it, that activity is listed as a problem for intervention. It is important to recognize that a person with a new illness may not have recognized or be ready to identify these issues. The therapist and the person can begin by working on identified issues and return later to see if other issues have emerged. After all of the occupational performance problems are identified, clients score the problems in terms of importance, their perception of current performance, and satisfaction with that performance. Reassessment is completed when the client and the therapist consider it appropriate (Fig. 3-1).

COPM, published by the Canadian Association of Occupational Therapists, is translated into 12 languages and used in more than 25 countries around the world. The mean length of administration time for *COPM* is 40 minutes and the median length of administration time is 30 minutes.

Test–retest reliability of the *COPM* is good to excellent, with intraclass correlations coefficients of .63, .79 and .80 for performance scores and .84, .75 and .89 for satisfaction scores (Law et al., 1998). For validity, research indicates that change in overall function as rated by caregivers, clients, and therapists correlates significantly with change scores on the *COPM*. In a sample of 139 adults, mean performance scores were 3.97 at initial assessment and 6.95 at reassessment, giving an average change score of 3.06 ($p < .0001$). Mean satisfaction score was 3.75 at initial assessment and 6.82 at reassessment, giving a change score of 3.23 ($p < .0001$). The size of these change scores is approximately 1.3 times the standard deviation of the scores, a large clinical change.

Another assessment that can be used to identify problems in roles and competence is the *Occupational Performance History Interview-II (OPHI-II)* (Kielhofner et al., 1998). *OPHI-II* is an assessment of occupational life

Through an interview, clients identify occupational performance activities that are important to them and which they are having difficulties performing satisfactorily. These are scored on a 1–10 scale.

Activity Problems:	Importance	Performance	Satisfaction
Doing up fasteners	9	3	1
Washing face and hands	10	1	1
Preparing sandwich	5	1	4
Holding a book	7	3	5
Visiting friends	9	2	4

Figure 3-1 Example of the scores for the *Canadian Occupational Performance Measure.*

history in work, leisure, and daily life activities, developed using the Model of Human Occupation. The *OPHI-II* interview explores organization of daily routines, life roles, interests, values, goals, perceptions of ability and responsibility; and environmental influences. An accompanying Life History Narrative Form is used to document qualitative information from the interview. *OPHI-II* can be used with all persons older than adolescence; it takes about 50 minutes to complete. Interrater reliability of *OPHI-II*, when there was a specific period between past and present specified, is adequate to good, ranging from .70 to .73 for past and .57 to .72 for present. Test–retest reliability, also using a specified time to mark past and present, is .80–.89 for past and .80–.88 for present (Kielhofner et al., 1991).

Assessing Roles and Community Integration

Trombly (1995b) outlines the taxonomy of three types of life roles. She describes self-maintenance roles as associated with the care of self and cites examples of parent, homemaker, caregiver, and home maintainer. Self-enhancement roles contribute to a person's accomplishment; they include friend, hobbyist, reader, and participant in organizations. Roles that support the productive activities of a person, self-advancement roles, include examples such as student, shopper, worker, volunteer, and voter. Relating this taxonomy to guidelines from AOTA, self-maintenance roles include self-care and care of the home and family. Self-enhancement roles include play and leisure, while self-advancement roles are closest to the occupational function area of work.

The most widely used role assessments in occupational therapy include the *OPHI-II*, already reviewed in this chapter; the *Role Checklist* (Oakley et al., 1986); and the *Occupational Role History* (Florey & Michelman, 1982).

The *Role Checklist* uses a self-report format for a person to record information about roles such as family member, worker, student, homemaker, caregiver, volunteer, and hobbyist. Information focuses on past, present, and future performance of these roles and their value to the person completing the assessment. This assessment has good evidence of reliability and validity (Barris, Oakley, & Kielhofner, 1988; Barris, Dickie, & Baron, 1988).

Community integration refers to the ability of a person to live, work and enjoy his or her free time within the community setting. Several assessments can be used to assess community integration:

▶ The *Craig Handicap Assessment and Reporting Technique* (CHART) (Whiteneck et al., 1992) reflects the language of the International Classification of Impairment, Disability and Handicap (WHO, 1981). Using 27 items, the CHART assesses a person's performance in the six roles of orientation, physical independence, mobility, occupation, social integration and economic self-sufficiency. The CHART has undergone extensive validation. Interrater reliability is .69–.84 between patient and family member ratings, and test–retest reliability is .80–.95. CHART scores correlate significantly with therapist ratings of level of handicap.

▶ The *Reintegration to Normal Living Index* (RNL) (Wood-Dauphinee et al., 1988) is an easy-to-use 11-item assessment that focuses on participation in community activities important to the person (Fig. 3-2). The RNL has evidence of good reliability and correlates significantly with other quality-of-life measures.

▶ The *Community Integration Measure* (CIM) (McColl et al., 2001) uses 10 items to gather information about a person's qualitative experience of living in a

---

I move around my living quarters as I feel necessary. (Wheelchairs, other equipment or resources may be used.)

I am comfortable with how my self-care needs (dressing, feeding, toileting, bathing) are met. (Adaptive equipment, supervision, and/or assistance may be used.)

I spend most of my days occupied in a work activity that is necessary or important to me. (Work activity could be paid employment, housework, volunteer work, school, etc. Adaptive equipment, supervision, and/or assistance may be used.)

In general, I am comfortable with my personal relationships.

I feel that I can deal with life events as they happen.

Each item is scored with a 10-cm visual analogue, with 10 as "fully describes my situation" and 1 as "does not describe my situation."

Figure 3-2 Example of items on the Reintegration to Normal Living Index. (Reprinted with permission from Wood-Dauphinee et al. [1988]. Assessment of global function: The Reintegration to Normal Living Index. *Archives of Physical and Medical Rehabilitation, 69,* 583–590.)

community. This easy-to-use measure was developed for use with persons who have a brain injury. The internal consistency of the CIM is excellent, although interrater and test–retest reliability has not been determined. The CIM correlates significantly with another measure of community integration and is able to differentiate persons with and without disabilities.

▶ Many assessments of health-related quality of life have been developed for use with persons with chronic illness. Examples of these that have excellent reliability and validity include the *Sickness Impact Profile* (SIP) (Bergner et al., 1981) and the *MOS (Medical Outcomes Study) Short Form 36 (SF-36)* (Jenkinson et al., 1994).

Assessing Tasks and Activities

Occupational therapists use a variety of assessment tools to measure baseline and discharge performance in tasks and activities of importance to the client, including ADL, instrumental ADL, work, and leisure.

Activities of Daily Living

ADL generally include mobility at home, feeding, dressing, bathing, grooming, toileting, basic communication, and personal hygiene (Trombly, 1995a). Observation of the activities identified by the patient as problems should be done at the time of day when these activities are normally done and if possible, in the place where the patient usually performs the tasks. Remember that many people may have strong feelings of modesty regarding personal care, and those feelings should be respected. If

many activities are evaluated, ADL are not done all at one time, because it is fatiguing. The therapist should discontinue the evaluation if the patient tires. Items that would be unsafe or obviously unsuccessful are postponed until the patient's physical status improves. If the patient is not independent in some required task at the time of discharge, plans must be developed to ensure that this task is done by others or that additional training is received.

Most standardized ADL evaluations were designed for program evaluation to document the level of independence achieved by patients as the result of a particular program. The most frequently cited standardized ADL tests used by occupational therapists are the *Katz Index* (Katz et al., 1963), the *Barthel Index* (Mahoney & Barthel, 1965), the *Functional Independence Measure (FIM)* (Granger & Hamilton, 1992), the *Functional Status Index* (Jette, 1980), and the *Klein–Bell ADL Scale* (Klein & Bell, 1982).

The Katz Index

The *Katz Index* evaluates six functions, including feeding, continence, transfer, toileting, dressing, and bathing; scoring is based on ontogenetic development of self-care skills (Gresham et al., 1980; Katz et al., 1963). Scoring is on a 3 point scale (independence, receives assistance, dependent). Interobserver reliability is reported to be low (Brorsson & Asberg, 1984), but the Katz has been found to predict length of stay in hospital, living situation 1 year after discharge, and mortality (Brorsson & Asberg, 1984; Asberg & Nydevik, 1991). The Katz is quick to use but does not provide detailed information for treatment planning.

The *Barthel Index*

The *Barthel Index* looks at 10 functions: feeding, bathing, grooming, dressing, bowel control, bladder control, toilet transfers, transfers between chair and bed, walking, and stair climbing. Total score can range from 0 to 100 (total independence) in increments of 5. Functions are weighted according to importance to independence (Gresham et al., 1980; Mahoney & Barthel, 1965). Actual scoring of the *Barthel* takes only 5 to 10 minutes, but observation of the tasks for scoring takes up to an hour. A score of 60 seems to be the transition point from dependency to assisted independence. Many research studies on the *Barthel* indicate that it has excellent reliability and validity (Fricke & Unsworth, 1996; Granger et al., 1979; Loewen & Anderson, 1988; Shah et al., 1989). The responsiveness of the *Barthel* has not been well tested. A modified version of the *Barthel Index* has been found to be reliable and valid when administered during a telephone interview (Shinan et al., 1987).

Functional Independence Measure

FIM uses a 7-point scale to evaluate 18 items in the areas of self-care, sphincter control, mobility, locomotion, communication, and social cognition (Fig. 3-3). *FIM* is intended to measure disability and as such is most useful for description of disability or for program evaluation of initial rehabilitation programs. It is part of a uniform data system that collects information about rehabilitation outcomes and effectiveness. *FIM* is scored according to information observed and derived from the patient directly and from the rehabilitation team. *FIM* has good to excellent reliability and has been the subject of extensive validation (Granger & Hamilton, 1992; Granger et al., 1993; Hamilton et al., 1994). *FIM* also predicts functional status at discharge and length of stay (Heinneman et al., 1994).

Klein–Bell Activities of Daily Living Scale

The *Klein–Bell Activities of Daily Living Scale* (Klein & Bell, 1982) is one of the most responsive ADL assessments because of its large number of items (Fig. 3-4). It documents basic ADL skills, including dressing, elimination, mobility, bathing, hygiene, eating, and emergency telephone communication. Each area is broken down into tasks, and each task is broken down into step-by-step simple behavioral items. There are 170 such items on the scale, which are scored achieved (no physical or verbal assistance) or failed (assistance needed). If the person can do the item with adapted equipment, he or she scores achieved. Interrater agreement of 92% has been determined from the scoring of 30 patients by three pairs of occupational therapists and three pairs of registered nurses, even without extensive training (Klein & Bell, 1982). Validity was established on 14 patients by com-

paring the total score at discharge against the hours of assistance required. A correlation of −0.86 was obtained, indicating that the amount of assistance decreases as the Klein-Bell score increases.

Functional Status Index

The *Functional Status Index* (Jette, 1980) assesses level of performance, degree of difficulty, and degree of pain in five ADL areas: mobility, hand activities, personal care, home chores, and social and role activities. The scale interview takes 20 to 30 minutes. Interobserver and test–retest reliability are good to excellent, and scores on this measure correlate from 0.71 to 0.95 with observed performance (Jette, 1987). This assessment provides an excellent overview of ADL but may not be as useful for treatment planning as assessments that include more ADL items.

SAFE and *SAFER*

Two assessments developed recently focus on evaluating functional performance and safety of ADL concurrently. The *Safety and Functional ADL Evaluation* (*SAFE*) (Morgan, 1992), which is in the process of standardization, assesses independence and degree of required supervision in bathing, dressing, feeding, bowel and bladder control, transfers, and mobility (Fig. 3-5). It is undergoing reliability and validity testing. The *Safety Assessment of Function and the Environment for Rehabilitation* (*SAFER*) (Oliver et al., 1993) assesses safety in 15 areas, such as living situation, mobility, ADL tasks, and recreation. The *SAFER* has evidence of good reliability and validity (Letts et al., 1998).

Instrumental Activities of Daily Living

Instrumental ADL, or IADL, include meal planning, preparation, service, and cleanup; marketing for food and clothing; and routine and seasonal care of the home and one's clothing. Yard work and other maintenance tasks may have been the responsibility of the patient and may be considered homemaking tasks. While there is an overabundance of ADL evaluations, there are fewer evaluations of IADL. IADL evaluations are more complex to develop and validate, and more attention is paid to basic ADL tasks in most rehabilitation programs. As occupational therapy services move into the community, there will be more need for IADL assessments.

Assessment of Motor and Process Skills

The *Assessment of Motor and Process Skills* (*AMPS*) (Fisher, 1993, 1995), is an innovative assessment through which the therapist can simultaneously assess performance of IADL tasks and the motor and process (organizational and adaptive) performance components that contribute to completion of these tasks. *AMPS* was

Case Example

ASSESSING OCCUPATIONAL NEEDS, ROLES, TASKS, AND ACTIVITIES AFTER STROKE

Patient Information

Mrs. K. is a 78-year-old woman recently admitted to the rehabilitation unit after a cerebral vascular accident 2 weeks ago. Her medical course in the acute-care hospital was difficult, and she is only now stable. Her cerebral vascular accident was right-sided, leaving her with left hemiplegia. She can be up approximately 2 hours at a time. Mrs. K. lives alone, having been widowed 2 years ago. She has continued to live in the family home, a bungalow close to the downtown of a small city. One of her two children lives about an hour away. Mrs. K.'s interests include gardening, hiking, volunteer work at her church, reading, and embroidering.

Description of Assessment

The occupational therapist met briefly with Mrs. K. during the morning, when she was up in a wheelchair. During the first meeting, the therapist introduced herself and described occupational therapy and its focus on the activities and tasks that a person does every day. She talked to Mrs. K. about where she lived and her interests. Since this meeting was very brief, the therapist and Mrs. K. agreed that they would meet again the next day. At the next meeting, the therapist used the *COPM* (Law et al., 1998) to gather information about the occupations that Mrs. K. wanted to do, needed to do, or was expected to do. Mrs. K. identified several activities that she wanted to perform but was having difficulty with. These activities included getting in and out of bed by herself, using the bathroom, getting dressed, moving about indoors and outdoors, resuming her gardening, volunteer, and other leisure activities, and returning to her home. The activities that she wanted to master included both short- and long-term goals. The therapist and Mrs. K. explored what she would have to do to return home; meal preparation, grocery shopping, and banking were then added to the *COPM* list. Using the *COPM* procedures, Mrs. K. rated the importance of each activity to her. These ratings indicated that getting in and out of bed, dressing, using the bathroom by herself, and holding a book were most important to her immediately. She indicated that when she was able to do these activities, she wanted to focus on performing tasks necessary for her to return home.

Because mobility, using the bathroom, and dressing were important to Mrs. K., the occupational therapist used the *Klein–Bell ADL Assessment* to gather further information about her specific performance in ADL. The results of this assessment indicated that Mrs. K. needed assistance in transfers between the bed and wheelchair and was unable to perform any dressing tasks requiring the use of two hands. Mrs. K. was eager to relearn these activities and was well aware of the need to learn methods to accomplish them safely. As part of the regular care process of the rehabilitation unit, the rehabilitation team completed the *FIM* (Hamilton et al., 1987) for Mrs. K. The therapist used information from the Klein–Bell assessment and information from nursing staff to assign *FIM* scores. Mrs. K.'s initial *FIM* motor score was 32 (of 91 possible) and the *FIM* cognitive score was 28 (of 35 possible). The *FIM* provided some information about Mrs. K.'s performance but little detail about her priorities for each activity.

Once these activities were accomplished, the occupational therapist planned to use the *Rabideau Kitchen Assessment* and the *SAFER* to assess Mrs. K.'s performance in meal preparation and her safety at home. Mrs. K. continued to receive home-based occupational therapy once discharged. The occupational therapist seeing her at home continued to use the *COPM* for identification of occupational performance issues and evaluation of outcome. As well, she used the revised *Activity Index* and *Meaningfulness of Activity Scale* to identify the leisure activities that Mrs. K. wanted to do and the meaning of these activities to her. This information enabled the therapist and Mrs. K. to explore what activities she could still do and what new activities she could begin that would be meaningful to her.

Analysis of Results

The results of the initial assessment using the *COPM* indicated that getting in and out of bed, dressing, using the bathroom by herself, and holding a book to read were most immediately important to her. The *FIM* results indicate that she has more significant motor than cognitive difficulties. Using the *Klein–Bell ADL Scale*, the therapist was able to observe performance of the basic ADL. It became clear that Mrs. K. knew how to perform each activity but was unable because of the physical limitations caused by the stroke. She could articulate the steps of each task. Lack of movement and postural control were important limiting factors. The therapist designed an intervention program using adaptive devices, adaptive techniques, and reeducation of movement to help Mrs. K. relearn these ADL.

CLINICAL REASONING
in Occupational Therapy Practice

Effects of Assessing Starting With Assessment of Occupation

The therapist working with Mrs. K. began the assessment process by interviewing Mrs. K. using the *COPM*. What effect did this have on the assessment process and use of further assessments? How did the results of the *COPM* differ from the results using the *FIM*?

FIM™ instrument

L **E** **V** **E** **L** **S**	7 Complete Independence (Timely, Safely) 6 Modified Independence (Device)	**NO HELPER**
	Modified Dependence 5 Supervision (Subject = 100%+) 4 Minimal Assist (Subject = 75%+) 3 Moderate Assist (Subject = 50%+) **Complete Dependence** 2 Maximal Assist (Subject =25%+) 1 Total Assist (Subject = less than 25%)	**HELPER**

	ADMISSION	DISCHARGE	FOLLOW-UP
Self-Care A. Eating B Grooming C. Bathing D. Dressing - Upper Body E. Dressing - Lower Body F. Toileting			
Sphincter Control G. Bladder Management H. Bowel Management			
Transfers I. Bed, Chair, Wheelchair J. Toilet K. Tub, Shower			
Locomotion L. Walk/Wheelchair M. Stairs	W Walk C Wheelchair B Both	W Walk C Wheelchair B Both	W Walk C Wheelchair B Both
Motor Subtotal Score			
Communication N. Comprehension O. Expression	A Auditory V Visual B Both V Vocal N Nonvocal B Both	A Auditory V Visual B Both V Vocal N Nonvocal B Both	A Auditory V Visual B Both V Vocal N Nonvocal B Both
Social Cognition P. Social Interaction Q. Problem Solving R. Memory			
Cognitive Subtotal Score			
TOTAL FIM Score			

NOTE: Leave no blanks. Enter 1 if patient not testable due to risk

Figure 3-3 Items and scoring for the *Functional Independence Measure* (*FIM*). Used with permission.

```
┌─────────────────────────────────────────────────────┐
│ Socks                                                │
│    8. Grasp sock                              (1)    │
│    9. Reach sock to R foot                    (2)    │
│   10. Reach sock to L foot                    (2)    │
│   11. Pull sock over R toes                   (2)    │
│   12. Pull sock over L toes                   (2)    │
│   13. Pull sock over R foot with heel to heel (2)    │
│   14. Pull sock over L foot with heel to heel (2)    │
│   15. Pull sock up to full extension on R leg (2)    │
│   16. Pull sock up to full extension on L leg (2)    │
│                                                      │
│                                                      │
│ Mobility through doors                               │
│   114. Operate doorknob                       (1)    │
│   115. Open door toward self                  (2)    │
│   116. Open door away from self               (2)    │
│   117. Close door toward self                 (2)    │
│   118. Close door away from self              (1)    │
│                                                      │
│ Scoring - Points in parentheses next to each item    │
│ (either 1 or 2) are given if person is able to       │
│ complete the activity. Use of equipment is allowed.  │
│ Total score equals the addition of points for each   │
│ item. Item is marked N/A if clearly not applicable.  │
└─────────────────────────────────────────────────────┘
```

Figure 3-4 Example of items and scoring information for the Klein-Bell ADL Scale. (Used with permission from University of Washington, Health Sciences for Educational Resources.)

developed to reveal the relation between an individual's performance of IADL tasks and the underlying process and motor components that contribute to that performance. During the *AMPS* evaluation, motor and process skills are assessed concurrently with observation of functional performance. The *AMPS* procedure entails six steps: client selection, interview, task selection by client, preparation of the client and test environment, administration of the assessment, and scoring. Tasks offered to clients present a challenge to them, are not overlearned, and are appropriate to the client's environment, age, and culture (Fisher, 1993). Administration of two tasks on *AMPS* usually takes 10 to 20 minutes, with assessment and scoring taking about 1 hour. Training requirements for the *AMPS* are extensive, and this has limited its clinical utility.

The authors of *AMPS* have used many-faceted Rasch analysis (Linacre, 1989), a scaling method designed to ensure a hierarchical equal-interval scale. The use of Rasch analysis allows adjustment of a score for the difficulty of the IADL item and for differences in raters observing performance. Information on functional tasks and motor and process skills can be obtained by having an individual perform a few tasks. Performance on a few tasks, once calibrated using the Rasch analysis, is used to predict performance on other tasks. Many tasks have been included in *AMPS* validation studies, so that a client can choose a few tasks that are culturally and environmentally appropriate. For example, a man who

does not perform complex meal preparation (perhaps because he lives with his wife) may choose tasks such as making toast and brewing coffee rather than making a grilled cheese sandwich or an omelet. The flexibility of including clients' choice in the tasks that are assessed is a significant advantage of *AMPS*.

Scoring for *AMPS*, which must be done by computer, and is available for therapists who have been trained to use *AMPS*. The goal of the research team is to have a computer program that therapists can use to score *AMPS* for individual clients. This program will be available when enough scores have been obtained for each *AMPS* task to satisfy criteria for reliability and validity. Interrater and test–retest reliability of *AMPS* range from .74 to .93 (Doble, 1991; Fisher, 1995). Bryze (1991) found correlations ranging from .62 to .85 between the *AMPS* scale and the *Scales of Independent Behaviour*. In a 1991 study of 162 persons aged 16 to 87, Fisher (1995) found that the data from the *AMPS* assessment conformed well to the Rasch model in terms of acceptable fit. The equivalent of Cronbach's alpha was .83 for motor tasks, .98 for motor skill items, .96 for process tasks, and .98 for process skill items. The correlation between *AMPS* IADL motor measures and *AMPS* IADL process measures was .58. *AMPS* has been shown to discriminate well between people without disabilities and those with cognitive impairments or physical disabilities. Doble et al. (1994), in a study of persons with multiple sclerosis, found that the subjects differed significantly in mean IADL motor and IADL process scores based on their overall level of independence in community living.

Structured Assessment of Independent Living Skills

The *Structured Assessment of Independent Living Skills* (SAILS) is an assessment of 10 areas of daily activities: fine motor skills, gross motor skills, dressing, eating, expressive language, receptive language, time and orientation, money-related skills, instrumental activities, and social interaction. SAILS includes 50 tasks scored on a scale of 0 to 3 after direct observation of performance of each task. Scores are achieved for each of the 10 subdomains as well as a combined motor score, combined cognitive score, and total score. To date, research with SAILS on individuals who have Alzheimer's disease has indicated that test–retest reliability is excellent and that the assessment significantly discriminates between different levels of ability in ADL (Mahurin et al., 1991).

Kitchen Tasks

Two assessments of the performance of kitchen tasks have recently been developed for use in occupational therapy. The *Kitchen Task Assessment (KTA)* (Baum & Edwards, 1993) uses the task of making a pudding to assess the cognitive support required by a person with

SPAULDING REHABILITATION HOSPITAL

Occupational Therapy Department

SAFE EVALUATION:

(Safety and Functional ADL Evaluation)

Adm. Date: _____

Onset Date: _____

Diagnosis: _____

FUNCTIONAL INTERPRETATION	SAFETY INTERPRETATION
0 to 7 = Max. Assist. to Dependent	0 to 7 = Constant Supervision
8 to 20 = Min. to Mod. Assistance	8 to 20 = Close Supervision
21 to 27 = Supervision	21 to 27 = Distant Supervision
28 = Independent	28 = Independent

ACTIVITY	TASKS	EVAL. DATE		EVAL. DATE		EVAL. DATE	
		$F = \frac{\quad}{28}$	$S = \frac{\quad}{28}$	$F = \frac{\quad}{28}$	$S = \frac{\quad}{28}$	$F = \frac{\quad}{28}$	$S = \frac{\quad}{28}$
I. BATHING	Washes face and hands						
	Washes upper torso						
	Washes back						
	Washes perineal area						
	Washes legs and feet						
	Brushes teeth						
	Combs hair						
	Shaving/Make-up	F	S	F	S	F	S
	÷ 8						
II. DRESSING	Undershirt/bra on/off						
	Underpants on/off						
	Front opening shirt/ sweater on/off						
	Pullover on/off						
	Pants/skirt on/off						
	Stockings on/off						
	Shoes/slippers on/off						
	Belt/fasteners on/off						
	Glasses on/off						
	Equipment - splints/ sling/prosthesis	F	S	F	S	F	S
	÷ 10						
III. FEEDING	Adequate reflexes/ musculature						
	Finger feed						
	Use of utensils						
	Pour from container						
	Drink (cup, glass, straw)	F	S	F	S	F	S
	÷ 5						

Figure 3-5 The Spaulding *Safety and Functional ADL Evaluation*. A facility-generated assessment in the process of standardization. (Reprinted with permission from Virginia Morgan, OTR, Director of Occupational Therapy, Spaulding Rehabilitation Hospital, 125 Nashua St., Boston, MA 02114.)

Alzheimer's disease to complete a cooking task. Thus, the *KTA* provides information about performance as well as components of function, such as initiation, sequencing, organization, and problem solving. Internal consistency of the *KTA* ranges from .87 to .96, and interrater reliability for the total score is .85. There is a significant relation between scores on the *KTA* and other neuropsychological assessments.

The *Rabideau Kitchen Evaluation—Revised* (Neistadt, 1992, 1994) is an assessment of meal preparation primarily developed for adults with brain injury. It uses preparing a sandwich and a hot beverage, and all aspects of the task are scored according to the level of assistance required for completion. Interrater reliability is .81, and test–retest reliability on a small sample indicated a reliability coefficient of .80. Results on the *Rabideau* correlate significantly with scores on other assessments of sequencing, such as the WAIS-R Block Design.

The *Kohlman Evaluation of Living Skills*

The *Kohlman Evaluation of Living Skills* (*KELS*) assesses daily activities in self-care, safety, health, money management, transportation, telephone, work, and leisure. *KELS* is administered through interview and direct observation. Individual items are scored as independent, needs assistance, or not applicable. Interrater reliability of *KELS* has been reported to be good to excellent, and construct validation has been studied (Kohlman Thomson, 1993).

Child Care

Child care and parenting include but are not limited to the physical care of children and use of age-appropriate activities, communication, and behavior to facilitate child development (AOTA, 1994). Because no standard evaluations exist, the therapist must analyze the tasks, taking the ages and personalities of the children into account to determine what assistance the patient may need in this area. The *Canadian Occupational Performance Measure* can be used to assess issues in these performance areas.

Work

Work is another area of concern to occupational therapists (AOTA, 1994). Employment evaluation includes determining whether an individual has the ability to perform the necessary job skills and is otherwise prepared for employment in terms of work habits; work quality; ability to learn or acquire new skills; and ability to work with others as a team member, supervisor, or supervisee. Velozo (1993) questioned whether work evaluations reflect occupational therapists' interest in

the meaning of work and focus on work environments. He described two categories of work evaluations: (1) standardized commercial evaluations and (2) evaluations of physical and work capacity.

Standardized vocational evaluation systems use job analysis or work samples to determine an individual's ability to perform tasks similar to those encountered at work. In the United States, the *Dictionary of Occupational Titles* (United States Department of Labor, 1991) provides a taxonomy for measurement of work performance that lists specific job requirements, including skills and equipment. An example of a work sample assessment system is the *VALPAR Component Work Samples*. The *VALPAR* system consists of work samples that simulate tasks required for specific jobs. Evidence of the reliability and validity of the *VALPAR* system is extensive. The disadvantage of a system such as the *VALPAR* is the expense. Occupational function evaluations of work commonly focus on work and physical capacity. Evaluation of work capacity entails assessment of tasks such as lifting, sitting, and standing that are necessary for a specific work setting. Physical capacity evaluations focus on physical components necessary for work, such as strength, endurance, and freedom from pain.

Occupational therapists have also made specific observations of behaviors that are important for work, such as punctuality, communication ability, ability to work with others, and grooming. The *Worker Role Interview* (Velozo et al., 1998) is a semistructured assessment designed to evaluate the psychosocial and environmental factors that influence return to work. This assessment, which takes 30 to 60 minutes to complete, has been found to have adequate test–retest and interrater reliability and construct validity. The *Feasibility Evaluation Checklist* (Matheson et al., 1985) evaluates required work-related behaviors such as attendance, timeliness, workplace tolerance, and ability to accept supervision. The assessment includes 21 items, takes 5 minutes, and has evidence of adequate reliability and validity.

Leisure

Leisure refers to performance and value in choosing, performing, or engaging in activities for amusement, relaxation, spontaneous enjoyment, and/or self-expression (Hersch, 1991). Some assessments evaluate leisure interests (Matsutsuyu, 1969; Rogers et al., 1978; Witt & Ellis, 1984); others evaluate performance and satisfaction with leisure activities (Beard & Ragheb, 1980; Gregory, 1983). Hersch (1991) pointed out that "the concept of leisure encompasses a multitude of meanings—the leisure event itself, the amount and frequency of the activity, its meaningfulness to the participant, and the social context" (p. 55). In fact, Hersch (1991) and Bundy (1993) have suggested that leisure, or the playfulness of an activity, depends on the characteristics of the activity rather than the classification of an activity as leisure. For an activity to be leisured or playful, it must be chosen by an individual and present a challenge, and the results must be under the individual's control.

The *Leisure Activities Inventory* by Havighurst (Mangen & Peterson, 1982) assesses the types of leisure activity in which an individual is engaged, the value of those activities, and the meaning of the activities to the person. In a pilot study with 10 subjects using the *Leisure Activities Inventory*, Hersch (1991) found a positive relation between high scores and a measure of life satisfaction. The revised *Activity Index* (Gregory, 1983) is a self-report assessment that determines involvement and frequency of involvement in a variety of activities, ranging from card games and theater to quiet hobbies at home. It has good test–retest reliability and is significantly correlated with life satisfaction.

Other assessments focus on what leisure activities mean to individuals. Using the activities in the revised *Activity Index*, the *Meaningfulness of Activity Scale* measures the motivation for involvement and sense of meaning derived from involvement in leisure activities (Gregory, 1983). Test–retest reliability has been reported to be excellent, and scores on this scale are significantly related to life satisfaction (Gregory, 1983).

The *Leisure Satisfaction Questionnaire* (Beard & Ragheb, 1980) uses a self-report format with scoring on a 5-point scale to measure the agreement of individuals with 51 items that reflect points of view about leisure. Items are sorted into six domains: psychological, educational, social, relaxation, physiological, and aesthetic. Internal consistency of this scale is .96 (Beard & Ragheb, 1980). There is limited reliability and validity information for the *Leisure Satisfaction Questionnaire*. The *Leisure Diagnostic Battery* (Witt & Ellis, 1984) assesses a person's perceived leisure competence. This measure has good test–retest reliability and appears to be responsive to changes in leisure performance after a recreation intervention (Ellis & Witt, 1986).

Summary Review Questions

1. Describe one method used to evaluate an individual's perception of his or her occupational performance. What are the advantages and disadvantages of this method?
2. Define IADL and basic ADL.
3. What are the three psychometric characteristics of standardized evaluation instruments? Define each.
4. What are the methods used to evaluate ADL, work, and leisure?
5. What is the relation between evaluation of occupational function and development of the occupational therapy treatment plan?
6. Choose one of the assessments described in this chapter. Describe the assessment and its psychometric characteristics and state its strengths and weaknesses.

Resources

Assessment of Motor and Process Skills

Dr. A. Fisher · Three Star Press, College of Applied Human Sciences, Colorado State University, 200 Occupational Therapy Building, Fort Collins, CO 80523.

Canadian Occupational Performance Measure

American Occupational Therapy Association · 4720 Montgomery Lane Bethesda. MD 20824. Outside the United States:Canadian Association of Occupational Therapists, Carleton Technology and Training Centre, Suite 3400, 1125 Colonel By Drive,Ottawa ON, Canada K1S 5R1.

Feasibility Evaluation Checklist

Dr. L. Matheson · Program in Occupational Therapy, Washington University School of Medicine, 4444 Forest Park Ave., St. Louis, MO 63108.

Functional Independence Measure

Data Management Service of the Uniform Data System for Medical Rehabilitation · State University of New York at Buffalo, 100 High Street, Buffalo, NY 14230.

Kitchen Task Assessment

Dr. C. Baum · Program in Occupational Therapy, Washington University School of Medicine, 4444 Forest Park Ave., St. Louis, MO 63108.

Klein-Bell Activities of Daily Living Scale

University of Washington Medical School · Health Sciences Learning Resource Center, Distribution, SB-56, Seattle, WA 98195.

Leisure Satisfaction Questionnaire

Idyll Arbor Inc. · 25119 SE 262nd St., PO Box 720, Ravensdale, WA 98051-9763.

Occupational Therapy Performance History Interview—II

American Occupational Therapy Association · 4720 Montgomery Lane, Bethesda, MD 20814-3425.

Rabideau Kitchen Evaluation—Revised

Neistadt, M. E. (1994) · A meal preparation treatment protocol for adults with brain injury. *American Journal of Occupational Therapy, 48,* 431–438.

Safety and Functional ADL Evaluation

Virginia Morgan · Director of Occupational Therapy, Spaulding Rehabilitation Hospital, 125 Nashua St., Boston, MA 02114.

Safety Assessment of Function and the Environment for Rehabilitation

Community Occupational Therapy Associates (COTA) · 3101 Bathurst St., Toronto, ON, Canada M6A 2A6.

Valpar Component Work Samples

VALPAR International Corp. · PO Box 5767, Tucson, AZ 85703.

Worker Role Interview

Model of Human Occupation Clearinghouse · Department of Occupational Therapy, College of Health and Human Development Sciences, University of Illinois at Chicago, 1919 W. Taylor St., 60612–7249.

Kohlman Evaluation of Living Skills

American Occupational Therapy Association · 4720 Montgomery Lane, Bethesda, MD 20824.

Leisure Diagnostic Battery

LDB Project · Division of Recreation and Leisure Studies, North Texas University, Denton, TX 76203.

References

American Occupational Therapy Association. (1994). *Uniform Terminology for Occupational Therapy and Application of Uniform Terminology to Practice*. Bethesda, MD: AOTA.

Asberg, K. H., & Nydevik, I. (1991). Early prognosis of stroke outcome by means of Katz Index of activities of daily living. *Scandinavian Journal of Rehabilitation Medicine, 23*(4), 187–191.

Asberg, K. H., & Sonn, U. (1989). The cumulative structure of personal and instrumental ADL: A study of elderly people in a health service district. *Scandinavian Journal of Rehabilitation Medicine, 21*, 171–177.

Barris, R., Oakley, F., & Kielhofner, G. (1988). The *Role Checklist*. In B. Hemphill (Ed.). *Mental Health Assessment in Occupational Therapy: An Integrative Approach to the Evaluation Process* (pp 73–91). Thorofare, NJ: Slack.

Barris, R., Dickie, V., & Baron, K. B. (1988). A comparison of psychiatric patients and normal subjects based on the Model of Human Occupation. *Occupational Therapy Journal of Research, 8*, 3–37.

Baum, C., & Edwards, D. F. (1993). Cognitive performance in senile dementia of the Alzheimer's type: The kitchen task assessment. *The American Journal of Occupational Therapy, 47*, 431–436.

Beard, J. G., & Ragheb, M. G. (1980). Measuring life satisfaction. *Journal of Leisure Research, 12*(1), 20–25.

Bergner, M., Bobbit, R. A., Carter, W. B., & Gilson, B. S. (1981). The Sickness Impact Profile: Development and final revision of health status measure. *Medical Care, 19*, 787–805.

Brorsson, B., & Asberg, K. (1984). *Katz Index* of independence in ADL: Reliability and validity in short term care. *Scandinavian Journal of Rehabilitation Medicine, 16*, 125–132.

Brown, C., Moore, W. P., Hemman, D., & Yunek, A. (1996). Influence of instrumental activities of daily living assessment method on judgments of independence. *American Journal of Occupational Therapy, 50*, 202–206.

Bryze, K. A. (1991). *Functional assessment of adults with developmental disabilities*. Unpublished Master's thesis, University of Illinois at Chicago, Chicago.

Bundy, A. C. (1993). Assessment of play and leisure: Delineation of the problem. *American Journal of Occupational Therapy, 47*, 217–222.

Collin, C., Wade, D. T., Davies, S., & Horne, V. (1988). The Barthel ADL index: A reliability study. *International Disabilities Studies, 10*, 61–63.

Doble, S. (1991). Test–retest and interrater reliability of a process skills assessment. *Occupational Therapy Journal of Research, 11*, 8–23.

Doble, S. E., Fisk, J. D., Fisher, A. G., Ritvo, P. G., & Murray, T. J. (1994). Functional competence of community-dwelling persons with multiple sclerosis using the assessment of motor and process skills. *Archives of Physical Medicine and Rehabilitation, 75*, 843–851.

Edwards, M. M. (1990). The reliability and validity of self-report activities of daily living scales. *Canadian Journal of Occupational Therapy, 57*, 273–278.

Ellis, G. D., & Witt, P. A. (1986). The *Leisure Diagnostic Battery*: Past, present and future. *Therapeutic Recreation Journal, 19*, 31–47.

Fisher, A. G. (1993). The assessment of IADL motor skills: An application of many-faceted Rasch analysis. *American Journal of Occupational Therapy, 47*, 319–329.

Fisher, A. G. (1995). *Assessment of Motor and Process Skills*. Fort Collins, CO: Three Star.

Florey, L. L., & Michelman, S. M. (1982). Occupational Role History: A screening tool for psychiatric occupational history. *American Journal of Occupational Therapy, 36*, 301–308.

Fricke, J., & Unsworth, C. A. (1996). Inter-rater reliability of the original and modified *Barthel Index* and a comparison with the *Functional Independence Measure*. *Australian Occupational Therapy Journal, 43*, 22–29.

Gitlin, L., Corcoran, M., & Leinmiller-Eckhardt, S. (1995). Understanding the family perspective: An ethnographic framework for providing occupational therapy in the home. *American Journal of Occupational Therapy, 49*, 802–809.

Granger, C. V., Albrecht, G. L., & Hamilton, B. B. (1979). Outcome of comprehensive medical rehabilitation: Measurement by PULSES Profile and the *Barthel Index*. *Archives of Physical Medicine & Rehabilitation, 60*(4), 145–153.

Granger, C. V., & Hamilton, B. B. (1992). The Uniform Data System for medical rehabilitation report of first admissions for 1990. *American Journal of Physical Medicine and Rehabilitation, 71*(4), 108–113.

Granger, C. V., Hamilton, B. B., Linacre, J. M., Heinemann, A. W., & Wright, B. D. (1993). Performance profiles of the Functional Independence Measure. *American Journal of Physical Medicine and Rehabilitation, 72*, 84–89.

Gregory, M. D. (1983). Occupational behavior and life satisfaction among retirees. *American Journal of Occupational Therapy, 137*(8), 548–553.

Gresham, G. E., Phillips, T. F., & Labi, M. L. C. (1980). ADL status in stroke: Relative merits of three standard indexes. *Archives of Physical Medicine & Rehabilitation, 61*(8), 355–358.

Hamilton, B. B., Granger, C. V., Sherwin, F. S., Zielezny, M., & Tashman, J. S. (1987). A uniform data system for medical rehabilitation. In Fuhrer, M. J. (Ed.). *Rehabilitation outcomes: Analysis and measurement*. Baltimore: Paul H. Brookes.

Hamilton, B. B., Laughlin, J. A., Fiedler, R. C., & Granger, C. V. (1994). Interrater reliability of the 7-level *Functional Independence Measure (FIM)*. *Scandinavian Journal of Rehabilitation Medicine, 26*, 115–119.

Harris, B. A., et al. (1986). Validity of self-report measures of functional disability. *Topics in Geriatric Rehabilitation, 1*(3), 31–41.

Hasselkus, B. R., & Safrit, M. J. (1976). Measurement in occupational therapy. *American Journal of Occupational Therapy, 30*, 429–436.

Heinemann, A. W., Linacre, J. M., Wright, B. D., Hamilton, B. B., & Granger, C. V. (1994). Prediction of rehabilitation outcomes with disability measures. *Archives of Physical Medicine and Rehabilitation, 75*, 133–143.

Hersch, G. (1991). Leisure and aging. *Physical and Occupational Therapy in Geriatrics, 9*, 55–78.

Jenkinson, C., Wright, L., & Coulter, A. (1994). Criterion validity and reliability of the SF-36 in a population sample. *Quality of Life Research, 3*, 7–12.

Jette, A. M. (1980). *Functional Status Index*: Reliability of a chronic disease evaluation instrument. *Archives of Physical Medicine & Rehabilitation, 61*, 395–401.

Jette, A. M. (1987). The functional status index: Reliability and validity of a self-report functional disability measure. *Journal of Rheumatology, 14*(Suppl 15), 15–19.

Katz, S., Ford, A. B., Moskowitz, R. W., Jackson, B. A., & Jaffe, M. W. (1963). Studies of illness in the aged: The index of ADL: A standardized measure of biological and psychosocial function. *JAMA, 185*(12), 94–99.

Kielhofner, G., Henry, A. D., Walens, D., & Rogers, E. S. (1991). A generalizability study of the *Occupational Performance History Interview. Occupational Therapy Journal of Research, 11*(5), 292–306.

Kielhofner, G., Mallinson, T., Crawford, D., Nowak, M., Rigby, M., & Henry, A. (1998). *User's manual for the OPHI-II.* Chicago, IL: Model of Human Occupation Clearinghouse (University of Illinois at Chicago, Department of Occupational Therapy).

Klein, R. M., & Bell, B. (1982). Self-care skills: Behavioral measurement with Klein-Bell ADL Scale. *Archives of Physical Medicine and Rehabilitation, 63,* 335–338.

Kohlman Thomson, L. (1993). *The Kohlman Evaluation of Living Skills* (3rd ed.). Rockville, MD: AOTA.

Law, M. (1987). Measurement in occupational therapy: Scientific criteria for evaluation. *Canadian Journal of Occupational Therapy, 54,* 133–138.

Law, M. (1991). The environment: A focus for occupational therapy. *Canadian Journal of Occupational Therapy, 58,* 171–179.

Law, M., editor. (1998). *Client-centered Occupational Therapy.* Thorofare, NJ: Slack Incorporated.

Law, M., Baptiste, S., Carswell, A., McColl, M., Polatajko, H., & Pollock, N. (1994). *Canadian Occupational Performance Measure* (2nd ed.). Toronto: CAOT.

Law, M., Baptiste, S., Carswell, A., McColl, M., Polatajko, H., & Pollock, N. (1998). *Canadian Occupational Performance Measure* (3rd ed.). Ottawa: CAOT.

Law, M., & Letts, L. (1989). A critical review of scales of activities of daily living. *American Journal of Occupational Therapy, 43,* 522–528.

Letts, L., Scott, S., Burtney, J., Marshall, L., & McKean, M. (1998). The reliability and validity of the Safety Assessment of Function and the Environment for Rehabilitation (SAFER). *British Journal of Occupational Therapy, 61,* 127–132.

Linacre, J. M. (1989). *Many-faceted Rasch measurement.* Chicago: MESA.

Loewen, S. C., & Anderson, B. A. (1988). Reliability of the modified motor assessment scale and the *Barthel Index. Physical Therapy, 68,* 1077–1081.

Long, K., Sudha, S., & Mutran, E. J. (1998). Elder-proxy agreement concerning the functional status and medical history of the older person: the impact of caregiver burden and depressive symptomatology. *Journal of the American Geriatric Society, 46,* 1103–1111.

Mahoney, F. I., & Barthel, D. W. (1965). Functional evaluation: The *Barthel Index. Maryland State Medical Journal, 14*(2), 61–65.

Mahurin, R. K., DeBettignies, B. H., & Pirozzolo, F. J. (1991). Structured assessment of independent living skills: Preliminary report of a performance measure of functional abilities in dementia. *Journal of Gerontology, 46,* 58–66.

Mangen, D. J., & Peterson, W. A. (1982). *Research instruments in social gerontology, Volume 2, Social Roles and Social Participation.* Minneapolis, MN: University of Minnesota Press.

Matheson, L., Ogden, L., Violette, K., & Schultz, K. (1985). Work hardening: Occupational therapy in industrial rehabilitation. *The American Journal of Occupational Therapy, 39*(5), 314–321.

Matsutsuyu, J. S. (1969). Interest checklist. *American Journal of Occupational Therapy, 23*(4), 323–328.

McColl, M., Davies, D., Carlson, P., Johnston, J., & Minnes, P. (2001). The community integration measure: Development and preliminary validation. *Archives of Physical Medicine and Rehabilitation, 82,* 429–434.

Morgan, V. J. (1992). *The Safety and Functional ADL Evaluation.* Poster presented at the annual conference of the American Occupational Therapy Association, Houston, TX.

Neistadt, M. E. (1994). A meal preparation treatment protocol for adults with brain injury. *American Journal of Occupational Therapy, 48,* 431–438.

Neistadt, M. E. (1992). The Rabideau Kitchen Evaluation Revised: An assessment of meal preparation skill. *Occupational Therapy Journal of Research, 12,* 242–255.

Oakley, F., Kielhofner, G., Barris, R., & Reichler, R. K. (1986). The Role Checklist: Development and empirical assessment of reliability. *The Occupational Therapy Journal of Research, 6,* 157–170.

Oliver, R., Blathwayt, J., Brockley, C., & Tamaki, T. (1993). Development of the *Safety Assessment of Function and the Environment for Rehabilitation (SAFER)* tool. *Canadian Journal of Occupational Therapy, 60,* 78–82.

Rogers, J. C., Weinstein, J. M., & Figone, J. J. (1978). The interest checklist: An empirical assessment. *American Journal of Occupational Therapy, 32,* 628–630.

Sagar, M. A., Dunham, N. C., Schwartes, A., Mecum, L., Halverson, K., & Harlowe, D. (1992). Measurement of activities of daily living in hospitalized elderly: A comparison of self-report and performance-based methods. *Journal of American Geriatric Society, 40,* 457–462.

Shah, S., Vanclay, F., & Cooper, B. (1989). Improving the sensitivity of the *Barthel Index* for stroke rehabilitation. *Journal of Clinical Epidemiology, 42,* 703–709.

Sinoff, G., & Ore, L. (1997). The Barthel activities of daily living index: self-reporting versus actual performance in the old-old ($\geq$ 75 years). *Journal of American Geriatric Society, 45,* 832–836.

Streiner, D. L., & Norman, G. R. (1989). *Health measurement scales: A practical guide to their development and use.* New York: Oxford University.

Trombly, C. A. (1995a). Retraining basic and instrumental activities of daily living. In C. A. Trombly (Ed.), *Occupational therapy for physical dysfunction* (4th ed.). Baltimore: Williams & Wilkins.

Trombly, C. A. (1995b). Occupation: purposefulness and meaningfulness as therapeutic mechanisms. 1995 Eleanor Clarke Slagle Lecture. *American Journal of Occupational Therapy, 49*(10), 960–972.

U.S. Department of Labor. (1991). *Dictionary of occupational titles.* (4th ed., Vol. I & II). Washington, DC: Author.

Velozo, C. A. (1993). Work evaluations: Critique of the states of the art of functional assessment of work. *American Journal of Occupational Therapy, 47,* 203–209.

Velozo, C., Kielhofner, G., & Fisher, G. (1998). *Worker Role Interview (WRI).* Chicago: Model of Human Occupation Clearinghouse.

Whiteneck, G., Charlifue, S., Gerhart, K., Overholser, D., & Richardson, G. (1992). Quantifying handicap: A new measure of long-term rehabilitation outcomes. *Archives of Physical Medicine and Rehabilitation, 73,* 519–526.

Witt, P. A., & Ellis, G. D. (1984). The *Leisure Diagnostic Battery*: Measuring perceived freedom in leisure. *Society and Leisure, 7,* 109–124.

Wood-Dauphinee, S., Opzoomer, A., Williams, J. I., Marchand, B., & Spitzer, W. O. (1988). Assessment of global function: The Reintegration to Normal Living Index. *Archives of Physical Medicine and Rehabilitation, 69,* 583–590.

World Health Organization. (1981). *International Classification of Impairment, Disability and Handicap.* Geneva, SW: Author.

World Health Organization. (2000). *ICIDH-2: International Classification of Functioning, Disability and Health.* Geneva, SW: Author.

4

Assessing Abilities and Capacities: Range of Motion, Strength, and Endurance

Catherine A. Trombly and Carolyn Robinson Podolski

LEARNING OBJECTIVES

After studying this chapter and practicing the skills described here, the reader will be able to do the following:

1. Evaluate range of motion of the upper extremity using a goniometer.
2. Use two different methods to determine the amount of edema of the hand.
3. Perform a manual muscle test to evaluate strength of the upper extremity.
4. Determine the functional strength of selected lower extremity musculature.
5. Determine functional endurance level.
6. Use a Visual Analogue Scale to determine pain level.
7. Interpret the findings of the evaluations in this chapter.

Sense of self-efficacy and self-esteem

Satisfaction with life roles
• Self-maintenance
• Self-advancement
• Self-enhancement

Competence in tasks of life roles

Activities and habits

Abilities and skills

Developed capacities

First-level capacities

Organic substrate

*T*he assessments presented in this chapter are appropriate for patients who are unable to do or are restricted in doing the occupational tasks and activities important to them because of impairments in range of joint motion, strength, or endurance. Being able to move (mobility, or range of motion); and use extremities against resistance (strength) for an extended period (endurance) is essential for the completion of most occupational tasks. For example, a person who cannot fully flex the elbow, is too weak to lift a spoon to the mouth, or is too fatigued to lift the utensil repeatedly cannot eat a meal independently. Since deficits in abilities and capacities may lead to

GLOSSARY

Active range of motion (AROM)—The amount of movement possible at a joint when the patient voluntarily moves the limb by muscle contraction.

Anatomical position—Standing straight with feet together and flat on the floor, arms by the sides with hands facing forward. The zero position for ROM measurement.

Calibrate—To set an instrument at a known value according to a standard.

Contracture—Inability to move a body part because of soft tissue shortening or bony ankylosis.

Limits of motion—The beginning and ending positions of movement at a joint.

Maximum heart rate reserve (MHRR)—The difference between resting and peak exercise heart rates; measured in beats per minute (Whaley et al., 1997).

Maximum voluntary contraction—The greatest amount of tension a muscle can generate and hold only for a moment, such as in muscle testing.

Mechanical advantage—The position in which the muscle is able to generate greatest tension, that is, when it is longer than the resting length of the muscle. In this position, the passive tension generated by the viscoelastic properties of the muscle and its tendon combine with the active tension generated by the contraction of the muscle fibers to produce a maximum voluntary contraction. When the muscle is fully lengthened or shortened, the viscoelastic, or passive, tension is reduced.

Passive range of motion (PROM)—The amount of movement possible at a joint when an outside force moves the limb.

Reliability—Characteristic of a measuring instrument, indicating the stability of the instrument's findings over time, between testers, and within its various parts when properly administered under similar circumstances (Johnston et al., 1992). Reliability is usually defined by a correlation coefficient (r) or an interclass correlation coefficient (ICC). An r or ICC of 1 indicates a perfect linear relation between one variable (e.g., rater A's scores) and another variable (e.g., rater B's scores). An r of .85 or ICC of .75 is considered acceptable for measuring instruments. Reliability can be increased by controlling all variables that affect the scores other than the one being measured (e.g., change in ROM). Control is gained by keeping everything the same or by deleting some variables.

Standard deviation (SD)—A measure of dispersion indicating the variability within a set of scores. Low variability within the scores of a set of therapists indicates that the therapists are following the same protocol and the phenomenon being measured is unchanging; high variability indicates that the phenomenon being measured is unstable or the therapists should control their test administration better.

To interpret a score, the therapist often compares it with norms (averages and standard deviations). The SD tells you where your patient's score falls in relation to the norm, because you can relate it to the normal curve. In the bell-shaped normal curve, ±1 SD is equal to approximately 68% of the area under the curve (34% on each side of the mean); ±2 SD is equal to approximately 95% of the area under the curve; and ±3 SD is equal to approximately 99% of the area under the curve. A score of 2 to 3 SD below the mean normative score indicates a limitation in need of treatment.

Tenodesis—The mechanical effect caused by the length of extrinsic finger flexors and extensors. When the wrist is flexed, the fingers tend to extend because the extensors are too short to allow full finger flexion and wrist flexion at the same time. Similarly, when the wrist is extended, the fingers tend to flex.

---

impaired occupational functioning, it is within the realm of occupational therapy to assess them. Keep in mind that occupational therapy assessments of mobility, strength, endurance, and pain focus on occupational functioning, not on these abilities and capacities per se.

Furthermore, besides an individual's abilities and capacities many variables, including environmental and contextual constraints, contribute to the ability to do an activity. Use of the assessments described in this chapter allows establishment of a baseline of the patient's abilities. Reassessment produces documentation of pro-gress. With the significant changes in health care delivery, it is essential that occupational therapists be efficient and accurate in their evaluations of patients.

Measurement of Range of Motion

Normally each joint can move in certain directions and to certain **limits of motion** determined by its structure and the integrity of surrounding tissues. Trauma or disease that affects joint structures or the surrounding tissues can decrease the amount of motion at the joint and limit occupational functioning.

Measurement of joint range may be done actively or passively. **Passive range of motion** (PROM) is the amount of motion at a given joint when the joint is moved by an outside force. **Active range of motion** (AROM) is the amount of motion at a given joint achieved by the patient using his or her own strength. If AROM is less than PROM, there is a problem of muscle weakness (or tendon integrity in hands). AROM measurement, used as a supplement to the measurement of the strength of muscles graded poor minus (2–) or fair minus (3–) indicates small gains that would otherwise not be noted by the muscle test.

Evaluation of ROM should start with a quick functional AROM scan (Box 4-1). If no limitations in ROM that would interfere with occupational functioning are found during the functional AROM scan, record the range as within normal limits; no further testing is required.

If limitations are observed, the therapist attempts to move the joint through its full ROM. If the joint is free to move to the end range, the problem is with active motion. The limited active range is measured and recorded. If the end range can not be attained when the therapist moves the limb, the problem is with passive motion, and the limitation is measured and recorded.

A goniometer is used for measuring joint motion. Every goniometer has a protractor, an axis, and two arms. The stationary arm extends from the protractor, on which the degrees are marked. The movable arm has a center line or pointer to indicate angle measurement. The axis is the point at which these two arms are riveted together. A full-circle goniometer, which measures 0 to 180° in each direction, permits measurement of motion in both directions, such as flexion and extension, without repositioning the tool. When using a half-circle goniometer, it is necessary to position the protractor opposite to the direction of motion so that the indicator remains on the face of the protractor. A finger goniometer is designed with a shorter movable arm and flat surfaces to fit comfortably over the finger joints. Figure 4-1 shows each of these types of goniometers.

The therapist must place the axis and arms appropriately to ensure accuracy and **reliability** (Box 4-2). The specific placement of the goniometer for each joint is described and demonstrated in this chapter.

In addition to goniometer placement, multiple patient-related and environmental factors can affect accuracy and reliability of ROM measurements. Patient-related factors include pain, fear of pain, fatigue, and feelings of stress or tension. For the most accurate and reliable results, every effort should be made to make the patient physically and emotionally comfortable, including talking to the patient and describing the procedure

---

BOX 4-1
PROCEDURES FOR PRACTICE

Functional Active Range of Motion Scan

- ▶ The patient should be seated if possible.
- ▶ The patient should perform the motions bilaterally if possible. If not, the more normal side should move first to set a baseline for normal for this person.
- ▶ Observe for complete movements, symmetry of movements, and timing of movements.
- ▶ Demonstrate the movements if the patient has a language barrier or cognitive deficits.

To estimate the amount of active movement in the following motions, give instructions such as these to the patient:

Motion	Examples of Instruction
Shoulder flexion (sagittal plane)	Lift your arms straight up in front and reach toward the ceiling.
Shoulder abduction (frontal plane)	Move your arms out to the side. Now reach over your head.
Shoulder horizontal abduction and adduction (horizontal plane)	Raise your arms forward to shoulder height. Move each arm out to the side, then back again.
External rotation	Touch the back of your head with your hand.
Internal rotation	Touch the small of your back with your hand.
Elbow flexion and extension	Start with your arms straight down by your sides. Now bend your elbows so your hands touch your shoulders.
Forearm supination and pronation	With your arms at your side and your elbows flexed to 90°, rotate your forearms so the palms of your hands face the floor and then the ceiling.
Wrist flexion and extension	Move one of your wrists up and down. Now, the other one.
Finger flexion and extension	Make a fist, then spread your fingers out.
Finger opposition	Touch your thumb to the tip of each finger one at a time.

---

that is to follow. Environmental factors include time of day, temperature of the room, type of goniometer used, and experience of the tester. For the most reliable pretest–posttest information, the same tester should use the same goniometer at the same time of day.

Reliability

Intrarater reliability is consistently higher than interrater reliability for ROM testing using the universal

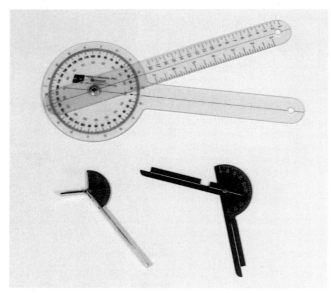

Figure 4-1 Three types of goniometers. The large full-circle goniometer (*top*) is used to measure large joints. The small finger goniometer (*bottom left*) has flat arms that fit over the fingers. The small half-circle goniometer (*bottom right*) is used to measure small joints, such as the wrist.

(full-circle) goniometer. In one study of shoulder motions, intrarater reliability ranged from .90 to .98, whereas interrater reliability ranged from .26 to .89 (Riddle et al., 1987). In a study of low-back ROM of people with and without back pain, intrarater reliability for flexion and extension was 0.97 and 0.95 respectively, while interrater reliability for the same positions was .86 and .93 (Chiarello & Savidge, 1993).

Active motion measurements are more reliable than passive ones (Gajdosik & Bohannon, 1987; Sabari et al., 1998). In one study, 30 adults were measured for both active and passive ROM for shoulder flexion and abduction in two positions, sitting and supine. The AROM measurements were more reliable than the PROM measurements for both positions (Sabari et al., 1998). Furthermore, the researchers found only a moderate range of agreement (.64 to .81) between goniometric measurements of shoulder movements with the patient sitting and supine. The authors concluded that the position of the patient can affect the ROM. Therefore, therapists should record the testing position, and the same position should be used each time the patient is retested. This chapter demonstrates measurement of shoulder ROM in a sitting patient because it measures shoulder mobility in the position more frequently used for functional task performance.

A multicenter study looked at the reliability of three goniometric techniques for measuring passive wrist flexion and extension: radial, ulnar and volar–dorsal approaches. This study found the volar–dorsal approach to be slightly more reliable. The interclass correlation

coefficient (ICC) was .93 for flexion and .84 for extension, .88 and .80 for the radial approach, and .89 and .80 for the ulnar approach (LaStayo & Wheeler, 1994). All three approaches are reliable, but they are not interchangeable. The therapist must be sure to document which approach is being used and use the same approach consistently to document progress.

It is commonly believed that experience plays a major role in the reliability of ROM measurements. A study of experience of the therapist and how it influences reliability of goniometric measurements found no dramatic difference in reliability between experienced and inexperienced therapists who were measuring foot position. All of the inexperienced therapists were uniformly trained on specific testing procedures (Somers et al., 1997). It may be inferred from this study that interrater reliability may be more dependent on training than experience.

Recording Range of Motion

Each measurement is accurately recorded on a ROM form, which the therapist signs and dates because a medical record is a legal document. Notation is made whether scores represent AROM or PROM. A sample form is provided in Table 4-1. Any form should allow for recording the starting and ending positions (limits of motion) for each movement. When reading the goniometer, always state your results as a range using two numbers. The first number is the starting position of the

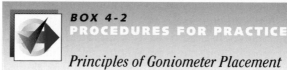

BOX 4-2
PROCEDURES FOR PRACTICE

Principles of Goniometer Placement

▶ Place the axis of the goniometer over the axis of motion. The axis of motion for some joints coincides with bony landmarks, but for others it must be found by observing movement and finding the point around which the movement occurs. In that case, the axis of motion can change position during movement, so it is acceptable for the goniometer to be repositioned at the end of range. When the two arms of the goniometer are placed correctly, they intersect at the axis of motion (Moore, 1978), so it is more important to have the arms line up correctly. The axis placement then automatically falls in line.
▶ Position the stationary arm parallel to the longitudinal axis of the body segment proximal to the joint being measured, although there are some exceptions.
▶ Position the movable arm parallel to the longitudinal axis of the body segment distal to the joint being measured, with some exceptions.

TABLE 4-1
Range of Motion

Patient's Name _____

Type of motion: AROM _____

PROM _____

LEFT			RIGHT	
DATE	**DATE**	**JOINT TO BE MEASURED**	**DATE**	**DATE**
		SHOULDER		
		Flexion	0–180		
		Extension	0–60		
		Abduction	0–180		
		Horizontal abduction	0–90		
		Horizontal adduction	0–45		
		Internal rotation	0–70		
		External rotation	0–90		
		Internal Rotation (alt)	0–80		
		External rotation (alt)	0–60		
		ELBOW AND FOREARM		
		Flexion–extension	0–150		
		Supination	0–80		
		Pronation	0–80		
		WRIST		
		Flexion	0–80		
		Extension	0–70		
		Ulnar Deviation	0–30		
		Radial Deviation	0–20		
		THUMB		
		CM flexion	0–15		
		CM extension	0–20		
		MP flexion–extension	0–50		
		IP flexion–extension	0–80		
		Abduction cm.			
		Opposition cm.			
		INDEX FINGER		
		MP flexion	0–90		
		PIP flexion–extension	0–100		
		DIP flexion–extension	0–90		
		Abduction	no norm		
		Adduction	no norm		
		MIDDLE FINGER		
		MP flexion	0–90		
		PIP flexion–extension	0–100		
		DIP flexion–extension	0–90		
		Abduction	no norm		
		Adduction	no norm		
		RING FINGER		
		MP flexion	0–90		
		PIP flexion–extension	0–100		
		DIP flexion–extension	0–90		
		Abduction	no norm		
		Adduction	no norm		
		LITTLE FINGER		
		MP flexion	0–90		
		PIP flexion–extension	0–100		
		DIP flexion–extension	0–90		
		Abduction	no norm		
		Adduction	no norm		

Therapist's signature: _____

Case Example

RANGE OF MOTION, STRENGTH AND ENDURANCE

Patient Information

Mrs. B. is a 58-year-old right-handed woman with a 5-year history of primary degenerative joint disease (DJD), or osteoarthritis. She complains of upper extremity weakness, stiffness, and Heberden's nodes over several DIP joints. She also complains of pain and fatigue that are limiting her self-maintenance, self-advancement, and self-enhancement roles.

She is a divorced fifth-grade teacher who lives alone in a one-story house. She has two grown children and enjoys gardening, reading, and antique shopping. She has a referral for occupational therapy services because of the occupational dysfunction and has been approved for four outpatient visits.

Description of Assessment

To determine Mrs. B.'s perception of her occupational dysfunction and her priorities, the therapist administered the *Canadian Occupational Performance Measure (COPM)*. To determine to what extent strength and endurance problems affected Mrs. B.'s occupational functioning, a manual muscle test on selected muscle groups, grip and pinch strength assessment using a Jamar dynamometer and B&L pinch meter, visual analogue pain rating scale, and the *Borg Perceived Exertion Scale* for endurance during activities were administered.

Results

Mrs. B. identified five problems concerning tasks and activities of self-care, productivity, and leisure and them put in order of importance. Mrs. B. also rated her performance and her satisfaction with her performance of these 5 tasks. The results of the COPM are as follows:

1. Difficulty writing on the chalk board, which she does 2 to 3 hours a day (performance 4, satisfaction 3)
2. Difficulty with morning activities of daily living, including showering and dressing. She has problems reaching overhead, manipulating bottle caps, doing buttons and zippers, and putting on jewelry (performance 6, satisfaction 5)
3. Difficulty decorating her classroom bulletin boards and doing arts and crafts at school because of the cutting and stapling (performance 5, satisfaction 5)
4. Inability to do many meal preparation activities, including manipulating kitchen appliances, cutting vegetables, and carrying dishes (performance 4, satisfaction 4)
5. Unable to garden as desired, specifically planting, digging with a trowel, and weeding (performance 3, satisfaction 2)

The results of Mrs. B.'s manual muscle test are displayed below. Grip strength using a Jamar dynamometer was 18 pounds on the right and 45 pounds on the left. Tip pinch strength was 3 pounds on the right, 9 pounds on the left. Lateral pinch was 5 pounds on the right, 12 pounds on the left. Palmar pinch was 4 pounds on the right, 13 pounds on the left.

Manual muscle strength	Right	Left
Shoulder flexion	3–	4–
Shoulder abduction	3–	4–
Shoulder external rotation	3–	4
Elbow flexion	4	4+
Elbow extension	3+	4
Forearm supination	3+	4+
Forearm pronation	4	4+
Wrist flexion	3+	4
Wrist extension	3+	4

Mrs. B. reported a 2 on the visual analog scale (VAS) for pain at rest but stated that pain in her hands and shoulders increases to 4 during morning activities of daily living, 5 during meal preparation, and 6 when she uses scissors or gardening tools.

Using the Borg Scale, Mrs. B. rated bathing and dressing this morning a 13; teaching an hour math lesson using the blackboard, a 14; and gardening for a half an hour, a 17.

Analysis of Results

The occupational therapist made the following conclusions: The manual muscle test shows significant weakness in the shoulder musculature of her left upper extremity and all of the muscle groups of the right upper extremity. The weakness of her right shoulder limits her ability to perform many desired occupational tasks because she is unable to reach overhead or take any resistance in most muscles of her right arm. She can take only moderate resistance or less with her left. This makes sustained writing on the blackboard and other tasks, such as washing and brushing her hair extremely difficult. The dynamometer test showed a significant decrease in grip strength for her right—dominant—hand, but was within normal limits for her left hand. Her right tip pinch, lateral pinch, and palmar pinch were also significantly limited compared to the left or to the norms. All three pinches of her left hand were within normal limits. The weakness in her right hand also contributes to her difficulty in many occupational tasks, such as using scissors or a stapler, opening jars, and manipulating garden tools.

Mrs. B.'s score on the VAS indicates increased pain in her hands and shoulders during many functional activities and decreased pain at rest. The results of the Borg Scale indicate low endurance, which contributes to her fatigue and decreased ability to perform a number of tasks, including standing while bathing, teaching, and gardening.

This patient would benefit from skilled occupational therapy services to remediate the deficient abilities and capacities that prevent performance and satisfaction with performance of important daily occupations.

Occupational Therapy Problem List

1. Decreased ability to perform morning activities of daily living, including bathing and dressing, because of shoulder weakness and low endurance.

2. Decreased ability to perform meal preparation tasks because of weak grasp and pinch.
3. Decreased ability to perform work-related tasks, including writing on the blackboard, decorating bulletin boards, and arts and crafts, because of weak shoulders bilaterally, poor endurance, and pain.
4. Decreased ability to garden because of weakness and pain.

---

extremity and the second number is the limit of motion at end range. Two columns can be used for recording of initial and retest information. Both columns should be dated to allow for tracking and easy analysis of the patient's progress.

The most common method of determining ROM is the Neutral Zero Method recommended by the Committee on Joint Motion of the American Academy of Orthopaedic Surgeons (Greene & Heckman, 1994). In this method, the **anatomical position** is considered to be 0, or if a given starting position is different from anatomical position, it is defined as 0. Measurement is taken from the stated starting position to the stated end position. If the patient cannot achieve the stated starting and end positions, the actual starting and end positions are recorded to indicate limitations in movement. An example of this, using elbow flexion, is as follows:

0 to 150°: No limitation

20 to 150°: A limitation in extension (problem with the start position)

0 to 120°: A limitation in flexion (problem with end position)

20 to 120°: Limitations in flexion and extension (problems with start and end positions)

To record hyperextension of a joint, which may be occasionally seen in metacarpophalangeal or elbow joints, the American Academy of Orthopaedic Surgeons recommends a separate measurement to describe the available ROM without confusion. For example, if 20° of elbow hyperextension (an unnatural movement) is noted, it should be recorded as follows:

0 to 150° of flexion

150 to 0° of extension

0 to 20° of hyperextension

If a joint is fused, the starting and end positions are the same, with no ROM. This is recorded as fused at $x°$. If a joint that normally moves in two directions cannot move in one direction, the ROM-limited motion is recorded as none. For example, if wrist flexion is 15 to 80° with a 15° flexion **contracture**, the wrist cannot be positioned at 0 or moved into extension; therefore, wrist extension is recorded as none.

Because there are various systems of notations, each having its own meaning, it is important to clarify the intended meaning to ensure consistency among therapists and physicians within the same facility.

Measurement of Range of Motion of the Upper Extremity

This chapter addresses ROM of the upper extremity, since most functional activities require upper extremity use and manipulation skills. Lower extremity ROM is typically measured by physical therapists who are interested in the ability to walk. References listed at the end of the chapter are good sources of information concerning measurement of lower extremity ROM.

For the measurements given here, unless otherwise noted, the patient is seated with trunk erect against the back of an armless straight chair, although the measurements can be taken with the patient standing or supine, if necessary. This procedure can be done actively or passively. For active movement, take special care to ensure that there are no substitutions of movement. For PROM, the tester supports both the body part and the goniometer proximal and distal to the joint, leaving the joint free to move. Practice is required for comfortable handling of the goniometer together with the movable body segment.

Shoulder Flexion

Movement of the humerus anteriorly in the sagittal plane (0–180°, which represents both glenohumeral and axio-scapular motion) (Figs. 4-2 and 4-3).

Goniometer Placement

Axis A point around which motion occurs through the lateral aspect of the glenohumeral joint; at the start of motion it lies approximately 1 inch below the acromion process. At the end position, the axis has moved and the goniometer must be repositioned.

Stationary Arm Parallel to the lateral midline of the trunk.

Movable Arm Parallel to the longitudinal axis of the humerus on the lateral aspect.

Possible Substitutions

Trunk extension, shoulder abduction.

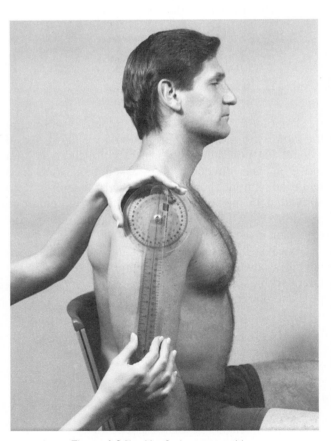

Figure 4-2 Shoulder flexion, start position.

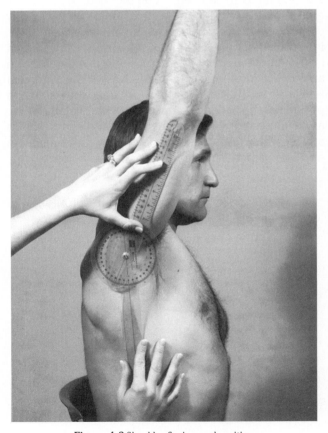

Figure 4-3 Shoulder flexion, end position.

Shoulder Extension

Movement of the humerus posteriorly in a sagittal plane (0–60°) (Figs. 4-4 and 4-5).

Goniometer Placement

Axis A point around which motion occurs; it lies approximately 1 inch below the acromion process through the lateral aspect of the glenohumeral joint.

Stationary Arm Parallel to the lateral midline of the trunk.
Movable Arm Parallel to the longitudinal axis of the humerus on the lateral aspect.

Possible Substitutions

Trunk flexion, scapular elevation and downward rotation, shoulder abduction.

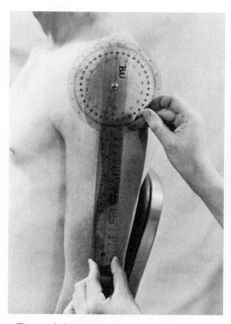

Figure 4-4 Shoulder extension, start position.

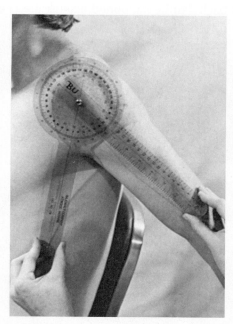

Figure 4-5 Shoulder extension, end position.

Shoulder Abduction

Movement of the humerus laterally in a frontal plane (0–180°, which represents both glenohumeral and axioscapular motion) (Figs. 4-6 and 4-7).

Goniometer Placement

Axis   A point through the anterior or posterior aspect of the glenohumeral joint. Some people consider measurement from the anterior aspect safer, because the patient's back can be supported against the chair, but it is preferable to measure women from the posterior aspect.

Stationary Arm Laterally along the trunk, parallel to the spine.

Movable Arm Parallel to the longitudinal axis of the humerus.

Possible Substitutions

Lateral flexion of trunk, scapular elevation, shoulder flexion or extension.

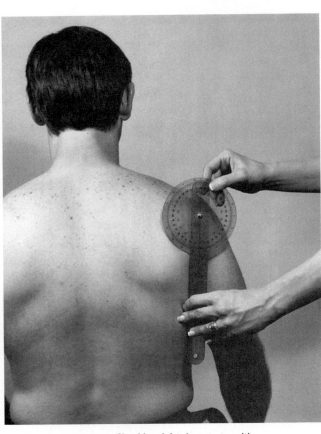

Figure 4-6 Shoulder abduction, start position.

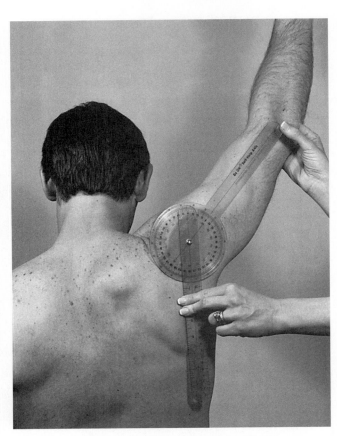

Figure 4-7 Shoulder abduction, end position.

Horizontal Abduction

Movement of the humerus on a horizontal plane from 90° of shoulder flexion to 90° of shoulder abduction and beyond to the limit of motion (0–90°) (Figs. 4-8 and 4-9).

Goniometer Placement

Axis On top of the acromion process.

Stationary Arm To start, the arm is parallel to the longitudinal axis of the humerus on the superior aspect and remains in that position, perpendicular to the body, although the humerus moves away. An alternative position of the stationary arm is across the shoulder, anterior to the neck and in line with the opposite acromion process. In this alternative position, the goniometer reads 90° at the start, and this must be considered when recording.

Movable Arm Parallel to the longitudinal axis of the humerus on the superior aspect.

Possible Substitution

Trunk rotation or trunk flexion.

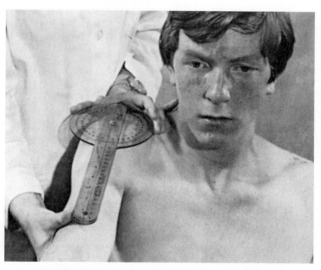

Figure 4-8 Shoulder horizontal abduction, start position.

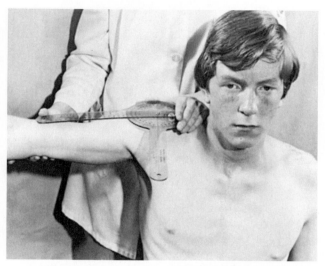

Figure 4-9 Shoulder horizontal abduction, end position.

Horizontal Adduction

Movement of the humerus on a horizontal plane from 90° of shoulder abduction through 90° of shoulder flexion, across the trunk to the limit of motion. The 90° of return motion from horizontal abduction is not measured. The motion is measured from 90° shoulder flexion across the trunk (0–45°) (Figs. 4-10 and 4-11).

Goniometer Placement

Axis On top of the acromion process.

Stationary Arm Parallel to the longitudinal axis on the superior aspect of the humerus in the starting position, it remains perpendicular to the body, although the humerus moves away. The alternative placement given for horizontal abduction also applies in this case.

Movable Arm Parallel to the longitudinal axis of the humerus on the superior aspect.

Possible Substitution

Trunk rotation.

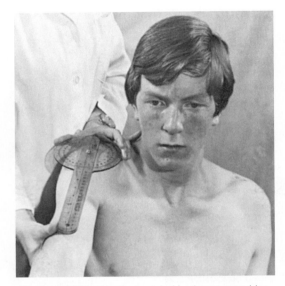

Figure 4-10 Shoulder horizontal adduction, start position.

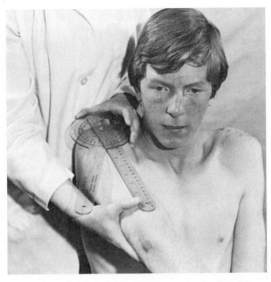

Figure 4-11 Shoulder horizontal adduction, end position.

Internal Rotation

Movement of the humerus medially around the longitudinal axis of the humerus (0–70°) (Figs. 4-12 and 4-13).

Goniometer Placement

Axis Olecranon process of the ulna.

Stationary Arm Perpendicular to the floor, which will be parallel to the lateral trunk if the patient is sitting up straight with hips at 90°. The goniometer reads 90° at the start, and this score must be deducted from the final score when recording ROM. *Note.* If the patient is supine with the shoulder abducted to 90° and the elbow flexed to 90°, the stationary arm is perpendicular to the floor, with the movable arm along the ulna. The goniometer reads 0° at the start (Moore, 1978).

Movable Arm Parallel to the longitudinal axis of the ulna.

Possible Substitutions

Scapular elevation and downward rotation, trunk flexion, elbow extension.

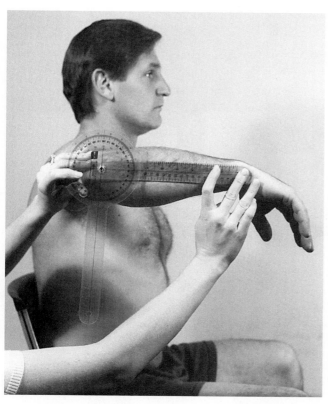

Figure 4-12 Shoulder internal rotation, start position.

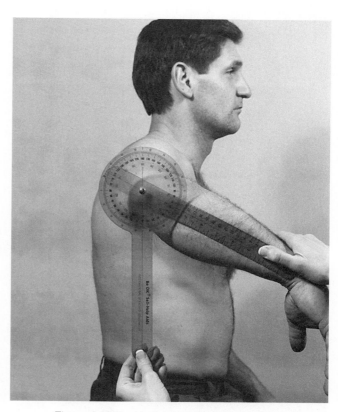

Figure 4-13 Shoulder internal rotation, end position.

External Rotation

Movement of the humerus laterally around the longitudinal axis of the humerus (0–90°) (Figs. 4-14 and 4-15).

Goniometer Placement

Axis Olecranon process of the ulna.
Stationary Arm Perpendicular to the floor. The goniometer will read 90° at the start, and this must be considered when recording the ROM score.

Movable Arm Parallel to the longitudinal axis of the ulna.

Possible Substitutions

Scapular depression and upward rotation, trunk extension, elbow extension.

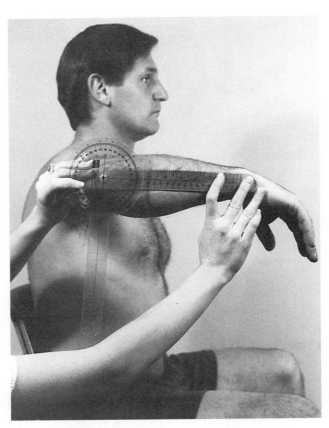

Figure 4-14 Shoulder external rotation, start position.

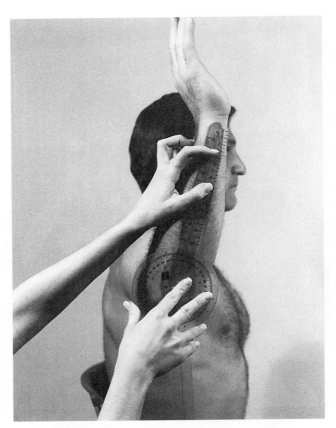

Figure 4-15 Shoulder external rotation, end position.

Internal and External Rotation: Alternative Method

If shoulder limitation prevents positioning for the previously described method, the patient may be seated with humerus adducted to the side and elbow flexed to 90° (Figs. 4-16 and 4-17). This method is inaccurate in internal rotation if the patient has a large abdomen. (Internal rotation, 0–80°; external rotation, 0–60°).

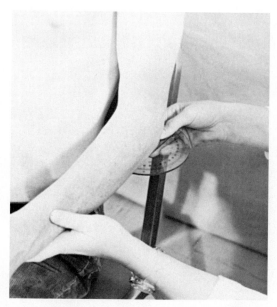

Figure 4-16 Shoulder internal and external rotation, alternative method, start position.

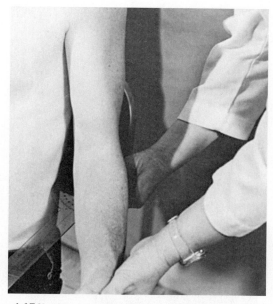

Figure 4-17 Shoulder external rotation, alternative method, end position.

Elbow Flexion-Extension

Movement of the supinated forearm anteriorly in the sagittal plane (0–150°) (Figs. 4-18 and 4-19).

Goniometer Placement

Axis Lateral epicondyle of the humerus.

Stationary Arm Parallel to the longitudinal axis of the humerus on the lateral aspect.

Movable Arm Parallel to the longitudinal axis of the radius.

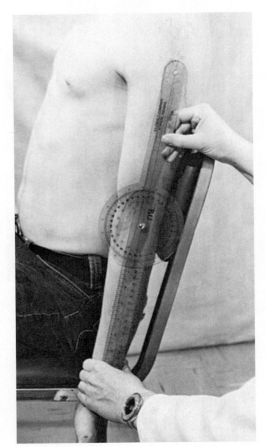

Figure 4-18 Elbow flexion, start position (elbow extension).

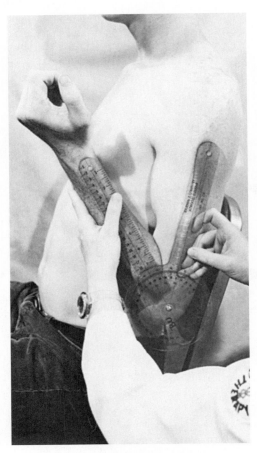

Figure 4-19 Elbow flexion, end position.

Forearm Supination

Rotation of the forearm laterally around its longitudinal axis from midposition so that the palm of the hand faces up (0–80°) (Figs. 4-20 and 4-21).

Goniometer Placement

Axis Longitudinal axis of the forearm displaced toward the ulnar side.

Stationary Arm Perpendicular to the floor.
Movable Arm Across the distal radius and ulna on the volar surface.

Possible Substitutions

Adduction and external rotation of the shoulder.

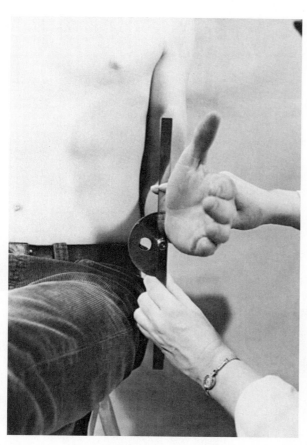

Figure 4-20 Supination, start position.

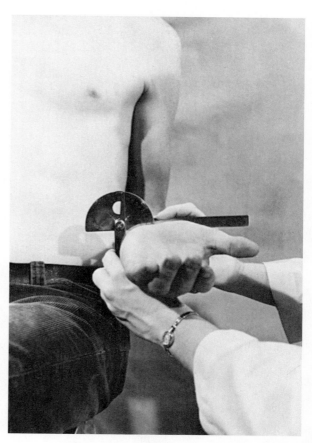

Figure 4-21 Supination, end position.

Forearm Pronation

Rotation of the forearm medially around its longitudinal axis from midposition so that the palm of the hand faces down (0–80°) (Figs. 4-22 and 4-23).

Goniometer Placement

Axis Longitudinal axis of forearm displaced toward the ulnar side.

Stationary Arm Perpendicular to the floor.
Movable Arm Across the distal radius and ulna on the dorsal surface.

Possible Substitutions

Abduction and internal rotation of the shoulder.

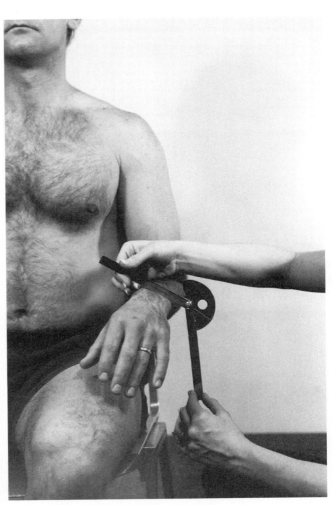

Figure 4-22 Pronation, start position.　　**Figure 4-23** Pronation, end position.

Wrist Flexion (Volar Flexion)

Movement of the hand volarly in the sagittal plane (0–80°) (Figs. 4-24 and 4-25).

Goniometer Placement

Axis On the dorsal aspect of the wrist joint in line with the base of the third metacarpal.

Stationary Arm Along the midline of the dorsal surface of the forearm.

Movable Arm Parallel to the longitudinal axis of the third metacarpal.

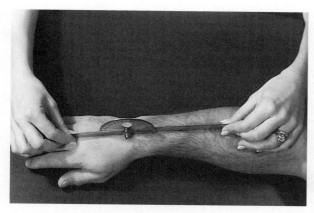

Figure 4-24 Wrist flexion, start position.

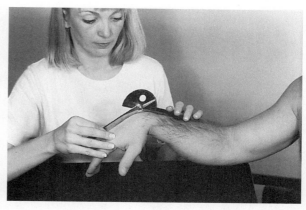

Figure 4-25 Wrist flexion, end position.

Wrist Extension (Dorsiflexion)

Movement of the hand dorsally in the sagittal plane (0–70°) (Figs. 4-26 and 4-27).

Goniometer Placement

Axis On the volar surface of the wrist in line with the insertion of the tendon of the palmaris longus.

Stationary Arm Along the midline of the volar surface of the forearm.
Movable Arm Parallel to the longitudinal axis of the third metacarpal.

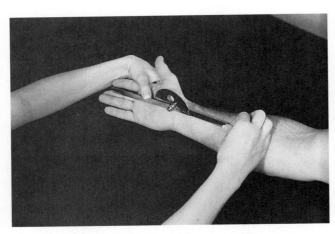

Figure 4-26 Wrist extension, start position.

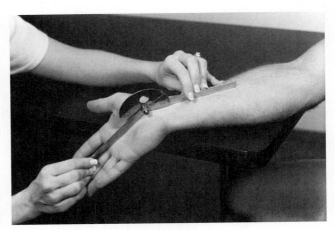

Figure 4-27 Wrist extension, end position .

Wrist Ulnar Deviation

Movement of the hand toward the ulnar side in a frontal plane (0–30°) (Figs. 4-28 and 4-29).

Goniometer Placement

Axis On the dorsal aspect of the wrist joint in line with the base of the third metacarpal.

One Arm Along the midline of the forearm on the dorsal surface.

Other Arm Along the midline of the third metacarpal.

Possible Substitutions

Wrist extension, wrist flexion.

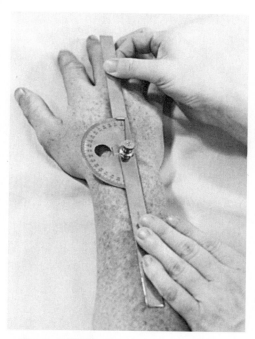

Figure 4-28 Wrist ulnar deviation, start position.

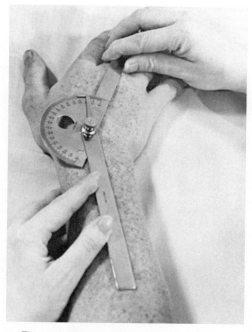

Figure 4-29 Wrist ulnar deviation, end position.

Wrist Radial Deviation

Movement of the hand toward the radial side in a frontal plane (0–20°) (Figs. 4-30 and 4-31).

Goniometer Placement

Axis On the dorsal aspect of the wrist joint in line with the base of the third metacarpal.

Stationary Arm Along the midline of the forearm on the dorsal surface.

Movable Arm Along the midline of the third metacarpal.

Possible Substitution

Wrist extension.

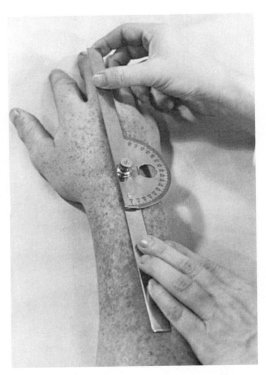

Figure 4-30 Wrist radial deviation, start position.

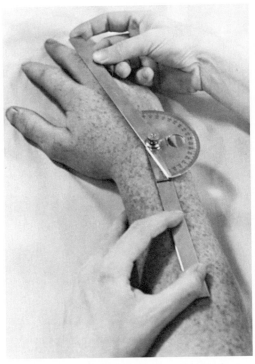

Figure 4-31 Wrist radial deviation, end position.

Thumb Carpometacarpal Flexion

Movement of the thumb across the palm in the frontal plane (0–15°) (Figs. 4-32 and 4-33).

Goniometer Placement

Axis On the radial side of the wrist at the junction of the base of the first metacarpal and the trapezium.

Stationary Arm Parallel to the longitudinal axis of the radius.

Movable Arm Parallel to the longitudinal axis of the first metacarpal. For accuracy, the arms of the goniometer must remain in full contact with skin surface over the bones. ***However, excessive pressure with the edge of a half-circle goniometer must be avoided***. These statements apply to all flexion–extension measurements of the thumb and fingers.

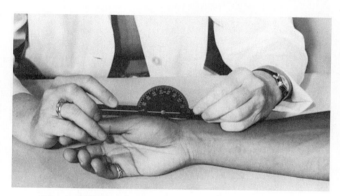

Figure 4-32 Thumb carpometacarpal flexion, start position.

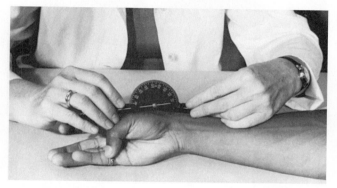

Figure 4-33 Thumb carpometacarpal flexion, end position.

Thumb Carpometacarpal Extension

Movement of the thumb away from the palm in the frontal plane (0–20°) (Figs. 4-34 and 4-35).

Goniometer Placement

Axis On the volar side of the wrist at the junction of the base of the first metacarpal and the trapezium.

One Arm Parallel to the longitudinal axis of the radius. Other Arm Parallel to the longitudinal axis of the first metacarpal.

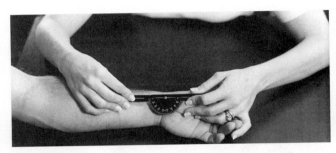

Figure 4-34 Thumb carpometacarpal extension, start position.

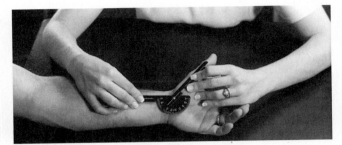

Figure 4-35 Thumb carpometacarpal extension, end position.

Thumb Metacarpophalangeal (MP) Flexion-Extension

Movement of the thumb across the palm in the frontal plane (0–50°) (Figs. 4-36 and 4-37).

Goniometer Placement

Axis On the dorsal aspect of the MP joint.

Stationary Arm On the dorsal surface along the midline of the first metacarpal.

Movable Arm On the dorsal surface along the midline of the proximal phalanx of the thumb.

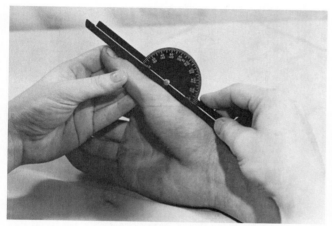

Figure 4-36 Thumb metacarpophalangeal flexion, start position (extension).

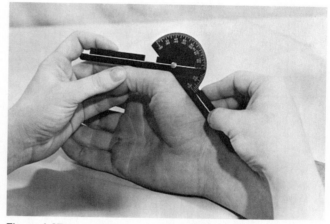

Figure 4-37 Thumb metacarpophalangeal flexion and extension, end position.

Thumb Interphalangeal (IP) Flexion-Extension

Movement of the distal phalanx of the thumb toward the volar surface of the proximal phalanx of the thumb (0–80°) (Figs. 4-38 and 4-39).

Goniometer Placement

Axis On the dorsal aspect of the IP joint.

Stationary Arm On the dorsal surface along the proximal phalanx.

Movable Arm On the dorsal surface along the distal phalanx. *Note.* If the thumbnail prevents full goniometer contact, shift the movable arm laterally to increase accuracy. Also, thumb MP and IP flexion and extension can be measured on the lateral aspect of the thumb using lateral aspects of the same landmarks.

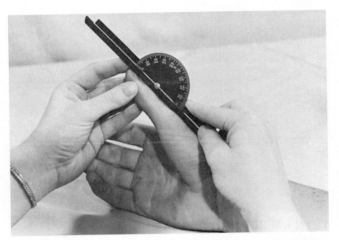

Figure 4-38 Thumb interphalangeal flexion, start position (extension).

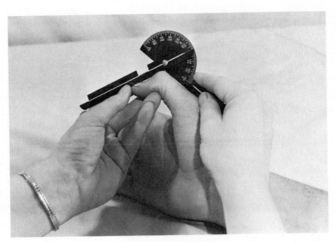

Figure 4-39 Thumb interphalangeal flexion, end position.

Thumb Abduction and Opposition: Ruler Measurements

Abduction

Take the measurement from the midpoint of the head of the first metacarpal to the midpoint of the head of the second metacarpal while the thumb is in full abduction (Fig. 4-40).

Opposition

The pad of the thumb rotates to meet the pad of each finger. The little finger rotates to better meet the pad of the thumb. As a summary measure of opposition, record the distance from the tip of the thumb (not the thumbnail) to the tip end of the little finger (Fig. 4-41).

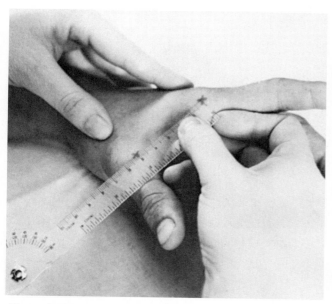

Figure 4-40 Measurement of thumb abduction using a centimeter ruler.

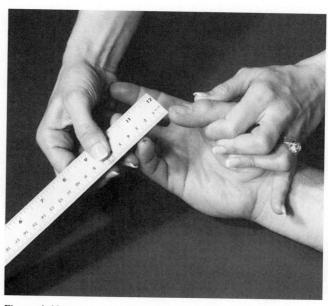

Figure 4-41 Measurement of opposition to the little finger using a centimeter ruler.

Finger Metacarpophalangeal Flexion-Extension

Movement of the finger at the MP joint in a sagittal plane (0–90°) (Figs. 4-42 and 4-43).

Goniometer Placement

Axis On the dorsal aspect of the MP joint of the finger being measured.

Stationary Arm On the dorsal surface along the midline of the metacarpal of the finger being measured.

Movable Arm On the dorsal surface along the midline of the proximal phalanx of the finger being measured.

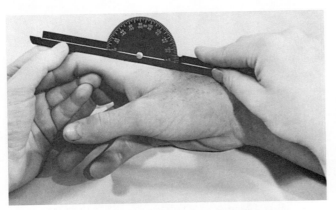

Figure 4-42 Finger metacarpophalangeal flexion, start position (extension).

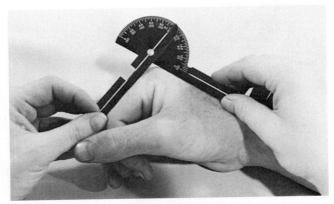

Figure 4-43 Finger metacarpophalangeal flexion, end position.

Finger Proximal Interphalangeal (PIP) Flexion-Extension

Movement of the middle phalanx toward the volar surface of the proximal phalanx in the sagittal plane (0–100°) (Figs. 4-44 and 4-45).

Goniometer Placement

Axis On the dorsal aspect of the PIP joint of the finger being measured.

Stationary Arm On the dorsal surface along the midline of the proximal phalanx of the finger being measured.

Movable Arm On the dorsal surface along the midline of the middle phalanx of the finger being measured.

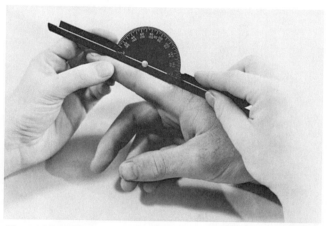

Figure 4-44 Proximal interphalangeal flexion, start position (extension).

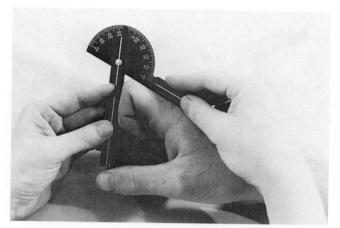

Figure 4-45 Proximal interphalangeal flexion, end position.

Finger Distal Interphalangeal (DIP) Flexion-Extension

Movement of the distal phalanx toward the volar surface of the middle phalanx in a sagittal plane (0–90°) (Figs. 4-46 and 4-47).

Goniometer Placement

Axis On the dorsal aspect of the DIP joint of the finger being measured.

Stationary Arm On the dorsal surface along the midline of the middle phalanx of the finger being measured.

Movable Arm On the dorsal surface along the midline of the distal phalanx of the finger being measured. *Note.* If the fingernail prevents full goniometer contact, shift the movable arm laterally to increase accuracy. Also, finger PIP and DIP flexion and extension can be measured from the lateral aspect of each finger using the lateral aspect of the same landmarks. This method may be more accurate when joints are enlarged.

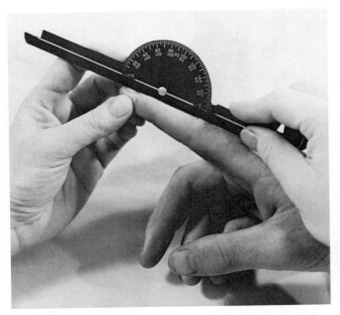

Figure 4-46 Distal interphalangeal flexion, start position (extension).

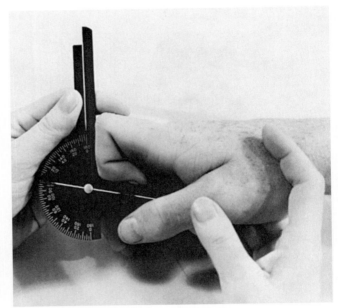

Figure 4-47 Distal interphalangeal flexion, end position.

Composite Measurement and Recording of Total Finger Flexion

A method of recording composite digital motion used by hand therapists is to sum the values for the degrees of flexion motion of the MP, PIP, and DIP joints, taking into consideration extension deficits (Fess, 1990). Total active motion (TAM) or total passive motion (TPM) can then be expressed by a single number. The formula for calculating these values is as follows: (MP + PIP + DIP flexion) – (MP + PIP + DIP extension deficits) = TAM or TPM.

Another method for measuring combined flexion of the PIP and DIP joints (Fig. 4-48) or combined flexion of the MP, PIP, and DIP joints (Fig. 4-49), using a centimeter ruler, is illustrated in the figures.

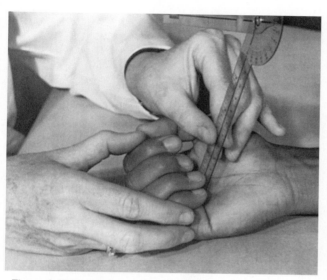

Figure 4-48 PIP and DIP combined finger flexion: ruler measurement.

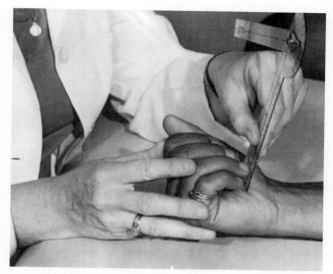

Figure 4-49 MP, PIP, and DIP combined finger flexion: ruler measurement.

Finger Abduction

Movement of the index, ring, and little fingers away from the midline of the hand in a frontal plane. The middle finger, which is the midline of the hand, abducts in both radial and ulnar directions (Figs. 4-50 and 4-51).

Goniometer Placement

Axis On the dorsal aspect of the MP joint of the finger being measured.

Stationary Arm Along the dorsal surface of the metacarpal of the finger being measured.

Movable Arm Along the dorsal surface of the proximal phalanx of the finger being measured.

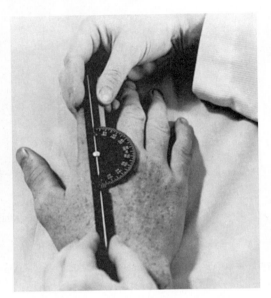

Figure 4-50 Finger abduction, start position.

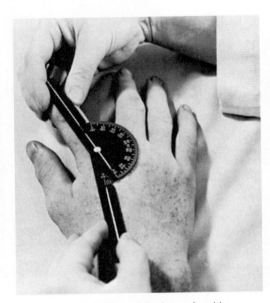

Figure 4-51 Finger abduction, end position.

Finger Adduction

Movement of the index, ring, and little fingers toward the midline of the hand in a frontal plane (Figs. 4-52 and 4-53).

Goniometer Placement

Axis On the dorsal aspect of the MP joint of the finger being measured.

One Arm Along the dorsal surface of the metacarpal of the finger being measured. The middle finger is not measured.

Other Arm Along the dorsal surface of the proximal phalanx of the finger being measured.

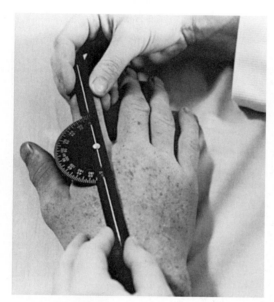

Figure 4-52 Finger adduction, start position.

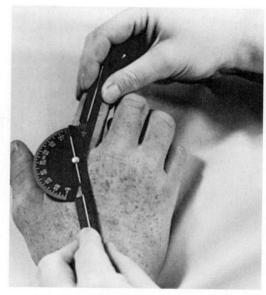

Figure 4-53 Finger adduction, end position.

MP Deviation Correction Measurement

When there is ulnar deviation deformity of the metacarpophalangeal joints, often seen in rheumatoid arthritis, this additional measurement is taken (Figs. 4-54 and 4-55).

The active range is compared with the passive range to determine whether muscle weakness is present. PROM is compared with the norm of 0° deviation to determine whether a fixed deformity exists.

Goniometer Placement

Axis Over the MP joint of the finger being measured.
One Arm Placed along the dorsal midline of the metacarpal.
Other Arm Placed along the dorsal midline of the proximal phalanx.

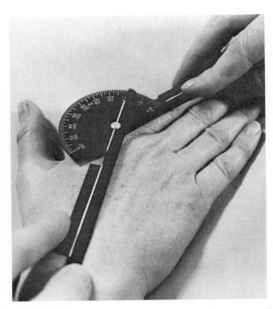

Figure 4-54 Metacarpophalangeal deviation correction, start position.

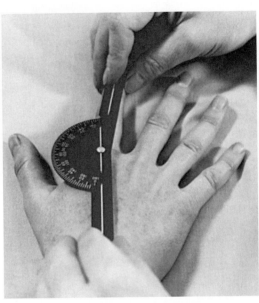

Figure 4-55 Metacarpophalangeal deviation correction, end position.

Interpreting the Results

The initial evaluation is interpreted by reviewing the recording form to identify which joints have significant limitation. A significant limitation is one that decreases functional performance or may lead to deformity. The therapist notes whether the limitation is the result of tissue changes (PROM < norms) or muscle weakness (AROM < PROM).

Limits of motion scores can be used in several ways. First, the therapist can compare the scores of the involved and the other extremities. However, a study of more than 1000 healthy male subjects found a significant difference in ROM between the dominant and nondominant sides. The nondominant side had greater range in many of the upper extremity joints tested (Gunal et al., 1996). This information should be kept in mind when comparing the two sides. The patient's scores can be compared with the average limits (norms) expected for each motion. The average limits stated by the Committee on Joint Motion of the American Academy of Orthopaedic Surgeons (Greene & Heckman, 1994) are commonly used and are included here. However, patients may be functional with less ROM than is noted in the norms for particular joints. The emphasis in occupational therapy is functional movement.

With the significant limitations and probable cause in mind, treatment goals that reflect the identified problem can be developed. For example, if skin, joint, and/or muscle tissues have shortened as a result of immobilization, the goal is to increase range by stretching these tissues. If the limitation is caused by edema, pain, spasticity, or muscle weakness, the primary goal is to reduce or correct the underlying problem, and the secondary goal is to prevent loss of ROM caused by the immobility imposed by the primary condition. If the cause is bony ankylosis or longstanding contracture, the goal is to teach the patient methods of compensation, since these conditions do not respond to nonsurgical treatment.

It is important to compare initial evaluation scores to mid and post treatment scores to assess the outcome and redirect treatment if necessary. However, interpretation of a reevaluation that shows improvement following treatment must be tempered with the realization that changes may occur simply as a result of remeasurement. According to Boone et al., (1978), for a difference in measurements of ROM to be considered to reflect actual change, the amount of change must exceed measurement error, which was found to be 5° for the upper extremity and 6° for the lower extremity. Horger (1990) found similar values for wrist motion. If in a reevaluation the patient has shown an increase of 10° in shoulder flexion, for example, that is a minimal improvement, since 5° may be accounted for by measurement error.

Edema

Edema, one cause of limited ROM, is quantified using circumferential or volumetric measurements. A millimeter tape is used to measure the circumference of a body part not easily submerged. It is essential to measure at exactly the same place from test to test.

Volumetric measures document changes in the mass of a body part by use of water displacement. It is most often used to measure hand edema. A water vessel that is large enough to allow submersion of the whole hand is used (Fig. 4-56). It has a spillover spout near the top of the water level. When the hand is placed in the vessel, water is displaced and spills out into a graduated beaker. An edematous hand displaces more water than an unswollen hand, so that a lower reading is considered an improvement. A study to determine the ability of therapists to orient the extremity consistently within the measuring device and to measure the displaced water correctly indicated high reliability over three repeated tests on 24 hands (DeVore & Hamilton, 1968). Sitting or

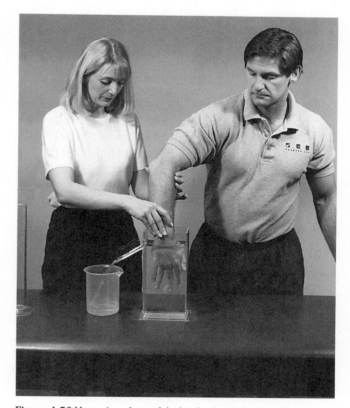

Figure 4-56 Measuring edema of the hand using a volumeter. Note the water being displaced into the graduated beaker as the hand is submerged.

standing significantly affects the score of volumetric measurement; 5.3 mL less volume was seen for seated patients. It is therefore important to standardize the administration procedure. Test–retest correlations of each posture were acceptable (r = .91–0.99) (Stern, 1991).

To interpret findings, compare the measurement of the affected part with that of its contralateral counterpart. If edema is present, the short-term goal of treatment may be, for example, to decrease edema more than 15 mL, which is slightly more than the identified within-patient variance of 10 mL (Waylett & Seibly, 1981) or to reduce measurement by x mL. The information gathered from this assessment tool is used to determine the effectiveness of the treatment, that is, before and after retrograde hand massage or other edema management techniques.

Pain

Pain is another possible cause of ROM limitations. Pain or fear of pain my affect a person's willingness to move. The International Association for the Study of Pain (IASP) defines pain as "an unpleasant sensory and emotional experience associated with actual or potential tissue damage" (Merskey & Bogduk, 1994). Because pain is subjective, self-report measures provide the most valid measure of the experience (Katz & Melzak, 1999). The several self-report measures include the Visual Analogue Scale (VAS), Faces Test, Color Scale, and the Adjective Test (Gordon et al., 1998). The most frequently used method to measure the intensity of pain is the VAS (Gordon et al., 1998; Katz & Melzak, 1999). It is quick and simple to use. It consists of a 10-cm line with 0 and 10 noted at each end of the line. The zero end is designated as "no pain at all"; the other end is designated "the worst pain I ever felt" (Fig. 4-57). The patient marks on the line the point that represents the intensity of the pain he or she feels. The score is obtained by measuring the line from the zero point to the patient's mark in cm. For example, if the mark is made at 4.6 cm on the 10-cm line, the score could be 4 or the more exact 4.6, depending on

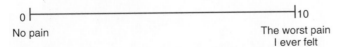

Figure 4-57 A visual analogue scale used to quantify the phenomenological experience of pain.

the practice at the facility. There are no norms for this scale, and it cannot be used to compare different patients, but it is useful in monitoring the progress of the same patient over time (Wittink & Michel, 1997).

Muscle Strength

The Quick Reference Dictionary for Occupational Therapy defines strength as "the ability to demonstrate a degree of power of a muscle when movement is resisted, as with objects or gravity" (Jacobs, 1999, p. 142). Weakness is a lack or reduction of the power of a muscle or muscle group. When weakness limits or impairs the individual's occupational functioning, it is necessary to determine the degree and distribution of weakness to establish an appropriate intervention plan. Treatment can be focused on remediating the weakness, or it can focus on alternative ways of accomplishing the task. Weakness can be manifested in several forms. It can be general, as with Guillain-Barré syndrome, or it can be local, such as with a peripheral nerve lesion. In the former case, muscles throughout the body are assessed; in the latter case just the muscles innervated by the involved nerve are tested. In both cases the muscles to be tested are the ones contributing to the functional limitations on which treatment will focus.

A **maximum voluntary contraction** (MVC), the maximum amount of tension that can be produced under voluntary control, is commonly used to measure strength (Wilmore & Costill, 1999). Because muscle testing is a measurement of voluntary contraction of an isolated muscle or muscle group, strength testing is inappropriate for patients who lack the ability to contract one muscle or a muscle group in isolation, such as patients who exhibit synergistic movement patterns.

In this chapter a technique called the break test is used. In the break test, the muscle to be tested is positioned at its greatest **mechanical advantage**. Once the extremity is positioned, the patient is asked to hold the position as the tester imparts an external force to overcome the contractile force of the muscle or muscle group using either his or her hand alone or a hand-held dynamometer. In other words, the therapist tries to break the patient's isometric contraction (Smidt & Rogers, 1982).

The term mechanical advantage refers to the length–tension relationship of a muscle. Total tension of a muscle is the sum of the passive tension exerted by the elastic components in the lengthened muscle and surrounding tissue and the active tension generated by the contractile elements of the contracting muscle (Gowitzke & Milner, 1980). A muscle is able to generate its greatest total tension or sustain the heaviest load when positioned at a length that gives it optimal mechanical advantage. This is usually slightly (10%) longer than resting length. Developed (active) tension, which is total tension minus the elastic contribution, is greatest at resting length but decreases as the muscle shortens or lengthens. The length–tension principle is used to elicit the best response from prime movers during muscle testing. Furthermore, this principle is used to reduce the contribution of synergist muscles when testing the prime mover. Synergist muscles are placed at mechanical disadvantage (either lengthened or shortened) while the prime mover is asked to resist the applied force (Howell et al., 1989).

For muscles or muscle groups too weak to resist an external force, muscle strength is evaluated by isotonic contraction, in which the muscle is required to move the mass of the body part against gravity without applied resistance or with the effect of gravity decreased (Daniels & Worthingham, 1986; Kendall & Kendall, 1983).

Gravity as resistance is considered an important variable and is used to test all motions when practical. Standard procedures for evaluation against gravity and with gravity eliminated are described in this chapter. Tests of the upper and lower extremities described here for the most part are motion tests for the purpose of evaluating strength in terms of ability to perform functionally. Tests of individual muscles in the wrist and hand are included because of the responsibility of the occupational therapist in rehabilitation of hand injuries.

The movements of the face, head, neck, and trunk, while important in the assessment of some patients, have not been included in the interest of conserving space; however, this information can be found in references listed at the end of this chapter.

Prior to the start of manual muscle testing (MMT), a passive ROM scan should be done to determine what ROM is available at each joint. The available range is considered to be full ROM for the purposes of muscle testing. However, make a notation of any limitation. The muscle or muscle group is assigned a grade, according to the amount of resistance it can take. Two grading systems are presented here; Table 4-2 equates the Medical Research Council (1976) Oxford system to the

TABLE 4-2
Muscle Testing Grading System

5	Normal	The part moves through full ROM against gravity and takes maximal resistance.
4	Good	The part moves through full ROM against gravity and takes moderate resistance.
4−	Good minus	The part moves through full ROM against gravity and takes less than moderate resistance.
3+	Fair plus	The part moves through full ROM against gravity and takes minimal resistance before it breaks.
3	Fair	The part moves through full ROM against gravity and is unable to take any added resistance.
3−	Fair minus	The part moves less than full range of motion against gravity.
2+	Poor plus	The part moves through full ROM in a gravity-eliminated plane and takes minimal resistance, then breaks.
2	Poor	The part moves through full ROM in a gravity-eliminated plane with no added resistance.
2−	Poor minus	The part moves less than full ROM in a gravity-eliminated plane.
1	Trace	Tension is palpated in the muscle or tendon but no motion occurs at the joint.
0	Zero	No tension is palpated in the muscle or tendon.

descriptive grading system (Daniels & Worthingham, 1986).

Box 4-3 shows the sequence of steps for testing every muscle or muscle group to ensure reliability and accuracy. There are additional considerations when performing a manual muscle test. First, although fatigue differs for each person and each muscle, a rest of 2 minutes between maximum effort of the same muscle is considered adequate (Milner-Brown et al., 1986). Second, for the comfort and convenience of the patient, all testing in one position is done before the patient changes to another position. Also, position of head, neck, and proximal parts are usually kept the same from test to test, although preliminary study results indicated that this does not affect tension development (Anderson & Bohannon, 1991; Bohannon et al., 1991).

BOX 4-3
PROCEDURES FOR PRACTICE

Muscle Testing Procedures

1. Explain the procedure and demonstrate the desired movement.
2. Position the patient so the direction of movement will be against gravity.
3. Stabilize proximal to the joint that will move to prevent substitutions.
4. Instruct the patient to move actively to the end position. If the patient cannot move actively against gravity, place the patient in a gravity-eliminated position and ask the patient to move actively in this position.
5. If the patient can move actively against gravity, tell the patient to hold the contraction at the end position.
6. Apply resistance:
   - to the distal end of the segment into which the muscle inserts
   - in the direction the movement came from
   - by starting with light resistance and increase to maximal resistance over a 2- to 3-second period
7. Palpate over the prime mover to determine whether the muscle is contracting or whether gravity and/or synergistic muscles are substituting.
8. Record the appropriate grade according to the resistance tolerated before the muscle broke or by the amount of movement achieved without resistance in an against-gravity or gravity-eliminated position.

CLINICAL REASONING
in OT Practice

Planning a Muscle-Testing Strategy

Testing of shoulder, elbow and lower extremity musculature may require the patient to lie prone or supine or sit up, depending on whether you are testing in an antigravity or gravity-eliminated position. It would be too tiring for the patient to keep switching postures between lying and sitting during a muscle test as presented in this chapter. Devise a practical strategy you will use in muscle testing that will be least fatiguing for a patient. The strategy will list the order of muscles to be tested and for what grade, according to position.

Reliability

Reliability is essential for meaningful evaluation. Most important to the reliability of the scores of repeated tests is strict adherence to the exact procedures of testing. In addition, reliability of muscle testing scores is affected by the interest and cooperation of the patient and by the experience and tone of voice of the tester (Johannson et al., 1983). The most suitable environment is free of distractions, is at a comfortable temperature, and has proper lighting. Other factors known to affect outcome are posture, fatigue, the patient's ability to understand directions, the therapist's operational definitions of various grades, and test positions. For reliability, these variables must be controlled from test to test and among therapists at the same facility. It is necessary for the inexperienced therapist to develop a kinesthetic sense of minimal, moderate, and maximal resistances by working with experienced therapists, each testing the same patient and discussing the grade to be assigned.

Manual muscle testing (MMT) is a valid and reliable procedure to measure muscle strength (Herbison et al., 1996; Marx et al., 1999; Schwartz et al., 1992). A study of reliability for testing intrinsic hand muscles found the correlation for intrarater reliability to range from .71 to .96 and from .72 to .93 for interrater reliability (Brandsma et al., 1995). Florence et al. (1992) performed MMT on patients with Duchenne's muscular dystrophy. Using a standard method of testing and the modified Medical Research Council grading scale (Table 4-2), reliability for muscle grades 0 to 5 ranged from .80 to .99. The most reliable grades were 3 and below, with the least reliable grades being 3+ (.80), 4– (.83), and 5– (.83), those that involve a developed kinesthetic sense of minimal, moderate, and maximal resistance.

Recording Muscle Strength Scores

The grade is accurately recorded in the appropriate place on a form that has columns to record grades for both the right and left sides of the body. The therapist must sign and date each test; if a test continues over several days, the form should reflect that. A sample form is presented in Table 4-3. On that form, the peripheral nerve and spinal segmental levels are listed beside each muscle to assist the therapist in interpreting the results of the muscle test.

TABLE 4-3
Sample Form for Recording Manual Muscle Strength

Patient's Name: _____ Age: _____

| LEFT | | | | RIGHT | |
DATE	DATE			DATE	DATE
		SCAPULA			
		ELEVATION			
		Upper trapezius (accessory) CN XI, C3-4			
		Levator scapulae (dorsal scapular) C5, C3-4			
		DEPRESSION			
		Lower trapezius (accessory) CN XI, C3-4			
		Latissimus dorsi (thoracodorsal) C6-8			
		ADDUCTION			
		Middle trapezius (accessory) CN XI, C3-4			
		Rhomboids (dorsal scapular) C5			
		ABDUCTION			
		Serratus anterior (long thoracic) C5-7			
		SHOULDER			
		FLEXION			
		Anterior deltoid (axillary) C5-6			
		Coracobrachialis (musculocutaneous) C5-6			
		Pectoralis major-clavicular (pectoral) C5-6			
		Biceps (musculocutaneous) C5-6			
		EXTENSION			
		Latissimus dorsi (thoracodorsal) C6-8			
		Teres major (lower subscapular) C5-6			
		Posterior deltoid (axillary) C5-6			
		Triceps-long head (radial) C7-8			
		ABDUCTION			
		Supraspinatus (suprascapular) C5-6			
		Middle deltoid (axillary) C5-6			
		ADDUCTION			
		Latissimus dorsi (thoracodorsal) C6-8			
		Teres major (lower subscapular) C5-6			
		Pectoralis major (pectoral) C5-T1			
		HORIZONTAL ABDUCTION			
		Posterior deltoid (axillary) C5-6			
		HORIZONTAL ADDUCTION			
		Pectoralis major (pectoral) C5-T1			
		Anterior deltoid (axillary) C5-6			
		EXTERNAL ROTATION			
		Infraspinatus (suprascapular) C5-6			
		Teres minor (axillary) C5-6			
		Posterior deltoid (axillary) C5-6			
		INTERNAL ROTATION			
		Subscapularis (upper, lower subscapular) C5-7			
		Teres major (lower subscapular) C6-7			
		Latissimus dorsi (thoracodorsal) C6-8			
		Pectoralis major (pectoral) C5-T1			
		Anterior deltoid (axillary) C5-6			
		ELBOW			
		FLEXION			
		Biceps (musculocutaneous) C5-6			
		Brachioradialis (radial) C5-7			
		Brachialis (musculocutaneous) C5-6 (radial) C7-8			
		EXTENSION			
		Triceps (radial) C6-8			

(continued)

TABLE 4-3
Sample Form for Recording Manual Muscle Strength *(Continued)*

Patient's Name: _____   Age: _____

LEFT			RIGHT	
DATE	**DATE**		**DATE**	**DATE**
		FOREARM		
		PRONATION		
		Pronator teres (median) C6-7		
		Pronator quadratus (median) C8-T1		
		SUPINATION		
		Supinator (radial) C5-6		
		Biceps (musculocutaneous) C5-6		
		WRIST		
		EXTENSION		
		Ext. carpi radialis longus (radial) C6-7		
		Ext. carpi radialis brevis (radial) C7-8		
		Ext. carpi ulnaris (radial) C7-8		
		FLEXION		
		Flexor carpi radialis (median) C6-7		
		Palmaris longus (median) C7-8		
		Flexor carpi ulnaris (ulnar) C8-T1		
		FINGERS		
		DIP FLEXION		
		1st flexor profundus (median) C8-T1		
		2nd flexor profundus (median) C8-T1		
		3rd flexor profundus (ulnar) C8-T1		
		4th flexor profundus (ulnar) C8-T1		
		5TH MP FLEXION		
		Flexor digiti minimi (ulnar) C8-T1		
		PIP FLEXION		
		1st flexor superficialis (median) C7-T1		
		2nd flexor superficialis (median) C7-T1		
		3rd flexor superficialis (median) C7-T1		
		4th flexor superficialis (median) C7-T1		
		ABDUCTION		
		1st palmar interosseus (ulnar) C8-T1		
		2nd palmar interosseus (ulnar) C8-T1		
		3rd palmar interosseus (ulnar) C8-T1		
		ABDUCTION		
		1st dorsal interosseus (ulnar) C8-T1		
		2nd dorsal interosseus (ulnar) C8-T1		
		3rd dorsal interosseus (ulnar) C8-T1		
		4th dorsal interosseus (ulnar) C8-T1		
		MP EXTENSION		
		1st extensor digitorum (radial) C7-8		
		2nd extensor digitorum (radial) C7-8		
		3rd extensor digitorum (radial) C7-8		
		4th extensor digitorum (radial) C7-8		
		Extensor digiti minimi (radial) C7-8		
		IP EXTENSION		
		1st lumbrical (median) C8-T1		
		2nd lumbrical (median) C8-T1		
		3rd lumbrical (ulnar) C8-T1		
		4th lumbrical (ulnar) C8-T1		

(continued)

TABLE 4-3
Sample Form for Recording Manual Muscle Strength *(Continued)*

Patient's Name: _____ Age: _____

DATE	DATE		DATE	DATE
		THUMB		
		EXTENSION		
		Extensor pollicis longus (radial) C7-8		
		Extensor pollicis brevis (radial) C7-8		
		FLEXION		
		Flexor pollicis longus (median) C8-T1		
		Flexor pollicis brevis (median) C8-T1		
		ABDUCTION		
		Abductor pollicis longus (radial) C7-8		
		Abductor pollicis brevis (median) C8-T1		
		ADDUCTOR		
		Adductor pollicis (ulnar) C8-T1		
		OPPOSITION		
		Opponens pollicis (median) C8-T1		
		Opponens digiti minimi (ulnar) C8-T1		
		HIP		
		FLEXION		
		Iliopsoas (femoral) L2-3		
		EXTENSION		
		Gluteus maximus (inf. gluteal) L5-S2		
		KNEE		
		FLEXION		
		Hamstrings (tibial) L5-S2		
		EXTENSION		
		Quadriceps (femoral) L2-4		
		ANKLE		
		DORSIFLEXION		
		Tibialis anterior (deep peroneal) L4-S1		
		Extensor digitorum longus (deep peroneal) L4-S1		
		Extensor hallucis longus (deep peroneal) L4-S1		
		PLANTARFLEXION		
		Gastrocnemius (tibial) S1-2		
		Soleus (tibial) S1-2		

Therapist's signature: _____ Date: _____

Reprinted with permission from Pansky, B. (1996). *Review of Gross Anatomy* (6th ed.). New York: McGraw-Hill.

Measurement of the Proximal Upper Extremity

Scapular Elevation

Prime Movers

> Upper trapezius
>
> Levator scapulae

Against-Gravity Position (Fig. 4-58)

Start Position Patient sitting erect with arms at side.
Stabilize Trunk is stabilized against the plinth or chair back.
Instruction "Lift your shoulders toward your ears. Don't let me push them down."
Resistance The therapist places his or her hands over each acromion and pushes down toward scapular depression. A normal trapezius of an adult cannot be broken.

Substitution A substitution is the use of an alternate muscle or position a patient may use to complete a motion. In this case, it could appear that the patient's shoulders elevated if he or she pushed on the knees with his or her hands.

Gravity-Eliminated Position (Fig. 4-59)

Start Position Prone with arms at side and therapist supporting under the shoulder.
Stabilize The trunk is stabilized against the mat.
Instruction "Lift your shoulder toward your ear."
Palpation The upper trapezius is palpated on the shoulder at the curve of the neck. The levator scapulae is palpated posterior to the sternocleidomastoideus on the lateral side of the neck.

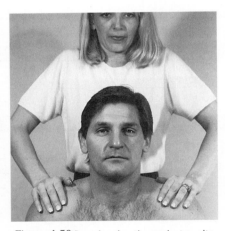

Figure 4-58 Scapular elevation against gravity.

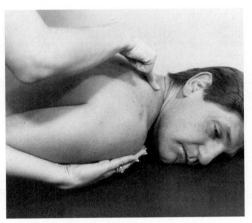

Figure 4-59 Scapular elevation, gravity eliminated.

Scapular Depression

Prime Mover

Lower trapezius.

Latissimus dorsi.

Resistance Test (Fig. 4-60)

Start Position This movement is tested in a gravity-eliminated position, since the patient cannot be positioned to move against gravity. The patient lies prone with arms by the sides.

Stabilize The trunk is stabilized by the mat.

Instruction "Reach your hand down toward your feet."

Resistance The therapist's hand cups the inferior angle of the scapula; the therapist pushes up toward scapular elevation. When the inferior angle is not easily accessible because of tissue bulk, apply resistance at the distal humerus if the shoulder joint is stable and pain free.

Palpation Palpate the lower trapezius lateral to the vertebral column as it passes diagonally from the lower thoracic vertebrae to the spine of the scapula. Palpate the latissimus dorsi along the posterior rib cage or in the posterior axilla as it attaches to the humerus.

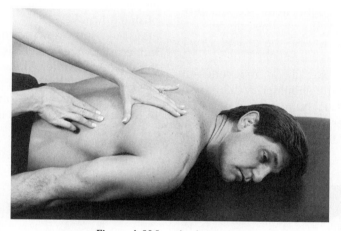

Figure 4-60 Scapular depression.

Scapular Adduction: Retraction

Prime Movers

    Middle trapezius

    Rhomboids

Against-Gravity Position for the Middle Trapezius (Fig. 4-61)

Start Position Prone on a mat with the shoulder abducted to 90° and the elbow flexed to 90°.

Stabilize The trunk is stabilized against the mat. Additional stabilization over the contralateral scapula provides counterpressure during action and resistance.

Instruction "Raise your elbow toward the ceiling. Don't let me push it down."

Resistance Apply resistance laterally at the vertebral border of the scapula or, if the shoulder is stable and pain free, downward at the distal humerus.

Palpation With your hand over the vertebral border of the scapula, feel to see whether the scapula stays adducted during resistance. Palpate the middle trapezius between the vertebral column and vertebral border of the scapula at the level of the spine of the scapula.

Against-Gravity Position for the Rhomboids (Fig. 4-62)

Start Position Prone on the mat with the shoulder internally rotated with the back of the hand resting on the lumbar region.

Stabilize The trunk is stabilized against the mat. Additional stabilization over the contralateral scapula will provide counterpressure during action and resistance.

Instruction "Lift your hand off of your back. Don't let me push it down."

Resistance Apply downward resistance against the distal humerus; if the shoulder is unstable or painful, against the vertebral border of the scapula in the direction of scapular abduction.

Palpation Palpate the rhomboids along the vertebral border of the scapula near the inferior angle.

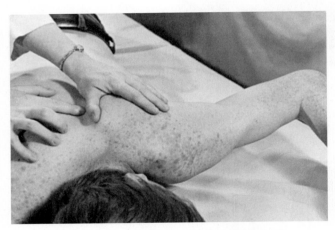

Figure 4-61 Scapular adduction, test for middle trapezius.

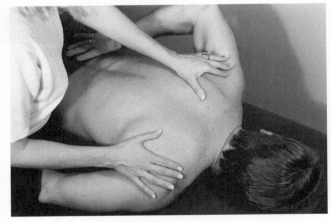

Figure 4-62 Scapular adduction, test for rhomboids.

Gravity-Eliminated Position for the Middle Trapezius and Rhomboids (Fig. 4-63)

Start Position Sitting erect with the humerus abducted to 90° and supported.
Stabilize The trunk is stabilized by the chair.
Instruction "Try to move your arm backward."

Grading If the scapula moves toward the spine, give a grade of 2. If no movement is noted, palpate the scapular adductors.
Palpation Same as previously described.

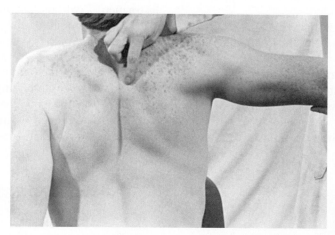

Figure 4-63 Scapular adduction, gravity eliminated. The therapist is pointing to the middle trapezius.

Scapular Abduction: Protraction

Prime Mover

Serratus anterior.

Against-Gravity Position (Fig. 4-64)

Start Position Supine with the humerus flexed to 90°. The elbow may be flexed or extended.

Stabilize The trunk is stabilized on the mat.

Instruction "Reach your arm toward the ceiling."

Resistance According to the rule, resistance should be applied along the axillary border of the scapula. Because it is difficult to apply resistance there, therapists often resist this motion either by grasping the distal humerus or by cupping the hand over the patient's elbow and pushing down or back toward scapular adduction. Of course, this method is not used if the glenohumeral joint is unstable or painful.

Gravity-Eliminated Position (Fig. 4-65)

Start Position Sitting erect with the humerus flexed to 90° and supported.

Stabilize The trunk is stabilized against the chair.

Instruction "Try to reach your arm forward."

Grading Movement of the scapula into abduction receives a grade of 2. If no movement occurs, palpate the serratus anterior.

Palpation Palpate the serratus anterior on the lateral ribs just lateral to the inferior angle of the scapula.

Substitution In the gravity-eliminated position, this motion can be achieved by inching the arm forward on a supportive surface using the finger flexors.

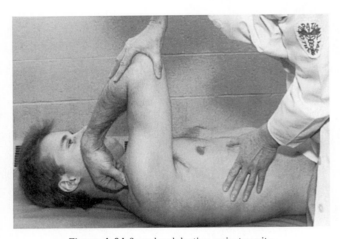

Figure 4-64 Scapular abduction against gravity.

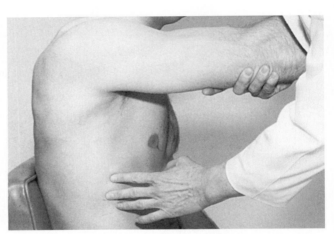

Figure 4-65 Scapular abduction, gravity eliminated.

Shoulder Flexion

Prime Movers

> Anterior deltoid
>
> Coracobrachialis
>
> Pectoralis major, clavicular head
>
> Biceps, both heads

Against-Gravity Position (Fig. 4-66)

Start Position Sitting in a chair with the arm down at the side in midposition.

Stabilize Over the clavicle and the scapula.

Instruction "Lift your arm in front of you to shoulder height. Don't let me push it down."

Resistance The therapist's hand, placed over the distal end of the humerus, pushes down toward extension. Movement above 90° involves scapular rotation; these motions are separated for muscle testing, although they are not separated for ROM measurement.

Substitutions Shoulder abductors, scapular elevation, or trunk extension.

Gravity-Eliminated Position (Fig. 4-67)

Start Position Side-lying with the arm along the side of the body in midposition; therapist supports the arm under the elbow.

Instruction "Try to move your arm so your hand is at the level of your shoulder."

Palpation Palpate the anterior deltoid immediately anterior to the glenohumeral joint. Coracobrachialis may be palpated medially to the tendon of the long head of the biceps, which is palpated on the anterior aspect of the humerus. The clavicular head of the pectoralis major may be palpated below the clavicle on its way to insert on the humerus below the anterior deltoid.

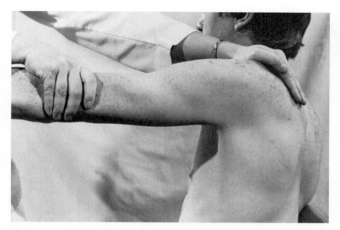

Figure 4-66 Shoulder flexion against gravity.

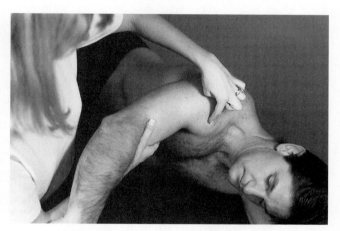

Figure 4-67 Shoulder flexion, gravity eliminated.

Shoulder Extension

Prime Movers

> Latissimus dorsi
>
> Teres major
>
> Posterior deltoid
>
> Triceps, long head

Against-Gravity Position (Fig. 4-68)

Start Position Sitting with the arm by the side and the humerus internally rotated.

Stabilize Over the clavicle and scapula; make sure the patient remains upright.

Instruction "Move your arm straight back as far as it will go. Keep your palm facing the back wall."

Resistance The therapist's hand, placed over the distal end of the humerus, pushes forward toward flexion.

Substitutions Shoulder abductors, tipping the shoulder forward, bending the trunk forward.

Gravity-Eliminated Position (Fig. 4-69)

Start Position: Side-lying with the arm along the side of the body and in internal rotation. Therapist supports the elbow during the motion.

Instruction "Try to move your arm backward."

Palpation The latissimus dorsi and teres major form the posterior border of the axilla. The latissimus dorsi is inferior to the teres major. The posterior deltoid is immediately posterior to the glenohumeral joint. The triceps are palpated on the posterior aspect of the humerus.

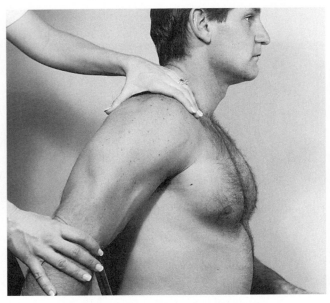

Figure 4-68 Shoulder extension against gravity.

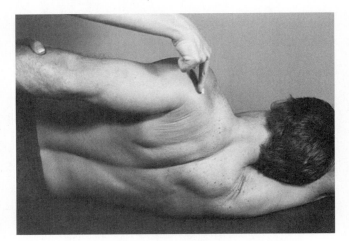

Figure 4-69 Shoulder extention, gravity eliminated.

Shoulder Abduction

Prime Movers

Supraspinatus

Middle deltoid

Against-Gravity Position (Fig. 4-70)

Start Position Sitting erect with the arm down at the side and in midposition.

Stabilize Over the clavicle and the scapula.

Instruction "Raise your arm out to the side to shoulder level. Don't let me push it down."

Resistance The therapist's hand, placed over the distal end of the humerus, pushes the humerus down toward

the body. Movement above 90° involves scapular rotation and is not measured.

Substitutions The long head of the biceps can substitute if the humerus is allowed to move into external rotation; trunk lateral flexion.

Gravity-Eliminated Position (Fig. 4-71)

Start Position Supine with the arm supported at the side in midposition. The therapist supports the elbow during the motion.

Instruction "Try to move your arm out to the side."

Palpation The supraspinatus lies too deep for easy palpation. Palpate the middle deltoid below the acromion and lateral to the glenohumeral joint.

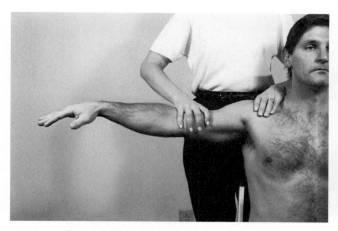

Figure 4-70 Shoulder abduction against gravity.

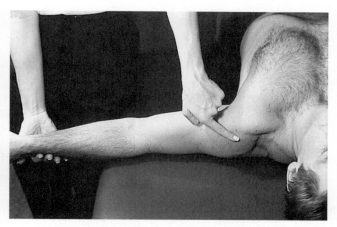

Figure 4-71 Shoulder abduction, gravity eliminated.

Shoulder Adduction

Prime Movers

Pectoralis major

Teres major

Latissimus dorsi

Gravity-Eliminated Position (Fig. 4-72)

The patient cannot be positioned for this motion against gravity.

Start Position Supine with the humerus abducted to 90° and the forearm in midposition.

Stabilize The trunk is stabilized by the mat.

Instruction "Bring your arm down to your side, and don't let me pull it away."

Resistance The therapist's hand, placed on the medial side of the distal end of the humerus, attempts to pull the humerus away from the patient's body.

Palpation The pectoralis major forms the anterior border of the axilla, where it may be easily palpated. Palpation of the teres major and the latissimus dorsi are described earlier in the chapter.

Grading Antigravity grades can only be estimated; a question mark should be entered beside the grade on the form. With experience, the therapist develops the skill to estimate reliably.

Substitutions On a supporting surface, the arm can be inched down using the finger flexors.

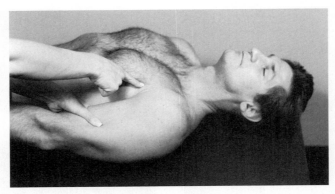

Figure 4-72 Shoulder adduction.

Shoulder Horizontal Abduction

Prime Mover

Posterior deltoid.

Against-Gravity Position (Fig. 4-73)

Start Position Prone with the arm over the edge of the plinth. The shoulder is abducted to 90° and the elbow flexed to 90°.

Stabilize The scapula and trunk are stabilized by the mat. Counterpressure over the contralateral scapula is helpful during action and resistance.

Instruction "Raise your elbow toward the ceiling."

Resistance The therapist's hand, placed on the posterior surface of the distal end of the humerus, pushes the arm down toward horizontal adduction.

Gravity-Eliminated Position (Fig. 4-74)

Start Position Sitting in a chair with the humerus supported in 90° of flexion and the elbow straight. The therapist supports the elbow.

Stabilize The trunk is stabilized against the back of the chair.

Instruction "Try to move your arm out to the side."

Palpation Palpate the posterior deltoid immediately posterior to the glenohumeral joint.

Substitution Trunk rotation.

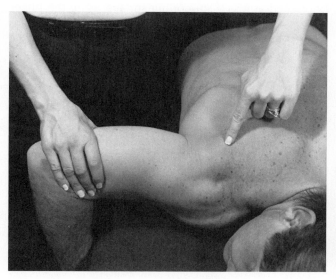

Figure 4-73 Shoulder horizontal abduction against gravity.

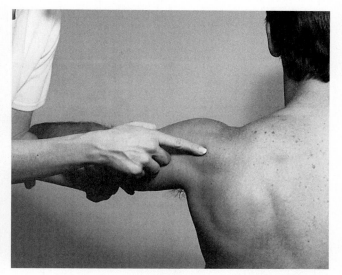

Figure 4-74 Shoulder horizontal abduction, gravity eliminated.

Shoulder Horizontal Adduction

Prime Movers

Pectoralis major

Anterior deltoid

Against-Gravity Position (Fig. 4-75)

Start Position Supine with the humerus abducted to 90° in neutral rotation and the elbow extended.

Stabilize The table stabilizes the scapula and trunk. If the elbow extensors are weak, be sure to support the distal end of the forearm so the hand doesn't fall into the patient's face during horizontal adduction.

Instruction "Move your arm in front of you and across your chest."

Resistance The therapist's hand, placed on the anterior surface of the distal end of the humerus, pulls the arm out toward horizontal abduction.

Gravity-Eliminated Position (Fig. 4-76)

Start Position Sitting in a chair with the arm abducted to 90°.

Stabilize The trunk is stabilized against the back of the chair. The therapist supports the arm under the elbow.

Instruction "Try to bring your arm across your chest."

Palpation Palpate the pectoralis major along the anterior border of the axilla. The anterior deltoid is immediately anterior to the glenohumeral joint below the acromion process and superior to the pectoralis major.

Substitutions Trunk rotation can substitute. The arm can be inched across a supporting surface using the finger flexors.

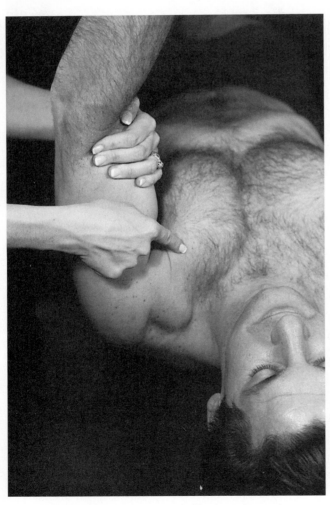

Figure 4-75 Shoulder horizontal adduction against gravity.

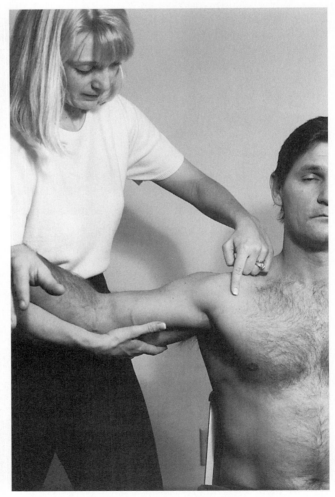

Figure 4-76 Shoulder horizontal adduction, gravity eliminated.

Shoulder External Rotation

Prime Movers

Infraspinatus

Teres minor

Posterior deltoid

Against-Gravity Position (Fig. 4-77)

Start Position Prone with the humerus abducted to 90° and supported by the mat. The elbow is flexed to 90° and is hanging over the edge of the table.

Stabilize The humerus is held just proximal to the elbow to allow only rotation.

Instruction "Lift the back of your hand toward the ceiling."

Resistance The therapist's hand, placed on the dorsal surface of the distal end of the forearm, pushes toward the floor. The therapist's other hand keeps the patient's elbow supported and flexed to 90° to prevent supination.

Substitutions Scapula adduction combined with downward rotation can substitute. The triceps may substitute when resistance is applied.

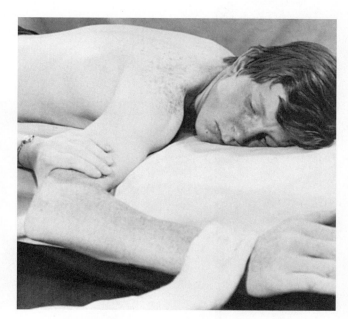

Figure 4-77 Shoulder external rotation against gravity.

Gravity-Eliminated Position (Fig. 4-78)

Start Position Prone with the entire arm hanging over the edge of the mat. The arm is in internal rotation.

Stabilize The trunk and scapula are stabilized on the plinth.

Instruction "Try to turn your palm outward."

Palpation Palpate the infraspinatus inferior to the spine of the scapula. Palpate the teres minor between the posterior deltoid and the axillary border of the scapula; it is superior to the teres major. Palpation of the posterior deltoid was described earlier.

Substitution Supination may be mistaken for external rotation in a gravity-eliminated position.

Alternative Gravity-Eliminated Position (Fig. 4-79)

Start Position Sitting in a chair with the humerus adducted to the side and the elbow flexed to 90°.

Stabilize The distal end of the humerus is held against the body to allow only rotation.

Instruction "Try to move the back of your hand out to the side."

Palpation Same as previously described.

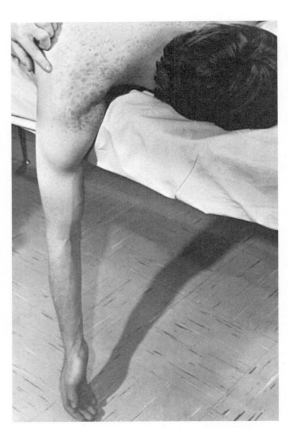

Figure 4-78 Shoulder external rotation, gravity eliminated.

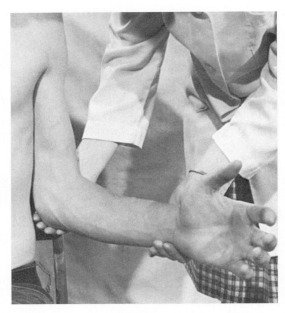

Figure 4-79 Shoulder external rotation, alternative position with gravity eliminated.

Shoulder Internal Rotation

Prime Movers

> Subscapularis
>
> Teres major
>
> Latissimus dorsi
>
> Pectoralis major
>
> Anterior deltoid

Against-Gravity Position (Fig. 4-80)

Start Position Prone with the humerus abducted to 90° and supported by the mat. The elbow is flexed to 90° and hangs over the edge of the mat.

Stabilize The humerus is held just proximal to the elbow to allow only rotation.

Instruction "Lift the palm of your hand toward the ceiling."

Resistance The therapist's hand, placed on the volar surface of the distal end of the forearm, pushes toward the floor. The therapist's other hand keeps the patient's elbow supported and flexed to 90° to prevent supination.

Substitutions Scapular abduction combined with upward rotation can substitute. The triceps can substitute as in external rotation.

Gravity-Eliminated Position (Fig. 4-81)

Start Position Prone with the entire arm hanging over the edge of the mat. The arm is in external rotation.

Stabilize The trunk and scapula are stabilized by the mat.

Instruction "Try to turn your palm inward."

Palpation The subscapularis is not easily palpated but may be found in the posterior axilla. Palpate the teres major, latissimus dorsi, pectoralis major, and anterior deltoid as previously described.

Substitutions Scapular abduction combined with upward rotation can substitute. Pronation may be mis-

taken for internal rotation in a gravity-eliminated position.

Alternative Gravity-Eliminated Position (Fig. 4-82)

Start Position Sitting in a chair with the humerus adducted to the side and the elbow flexed to 90°.

Stabilize The distal end of the humerus is held against the body to allow only rotation.

Instruction "Try to move the palm of your hand in toward your stomach."

Palpation Same as previously described.

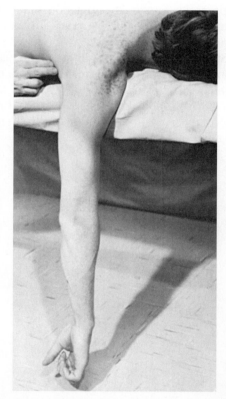

Figure 4-81 Shoulder internal rotation, gravity eliminated.

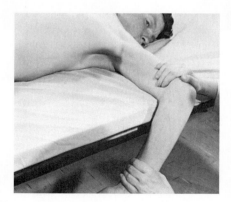

Figure 4-80 Shoulder internal rotation against gravity.

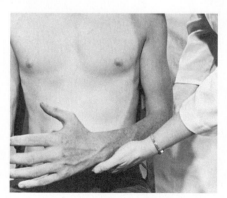

Figure 4-82 Shoulder internal rotation, alternative position with gravity eliminated.

Elbow Flexion

Prime Movers

Biceps

Brachialis

Brachioradialis

Against-Gravity Position (Fig. 4-83)

Start Position Sitting in a chair with the arm at the side. The position of the forearm determines which muscle is working primarily: forearm in supination, biceps brachii; forearm in pronation, brachialis; forearm in midposition, brachioradialis.

Stabilize Stabilize the distal end of the humerus during the action. While applying resistance, provide counter-pressure at the front of the shoulder.

Instruction While the patient is in each of the three forearm positions, say, "Bend your elbow to touch your shoulder and don't let me pull it back down."

Resistance For each of the three positions the therapist's hand is placed on the distal end of the forearm and pulls out toward extension.

Gravity-Eliminated Position (Fig. 4-84)

Start Position Sitting with the arm supported by the therapist in 90° of abduction and elbow extension. The position of the forearm determines which muscle is working, as described earlier.

Stabilize Distal humerus.

Instruction "Try to move your hand toward your shoulder."

Palpation The biceps is easily palpated on the anterior surface of the humerus. With the biceps relaxed and the forearm pronated, palpate the brachialis just medial to the distal biceps tendon. With the forearm in midposition, palpate the brachioradialis along the radial side of the proximal forearm.

Substitution In a gravity-eliminated plane, the wrist flexors may substitute.

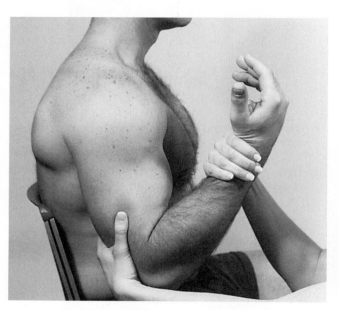

Figure 4-83 Elbow flexion against gravity.

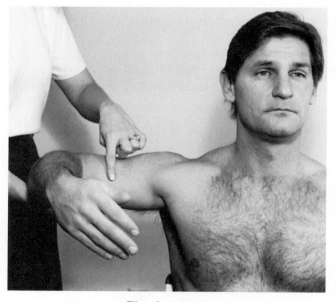

Figure 4-84 Elbow flexion, gravity eliminated.

Elbow Extension

Prime Mover

Triceps

Against-Gravity Position (Fig. 4-85)

Start Position Prone with humerus abducted to 90° and supported on the table. The elbow is flexed and the forearm is hanging over the edge of the table.

Stabilize Support the arm under the anterior surface of the distal humerus.

Instruction "Straighten your arm, and don't let me push it back down."

Resistance Apply resistance with the elbow at 10 to 15° less than full extension so that the elbow does not lock into position, which may indicate greater strength than the patient actually has. The therapist's hand, placed on the dorsal surface of the patient's forearm, pushes toward flexion.

Gravity-Eliminated Position (Fig. 4-86)

Start Position Sitting, with the humerus supported by the therapist in 90° of abduction. The elbow is fully flexed.

Stabilize The humerus is supported and stabilized.

Instruction "Try to straighten your elbow."

Palpation The triceps are easily palpated on the posterior surface of the humerus.

Substitutions In the gravity-eliminated position, no external rotation of the shoulder is permitted, so as to avoid letting the assistance of gravity produce extension. On a supporting surface, finger flexion may be used to inch the forearm across the surface.

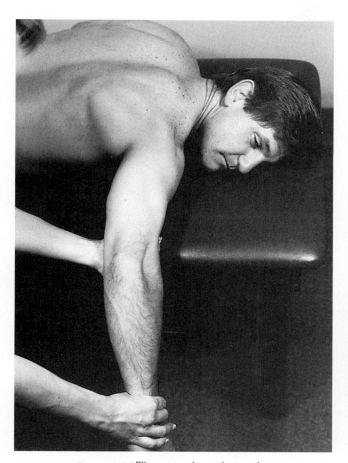

Figure 4-85 Elbow extension against gravity.

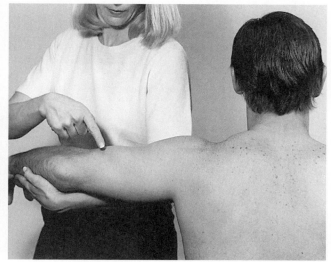

Figure 4-86 Elbow extension, gravity eliminated.

Pronation

Prime Movers

Pronator teres

Pronator quadratus

Against-Gravity Position (Fig. 4-87)

Start Position Sitting with the humerus adducted, elbow flexed to 90° and forearm supinated. The wrist and fingers are relaxed.

Stabilize The distal humerus is stabilized to keep it adducted to the body.

Instruction "Turn your palm to the floor, and don't let me turn it back over."

Resistance The therapist's hand encircles the patient's volar wrist with the therapist's index finger extended along the forearm. The therapist applies resistance in the direction of supination.

Substitutions Shoulder abduction or wrist and finger flexion may substitute.

Gravity-Eliminated Position (Fig. 4-88)

Start Position Sitting with the humerus flexed to 90° and supported. The elbow is flexed to 90° and the forearm is in full supination. The wrist and fingers are relaxed.

Stabilize The humerus is stabilized.

Instruction "Try to turn your palm away from your face."

Palpation The pronator teres is palpated medial to the distal attachment of the biceps tendon on the volar surface of the proximal forearm. Pronator quadratus is too deep to palpate.

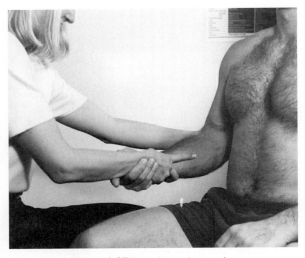

Figure 4-87 Pronation against gravity.

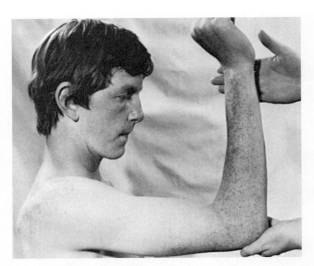

Figure 4-88 Pronation, gravity eliminated.

Supination

Prime Movers

Supinator

Biceps

Against-Gravity Position (Fig. 4-89)

Start Position Sitting with the humerus adducted, elbow flexed to 90° and forearm pronated. The wrist and fingers are relaxed. To differentiate the supinator from the supination function of the biceps, test the supinator with elbow extended. The biceps does not supinate the extended arm unless resisted (Basmajian & DeLuca, 1985).

Stabilize The distal humerus is stabilized.

Instruction "Turn your palm up toward the ceiling, and don't let me turn it back over."

Resistance Same as for pronation except that resistance is in the direction of pronation.

Substitutions The wrist and finger extensors may substitute.

Gravity-Eliminated Position (Fig. 4-90)

Start Position Sitting with the humerus flexed to 90° and supported. The elbow is flexed to 90° and the forearm is in full pronation. The wrist and fingers are relaxed.

Stabilize The humerus is stabilized and supported.

Instruction "Try to turn your palm toward your face."

Palpation The supinator is palpated on the dorsal surface of the proximal forearm just distal to the head of the radius. Palpation of the biceps was described earlier.

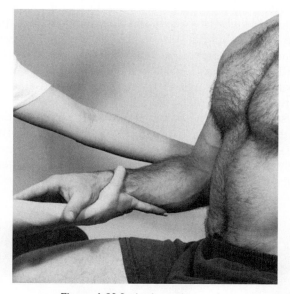

Figure 4-89 Supination against gravity.

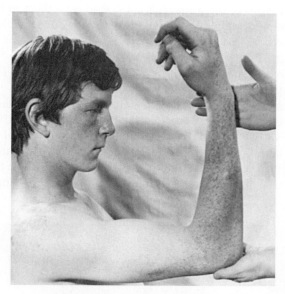

Figure 4-90 Supination, gravity eliminated.

Measurement of the Wrist and Hand

Many tendons of the wrist and hand cross more than one joint. For this reason, test positions for individual muscles must include ways to minimize the effect of other muscles crossing the joint. As a general rule, to minimize the effect of a muscle, place it opposite the prime action. For example, to minimize the effect of the extensor pollicis longus on extension of the proximal joint of the thumb, flex the distal joint.

Wrist Extension

Prime Movers

> Extensor carpi radialis longus (ECRL)
>
> Extensor carpi radialis brevis (ECRB)
>
> Extensor carpi ulnaris (ECU)

Against-Gravity Position (Figs. 4-91 and 4-92)

Start Position The forearm is supported on a table in full pronation with fingers and thumb relaxed or slightly flexed.

Stabilize The forearm is stabilized on the table.

Instruction "Lift your wrist as far as you can, and don't let me push it down."

Resistance To test ECRL, which extends and radially deviates, apply resistance to the dorsum of the hand on the radial side in the direction of flexion and ulnar deviation (Fig. 4-91). To test the ECRB, apply resistance on the dorsum of the hand and push into flexion. To test the ECU, which extends and ulnarly deviates, apply resistance to the dorsum of the hand on the ulnar side and push in the direction of flexion and radial deviation (Fig. 4-92).

Substitutions Extensor pollicis longus, extensor digitorum.

Gravity-Eliminated Position

Start Position The forearm is supported on the table in midposition with the wrist in a slightly flexed position.

Instruction "Try to bend your wrist backward."

Palpation Palpate the tendon of the ECRL on the dorsal surface of the wrist at the base of the second metacarpal. The muscle belly is on the dorsal proximal forearm adjacent to the brachioradialis. Palpate the tendon of the ECRB on the dorsal surface of the wrist at the base of the third metacarpal adjacent to the ECRL. The muscle belly of the ECRB is distal to the belly of the ECRL on the dorsal surface of the proximal forearm. Palpate the ECU on the dorsal surface of the wrist between the head of the ulna and the base of the fifth metacarpal. The muscle belly is approximately 2 inches distal to the lateral epicondyle of the humerus (Lehmkuhl & Smith, 1983).

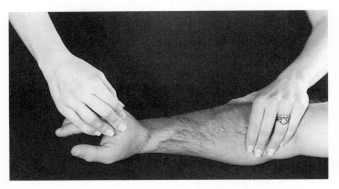

Figure 4-91 Wrist extension. Resistance is being given to the extensor carpi radialis.

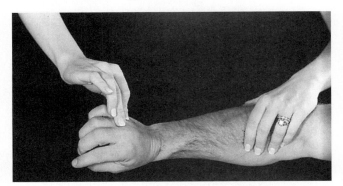

Figure 4-92 Wrist extension. Resistance is being given to the ECU.

Wrist Flexion

Prime Movers

Flexor carpi radialis (FCR)

Palmaris longus

Flexor carpi ulnaris (FCU)

Against-Gravity Position (Figs. 4-93 and 4-94)

Start Position The forearm is supinated, the wrist extended, and fingers and thumb relaxed.

Stabilize The forearm is stabilized on the table with the back of the hand raised off the table to allow the wrist to go into slight extension.

Instruction "Bend your wrist all the way forward, and don't let me push it back."

Resistance To test the FCR and palmaris longus, the therapist applies resistance over the heads of the metacarpals on the volar surface of the hand toward extension. To test for the FCU, the therapist applies resistance over the head of the fifth metacarpal on the volar surface of the hand toward wrist extension and radial deviation.

Substitutions Abductor pollicis longus, flexor pollicis longus, flexor digitorum superficialis, and flexor digitorum profundus.

Gravity-Eliminated Position

Start Position Forearm in midposition, wrist extended, and fingers and thumb relaxed.

Stabilize The forearm rests on the table.

Instruction "Try to bend your wrist forward."

Palpation Palpate the FCR on the volar surface of the wrist in line with the second metacarpal and radial to the palmaris longus (if present) (Fig. 4-93). Palpate the FCU on the volar surface of the wrist just proximal to the pisiform bone (Fig. 4-94). The palmaris longus is a weak wrist flexor. The tendon crosses the center of the volar surface of the wrist (Fig. 4-95). It is not tested for strength and may not even be present. However, if it is present, it will stand out prominently in the middle of the wrist when wrist flexion is resisted or the palm is cupped.

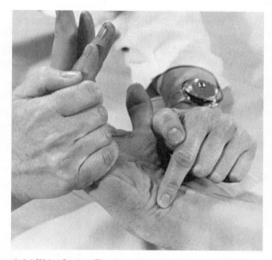

Figure 4-94 Wrist flexion. The therapist is pointing to the FCU tendon as she gives resistance.

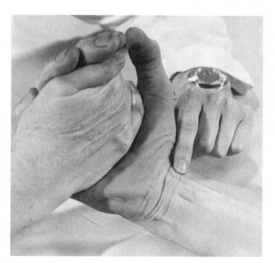

Figure 4-93 Wrist flexion. The therapist is pointing to the flexor carpi radialis longus tendon as she gives resistance.

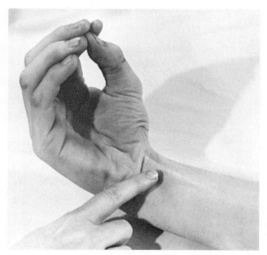

Figure 4-95 The therapist is pointing to the tendon of the palmaris longus as the patient cups his hand in an effort to make this tendon stand out.

Finger MP Extension

Prime Movers

Extensor digitorum (ED)

Extensor indicis proprius

Extensor digiti minimi

Against-Gravity Position (Fig. 4-96)

Start Position The forearm is pronated and supported on the table. The wrist is supported in neutral position and the finger MP and IP joints are in a relaxed flexed posture.

Stabilize Wrist and metacarpals.

Instruction "Lift this knuckle straight as far as it will go [touch the finger that is to be tested]. Keep the rest of your fingers bent. Don't let me push your knuckle down." (Be sure to demonstrate this action.)

Resistance Using one finger, the therapist pushes the head of each proximal phalanx toward flexion, one at a time.

Substitution Apparent extension of the fingers can result from the rebound effect of relaxation following finger flexion. Flexion of the wrist can cause finger extension through **tenodesis** action.

Gravity-Eliminated Position

Start Position Forearm supported in midposition, wrist in neutral position, and fingers flexed.

Stabilize Wrist and metacarpals.

Instruction "Try to move your knuckles back as far as they will go, one at a time. Keep the rest of your fingers bent."

Palpation Palpate the muscle belly of the ED on the dorsal-ulnar surface of the proximal forearm. Often the separate muscle bellies can be discerned. The tendons of this muscle are readily seen and palpated on the dorsum of the hand. The extensor indicis proprius tendon is ulnar to the extensor digitorum tendon. Palpate the belly of this muscle on the mid to distal dorsal forearm between the radius and ulna. Palpate the extensor digiti minimi tendon ulnar to the ED. Actually, it is the tendon that looks as if it were the ED tendon to the little finger, because the ED to the little finger is only a slip from the ED tendon to the ring finger.

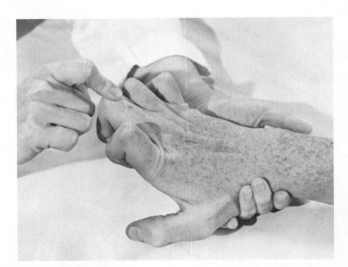

Figure 4-96 Finger metacarpophalangeal extension. The tendons of the extensor digitorum can be seen on the back of the patient's hand.

Finger Interphalangeal Extension

Prime Movers

Lumbricales

Interossei

Extensor digitorum

Extensor indicis proprius

Extensor digiti minimi

According to electromyographic evidence, the intrinsics, especially the lumbricales, are the primary extensors of the interphalangeal joints (Long, 1968; Long & Brown, 1962). Except for the lumbricales and interossei, the other muscles have been discussed. The interossei are discussed under their alternative action of finger abduction and adduction. The lumbricales, arising as they do from the flexor profundus and inserting on the extensor digitorum, have a unique action in regard to finger extension. Contracting against the noncontracting flexor profundus, the lumbricales pull the tendons of the profundus toward the fingertips. This slackens the profundus tendons distal to the insertion of the lumbricales, allowing the extensor digitorum to extend the interphalangeal joints fully, regardless of the position of the MP joints (Landsmeer & Long, 1965; Long, 1968). The interossei flex the MP joints while extending the inter-phalangeal joints and in fact operate to extend only when the MP joints are flexed or flexing (Long, 1968).

Against-Gravity Position for the Lumbricales

There is no reliably good test for lumbrical function. Test 1, following, is traditional. Test 2 is suggested in accordance with electromyographic evidence.

Start Position The forearm is supinated and supported. The wrist is in neutral position. Test 1: MPs are extended with the IPs flexed. Test 2: MPs are flexed with the IPs extended.

Stabilize Metacarpals and wrist.

Instruction Test 1: "Bend your knuckles and straighten your fingers at the same time." (Be sure to demonstrate this movement.) Test 2: "Straighten your knuckles and keep your fingers straight at the same time."

Resistance Test 1. The therapist holds the tip of the finger being tested and pushes it toward the starting position. Test 2. The therapist places one finger on the patient's fingernail and pushes toward flexion (Fig. 4-97).

Substitution Nothing substitutes for DIP extension in the event of the loss of lumbrical function when the MP joint is extended. Other muscles of the dorsal expansion can substitute for DIP extension when the MP joint is flexed.

Palpation Lumbricales lie too deep to be palpated.

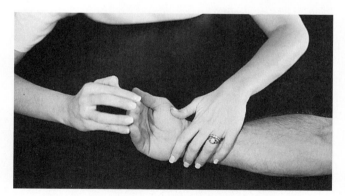

Figure 4-97 Finger interphalangeal extension. Resistance is given to the lumbricales as described for test 2.

Finger DIP Flexion

Prime Mover

Flexor digitorum profundus (FDP)

Against-Gravity Position (Fig. 4-98)

Start Position Forearm supinated and supported on a table; wrist and interphalangeal joints relaxed.

Stabilize Firmly support the middle phalanx of each finger as it is tested to prevent flexion of the proximal interphalangeal joint; wrist should remain in neutral position.

Instruction "Bend the last joint on your finger as far as you can."

Resistance The therapist places one finger on the pad of the patient's finger and applies resistance toward extension.

Substitutions Rebound effect of apparent flexion following contraction of extensors. Wrist extension causes tenodesis action.

Gravity-Eliminated Position

Start Position The forearm is in midposition, resting on the ulnar border on a table. The wrist and interphalangeal joints are relaxed in neutral position.

Stabilize Same as previously described.

Instruction Same as previously described.

Palpation Palpate the belly of the FDP just volar to the ulna in the proximal third of the forearm. The tendons are sometimes palpable on the volar surface of the middle phalanges.

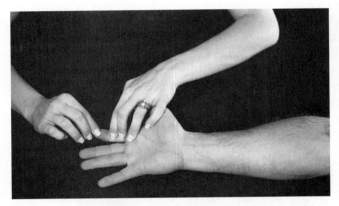

Figure 4-98 Finger distal interphalangeal flexion. The other joints of the finger are prevented from flexing.

Finger PIP Flexion

Prime Movers

Flexor digitorum superficialis (FDS)

Flexor digitorum profundus

Against-Gravity Position for the Flexor Digitorum Superficialis (Fig. 4-99)

Start Position Forearm supinated and supported on the table; wrist and metacarpophalangeal joints relaxed and in zero position. To rule out the influence of the profundus when testing the superficialis, hold all interphalangeal joints of the fingers not being tested in full extension. Because the profundus is essentially one muscle with four tendons, preventing its action in three of the four fingers prevents it from working in the tested finger. In fact, the patient cannot flex the distal joint of the tested finger at all. In some people, the profundus slip to the index finger is such that this method cannot rule out its influence on the PIP joint of the index finger. This should be noted on the test form.

Stabilize All IP joints of the other digits of the hand.

Instruction Point to the PIP joint and say "Bend just this joint."

Resistance Using one finger, the therapist applies resistance to the head of the middle phalanx toward extension.

Substitutions Flexor digitorum profundus. Wrist extension causes tenodesis action.

Gravity-Eliminated Position

Start Position Forearm supported in midposition, with the wrist and MP joints relaxed in neutral position. Again, rule out the influence of the FDP by holding all the joints of the untested fingers in extension.

Stabilize Proximal phalanx of the finger being tested as well as all IP joints of the other digits of the hand.

Instruction Point to the PIP joint and say, "Try to bend just this joint."

Palpation Palpate the superficialis on the volar surface of the proximal forearm toward the ulnar side. Palpate the tendons at the wrist between the palmaris longus and the flexor carpi ulnaris.

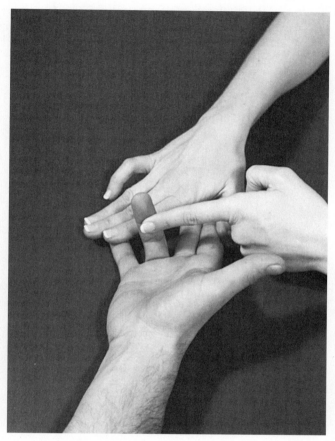

Figure 4-99 Finger proximal interphalangeal flexion. The flexor profundus is prevented from substituting because the therapist is holding in extension all fingers not being tested.

Finger MP Flexion

Prime Movers

  Flexor digitorum profundus

  Flexor digitorum superficialis

  Dorsal interossei

  Volar (palmar) interossei

  Flexor digiti minimi

The tests for the first four muscles are discussed under their alternative actions. The flexor of the little finger has no other action and is described here.

Against-Gravity Position for the Flexor Digiti Minimi (Fig. 4-100)

Start Position Forearm supported in supination.
Stabilize Other fingers in extension.

Instruction "Bend the knuckle of your little finger toward your palm while you keep the rest of the finger straight."
Resistance Using one finger, the therapist pushes the head of the proximal phalanx toward extension. The therapist must be sure the interphalangeal joints remain extended.
Substitutions The flexor digitorum profundus, flexor digitorum superficialis, or third volar interosseus may substitute.

Gravity-Eliminated Position

Start Position Forearm supported in midposition.
Stabilize Other fingers in extension.
Instruction "Try to bend the knuckle of your little finger toward your palm while you keep the rest of the finger straight."
Palpation The flexor digiti minimi is found on the volar surface of the hypothenar eminence.

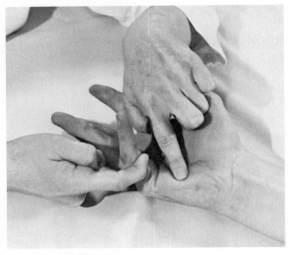

Figure 4-100 Flexor digiti minimi. The therapist is pointing to the muscle belly.

Finger Abduction

Prime Movers

Dorsal interossei (4)

Abductor digiti minimi

Gravity-Eliminated Position (Fig. 4-101)

Start Position The pronated forearm is supported with the wrist neutral. The fingers are extended and adducted. Be sure the MP joints are in neutral or slight flexion.

Stabilize The wrist and metacarpals are gently supported.

Instruction "Spread your fingers apart, and don't let me push them back together."

Action Because the midline of the hand is the third finger and abduction is movement away from midline, the action of each finger is different. It is important to know which dorsal interossei (DAB) you are testing. The first dorsal interosseus (DAB 1) abducts the index finger toward the thumb. The DAB 2 abducts the middle finger toward the thumb. The DAB 3 abducts the middle finger toward the little finger. The DAB 4 abducts the ring finger toward the little finger. The abductor digiti minimi abducts the little finger ulnarly.

Resistance Using the thumb and index finger to form a pincer, the therapist applies resistance at the radial or ulnar side of the head of the proximal phalanx in an attempt to push the finger toward midline. Applying resistance to the radial side of the heads of the index and middle finger tests DABs 1 and 2. Applying resistance to the ulnar side of the middle, ring, and little fingers tests DABs 3 and 4 and the abductor digiti minimi.

Substitutions Extensor digitorum.

Grading Normal finger abductors do not tolerate much resistance. If the fingers give way to resistance but spring back when the resistance is removed, the grade is 5. The grade is 4 if the muscle takes some resistance. The grade is 3 when there is full AROM. The grade is 2 if there is partial AROM. The grade is 1 when contraction is felt with palpation. The grade is 0 when no contractile activity is palpable.

Palpation DAB 1 fills the dorsal web space and is easy to palpate there. Palpate the abductor digiti minimi on the ulnar border of the fifth metacarpal. The other interossei lie between the metacarpals on the dorsal aspect of the hand, where they may be palpated; on some people, the tendons can be palpated as they enter the dorsal expansion near the heads of the metacarpals. When the DABs are atrophied, the spaces between the metacarpals on the dorsal surface appear sunken.

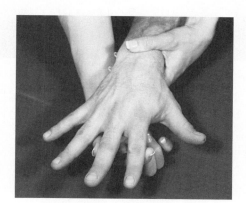

Figure 4-101 Finger abduction.

Finger Adduction

Prime Movers

Volar (palmar) interossei (3).

Gravity-Eliminated Position (Fig. 4-102)

Start Position The forearm is pronated and the MPs are abducted and in extension.

Stabilize Both of the therapist's hands are needed for resistance. The forearm and wrist can be supported on a table.

Instruction "Bring your fingers together and hold them. Don't let me pull them apart."

Action Because the midline of the hand is the third finger and adduction is movement toward midline, the action of each finger is different. Palmar interosseus (PAD) 1 adducts the index finger toward the middle finger. PAD 2 adducts the ring finger toward the middle finger. PAD 3 adducts the little finger toward the middle finger.

Resistance The therapist holds the heads of the proximal phalanx of two adjoining fingers and applies resistance in the direction of abduction to pull the fingers apart. For the index and middle finger pair, PAD 1 is tested. For the middle and ring finger pair, PAD 2 is tested. For the ring and little finger pair, PAD 3 is tested.

Substitutions Extrinsic finger flexors.

Grading Same as with the finger abductors.

Palpation The palmar interossei are usually too deep to palpate with certainty. When these muscles are atrophied, the areas between the metacarpals on the volar surface appear sunken.

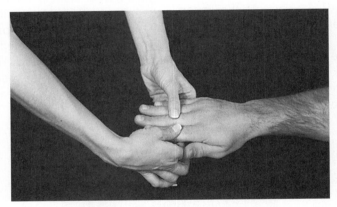

Figure 4-102 Finger adduction.

Thumb IP Extension

Prime Mover

Extensor pollicis longus (EPL)

Against-Gravity Position (Fig. 4-103)

Start Position Forearm supported in midposition, wrist flexion of 10 to 20° and thumb MP and IP flexion.
Instruction "Straighten the end of your thumb."
Stabilize Proximal phalanx into MP flexion.
Resistance The therapist places one finger over the dorsum of the distal phalanx (thumbnail) and pushes only the DIP toward flexion.
Substitutions Relaxation of the flexor pollicis longus produces apparent extensor movement as a result of rebound effect. Because the abductor pollicis brevis, adductor pollicis, and flexor pollicis brevis insert into the lateral aspects of the dorsal expansion, they may produce thumb IP extension when the extensor pollicis longus is paralyzed. To prevent this, the position of maximal flexion of the carpometacarpal and MP joints, wrist flexion of 10° to 20°, and full forearm supination are used to put these synergists in a shortened, disadvantaged position while testing the EPL (Howell et al., 1989).

Gravity-Eliminated Position

Start Position Forearm supinated, thumb flexed.
Instruction "Try to straighten the end of your thumb."
Palpation The tendon of the EPL may be palpated on the ulnar border of the anatomical snuffbox and on the dorsal surface of the proximal phalanx of the thumb.

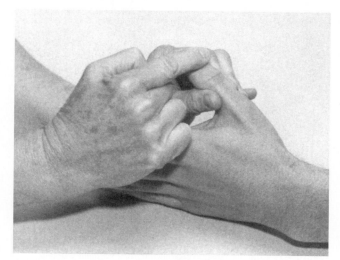

Figure 4-103 The therapist is resisting the extensor pollicis longus, whose tendon is prominent.

Thumb MP Extension

Prime Movers

Extensor pollicis brevis (EPB)

Extensor pollicis longus

Against-Gravity Position for the Extensor Pollicis Brevis (Fig. 4-104)

Start Position Forearm supported in midposition, MP and IP joints flexed.

Stabilize Firmly support the first metacarpal in abduction.

Instruction "Straighten the knuckle of your thumb while keeping the end joint bent." You may have to move the thumb passively a few times for the patient to get the kinesthetic input regarding the movement.

Resistance The therapist's index finger, placed on the dorsal surface of the head of the proximal phalanx, pushes toward flexion.

Substitution Extensor pollicis longus.

Gravity-Eliminated Position

Start Position Forearm supinated, MP and IP joints flexed.

Stabilize First metacarpal in abduction.

Instruction "Try to straighten the knuckle of your thumb while keeping the end joint bent."

Palpation Palpate the tendon of the EPB on the radial border of the anatomical snuffbox medial to the tendon of the abductor pollicis longus. The EPB may not be present.

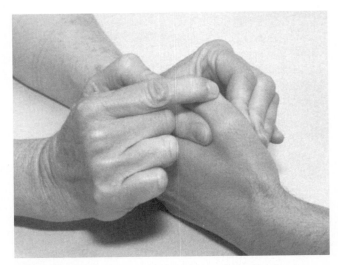

Figure 4-104 The therapist is resisting the extensor pollicis brevis, whose tendon can be seen.

Thumb Abduction

Prime Movers

Abductor pollicis longus

Abductor pollicis brevis

Against-Gravity Position for the Abductor Pollicis Longus (Fig. 4-105)

Start Position Forearm supinated, wrist in neutral position, thumb adducted.

Stabilize Support the wrist on the ulnar side and hold it in neutral position.

Instruction "Bring your thumb away from your palm. Don't let me push it back in."

Action Patient abducts the thumb halfway between thumb extension and palmar abduction. The therapist may have to demonstrate this action while giving the instructions.

Resistance The therapist's finger presses the head of the first metacarpal toward adduction.

Substitutions Abductor pollicis brevis, extensor pollicis brevis.

Gravity-Eliminated Position

Start Position Forearm in midposition, wrist in neutral position, thumb adducted.

Stabilize Support the wrist on the ulnar side and hold it in neutral position.

Instruction "Try to bring your thumb away from your palm."

Palpation Palpate the tendon of the abductor pollicis longus at the wrist joint just distal to the radial styloid and lateral to the EPB.

Against-Gravity Position for the Abductor Pollicis Brevis (Fig. 4-106)

Start Position Forearm is supported in supination, wrist in neutral position, thumb adducted.

Stabilize Support the wrist in neutral position by holding it on the dorsal and ulnar side.

Instruction "Lift your thumb directly out of the palm of the hand. Don't let me push it back in."

Resistance The therapist's finger presses the head of the first metacarpal toward adduction.

Substitution Abductor pollicis longus.

Gravity-Eliminated Position

Start Position Forearm is supported in midposition, wrist in neutral position, thumb adducted.

Stabilize Support the wrist in neutral position by holding it on the dorsal and ulnar side.

Instruction "Try to move your thumb away from the palm of your hand."

Palpation Palpate the abductor pollicis brevis over the center of the thenar eminence.

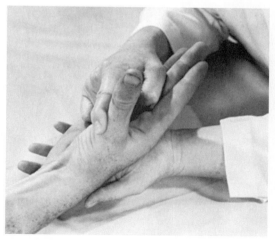

Figure 4-105 The therapist is resisting the abductor pollicis longus, which moves the thumb away from the palm halfway between extension and palmar abduction.

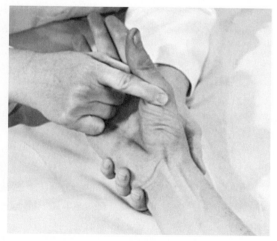

Figure 4-106 The therapist is resisting the abductor pollicis brevis, which moves the thumb directly up from the palm of the hand (palmar abduction).

Thumb IP Flexion

Prime Mover

Flexor pollicis longus

Against-Gravity Position (Fig. 4-107)

Start Position Elbow flexed and supported on a table. Forearm supinated so that the palmar surface of the thumb faces the ceiling; thumb extended at the MP and IP joints.
Stabilize Proximal phalanx, holding MP joint in extension.
Instruction "Bend the tip of your thumb as far as you can, and don't let me straighten it."

Resistance The therapist's finger pushes the head of the distal phalanx toward extension.
Substitution Relaxation of the extensor pollicis longus causes apparent rebound movement.

Gravity-Eliminated Position

Start Position Forearm supinated to 90° so that the thumb can flex across the palm.
Stabilize Proximal phalanx, holding MP joint in extension.
Instruction "Try to bend the tip of your thumb as far as you can."
Palpation Palpate the flexor pollicis longus on the palmar surface of the proximal phalanx.

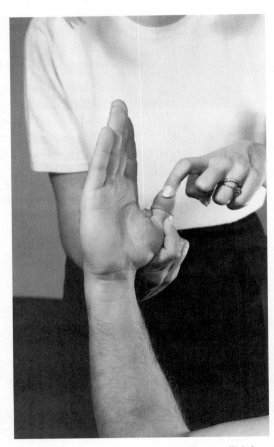

Figure 4-107 The therapist is resisting the flexor pollicis longus.

Thumb MP Flexion

Prime Movers

Flexor pollicis brevis

Flexor pollicis longus

Against-Gravity Position for the Flexor Pollicis Brevis (Fig. 4-108)

Start Position Elbow flexed and supported on the table. Forearm supinated so that the palmar surface of the thumb faces the ceiling; thumb is extended at both the MP and IP joints.

Stabilize Firmly support the first metacarpal.

Instruction "Bend your thumb across your palm, keeping the end joint of your thumb straight. Don't let me pull it back out."

Resistance The therapist's finger pushes the head of the proximal phalanx toward extension.

Substitution Flexor pollicis longus; the abductor pollicis brevis and the adductor pollicis through insertion into the extensor hood. To rule out the effect of the flexor pollicis longus when testing the flexor pollicis brevis, a test position of maximal elbow flexion, maximal pronation, and maximal wrist flexion has been recommended (Howell et al., 1989).

Gravity-Eliminated Position

Start Position Forearm supinated to 90° so that the thumb can flex across the palm.

Stabilize First metacarpal.

Instruction "Try to bend your thumb into your palm, keeping the end joint of your thumb straight."

Palpation Palpate the flexor pollicis brevis on the thenar eminence just proximal to the MP joint and medial to the abductor pollicis brevis.

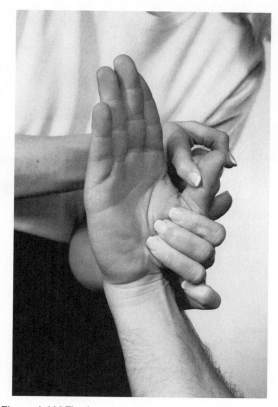

Figure 4-108 The therapist is resisting the flexor pollicis brevis.

Thumb Adduction

Prime Mover

Adductor pollicis

Against-Gravity Position (Fig. 4-109)

Start Position Forearm pronated, wrist and fingers in neutral position, thumb abducted, and MP and IP joints of the thumb in extension.
Stabilize Metacarpals of fingers, keeping the MP joints in neutral.
Instruction "Lift your thumb into the palm of your hand, and don't let me pull it out."

Resistance The therapist grasps the head of the proximal phalanx and tries to pull it away from the palm toward abduction.
Substitutions The extensor pollicis longus, flexor pollicis longus, or flexor pollicis brevis may substitute.

Gravity-Eliminated Position

Start Position Same except forearm in midposition.
Stabilize Metacarpals of fingers, keeping the MP joints in neutral.
Instruction "Try to bring your thumb into the palm of your hand."
Palpation Palpate the adductor pollicis on the palmar surface of the thumb web space.

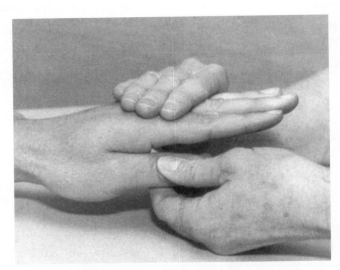

Figure 4-109 The therapist is resisting the adductor pollicis.

Opposition

Prime Movers

Opponens pollicis

Opponens digiti minimi

Against-Gravity Position (Fig. 4-110)

Start Position Forearm supinated and supported, wrist in neutral position, thumb adducted and extended.

Stabilize Hold the wrist in a neutral position.

Instruction "Touch the pad of your thumb to the pad of your little finger. Don't let me pull them apart."

Resistance The therapist holds along the first metacarpal and derotates the thumb or holds along the fifth metacarpal and derotates the little finger. These can be resisted simultaneously using both hands.

Substitutions The abductor pollicis brevis, flexor pollicis brevis, or flexor pollicis longus may substitute.

Gravity-Eliminated Position

Start Position Elbow resting on the table with forearm perpendicular to the table, wrist in neutral position, thumb adducted and extended.

Stabilize Hold the wrist in a neutral position.

Instruction "Try to touch the pad of your thumb to the pad of your little finger."

Palpation Place fingertips along the lateral side of the shaft of the first metacarpal where the opponens pollicis may be palpated before it becomes deep to the abductor pollicis brevis. The opponens digiti minimi can be palpated volarly along the shaft of the fifth metacarpal.

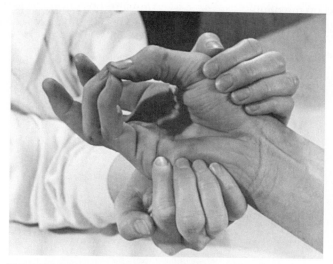

Figure 4-110 The therapist is resisting both the opponens pollicis and the opponens digiti minimi.

Measurement of Selected Lower Extremity Muscle Groups

Muscle testing of the flexors and extensors of the three major joints of the lower extremity are described here because of their importance to functions required for completion of certain activities of daily living, such as climbing stairs and curbs, dressing, bathing, sitting, standing, and transferring. Only against-gravity testing is described. Muscles weaker than 3 (fair) are too weak for functional activities in occupational therapy, and in these cases adaptive methods of doing activities of daily living are the most efficient therapeutic intervention.

Hip Flexion

Prime Mover

> Iliopsoas:
>
>> Iliacus
>>
>> Psoas major

Against-Gravity Start Position Sitting on the plinth with lower leg hanging down.
Stabilize The pelvis is stabilized on the plinth.

Instruction "Lift your knee toward the ceiling, keeping your knee bent. Don't let me push your leg back down."
Resistance The therapist presses the distal anterior thigh down toward extension (Fig. 4-111).
Palpation The iliacus is too deep to be palpated. With the patient sitting, the psoas major can be palpated if the patient bends forward and relaxes the abdominal muscles. The therapist's fingers lie at the waist between the ribs and the iliac crest, and the therapist applies pressure posteriorly to feel the contraction of the psoas major as the hip flexes (Lehmkuhl & Smith, 1983).

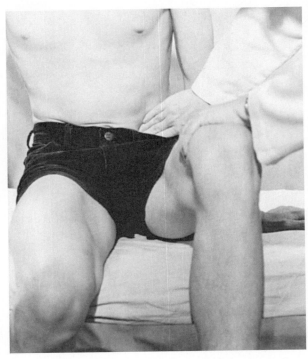

Figure 4-111 The therapist is attempting to palpate the psoas major while resisting hip flexion.

Hip Extension

Prime Movers

Gluteus maximus

Biceps femoris

Against-Gravity Start Position for the Gluteus Maximus The patient lies prone with the knee flexed to 90° or more (Daniels & Worthingham, 1986).

Stabilize The pelvis and lumbar spine are stabilized on the plinth.

Instruction "Lift your leg off the table as high as you can. Keep your knee bent."

Resistance The therapist presses the distal posterior thigh down toward flexion (Fig. 4-112).

Palpation The gluteus maximus, the large muscle of the buttocks, can be easily palpated.

Substitutions Extension of the lumbar spine. The other hamstrings, the semimembranosus and the semitendino-sus, assist resisted hip extension if the hip is abducted (Basmajian & DeLuca, 1985).

Start Position for Combined Gluteus Maximus and Biceps Femoris Action The patient lies supine with the leg to be tested in full extension and holds the other leg in flexion at the hip and knee (Diekmeyer, 1978).

Stabilize The pelvis and lumbar spine are stabilized by the plinth.

Instruction "Do not let me lift your leg off the plinth."

Resistance The therapist holds the thigh just above the knee and attempts to raise the leg off the plinth (Fig. 4-113).

Grading Hip extension is graded 5 (normal) if the trunk rather than the leg comes up off the plinth and a 3 (fair) if the hip gives as the trunk begins to come up off the table.

Palpation Palpate the biceps femoris on the posterior aspect of the thigh; its tendon bounds the popliteal fossa laterally (Basmajian & DeLuca, 1985).

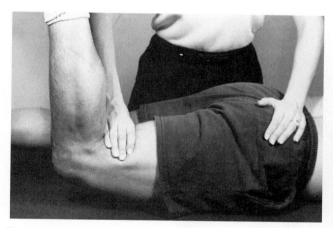

Figure 4-112 The therapist is resisting hip extension with the knee flexed to test the gluteus maximus.

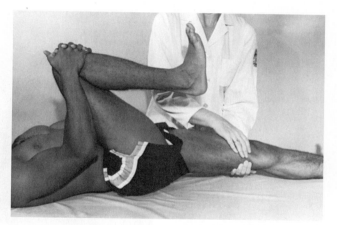

Figure 4-113 During testing of the gluteus maximus and the biceps femoris together, the patient lies supine and holds the hip and knee of the untested leg flexed. The therapist tries to lift the extended leg off the plinth.

Knee Flexion

Prime Movers

Hamstrings:

Semimembranosus

Semitendinosus

Biceps femoris

Against-Gravity Start Position The patient lies prone with both hips and knees extended.

Stabilize The thigh is stabilized against the plinth.

Instruction "Bend your knee. Hold it. Don't let me push it back to the plinth."

Resistance The therapist's hand, placed on the distal end of the posterior surface of the tibia, pushes toward extension. If resistance is applied to one side, medially or laterally, either the lateral or medial hamstrings will contract more strongly (Fig. 4-114).

Grading In deciding between a 3– and 3 grade, the therapist must make an educated guess unless the patient can stand up and demonstrate knee flexion to 120°, that is, full flexion, against gravity.

Palpation Palpate these three muscles on the posterior surface of the thigh. Palpate the tendon of the biceps femoris on the lateral side of the popliteal space and the tendon of the semitendinosus on the medial side of the popliteal space. Both tendons become prominent when resistance is applied (Lehmkuhl & Smith, 1983). Isolate the biceps femoris from the other muscles by rotating the lower leg externally with respect to the femur. The semitendinosus contracts more prominently if the lower leg is rotated internally with respect to the femur. The semimembranosus lies deep to the semitendinosus, but its lower portion is palpable on both sides of the semitendinosus tendon.

Substitutions When the patient is prone, gravity assists flexion beyond 90°. When the patient is sitting, gravity can flex the knee.

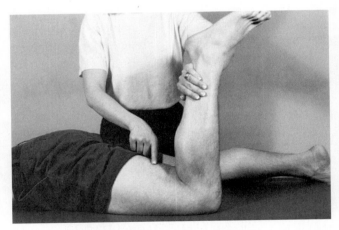

Figure 4-114 Knee flexion against gravity.

Knee Extension

Prime Movers

Quadriceps:

Rectus femoris

Vastus medialis

Vastus intermedius

Vastus lateralis

Against-Gravity Start Position The patient sits on the plinth with the knee flexed and lower leg hanging down.
Stabilize The thigh is stabilized on the plinth.
Instruction "Straighten your knee. Don't let me bend it."
Resistance After the patient achieves full extension, the knee is flexed approximately 10 to 15° before resistance is applied. The therapist's hand is placed at the distal end of the anterior surface of the tibia (Fig. 4-115). Resistance is applied slowly to build up to the patient's maximum to avoid injury to the knee. ***Applying sudden or excessive resistance can injure the knee***. It is almost impossible to break a normal quadriceps (Hines, 1965).
Palpation Palpate the tendon of the quadriceps as it approaches the patella. Except for the vastus intermedius, the muscle bellies can be palpated on the anterior surface of the thigh: The rectus femoris is in the center and lies over the vastus intermedius. Palpate the other vasti medially and laterally to the rectus femoris.
Substitutions None.

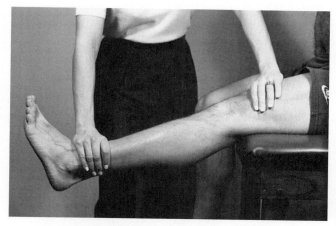

Figure 4-115 Knee extension against gravity.

Ankle Dorsiflexion

Prime Movers

Tibialis anterior

Extensor hallucis longus

Extensor digitorum longus

Against-Gravity Start Position The patient sits on the plinth with the lower leg hanging down. The foot is perpendicular to the lower leg.

Stabilize Lower leg just proximal to the ankle.

Instruction "Lift your foot up so your toes point to the ceiling."

Resistance The therapist's hand lies on the forefoot and pushes toward plantar flexion without allowing the foot to invert or evert (Fig. 4-116).

Palpation Palpate the belly of the tibialis anterior immediately lateral to the shaft of the tibia. Palpate its large tendon on the anterior surface of the ankle, medial to the tendon of the extensor hallucis longus. Palpate the latter in the middle of the anterior surface of the ankle. The extensor digitorum longus tendon is prominent on the lateral side of the anterior aspect of the ankle. The tendons of the extensor hallucis longus and extensor digitorum longus can be traced to their insertions on the toes.

Substitutions None.

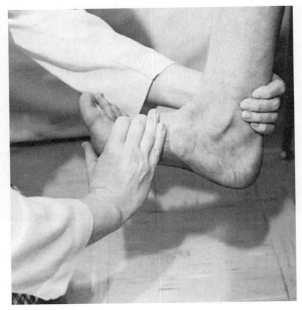

Figure 4-116 Ankle dorsiflexion against gravity.

Ankle Plantar Flexion

Prime Movers

Gastrocnemius

Soleus

Against-Gravity Start Position There are two ways to test plantar flexion: (1) The patient stands. (2) The patient who cannot stand lies prone on the plinth with the foot off the end of the plinth.

Stabilize In the standing test, the patient may have to hold onto something for balance. In the prone test, stabilize the lower leg just above the ankle.

Instruction (1) "Stand on your tiptoes. Do it 20 times." (2) "Press down with your foot as if you were pressing on the gas pedal of a car. Don't let me push it back."

Resistance In the standing test, the full body weight resists these muscles (Fig. 4-117). In the prone test, the therapist applies manual resistance against the distal portion of the foot and pushes the foot toward dorsiflexion (Fig. 4-118).

Grading According to Hislop and Montgomery (1995), the grade is 5 (normal) if the patient completes 20 heel raises through full ROM without rest or fatigue. Other therapists grade 5 if the person can go up on tiptoes and maintain the position longer than momentarily. Hislop and Mont-

gomery grade 4 (good) if the patient completes 10 to 19 heel raises through full ROM without rest or fatigue. The grade is 3 (fair) if 1 to 9 heel raises are completed correctly without rest or fatigue. If the patient is unable to complete full ROM in any one repetition, the grade drops automatically to the next lower level. If the patient cannot complete one heel raise, the grade must be less than 3 and the patient is tested prone. In the prone test, the grade is 2+ (poor plus) if the patient can complete full range and hold against maximal resistance. If the patient completes full range but cannot take any resistance, the grade is 2 (poor).

Palpation The soleus is palpable at the distal portion of the lower leg. The gastrocnemius is the superficial muscle of the calf; the two heads can be palpated at their origin on either side of the posterior femur. The Achilles tendon is the insertion of both the soleus and gastrocnemius and is readily palpable at the back of the ankle. To minimize the influence of the gastrocnemius when testing for the soleus, the patient lies prone with the knee flexed. Slight resistance is applied to plantar flexion (Lehmkuhl & Smith, 1983).

Substitutions Gravity substitutes when the person is lying supine or is sitting with feet off the supporting surface. The extrinsic toe flexors substitute weakly.

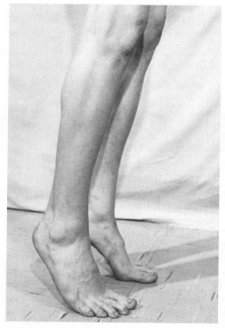

Figure 4-117 Ability to stand on tiptoe indicates grade 5 ankle plantar flexion.

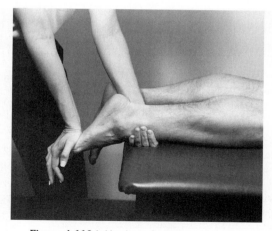

Figure 4-118 Ankle plantarflexion against gravity.

Interpreting the Muscle Test

After recording all muscle test scores, the therapist reviews the scores and looks for the weak muscles and the distribution and significance of the weakness. Any muscle that grades good minus (4–) or below is considered weak. Good plus (4+) muscles are functional and usually require no therapy. Good (4) muscles may or may not be functionally adequate for the patient, depending on his or her occupational task requirements. The pattern of muscle weakness is important. The pattern may indicate general weakness caused by disuse secondary to immobilization, or it may reflect the level of spinal innervation in a patient after spinal cord injury or the distribution of a peripheral nerve in the case of peripheral nerve injury. A pattern of imbalance of forces in agonist and antagonist muscles may be deforming; therefore, counterpositioning or splinting should be considered along with strengthening of the weak muscles.

The pattern of significant strengths is also important. For example, a muscle test of a patient with injured spinal cord that indicates some strength in a muscle innervated by a segment below the diagnosed level of injury is hopeful for more recovery. Or, because muscles are reinnervated proximally to distally after peripheral nerve injury, findings showing beginning return of strength in particular muscles help to track the progress of nerve regeneration.

Short-term goals move the patient from the level of strength determined by testing to the next higher level; for example, if a muscle grades 3, the short-term goal is to improve strength to 3+; if it grades 3+, the goal is to increase strength to 4–, and so on. The required strength for occupational function must always be kept in mind when establishing goals.

If the muscle test is a reevaluation, the scores are compared with those of the previous test. The frequency of reevaluation depends on the nature of expected recovery. Expected rapid recovery requires frequent reevaluation. If the repeated muscle test shows that the patient is making gains, the program is considered beneficial and its demands are upgraded. If repeated muscle tests show no gains despite program adaptations, the patient is considered to have reached a plateau and no longer to benefit from remedial therapy. In that case, the focus of treatment shifts to teaching the patient compensatory strategies to enable participation in desired tasks and activities.

Patients with degenerative diseases are expected to get weaker; therefore, therapy is aimed at maintaining their strength and function for as long as possible. Repeated muscle tests confirm that effect of therapy. A plateau for these patients is desirable; it indicates that the therapy is effective for maintaining strength and should be continued.

Measurement of Grasp and Pinch Strength

Therapists supplement manual strength testing with dynamometric evaluations of grip and pinch strength that are valid and reliable (Mathiowetz, 1991; Mathiowetz et al., 1984) and for which norms have been established (Mathiowetz et al., 1985). Abbreviated versions of the norms are listed in Tables 4-4 and 4-5.

As with any tool of measurement, the instrument must be **calibrated** and set at 0 to start. Dynamometers and pinch meters can be calibrated by placing known weights on or suspending them from the compression

---

TABLE 4-4
Jamar Grasp Dynamometer Norms in Pounds: Mean of Three Trials

	Norms at Age	20	25	30	35	40	45	50	55	60	65	70	75+
Men	Right	121	121	122	120	117	110	114	101	90	91	75	66
	SD	21	23	22	24	21	23	18	27	20	21	21	21
	Left	104	110	110	113	113	101	102	83	77	77	65	55
	SD	22	16	22	22	19	23	17	23	20	20	18	17
Women	Right	70	74	79	74	70	62	66	57	55	50	50	43
	SD	14	14	19	11	13	15	12	12	10	10	12	11
	Left	61	63	68	66	62	56	57	47	46	41	41	38
	SD	13	12	18	12	14	13	11	12	10	8	10	9

N = 628; age range = 20–94.
Reprinted with permission from Mathiowetz, V., Kashman, N., Volland, G., Weber, K., Dowe, M., & Rogers, S. (1985). Grip and pinch strength: Normative data for adults. *Archives of Physical Medicine and Rehabilitation, 66*(2), 69–74.

TABLE 4-5
B&L Pinch Meter in Pounds: Mean of Three Trials

		Norms at Age	20	30	40	50	60	70	75+
Tip	Men	Right	18	18	18	18	16	14	14
		Left	17	18	18	18	15	13	14
	Women	Right	11	13	11	12	10	10	10
		Left	10	12	11	11	10	10	9
Lateral	Men	Right	26	26	26	27	23	19	20
		Left	25	26	25	26	22	19	19
	Women	Right	18	19	17	17	15	14	13
		Left	16	18	16	16	14	14	11
Palmar	Men	Right	27	25	24	24	22	18	19
		Left	26	25	25	24	21	19	18
	Women	Right	17	19	17	17	15	14	12
		Left	16	18	17	16	14	14	12

Tip pinch average standard deviation (SD): Men, 4.0; Women, 2.5.
Lateral pinch average SD: Men, 4.6; Women, 3.0.
Palmar pinch average SD: Men, 5.1; Women, 3.7.
N = 628; age range = 20–94.
Reprinted with permission from Mathiowetz, V., Kashman, N., Volland, G., Weber, K., Dowe, M., & Rogers, S. (1985). Grip and pinch strength: Normative data for adults. *Archives of Physical Medicine and Rehabilitation*, 66(2), 69–74.

part of the meter (Fess, 1987). With this procedure, the Jamar dynamometer, designed by Bechtol (1954), was found to be accurate to within ±5%, and the B & L pinch meter to within ±1% (Mathiowetz, 1990; Mathiowetz et al., 1984).

The standard method of measurement used in the study from which the norms were established reflects the recommendations of the American Society of Hand Therapists (1981). Test–retest (1 week) reliability of this method using the Jamar hydraulic dynamometer was found to be .88; interrater reliability (two raters, same time) was .99. Interrater (two raters, same time) reliability of averaged B & L pinch meter scores was .98; test–retest (1 week) reliability was .81 (Mathiowetz et al., 1984).

Flood-Joy and Mathiowetz (1987) reported significant discrepancies among three different models of the Jamar hydraulic grasp meter. For this reason, it is essential that the exact same dynamometer be used when reevaluating gains as during the initial evaluation. Until the normative study is replicated, the data in Table 4-4 can be used with confidence if you use model 6420, the one used in the study, which can be recognized by its off-center calibration screw. However the scores of patients older than 50 years cannot be used with confidence because 25% of the measurements were taken with a different dynamometer. Newer versions of the dynamometer have less friction; therefore, patients

score higher and appear to be doing better than if they had been measured on the original instrument.

A vigorometer is an acceptable alternative hand strength–measuring device for patients whose diagnoses contraindicate stress on joints and/or skin. It requires the patient to squeeze a rubber bulb rather than a steel handle. The vigorometer is a commercially available instrument for which norms have been published (Fike & Rousseau, 1982).

Another adapted sphygmomanometer for measuring grip strength of patients with rheumatoid arthritis was found to have a strong linear relationship ($r = .83$ for the right hand; $r = .84$ for the left) to the Jamar when tested on 88 patients. Agnew & Maas (1991) used linear regression equations to develop conversion tables to relate scores of the Jamar to the sphygmomanometer.

The power grip attachment of the Baltimore Therapeutic Equipment Work Simulator has been evaluated for test–retest reliability on 30 right-dominant men and women aged 20 to 45 years (Trossman et al., 1990) and found to be .98. The mean of three trials was the most reliable score. Day-to-day variability was 5% for the right hand and 3% for the left hand.

Position can be a factor in the results of a grip strength test. Su et al. (1994) examined the effects of different positions of the elbow and shoulder on grip strength using the Jamar dynamometer. The researchers found significant differences in the highest mean grip strength recorded in various positions. This study demonstrates the importance of consistency in the position used for grip testing. If the shoulder or elbow is positioned differently from test to test, the scores will not be reliable, and if the patient is not positioned as in the study that established the norms, the norms are unusable.

Lamoreaux and Hoffer (1995) looked at wrist deviation and its effects on grip and pinch strength. They found no statistical difference in pinch strength when the wrist was deviated, but wrist radial and ulnar deviation significantly decreased grip strength. This research is clinically relevant because certain patients in occupational therapy practice, such as those with Colles' fractures and rheumatoid arthritis, are prone to develop wrist deviations.

A study by Nitschke et al. (1999) addressed how much change in a grip score is necessary to result in a functional change. The study consisted of 42 female participants, 32 healthy and 10 with nonspecific regional pain. The authors concluded that at least a 13-pound change in grip strength was necessary to be sure the improvement was not a chance occurrence.

With practices moving into the community and home, the need for valid tools that are quick, portable, and easy to use is increasing. Bohannon (1998) looked at the validity of using the Jamar dynamometer to assess upper extremity strength as compared to manual muscle testing in adult home care patients. There were significant correlations between grip dynamometry and manual muscle testing, with the highest correlation between the dynamometer and manual tests of grip ($r = .80$) for the left hand and ($r = .78$) for the right hand. Therefore, the handgrip dynamometer was found to be a good predictor of overall strength.

Grasp (Fig. 4-119; Table 4-4)

The patient should be seated with his or her shoulder adducted and neutrally rotated, elbow flexed at 90°, and the forearm and wrist in neutral position. Grip strength varies with elbow position, so a standardized position is necessary (Kuzala & Varga, 1992; Su et al., 1994). The handle of the Jamar dynamometer is set at the second position (Mathiowetz et al., 1984, 1985). The task is demonstrated to the patient. After the dynamometer is positioned in the patient's hand, the therapist says, "Ready? Squeeze as hard as you can," and urges the patient on throughout the attempt. The patient squeezes the dynamometer with as much force as he or she can, three times with a 2- to 3-minute rest between trials. The score is the average of the three trials.

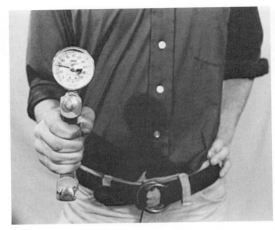

Figure 4-119 Measuring grasp using a dynamometer. The patient's upper arm is close to his body and the elbow is flexed to 90°.

Pinch

Three types of pinch are typically evaluated because they are involved in accomplishing occupational tasks and activities efficiently.

Tip Pinch (Fig. 4-120; Table 4-5)

The patient pinches the ends of the B & L pinch meter between the tips of the thumb and index finger (Mathiowetz et al., 1985) or between the thumb and the index and middle fingers (Kellor et al., 1971). The test is administered by first giving the patient instructions and a demonstration. Then the therapist says, "Ready? Pinch as hard as you can." The patient is urged on as he or she attempts to pinch. Three trials, with a rest between each trial, are completed. The average of three trials is recorded.

Lateral Pinch (Fig. 4-121; Table 4-5)

The patient pinches the meter between the pad of the thumb and the lateral surface of the index finger. The instructions and procedure are the same as for tip pinch.

Palmar Pinch: Three-Jaw Chuck (Fig. 4-122; Table 4-5)

The patient pinches the meter between the pad of the thumb and the pads of the index and middle fingers. The instructions and procedure are the same as for tip pinch.

Interpretation of Grasp and Pinch Scores

Scores are compared with those of the other hand or to norms to ascertain whether the patient has a significant limitation. The accuracy of the Jamar dynamometer was found to be ±5%, which means that if the patient scored 50 pounds, the actual strength may range from 47.5 to

52.5 pounds (Mathiowetz, 1990). Grasp and pinch scores are considered abnormal if they are associated with a functional limitation and/or if they are ±3 **standard deviations** (SD) from the mean (Mathiowetz, 1990). For example, suppose a 40-year-old man had a grasp score of 55 pounds when you averaged the three trials for his dominant right hand. Table 4-4 shows that the average score for his age group is 117 pounds, so the patient's grasp score was 62 pounds less than the mean normal score on the table. When you divide the difference in his score (62) by the SD given in the table (21), you find that he is 2.95 SD below the mean. This is close enough to −3 SD to consider that he has a significant limitation. Grasp and pinch measurements can be quickly and easily reevaluated over time to monitor the progress of the patient and the effectiveness of the treatment plan.

Measurement of Endurance

Endurance is the ability to sustain effort and to resist fatigue (Wilmore & Costill, 1999). It is related to cardiopulmonary and muscular function. The better cardiopulmonary and muscular function a person has, the better the endurance. Many of the patients seen in occupational therapy have endurance limitations. A variety of conditions, including cardiac or pulmonary impairments, a major trauma or illness requiring bed rest, loss

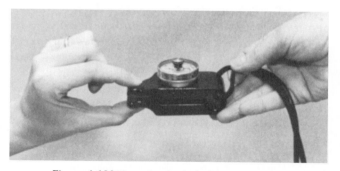

Figure 4-120 Measuring tip pinch with a pinch meter.

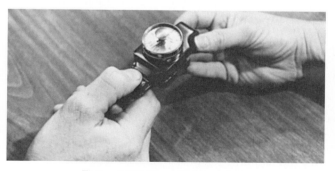

Figure 4-121 Measuring lateral pinch.

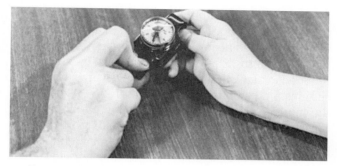

Figure 4-122 Measuring palmar pinch or three-jaw chuck pinch.

of significant muscle function, or the need to use prostheses or adapted equipment, can affect one's endurance.

Cardiopulmonary Aspects of Endurance

Cardiopulmonary endurance is the ability of the whole body to sustain prolonged rhythmical activity (Wilmore & Costill, 1999). Muscular work creates a demand for oxygen (Astrand & Rodahl, 1986). As an immediate effect of activity, the heart rate and stroke volume increase. Heart rate increases to deliver the required amount of oxygenated blood to the active muscles. Stroke volume, or amount of blood pumped per heartbeat, increases because of increased venous flow into the heart during diastole (the period of relaxation when the chambers fill) (Ellestad, 1986). As the intensity of muscular work increases, more oxygen is required. There is, however, a maximal amount of oxygen that a person can take in and dispense to muscles during exercise. Termed maximal oxygen uptake, it is abbreviated VO_{2max}. VO_{2max} is a standard measure of cardiovascular fitness (Taylor et al., 1955). It increases with physical training and decreases with bed rest and age. With physical training, the heart rate becomes lower for the same level of work, referred to as the training effect. The training effect indicates improvement in efficiency of the circulatory system (McArdle et al., 1994).

There is a linear relationship between oxygen uptake and heart rate for various intensities of light to moderately heavy exercise. Therefore, heart rate can be used to estimate VO_2. However, the heart rate of those who are physically unfit increases faster for a given level of oxygen uptake; therefore, the relationship is individual (McArdle et al., 1994).

Muscular Aspects of Endurance

Endurance of a muscle or muscle group is its ability to sustain intensive activity (Wilmore & Costill, 1999); endurance may be decreased because of local trauma or reduction of innervation. In normal muscle contraction against low resistance, only a few of the available motor units are needed at any one time. The active and resting units take turns. Fatigue rarely occurs in conditions required for activities of daily life. However, if the person sustains a contraction that exceeds 15 to 20% MVC for the muscle group involved, blood flow to the working muscle decreases, causing a shift to anaerobic metabolism, which limits duration of contraction (Dehn, 1980). The limitation is signaled by symptoms of muscle fatigue (cramping, burning, and tremor, which are secondary to the accumulation of lactic acid) and slowed nerve conduction velocity to the muscle fibers, which reduce tension and eventually result in inability to hold the contraction (Basmajian & DeLuca, 1985). Strength and endurance are closely related. As a muscle gains strength, its endurance for a given level of work also increases.

For neurologically disadvantaged muscle, such as after a spinal cord injury, peripheral nerve injury, or stroke, fewer motor units or muscle fibers may be available than are required for daily activity. Such muscles work at as much as 50 to 75% MVC to do otherwise low-intensity work (Trombly & Quintana, 1985).

The Evaluation

Endurance can be measured dynamically or statically. Dynamic assessments include (1) the number of repetitions per unit of time, (2) the percent of maximal heart rate generated by an aerobic activity or exercise or (3) metabolic equivalent (MET) level. Static assessment is the amount of time a contraction can be held (Milner-Brown et al., 1986).

Intensity, duration, and frequency of the activity are considerations in evaluation of endurance. Intensity is related to both resistance and speed. The heavier the resistance or the faster the pace, the higher the intensity. The intensity of the test activity must be kept constant from test to test to gauge improvement.

Intensity of an activity is estimated in terms of light, moderate, or heavy work or number of METs. One MET equals basal metabolic rate (Erb et al., 1979). Basal metabolic rate is the amount of oxygen consumption necessary to maintain metabolic processes (e.g., respiration, circulation, peristalsis, temperature regulation, glandular function) of the body at rest and is quantified as 3.5 mL oxygen per kilogram of body weight per minute. The energy cost of activities or exercise can be rated using multiples of METs. An exercise that is rated 4 METs requires 4 times the amount of oxygen per kilogram of body weight per minute than the basal rate. Oxygen consumption of daily living, recreational, and vocational tasks has been measured for normal subjects,

and the METs required for each task have been calculated (Box 4-4). These costs are estimates that vary with environmental conditions such as humidity and temperature and personal conditions such as anger.

Heart rate is a simple means to quantify the physiological demand of a dynamic activity for a particular person (McArdle et al., 1994). Because heart rate relates linearly to VO_{2max} except at the upper limits (80–90%) of maximal capacity, if a person's heart rate is 70% of maximal heart rate (HR_{max}), he or she is using approximately 70% of VO_{2max}. HR_{max} is estimated by subtracting the person's age from 220. The pulse taken immediately after aerobic large-muscle exercise is then related to the person's HR_{max} as percent of maximum. A constant heart rate obtained during exercise indicates a steady state, that is, balance of oxygen intake and consumption (Ellestad, 1986). Heart rate is measured by placing the index and middle fingers lightly but firmly over the radial artery at the wrist (lateral to the flexor carpi radialis) and counting the number of beats per minute (bpm). It is most accurate to count for a full minute, but an exercise heart rate can be counted for only 10 to 15 seconds, as the return to resting rate occurs quickly after stopping exercise. In that case, the obtained value is multiplied by 6 for 10 seconds or 4 for 15 seconds to arrive at the bpm (Lunsford, 1978). ***The relation between heart rate and oxygen uptake does not hold for patients with chronic obstructive pulmonary disease, who because of reduced expiration and expulsion of carbon dioxide waste have greater ventilatory requirements (Whipp & Ward, 1986). These patients have limited exercise capacity (Hansen, 1986)***.

Whether to measure dynamically or statically depends on the functional goal of the patient and his or her cardiopulmonary status. If the patient's work and hobbies require mostly isotonic activity, endurance should be evaluated dynamically. To measure endurance in terms of number of repetitions, use a light repetitive activity such as the *Box and Block Test*, described in Chapter 42. It can be adapted to measure upper extremity endurance for light work by counting the number of blocks the patient can transfer before becoming fatigued.

If the patient expects to return to a job or hobby that requires maintained grasp or holding loads (isometric contractions), static endurance should be tested. To measure statically, the amount of time a person can hold an object or position requiring a certain level MVC is noted. Normally, a person can hold 25% MVC for 5 to 6 minutes, 50% MVC for 1 to 2 minutes, and 100% MVC only momentarily (Dehn & Mullins, 1977).

Isometric holding increases blood pressure and stresses the cardiopulmonary system (Dehn, 1980;

BOX 4-4
Metabolic Equivalents

Energy Level	Activities of Daily Living	Occupational Activities	Recreational Activities
1–2 MET	Eating Dressing and undressing Washing hands and face Sweeping the floor	Desk and phone work Keyboard operation Riding in a car Watch repair	Standing Walking (strolling 1mile/hr) Playing cards and board games Painting
2.5–3.5 MET	Showering Food preparation Making beds Ironing Cleaning windows	Welding Small-parts assembly Bricklaying and plastering Playing a musical instrument	Walking (2 miles/hr) Cycling (5.5 miles/hr) Horseback riding (walk) Billiards Bowling Golf (pulling bag cart)
4–5 MET	Raking leaves Hoeing Walking downstairs Beating carpets	Heavy assembly work Painting Light carpentry Paperhanging	Walking (3 miles/hr) Cycling (9 miles/hr) Golf (carrying clubs) Ballroom dancing Table tennis
5.5–6.5 MET	Walking with braces and crutches Mowing lawn by hand mower	Carpentry Chopping wood	Walking (4 miles/hr) Tennis Horseback riding (trot) Folk dancing Ice or roller skating
7–8 MET		Shoveling (22 pounds for 10 minutes) Digging	Jogging (5 miles/hr) Skiing (vigorous) Horseback riding (gallop)
8.5–9.5 MET		Shoveling (31 pounds for 10 minutes)	Running (7.5 miles/hr) Squash Fencing Football Basketball

MET, metabolic equivalents.
Adapted with permission from Wilmore, J. H., & Costill, D. L. (1999). *Physiology of Sport and Exercise* (2nd ed.). Champaign IL: Human Kinetics.

Ellestad, 1986) (Box 4-5). This is true especially if the person holds his or her breath (Valsalva maneuver) while holding the contraction. Therefore, persons being tested should talk (e.g., count or sing) while doing an isometric contraction to preclude breath holding. Isometric testing can produce arrhythmias, and therefore, electrocardiogram and blood pressure should be monitored during isometric testing of patients with heart disease or abnormalities. The results of isometric testing cannot be extrapolated to gauge isotonic aerobic exercise capacity (Ellestad, 1986).

Another way to assess dynamic endurance is to ascertain the individual's perception of how hard he or she is working. Scales of ratings of perceived exertion (RPE), such as the *Rating of Perceived Exertion* (Borg, 1985), are based on psychophysics or the relating of a physical property to a subjective property via scaling procedures (Russell, 1997). The Borg (15- point) *Scale of Perceived Exertion* ranges from 6 (no exertion at all) to 20 (maximal exertion) (Wilmore & Costill, 1999). This scale

BOX 4-5
SAFETY BOX

Precautions for Isometric Testing

▶ If the patient exhibits dyspnea, weakness, changes in sensorium, angina, decreased HR for increased workload, increased ventricular arrhythmias, pallor, or cyanosis, his or her cardiopulmonary capacity has been exceeded (Dehn & Mullins, 1977).

▶ Endurance testing in occupational therapy should not reach this level, but if any of these symptoms are observed or reported by the patient, the intensity of work should be immediately reduced to a comfortable level.

allows the person to assign one of a consecutive set of numbers with a corresponding descriptor of amount of exertion to the ongoing activity (e.g. 11, fairly light, or 17, very hard). The American Heart Association (1990) and the American College of Sports Medicine (1995) suggest that an RPE of 12 to 16 on the 15-point *Borg Scale* is associated with a physiological training effect (Whaley et al., 1997). Therapists should be aware, however, that perceived exertion for a given level of oxygen uptake is higher for arm work than leg work (Russell, 1997). For dynamic activities, the *Borg Scale* has been found over the years to correlate validly to heart rate, oxygen uptake, and blood lactate levels (Russell, 1997). More recent studies question that validity because of poor reliability when the actual scores of each subject during the trial and the retrial are tested. Lamb et al. (1999) looked at test–retest reliability and found it to differ as much as 3 RPE when level of agreement between trials was examined and the scores of the two trials were not merely correlated. Whaley et al. (1997) tested the validity of the oxygen consumption associated with each score on the 15-point *Borg Scale*. They found interindividual differences that ranged from a rating of 6 to 20 for 60% **maximum heart rate reserve (MHRR)** and from 8 to 20 for 80% MHRR in both normal healthy adults and cardiac patients. Nevertheless, these scales provide a good estimate when used repeatedly for the same patient and therefore may be used clinically during ongoing continuous activity, such as walking, bicycling, scrubbing floors, painting a wall, mowing the lawn, raking leaves, and calisthenic exercises. These scales do not apply to activities composed of sporadic variable movements.

The therapist should orient the person to the scale using standardized instructions published by Borg (1985) prior to the start of the activity. The scale should be enlarged and posted so that it can be seen easily from where the person is exercising. At 1- or 2-minute intervals, the therapist prompts the patient to rate exertion at that moment. The decision to continue depends on the goal and precautions for the particular patient.

Summary Review Questions

1. Describe in general the correct placement of a goniometer.
2. What does it mean if AROM is less than PROM?
3. ROM limitations can be caused by a number of underlying conditions. State the short-term goal for treatment of elbow flexion contracture after removal of a cast used to immobilize a fractured humerus.
4. How is a break test used to determine strength?
5. Of what importance is the length/tension relationship of a muscle in manual muscle testing?
6. Describe the standardized procedures for testing muscle strength.
7. For what muscle test grades is treatment to increase strength an appropriate goal?
8. How is dynamic endurance measured?
9. How is static endurance measured?
10. What is your maximum heart rate? What percentage of VO_{2max} do you use to vacuum a room? take a shower? wash the dishes?

Acknowledgments

Over the many editions of this textbook, several photographers have contributed to this chapter. They are Anne Fisher, ScD, OTR; Lucia Grochowska-Littlefield; Judith La Drew; and Keith Weaver. The models for the photographs are Brian Despres, OTR; Mark Erikson; Sam Fitzpatrick, Jim Morando; and Christopher Trombly. To all of these people, without whom we could not have produced this chapter, we give our deepest thanks. We also extend our thanks to Tracey Proano for her help with the chapter for this edition.

References

Agnew, P. J., & Maas, F. (1991). Jamar dynamometer and adapted sphygmomanometer for measuring grip strength in patients with rheumatoid arthritis. *Occupational Therapy Journal of Research, 11*, 259–270.

American College of Sports Medicine. (1995). *Guidelines for Exercise Testing and Prescription* (5th ed.). Baltimore: Williams & Wilkins.

American Heart Association. (1990). Exercise standards: A statement for health care professionals from the American Heart Association. *Circulation, 82*, 2286–2322.

American Society for Hand Therapists. (1981). *Clinical Assessment Recommendations*. Indianapolis: American Society for Hand Therapists.

Anderson, L. R. III, & Bohannon, R. W. (1991). Head and neck position does not influence maximum static elbow extension force measured in healthy individuals tested while prone. *Occupational Therapy Journal of Research, 11*, 121–126.

Astrand, P. O., & Rodahl, K. (1986). *Textbook of Work Physiology: Physiological Basis of Exercise* (3rd ed.). New York: McGraw-Hill.

Basmajian, J. V., & DeLuca, C. J. (1985). *Muscles Alive: Their Functions Revealed by Electromyography* (5th ed.). Baltimore: Williams & Wilkins.

Bechtol, C. O. (1954). Grip test: Use of a dynamometer with adjustable handle spacing. *Journal of Bone and Joint Surgery, 36A*(7), 820–824, 832.

Bohannon, R. W. (1998). Hand-grip dynomometry provides a valid indication of upper extremity strength impairment in home care patients. *Journal of Hand Therapy, 11*(4), 258–260.

Bohannon, R. W., Warren, M., & Cogman, K. (1991). Influence of shoulder position on maximum voluntary elbow flexion force in stroke patients. *Occupational Therapy Journal of Research, 11*, 73–79.

Boone, D. C., Azen, S. P., Lin, C.-M., Spence, C., Baron, C., & Lee, L. (1978). Reliability of goniometric measurements. *Physical Therapy, 58*, 1355–1360.

Borg, G. A. V. (1985). *An Introduction to Borg's RPE-Scale*. New York: Mouvement.

Brandsma, J. W., Schreuders, T. R., Birke, J. A., Piefer, A., & Oostendorp, P. (1995). Manual muscle strength testing: Intraobserver and interobserver reliabilities for the intrinsic muscles of the hand. *Journal of Hand Therapy, 8*, 185–190.

Chiarello, C. M., & Savidge, R. (1993). Interrater reliability of the Cybex EDI-320 and fluid goniometer in normals and patients with low back pain. *Archives of Physical Medicine and Rehabilitation, 74*, 32–37.

Daniels, L., & Worthingham, C. (1986). *Muscle testing: Techniques of manual examination* (5th ed.). Philadelphia: Saunders.

Dehn, M. M. (1980). Rehabilitation of the cardiac patient: The effects of exercise. *American Journal of Nursing, 80*, 435–440.

Dehn, M. M., & Mullins, C. B. (1977, April). Physiologic effects and importance of exercise in patients with coronary artery disease. *Cardiovascular Medicine 2*, 365–371, 377–387.

DeVore, G. L., & Hamilton, G. F. (1968). Volume measuring of the severely injured hand. *American Journal of Occupational Therapy, 22*, 16–18.

Diekmeyer, G. (1978). Altered test position for hip extensor muscles. *Physical Therapy, 58*(11), 1379.

Ellestad, M. H. (1986). *Stress testing: Principles and practice* (3rd ed.). Philadelphia: Davis.

Erb, B. D., Fletcher, G. F., & Sheffield, T. L. (1979). AHA Committee report: Standards for cardiovascular exercise treatment programs. *Circulation, 59*, 1084A–1090A.

Fess, E. E. (1987). A method of checking Jamar dynamometer calibration. *Journal of Hand Therapy, 1*, 28–32.

Fess, E. E. (1990). Assessment of the upper extremity: Instrumentation criteria. *Occupational Therapy Practice, 1*(4), 1–11.

Fike, M. L., & Rousseau, E. (1982). Measurement of adult hand strength: A comparison of two instruments. *Occupational Therapy Journal of Research, 2*, 43–49.

Flood-Joy, M., & Mathiowetz, V. (1987). Grip-strength measurement: A comparison of three Jamar dynamometers. *Occupational Therapy Journal of Research, 7*(4), 235–243.

Florence, J. M., Pandya, S., & King, W. M. (1992). Intrarater reliability of manual muscle test grades in Duchenne's muscular dystrophy. *Physical Therapy, 72*, 115–126.

Gajdosik, R. L., & Bohannon, R. W. (1987). Clinical measurement of range of motion: Review of goniometry emphasizing reliability and validity. *Physical Therapy, 67*, 1867–1872.

Gordon, M., Greenfield, E., Marvin, J., Hester C., & Lauterbach, S. (1998). Use of pain assessment tools: Is there a preference? *Journal of Burn Care Rehabilitation, 19*, 451–454.

Gowitzke, B. A., & Milner, M. (1980). *Understanding the Scientific Bases of Human Movement* (2nd ed.). Baltimore: Williams & Wilkins.

Greene, W. B., & Heckman, J. D. (Eds.). (1994). *The Clinical Measurement of Joint Motion.* Rosemont, IL: American Academy of Orthopaedic Surgeons.

Gunal, I., Kose, N., Erdogan, O., Gokturk, E., & Seber, S. (1996). Normal range of motion of the joints of the upper extremity in male subjects, with special reference to side. *Journal of Bone and Joint Surgery, 78–A*, 1401–1404.

Hansen, J. E. (1986). Respiratory abnormalities: Exercise evaluation of the dyspneic patient. In A. R. Leff (Ed.), *Cardiopulmonary Exercise Testing* (pp. 69–88). New York: Grune & Stratton.

Herbison, G. J., Issac, Z., Cohne, M. E., & Ditunno, J. F. (1996). Strength post-spinal cord injury: Myometer versus manual muscle test. *Spinal Cord, 34*, 543–548.

Hines, T. (1965). Manual muscle examination. In S. Licht (Ed.), *Therapeutic Exercise* (2nd ed., pp. 163–256). Baltimore: Waverly.

Hislop, H., & Montgomery, J. (Eds.). (1995). *Daniel's and Worthingham's Muscle Testing* (6th ed.). Philadelphia: W. B. Saunders Co.

Horger, M. M. (1990). The reliability of goniometric measurements of active and passive wrist motions. *American Journal of Occupational Therapy, 44*, 342–348.

Howell, J. W., Rothstein, J. M., Lamb, R. L., & Merritt, W. H. (1989). An experimental investigation of the validity of the manual muscle test positions for the extensor pollicis longus and flexor pollicis brevis muscles. *Journal of Hand Therapy, 3*, 20–28.

Jacobs, K. (Ed.). (1999). *Quick Reference Dictionary for Occupational Therapy* (2nd ed.). Thorofare, NJ: Slack.

Johannson, C. A., Kent, B. E., & Shepard, K. F. (1983). Relationship between verbal command volume and magnitude of muscle contraction. *Physical Therapy, 63*,1260–1265.

Johnston, M. V., Keith, R. A., & Hinderer, S. R. (1992). Measurement standards for interdisciplinary medical rehabilitation. *Archives of Physical Medicine and Rehabilitation, 73*, S1–S22.

Katz, J, & Melzach, R. (1999). Measurement of pain. *Surgical Clinics of North America, 79*, 231–252.

Kellor, M., Frost, J., Silverberg, N., Iverson, I., & Cummings, R. (1971). Hand strength and dexterity. *American Journal of Occupational Therapy, 25*(2),77–83.

Kendall, F. P., & Kendall, E. (1983). *Muscles: Testing and function* (3rd ed.). Baltimore: Williams & Wilkins.

Kuzala, E. A., & Vargo, M. C. (1992). The relationship between elbow position and grip strength. *American Journal of Occupational Therapy, 46*, 509–512.

Lamb, K. L., Eston, R. G., & Corns, D. (1999). Reliability of ratings of perceived exertion during progressive treadmill exercise. *British Journal of Sports Medicine, 33*, 336–339.

Lamoreaux, L., & Hoffer, M. M. (1995). The effect of wrist deviation on grip and pinch strength. *Clinical Orthopaedics and Related Research, 314*, 152–155.

Landsmeer, J. M. F., & Long, C. (1965). The mechanism of finger control based on electromyograms and location analysis. *Acta Anatomica (Basel), 60*, 330–347.

LaStayo, P. C., & Wheeler, D. L. (1994). Reliability of passive wrist flexion and extension goniometric measurements: A multi center study. *Physical Therapy, 74*, 162–176.

Lehmkuhl, L. D., & Smith, L. K. (1983). *Brunnstrom's Clinical Kinesiology* (4th ed.). Philadelphia: Davis.

Long, C. (1968). Intrinsic-extrinsic muscle control of the fingers. *Journal of Bone and Joint Surgery, 50A*, 973–984.

Long, C., & Brown, M. E. (1962). EMG kinesiology of the hand. Part III. Lumbricales and flexor digitorum profundus to the long finger. *Archives of Physical Medicine and Rehabilitation, 43*, 450–460.

Lunsford, B. R. (1978). Clinical indicators of endurance. *Physical Therapy, 58*(6), 704–709.

Marx, R. G., Bombardier, C., & Wright, J. G. (1999). What do we know about the reliability and validity of physical examination tests used to examine the upper extremity? *Journal of Hand Surgery, 24-A*, 185–193.

Mathiowetz, V. (1990). Grip and pinch strength measurements. In L. R. Amundsen (Ed.), *Muscle Strength Testing: Instrumented and Non-instrumented Systems* (pp. 163–177). New York: Churchill Livingstone.

Mathiowetz, V. (1991). Reliability and validity of grip and pinch strength measurements. *Critical Reviews in Physical and Rehabilitation Medicine, 2*(4), 201–212.

Mathiowetz, V., Kashman, N., Volland, G., Weber, K., Dowe, M., & Rogers, S. (1985). Grip and pinch strength: Normative data for adults. *Archives of Physical Medicine and Rehabilitation, 66*(2), 69–74.

Mathiowetz, V., Weber, K., Volland, G., & Kashman, N. (1984). Reliability and validity of grip and pinch strength evaluations. *Hand Surgery, 9A*(2), 222–226.

McArdle, W. D., Katch, F. I., & Katch, V. L. (1994). *Essentials of Exercise Physiology.* Baltimore: Williams & Williams.

Medical Research Council (1976). *Aids to the Examination of the Peripheral Nervous System.* London: Her Majesty's Stationary Office.

Merskey, H., & Bogduk, N. (1994). *Classification of chronic pain* (2nd ed.). Seattle: International Association for the Study of Pain.

Milner-Brown, H. S., Mellenthin, M., & Miller, R. G. (1986). Quantifying human muscle strength, endurance and fatigue. *Archives of Physical Medicine and Rehabilitation, 67,* 530–535.

Moore, M. L. (1978). Clinical assessment of joint motion. In J. V. Basmajian (Ed.), *Therapeutic Exercise* (3rd ed., pp. 151–190). Baltimore: Williams & Wilkins.

Nitschke, J. E., McMeeken, J. M., Burry, H. C., & Matyas, T. A. (1999). When is a change a genuine change? A clinically meaningful interpretation of grip strength measurements in healthy and disabled women. *Journal of Hand Therapy, 12,* 25–30.

Riddle, D. L., Rothstein, J. M., & Lamb, R. L. (1987). Goniometric reliability in a clinical setting. *Physical Therapy, 67,* 668–673.

Russell, W. D. (1997). On the current status of rated perceived exertion. *Perceptual and Motor Skills, 84,* 799–808.

Sabari, J. S., Maltzev, I., Lubarsky, D., Liszkay, E., & Homel, P. (1998). Goniometric assessment of shoulder range of motion: Comparison of testing in supine and sitting positions. *Archives of Physical Medicine and Rehabilitation, 79,* 647–651.

Schwartz, S., Cohen, M. E., Herbison, G. J., & Shah, A. (1992). Relationship between two measures of upper extremity strength: Manual muscle testing compared to hand held myometry. *Archives of Physical Medicine and Rehabilitation, 73,* 1063–1068.

Smidt, G. L., & Rogers, M. W. (1982). Factors contributing to the regulation and clinical assessment of muscular strength. *Physical Therapy, 62,* 1283–1290.

Somers, D. L., Hanson, J. A., Kedzierski, C. M., Nestor, K. L., & Quinlivan, K. Y. (1997). The influence of experience on the reliability of

goniometric and visual measurement of forefoot position. *Journal of Orthopedic Sports Physical Therapy, 25,* 192–202.

Stern, E. (1991). Volumetric comparison of seated and standing postures. *American Journal of Occupational Therapy, 45*(9), 801–804.

Su, C-Y., Lin, J-H., Chien, T-H., Cheng, K-F., & Sung, Y-T. (1994). Grip strength in different positions of elbow and shoulder. *Archives of Physical Medicine and Rehabilitation, 75,* 812–815.

Taylor, H. L., Buskirk, E., & Henschel, A. (1955). Maximal oxygen uptake as objective measure of cardiorespiratory performance. *Journal of Applied Physiology, 8,* 73–80.

Trombly, C. A., & Quintana, L. A. (1985). Differences in response to exercise by post-CVA and normal subjects. *Occupational Therapy Journal of Research, 5*(1), 39–58.

Trossman, P. B., Suleski, K. B., & Li, P.-W. (1990). Test-retest reliability and day-to-day variability of an isometric grip strength test using the work simulator. *Occupational Therapy Journal of Research, 10*(5), 266–279.

Waylett, J., & Seibly, D. (1981). A study to determine the average deviation accuracy of a commercially available volumeter. *Journal of Hand Surgery, 6,* 300.

Whaley, M. H., Brubaker, P. H., Kaminsky, L. A., & Miller, C. R. (1997). Validity of rating of perceived exertion during graded exercise testing in apparently healthy adults and cardiac patients. *Journal of Cardiopulmonary Rehabilitation, 17,* 261–267.

Whipp, B. J., & Ward, S. (1986). The normal respiratory response in exercise. In A. R. Leff (Ed.), *Cardiopulmonary exercise testing* (pp. 45–68). New York: Grune & Stratton.

Wilmore, J. H., & Costill, D. L. (1999). *Physiology of sport and exercise* (2nd ed.). Champaign, IL: Human Kinetics.

Wittink, H., & Michel, T. (1997). *Chronic Pain Management for Physical Therapists.* Boston: Butterworth-Heinemann.

5

Assessing Abilities and Capacities: Motor Behavior

Virgil Mathiowetz and Julie Bass-Haugen

LEARNING OBJECTIVES

After studying this chapter, the reader will be able to do the following:

1. Contrast the reflex-hierarchical and systems models of motor control.
2. Describe various types of motor dysfunction seen in persons with central nervous system lesions.
3. Compare the neuromaturational and systems theories of motor development.
4. Contrast the assumptions of the neurophysiological and task-related approaches to treatment.
5. Describe the different evaluation strategies that would be used by the neurophysiological and task-related approaches.

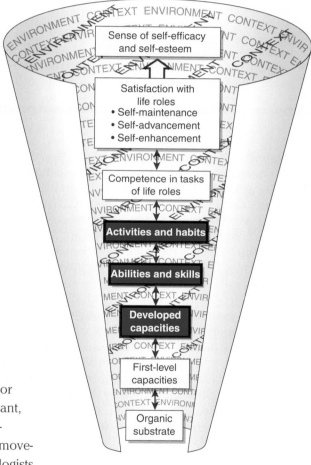

*O*ur understanding of motor behavior—motor control, motor development, and motor learning—continues to evolve (VanSant, 1991a). Sophisticated technology has led to an explosion of information about the control, development, and acquisition of movement (Lister, 1991). Human movement scientists, neurophysiologists, neuropsychologists, and others contribute to this effort. In an attempt to impose order on the many pieces of information, they deduce models and theories of motor behavior. As these models and theories change, therapeutic approaches also must change.

As a result of changes in the motor behavior literature, some (e.g., Gordon, 1987; Shumway-Cook & Woolacott, 1995) have questioned the assumptions underlying the neurophysiological approaches, which include Rood's (1954) sensorimotor approach, Knott & Voss' (1968) proprioceptive neuromuscular facilitation, Brunnstrom's (1970) movement therapy, and Bobath's (1978, 1990) neurodevelopmental treatment. Two task-related approaches, a task-oriented approach (Horak, 1991; Mathiowetz & Bass Haugen, 1994) (see Chapter 21) and Carr and Shepherd's (1987) approach (see Chapter 22), are being proposed as alternatives to the neurophysiological approaches. The assumptions of these new approaches are derived from a systems model of motor control, systems theories of motor development, and recent motor learning theories.

Box 5-1 provides an overview of this chapter, which contrasts the assumptions of the neurophysiological and task-related approaches, the models and theories of motor behavior that they are based on, and the evaluation strategies associated with each approach. We believe the evaluation strategies used by the neurophysiological approaches still continue to have a major influence on clinical practice. However, we expect that task-related evaluation strategies will have a greater influence on practice in the future.

Neurophysiological Approaches

Assumptions of the Neurophysiological Approaches

Box 5-1 includes the assumptions of the four neurophysiological approaches as described by their original proponents. Although there have been recent efforts to update the theoretical rationale of the neurophysiological approaches (e.g., Bly, 1991; Ryerson & Levit, 1997),

many of the original treatment techniques remain the same. To understand the neurophysiological approaches, one must understand the reflex-hierarchical model of motor control and neuromaturational theories of motor development from which these treatment approaches originated. A discussion of the motor learning theories that influenced the neurophysiological and task-related approaches is covered in Chapter 12.

Reflex and Hierarchical Models of Motor Control

The integration of the earlier reflex model with the **hierarchical** model resulted in the reflex-hierarchical model of motor control. This combined model explains a broader range of motor behaviors than the earlier models could explain individually. To provide an historical perspective, we briefly discuss the earlier reflex and hierarchical models before explaining in more detail an integrated reflex-hierarchical model of motor control.

Reflex Models

The idea that sensory input could elicit movement originated with reflex models of motor control. For example, Sherrington (1906) viewed the central nervous system CNS) as a black box through which specific sensory input would elicit reflexes or stereotyped motor output. In addition, the sensory feedback from the motor output could trigger other reflexes or stereotyped movements. This model suggested that human movement was the summation of reflexes and that peripheral sensory

---

BOX 5-1
Comparison of the Neurophysiological and OT Task-Oriented Approaches

Neurophysiological Approaches   **OT Task-Oriented Approach**

Models of Motor Control

Reflex-Hierarchical

- ▶ Movements are elicited by sensory input or controlled by central programs.
- ▶ Open-loop and closed-loop control is used.
- ▶ Feedback and feed-forward influence movements.
- ▶ CNS is hierarchically organized, with higher centers controlling lower centers.
- ▶ Reciprocal innervation is essential for coordinated movement.

Systems

- ▶ Personal and environmental systems interact to achieve functional goals.
- ▶ Movement emerges from the interaction of many systems.
- ▶ Systems are dynamical, self-organizing, and heterarchical.
- ▶ Movement used for a task is the preferred means for achieving a functional goal.
- ▶ Changes in one or more systems can alter behavior.

Theories of Motor Development

Neuromaturational

- ▶ Changes are due to CNS maturation.
- ▶ Development follows a predictable sequence (e.g., cephalo-caudal, proximal-distal).
- ▶ CNS damage leads to regression to lower levels and more stereotypical behaviors.

Systems

- ▶ Changes due to interaction of multiple systems
- ▶ Progression varies because person and environmental contexts are unique.
- ▶ CNS damage leads to attempts to use remaining resources to achieve functional goals.

Assumptions of Therapeutic Approaches

- ▶ CNS is hierarchically organized.
- ▶ Sensory stimuli inhibit spasticity and abnormal movement and facilitate normal movement and postural responses.
- ▶ Repetition of movement results in positive permanent changes in CNS.
- ▶ Recovery from CNS damage follows a predictable sequence.
- ▶ Behavioral changes after CNS damage have a neurophysiological basis.

- ▶ Personal and environmental systems, including the CNS, are heterarchically organized.
- ▶ Functional tasks help organize behavior.
- ▶ Occupational performance emerges from the interaction of persons and their environment.
- ▶ Experimentation with various strategies leads to optimal solutions to motor problems.
- ▶ Recovery is variable because personal characteristics and environmental contexts are unique.
- ▶ Behavioral changes reflect attempts to compensate and to achieve task performance.

Evaluation

Primary focus on performance components

- ▶ Abnormal muscle tone
- ▶ Abnormal reflexes and stereotypical movement patterns lead to incoordination.
- ▶ Postural control
- ▶ Sensation and perception
- ▶ Memory and judgment
- ▶ Stage of recovery or developmental level

Secondary focus on occupational performance

Primary focus on role & occupational performance using a client-centered view

- ▶ Task analysis to determine performance components and contexts that limit function and to identify preferred movement patterns for specific tasks in varied contexts.
- ▶ Variables that cause transitions to new patterns.

Secondary focus on selected occupational performance components and contexts that limit function

---

feedback controlled movement. An example of using sensory input to elicit a motor output is when therapists use vibration or tapping over the triceps muscle to elicit elbow extension.

A number of studies have revealed the limitations of the reflex models. Deafferented animals have demonstrated coordinated movement without sensory input (Taub, 1976). Lashley (1917) reported the case of a human with severe lower extremity sensory loss who had minimal problems with coordinated movement. Thus, sensory input is not necessary for all types of motor

behavior. In addition, the reflex model cannot account for preprogrammed instructions or anticipatory control of movement, key components of the hierarchical model. In conclusion, the reflex model of motor control by itself has significant limitations and is an inadequate model for explaining human motor control.

Hierarchical Models

The idea that central programs control movement originated with hierarchical models of motor control. One of the earliest models (Jackson & Taylor, 1932) proposed

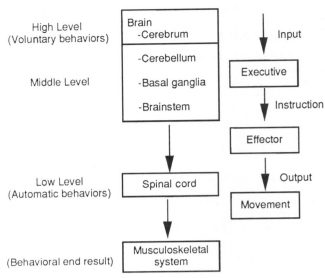

Figure 5-1 Hierarchical models of motor control, which emphasize central or top-down control of movement. The left side is an adaptation of VanSant (1991a), and the right side is an adaptation of Schmidt (1988). [Reprinted with permission from Mathiowetz V. & Bass Haugen J. (1994). Motor behavior research: Implications for therapeutic approaches to CNS dysfunction. *American Journal of Occupational Therapy, 48*, 733–744. Copyright 1994 by American Occupational Therapy Association, Inc.]

that movements are controlled centrally from the top down: the highest level of the nervous system controls the middle level, and the middle level in turn controls the lowest level (Fig. 5-1, left side). Some hierarchical models of motor control (e.g., Schmidt, 1988) suggest that control of movement originates centrally with the executive selecting, planning, and initiating a motor program to respond to specific input (Fig. 5-1, right side). The motor program contains the instructions for the **effector**, which carries them out without the possibility of modification if something goes wrong. The output is the movement that can be observed.

The hierarchical model incorporates an **open-loop system** of control rather than a **closed-loop system**. Fast movements (approximately 160 msec or less) are under open-loop control. In these cases, there isn't time to use feedback information for monitoring and correcting because the movement has ended before the feedback can be used. When a baseball player decides to swing at a pitch, it is impossible or extremely difficult to adjust the swing for an unanticipated pitch, because the movement is under open-loop control.

Many postural adjustments, which were thought to be reflexive reactions in response to sensory input, have been shown to be anticipatory adjustments prior to self-initiated limb movements (Horak et al., 1984). For example, Belen'kii et al. (1967) demonstrated that in a reaching task, electromyographic (EMG) activity occurred in the opposite leg about 60 msec before any

EMG activity in the arm. Thus, the subjects made postural adjustments in anticipation of changes in the center of gravity. In the hierarchical model of motor control, these types of anticipatory adjustments are thought to be part of the motor program.

However, hierarchical models without feedback loops cannot explain closed-loop movements that require feedback. This limitation resulted in an integration of these two models of motor control.

Reflex-Hierarchical Model of Motor Control

Figure 5-2 illustrates a reflex-hierarchical model that is an adaptation of Trombly's (1989) model and that synthesizes the basic science literature of the 1970s and 1980s. Each step of the model is discussed conceptually, using the example of a person reaching for a bottle of water. See the references listed at the end of this chapter for greater detail.

Motivation to Move Is Generated. Purposeful movement does not occur in the absence of a need to move, which is generated from within the person or as a response to external stimuli (Marsden, 1982). Thus, a person who is thirsty (internal stimulus) or sees a cold bottle of water (external stimulus) becomes motivated to reach for the bottle.

Long-Term Memory Is Searched. Once the person is motivated, the executive or programming center searches long-term memory (LTM) for a pattern of movement that would enable reaching for the bottle. All previous efforts to

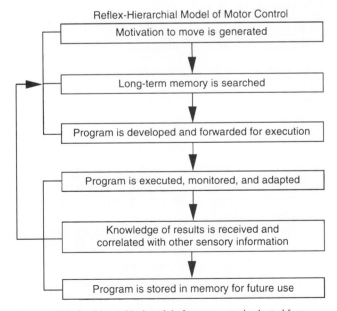

Figure 5-2 Reflex-hierarchical model of motor control, adapted from Trombly (1989), includes both open-loop and closed-loop control.

reach a bottle were stored in a generalized motor program that contains an abstract representation about the order, relative timing, and relative force of the reaching movement (Schmidt, 1988). It also includes the postural adjustments that will be needed, so that the person does not overbalance while reaching for the bottle.

A Program Is Developed and Forwarded for Execution. Using the selected generalized motor program, the reaching movement is organized and planned (Marsden, 1982). The program is adapted to take into account environmental factors and to designate the specific muscles needed, the force of the contractions, and the overall duration of the movement. In this way the generalized motor program is modified to meet the requirements of this specific action (reaching for a bottle of water on a table in front of the person).

Postural muscles are activated automatically as part of the program to provide a stable base from which movement may occur. In addition, the γ-motor neurons are programmed so that spindle sensitivity is set and accurate information concerning the length and speed of length change can be continually monitored (Fredericks & Saladin, 1996). Different types of movements and environmental factors require different control strategies (Brooks, 1986). Strategies also differ among people and between trials by the same person.

Program Is Executed, Monitored, and Adapted. As the program for reaching a bottle of water is executed, the movements are monitored via cutaneous input, visual and auditory cues, and ongoing proprioceptive input (Brooks, 1986). If the movement appears to be progressing successfully (the bottle of water is reached and picked up), the program is continued as planned. If the movement is sensed to be wrong (e.g., the hand misses the target) or an unexpected event occurs (e.g., the bottle is empty instead of full), an adjustment is made while the movement is still in progress. In the latter case, it is the α-γ coactivation that keeps the muscle spindle sensitive to the unexpected event. The agonist lifter muscles were programmed to lift a full bottle. The antagonist muscles were programmed to relax enough to allow the movement and then to contract to brake the movement as the bottle reached the mouth. Because the bottle was lighter than expected, the person lifted faster initially than was programmed. As a result, the muscle spindles of the agonist muscles went slack because they shortened faster than expected, while the muscle spindles of the antagonist muscles stretched because they lengthened faster than was programmed. This information was returned to various levels of the CNS, which made adjustments for this unexpected event.

It is important to understand how the CNS adjusts for unexpected events because it is the basis of some therapeutic procedures and because it illustrates why active rather than passive movement is used for therapy. When the motor program is executed, the α- and γ-motor neurons are coactivated and excite the extrafusal and intrafusal muscle fibers according to the plan. When active movement is stopped by an unexpectedly full bottle of water or a therapist's hand (i.e., external stretch), the extrafusal muscle fibers are mechanically prevented from shortening as programmed. Meanwhile, the intrafusal fibers keep contracting as programmed. Soon the discrepancy between their length and the length of the extrafusal fibers is signaled to higher centers. Because the muscle spindle is held in place by connective tissue attached to the extrafusal muscle fibers, the spindle is mechanically prevented from shortening despite the intrafusal muscle contractions (i.e., internal stretch). As a result, external and internal stretch of the midportions of the spindle fibers add together and stretch reflexes are activated (Brooks, 1986). Therapists use this technique to increase the strength of muscle contraction.

Knowledge of Results Is Received and Correlated With Other Sensory Information. *Knowledge of results* (KR) is awareness of the outcome of movement in relation to the goal. Open-loop movements are learned first as closed-loop movements in which attention is focused on the sensory feedback during the movement. Then the feedback is correlated to the outcome of the movement—KR—and the plan is modified for future movements. An open-loop movement can be executed exactly as programmed and yet be inaccurate for accomplishing the goal (Schmidt, 1988). For example, the person reaching for the bottle of water may miss the target, which illustrates the importance of KR and sensory feedback for improving motor learning.

The Program Is Stored in Memory for Future Use. Movements are generated from past experiences if success has been recognized (Brooks, 1986). Memories of successful movement are stored in LTM. "Successful" indicates that the sensory feedback generated by the movement matched the sensory outflow at the time the program was generated and accomplished the goal (Gentile, 1972). If attention is directed to the movement so that information concerning it remains in short-term memory (STM) for a time, the memory becomes stored in LTM for future use. However, if the information is lost from STM, it does not become part of LTM, and learning does not take place (Schmidt, 1988). The learned motor skill must be practiced to be retained at the same level of expertise (Brooks, 1986). Expertise is improved by practice with intention to improve.

Reflex-hierarchical models of motor control have been challenged by three interrelated questions: (1) How can the CNS control the many **degrees of freedom** of each movement (i.e., the large number of joints, planes of motion within each joint, muscles that control each joint, and single motor units within each muscle) without specifying the details of the muscle activation pattern? (Bernstein, 1967). If the CNS does specify the details, each motor program would be extremely complex. (2) How many motor programs would be needed to perform the numerous tasks that humans perform in everyday life? It is likely that an extremely large number would be necessary, which creates a storage problem for the brain. (3) How many motor programs would be needed to perform a given task in varied contexts? Studies (Marteniuk et al., 1987; Mathiowetz & Wade, 1995) have demonstrated that small changes in environmental context can result in unique movement patterns during simple reaching tasks. Thus, the environment has a larger role in motor control than the reflex-hierarchical model would suggest, and it seems that an incomprehensible number of motor programs would be necessary to respond to various contexts. Does the brain have unlimited storage capacity to accommodate all of the motor programs, even generalized motor programs? Probably not. An alternative explanation of motor behavior is explored after the neurophysiological approach is fully presented.

Neuromaturational Theory of Motor Development

The neuromaturational theory of motor development (McGraw, 1945; Gesell, 1954) has influenced the neurophysiological approaches in various ways (Heriza, 1991). It suggests that changes in motor development are due to maturation of the nervous system. In other words, changes in neural structures cause changes in motor function (McGraw, 1945). This implies that the environment plays a minimal role in motor development. If this were true, a child's experiences and therapist's interventions would have little influence on motor development.

Developmental sequences are also an integral part of neuromaturational theory. Gesell (1954) proposed that development progresses through a particular sequence. Although he acknowledged that the rate of development was variable among children, he believed that the sequence was invariant and that it followed a particular direction: cephalic to caudal and proximal to distal.

When neuromaturational theory and its developmental sequences are used as a guide in therapy, it is assumed that treatment must start at the patient's current developmental level. Developmental and reflex testing serve as primary assessment tools (Bobath, 1978; Fiorentino, 1973). For treatment, it is assumed a patient

must master the current developmental level before progressing to the next level (Rood, 1954). If patients master the developmental sequence, these motor skills are assumed to generalize to task performance. It is thought that working on specific functional tasks will result in **splinter skills**, which will not generalize and may in fact interfere with a child's progression through the developmental sequence. As a result, the development of movement skills is emphasized at the expense of functional performance.

Neuromaturational theories have also been used to explain motor problems seen in adults with CNS damage. It is believed that CNS damage frees lower centers from higher-level control, resulting in a release of primitive reflexes and abnormal muscle tone (Bobath, 1990). Neurophysiological approaches focus on a progression through the developmental sequence, inhibition of primitive reflexes and spasticity, and facilitation of higher-level control. Some of these concepts are still used in practice; others have been modified or discarded.

Motor Dysfunction Due to CNS Lesions

The view of the neurophysiological approaches is that motor dysfunctions that follow CNS damage (Box 5-2) are understood best by knowing the site and extent of the lesions (Cheney, 1985). It is assumed that specific areas of the brain serve specific functions. Therefore, if a given area of the brain is damaged, its associated function is expected to be impaired.

Cortical Lesions

Local cortical lesions, such as occur as a result of cerebrovascular accident or penetrating injury, result in deficits in motor planning or execution of voluntary goal-directed movement, depending on the particular cortical area damaged. Although patients may be unable to move a segment of a limb in isolation, they are often able to move the whole limb in a stereotyped way because lower levels of the CNS that control this function are spared. However, even in patients who seem to have similar lesions, dysfunction varies because of the complexity of the control options available to the CNS and the way each individual uses them (Scholz & Campbell, 1980). Diffuse lesions such as those seen after closed head injury can result in extensive damage to cortical areas and deeper structures of the brain. The motor dysfunction includes deficits described earlier plus any deficits associated with the lower level areas involved.

The motor deficits of cortical damage can be described as both positive and negative (Burke, 1988). The positive features are phenomena that are released from the inhibitory control of the cortex: exaggerated reflexes, spasticity, and the hemiplegic posture. The

BOX 5-2
Motor Dysfunction Due to CNS Lesions

Cortical Lesions

► *Hemiplegic posture or pattern of spasticity* includes retraction and depression of the scapula; internal rotation of the shoulder; flexion of the elbow, wrist, and fingers; pronation of the forearm; lateral flexion of the trunk toward the involved side; elevation and retraction of the pelvis; internal rotation of the hip; extension of the hip and knee; supination of the foot; and plantar flexion of the ankle and toes (Bobath, 1990).

► *Hypotonia* (decreased muscle tone or flaccidity) is less than normal resistance to passive elongation; the affected limb feels limp and heavy.

► *Hypertonia* (increased muscle tone) is more than normal resistance of a muscle to passive elongation. Both neural (spasticity) and mechanical (soft tissue stiffness) factors cause it.

► *Spasticity*, the neural component of hypertonus, is characterized by a velocity-dependent increase in tonic stretch reflexes and exaggerated tendon reflexes (Katz & Rymer, 1989). It is commonly accompanied by muscle clonus and the clasp knife reflex.

► *Clonus* is the oscillating contraction and relaxation of a limb segment due to the alternating pattern of stretch reflex and inverse stretch reflex of a spastic muscle.

► *Clasp knife phenomenon or reflex* is resistance to passive stretch of a spastic muscle that suddenly gives way, like the blade of a jackknife.

► *Weakness* is the inability to generate the necessary force for effective motor action.

► *Loss of fractionation* is the inability to move a single joint without producing unnecessary movements in other joints resulting in stereotyped movement patterns instead of selective, flexible movement patterns.

► *Apraxia* is the inability to perform goal-directed motor activity in the absence of paresis, ataxia, sensory loss, or abnormal muscle tone. Apraxia is characterized by omissions, disturbed order of submovements within a sequence, clumsiness, perseveration, and inability to gesture or use common tools or utensils.

► *Lead pipe rigidity* is characterized by hypertonus in both agonist and antagonist muscles, with resistance to movement that is not velocity dependent and that is felt throughout the range of motion.

Cerebellar Lesions

► *Intention tremor* is the rhythmic oscillating movement that develops during precise intentional movements due to involuntary alternating contractions of opposing muscles.

► *Dysmetria* is the inability to judge distances accurately; it results in overshooting or undershooting a specific target.

► *Decomposition of movement*, or *dyssynergia*, is characterized by movements that are broken up into a series of successive simple movements rather than one smooth movement involving multiple joints.

► *Dysdiadochokinesia* is impairment in the ability to perform repeated alternating movements, such as pronation and supination, rapidly and smoothly.

► *Adiadochokinesia* is the loss of ability to perform rapid alternating movements.

► *Ataxia* is unsteadiness, incoordination, or clumsiness of movement.

► *Ataxic gait* is a wide-based, unsteady, staggering gait with a tendency to veer from side to side.

Lesions of the Basal Ganglia

► *Tremors at rest*, or *non–intention tremors*, stop at the initiation of voluntary movement but resume during the holding phase of a motor task when attention wanes or is diverted to another task. Tremors at rest are fatiguing.

► *Cogwheel rigidity* is characterized by rhythmic interrupted resistance of the muscles being stretched when the wrist or elbow is flexed quickly.

► *Hypokinesia* is slowness or poverty of movement. It includes *akinesia*, difficulty initiating voluntary movements, and *bradykinesia*, slowness in carrying out movements. These symptoms are reflected in lack of facial expression, monotone speech, reduced eye movements, diminished arm swing during walking, decreased balance and equilibrium responses seen in Parkinson's disease.

► *Festinating gait* is characterized by small, fast, shuffling steps that propel the body forward at an increasing rate and by difficulty stopping or changing directions.

► *Athetosis* is characterized by slow, writhing involuntary movements, particularly in the neck, face, and extremities. Athetosis ceases during sleep. Muscle tone may be increased or decreased.

► *Dystonia* is characterized by powerful, sustained contractions of muscles that cause twisting and writhing of a limb or of the whole body, often resulting in distorted postures of the trunk and proximal extremities.

► *Chorea* is characterized by sudden involuntary purposeless, rapid, jerky movements and/or grimacing, primarily in the distal extremities and face (e.g., Huntington's chorea).

► *Hemiballismus* is unilateral chorea in which there are violent, forceful, flinging movements of the extremities on one side of the body, particularly involving the proximal musculature.

Primary source: Fredericks & Saladin, 1996.

negative features are weakness and abnormal coordination. The neurophysiological approaches assume that the positive symptoms have the most devastating effect on the motor function of cortically damaged patients. They also assume that until the positive symptoms are corrected, the negative deficits cannot be improved (Bobath, 1978). There is growing evidence to doubt these assumptions (Bourbonnais et al., 1989; Nwaobi,

1983). In fact, Burke (1988) suggested that the negative features affect function more than the positive features.

Motor control is abnormal not only because of the motor deficits but also because of deficits in sensation, cognition, and perception. Patients with sensory loss due to a cortical lesion cannot use the affected limb spontaneously. However, they can compensate for the loss using intact sensory systems when directed to do so (Jeannerod et al., 1984). The sensory loss seriously affects the ability to sustain a constant level of force needed to hold an object or to maintain a posture. In the case of impaired sensation, movement is affected by the distortion, and the patient needs to relearn the meaning of the new sensations through active movement. No relearning occurs during passive movement, even if the patient watches the movement (Gentile, 1972). Sensory problems are covered in more detail in Chapters 6 and 27.

Deficits in cognitive and perceptual processing can affect motor control as well. Perceptual processing entails accurate interpretation of sensory stimuli from the internal and external environment. A patient with poor depth perception has problems in reaching for objects. Cognitive processing involves orientation, attention span, memory, and problem solving. Patients with impaired memory have problems learning new tasks because they can't remember how they were instructed to perform them or the task itself. Cognition and perception are covered in more detail in Chapters 7, 8, 28 and 29.

Cerebellar Lesions

Symptoms of cerebellar lesions (Box 5-2) reflect timing abnormalities and problems with the rate, range, and force of a movement. The basis for these deficits is a combination of delayed initiation of preprogrammed patterns and delayed termination of agonistic muscular activity, which result in delayed or missing initiation of the antagonist (Brooks, 1986). These patients are able to carry out voluntary programmed movement of a limb but lack the fine adjustments needed for end-point accuracy.

Basal Ganglia Lesions

The basal ganglia control automatic rhythmical patterned movements and the initiation of automatic (learned) movements. Lesions of the basal ganglia (e.g., Parkinson's disease) result in problems of voluntary movement, such as akinesia and bradykinesia, and of involuntary movements, such as tremor at rest and rigidity (Phillips & Stelmach, 1996).

For the most part, diseases of the cerebellum or basal ganglia are degenerative, and recovery arising from neural changes is not expected. Therefore, treatment focuses on compensation for the deficits. In contrast, some recovery is expected after traumatic injury to the cerebellum and basal ganglia.

View of Recovery After CNS Lesions

The view of the neurophysiological approaches is that recovery after CNS lesions is due to changes in the CNS. Recovery from cortical lesions is believed to follow a developmental sequence from reflex to voluntary control, from mass to discrete movements, and from proximal to distal control. Recovery can stop at any level along the continua, and this is not totally predictable. The speed of early spontaneous recovery offers a clue to the ultimate level of function to be gained (Twitchell, 1951).

There is insufficient evidence to determine what exactly is responsible for recovery (Craik, 1991; Moore, 1986). Some believe that the changes after CNS damage are due to natural neurological recovery only (i.e., changes that occur when there is no therapeutic intervention), while others believe they are due to therapeutic interventions. Recovery probably results from both (Bach-y-Rita, 1993). However, that does not explain the underlying mechanisms that account for these changes.

Bishop (1982) suggested neuronal plasticity as an explanation for the recovery seen after CNS damage. Some examples of plasticity include use of remaining pathways in systems with bilateral tracts, recruitment of silent synapses or latent pathways, and sprouting of axonal branches to form new synapses (Craik, 1991; Moore, 1986). Thus, recovery can occur because of a takeover of function by spared tissue and/or by morphological reorganization. None of the recovery mechanisms seem universal for a specific type of lesion. People recover differently, because no two brains are alike structurally or functionally (Moore, 1986). Therapists attempt to enhance neuronal plasticity in the rehabilitation of patients with CNS lesions.

Evaluations Used by Neurophysiological Approaches

Given the assumptions of the neurophysiological approaches (Box 5-1), the evaluations of patients focus primarily on abilities and capacities impaired by CNS damage. These include muscle tone, abnormal reflexes and movement patterns, postural control, sensation (see Chapter 6), perception (see Chapter 7), and cognition (see Chapter 8). In addition, it is important to determine the patient's stage of recovery or developmental level. Finally, occupational performance (see Chapter 3) is evaluated secondarily on the assumption that any deficits in these areas are due to impaired performance components. This bottom-up evaluation framework is not consistent with the model of occupational functioning (see Chapter 1).

Muscle Tone Evaluations
Muscle Tone and Associated Factors
Muscle tone is defined as the resistance of a muscle to passive elongation or stretching (Stolov, 1966). Slight resistance in response to passive movement characterizes normal muscle tone. When the therapist moves the arm, it feels relatively light, and if the therapist lets go of it, it is able to maintain the position. *Hypotonia* is less than normal resistance to passive elongation. When the therapist moves the arm, it feels floppy and heavy. If the therapist lets go of it, it cannot maintain the position or resist the effects of gravity. *Hypertonia*, more than normal resistance of a muscle to passive elongation, is due to neural and mechanical factors. The neural factor (i.e., spasticity) is due to hyperactive stretch reflexes frequently seen after CNS damage. In a spastic muscle, there is a range of free movement, then a strong contraction of the muscle in response to stretch (i.e., stretch reflex), and free movement again when the muscle suddenly relaxes (i.e., clasp knife phenomenon or reflex) (Fredericks & Saladin, 1996). Thus, spasticity is not synonymous with hypertonus. The mechanical factors of hypertonus are the elastic properties of connective tissue and the viscoelastic properties of muscle. The mechanical factors change if a muscle is immobilized in a shortened or lengthened position (i.e., there is increased or decreased resistance to passive elongation) (Stolov, 1966). The neural changes after CNS damage—spasticity—contribute to abnormal positioning of limbs, which causes secondary changes in the mechanical factors. Together the neural and mechanical factors account for increased resistance to passive elongation—hypertonus—that is seen after CNS damage.

Muscle tone is measured clinically by observing the response of a muscle to passive stretch. A problem in measuring hypertonus, especially the neural factor, is the high variation in spasticity from day to day in the same subject. The reliability of a test is affected by the speed of the passive test movement because the tonic stretch reflexes are velocity dependent (Katz & Rymer, 1989). Reliability is also affected by effort, emotional stress, temperature, fatigue, changes in concurrent sensory stimulation, urinary tract infections, and head position (Sloan et al., 1992). Rigid standardization of the test procedure must be the rule; otherwise the findings may be misleading. Poor evaluation techniques that allow high test–retest variability may obscure therapeutic effectiveness.

Modified Ashworth Scale
Ashworth (1964) proposed a qualitative scale for assessing the degree of spasticity as part of a drug study. The resistance encountered to passive movement through the full available range was rated on a five-point scale ranging from "no increase in muscle tone" to "limb rigid in flexion and extension." Although it was described as a measure of spasticity, it is a measure of muscle tone. Bohannon and Smith (1987) modified the *Ashworth Scale* (Box 5-3) by adding an additional level (1+), by incorporating the angle at which resistance first appeared, and by controlling the speed of the passive movement with a one second count. The examiner performs five to eight repetitions of the movement before assigning the rating.

There have been several studies of the reliability of the *Modified Ashworth Scale*. Bohannon and Smith (1987) reported an 86.7% agreement between two raters and a very high correlation, $\tau = .847$, which support the interrater reliability of the modified scale for assessing elbow flexors of persons with CNS dysfunction (N = 30). Sloan et al. (1992) reported the interrater reliability for elbow flexion ($r_s = .67$), elbow extension ($r_s = .73$), and knee flexion ($r_s = .45$) in 34 persons who had had a stroke. The high correlations for the elbow suggest adequate reliability, whereas the moderate correlation for the knee suggests inadequate reliability. Allison et al.

BOX 5-3
PROCEDURES FOR PRACTICE

Modified Ashworth Scale for Grading Spasticity

Grade	Description
0	No increase in muscle tone
1	Slight increase in muscle tone manifested by a catch and release or by minimal resistance at the end of the range of motion when the affected part or parts are moved in flexion or extension
1+	Slight increase in muscle tone manifested by a catch, followed by minimal resistance throughout the remainder (less than half) of the ROM
2	Marked increase in muscle tone through most of the ROM, but affected parts are easily moved
3	Considerable increase in muscle tone; passive movement difficult
4	Affected part or parts rigid in flexion or extension

Reprinted with permission from Bohannon, R. W., and Smith, M. B. (1987). Interrater reliability of a *Modified Ashworth Scale* of muscle spasticity. *Physical Therapy, 67,* p. 207. Copyright 1987 by American Physical Therapy Association.

(1996) assessed plantar flexion spasticity in patients with traumatic brain injury. They reported interrater reliability (r_s = .73 and 55% agreement), intrarater reliability (rater 1, r_s = .74 and 53% agreement; rater 2, r_s = .55 and 48% agreement), and test–retest reliability (r_s = .82 and 58% agreement). The high correlations for interrater and test–retest reliability suggest adequate reliability, but the low percent agreements throughout suggest marginal reliability. In conclusion, reliability of the *Modified Ashworth Scale* is adequate for the elbow but is questionable for the knee and ankle.

Efforts to establish the concurrent validity of the *Modified Ashworth Scale* are limited by the lack of a gold standard with which to compare it (Katz & Rymer, 1989). Skold et al. (1998) compared it to EMG recordings in persons with spinal cord injury. Although the results overall were mixed, they provided some evidence of concurrent validity with EMG recordings. Allison and Abraham (1995) compared the *Modified Ashworth Scale* with three possible quantitative measures of spasticity on patients with traumatic brain injury. They reported low to moderate correlations (r_s = .39–.49), which indicates that only 15 to 24% of the variance is held in common. In conclusion, additional studies on the validity of the *Modified Ashworth Scale* are needed. Despite its limitations, the *Modified Ashworth Scale* is the best available measure of muscle tone and the most widely cited in the literature (Sloan et al., 1992).

Evaluation of Motor Function and Balance
Fugl-Meyer Assessment
The *Fugl-Meyer Assessment* (*FMA*) was developed to evaluate motor function, balance, some aspects of sensation, and joint function in persons post stroke (Fugl-Meyer et al., 1975). The items were based on earlier studies on the sequential stages of motor recovery post stroke (e.g., Brunnstrom, 1970; Twitchell, 1951). Most items are scored on a three-point ordinal scale (0, cannot be performed; 1, performed partly; 2, performed faultlessly). The maximum points are 66 for the upper extremity, 34 for lower extremity, 14 for balance, 24 for sensation, 24 for position sense, 44 for range of motion, and 44 for joint pain (total possible score, 250). Each section can be scored separately. See Fugl-Meyer et al. (1975) for test procedures and scoring criteria. The procedures for the upper extremity subtest are described in Chapter 24.

Duncan et al. (1983) reported that the interrater reliability of the upper and lower extremity subtests ranged from r = .79 to .99 and intrarater reliability ranged from .86 to .99. These data support the reliability of *FMA* for poststroke evaluation. A number of studies have provided evidence in support of the content and construct validity of the *FMA*. For example, actual motor recovery post stroke parallels the test items (Fugl-Meyer et al., 1975). Wood-Dauphinee et al. (1990) reported significant correlations between the *FMA* and the *Barthel Index*, a measure of self-care abilities. Duncan et al. (1994) used the *FMA* to document that recovery of motor function for the upper and lower extremities is similar. The *FMA* is widely used in outcome studies and is a recommended assessment of motor function in the Agency for Health Care Policy and Research (AHCPR) clinical practice guidelines for poststroke rehabilitation (Gresham et al., 1995).

The *FMA* has some limitations. The test is long (30 to 45 minutes for the upper and lower extremity sections alone). The items of the *FMA* appear to have little relevance to everyday activities, in contrast to the *Motor Assessment Scale* (*MAS*), an alternative measure of motor function described later in the chapter. Malouin et al. (1994) questioned the validity of testing balance in static positions only when most functional activities require dynamic balance.

Tests of Balance and Other Automatic Protective Reactions
Bobath (1990) suggested that abnormal postural tone and movement patterns that follow CNS lesions are due to "disinhibition" (i.e., the release of lower level reflex activity from higher level inhibitory control). She suggested that associated reactions, asymmetrical tonic neck reflex, and positive supporting reactions specifically interfere with normal balance and movement. Thus, in her qualitative tests of balance and other reactions, she is looking for evidence of these reflex responses. Patients are asked or assisted in assuming developmental positions—supine, prone on elbows, on hands and knees, kneeling, half-kneeling, sitting, and standing—to observe their responses to the position, to self-initiated movement, and to being pushed by the therapist. (Bobath [1990] describes this in detail.) Scoring entails checking whether the patient's response was normal or not. A major limitation of these tests is the lack of reliability and validity data.

Task-Related Approaches
Assumptions of the Task-Related Approaches

The assumptions of the occupational therapy (OT) task-oriented approach are listed in Box 5-1. They originate from recent motor behavior and movement science literature, specifically a systems model of motor behavior, a systems view of motor development, and recent motor learning theories. Carr and Shepherd's (1987) *Motor Relearning Programme for Stroke* (see Chapter 22) is also based on recent motor behavior research. The assumptions of their program (p. 5):

▶ Regaining the ability to perform motor tasks such as walking, reaching, and standing up is a learning process, and the disabled have the same learning needs as the undisabled; that is, they need to practice, get feedback, understand goals, and so on.

► Motor control is exercised in both anticipatory and ongoing modes, and postural adjustments and focal limb movements are interrelated.

► Control of a specific motor task can best be regained by practice of that specific motor task, and such tasks should be practiced in their various environmental contexts.

► Sensory input related to the motor task helps modulate action.

To understand the evaluation framework of the task-related approaches, it is important to understand the origins of their assumptions.

Systems Model of Motor Control

Over the past 30 years, a new model of motor control has evolved from the ecological approach to perception and action (Gibson, 1979; Turvey, 1977) and from the study of complex dynamical systems in mathematics and the sciences (Gleick, 1987). The new model emphasizes the interaction between persons and environments and suggests that motor behavior emerges from persons' multiple systems interacting with unique task and environmental contexts (Newell, 1986). Thus, the systems model of motor control is more interactive or **heterarchical** and emphasizes the role of the environment more than the reflex-hierarchical model.

In the systems model, the nervous system is only one system among many that influence motor behavior. The nervous system itself is organized heterarchically so that higher centers interact with the lower centers but do not control them. Closed-loop and open-loop systems work cooperatively, and both feedback and feed-forward control are used to achieve task goals. The CNS interacts with multiple personal and environmental systems as a person attempts to achieve a goal.

Ecological Approach to Perception and Action

The ecological approach to perception and action emphasizes the study of interaction between the person and the environment during everyday functional tasks and the close linkage between perception and action (i.e., purposeful movement). Gibson recognized the role of functional goals and the environment in the relationship between perception and action. He stated that direct perception entails the active search for *affordances* (Gibson, 1977), defined as the functional utility of objects for a person and his or her unique characteristics (Warren, 1984). Thus, Gibson's concept of affordances explains the close relationship between perception and action in terms of what the information in the environment means to a specific person.

Bernstein (1967) recognized the importance of the environment and personal characteristics other than the CNS in motor behavior. He suggested that the role a particular muscle plays in a movement depends on the context or circumstances. Bernstein identified three possible sources of variability in muscle function. First is anatomical factors. For example, from kinesiology you know that the pectoralis major muscle will either flex or extend the shoulder, depending on the initial position of the arm. Another example relates to adducting the shoulder. If you want to adduct it quickly or against resistance, the latissimus dorsi contracts. In contrast, if you adduct the shoulder slowly against no resistance, the deltoid muscles contract eccentrically and the latissimus dorsi does not contract. In both cases, the role of the muscle depends on the context in which it is used. A second source of variability is mechanical factors. Many nonmuscular forces, such as gravity and inertia, determine the degree to which a muscle must contract. For example, a muscle must exert much more force to contract against gravity than in a gravity-eliminated plane. Likewise, because of the effects of inertia, the contraction of the elbow flexor muscles is different if the shoulder is flexing or extending at the same time. Again, the effect of a muscle contraction depends on the context. A third source of variability is physiological factors. When higher centers send down a command for a muscle to contract, middle and lower centers have the opportunity to modify the command. Lower and middle centers receive peripheral sensory feedback. Thus, the effect of the command on the muscle varies depending on the context and degree of influence of the middle and lower centers. As a result, the relationship between higher center or executive commands and muscle action is not one-to-one. Trombly and Wu (1999) demonstrated the influence of context on movement. They reported that goal-directed, object-present activity elicited different and more efficient movement patterns than non–goal-directed exercise.

Coordinative structures were proposed as a solution to the degrees-of-freedom problem discussed earlier. *Coordinative structures* are groups of muscles, usually spanning several joints, that are constrained to act as a single functional unit (Turvey, 1977). When learning a new task, a person tends to constrain or stiffen many joints to reduce the degrees of freedom to be controlled. This use of a coordinative structure enables the person to focus on controlling a limited number of joints. Natural tenodesis grasp and release is another example of a coordinative structure. The long flexor and extensor muscles of the forearm are constrained to work together

Case Example

ASSESSMENT USING AN OT TASK-ORIENTED APPROACH

Patient Information

Mr. B. is a 55-year-old man who worked as an administrator at a junior college until a week ago, when he had a left cerebral vascular accident with resultant right hemiparesis. His medical history includes insulin-dependent diabetes mellitus and two heart attacks in the past 5 years. He lives with his wife in a ranch-style house. She works as a middle manager at an electronics firm. They have two adult children who do not live nearby.

The acute-care occupational therapist reported that he is independent in feeding, grooming, oral hygiene, and wheelchair mobility for short distances. He needs assistance with bathing, toilet hygiene, and dressing. Other occupational performance areas were not assessed in acute care. He has weakness throughout his dominant right arm, with grade 2 spasticity on the *Modified Ashworth Scale* for scapular depression, shoulder internal rotation, and elbow, wrist, and finger flexors. PROM is within normal limits except for a 20° limitation in shoulder external rotation and elbow extension.

Description of Assessment

The primary aim of the assessment in the rehabilitation unit was to determine which roles and occupational performance tasks were most important to Mr. B. and to determine his ability on those tasks. The *Role Checklist* was used to identify which roles were most important to him and to identify the tasks and activities that are associated with those roles. The *COPM* was used to determine the occupational performance tasks he wanted or needed to do and to determine his perception of his ability. Task analysis was used with specific tasks he perceived as difficult or impossible. The therapist observed him for performance component deficits that might be limiting function and explored environmental factors that could support or limit his performance.

Results

It was clear from the *Role Checklist* that Mr. B.'s work role was important to him. His concerns about returning to work included problems with writing, word processing, and removing heavy manuals from shelves above his desk. His wife, however, was pushing him to consider early retirement because of his increasing health problems. He and his wife enjoyed entertaining friends at home, for which he was the primary chef. This was an important activity for both of them. Although he was responsible for many home and yard maintenance tasks, these were not important to him. He

thought friends would help them or they could hire help. On the *COPM*, return to work was ranked as most important, followed by cooking, toilet hygiene, dressing, and driving. He rated his performance and satisfaction for all of these tasks as very low.

His performance on several work-related, cooking, and self-care tasks were observed. He had difficulty holding a regular pen. However, a trial with an enlarged pen with a rubber grip enabled him to hold a pen for about 3 minutes and write with very poor legibility. He was unable to use his right hand for keyboarding because he could not isolate individual fingers. He became frustrated while performing a simple cooking task (i.e., making pudding) because he could not walk and had difficulty using his right hand for bilateral tasks. He was able to toilet himself with verbal cueing and standby assistance. During dressing he had difficulty raising his right arm, reaching down to put on his socks (concerned appropriately about balance), and difficulty performing bilateral tasks (e.g., tying his shoelaces). He complained about the time and energy needed to complete functional tasks. He used his right hand in half of the bilateral tasks he attempted. Thus, it appeared that sensorimotor factors might be the cause of the difficulty performing functional tasks, so these were evaluated further.

There was no evidence of unilateral visual neglect on a line bisection test. Sensory testing indicated loss of protective sensation and diminished light touch in the right hand (Semmes-Weinstein monofilaments) and impaired proprioception in the wrist and fingers only. Selective muscle testing indicated grade 3+ in scapular elevation, elbow flexion, and extension; 3– in shoulder flexion, abduction, and external rotation; and wrist flexion and extension. Grip strength in the right hand was 5 pounds, and in the left hand, 80 pounds; key pinch on the right was 3 pounds and on the left, 19 pounds.

Analysis of Findings

The occupational therapist concluded that work and cooking tasks were priorities for this client, followed by self-care tasks. It is not yet clear whether he will be able to return to work. Decreased strength and impaired sensation are limiting the function of the right hand. Decreased PROM of the shoulder external rotation is a concern because it is often associated with development of a painful shoulder. There is no evidence of cognitive or perceptual deficits. Additional information is needed from the client and employer about job requirements and work environment. In addition, more details about the home environment, home management roles and responsibilities, and other leisure interests are necessary.

Occupational Therapy Problem List

1. Decreased ability to perform work, cooking, and self-care tasks because of sensorimotor impairments
2. Decreased strength, PROM, sensibility, and dexterity in his right upper extremity; decreased endurance for activity; mild impairment of sitting balance
3. Insufficient information on home environments to prepare adequately for discharge

CLINICAL REASONING
in OT Practice

Why is Mr. B. not using his right arm and hand as much as he could be?

How can the therapist help Mr. B. and his wife deal with the decision to retire or return to work?

How would the assumptions and assessment differ if you used a neurophysiological approach?

Would that make a difference in the problems you identified?

---

for functional grasp and release. Fitch et al. (1982) suggested that perceptual information could modulate or tune the coordinative structures without intervention from the executive or higher centers. Reed (1982) suggested that postures and movements are modulated as needed by updated perceptual information to achieve the functional goal. Thus, postures and movements are not triggered by external stimulation or central commands, as suggested by the reflex and hierarchical models, but are coordinative structures, capable of adapting to changing circumstances. Thus, the study of motor behavior or action evolved into "the study of how organisms use available information to modulate their actions" (Reed, 1982, p. 110). Turvey (1977) and others have looked to the dynamical systems view as a means to explain the complex interactions between the person and the environment.

Dynamical Systems Theory

The study of dynamical systems originated in mathematics, physics, biology, chemistry, psychology, and kinesiology, and it has been applied to OT, physical therapy, nursing, adapted physical education, and some areas of medicine (Burton & Davis, 1992; Lister, 1991). It has influenced the systems model of motor control as well. Dynamical systems theory proposes that behaviors emerge from the interaction of many systems. Because the behavior is not specified but emergent, it is considered to be self-organizing (Kamm et al., 1990). This concept of **self-organization** is not compatible with the assumptions of the reflex-hierarchical model, which suggests that higher centers or motor programs prescribe movements. Evidence of self-organization is seen in the relatively stable patterns of motor behavior seen in many tasks in spite of the many degrees of freedom available to a person (Thelen & Ulrich, 1991). When we eat or write, we have many choices of ways to perform these tasks, yet we tend to use preferred patterns.

Behavior can change from stable to less stable as a result of aging or CNS damage. In fact, throughout life

behaviors shift between periods of stability and instability. It is during unstable periods, characterized by a high variability of performance, that new types of behaviors may emerge, either gradually or abruptly. These transitions in behavior, called **phase shifts**, are changes from one preferred pattern of coordinated behavior to another. A gradual phase shift occurs when an infant decreases automatic stepping between 2 and 4 months of age. An abrupt phase shift occurs when a person in a hurry walks faster and faster and suddenly changes to a running pattern. How can these changes in behavior be explained?

In the dynamical systems view, **control parameters** are variables that shift behavior from one form to another. They do not control the change but act as agents for reorganization of the behavior to a new form (Heriza, 1991). Control parameters are gradable in some way. In the case of the infant, Thelen and Fisher (1982) demonstrated that the decrease in automatic stepping was due in part to the rapid weight gain during this time. Because infants' muscles are not strong enough to move the heavier legs, automatic stepping decreases. This control parameter, the increase in body weight, shifts the behavior from automatic stepping to no stepping. In the other example, increasing the speed of locomotion elicits the change from a walking to a running pattern. Consequently, speed is considered a control parameter as well.

Explanations of changes in motor behavior in the systems model of motor control are quite different from earlier models. Thelen (1989) stated that an important characteristic of a system perspective is that the shift from one preferred movement pattern to another is marked by discrete, discontinuous transitions. These transitions in motor behavior are the result of changes in only one or a few personal or environmental systems (i.e., control parameters) (Davis & Burton, 1991). Thus, important points are that systems themselves are subject to change and that there is no inherent ordering of systems in terms of their influence on motor behavior.

Systems View of Motor Development

A systems view of motor development suggests that changes over time are due to multiple factors or systems such as maturation of the nervous system, biomechanical constraints and resources, and the influences of the physical and social environment (Heriza, 1991). A systems view also suggests that normal development does not follow a rigid intertask sequence, as the motor milestones suggest (VanSant, 1991b). In fact, children follow variable developmental sequences arising from their unique personal characteristics and environmental contexts. If the traditional intertask developmental sequences are no longer sufficient as a guide for working with children, then they are certainly not appropriate as a guide for working with adults with CNS dysfunction (VanSant, 1991b). In contrast, intratask sequences—developmental sequences within a single skill, such as rising without assistance or reaching to grasp an object—do provide guides for age-appropriate movement patterns (VanSant, 1991b).

Systems Model of Motor Behavior

Figure 5-3 depicts the theoretical basis of the OT task-oriented approach. It illustrates the interaction between the performance components or systems of the person and the performance context or systems of the environment. Occupational performance tasks (i.e., activities of daily living (ADL), work, and play–leisure) and role performance emerge from the interaction between performance components (cognitive, psychosocial, and sensorimotor) and performance contexts (physical, socioeconomic, and cultural). Changes in any one of these systems can affect occupational performance tasks and ultimately role performance. In some cases, only one primary factor may determine occupational performance. In most cases, occupational performance tasks emerge from the interaction of many systems. The ongoing interactions among all components of the model reflect its heterarchical nature.

In addition, any occupational performance task affects the environment in which it occurs and the person acting. For example, a client with hemiplegia who has just become independent in making his own lunch may free his spouse from coming home from work during her lunch hour. It also may mean that certain objects in the kitchen must be kept in accessible places, and the kitchen may not be as orderly as the spouse is used to. Thus, the task of making lunch affects people and objects in the environment. It also affects the person and the associated performance components. The ability to be less dependent on his spouse may improve the client's self-esteem (i.e., psychosocial subsystem). The

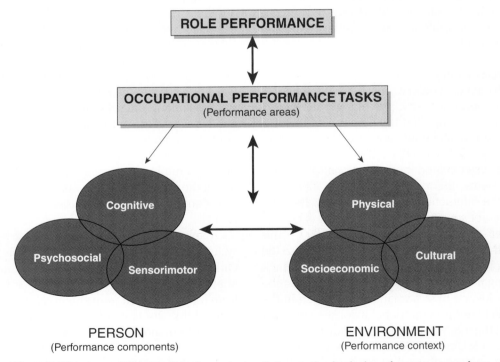

Figure 5-3 Systems model of motor behavior emphasizes that occupational and role performance emerge from an interaction of the person and the environment and that any occupational performance affects the environment and the person in return. There is also an ongoing interaction between occupational and role performance. All of these interactions are continuous across time.

process of making lunch provides the client the opportunity to solve problems and to discover optimal strategies for performing tasks. This influences a client's cognitive and sensorimotor subsystems and the ability to perform other functional tasks.

The specific components of the systems (i.e., subsystems) that influence occupational performance tasks may be framed in OT terminology (AOTA, 1994). Strength, endurance, range of motion, coordination, sensory awareness, postural control, and perceptual skills are subsystems associated with the sensorimotor system. The psychosocial system includes a person's values, interests, self-concept, social interactions, and self-management skills that can affect occupational performance tasks. Orientation, attention span, memory, problem-solving skills, and learning ability are components of the cognitive system. The performance context includes physical, socioeconomic, and cultural characteristics of the task itself and the broader environment. The physical environment system includes objects, tools, and the natural and built environment, which may limit or enhance task performance. Societal standards (customs, beliefs, values, and behavioral standards) and societal (legal and educational) supports are subsystems of the cultural system, which also could affect occupational performance tasks. Finally, the socioeconomic system includes social supports provided by the family, friends, caregivers, social groups, and community and financial resources, which may influence choice in activities.

The inclusion of role performance in this model reflects a perspective of OT, not motor behavior. Occupational therapists believe the roles that persons want and need to fulfill determine the occupational performance (i.e., the tasks and activities) they need to do. Conversely, the tasks and activities persons are able to do determine what roles they are able to fulfill. Although this model may have applications to all areas of OT practice and to OT theory development, the focus of this chapter is its application to individuals with CNS dysfunction.

View of Recovery After CNS Dysfunction

A client with a damaged CNS attempts to compensate for the lesion to achieve functional goals. Recovery from brain damage is a process of discovering what abilities and capacities remain to enable performance of activities and tasks. CNS damage affects each system differently relative to occupational performance. Therapists must consider all systems as potential variables to explain behavior of each client at a specific time. For example, the flexor pattern of spasticity commonly seen after a stroke is due to various factors in addition to spasticity, such as inability to recruit appropriate

muscles, weakness, soft tissue tightness, and perceptual deficits (Bourbonnais & Vanden Noven, 1989). This pattern may become obligatory because of abnormal positioning and decreased use in functional contexts. Because each client is a unique person and functions in a unique environment, therapists should expect recovery for each client to vary even if the CNS damage is similar.

There is increasing evidence that neural reorganization after a brain lesion reflects the functional demands on the CNS. For example, forced use of the involved limb has improved functional performance in persons more than a year post stroke (Taub et al., 1993). These changes can hardly be attributed to spontaneous recovery. Thus, providing appropriately challenging tasks and environments for those with CNS dysfunction, both in the hospital and at home, appears critical to the maximal rehabilitation of our clients (Bach-y-Rita, 1993).

Evaluations

Evaluation Using the OT Task-Oriented Approach

Evaluation is conducted using a top-down approach consistent with the model of occupational functioning (see Chapter 1). A framework for evaluation is described in Box 5-4. Evaluation efforts focus initially on role and occupational performance because they are the goals of motor behavior. A thorough understanding of the roles that a client wants, needs, or is expected to perform and of the tasks needed to fulfill those roles enables therapists to plan meaningful and motivating treatment programs. After a client has identified the most important role and occupational performance limitations, therapists use task analysis to identify which performance components and/or performance contexts are limiting functional performance. This process may indicate the need for evaluation of selected performance components and/or performance contexts (Fisher & Short-DeGraff, 1993). The emphasis on role and occupational performance in the OT task-oriented approach suggests that evaluation in OT should be primarily at the participation and activities levels rather than the impairment level, using the World Health Organization (1998) terminology. The evaluation process necessitates use of both qualitative and quantitative measures (VanSant, 1990). Therefore, therapists use interviews, skilled observations, and standardized assessments to evaluate their clients. Although the client is the primary source of information, other sources, including the client's records, caregivers, family members, and the physical environment, contribute as well. Next, each step of the evaluation framework is described in more detail.

The first step in evaluation is the assessment of role performance. Trombly (1993) states that satisfactory

BOX 5-4
PROCEDURES FOR PRACTICE

Evaluation Framework for the OT Task-Oriented Approach Based on a Systems Model of Motor Behavior

1. Role Performance
- Identify past roles and whether they can be maintained or must be changed.
- Determine how future roles will be balanced:

Worker, student, volunteer, home maintainer, hobbyist, amateur, participant in organizations, friend, family member, caregiver, religious participant, other?

2. Occupational Performance Tasks: Performance Areas
- ADL: feeding, grooming, functional communication and mobility, dressing, oral and toilet hygiene, bathing, and medications
- Work: home management, care of others, and educational and vocational activities
- Play–leisure: exploration and performance

3. Task Selection and Analysis
- What performance components and/or performance contexts limit or enhance occupational performance?

4. Person: Performance Components
- Cognitive: orientation, attention span, memory, problem solving, learning, and generalization
- Psychosocial: values, interests, self-concept, interpersonal skills, self-expression, coping skills, time management, and self-control
- Sensorimotor: strength, endurance, range of motion, sensory awareness and processing, perceptual processing, and postural control

4. Environment: Performance Context
- Physical: objects, tools, devices, animals, and built and natural environment
- Socioeconomic: social supports, including family, friends, caregivers, social groups, and community and financial resources
- Cultural: societal standards, including customs, beliefs, behavioral standards, and societal supports—legal, educational, and economic

fulfillment of roles is necessary for clients to achieve a sense of efficacy (i.e., competence and self-esteem). These roles may serve a variety of purposes, including development and maintenance of self (self-care), advancement of self or productivity (work), and enhancement of self (leisure). Therapists must determine which roles clients had prior to the onset of disability and which roles they can and cannot do at this time. A discussion of which roles clients want or need to perform in the future helps therapists to determine which roles are most important to their clients. In addition, therapists must explore how any role changes have affected or will affect their client and their families, especially the primary caregivers. Jongbloed et al. (1993) suggested that therapists ask questions such as these: "How have roles changed since the disability? How have family members reacted to these changes? Is there role flexibility when needed? How competently do members perform roles?" (p. 76). These questions may have to be adapted to the respondent's level of understanding. The evaluation of role performance must include both the client and significant others.

Although role performance can be assessed using a nonstandardized, semistructured interview, a standardized assessment tool such as the *Role Checklist* (Barris et al., 1988) is recommended. The *Role Checklist* is a written inventory designed for adolescents and adults with physical dysfunction. In part 1, clients indicate which of 10 roles (Box 5-4) they have performed in the past, are performing in the present, and plan to perform in the future. In part 2, clients indicate the value of each role to them. Other role assessment tools may be appropriate depending on the type of client and the setting. For example, if a client is undergoing major role changes and there is sufficient time for a comprehensive assessment, the *Role Change Assessment* for older adults (Rogers & Holm, 1999) is recommended. Detailed information on the assessment of role performance and other role assessment tools is presented in Chapter 3. After clients have identified the roles that they want or need to perform, it is easier for them to identify the tasks and activities needed to fulfill each role.

The second step in the evaluation process is the assessment of occupational performance tasks: ADL, work, and play–leisure (Box 5-4). Because roles, tasks, activities, and their contexts are unique to each person, a client-centered assessment tool such as the *Canadian Occupational Performance Measure* (*COPM*) (Law et al.,

1998) is recommended. It was designed to measure a client's perception of his or her occupational performance over time. A semistructured interview is used to administer the *COPM*. First, clients are asked to identify problem areas in self-care, productivity, and leisure. Second, the importance of each problem area is rated. Third, clients rate their own performance and their satisfaction with the performance. The importance ratings assist therapists in setting treatment priorities. The performance and satisfaction ratings can be used as outcome measures to assess change across time. When therapists are concerned that a client may not provide accurate information because of a cognitive impairment or age, a caregiver may be interviewed, or direct observation of selected activities can be used to validate the information. The information elicited by the *COPM* is unique to each client and his or her environmental context, which is critical to the OT task-oriented approach.

The *Assessment of Motor and Process Skills (AMPS)* is another recommended measure of occupational performance, specifically personal and instrumental ADL (Fisher, 1999). It is a client-centered assessment because the person chooses two or three ADL tasks to be performed, which ensures familiarity and relevance to the person being evaluated. The purpose of the *AMPS* is "to determine whether or not a person has the necessary motor and process skills to effortlessly, efficiently, safely and independently perform the ADL tasks needed for community living" (Fisher, 1999, p. 4). Because the *AMPS* has been standardized internationally and cross-culturally, it is appropriate for persons from diverse backgrounds and with diverse needs and interests. A unique feature of the *AMPS* is that it can adjust, through Rasch analysis, for the difficulty of tasks performed and the severity of the rater who scores the client's performance. In addition, it allows a therapist to compare the performance of clients who performed one set of tasks on initial evaluation with the results of a reevaluation on a different set of tasks. A limitation of the *AMPS* is that it requires a 5-day training and calibration workshop to learn how to administer the assessment reliably and validly. Computer software, which is required to score the *AMPS*, is provided with the workshop. Because the *AMPS* requires observation of clients performing occupational performance tasks, it also assists the third step in the evaluation process.

While evaluating occupational performance, therapists must observe both the outcome and the process (i.e., the preferred movement patterns, their stability or instability, the flexibility to use other patterns, efficiency of the patterns, and ability to learn new strategies) to understand the motor behaviors used to compensate and to achieve functional goals. It is important to determine the stability of the motor behavior, because it will help determine the feasibility of achieving behavioral change in treatment. Behaviors that are very stable require a great amount of time and effort to change. Behaviors that are unstable are in transition, the optimal time for eliciting behavioral change. Thus, a compensatory approach may be most appropriate when behaviors are stable, and a remediation approach may be more appropriate when behaviors are unstable. Evaluation of the process of task performance is likely to require use of both quantitative and qualitative measures. We expect development of clinical process measures to occur in the next decade.

The third step is task selection and analysis. The tasks selected for observation should be ones that clients have identified as important but difficult. Task analysis requires therapists to observe their clients performing one or more occupational performance tasks. In most cases, observation of performance will happen as part of the second step. Therapists use task or activity analysis (see Chapter 11) to evaluate task requirements and personal characteristics to determine whether there is a match that enables task performance within a relevant environment. If not, therapists attempt to determine which performance components and/or performance contexts are interfering with occupational performance. In dynamical systems theory, these are considered the critical control parameters, or the variables that have the potential to shift behavior to a new level of task performance. Each person with CNS dysfunction has unique strengths, limitations, and environmental context. As a result, the critical control parameters that limit or support occupational performance are also unique. As persons and their environments change over time, the critical control parameters also change.

The identification of critical control parameters is the most challenging part of the evaluation. However, there is evidence in the research literature that some performance components and/or environmental variables may be critical control parameters for persons with CNS dysfunction. Gresham et al. (1979) reported that psychosocial and environmental factors were significant determinants of functional deficits long after stroke. In a review, Gresham et al. (1995) reported that 11 to 68% of individuals post stroke have depression, with 10 to 27% meeting the criteria for major depression. In the cognitive area, Rao et al. (1991) reported that 43% of those with multiple sclerosis had cognitive impairments of recent memory and sustained attention. In the sensorimotor area, weakness (Olsen, 1990), fatigue (Ingles et al., 1999), impaired motor function (Bernspang et al., 1987), and visuospatial deficits (Titus et al., 1991) are associated with poorer functional outcomes. For example, Bernspang et al. (1987) reported that motor function measured with the *FMA* was moderately correlated ($r = .64$) with self-care ability.

One caution is that most of these studies were correlational, which indicate relationships between these variables and functional performance but do not establish a causal link. Also, most correlations were moderate or low, which indicates that any one variable explains a relatively small percentage of the variance associated with functional performance. However, Reding and Potes (1988) provided evidence that as the number of performance component impairments increased, functional outcomes decreased. Thus, multiple variables contribute to functional performance for most individuals with CNS dysfunction. The challenge is to identify the variables that are most important to your clients.

Bobath (1990) suggested that spasticity is the primary cause of motor deficits in individuals with CNS dysfunction and that weakness and decreased range of motion are due to spastic antagonists. However, there is increasing evidence that spasticity is not a critical control parameter (Bourbonnais & Vanden Noven, 1989). For example, Sahrmann and Norton (1977) reported EMG findings indicating that movements were limited not by antagonist stretch reflexes (spasticity) but by delayed initiation and cessation of agonist contraction. Similarly, Fellows et al. (1994) found no relation between movement impairments and passive muscle hypertonia in the antagonist muscles. O'Dwyer et al. (1996) found no relation between spasticity and either weakness or loss of dexterity. Thus, research evidence challenges the assumption that spasticity causes the weakness and decreased range of motion often seen in individuals with CNS dysfunction.

After identifying the variables that support or constrain occupational performance, the therapist must assess the interactions of these systems. Consider two clients who have small limitations in shoulder flexion. The role and tasks of client as worker may or may not be affected. If the worker is a carpenter, the interaction of this personal limitation with the demands of the work environment is likely to make nailing overhead, installing cabinets, and hanging doors difficult or impossible. However, a worker who is a word processor probably can do most tasks adequately, because the interaction of personal characteristics and the performance context does not interfere with task performance. This part of the evaluation requires a qualitative assessment and clinical reasoning by the therapist using the information gathered.

The fourth step in the evaluation process is to perform specific assessments of the performance components and/or performance contexts, which are thought to be critical control parameters. The critical control variables are the only ones that must be evaluated. The evaluation of selected variables according to the OT task-oriented approach contrasts with bottom-up approaches that evaluate all component variables. This selective approach eliminates the need to evaluate variables that have little functional implication and saves therapists' time, which is critical for cost containment.

It is likely that occupational therapists will use a variety of measures in their evaluation of the performance components and/or performance contexts that constrain or support occupational performance. Some assessments are designed to examine one or more components within the context of occupational performance. The *Fatigue Impact Scale* (Fisk et al., 1994) was developed to evaluate the perceived effect of fatigue on the everyday lives of those with multiple sclerosis. Assessment of cognitive function through a functional task is the focus of the *Allen Cognitive Level Scale* (Allen, 1985). The *A-One Evaluation* (Arnadattoir, 1990) facilitates evaluation of perceptual and cognitive systems within the context of ADL. From a task-oriented perspective, these are preferred assessment tools because they closely link performance components to occupational performance. In contrast, most assessments of performance components are conducted independent of occupational performance (See Chapters 4 and 6–8 for specific assessments).

Evaluation of critical performance contexts is an important part of the fourth step of the evaluation. The inclusion of physical, social, and cultural environments in AOTA (1994) uniform terminology acknowledges their important influence on occupational performance. Dunn (1993) and Spencer et al. (1993) emphasized the importance of assessing environmental context as part of the overall evaluation process. Chapters 9 and 10 review assessments for these variables.

Evaluation Using Carr and Shepherd's Approach

Carr and Shepherd (1987, 1998) developed their approach in response to disillusionment with the neurophysiological approaches and attempts to apply recent motor behavior research to clinical practice. Although Carr and Shepherd are physical therapists, their approach to optimizing motor performance is relevant to occupational therapy because it emphasizes the relearning of daily activities and provides a task-related strategy for improving motor control (Sabari, 1995). Their most recent book (Carr & Shepherd, 1998) describes in detail how they approach evaluation. Their most important contribution to evaluation is their *MAS*, a recommended test of motor function in the AHCPR clinical practice guidelines for poststroke rehabilitation (Gresham et al., 1995). In addition, they deserve credit for their strong emphasis on task analysis as part of the evaluation (see Chapter 22).

Motor Assessment Scale

Carr et al. (1985) developed the *MAS* as an easily administered and relatively brief (15–30 minutes) assessment relevant to everyday motor activities (Box 5-5). Carr et al. reported very high interrater reliability ($r = .95$ and overall average of 87% agreement between raters) and test–retest reliability ($r = .98$) on clients post stroke. Poole and Whitney (1988) confirmed the very high interrater reliability ($r_s = .99$) and established concurrent validity for the total *MAS* score with the total *FMA* score (Fugl-Meyer et al., 1975) ($r_s = .88$) on clients averaging 12 months post stroke. The concurrent validity of selected items of the two assessments ranged from $r_s = .28$ for balance in sitting to $r_s = .91$ for total upper extremity. A low correlation was expected for balance in sitting because the *MAS* measures dynamic balance, whereas the *FMA* measures static balance (Poole & Whitney, 1988). Malouin et al. (1994) reported remarkably similar concurrent validity data on individuals averaging 2 months post stroke. With the exception of balanced sitting, these results support the concurrent validity of these two assessments of motor function on clients post stroke. One limitation of the *MAS* is that several studies (Dean & Mackey, 1992; Malouin et al., 1994; Poole & Whitney, 1988) provided evidence that the scoring hierarchy for the advanced hand activities may not be sequenced correctly. A second limitation is that the *MAS* is less sensitive to change than the *FMA* in those with severe strokes (Malouin et al., 1994). In contrast, the

balance and locomotion subtests of the *MAS* were more closely associated with sensory recovery than the *FMA* (Malouin et al., 1994). Items from the *MAS* are predictive of motor outcomes of clients post stroke. For example, the score for arm function at 1 week ($r_s = .84$) and at 1 month ($r_s = .91$) are good predictors of arm function at discharge (Loewen & Anderson, 1990). Because reliability and validity data for individual subtests of the *MAS* are available, one or more subtests can be used with each client. However, the *MAS* total score across the subtests should not be used because it is an ordinal scale (Carr & Shepherd, 1998). Dean and Mackey (1992) demonstrated the sensitivity of the *MAS* by reporting significant improvements for clients post stroke on all subtests as a result of an inpatient rehabilitation program. *MAS* has been successfully used as an outcome measure in other published efficacy studies of clinical intervention (e.g., Ada & Westwood, 1992).

Balance Scale

The *Balance Scale* (Berg et al., 1992) is not associated with a particular neurophysiological or task-related approach. It is compatible with the task-related approaches because it evaluates clients' performance on 14 items common in everyday life. The items include "the subject's ability to maintain positions of increasing difficulty by diminishing the base of support from sitting, to comfortable stance, to standing with feet together, and finally tandem standing (i.e., one foot in front of the other) and single leg stance, the two most difficult items. Other items assess how well the subject is able to change positions from sitting to standing, transfer from chair to chair, turn, pick up an object from the floor, and sit down. All items are graded on a five-point scale, 0 to 4. Points are based on the time the position can be maintained, the distance the arm is able to reach forward, or the time to complete the task" (Berg et al., 1992, p. 1074–1075). The test takes about 15 minutes to administer and requires only a watch and ruler.

Berg et al. (1989) assessed the reliability of the *Balance Scale* using 5 raters, who scored the videotaped performances of 14 subjects on two occasions. They reported very high intraclass correlation coefficients (ICC = .98) for both intrarater and interrater reliability, which demonstrates excellent agreement. In addition, internal consistency was high (Cronbach's $\alpha = .96$), which means the scale measures one construct.

Berg et al. (1992) provided evidence of the test's validity. They reported high to very high correlations between the *Balance Scale* and other clinical measures: *Barthel Mobility* ($r = .67$), *Timed Up-and-Go Test* (Podsiadlo & Richardson, 1991) ($r = .76$), and the *Tinetti Balance Subscale* (r = .91) (Tinetti, 1986). The *Balance Scale* correlated moderately (average $r = -.55$)

with 8 of 10 laboratory tests of balance. These results support the concurrent validity of the scale. Finally, the *Balance Scale* was the most efficient measure for discriminating among participants according to their use of walking aids. This result supports the discriminant validity of the test. The sensitivity of the test as an outcome measure should be studied further. Nevertheless, the *Balance Scale* is a recommended assessment of balance in the AHCPR clinical practice guidelines for poststroke rehabilitation (Gresham et al., 1995). For a broader review of balance assessments, see Whitney et al. (1998).

Summary Review Questions

1. How do the reflex-hierarchical and systems models of motor control differ?
2. How do neuromaturational and systems theories of motor development differ?
3. What types of motor dysfunction are associated with cortical, cerebellar, and basal ganglia lesions of the CNS?
4. What might account for the recovery seen after CNS damage?
5. What are at least four assumptions of the neurophysiological approaches?
6. How would you evaluate abnormal muscle tone and movement patterns?
7. What are at least four assumptions of the OT task-oriented approach?
8. How do evaluations used by the neurophysiological and task-related approaches differ?

Acknowledgment

Thanks to Nancy Flinn, MA, OTR, who uses the OT task-oriented approach in her clinical practice and has provided constructive feedback

References

Ada, L., & Westwood, P. (1992). A kinematic analysis of recovery of the ability to stand up following stroke. *Australian Physiotherapy, 38*, 135–142.

Allen, C. (1985). *Occupational Therapy for Psychiatric Diseases: Measurement and Management of Cognitive Disabilities*. Boston: Little, Brown.

Allison, S. C., & Abraham, L. D. (1995). Correlation of quantitative measures with the *Modified Ashworth Scale* in the assessment of plantar flexor spasticity in patients with traumatic brain injury. *Journal of Neurology, 242*, 699–706.

Allison, S. C., Abraham, L. D., & Petersen, C. L. (1996). Reliability of the *Modified Ashworth Scale* in the assessment of plantar flexor muscle spasticity in patients with traumatic brain injury. *International Journal of Rehabilitation Research, 19*, 67–78.

American Occupational Therapy Association. (1994). Uniform termi-

nology for occupational therapy (3rd ed.). *American Journal of Occupational Therapy, 48*, 1047–1054.

Arnadattoir, G. (1990). *The Brain and Behavior: Assessing Cortical Dysfunction Through Activities of Daily Living*. St. Louis: Mosby.

Ashworth, B. (1964). Preliminary trial of carisoprodol in multiple sclerosis. *Practitioner, 192*, 540–542.

Bach-y-Rita, P. (1993). Recovery from brain damage. *Journal of Neurological Rehabilitation, 6*, 191–199.

Barris, R., Oakley, F., & Kielhofner, G. (1988). The *Role Checklist*. In B. J. Hemphill (Ed.), *Mental Health Assessment in Occupational Therapy* (pp. 73–91). Thorofare, NJ: Slack.

Belen'kii, V., Gurfinkel, V., & Pal'tsev, Y. (1967). Elements of control of voluntary movements. *Biophysics, 12*, 135–141.

Berg, K., Maki, B., Williams, J. I., Holliday, P. J., & Wood-Dauphinee, S. (1992). Clinical and laboratory measures of postural balance in an elderly population. *Archives of Physical Medicine & Rehabilitation, 73*, 1073–1080.

Berg, K., Wood-Dauphinee, S., Williams, J. I., & Gayton, D. (1989). Measuring balance in the elderly: Preliminary development of an instrument. *Physiotherapy Canada, 41*, 301–311.

Bernspang, B., Asplund, K., Eriksson, S., & Fugl-Meyer, A. R. (1987). Motor and perceptual impairments in acute stroke patients: Effects on self-care ability. *Stroke, 18*, 1081–1086.

Bernstein, N. (1967). *The Coordination and Regulation of Movements*. Elmsford, NY: Pergamon.

Bishop, B. (1982). Neural plasticity: Part IV. Lesion-induced reorganization of the CNS. *Physical Therapy, 62*, 1442–1451.

Bly, L. (1991). A historical and current view of the basis of NDT [neurodevelopmental treatment]. *Pediatric Physical Therapy, 3*, 131–135.

Bobath, B. (1978). *Adult hemiplegia: Evaluation and Treatment* (2nd ed.). London: Heinemann Medical.

Bobath, B. (1990). *Adult Hemiplegia: Evaluation and Treatment* (3rd ed.). Oxford: Butterworth Heinemann.

Bohannon, R. W., & Smith, M. B. (1987a). Interrater reliability of a modified Ashworth scale of muscle spasticity. *Physical Therapy, 67*, 206–207.

Bourbonnais, D., & Vanden Noven, S. (1989). Weakness in patients with hemiparesis. *American Journal of Occupational Therapy, 43*, 313–319.

Brooks, V. B. (1986). *The Neural Basis of Motor Control*. New York: Oxford University.

Brunnstrom, S. (1970). *Movement therapy in hemiplegia*. New York: Harper & Row.

Burke, D. (1988). Spasticity as an adaptation to pyramidal tract injury. In S. G. Waxman (Ed.), *Advances in Neurology. Vol. 47: Functional Recovery in Neurological Disease* (pp. 401–423). New York: Raven.

Burton, A. W., & Davis, W. E. (1992). Optimizing the involvement and performance of children with physical impairments in movement activities. *Pediatric Exercise Science, 4*, 236–248.

Carr, J. H., & Shepherd, R. B. (1987). *A motor relearning programme for stroke* (2nd ed.). Rockville, MD: Aspen.

Carr, J. H., & Shepherd, R. B. (1998). *Neurological Rehabilitation:Optimizing Motor Performance*. Oxford: Butterworth Heinemann.

Carr, J. H., Shepherd, R. B., Nordholm, L., & Lynne, D. (1985). Investigation of a new *Motor Assessment Scale* for stroke patients. *Physical Therapy, 65*, 175–180.

Cheney, P. D. (1985). Role of cerebral cortex in voluntary movements: A review. *Physical Therapy, 65*, 624–635.

Craik, R. L. (1991). Recovery processes: Maximizing function. In M. J. Lister (Ed.), *Contemporary Management of Motor Control Problems: Proceedings of the II STEP Conference* (pp. 165–173). Alexandria, VA: Foundation for Physical Therapy.

Davis, W. E., & Burton, A. W. (1991). Ecological task analysis: Translating movement behavior theory into practice. *Adapted Physical Activity Quarterly, 8*, 154–177.

Dean, D., & Mackey, F. (1992). *Motor Assessment Scale* scores as a measure of rehabilitation outcome following stroke. *Australian Journal of Physiotherapy, 38*, 31–35.

Duncan, P. W., Propst, M., & Nelson, S. G. (1983). Reliability of the *Fugl-Meyer Assessment* of the sensorimotor recovery following cerebrovascular accident. *Physical Therapy, 63*, 1606–1610.

Duncan, P. W., Goldstein, L., Horner, R., Landsman, P., Samsa, G., & Matchar, D., (1994). Similar motor recovery of upper and lower extremities after stroke. *Stroke, 25*,1181–1188.

Dunn, W. (1993). Measurement of function: Actions for the future. *American Journal of Occupational Therapy, 47*, 357–359.

Fellows, S. J., Kaus, C., & Thilmann, A. (1994). Voluntary movement at the elbow in spastic hemiparesis. *Annals of Neurology, 36*, 397–407.

Fiorentino, M. R. (1973). *Reflex testing methods for evaluating CNS development* (2nd ed.). Springfield, IL: Charles C. Thomas.

Fisher, A. (1999). *Assessment of Motor and Process Skills* (3rd ed.). Fort Collins, CO: Three Star.

Fisher, A. G., & Short-DeGraff, M. (1993). Improving functional assessment in occupational therapy: Recommendations and philosophy for change. *American Journal of Occupational Therapy, 47*, 199–201.

Fisk, J. D., Pontefract, A., Ritvo, P., Archibald, C., & Murray, T. (1994). The impact of fatigue on patients with multiple sclerosis. *Canadian Journal of Neurological Science, 21*, 9–14.

Fitch, H. L., Tuller, B., & Turvey, M. T. (1982). The Bernstein perspective: III. Tuning of coordinative structures with special reference to perception. In J. A. S. Kelso (Ed.), *Human Motor Behavior: An Introduction* (pp. 271–281). Hillsdale, NJ: Erlbaum.

Fredericks, C. M., & Saladin, L. K. (Eds.). (1996). *Pathophysiology of the motor systems: Principles and Clinical Presentations*. Philadelphia: Davis.

Fugl-Meyer, A. R., Jääskö, L., Leyman, I., Olsson, S., & Steglind, S. (1975). The post-stroke hemiplegic patient: A method for evaluation of physical performance. *Scandinavian Journal of Rehabilitation Medicine, 7*, 13–31.

Gentile, A. M. (1972). A working model of skill acquisition with application to teaching. *Quest, 17*, 3–23.

Gesell, A. (1954). The ontogenesis of infant behavior. In L. Carmichael (Ed.), *Manual of Child Psychology* (2nd ed., pp. 335–373). New York: Wiley.

Gleick, J. (1987). *Chaos: Making a New Science*. New York: Penguin.

Gibson, J. J. (1977). The theory of affordances. In R. Shaw & J. Bransford (Eds.), *Perceiving, Acting, and Knowing* (pp. 67–82). Hillsdale, NJ: Erlbaum.

Gibson, J. J. (1979). *The Ecological Approach to Visual Perception*. Boston: Houghton Mifflin.

Gordon, J. (1987). Assumptions underlying physical therapy interventions: Theoretical and historical perspectives. In J. H. Carr, R. B. Shepherd, J. Gordon, A. M. Gentile, & J. M. Held (Eds.), *Movement Science: Foundations for Physical Therapy in Rehabilitation* (pp. 1–30). Rockville, MD: Aspen.

Gresham, G. E., Phillips, T. Wolf, P., McNamara, P., Kannel, W., & Dawber, T. (1979). Epidemiologic profile of long-term stroke disability: The Framingham study. *Archives of Physical Medicine & Rehabilitation, 60*, 487–491.

Gresham G. E., Duncan, P. W., Stason, W. B., et al. (1995). *Post-Stroke Rehabilitation: Clinical Practice Guidelines No. 16*. Rockville, MD: U.S. Department of Health and Human Services. AHCPR Publication 95-0662.

Heriza, C. (1991). Motor development: Traditional and contemporary theories. In M. J. Lister (Ed.), *Contemporary Management of Motor Control Problems: Proceedings of the II STEP Conference* (pp. 99–126). Alexandria, VA: Foundation for Physical Therapy.

Horak, F. B., Anderson, M., Esselman, P., & Lynch, K. (1984). The effects of movement velocity, mass displaced and task certainty on associated postural adjustments made by normal and hemiplegic individuals. *Journal of Neurology, Neurosurgery, & Psychiatry, 47*, 1020–1028.

Horak, F. B. (1991). Assumptions underlying motor control for neurologic rehabilitation. In M. J. Lister (Ed.), *Contemporary Management of Motor Control Problems: Proceedings of the II Step Conference* (pp. 11–27). Alexandria, VA: Foundation for Physical Therapy.

Ingles, J. L., Eskes, G. A., & Phillips, S. J. (1999). Fatigue after stroke. *Archives of Physical Medicine & Rehabilitation, 80*, 173–178.

Jackson, J. H., & Taylor, J. (Eds.). (1932). *Selected writings of John B. Hughlings, I and II*. London: Hodder & Stoughter.

Jeannerod, M., Michel, F., & Prablanc, C. (1984). The control of hand movements in a case of hemianesthesia following a parietal lesion. *Brain, 107*, 899–920.

Jongbloed, L., Stanton, S., & Fousek, B. (1993). Family adaptation to altered roles following stroke. *Canadian Journal of Occupational Therapy, 60*, 70–77.

Kamm, K., Thelen, E., & Jensen, J. L. (1990). A dynamical systems approach to motor development. *Physical Therapy, 70*, 763–775.

Katz, R. T., & Rymer, W. Z. (1989). Spastic hypertonia: Mechanism and measurement. *Archives of Physical Medicine & Rehabilitation, 70*, 144–155.

Knott, M., & Voss, D. E. (1968). *Proprioceptive neuromuscular facilitation* (2nd ed.). New York: Harper & Row.

Law, M., Baptiste, S., Carswell, A., McColl, M., Polatajko, H., & Pollock, N. (1998). *Canadian Occupational Performance Measure* (3rd ed.). Ottawa: CAOT.

Law, M., Cooper, B., Strong, S., Stewart, D., Rigby, P., & Letts, L. (1997). Theoretical contexts for the practice of occupational therapy. In C. Christiansen & C. Baum (Eds.), *Occupational Therapy: Enabling Function and Well-Being* (2nd ed., pp. 72–102). Thorofare, NJ: Slack.

Lashley, K. S. (1917). The accuracy of movement in the absence of excitation from the moving organ. *American Journal of Physiology, 43*, 169–194.

Lister, M. J. (Ed.). (1991). *Contemporary Management of Motor Control Problems: Proceedings of the II STEP Conference*. Alexandria, VA: Foundation for Physical Therapy.

Loewen, S. C., & Anderson, B. A. (1990). Predictors of stroke outcome using objective measurement scales. *Stroke, 21*, 78–81.

Malouin, F., Pickard, L., Bonneau, C., Durand, A., & Corriveau, D. (1994). Evaluating motor recovery early after stroke: Comparison of the *Fugl-Meyer Assessment* and the *Motor Assessment Scale*. *Archives of Physical Medicine & Rehabilitation, 75*, 1206–1212.

Marsden, C. D. (1982). The mysterious motor function of the basal ganglia: the Robert Wartenberg lecture. *Neurology, 32*, 514–539.

Marteniuk, R. G., MacKenzie, C. L., & Jeannerod, M. (1987). Constraints on human arm trajectories. *Canadian Journal of Psychology, 41*, 365–368.

Mathiowetz, V., & Bass Haugen, J. (1994). Motor behavior research: Implications for therapeutic approaches to CNS dysfunction. *American Journal of Occupational Therapy, 48*, 733–745.

Mathiowetz, V. G., & Wade, M. (1995). Task constraints and functional motor performance of individuals with and without multiple sclerosis. *Ecological Psychology, 7*, 99–123.

McGraw, M. B. (1945). *The neuromuscular maturation of the human infant*. New York: Hafner.

Moore, J. C. (1986). Recovery potentials following CNS lesions: A brief historical perspective in relation to modern research data on neuroplasticity. *American Journal of Occupational Therapy, 40,* 459–463.

Newell, K. M. (1986). Constraints on the development of coordination. In M. G. Wade & H. T. A. Whiting (Eds.), *Motor Development in Children: Aspects of Coordination and Control* (pp. 341–360). Dordrecht: Martinus Nijhoff.

Nwaobi, O. M. (1983). Voluntary movement impairment in upper motor neuron lesions: Is spasticity the main cause? *Occupational Therapy Journal of Research, 3,* 131–140.

O'Dwyer, N. J., Ada, L., & Neilson, P. D. (1996). Spasticity and muscle contracture following stroke. *Brain, 119,* 1737-1749.

Olsen, T. S. (1990). Arm and leg paresis as outcome predictors in stroke rehabilitation. *Stroke, 21,* 247–251.

Phillips, J. G., & Stelmach, G. E. (1996). Parkinson's disease and other involuntary movement disorders of the basal ganglia. In C. M. Fredericks & L. K. Saladin (Eds.), *Pathophysiology of the Motor Systems: Principles and Clinical Presentations* (pp. 203–216). Philadelphia: Davis.

Podsiadlo, D., & Richardson, S. (1991). The timed "up and go" a test of basic mobility for frail elderly persons. *Journal of the American Geriatrics Society, 39,* 142–148.

Poole, J. L., & Whitney, S. L. (1988). *Motor Assessment Scale* for stroke patients: Concurrent validity and interrater reliability. *Archives of Physical Medicine & Rehabilitation, 69,* 195–197.

Rao, S. M., Leo, G., Bernardin, L., & Unverzagt, F. (1991). Cognitive dysfunction in multiple sclerosis: I. Frequency, patterns, and prediction. *Neurology, 41,* 685–691.

Reding, M. J., & Potes, E. (1988). Rehabilitation outcomes following initial unilateral hemispheric stroke: Life table analysis approach. *Stroke, 19,* 1354–1358.

Reed, E. S. (1982). An outline of a theory of action systems. *Journal of Motor Behavior, 14,* 98–134.

Rogers, J. C., & Holm, M. B. (1999). *Role Change Assessment:* An interview tool for older adults. In B. J. Hemphill-Pearson (Ed.). *Assessments in Occupational Therapy Mental Health: An Integrated Approach* (pp. 73–82). Thorofare, NJ: Slack.

Rood, M. S. (1954). Neurophysiological reactions as a basis for physical therapy. *Physical Therapy Review, 34,* 444–449.

Ryerson, S., & Levit, K. (1997). *Functional Movement Reeducation: A Contemporary Model of Stroke Rehabilitation.* New York: Churchill Livingstone.

Sabari, J. C. (1995). Carr and Shepherd's motor relearning programme for individuals with stroke. In C. Trombly (Ed.), *Occupational Therapy for Physical Dysfunction* (4th ed., pp. 501–509). Baltimore: Williams & Wilkins.

Sahrman, S. A., & Norton, B. J. (1977). The relationship of voluntary movement to spasticity in the upper motor neuron syndrome. *Annals of Neurology, 2,* 460–465.

Schmidt, R. A. (1988). *Motor control and learning: A behavioral emphasis* (2nd ed.) Champaign, IL: Human Kinetics.

Scholz, J. P., & Campbell, S. K. (1980). Muscle spindles and the regulation of movement. *Physical Therapy, 60,* 1416–1424.

Sherrington, C. S. (1906). *The integrative action of the nervous system.* New Haven: Yale University.

Shumway-Cook, A., & Woolacott, M. (1995). *Motor Control: Theory and Practical Application.* Baltimore: Williams & Wilkins.

Skold, C., Harms-Ringdahl, K., Hultling, C., Levi, R., & Seiger, A. (1998). Simultaneous Ashworth measurements and electromyographic recordings in tetraplegic patients. *Archives of Physical Medicine & Rehabilitation, 79,* 959–965.

Sloan, R. L., Sinclair, E., Thompson, J., Taylor, S., & Pentland, B. (1992). Inter-rater reliability of the Modified Ashworth Scale for spasticity in hemiplegic patients. *International Journal of Rehabilitation Research, 15,* 158–161.

Spencer, J., Krefting, L., & Mattingly, C. (1993). Incorporation of ethnographic methods in occupational therapy assessment. *American Journal of Occupational Therapy, 47,* 303–309.

Stolov, W. C. (1966). The concept of normal muscle tone, hypotonia, and hypertonia. *Archives of Physical Medicine & Rehabilitation, 47,* 156–168.

Taub, E. (1976). Motor behavior following deafferentation in the developing and motorically mature monkey. *Advances in Behavioral Biology, 18,* 675–705.

Taub, E., Miller, N. E., Novack, T. A., Cook, E. W., Fleming, W., Nepomuceno, C., Connell, J., & Crago, J. (1993). Technique to improve chronic motor deficit after stroke. *Archives of Physical Medicine & Rehabilitation, 74,* 347–354.

Thelen, E. (1989). Self-organization in developmental processes: Can systems approaches work? In M. R. Gunnar & E. Thelen (Eds.), *Systems and Development* (pp. 77–117). Hillsdale, NJ: Erlbaum.

Thelen, E., & Fisher, D. M. (1982). Newborn stepping: An explanation for a "disappearing reflex." *Developmental Psychology, 18,* 760–775.

Thelen, E., & Ulrich, B. D. (1991). Hidden skills. *Monograph of the Society for Research in Child Development, 56* (Serial 223). Chicago: University of Chicago.

Titus, M. N., Gall, N. G., Yerxa, E. J., Roberson, T. A., & Mack, W. (1991). Correlation of perceptual performance and activities of daily living in stroke patients. *American Journal of Occupational Therapy, 45,* 410–418.

Tinetti, M. E. (1986). Performance-oriented assessment of mobility problems in elderly patients. *Journal of American Geriatrics Society, 34,* 119–126.

Trombly, C. A. (1989). Motor control therapy. In C. Trombly (Ed.), *Occupational Therapy for Physical Dysfunction* (3rd ed., pp. 72–95). Baltimore: Williams & Wilkins.

Trombly, C. A. (1993). The issue is—anticipating the future: Assessment of occupational function. *American Journal of Occupational Therapy, 47,* 253–257.

Trombly, C. A., & Wu, C. (1999). Effect of rehabilitation tasks on organization of movement after stroke. *American Journal of Occupational Therapy, 53,* 333–344.

Turvey, M. T. (1977). Preliminaries to a theory of action with reference to vision. In R. Shaw & J. Bransford (Eds.), *Perceiving, Acting, and Knowing* (pp. 211–265). Hillsdale, NJ: Erlbaum.

Twitchell, T. E. (1951). The restoration of motor function following hemiplegia in man. *Brain, 74,* 443–480.

VanSant, A. (1990). Life-span development in functional tasks. *Physical Therapy, 70,* 788–798.

VanSant, A. (1991a). Motor control, motor learning, and motor development. In P. C. Montgomery & B. H. Connolly (Eds.), *Motor Control and Physical Therapy: Theoretical Framework and Practical Applications* (pp. 13–28). Hixson, TN: Chattanooga Group.

VanSant, A. (1991b). Should the normal motor developmental sequence be used as a theoretical model to progress adult patients? In M. J. Lister (Ed.), *Contemporary Management of Motor Control Problems: Proceedings of the II STEP Conference* (pp. 95–97). Alexandria, VA: Foundation for Physical Therapy.

Warren, W. H. (1984). Perceiving affordances: Visual guidance of stair climbing. *Journal of Experimental Psychology: Human Perception and Performance, 10,* 683–703.

Whitney, S. L., Poole, J. L., & Cass, S. P. (1998). A review of balance instruments for older adults. *American Journal of Occupational Therapy, 52,* 666–671.

Wood-Dauphinee, S. L., Williams, J. I., & Shapiro, S. H. (1990). Examining outcome measures in a clinical study of stroke. *Stroke, 21,* 731–739.

World Health Organization. (1998). *Toward a Common Language for Functioning and Disablement: ICIDH-2 International Classification of Impairments, Activities, and Participation.* Geneva: Author.

6

Assessing Abilities and Capacities: Sensation

Karen Bentzel

LEARNING OBJECTIVES

After studying this chapter, the reader will be able to do the following:

1. Describe the effects of sensory loss on occupational function.
2. Predict the pattern of sensory loss based on diagnosis or described lesion in the somatosensory system.
3. Demonstrate appropriate sensory testing techniques for tactile sensation when provided with appropriate tools or equipment.
4. Differentiate standardized and nonstandardized tactile tests.
5. Choose appropriate sensory testing techniques for a given patient or situation.
6. Correctly interpret the results of sensory testing for treatment planning.

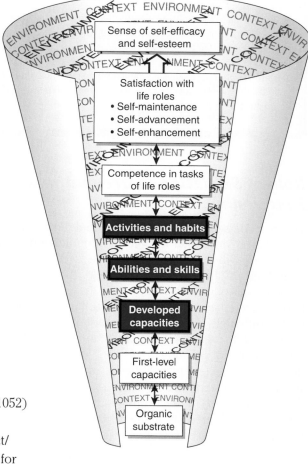

*T*he American Occupational Therapy Association (1994, p. 1052) defines tactile sensory processing as "interpreting light touch, pressure, temperature, pain, and vibration through skin contact/ receptors." The tactile sense is necessary throughout the body for occupational functioning but is especially important in the hands. Moberg described hands without sensation as being like eyes without vision (Dellon, 1988).

Immediately after birth, an infant is bombarded with tactile sensations that are different from those in utero. Within a few months, the infant learns to interpret a multitude of tactile stimuli, such as soothing touch from a parent that brings comfort and contentment. This developed capacity supports further development of abilities and skills, as the infant uses touch to grasp an object, bring two hands together at midline, and perform other skills. These abilities are necessary for self-maintenance, self-enhancement, and self-advancement roles in childhood and throughout adulthood.

GLOSSARY

Aesthesiometer—Instrument designed for sensory testing. The term usually indicates a tool consisting of a ruler type of scale and two prongs that can be moved progressively closer or farther apart, used for assessing two-point discrimination. Monofilaments are occasionally called pressure aesthesiometers in the literature.

Hemianesthesia—complete loss of sensation on the left or right side of the body.

Hypersensitivity, hyperesthesia—A condition in which an exaggerated or unpleasant sensation is experienced in response to ordinary stimuli.

Kinesthesia—The ability to identify "the excursion and direction of joint movement" (American Occupational Therapy Association, 1994, p. 1053).

Monofilament—Thin nylon strand resembling fishing line, of graded thicknesses, attached to a handle and used in testing the threshold of light touch sensation.

Paresthesia—An abnormal sensation such as a feeling of pins and needles, tingling, or tickling in the absence of tactile stimulation or in response to tactile stimuli that ordinarily do not evoke tingling or tickling.

Proprioception—"Interpreting stimuli originating in muscles, joints, and other internal tissues that give information about the position of one body part in relation to another" (American Occupational Therapy Association, 1994, p. 1052).

Stereognosis—The ability to identify objects through proprioception, cognition, and the sense of touch (American Occupational Therapy Association, 1994). Astereognosis is the term used to describe the absence of this ability.

Vibrometer—Instrument designed to test the threshold of vibration sensation. It consists of a vibrating head that is applied to the patient's skin and a control unit that allows for gradual changes in the amplitude and frequency of vibration.

Role of Sensation in Occupational Functioning

The role of sensation in occupational functioning is dramatically described in Cole's (1991) account of Ian Waterman, who at 19 years of age acquired a rare neurological illness that resulted in the loss of all sensation of touch in his body from the neck down. He had no awareness of the positions of his arms, legs, or body. Although his muscles were not affected, any attempt at movement was wildly uncontrolled. Ian's initial attempt at standing up resulted in him falling "in a heap . . . like a pile of wet clothes" (Cole, 1991, p. 11). He was unable to feed himself, get dressed, or do any functional activity requiring control of movement. Over several years, Waterman learned how to complete functional activities by substituting vision for his lost sensation. Every movement had to be carefully watched and consciously controlled. The high level of concentration required and the energy expended to complete daily self-care and work activities led Cole to name the account of Waterman's life *Pride and a Daily Marathon*.

Although a loss of sensation like Waterman's without any motor loss is unusual, it exemplifies the close connection between the motor and sensory systems. With sensory loss in the hand, fine motor coordination is impaired, and manipulative ability is decreased (Chapman et al., 1996; Jones, 1996). The risk of falling increases in association with decreased **proprioception** (awareness of joint position) in the lower extremities (Kaplan et al., 1985).

The amount of force needed to maintain grasp on an object also depends on sensory feedback. Usually, we use force that is just sufficient to overcome the pull of gravity, taking into account the amount of friction afforded by the surface texture. Without adequate tactile sensation, the force used to grip an object is either lower or higher than the force needed, resulting in objects slipping from grasp, delicate objects (such as a plastic foam cup) being crushed by excessive grip force, or muscles developing fatigue from overactivity (Johansson, 1996).

Some activities require sensory feedback because they depend on the sense of touch, such as determining the temperature of a bowl taken from the microwave. Tactile sensations let us know whether the food is warm and whether the bowl is too hot to carry to the table. Finding coins or other objects in a pocket and fastening a necklace or closing a back zipper are examples of activities for which vision is not used; therefore, we rely entirely upon sensory feedback. It is the tactile sense that tells us when our new shoes are a bit too tight and we had better remove them or we will get a blister. Impairment in the somatosensory system not only hinders movement but also increases the risk of injury.

Purposes of Sensory Evaluation

The purposes of sensory testing, as defined by Cooke (1991), are as follows:

► Assess the type and extent of sensory loss.
► Evaluate and document sensory recovery.
► Assist in diagnosis.
► Determine impairment and functional limitation.
► Provide direction for occupational therapy intervention.
  a. Determine time to begin sensory reeducation.
  b. Determine need for education to prevent injury during occupational functioning.
  c. Determine need for desensitization.

Before considering sensory evaluation, therapists need a good understanding of the neural structures responsible for tactile sensation.

Neurophysiological Foundations of Tactile Sensation

Receptors for tactile sensation are present within skin, muscles, and joints. Each tactile receptor is usually specialized for a single type of sensory stimulation such as touch, temperature, or pain (Fredericks, 1996a). The types of sensation, specific kinds of receptors, and corresponding neurons that connect the sensory receptors with the spinal cord and ultimately with the cerebral cortex appear in Table 6-1. Neural impulses follow the described pathways to the brain, where the sensations are perceived and interpreted.

Each sensory neuron and its distal and proximal terminations can be considered a sensory unit. Each sensory unit has an area of skin that encompasses its defined receptive field. A stimulus anywhere in the field may evoke a response, but stimuli applied to the center of the receptive field produce sensations more easily. In other words, the center of a receptive field has a lower threshold than the periphery. Adjacent receptive fields overlap; therefore, a single stimulus evokes a profile of responses from overlapping sensory units.

The variation in the number of sensory units in a given area of skin is called innervation density. The face, hand, and fingers have high innervation densities. Areas with high innervation density are highly sensitive and have a proportionately large representation area within the somatosensory area of the cortex, the postcentral

TABLE 6-1
Neural Pathways of Sensory Stimuli

Type of Sensation	Sensory Receptor	Type of Afferent Neuron	Pathway	Termination of Pathway
Constant touch or pressure	Merkel's cell Ruffini's end organ	Type A-beta slowly adapting I and II myelinated neurons	Ascend in dorsal column and medial lemniscus of spinal cord in posterior pyramidal tract, cross to opposite side in medulla	Thalamus and somatosensory cortex
Moving touch or vibration	Meissner's corpuscles Pacinian corpuscles Hair follicles	Type A-beta rapidly adapting I and II myelinated neurons		
Proprioception and kinesthesia	Same as both moving and constant touch or vibration plus touch receptors found in skin and joint structures Muscle spindles Golgi tendon organs	Same as for moving touch or vibration plus A-alpha myelinated neurons	Same as for moving touch or vibration plus spinocerebellar tract	Same as for moving touch or vibration plus cerebellum
Pain (pinprick)	Free nerve endings	Type A-delta myelinated neurons	Immediately cross to opposite side and pass upward in anterior spinothalamic tracts of spinal cord	Brainstem, thalamus, and somatosensory cortex
Pain (chronic)	Free nerve endings	Type C unmyelinated fibers		
Temperature	Free nerve endings Warm receptors Cold receptors	Type A-delta myelinated neurons and type C unmyelinated fibers		

Based on information in Dellon, A. L. (1997). *Somatosensory Testing and Rehabilitation.* Bethesda, MD: American Occupational Therapy Association; Chapman, C. E., Tremblay, F., & Ageranioti-Bélanger, A. (1996). Role of primary somatosensory cortex in active and passive touch. In A. M. Wing, P. Haggard, & J. R. Flanagan (Eds.), *Hand and Brain: The Neurophysiology of Hand Movements* (pp. 329–347). San Diego: Academic; Fredericks, C. M. (1996). Basic sensory mechanisms and the somatosensory system. In C.M. Fredericks & L. K. Saladin (Eds.), *Pathophysiology of the Motor Systems: Principles and Clinical Presentations* (pp. 78–106). Philadelphia: Davis; and Fredericks, C. M. (1996). Disorders of the spinal cord. In C. M. Fredericks & L. K. Saladin (Eds.), *Pathophysiology of the Motor Systems: Principles and Clinical Presentations* (pp. 394–423). Philadelphia: Davis.

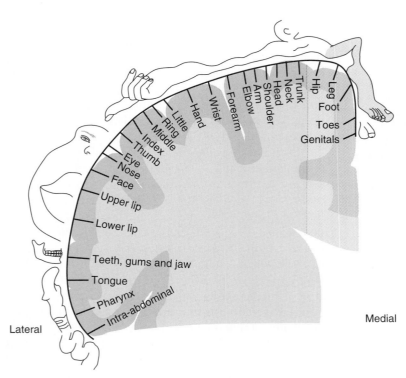

Figure 6-1 The areas responsible for sensation of body parts within the postcentral gyrus of the cerebral cortex. (Reprinted with permission from Kingsley, R. E. [1996]. *Concise Text of Neuroscience* [p. 185]. Baltimore: Williams & Wilkins.)

gyrus of the parietal lobe (Fredericks, 1996a). Figure 6-1 shows the organization within the cortex of sensory receptors from various regions of the body.

Table 6-1 and the description of sensory pathways simplify a complex process. For example, tactile stimuli of sufficient strength elicit responses from both constant and moving touch receptors and perhaps also from the pain receptors (Fredericks, 1996a). Extremes of hot and cold stimuli activate the pain receptors rather than the temperature receptors (Lindblom, 1994). Perception of joint motion (**kinesthesia**) and joint position (proprioception) appear to be a result of information from multiple kinds of receptors. Researchers disagree about the relative contributions of joint, muscle, and skin receptors to proprioception and kinesthesia (Fredericks, 1996a; Jones, 1996).

Therapists use a solid understanding of the neurophysiology of the tactile system to choose evaluation and treatment techniques for sensory deficits.

Somatosensory Deficit Patterns

Any interruption along the ascending sensory pathway or in the sensory areas of the cortex can lead to a decrease or loss of sensation. The extent and severity of the sensory deficit can generally be predicted in accordance with the mechanism and location of the lesion or injury. Patterns of sensory impairment are directly related to the involved neuroanatomical structures.

Individual sensory distributions sometimes vary from the illustrations of typical sensory distributions included in this and other texts. Furthermore, although there are clear lines of demarcation on the illustrations, humans generally have some overlapping areas of innervation along the borders of sensory receptive areas (Adams et al., 1997).

Cortical Injury

Patients with brain lesions caused by cerebrovascular accident (CVA) or head trauma demonstrate sensory losses related to loss of functioning of neurons within the central nervous system. Effects of CVA on sensation depend on specific disruption of blood supply. For instance, occlusion of the middle cerebral artery (the most common site of CVA) is often associated with contralateral impairment of all sensory modalities on the face, arm, and leg. Occlusion of the anterior cerebral artery tends to cause more loss of sensation in the contralateral leg than in the arm, because of this artery's supply to the medial aspect of the cerebral cortex (Fig. 6-1) (Saladin, 1996a). Approximately 60% of patients with stroke in the carotid artery system, which includes the anterior and middle cerebral arteries, have sensory deficits (Garrison et al., 1988). Patterns of sensory loss following head trauma are less predictable because of the more diffuse areas of brain damage associated with this condition (Saladin, 1996b). For patients with either CVA or head injury, perception of fine touch and proprioception are most affected, temperature sensation is affected less, and pain sensibility least (Fredericks, 1996a).

Sterzi et al. (1993) compared patients with left and right CVA and found that loss of proprioception and pain perception were more common following right CVA than left CVA. Left neglect, an inability to recognize and use perceptions from the left side of the body and environment, was proposed as a factor underlying this difference. The study of Beschin et al. (1996) provides evidence to support the existence of tactile neglect; patients with right brain damage tend to ignore left space during active tactile exploration.

Partial recovery of sensation following cortical injury is attributed to decreased edema, improved vascular flow, cortical plasticity (adaptability of neurons to assume new functions), and relearning (Carr & Shepherd, 1998). Recovery of pain and temperature perception usually precedes recovery of proprioception and light touch (Fredericks, 1996a).

Spinal Cord Injury

Patients with complete lesions of the spinal cord demonstrate a total absence of sensation in the dermatomes (Fig. 6-2) below the level of the lesion. **Paresthesia** (tingling or pins and needles sensation) may occur in the dermatome associated with the level of the lesion. The level of the lesion determines the extent of the sensory loss, with the greatest loss occurring in patients with the lesions in the highest cervical regions of the spinal cord (Fredericks, 1996c).

Incomplete spinal cord lesions result in sensory losses that are related to damage within specific spinal tracts. For instance, damage to the anterior part of the spinal cord usually results in loss of pain and temperature sensation below the level of the lesion, whereas touch, vibration, and proprioception remain intact. Conversely, patients who have damaged the posterior portion of the spinal cord cannot feel light touch and vibration but can feel differences in temperature and

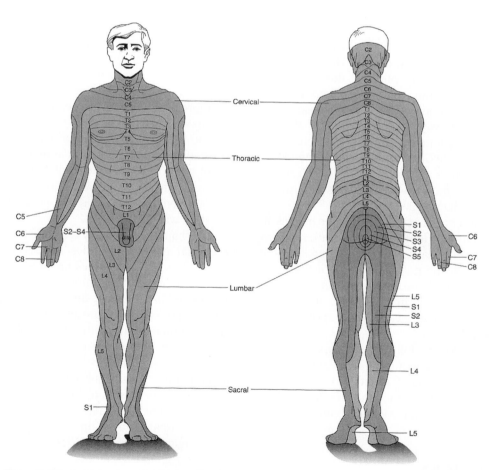

Figure 6-2 Typical dermatome distribution. (Reprinted with permission from Bear, M. F., Connors, B. W., & Paradiso, M. A. (1996). *Neuroscience: Exploring the Brain* [p. 322]. Baltimore: Williams & Wilkins.)

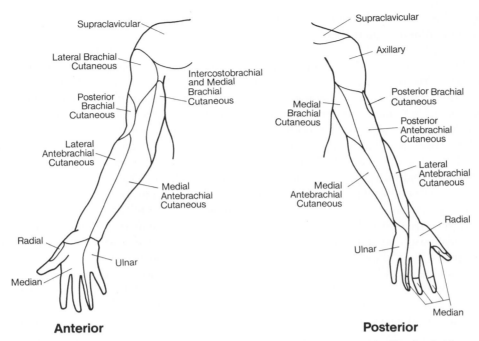

Figure 6-3 Typical sensory distribution of peripheral nerves within the upper extremity. (Reprinted with permission from Sieg, K. W., & Adams, S. R. [1996]. *Illustrated Essentials of Musculoskeletal Anatomy* [3rd ed., p. 79.]. Gainesville, FL: Megabooks.)

painful stimuli. Patients with damage to one side of the spinal cord (Brown Séquard syndrome) display loss of touch, vibration, and proprioception on the side of the lesion and loss of temperature and pain sensation on the side opposite the lesion. This occurs because of the differences in the pathways of the ascending sensory fibers; neurons carrying temperature and pain sensations cross to the opposite side of the spinal cord immediately after entering it, whereas neurons carrying touch sensations ascend to the medulla before crossing to the opposite side (Fredericks, 1996c).

Damage to the central spinal cord often results in bilateral loss of pain and temperature sensation below the level of the lesion because the neurons cross to the opposite side through the central portion of the cord. Compression of the spinal cord may result in decreased or absent sensation in the dermatome at the level of the compression and/or dermatomes below the compressed area (Fredericks, 1996c).

Any sensory recovery following traumatic spinal cord injury usually occurs within the first year, with the greatest recovery in the first 6 months (Waters et al., 1993). Recovery of sensation is thought to occur because of resolution of ischemia and edema within the spinal cord.

Peripheral Nerve Injury

Patterns of sensory loss following peripheral nerve injury vary with the nerve or nerves involved as well as the extent of the damage. Damage to a single nerve root as it exits the spinal cord affects sensation on one side of the body within a single dermatome (Fig. 6-2), whereas damage to a peripheral nerve affects sensation within the appropriate peripheral nerve distribution (Fig. 6-3) (Adams et al., 1997).

The extent of the sensory loss can vary widely. A mild nerve compression, such as in early stages of carpal tunnel syndrome, produces a slightly elevated threshold for sensing light touch or vibration. A complete transection of a peripheral nerve results in a total loss of tactile sensation within the region.

The pattern of sensory loss occurring as a result of peripheral polyneuropathies, associated with chronic conditions such as diabetes mellitus and alcoholism, is typically bilateral and symmetrical, usually beginning in the feet and hands (glove-and-stocking distribution) and spreading proximally. Paresthesia and pain may accompany peripheral neuropathy (Fredericks, 1996b).

Recovery of sensation following release of a nerve from compression is very likely if the compression was brief and mild. Significant recovery following prolonged compression is common, but sensory perception does not always reach normal levels. Recovery of sensation following total transection of a nerve is possible only with surgical intervention and adequate regrowth of neurons (Smith, 1995). Sensation of temperature and pain generally (but not always) recovers first, followed by touch sensation, because regrowth of pain fibers averages 1.08 mm per day, and regrowth of touch fibers averages 0.78 mm per day (Waylett-Rendall, 1988). Because of the chronic conditions associated with peripheral neuropathy, recovery of sensation is generally not expected (Fredericks, 1996b).

Evaluation Techniques

There are numerous methods of testing sensation. Some are intended to evaluate a specific type of sensory receptor, such as the test for vibration awareness using a tuning fork that is believed to be specific to the Meissner's and Pacinian corpuscles (Dellon, 1997). Some are intended to evaluate the use of sensation in skills that support occupational functioning, such as the use of the hand to identify objects by touch in the test of **stereognosis**. Some are designed to detect very small changes in sensory perception, such as the touch threshold test using **monofilaments** (fine nylon strands).

The principles of sensory testing optimize the reliability of the testing results. These are listed in Box 6-1. Specific descriptions of the administration of commonly

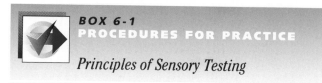

BOX 6-1
PROCEDURES FOR PRACTICE

Principles of Sensory Testing

- ▸ Choose an environment with minimal distractions.
- ▸ Ensure that the patient is comfortable and relaxed.
- ▸ Ensure that the patient can understand and produce spoken language. If the patient cannot, modify testing procedures to ensure reliable communication.
- ▸ Determine areas of the body to be tested.
- ▸ Stabilize the limb or body part being tested (Fig. 6-4).
- ▸ Note any differences in skin thickness, calluses, and so on. Expect sensation to be decreased in these areas.
- ▸ State the instructions for the test.
- ▸ Demonstrate the test stimulus on an area of skin with intact sensation while the patient observes.
- ▸ Ensure that the patient understands the instructions by eliciting the correct response to the demonstration.
- ▸ Occlude the patient's vision for administration of the test. Place a screen (Fig. 6-5) or a file folder between the patient's face and area being tested, blindfold the patient, or ask the patient to close his or her eyes.
- ▸ Apply stimuli at irregular intervals or insert catch trials in which no stimulus is given.
- ▸ Avoid giving inadvertent cues, such as auditory cues or facial expressions, during stimulus application.
- ▸ Carefully observe the correctness, confidence, and promptness of the responses.
- ▸ Observe the patient for any discomfort relating to the stimuli that may signal hypersensitivity.
- ▸ Ensure that the therapist who does the initial testing does any reassessment.

Sources: Brand & Hollister, 1993; Callahan, 1995; Reese, 1999.

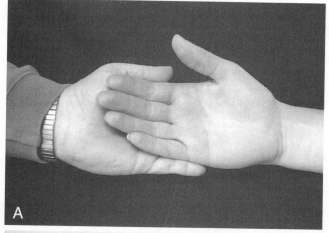

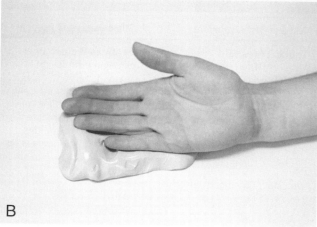

Figure 6-4 Hand support during testing. **A.** Fingers must be carefully stabilized and supported during testing so that motion is prevented, avoiding inadvertent cues to the patient. **B.** A cushion of therapy putty can be used to provide the stabilization.

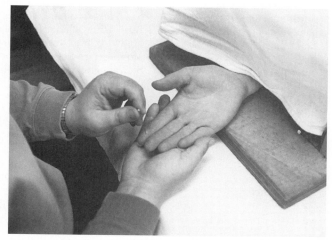

Figure 6-5 Vision must be occluded during testing. Using a screen such as this is usually more comfortable for patients than closing their eyes or being blindfolded.

used sensory evaluations are shown in Tables 6-2 and 6-3. The more standardized evaluations of sensation appear in Table 6-2, and the less standardized evaluations are shown in Table 6-3. Computerized evaluations of sensation are available for research and are becoming available in a limited number of areas for clinical use (Benton, 1994; Dellon, 1997; Riggle, 1999). The *Automated Tactile Tester*, for instance, measures touch, two-point discrimination, temperature, vibration, and pinprick thresholds (Horch et al., 1992).

Interpretation of Evaluation Findings

Sensory evaluation findings are often reported as absent, intact, or impaired. *Absent* describes a total loss of sensation or inability to detect a specific sensory modality. *Intact* describes normal sensation. Sensation is impaired when the patient is able to detect some but not all of the stimuli or when the perception of the stimulus is different from that of an area of skin that has intact sensation.

TABLE 6-2
Standardized Sensory Testing Techniques

Test and Test Instruments	Stimulus (S) and Response (R)	Scoring and Expected Results
Touch Threshold Measures threshold of light touch sensation (Bell-Krotoski, 1995; Tomancik, 1987; Weinstein et al., 1997) **Test Instruments** Semmes-Weinstein monofilaments OR Weinstein Enhanced Sensory Test (WEST)	**Semmes-Weinstein** **S:** Begin testing with filament marked 2.83; hold filament perpendicular to skin, apply to skin until filament bends (Fig. 6-6). Apply in 1.5 seconds, hold 1.5 seconds, and remove in 1.5 seconds. Repeat three times at each testing site, using thicker filaments if the patient does not perceive thin ones (except for filaments marked >4.08, which are applied one time to each site). **R:** Patient says yes upon feeling the stimulus. **WEST** **S:** Patient is prompted to stimulus, then filament is slowly applied perpendicular to skin and held for 1 sec, then slowly lifted. Catch trials consisting of prompt without filament application are randomly inserted within test sequence. **R:** Patient responds with yes or no to indicate whether stimulus was felt	**Semmes-Weinstein** Score is either the marking number or the actual force of the thinnest filament detected at least once in three trials; results are usually recorded according to a standard color key using colored pencils or markers and a diagram of the hand (Table 6-5 and Fig. 6-7). Normal touch threshold for adults is perception of the filament marked 2.83 (force 0.08 g) except for the sole of the foot, where the normal threshold is the filament marked 3.61 (force 0.21 g). **WEST** Results are recorded according to the color of the filament. Normal touch threshold is perception of the thinnest monofilament. There are two WEST devices, one for the hand and another for the foot.
Two-Point Discrimination **Static** Measures innervation density of slowly adapting fibers of the hand (Callahan, 1995; Dellon, 1997) **Moving** Measures innervation density of quickly adapting fibers of fingertips (Callahan, 1995; Dellon, 1988, 1997) **Test Instruments** (Fig. 6-8): Disk-Criminator OR Aesthesiometer	**Static Two-Point Discrimination** Begin with a 5-mm separation of points. Lightly (just to the point of blanching) apply one or two points (randomly sequenced) in a transverse or longitudinal orientation on the hand; hold for at least 3 sec or until patient responds. **Moving Two-Point Discrimination** **S:** Beginning with a 5- to 8-mm distance, move one or two points randomly from proximal to distal on the distal phalanx with points side by side and parallel to the long axis of the finger; use just enough pressure for the patient to appreciate the stimulus. **Both Static and Moving** Gradually adjust distance of separation to find least distance that patient can correctly perceive. **R:** Patient responds by saying 1, 2, or I can't tell.	Score is smallest distance at which perception of one or two points is better than chance. When the patient's responses become hesitant or inaccurate, require 2 of 3, 4 of 7, or 7 of 10 correct responses. **Static Two-Point Discrimination Norms** 3–5 mm in fingertips ages 18–70 (Bell-Krotoski, 1997) 5–6 mm in fingertips ages 70 and above (Desrosiers et al., 1996) 5–9 mm for middle and proximal phalanges in adults age 18–60, 0–12 mm middle and proximal phalanges of those age 60 and above (Shimokata & Kuzuya, 1995) **Moving Two-Point Discrimination Norms** 2–4 mm for ages 4–60 (Dellon, 1997; Hermann et al., 1995) 4–6 mm for ages 60 and above (Dellon, 1997, Desrosiers et al., 1996)

(continued)

TABLE 6-2
Standardized Sensory Testing Techniques *(Continued)*

Test and Test Instruments	Stimulus (S) and Response (R)	Scoring and Expected Results
Touch Localization Measures spatial representation of touch receptors in the cortex (Nakada, 1993) **Test Instruments** Semmes-Weinstein Monofilament number 4.17 or pen, pencil eraser	**S:** Apply touch to patient's skin **R:** Patient remembers location of stimulus. With vision no longer occluded, patient uses index finger or marking pen to point to spot just touched	Score is the measured distance in millimeters between location of stimulus and location of response. Normal response is approximately 3–4 mm in digit tips, 7–10 mm in palm of hand, 15–18 mm in forearm (Schady, 1994; Sieg & Williams, 1986).
Vibration Threshold Measures threshold of rapidly adapting fibers (Callahan, 1995; Dellon, 1997; Horch et al., 1992) **Test Instruments** Vibrometer: Biothesiometer, Sensortek II, Automated Tactile Tester, Case IV System, Force-Defined Vibrometer	Protocols vary with instrument. **S:** Generally, vibrating head is applied to area to be tested. Stimulus intensity is gradually increased or decreased **R:** Patient indicates when vibration is first felt or no longer felt.	Scoring varies with instrument; norms usually provided by manufacturer.
Dellon's *Picking-Up Test* Dellon's modification of Moberg's *Picking Up* test measures the interpretation of sensation in the distribution of the median nerve (Dellon, 1988) **Test Instruments** A small box and 12 standard metal objects: wing nut, screw, key, nail, large nut, nickel, dime, washer, safety pin, paper clip, small hex nut, and small square nut	**Part 1** **S:** Tape small and ring digits to palm to prevent use. With patient using vision, have him or her pick up and place objects in a box as quickly as possible; time performance on two trials. **R:** Patient picks up each object and deposits it in the box as quickly as possible. **Part 2** **S:** With patient's vision occluded, place one object at a time between three-point pinch in random order and measure speed of response **R:** Patient manipulates object and names it as rapidly as possible	**Part 1** Score is total time to pick up and place all 12 objects in the box for each of 2 trials. **Normal response** Trial 1, 10–19 sec Trial 2, 9–16 seconds **Part 2** Score is time to recognize each object on each of two trials (up to a maximum of 30 seconds) Normal response: 2 seconds per object

For standardized tests, results can be compared with norms; however, age should be taken into account because studies show a decline in sensation with age (Derosiers et al., 1996). For nonstandardized tests, results from the affected area of the patient can be compared with results from an unaffected area.

Monofilament testing usually results in a numerical rating that for patients under age 60 can be interpreted according to Table 6-4. Normative data for patients over age 60 are shown in Table 6-5. The test results indicate not only a rating of the severity of the deficit but also whether protective sensation is impaired or absent.

In planning treatment, diminished or lost protective sensation or absence of sensation indicates that the patient is at risk for injury of the affected body part or parts. The patient must be taught to use vision and an adapted environment to compensate for lost sensation and avoid injury. Results that indicate impaired sensation need further investigation to determine the appropriate course of intervention. If there is **hypersensitivity** (exaggerated or unpleasant sensation) of the body part,

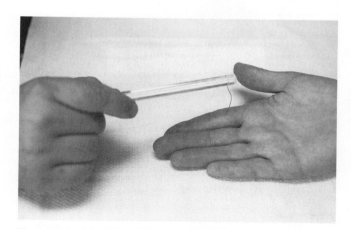

Figure 6-6 Testing of the median nerve distribution using Semmes-Weinstein monofilaments.

a program of desensitization is indicated. If there is a decrease but not total loss of sensation within an area, the patient may be a candidate for sensory retraining, as long as the diagnostic prognosis indicates that there is a

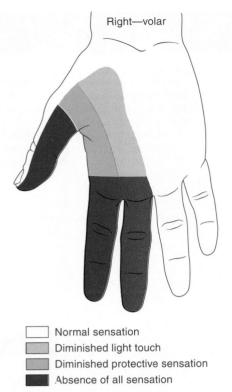

Right—volar

☐ Normal sensation
▨ Diminished light touch
▨ Diminished protective sensation
■ Absence of all sensation

Figure 6-7 Results of monofilament testing for Mr. T. (see case example) six weeks following median nerve laceration and surgery.

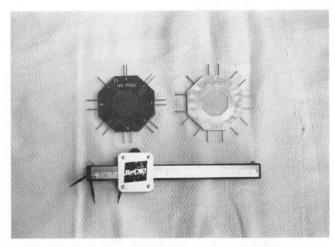

Figure 6-8 Tools used in two-point discrimination tests: a Disk-Criminator (*top*) and an aesthesiometer (*bottom*).

potential for improvement. Chapter 27 describes each of these interventions in detail.

Choosing Evaluation Methods

Therapists use a process of clinical reasoning to select appropriate sensory evaluation techniques for each patient. Diagnostic and procedural reasoning suggest

that certain tests are best at answering certain kinds of clinical questions. Ethical reasoning suggests that the tests should be the best available for each patient and that the practitioner has developed competence in test administration and interpretation. Pragmatic reasoning suggests that tests should be readily available and quickly administered.

Standardization, Reliability, and Validity

Fess (1995), in her article "Guidelines for Evaluating Assessment Instruments," describes four essential criteria for all assessment instruments. The first is reliability, which includes reliability of the instrument measurements as well as test–retest and interrater reliability. Second, she describes validity as the tool's ability to measure the sensory modality for which it was designed. Third, standards for the manufacture, administration, and scoring of the assessment and interpretation of the results must be set and followed. Finally, there must

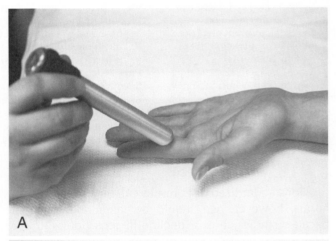

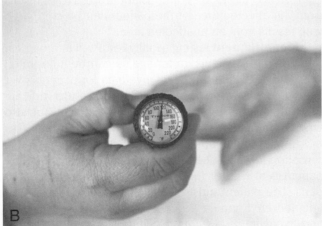

Figure 6-9 Temperature awareness testing. **A.** Metal probe is heated or cooled in water. **B.** The thermometer at the top helps to maintain consistency in testing.

TABLE 6-3
Nonstandardized Sensory Testing Techniques

Test and Test Instruments	Stimulus (S) and Response (R)	Scoring and Expected Results
Touch Awareness General awareness of touch input (Adams, 1997) **Test Instruments** Cotton ball or swab, fingertip, pencil eraser	**S:** Light touch to a small area of the patient's skin. **R:** Patient says yes or makes agreed-upon nonverbal signal each time stimulus is felt.	Score is number of correct responses in relation to number of applied stimuli. Expected score is 100%.
Pinprick or Pain Awareness Measures discrimination of sharp and dull stimuli, which indicates protective sensation (Brand & Hollister, 1993; Callahan, 1995; Reese, 1999) **Test Instrument** New or sterilized safety pin	**S:** Randomly apply sharp and blunt ends of safety pin, perpendicular to skin, at pressure necessary to elicit correct response on uninvolved side of body. **R:** Patient says "sharp" or "dull" after each stimulus.	Score is number of correct responses divided by number of stimuli. Expected score is 100%. Correct responses to sharp stimuli indicate intact protective sensation; incorrect responses to sharp stimuli indicate some awareness of pressure but absent protective sensation.
Temperature Awareness (Fig. 6-9) Measures discrimination of warm and cool stimuli (Waylett-Rendall, 1988) **Test Instrument** *Hot and Cold Discrimination Kit* or glass test tubes filled with warm and cool water	**S:** Apply cold (40°F) or warm (115–120°F) stimulus to patient's skin. **R:** Patient indicates hot or cold after each stimulus.	Score is number of correct responses divided by number of stimuli. Normal response is 100%.
Vibration Awareness Measures awareness of input to rapidly adapting A-beta fibers (Dellon, 1988) **Test Instrument:** Tuning forks: 30 cycles per second 256 cycles per second	**S:** Strike tuning fork with force to cause vibration; place prong tangentially to fingertip of injured and then uninjured hand; ask patient, "Does this feel the same or different?" **R:** Patient responds same or different and describes difference in perception.	Scoring is normal if stimuli to both hands feel the same, altered if stimuli feel different. The 30-cps tuning fork is used to test the Meissner afferents, and the 256-cps tuning fork is used to test the Pacinian afferents.
Stereognosis Measures the ability to identify objects, which requires interpretation of sensory input. Motor function is prerequisite. (Eggers, 1984). **Test Instrument** A number of small objects known to the patient	**S:** Place a small object in the hand to be tested. **R:** Patient may manipulate object within the hand, patient names object.	Scoring is number of correct responses divided by total number of objects presented or time to identify each object. Normal response is correct identification of almost all objects within 2–3 sec (Lederman & Klatzky, 1996).
Moberg's *Picking-up Test* Measures the function of slowly adapting A-beta fibers in medial nerve injury (Callahan, 1995; Dellon, 1988) **Test Instruments** An assortment of small objects and a small box	**S:** Instruct patient to pick up objects as rapidly as possible and place them In the box, using right and left hands, with and without vision. **R:** Patient quickly picks up objects and places them in box.	Scoring is total time to pick up objects. Compare scores of left and right hands and those with and without vision. Norms have not been established.
Proprioception Measures sense of joint position, which relies upon input from an unknown combination of muscle, joint, and skin receptors (Adams et al., 1997) **Test Instrument** None	**S:** Hold body segment being tested on the lateral surfaces; move the part into different positions and hold. **R:** Patient duplicates position with opposite extremity.	Graded as intact, impaired, or absent. Usually, reproduction of position can be accomplished within a few degrees. One study of the knee joint found on average 4° of error in subjects under age 30 and 7° of error in subjects over age 60 (Kaplan et al., 1985).
Kinesthesia Measures sense of joint motion, which relies on input from an unknown combination of muscle, joint, and skin receptors (Adams et al., 1997) **Test Instrument** None	**S:** Hold body segment being tested on the lateral surfaces; move the part through angles of varying degrees **R:** Patient indicates whether part moved up or down	Graded as intact, impaired, or absent. Nearly 100% correct identification is expected.

TABLE 6-4
Semmes-Weinstein and West Hand Monofilaments

Filament Number	Diameter (mm)	Mean Force (g)	Color Code	Interpretation	Hand Function and Use
2.83	0.127	0.076	Green	Normal	Normal
3.61	0.178	0.209	Blue	Diminished light touch	Stereognosis and perception of temperature and pain are good, close to normal use of hand.
4.31	0.305	2.35	Purple	Diminished protective sensation	Decreased recognition of objects and painful stimuli, difficulty in manipulating objects.
4.56	0.356	4.55	Red	Loss of protective sensation	Greatly impaired perception of pain, temperature and object recognition. No manipulation of object without vision. Marked decrease in spontaneous hand use.
6.65	1.143	235.61	Red-orange	Loss of all sensation except deep pressure	Unable to identify objects and temperature. Hand use only with visual guidance.
No response to 6.65	—	—	Red lines	Absence of all sensation	Unable to identify objects, temperature, and pain. Minimal hand use.

Based on information in Bell-Krotoski, J., & Tomancik, E. (1987). Repeatability of testing with Semmes-Weinstein monofilaments. *Journal of Hand Surgery, 12A*, 155–161; Tomancik, L. (1987). *Directions for using Semmes-Weinstein monofilaments.* San Jose, CA: North Coast Medical; Bell-Krotoski, J. A. (1997). Correlating sensory morphology and tests of sensibility with function. In J. M. Hunter, L. H. Schneider, & E. J. Mackin (Eds.), *Tendon and Nerve Surgery in the Hand: A Third Decade* (pp. 49–62). St. Louis: Mosby.

be normative data and ideally, diagnosis-specific data. Fess states, "unfortunately, very few assessment tools in hand rehabilitation meet even the most basic measurement criteria" (p. 144).

Sensory testing tools have been the target of much criticism for their lack of standardization, reliability, and validity. Although the sensory tests were divided into standardized and nonstandardized tests in Tables 6-2 and 6-3, few of the tests in Table 6-2, presented as standardized, meet all of the criteria described by Fess (1995).

One important criterion that has historically been overlooked in sensory testing is the amount of force with which sensory stimuli are applied to the skin. Larger amounts of force are known to stimulate larger numbers of sensory receptors; therefore, results can be significantly affected by varying amounts of force in stimulus applications. Recently, Bell-Krotoski and Buford (1988, 1997) have shown that using hand-held instruments for assessing two-point discrimination results in a wide range of variation in force produced and a tendency for the force to be greater when two points are applied than when one point is applied. Their conclusion was that patients may be able to

differentiate one and two points by the amount of force rather than the number of points touching the skin.

Bell-Krotoski and Buford's studies also showed that the Semmes-Weinstein monofilaments of identical measurements (length, 38 mm; diameters according to Table 6-4) deliver a consistently repeatable application force, as long as the evaluation protocols are followed carefully and the monofilaments are cared for properly. Monofila-

TABLE 6-5
Semmes-Weinstein Results for Subjects Over 60: Median Monofilament Marking Number by Gender and Age

Age	Women	Men
60–69	3.22	3.61
70–79	3.61	3.61
80+	3.61	3.84

Based on information from Desrosiers, J., Hébert, R., Bravo, G., & Dutil, É. (1996). Hand sensibility of healthy older people. *Journal of the American Geriatrics Society, 44*, 974–978.

ments should be stored in a dry place and in manner that will prevent bending. When testing, filaments should be slowly applied and removed, not bounced on the skin (Bell-Krotoski & Buford, 1988, 1997). Duration of skin contact has been shown to alter touch threshold measurements (van Vliet et al., 1993).

Bell-Krotoski and Tomancik (1987) studied the forces of the Semmes-Weinstein monofilaments in the 20-piece set and demonstrated some areas of overlap in the range of forces supplied by adjacent monofilaments. They also found some manufacturing errors, so that not all filaments delivered the expected amount of force. As a result, they recommend using the 5-piece minikit of monofilaments and measuring the diameter of the monofilaments with a micrometer.

Interrater reliability has been studied for some tactile assessments. Novak et al. (1993) report the following results for interrater reliability:

Object identification	.994
Moving two-point discrimination	.991
Static two-point discrimination	.989
Vibration threshold	.982
Semmes-Weinstein monofilaments	.965
Texture identification	.768

These results show high evidence of reliability except for the texture identification test. Halar et al. (1987) found no significant day-to-day variability in testing using Semmes-Weinstein monofilaments and an **aesthesiometer** for two-point discrimination, although the testing protocols used in that study were different from those described in this chapter. Sieg and Williams (1986) reported an interrater reliability (Pearson's r) of .98 and a test–retest reliability between .36 and .71 for the touch localization test.

Weinstein (1993) advised that sensitivity should also be considered in evaluating the usefulness of testing methods. The instrument and scoring must be sensitive enough to detect significant clinical changes. Two-point discrimination has been found more sensitive than stereognosis (Bolanos et al., 1989) but less sensitive than touch thresholds using monofilaments (Gellman et al., 1986). Vibration threshold seems to be slightly more sensitive to minor changes, such as those seen in early changes of carpal tunnel syndrome, than monofilament testing (Szabo et al., 1984). Testing vibration awareness using a tuning fork is less sensitive than either the vibration threshold or monofilament test (Szabo et al, 1984).

For optimum standardization, reliability, validity, and sensitivity, choose the monofilament test, the two-point discrimination test, and/or the vibration threshold test from those listed in Tables 6.2 and 6.3. The Auto-

mated Tactile Tester, a new computer-based assessment, has been reported to have moderate to high test–retest reliability (r >.659) (Horch et al., 1992) and greater sensitivity than monofilament testing (Hardy et al., 1992). This device, or a similar one, would be the best choice in clinics where it is available.

Matching Methods with Purpose of Evaluation

Before choosing an evaluation method, decide why the test is necessary and what information is needed. Consider the diagnosis and the patient's description of the problem. For instance, for a patient with spinal cord injury, it is important to know whether sensation is present or absent in each region of skin. A touch awareness or pinprick test is common, with the results recorded on a drawing of the body (Waters, 1993).

If the purpose is to assist in the diagnosis of a nerve compression, such as carpal tunnel syndrome, it is necessary to use a highly sensitive test, such as a monofilament test. Sensation can be evaluated in positions that are likely to provoke more symptoms, for example with the wrist flexed (Szabo et al., 1999). A self-report of sensory loss has also been found useful in the diagnosis of carpal tunnel syndrome (Katz & Stirrat, 1990).

During observation of dressing or grooming by a patient with a diagnosis of CVA, a suspicion may arise that the observed errors are related to a loss of proprioception. An evaluation of proprioception can confirm or refute this hypothesis. For this same patient, it is important to know whether there is risk of injury because of a loss of pain and temperature sensation (protective sensation). Either a pinprick and temperature test or monofilament test can provide this information. The monofilament test is more standardized and therefore a better choice, although it usually takes more time.

A test of stereognosis is most appropriate to predict, for example, whether a patient with a hand injury who is a mechanic can feel for and locate unseen automobile parts,. The result of a two-point discrimination test or a monofilament test correlates with but does not totally predict the ability to identify objects (Bell-Krotoski, 1997; Van Heest et al., 1993).

Pragmatic Constraints

Ideally, patients are thoroughly evaluated using standardized, reliable assessments that are easy to perform and that provide a complete understanding of sensation. A battery of tests is recommended if it is desirable to get a complete understanding of tactile sensation, because no one test can assess this complex sense (Callahan, 1995; Lundborg & Rosén, 1994; Rosén, 1996). In clinical practice, however, therapists must sometimes balance

Case Example

SENSORY PROBLEMS FOLLOWING MEDIAN NERVE LACERATION

Patient Information

Mr. T. is a 25-year-old married man with a son aged 2. Mr. T.'s right wrist was injured by a broken window, resulting in a complete laceration of the median nerve and the flexor digitorum superficialis tendons to the middle and ring fingers. Both the nerve and tendons were repaired surgically the day after the injury, and Mr. T. was referred to occupational therapy 2 days later.

Description of Assessment

Mr. T.'s initial evaluation revealed that he graduated from vocational–technical school with training in major appliance repair. At the time of his injury, he was working for a local company doing in-home repairs of refrigerators, freezers, washers, and dryers. He stated that his wife was working in a secretarial position. He is right-handed, but he reported that since the injury, he had been using his left hand successfully in basic activities of daily living, such as feeding, dressing, and hygiene. These activities were being completed slowly, and he occasionally required assistance from his wife. He had not attempted any work, home management, or child care since the injury.

Findings of the initial evaluation of abilities and capacities revealed a total absence of sensation in the median nerve distribution in the palm and the palmar surface of the thumb, index, and middle fingers. Movement was restricted throughout the hand due to tendon healing precautions and loss of innervation to the thenar muscles. A sutured scar measuring 3 inches on the volar wrist area was slightly pink, with no drainage. As a result of the performance component deficits, Mr. T. had no functional use of the right hand in any activities of daily living.

A dorsal blocking splint was fabricated and fitted to protect the surgically repaired tendons and nerve. The splint had a dynamic component that allowed for some movement during the day to promote tendon gliding while still protecting the surgical repair. Over the next 6 weeks, Mr. T. participated in a program of occupational therapy that included the following:

► Training in basic activities of daily living
► Protected, progressive passive and active range-of-motion exercises
► Education in edema prevention and management techniques
► Scar management techniques to promote good healing

At 6 weeks after injury, protective splinting was discontinued, and Mr. T. was allowed to begin to use his right hand in functional activities with light resistance. At that time, the occupational therapist performed a comprehensive reassessment to determine the level of motor and sensory recovery of the median nerve, the sensibility and sensitivity around the area of the scar, and Mr. T.'s ability to use his right hand in functional activities. Therefore, the occupational therapist selected the following sensory evaluation tools:

► Touch threshold test using Semmes-Weinstein monofilaments
► Static and moving two-point discrimination
► Touch localization
► Dellon's modification of the Moberg picking-up test

Results of Sensory Tests

The results of the Semmes-Weinstein monofilament test for the right palm and fingers are shown in Figure 6-7. Touch pressure threshold testing over the area of the scar revealed that Mr. T. disliked touch directly on the scar. The area was rubbed with textured items, and Mr. T. reported a marked preference for soft textures and no tolerance for rough textures, such as burlap and Velcro. Mr. T. was unable to feel the Disk-Criminator anywhere on the fingers or thumb in the static test nor on the fingertips in the moving test. Touch localization in the radial portion of the right palm measured 18 to 25 mm. Mr. T.'s scores on Dellon's modification of the *Picking Up Test* were as follows:

Part 1	Left	Right
Trial 1	17 seconds	55 seconds
Trial 2	15 seconds	60 seconds
Part 2	No objects could be identified without vision.	

Analysis of Results

The occupational therapist concluded that sensation was returning as expected considering the nature of the median nerve lesion. Return of some protective sensation in the palm was a positive sign that neuron regrowth was occurring. Absence of sensation in the fingertips was expected, because the average rate of neural regrowth was known by the therapist to be approximately 1 mm per day, or an inch per month. Mr. T. could use visual guidance to pick up small objects despite the sensory loss, but his movements were awkward. Because of lack of sensation in the fingertips, object identification was not possible. Mr. T. is probably at some risk for injury to the fingertips, because he can now start using his hand in more functional tasks but lacks any protective sensation in the digit tips, a likely place for thermal injuries or lacerations. The presence of some protective sensation in the palm and the mislocalization of touch stimuli suggests that retraining of sensation in this area can now be started. The presence of hypersensitivity around the area of the scar suggests that intervention to decrease this is required.

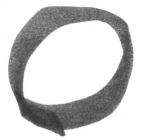

CLINICAL REASONING
in OT Practice

Interpretation and Treatment Planning for Peripheral Sensory Problem

Mr. T.'s touch threshold test performed 6 weeks post injury is shown in Fig. 6-7. How will the mapping likely change when Mr. T. is reassessed after 6 more weeks? What kind of sensation, pain or touch, will he be able to feel first in his fingertips? Compare his current functional hand use with his expected hand use when his fingertips regain touch sensation.

...sation in the thumb,

...the radial portion of

...r

...ability to pick up and manipulate objects

► Decreased use of the right hand in functional activities

---

the ideal with practical constraints. Schell (1998) described pragmatic constraints that affect assessment and treatment, including sensory testing, in occupational therapy. These include the availability of equipment and supplies, the availability of treatment time, team roles and responsibilities, reimbursement, trends within the profession, culture of the health care organization, and the therapist's clinical competencies or preferences.

Therapists should carefully assess their practices periodically to ensure that they are providing intervention that is as close to the ideal as possible despite pragmatic constraints. Brand and Hollister (1993) charge that much time is wasted in sensory testing and the results are open to question. Great improvements can and should be made in tests of sensation so that they are meaningful, quantitative, and meet the criteria for good test instruments (Peripheral Neuropathy Association, 1993).

Summary Review Questions

1. What pattern of sensory loss would be expected in a patient with a T10 complete spinal cord injury?
2. What pattern of sensory loss would be expected in a patient with peripheral polyneuropathy?
3. Which patient will have a better prognosis for recovery of sensation, one with a peripheral nerve compression or one with a middle cerebral artery stroke?
4. Name and describe the purposes of at least three standardized and three nonstandardized sensory tests.
5. Describe or demonstrate the administration and scoring of a touch threshold test, a pain awareness test, and a touch localization test.

6. Which sensory test or tests would you select for a patient with peripheral polyneuropathy? Justify your response.
7. What type of intervention is needed for a patient with lost or absent protective sensation?
8. Which dressing tasks will be most difficult for a woman who has **hemianesthesia** (loss of sensation on one side of the body)?

Acknowledgment

I extend my appreciation to Paul Petersen and Melanie Seltzer for their assistance with the photography for this chapter.

Resources

Sensory Evaluation Instrument Suppliers

Biomedical Instrument Co. (Biothesiometer vibrometer) · 15764 Munn Road, Newbury, OH 44065. 216-543-9443

Connecticut Bioinstruments (Weinstein Enhanced Sensory Test: WEST-Hand and WEST-Foot) · 36 Mill Plain Road, Danbury, CT 06811. 203-744-7488
www.cbi-pace.com

NeuroRegen, LLC (Disk-Criminator, force-defined vibrometer, pressure-specified sensory device) · 2328 West Joppa Road, Suite 325, Lutherville, MD 21093. 410-538-0200. Fax 410-583-0201

North Coast Medical (monofilaments, Disk-Criminator, aesthesiometer, testing shield) · 187 Stauffer Boulevard, San Jose, CA 95125-1042. 800-821-9319. Fax 408-283-1950
www.ncmedical.com

Sammons Preston (monofilaments, Disk-Criminator, aesthesiometer, tuning forks, *Picking Up Test*) · P.O. Box 5071, Bolingbrook, IL 60440-5071. 800-323-5547. Fax 800-547-4333

Smith & Nephew, Inc. (monofilaments, Disk-Criminator, aesthesiometer, hot and cold probes, tuning forks, testing shield) · One Quality Drive, P.O. Box 1005, Germantown, WI 53022-8205. 800-558-8633. Fax 800-545-7758
www.easy-living.com

Ztech, L.C. (Automated Tactile Tester) · P.O. Box 581215, Salt Lake City, UT 84148. 801-581-5928

References

Adams, R. D., Victor, M., & Ropper, A. H. (1997). *Principles of Neurology* (6th ed.). New York: McGraw-Hill.

American Occupational Therapy Association. (1994). Uniform terminology for occupational therapy (3rd ed.). *American Journal of Occupational Therapy, 48,* 1047–1054.

Bell-Krotoski, J. A. (1995). Sensibility testing: Current concepts. In J. M. Hunter, E. J. Mackin, & A. D. Callahan (Eds.), *Rehabilitation of the Hand: Surgery and Therapy* (4th ed., pp. 109–128). St. Louis: Mosby.

Bell-Krotoski, J. A. (1997). Correlating sensory morphology and tests of sensibility with function. In J. M. Hunter, L. H. Schneider, & E. J. Mackin (Eds.), *Tendon and Nerve Surgery in the Hand: A Third Decade* (pp. 49–62). St. Louis: Mosby.

Bell-Krotoski, J., & Buford, W. (1988). The force/time relationship of clinically used sensory testing instruments. *Journal of Hand Therapy, 1,* 76–85.

Bell-Krotoski, J. A., & Buford, W. L. (1997). The force/time relationship of clinically used sensory testing instruments. *Journal of Hand Therapy, 10,* 297–309.

Bell-Krotoski, J., & Tomancik, E. (1987). Repeatability of testing with Semmes-Weinstein monofilaments. *Journal of Hand Surgery, 12A,* 155–161.

Benton, S. (1994). Computerized assessment holds promise. *Rehab Management, 7,* 37.

Beschin, N., Cazzani, M., Cubelli, R., Sala, S. D., & Spinazzola, L. (1996). Ignoring left and far: an investigation of tactile neglect. *Neuropsychologia, 34,* 41–49.

Bolanos, A., Bleck, E., Firestone, P., & Young, L. (1989). Comparison of stereognosis and two-point discrimination testing of the hands of children with cerebral palsy. *Developmental Medicine and Child Neurology, 31,* 371–376.

Brand, P. W., & Hollister, A. (1993). *Clinical Mechanics of the Hand* (2nd Ed.). St Louis: Mosby.

Callahan, A. D. (1995). Sensibility assessment: Prerequisites and techniques for nerve lesions In continuity. In J. M. Hunter, E. J. Mackin, & A. D. Callahan (Eds.), *Rehabilitation of the Hand: Surgery and Therapy* (4th ed., pp. 129–152). St. Louis: Mosby.

Carr, J., & Shepherd, R. (1998). *Neurological Rehabilitation: Optimizing Motor Performance.* Oxford: Butterworth-Heinemann.

Chapman, C. E., Tremblay, F., & Ageranioti-Bélanger, A. (1996). Role of primary somatosensory cortex in active and passive touch. In A. M. Wing, P. Haggard, & J. R. Flanagan (Eds.), *Hand and Brain: The Neurophysiology of Hand Movements* (pp. 329–347). San Diego: Academic.

Cole, J. (1991). *Pride and a Daily Marathon.* Cambridge: MIT.

Cooke, D. (1991). Sensibility evaluation battery for the peripheral nerve injured hand. *Australian Occupational Therapy Journal, 38,* 241–245.

Dellon, A. (1988). *Evaluation of Sensibility and Re-education of Sensation in the Hand.* Baltimore: Lucas.

Dellon, A. L. (1997). *Somatosensory Testing and Rehabilitation.* Bethesda, MD: American Occupational Therapy Association.

Desrosiers, J., Hébert, R., Bravo, G., & Dutil, É. (1996). Hand sensibility of healthy older people. *Journal of the American Geriatrics Society, 44,* 974–978.

Eggers, O. (1984). *Occupational Therapy in the Treatment of Adult Hemiplegia.* Rockville, CO: Aspen Systems.

Fess, E. E. (1995). Guidelines for evaluating assessment instruments. *Journal of Hand Therapy, 8,* 144–148.

Fredericks, C. M. (1996a). Basic sensory mechanisms and the somatosensory system. In C.M. Fredericks & L. K. Saladin (Eds.), *Pathophysiology of the Motor Systems: Principles and Clinical Presentations* (pp. 78–106). Philadelphia: Davis.

Fredericks, C. M. (1996b). Disorders of the peripheral nervous system: The peripheral neuropathies. In C.M. Fredericks & L.K. Saladin (Eds.), *Pathophysiology of the Motor Systems: Principles and Clinical Presentations* (pp. 346–372). Philadelphia: Davis.

Fredericks, C. M. (1996c). Disorders of the spinal cord. In C. M. Fredericks & L. K. Saladin (Eds.), *Pathophysiology of the Motor Systems: Principles and Clinical Presentations* (pp. 394–423). Philadelphia: Davis.

Garrison, S. J., Rolak, L. A., Dodaro, R. R., & O'Callaghan, A. J. (1988). Rehabilitation of the stroke patient. In J. A. DeLisa, D. M. Currie, B. M. Gans, P. F. Gatens, J. A. Leonard, & M. C. McPhee (Eds.), *Rehabilitation Medicine: Principles and Practice* (pp. 565–584). Philadelphia : Lippincott.

Gellman, H., Gelberman, R. H., Tan, A. M., & Botte, M. J. (1986). Carpal tunnel syndrome: Evaluation of the provocative diagnostic test. *Journal of Bone and Joint Surgery, 68A,* 735–737.

Halar, E. B., Hammond, M. C., LaCava, E. C., Camann, C., & Ward, J. (1987). Sensory perception threshold measurement: An evaluation of semiobjective testing devices. *Archives of Physical Medicine and Rehabilitation, 68,* 499–507.

Hardy, M., Jiminez, S., Jabaley, M., & Horch, K. (1992). Evaluation of nerve compression with the Automated Tactile Tester. *Journal of Hand Surgery, 17A,* 838–842.

Hermann, R. P., Novak, C. B., & Mackinnon, S. E. (1995). Establishing normal values for moving two-point discrimination in children and adolescents. *Southern Medical Journal, 88(10),* S97 (abstract).

Horch, K., Hardy, M., Jiminez, S., & Jabaley, M. (1992). An Automated Tactile Tester for evaluation of cutaneous sensibility. *Journal of Hand Surgery, 17A,* 829–837.

Johansson, R. S. (1996). Sensory control of dexterous manipulation in humans. In A. M. Wing, P. Haggard, & J. R. Flanagan (Eds.), *Hand and Brain: The Neurophysiology of Hand Movements* (pp. 381–414). San Diego: Academic.

Jones, L. (1996). Proprioception and its contribution to manual dexterity. In A. M. Wing, P. Haggard, & J. R. Flanagan (Eds.), *Hand and Brain: The Neurophysiology of Hand Movements* (pp. 349–362). San Diego: Academic.

Kaplan, F. S., Nixon, J. E., Reitz, M., Rindfleish, L., & Tucker, J. (1985). Age-related changes in proprioception and sensation of joint position. *Acta Orthopaedica Scandinavia, 56,* 72–74.

Katz, J. N., & Stirrat, C. R. (1990). A self-administered hand diagram for the diagnosis of carpal tunnel syndrome. *Journal of Hand Surgery, 15A,* 360–363.

Lederman, S. J., & Klatzky, R. L. (1996). Action for perception: Manual exploratory movements for haptically processing objects and their features. In A. M. Wing, P. Haggard, & J. R. Flanagan (Eds.), *Hand and Brain: The Neurophysiology of Hand Movements* (pp. 431–446). San Diego: Academic.

Lindblom, U. (1994). Analysis of abnormal touch, pain, and temperature sensation in patients. In J. Boivie, P. Hansson, & U. Lindblom (Eds.), *Touch, Temperature, and Pain in Health and Disease: Mechanisms and Assessment* (pp. 63–84). Seattle: IASP.

Lundborg, G., & Rosén, B. (1994). Rationale for quantitative sensory tests in hand surgery. In J. Boivie, P. Hansson, & U. Lindblom (Eds.), *Touch, Temperature, and Pain in Health and Disease: Mechanisms and Assessment* (pp. 151–162). Seattle: IASP.

Nakada, M. (1993). Localization of a constant-touch and moving-touch stimulus in the hand: A preliminary study. *Journal of Hand Therapy, 6,* 23–28.

Novak, C. B., Mackinnon, S. E., Williams, J. I., & Kelly, L. (1993).

Establishment of reliability in the evaluation of hand sensibility. *Plastic and Reconstructive Surgery, 92*, 311–322.

Peripheral Neuropathy Association (1993). Quantitative sensory testing: A consensus report from the Peripheral Neuropathy Association. *Neurology, 43*, 1050–1052.

Reese, N.B. (1999). *Muscle and Sensory Testing*. Philadelphia: Saunders.

Riggle, M. (1999). [Review of the book *Somatosensory Testing and Rehabilitation*]. *American Journal of Occupational Therapy, 53*, 412.

Rosén, B. (1996). Recovery of sensory and motor function after nerve repair: A rationale for evaluation. *Journal of Hand Therapy, 9*, 315–327.

Saladin, L. K. (1996a). Cerebrovascular disease: Stroke. In C. M. Fredericks & L. K. Saladin (Eds.), *Pathophysiology of the Motor Systems: Principles and Clinical Presentations* (pp. 486–512). Philadelphia: Davis.

Saladin, L. K. (1996b). Traumatic brain injury. In C. M. Fredericks & L. K. Saladin (Eds.), *Pathophysiology of the Motor Systems: Principles and Clinical Presentations* (pp. 467–485). Philadelphia: Davis.

Schady, W. (1994). Locognosia: Normal precision and changes after peripheral nerve injury. In J. Boivie, P. Hansson, & U. Lindblom (Eds.), *Touch, Temperature, and Pain in Health and Disease: Mechanisms and Assessment* (pp. 143–150). Seattle: IASP.

Schell, B. B. (1998). Clinical reasoning: The basis of practice. In: M. E. Neistadt & E. B. Crepeau (Eds.), *Willard & Spackman's Occupational Therapy, 9th ed.* (pp. 90–100). Philadelphia: Lippincott.

Shimokata, H., & Kuzuya, F. (1995). Two-point discrimination test of the skin as an index of sensory aging. *Gerontology, 41*, 267–272.

Sieg, K., & Williams, W. (1986). Preliminary report of a methodology for determining tactile location in adults. *Occupational Therapy Journal of Research, 6*, 195–206.

Smith, K. L. (1995). Nerve response to injury and repair. In J. M. Hunter, E. J. Mackin, & A. D. Callahan (Eds.), *Rehabilitation of the Hand: Surgery and Therapy* (4th ed., pp. 609–626). St. Louis: Mosby.

Sterzi, R., Bottini, G., Celani, M. G., Righetti, E., Lamassa, M., Ricci, S., & Vallar, G. (1993). Hemianopia, hemianesthesia, and hemiplegia after right and left hemisphere damage: A hemispheric difference. *Journal of Neurology, Neurosurgery, and Psychiatry, 56*, 308–310.

Szabo, R., Gelberman, R., & Dimick, M. (1984). Sensibility testing in patients with carpal tunnel syndrome. *Journal of Bone and Joint Surgery, 66A*, 60–64.

Szabo, R. M., Slater, R. R., Farver, T. B., Stanton, D. B., & Sharman, W. K. (1999). The value of diagnostic testing in carpal tunnel syndrome. *Journal of Hand Surgery, 24A*, 704–714.

Tomancik, L. (1987). *Directions for using Semmes-Weinstein monofilaments*. San Jose, CA: North Coast Medical.

van Vliet, D., Novak, C. B., & Mackinnon, S. (1993). Duration of contact time alters cutaneous pressure threshold measurements. *Annals of Plastic Surgery, 31*, 335–339.

Van Heest, A., House, J., & Putnam, M. (1993). Sensibility deficiencies in the hands of children with spastic hemiplegia. *Journal of Hand Surgery, 18A*, 278–281.

Waters, R., Adkins, R., Yakura, J., & Sie, I. (1993). Motor and sensory recovery following complete tetraplegia. *Archives of Physical Medicine and Rehabilitation, 74*, 242–247.

Waylett-Rendall, J. (1988). Sensibility evaluation and rehabilitation. *Orthopedic Clinics of North America, 19*, 43–56.

Weinstein, S., Drozdenko, R., Weinstein, C. (1997). Evaluation of sensory measures in neuropathy. In J. M. Hunter, L. H. Schneider, & E. J. Mackin (Eds.), *Tendon and Nerve Surgery in the Hand: A Third Decade* (pp. 63–76). St. Louis: Mosby.

Weinstein, S. (1993). Fifty years of somatosensory research: From the Semmes-Weinstein monofilaments to the Weinstein Enhanced Sensory Tests. *Journal of Hand Therapy, 6*, 11–22.

7

Assessing Abilities and Capacities: Vision, Visual Perception, and Praxis

Lee Ann Quintana

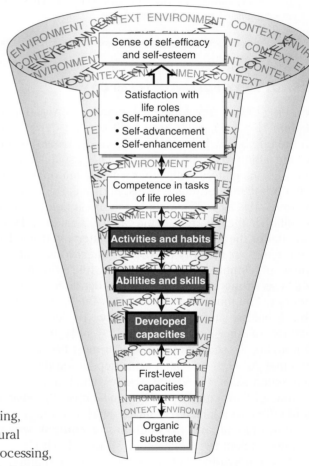

LEARNING OBJECTIVES

After studying this chapter, the reader will be able to do the following:

1. Understand the importance of evaluating the visual foundation skills prior to higher-level visual cognitive skills.
2. Identify and describe evaluation techniques for visual acuity, visual fields, and ocular motor control.
3. Describe and evaluate the two subtypes of unilateral neglect, sensory and motor.
4. Describe and evaluate apraxia.

*V*ision is a critical channel by which we gather information from the environment. We depend heavily on vision for learning, decision making, social interactions, motor control, and postural control because of its critical role in attention, information processing, and movement detection (Titcomb et al., 1997; Warren, 1999). It is the means by which we register information and decide what will happen next (e.g., move out of the way of a moving car, comfort a friend who is crying, pick up a tool lying on the table). Because of its importance to almost all activities of daily living, occupational therapists must know the basic status of the visual system of their patients.

The purpose of this chapter is to review evaluation of the visual system with emphasis on **visual foundation skills** and less on the higher-level visual cognitive skills. In addition, the chapter discusses assessment of praxis (motor planning).

Visual Perceptual Hierarchy

Warren (1993a) developed a hierarchy of visual perception (Fig. 7-1), each level built on and dependent on the one below it. Visual cognition, the highest level, is "the ability to mentally manipulate visual information and integrate it with other sensory information to solve problems, formulate plans, and make decisions" (Warren, 1993a, p. 43). Visual memory is below visual cognition in the hierarchy. If the car doesn't start and you look under the hood to check the battery, you need a picture in your memory of what a battery looks like, or you would fumble around for quite a while trying to find what was wrong. Likewise, pattern recognition subserves memory. You must be able to identify the features of an object before storing it in memory. To identify the features of an object, you must be able to scan it thoroughly. To scan thoroughly, you must be alert and attentive. All of these higher skills depend on the visual foundation skills: (1) **visual acuity**, which assures the accuracy of information sent to the brain; (2) **visual fields** (VF), which let the brain know what's going on in the environment; and (3) **oculomotor control**, which ensures efficient eye movements (Warren, 1993a).

Visual impairment changes the quality and amount of visual input to the brain and therefore decreases the ability to use vision to adapt (Warren, 1999) (Box 7-1). If a person has poor contrast sensitivity, he or she may no longer want to go out in the evening because of the difficulty of maneuvering in poor light. Patients generally have the most difficulty in dynamic environments. At home we are best able to control and compensate for the deficits; community activities such as shopping and driving present more of a problem.

In the past, therapists often evaluated higher-level visual perceptual skills without a good understanding of

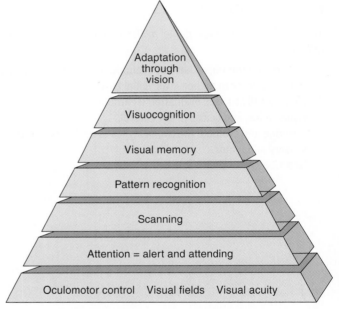

Figure 7-1 Hierarchy of visual perception. (From Warren, M. [1993]. A hierarchical model for evaluation and treatment of visual perceptual dysfunction in adult acquired brain injury, part 1. *American Journal of Occupational Therapy*, *47*, p. 43. Copyright 1993 by the American Occupational Therapy Association, Inc. Reprinted with permission.)

the optical system and how it provides the foundation for these skills (Warren 1999). A deficit in one of the higher-level visual perceptual skills, such as figure–ground or spatial relations, may be the result of a problem in one of the foundation skills. For example, patients who do poorly on a figure–ground test may have decreased visual acuity and be unable to get a clear picture of what they see or have poor convergence and therefore difficulty with any close work.

BOX 7-1
Definitions and Descriptions of Vision, Visual Perception, and Praxis Deficits

Area of Deficit	Definition	Functional Description of Deficit
Visual acuity	Ability of the eyes to make what is seen sharp and clear.	Complaints: blurred near or far vision; print too small, too faint; headaches, squinting. Effect on function: holds objects too close to face; loss of facial recognition; fear of new environments; lack of interest in environment; difficulty finding objects; loss of interest in reading; vision fluctuating throughout the day; bumps into low-contrast objects.
Visual field	Area that one sees when looking out into the environment. Central visual field: central 30 degrees where vision is clear and focused. Peripheral visual field: area seen other than central where vision is not as clear, but used for motion detection and orientation.	Complaints: bumps into objects; can't find things; difficulty reading. Effect on function: difficulty moving in crowded or busy environments; anxiety; startle response; difficulty with self-care; unsafe.
Binocular vision	Ability to resolve the images from the two eyes into one. Motor component: muscles and nerves align the eyes with the object. Sensory component: activity within the cortex allowing perception of one image.	Complaints: double vision; difficulty sustaining visual work effort; eye fatigue with sustained work; eyes look crossed; blurred vision; headaches. Effect on function: poor eye contact, inability to concentrate, avoidance of activities at near distance, loss of vision, difficulty with activities requiring depth perception.
Accommodation	Ability to adjust focus for distance.	Complaints: headaches; eye strain; difficulty with sustained activity at near distance; print moves while reading. Effect on function: underreaching and overreaching; frustration when maneuvering in visually stimulating environments; road fatigue.
Ocular motility	Ability of eyes to move smoothly and with coordination through full range of motion.	Complaints: headaches; difficulty keeping eyes focused; dizziness; balance problems. Effect on function: excessive head movements; frequent loss of place and skipping lines when reading.
Anosognosia	Unawareness or denial of deficits.	Functional activities unsafe; unable to learn compensatory techniques.
Unilateral neglect	Neglect of one side of the body or space. Types: motor (output, or intentional) and perceptual (input, or attentional).	Shaves only one side of face, dresses only one side of body; eats food from only half of the plate; reads only half of a page or word; transfers and functional mobility unsafe; bumps into objects on neglected side.
Body scheme	Awareness of body parts, position of body and its parts in relation to themselves and environment.	May result in dressing apraxia; may not recognize body parts or relations between them; transfers may be unsafe.
Right–left discrimination	Ability to understand the concepts of right and left. With right brain damage (RBD), problems may be caused by visuo-spatial deficit. With left brain damage (LBD) and aphasia, problems may be caused by language deficits or general mental impairment.	May have difficulty dressing and understanding concepts of right and left.
Body part identification	Ability to identify parts on self and/or others.	May respond incorrectly when told to move a specific body part.
Position in space	Ability to understand such concepts as over and under, above and below.	Difficulty moving through a crowded area; difficulty with dressing; difficulty following directions using these terms.
Spatial relations	Ability to perceive self in relation to other objects.	Difficulty moving through a crowded area; difficulty with dressing; difficulty following directions using these terms; transfers unsafe.
Topographical orientation	Ability to find one's way from one place to another.	Difficulty finding the way to a room, to therapy, or from one room to another.
Figure and ground perception	Ability to distinguish foreground from background.	Unable to find object in cluttered drawer, white washcloth on white sheet, brakes on wheelchair, food in refrigerator, etc.

continued

BOX 7-1
Definitions and Descriptions of Vision, Visual Perception, and Praxis Deficits (Continued)

Area of Deficit	Definition	Functional Description of Deficit
Limb apraxia	Inability to carry out purposeful movement in the presence of intact sensation, movement, and coordination.	May have difficulty with functional tasks involving objects, as patient does not know how to use objects or attempts to use incorrect object (e.g., uses knife to eat soup); difficulty producing and understanding gestures; may be clumsy, have poor fine coordination (e.g., trouble writing, knitting).
Constructional apraxia	Deficit in constructional activities: graphic and assembly RBD—drawings are complex but exhibit disorganized spatial relations and poor orientation in space LBD—drawings are simple, with few details	May result in dressing apraxia; difficulty setting a table, making a dress, wrapping a gift, arranging numerical figures for mathematical processing, making a sandwich, assembling a craft project from a kit, etc.
Dressing apraxia	Inability to dress oneself	Attempts to put clothes on inside out, backward, or in the wrong order; dresses only half of the body.

Assessing Vision and Visual Perception

If higher-level visual cognitive skills are the result of the integration of the skills that subserve them in the visual hierarchy, it seems that the therapist's limited time is best spent evaluating the foundation skills rather than higher-level visual cognitive skills (Warren, 1993b). Evaluation includes the following:

▶ A basic eye history, including premorbid visual conditions (e.g., congenital strabismus, ocular trauma)
▶ Interviews with the patient and/or family as to complaints or symptoms (e.g., difficulty concentrating, double vision, eyestrain, bumping into objects on one side)
▶ Observation of the patient during functional activities
▶ Screening of the foundation skills

The therapist bases plans for further evaluation and treatment on the results and the patient's goals and lifestyle. For example, if the 35-year-old stroke patient works as a mechanic, the therapist may evaluate his constructional abilities in depth. If the patient is 75 years old and retired and spends his time reading and watching television, detailed evaluation of constructional abilities may not be indicated. This idea is carried over into treatment as well. The 35-year-old mechanic needs a higher level of constructional skills than does the 75-year-old retiree. In addition, the therapist may find that the patient performs adequately on a test but exhibits difficulty in a functional situation. This also indicates the need for further evaluation.

All neurologically impaired patients should have their visual foundation skills screened. Screening is also considered for patients whose vision may have been affected by age. How much screening may depend on the team members who care for the patient. If working in a rehabilitation facility with the services of an eye care professional, the occupational therapist may only refer the patient to that professional and collaborate on the findings and development of a treatment plan. On the other hand, the occupational therapist may be the only one on the team to look specifically at vision and its effects on functional activities. In this case, the occupational therapist may choose to screen all patients and at any sign of difficulty refer the patient to an eye care professional.

Eye Care Professionals

The eye care professionals include the ophthalmologist and optometrist. The ophthalmologist is a medical doctor whose major concern is eye health (e.g., cataracts, macular degeneration, infections). Generally, "ophthalmologists are rarely trained, experienced or interested in visual system rehabilitation or function" (Gianutsos, 1997, p. 273). Optometrists receive 4 years of postgraduate training on diagnosis and treatment of eye disease focused mainly on function and how vision affects performance and quality of life (Scheiman, 1999). Even with this focus, most optometrists specialize in refraction and contact lenses, and only approximately 5% of optometrists do vision therapy (Scheiman, 1999). To find eye care professionals with a similar frame of reference, ask them questions such as these (Scheiman, 1997, p. 115):

▶ Do you have experience working with patients with acquired brain injury?
▶ Do you test accommodative amplitude and facility?
▶ Do you evaluate fusional vergence and facility?

► Do you evaluate visual information processing skills?
► Do you offer vision therapy as a service in your practice?

Once the decision has been made to refer the patient to an eye care professional, therapists ideally go to the appointment with the patient or send information such as this:

► Practical information: diagnosis, method of communication, reliability of responses, ability to transfer, medications
► Description of functional behaviors that may indicate a problem with vision
► Vision history

If the therapist is able to attend the appointment, he or she can take notes, act as an interpreter between the patient and family and the eye doctor, and interact with the doctor to discuss treatment plans (Gianutsos, 1997). The therapist provides input on function and follows through with recommendations. If unable to attend the appointment, the therapist may send a form with the patient for the doctor to complete, requesting information such as this (Warren, 1999):

► Visual acuity
► Ocular motility
► Visual fields
► Pertinent ocular diagnoses
► Recommendations for follow-up and treatment

Visual Foundation Skills

The visual foundation skills include visual acuity, visual fields, and oculomotor control. While deficits in these areas can affect function, patients may not complain of any problems, or they may make complaints that appear unrelated to vision and/or appear to be due to something else (Box 7-1). It is therefore important that these areas be screened even if the patient denies difficulty seeing things.

Visual Acuity

Visual acuity is the ability of the eyes to make what is seen sharp and clear. Most of us are familiar with the concept of 20/20 vision. The numerator denotes the distance at which the patient recognizes the stimulus and the denominator is the distance at which it would be recognized by someone with normal vision. For instance, a person with 20/200 vision can recognize at 20 feet a stimulus that a person with normal vision can recognize at 200 feet. Deficits in visual acuity may be the result of refractive errors, poor eye health with inability to process the image (e.g., cataract, macular degenera-

tion, diabetic retinopathy) or poor transmission of the image by the optic nerve (Warren, 1999).

Visual acuity is most often screened using conventional letter charts (e.g., *Snellen Chart*). Test cards are available that use symbols rather than letters for use with aphasic, non–English-speaking, and severely impaired patients (e.g., *Lea Symbol Test*). Acuity should be examined in each eye for both near (16 inches or less) and far (20 feet or more) vision. Near acuity is important for any tabletop activity, and far vision is especially important for activities such as driving. Testing of visual acuity should be carried out with the best correction available: patients should wear their glasses. If the glasses are not available, have the patient look through a pinhole in a piece of paper, as this helps the focusing power of the eye (Simon, Aminoff, & Greenberg, 1999).

Since conventional letter charts measure acuity by determining the smallest high-contrast detail a person can perceive at a given distance and most settings do not provide such high contrast, **contrast sensitivity** should be evaluated as well. It indicates the person's ability to see objects in various levels of contrast and how he or she will perform functionally. The tester presents a series of sine wave gratings that vary in orientation, contrast, and frequency. The patient must indicate the orientation of the grating: the poorer the acuity, the more contrast required to detect the orientation of the grating (Fig. 7-2). In addition, Warren (1996), in *Brain Injury Visual Assessment Battery for Adults (biVABA)*, presents some clinical tasks and observations that can indicate a person's level of contrast sensitivity.

Visual Fields

Confrontation testing is typically used to screen for visual field deficits (Fig. 7-3). Visual fields are measured one

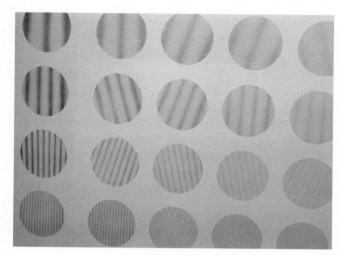

Figure 7-2 Contrast sensitivity test. (Reprinted with permission from Vistech Consultants, Inc., Dayton, Ohio.)

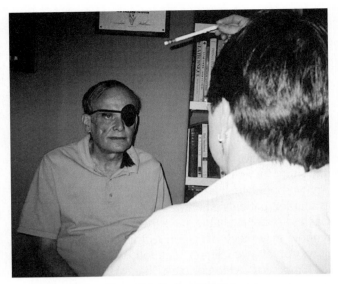

Figure 7-3 Confrontation test.

eye at a time, and the patient's visual fields are compared to the examiner's supposedly normal visual fields (Box 7-2). The normal limits of visual field are 60° superior, 75° inferior, 60° nasal and 100° temporal (Simon et al., 1999). Confrontation testing has been found to be relatively unreliable (Trobe, Acosta, Krischer, & Trick, 1981) and should therefore be used in conjunction with functional observations. Warren (1999) suggests observation of the patient during a dynamic functional activity, such as walking through a crowded area with moving objects, as a means of screening for visual field deficit. She also presents some other methods of confrontation testing as part of the *biVABA* (1996).

Automated perimetry provides a more accurate description and printout of the patient's visual field deficit. Figure 7-4 shows the results of a patient with visual field deficit. The results of the test are effectively used to teach the family and patient about visual field losses. There are several limitations:

1. The test can require up to 20 minutes of sustained concentration if there are significant deficits, and therefore, patients unable to maintain that level of concentration cannot be accurately tested.
2. The test requires a motor response to push a button within 1 to 3 seconds of the presentation, which may exclude evaluation of patients with significantly delayed motor responses or motor planning deficits.
3. The equipment is expensive.

The patient is generally referred to an eye care professional for perimetry testing. If the automated perimetry results are not available, the therapist can use the confrontation test along with close observation of the patient during daily activities.

Oculomotor Control

Control of eye movements depends on a complex interaction at cortical and subcortical levels. The role of the occupational therapist in screening oculomotor function is "not to diagnose the deficit, but to describe its functional effect and formulate the critical questions for the ophthalmologist or optometrist" (Warren, 1993b, p. 68). **Binocular vision** allows us to resolve two images, one from each eye, into one. It depends on good eye alignment and the ability of the eyes to converge and adjust focus at a range of distances. The therapist screens binocular vision, including eye alignment and convergence, and **accommodation**, smooth pursuits, and saccades.

Eye Alignment

Eye alignment is generally measured by observation of the reflection of light on the cornea. Seated in front of the patient, the therapist asks the patient to gaze at a penlight held in the quadrants of the visual field. The therapist observes the light reflection in each eye: the reflection should be in the same position in both eyes. Direction that the eye or eyes turn are noted (Box 7-3). Scheiman

---

BOX 7-2
PROCEDURES FOR PRACTICE

Screening Visual Field Deficits:
Confrontation Testing

Equipment
▸ Eye patch or patches
▸ Interesting target mounted on a wand

Setup
▸ Patient seated directly opposite examiner, approximately 20 inches eye to eye.
▸ Background behind examiner should be dark and distraction free.

Procedure
▸ Patch the patient's left eye and close or patch your own right eye.
▸ Instruct patient to look at your left eye and tell him or her you will be moving a target in from the side and the patient is to indicate when the target is first seen.
▸ Move target in from all angles (e.g., begin at 12 o'clock, then 2, 4, 6, 8, 10).
▸ Compare the patient's response with yours.
▸ Position hands at 3 and 9 o'clock so that you can just see your fingers. Ask the patient how many fingers you are holding up.
▸ Patch the patient's right eye and close or patch your own left eye. Repeat the previous 4 steps.
▸ A problem is indicated if the patient cannot see the target when you do or does not see both fingers simultaneously.

Adapted from Scheiman (1997).

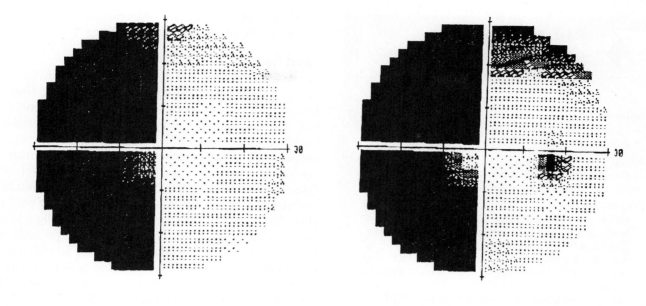

Left eye   Right eye

Figure 7-4 Automated perimetry results of a patient with RBD. The patient is unable to see anything in darkened areas (almost entire left visual field). There is some macular sparing on the left and a loss in the superior visual field in the right eye.

BOX 7-3
Definitions: Eye Movement

Accommodation
Ability of the eye to adjust focus at various distances.

Accommodative facility
Speed of response and ability to maintain response over time.

Accommodative amplitude
Amount of accommodation available (decreases with age).

Convergence
Ability to maintain focus as an object moves toward you.

Convergence insufficiency
Inability to focus on a near object because of exophoria at near distance.

Diplopia
Double vision.

Phoria
Tendency for the eyes to turn that is controlled with muscular effort.

   Esophoria
   Tendency of the eye to turn inward.

   Exophoria
   Tendency of the eye to turn outward.

   Hyperphoria
   Tendency of the eye to turn up.

   Hypophoria
   Tendency of the eye to turn down.

Presbyopia
Age-related loss of accommodation.

Saccades
Quick eye movements that change the fixation from one point to another and allow redirection of the line of sight.

Smooth pursuits
Eye movements that maintain continued fixation on a moving target.

Stereopsis
Depth perception; visual perception of three-dimensional space.

Strabismus
Misalignment of the eyes.

Suppression
Ignoring visual information from one eye, usually when there is a discrepancy between the two eyes.

Tropia
Synonym for strabismus.

   Esotropia
   Strabismus in which the eye turns inward.

   Exotropia
   Strabismus in which the eye turns outward.

   Hypertropia
   Strabismus in which the eye turns up.

   Hypotropia
   Strabismus in which the eye turns down.

BOX 7-4
PROCEDURES FOR PRACTICE
Screening: Convergence

Equipment
- Penlight or target
- Ruler

Set up
- Patient seated directly opposite the therapist.
- Patient's head should be vertically erect.

Procedure
- Slowly move the penlight or target toward patient at eye level (do not shine light directly into the patient's eyes; direct it at the brow slightly above eye level).
- Ask patient to keep eyes on the light and to report when two lights are seen. Note the distance at which diplopia occurs.
- Once two are seen, move the target in another inch or so and begin to move it away from the patient.
- Ask patient to let you know when he or she can see one light again. Note the distance at which the patient reports single vision.

Adapted from Scheiman (1997).

(1997) describes a method of evaluation of alignment using phoria cards (near and far), penlight, and a red Maddox rod. Using this method, the therapist should be able to determine the amount of strabismus present.

Convergence

Convergence is tested by having the patient follow a target moving slowly toward and away from the face (Box 7-4). Double vision normally occurs when the target is within 2 to 4 inches of the face, and recovery of a single image takes place at 4 to 6 inches. The patient may not report double vision because of suppression of vision from one eye. It is therefore important to observe the eyes and note when one eye drifts out during convergence and pulls back in with fusion.

Accommodation

Accommodation is the ability to adjust the focus of vision at a range of distances, such as the automatic refocusing of the eyes when you look up from the speedometer to the road while driving. It decreases with age. Presbyopia, a condition of decreased near vision secondary to decreased accommodative ability, sets in at 40 to 45 years of age. Information regarding the patient's accommodative ability is typically picked up by observing and listening to the patient's complaints. If the patient is over 40 to 45, expect accommodation to be decreased. With younger patients, Scheiman (1997)

presents a method for the occupational therapist to determine the patient's accommodation.

Visual Tracking

Visual tracking (smooth pursuits) are eye movements that maintain continued fixation on a moving target. Smooth pursuits, which are influenced by age, attention, and motivation, play a significant role in activities entailing movement of either the person or the object of regard (e.g., driving, playing sports). If smooth pursuits are impaired, acuity is impaired when motion is involved (Haarmeier & Thier, 1999). Smooth pursuits are usually evaluated by asking the patient to track a moving object (Box 7-5). Warren (1999) suggests using a penlight in a slightly darkened room. Scheiman (1997) presents a method of scoring in which performance is scored on (1) ability to complete two rotations in both directions, (2) accuracy (number of refixations required), and (3) head and body movement during the test.

Saccades

Saccades are quick eye movements that change fixation from one point to another and allow us to redirect our line of sight. These eye movements are more closely related to reading and close work and may appear more problematic following brain injury (Gianutsos, 1997). Saccades are tested by holding up two targets and asking the patient to keep looking from one target to another (Box 7-6). Performance of saccades is scored on (1)

BOX 7-5
PROCEDURES FOR PRACTICE
Screening: Smooth Pursuits and Visual Tracking

Equipment
- Small, interesting target

Setup
- Patient seated directly in front of the examiner.
- Hold target approximately 16 inches from the patient's face.

Procedure
- Give no instructions regarding head movement.
- Tell patient, "Watch the target and don't take your eyes off it."
- Move target clockwise two rotations and counterclockwise two rotations.
- Observe:
  - Number of rotations the patient can complete.
  - Ability to maintain fixation, that is, the number of times the patient has to refixate.
  - Movement of the head or body.

Adapted from Scheiman (1997).

BOX 7-6
PROCEDURES FOR PRACTICE

Screening: Saccades

Equipment
- Two interesting targets (e.g., 2 tongue depressors, one with a green circle on the end and the other with a red circle on the end).

Setup
- Patient seated directly in front of the examiner.

Procedure
- Hold wands approximately 16 inches from the face, separated by approximately 8 inches.
- Give no instructions regarding head movement.
- Tell patient, "Look at the red dot when I say red. Look at the green when I say green, and remember to *wait* until I say to look."
- Tell patient to look from one target to the other for a total of 10 fixations, 5 round trips.
- Observe:
  - Ability to complete 5 round trips
  - Accuracy of eye movements (overshooting or undershooting target)
  - Movement of head or body

Adapted from Scheiman (1997).

ability to complete five round trips, (2) accuracy (amount of overshooting and undershooting), and (3) head and body movement during the test (Scheiman, 1997).

Considerations for the Minimally Responsive Patient

Because visual testing requires attention and cooperation, it is often put off until patients have recovered and their neurological systems have settled down. It is imperative that we begin to look at the visual system as early as possible. How much better may patients do in therapy if corrective action is taken early in their stay? Whyte and DiPasquale (1995) present a method of assessing vision in minimally responsive patients (Box 7-7). The evaluation takes only a short time to administer and can be given frequently by various team members to provide a pattern of responses that are "more interpretable than clinicians' unstructured observations" (p. 810). The relationship between side, stimulus, and frequency of eye movements is analyzed: (1) total number of eye movements in each direction (unequal distribution of eye movements suggests gaze preference, asymmetrical visual fields, or visual attention deficit), (2) frequency of eye movement to stimulus side (contingent orienting), (3) difference in orienting to photos versus cards (as evidence of visual perception), and (4) comparison of bilateral to unilateral presentations. The authors found that they could identify hemifield deficits, extinction, and monocular pathology with this method (Whyte & DiPasquale, 1995).

Unilateral Neglect

Visual attention allows us to determine the what (object identification) and where (orientation in space) of things in our environment (Warren, 1999). Visual attention is influenced by general alertness, both nonspatial and spatial. It is evaluated through scanning tasks because a change in visual attention is manifested as a change in visual search (Warren, 1999). Visual attention can be influenced by the perceptual load, whether it be visual, tactile, or auditory (Mattingley et al., 1997; Robertson et al., 1997).

Unilateral neglect, a constellation of symptoms affecting both perceptual and exploratory behavior, has been variously called unilateral neglect, hemispatial neglect, and hemi-inattention. It is a heterogeneous

BOX 7-7
PROCEDURES FOR PRACTICE

Assessment of Vision in Minimally Responsive Patients

Equipment
- Six brightly colored snapshots from patient's family
- Plain white card, same size as photos
- Eye patch as needed

Setup
- Examiner stands 6 feet in front of patient, at the visual midline.
- Use eye patch for patients with dysconjugate gaze.

Procedure
- Present pictures at ear level, 30–40° lateral to midline.
- May give alerting stimulation prior to presentation as needed.
- Present pictures in 6 combinations (order can be varied from session to session):

Left Field	Right Field
Photo	—
—	Photo
Card	—
—	Card
Photo	Card
Card	Photo

Record the direction of the first lateral eye movement for each presentation. Record "no response" if there is no movement in 5 seconds.

Source: Whyte & DiPasquale (1995).

Case Example

ASSESSING VISUAL AND VISUAL PERCEPTUAL ABILITIES AND CAPACITIES AFTER STROKE

Patient Information

Mr. D. is a 21-year-old man who had a right CVA as a result of an arterial malformation 15 months ago. He was in a coma for 4 months. Following this he was in acute rehabilitation for 2 months and subsequently in outpatient therapy. Mr. D. attended college, where he was a math major and prior to the CVA, a basketball player. He is living with his family and taking one class at college and is beginning to assist in coaching sports at a local school. He has a personal care attendant who assists with self-care activities 2 to 4 hours a day.

Mr. D. has left hemiplegia, moderate tone throughout the left side, and little controlled movement in either extremity. He cannot walk and uses the wheelchair for all mobility. He has left neglect and mild cognitive deficits, especially in short-term memory. He was referred to occupational therapy at the Eye Institute by his physiatrist, as Mr. D.'s vision and left neglect were limiting his studies and mobility.

Description of Assessment

The occupational therapist wanted to determine the status of Mr. D.'s visual system and how it affected his daily functioning. The therapist used a questionnaire to determine the patient's symptoms and complaints and an interview to determine his level of daily functioning. She then evaluated the visual foundation skills, including acuity near and far, visual fields, and ocular motility, including convergence, scanning, saccades, and pursuits.

Results

During the interview, Mr. D. indicated that he had difficulty with eating (missing items on his plate), mobility, reading, doing his homework, and being able to track the children he was coaching. The symptom questionnaire appeared to indicate problems with accommodation, ocular motility, and visual fields.

▶ Acuity: Near and far vision were within normal limits when he wore his glasses.
▶ Visual fields: On confrontation testing he exhibited moderate difficulty with stimuli on the left, especially in the lower left quadrant.
▶ Convergence: 5 Trials. Right eye broke at 8 inches, 3 inches, and three times at 6 inches, which indicates convergence insufficiency.
▶ Scanning: During all scanning tasks he exhibited an inefficient scanning pattern. During tabletop activities he missed 75% of items on the left side of the page, and when scanning the room for specific sequential numbers, while he located all numbers, he required maximum cues and increased time.
▶ Pursuits: Scored 3 on ability, 3 on accuracy and 2 on head and body movement. He demonstrated a lag and occasionally lost the item, especially in lower left quadrant.
▶ Saccades: Scored 5 on ability, 1 on accuracy, and 2 on head and body movement.

Throughout testing he was cooperative and well motivated. He demonstrated awareness of his neglect but still required maximum cues and increased time to compensate.

Analysis of Results

Mr. D. exhibited convergence insufficiency, which may explain his difficulty with near activities such as reading, with accommodation, and being able to copy work from blackboard to tabletop. In addition, he exhibited left visual neglect, which affected all functional activities. When attempting to compensate for the neglect, he was only partially successful and required cueing and inordinate amounts of time to complete tasks. His inefficient scanning and left neglect interfered with his mobility and ability to coach sports.

Occupational Therapy Problem List

The following problem areas interfere with full resumption of self-care, student, and coaching roles:

▶ Appears to have a field cut on the left, especially lower left visual field
▶ Decreased ocular motor skills:
  ▶ Decreased convergence
  ▶ Decreased accommodation
  ▶ Inefficient saccades and smooth pursuits
▶ Left visual neglect

CLINICAL REASONING
in OT Practice

Effects of Functional Roles on Assessment of Vision, Visual, Perception, and Praxis

Mr. D. was 21 years old, a math major in college, and involved in playing basketball at the time of his CVA. How might the evaluation have differed if he had been 71 years old, retired, and enjoyed watching TV? 30 years old, working as a firefighter? 45 years old with an active dental practice?

TABLE 7-1
Unilateral Neglect Syndrome

Main Behavioral Components	
Hemi-inattention	Inability to orient to or respond to stimuli from one side of the environment, irrespective of the modality.
Hemispatial visual neglect	Inability to orient to relevant contralateral visual stimuli.
Extinction	Failure to report a contralesional stimulus when it occurs simultaneously with a more ipsilateral stimulus, even though able to do so if either is presented alone.
Allesthesia	Consistently attributing sensory stimuli on one side of the body to the other side, or moving limbs on one side when requested to move the limb on the other side.
Hemiakinesia	Motor neglect.
Related Disorders	
Anasognosia	Lack of awareness or denial of hemiparesis
Gaze paresis **Visual field deficit**	

Sources: Stone et al. (1993, 1998).

condition that includes both behavioral components and related disorders (Table 7-1). Unilateral neglect manifests as a failure to respond or orient to stimuli presented contralateral to a brain lesion (Heilman, et al., 1993). It is observed functionally in the patient who eats the food on only half of the plate, shaves only one side of his face, and so on. It is most commonly caused by a lesion in the right hemisphere; it does occur following left brain damage (LBD), although the deficit is usually not as severe as for right brain damage (RBD) (Heilman, Watson, & Valenstein, 1997; Mennemeier et al., 1997; Stone et al., 1993).

The incidence of neglect varies widely in the literature. This is most likely because of lack of a common definition, differences among tests used to evaluate neglect, and/or laterality of motor response (Mercier et al., 1995).

While it is generally agreed that neglect is related to a deficit in attention, just how this happens is still under discussion. Kinsbourne (1993) proposes a model in which attention to right and left space is controlled by the contralateral hemisphere. When one hemisphere is damaged, the other becomes disinhibited and biases

attention toward the contralateral side. Another view focuses on the hyporesponsiveness of the damaged hemisphere (Heilman & Watson, 1977). Posner and Rafal (1987) suggest that the problem is inability to disengage attention from objects in ipsilateral space.

Visual field deficits and unilateral neglect frequently occur together and are difficult to separate. Warren (1999) suggests that it is possible to differentiate the two by observing how patients organize their search patterns during a scanning task (Table 7-2). A patient who exhibits the behaviors listed for visual field deficit probably has no more than mild neglect, whereas if he or she demonstrates the neglect behaviors, you cannot assume that there are no field cuts.

Sensory Neglect

Two major subtypes of unilateral neglect have been described: sensory (input or attentional) and motor (output or intentional) (Bisiach et al., 1990; Coslett et al., 1990; Tegner & Levander, 1991). Sensory neglect can include awareness of all stimuli on one side of the space (spatial neglect) or be confined to one side of the body (personal neglect) (Heilman, Watson, & Valenstein, 1997). It may be evident in any of the modalities, including auditory, tactile, and visual. Historically, neglect has generally been referred to in the horizontal (right–left) dimension. More recently, research is being done on neglect in the vertical and radial (near and far space) dimensions (Cowey et al., 1994; Kageyama et al., 1994; Ladavas et al., 1994). There is also neglect of visual imagery (e.g., mental images of familiar places, spelling, drawing from memory), termed representational neglect (Beschin et al. 1997).

TABLE 7-2
Scanning: Visual Field Deficit Versus Unilateral Neglect

Visual Field Deficit	Unilateral Neglect
Abbreviated scanning pattern	Disorganized random scanning pattern
Scanning pattern organized	Asymmetrical search pattern in hemispace
Rescanning observed	Scanning pattern carried out with reduced effort and little or no rescanning
Length of time and effort appropriate for the task	Task completed swiftly, or if patient is aware of deficit, takes inordinate amount of time in attempt to compensate

Source: Warren (1999).

Evaluating neglect can be confusing, because the patient may exhibit neglect in one situation but not in another (Halligan & Marshall, 1998; Riddoch & Humphreys, 1994). Neglect can vary thus:

▶ Locus of lesion: Inferior and posterior parietal cortex are critical for monitoring and directing attention in the visual environment; anterior and frontal lesions result in difficulty executing movement in or toward the side contralateral to the lesion.

▶ Task: for example, verbal tasks versus spatial tasks; complexity and perceptual load of the task (e.g. one object versus several objects).

▶ Mode of response: verbal versus contralateral extremity versus ipsilateral extremity.

▶ Modality: visual, auditory, tactile.

Unilateral neglect has traditionally been evaluated in a variety of ways, including drawing tasks, cancellation tasks, line bisection, reading, and double simultaneous stimulation (Chatterjee & Mennemeier, 1997) (Table 7-3). In addition, the occupational therapist is in a position to observe the patient in a variety of functional activities in a variety of conditions that can provide vital information for the team. A patient is likely to perform differently in a quiet test room than in an everyday situation, such as preparing a simple meal.

Drawing and Copying Tasks

Drawing and copying tasks, while easy to give, are subjective in their scoring. In all such tasks the therapist looks for omissions and errors concentrated to one side (Fig. 7-5). These tasks can alert you to moderate or severe neglect but should be used in conjunction with other tests of neglect and functional activities to provide a clear picture of mild neglect.

Cancellation Tasks

Another common method of evaluation is cancellation tasks. These tests are easy to administer and score and are sensitive to mild neglect (Sea et al., 1993; Stam & Bakker, 1990). Cancellation tasks can be varied in many ways, including overall density, whether the display is organized or random, density of stimuli in ipsilateral space, complexity of stimuli in ipsilateral space, and

---

TABLE 7-3
Evaluation of Unilateral Neglect

Task	Description	Scoring
Drawing or copying	Patient is asked to draw and/or copy objects (e.g., person, clock, flower, geometric figures).	Observe how patient approaches task. Note variations between copying and free drawing; note missing elements on one side of picture or one side of objects in picture.
Line bisection	Patient is presented with a line or group of lines and asked to bisect it or them into 2 equal parts (Schenkenberg et al. [1980]).	Note direction and measure amount of deviation from center. Van Deusen (1983) standardized the scoring and suggested these norms: slight (± 1 standard deviation [SD]), moderate (± 2 SD), and severe (± 3 SD) neglect.
Cancellation tasks	Patient is presented with a page with several lines of letters or shapes and asked to mark a specific stimulus letter or shape that is scattered randomly throughout the array.	Based on the number of omissions (targets not marked) and commissions (cancellations of items other than the target) and where on the page the errors are made. Generally, the greater the number of errors, the greater the visual scanning deficit.
	Star Cancellation subtest of the *Rivermead Behavioral Inattention Test* (Wilson et al., 1987).	For the *Star Cancellation* subtest, cancelling fewer than 44 of 54 stars indicates neglect in post-CVA patients (Freidman, 1992).
Functional tasks	*Rivermead Behavioral Inattention Test* (Wilson et al., 1987).	Score during activities including eating a meal (simulation), dialing a phone, reading a menu, telling and setting the time, sorting coins, copying an address, and following a map.
	Several subtests of the *biVABA* (Warren, 1996).	Patient is scored on scanning while walking down a hall, using a scan board, and copying telephone numbers.
	Comb and Razor/Compact Test: Patient is asked to comb the hair and shave (men) or use a compact (women) for 30 seconds (Beschin & Robertson, 1997).	Count number of times patient strokes the right, left, ambiguous. Determine percent of time to the left by dividing number of strokes on left by total of all strokes. Cutoff of 0.35 identifies patients with personal neglect.

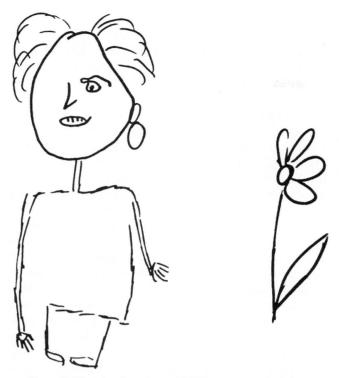

Figure 7-5 Drawings by patients with RBD and unilateral neglect.

amount of similarity between the target and distracters (Dawson & Tanner-Cohen, 1997; Heilman, Watson, & Valenstein, 1997; Kartsounis & Findley, 1994). Because of these many variations, it is important not to draw conclusions from one cancellation task.

Line Bisection

Line bisection, another traditional test, requires the patient to divide a line or lines in the center. The following factors can increase the percentage of error on line bisection tests: longer line, line placement in contralesional space, and cues placed on the ipsilateral end of the line (Heilman, Watson, & Valenstein, 1997).

Functional Tests

The traditional tests of unilateral neglect tend to be tabletop paper and pencil tasks. However, several standardized functional tests, including the *Rivermead Behavioral Inattention Test* (Wilson et. al., 1987) and subtests of the *biVABA* (Warren, 1996) address scanning in a functional situation. The *Comb and Razor/Compact Test* (Table 7-3) was developed to evaluate personal neglect (Beschin & Robertson, 1997).

Motor Neglect

Motor neglect presents as impaired initiation or execution of movement into contralateral hemispace by either limb (Bisiach et al., 1990; Tegner & Levander, 1991). Heilman, Watson, & Valenstein (1997) describe several

types of motor neglect (Box 7-8). It is often difficult to differentiate between sensory and motor neglect because tests of motor neglect typically entail some form of sensory input. Consequently, therapists wonder whether patients fail to respond to a stimulus on the involved side because they don't see it or because they cannot initiate movement toward it. If motor neglect is suspected, one method to distinguish between the two entails contrasting a task that requires a hand response with one that has minimal motor response (e.g., naming letters on the involved side as opposed to pointing to the same letters). In other words, the stimulus (letters on the involved side) stays the same and the motor response varies (Riddoch & Humphreys, 1994).

Observations of patients and how they use the extremity can provide insight into motor neglect. One may note reluctance to move the arm and movement only after a delay (hypokinesia), movement only with strong encouragement (akinesia), a tendency to undershoot a target when asked to move along a given line (hypometria), or inability to sustain a posture (impersistence) (Heilman, Watson, & Valenstein, 1997). Different limbs can be observed, as can the direction of the movement required (ipsilateral versus contralateral) and hemispace in which the movement is to occur (ipsilateral versus contralateral).

Assessing Praxis

People rapidly conceive of and plan motor acts in response to the environment (Crepeau, 1998). This innate capacity is referred to as praxis. **Apraxia** is the inability to carry out skilled movement in the presence of intact sensation, movement, and coordination (Heilman & Rothi, 1993). Apraxia is generally seen in patients with

---

BOX 7-8
Definitions: Motor Neglect

Limb akinesia
Failure to move limb.

Hypokinesia
Limb moves, but only after a long delay and much encouragement.

Hypometria
Decreased amplitude of movements.

Impersistence
Inability to maintain a movement or posture.

Motor perseveration
Inability to disengage from a motor activity.

Motor extinction
Delay or failure to move the contralesional limb when also required to move the ipsilateral limb.

Source: Heilman, Watson, & Valenstein (1997).

LBD (Goodglass & Kaplan, 1972; Haaland et al., 1987; Poeck, 1985). These patients generally can spontaneously use the extremity in such everyday tasks as eating, shaving, or opening a door, but if they are asked to pantomime an activity or carry out a series of steps, their performance is not correctly or smoothly executed.

Research has shown that LBD patients are clumsy, with more dexterity errors than normal controls (Sunderland et al., 1999). When mealtime eating behavior of apraxic patients was compared to that of normal subjects, the patients were found to be less efficient, be less well organized when sequencing activities, and produce more action errors (Foundas et al., 1995). These findings suggest that limb apraxia can affect activities of daily living. How it affects a particular patient depends on his or her goals and lifestyle. For instance, if the patient is aphasic as well, understanding and production of gestures is an important part of communication with others, and apraxia may have to be considered more closely.

There are five types of apraxia: verbal, buccofacial, limb, constructional, and dressing. The first two, which are usually evaluated by a speech and language pathologist, are not discussed in this chapter.

Limb Apraxia

Limb apraxia is usually associated with LBD in right-handed patients and RBD in left-handed patients (Heilman, Rothi, & Watson, 1997), although variations have been described (Marchetti & Della Sala, 1997). According to Heilman, Rothi, and Watson (1997), there are six types of limb apraxia: limb kinetic, ideomotor, ideational, dissociation, conduction, and conceptual (Table 7-4). Limb kinetic apraxia is characterized by loss of ability to make finely graded precise finger movements and is thought to be a motor problem rather than a true apraxia (Heilman, Watson, & Rothi, 1997).

Testing has traditionally consisted of gesture production. The patient is asked to pantomime a task on command (e.g., "Show me how you comb your hair"), to imitate the tester, or to use an object. These assessments require various types of gestures, including transitive gestures that entail object use (e.g., "Show me how a man shaves"), intransitive gestures that are meant to express ideas or feelings (e.g., "Show me how you wave good-bye"), meaningless or nonsymbolic gestures (e.g., "Put your hand under your chin"), proximal gestures (e.g., "Show me how you bounce a ball"), and distal

---

TABLE 7-4
Types of Limb Apraxia

Type of Apraxia	Error Type	How Elicited	Functional Example
Ideomotor	Production errors	Most errors on pantomiming transitive tasks; improves with imitation; usually does best with actual object.	Movements awkward but bear a resemblance to intended movement. Able to use tools to complete tasks but may appear clumsy or awkward.
Conceptual	Content errors Tool action knowledge Tool association knowledge Mechanical knowledge Tool fabrication	Use of tools; actions associated with specific tools, association between tool and object.	Obvious difficulty with tool use, e.g., may use tube of toothpaste to brush teeth, comb hair with fork.
Disassociation	Thought to be a disconnection between hemispheres; therefore, no recognizable movement on command.	Pantomime to command is impaired; imitation and use of object much better.	Unable to pantomime movements, but able to imitate and use tools, so minimal effect on functional activities.
Conduction	Difficulty decoding and understanding gestures.	Impaired imitation of gestures; does better when asked to pantomime.	May have difficulty understanding and using gestures.
Ideational	Difficulty with a series of tasks	Tasks requiring series of activities (e.g., clean pipe, put in tobacco, light pipe).	May complete task more skillfully than with ideomotor apraxia but difficulty sequencing steps in the correct order. (e.g., may try to light empty pipe, then put tobacco in, then clean it).

Source: Heilman, Watson, & Rothi (1997).

TABLE 7-5
Apraxia Tests

Test	Example
Gesture to command: Should include both transitive movements (tool use) and intransitive movements (nonverbal communication).	Transitive: "Show me how you would open the door with a key"; "use a hammer." Intransitive: "Show me how you hitchhike, salute, wave good-bye."
Gesture to imitation	Examiner produces a gesture and asks the patient to "do it the same way I do it; don't name the gesture, and don't start until I'm finished"; can be familiar gestures or nonsense gestures (e.g., hand to the forehead).
Gesture in response to tool	Visual: Examiner shows tool and says, "Show me how you use this." Tactile: Eyes closed or covered, patient examines tool by hand and examiner says, "Show me how you use this."
Gesture in response to seeing object on which the tool acts: tool selection task.	Examiner presents patient with object representing an incomplete action (e.g., if target is sawing, patient is shown a partially cut piece of wood); patient must choose correct tool from a choice of three, one of which is the saw.
Actual tool use	Patient is given a tool (e.g., hammer) and asked, "Show me how you use this."
Gesture decision—discrimination between correctly and incorrectly pantomimed movements.	Examiner makes a gesture and asks the patient, "Is this the correct way to . . ." (e.g., use a pair of scissors).
Gesture comprehension	Examiner makes a gesture and asks patient, "Tell me what I am doing." "What tool am I using?" "Am I using a hammer or a saw?"
Serial acts	Examiner tells patient, "Fold letter, put it in envelope, seal envelope, and place stamp on it."

Sources: Heilman & Rothi (1993); Rothi et al. (1997).

gestures (e.g., "Show me how you would use a telegraph key"). Transitive gestures are especially sensitive to apraxia (Haaland, 1993). Generally patients with apraxia have least difficulty with proximal intransitive gestures away from the body (e.g., waving good-bye) and most difficulty with distal transitive gestures on the body (e.g., putting on makeup) (Haaland, 1993; Helm-Estabrooks & Albert, 1991). More recently, gesture comprehension and discrimination have been added to the list of apraxia tests (Heilman & Rothi, 1993; Heilman, Watson, & Rothi, 1997; Joseph, 1996; York & Cermak, 1995) (Table 7-5).

Apraxia often occurs in conjunction with aphasia, and it is sometimes difficult to distinguish between the two. Therefore, it is important when evaluating a patient with aphasia to include (besides the regular commands, e.g., "show me how you would. . .") questions that can be answered by yes–no responses and by pointing at the correct answers (Heilman & Rothi, 1993). If the patient performs poorly but can answer yes–no questions, he or she may be apraxic. Similarly, if the patient cannot respond to yes–no questions, failure to make the appropriate movement to command may be due to a language problem rather than apraxia. If the patient has only a mild language deficit but uses a body part as object or makes a clumsy but recognizable response, it is probably due to apraxia rather than language. When assessing people with severe asphasia, provide a model for the

TABLE 7-6
Sample Items From the *Florida Apraxia Screening Test (Revised)*

Show me:
How you salute.
How to use a saw to cut a piece of wood in front of you.
How you hitchhike.
Stop.
How to use a salt shaker to salt food on a table in front of you.

Source: Rothi et al. (1997).

patient to imitate or place the object out of reach and ask the patient to pantomime its use. Use the tactile modality in testing by having the patient handle the object while blindfolded and then show how it is used.

There are few standardized tests for limb apraxia. Rothi and her colleagues have developed the *Florida Apraxia Screening Test—Revised* (*FAST-R*) for use in the research of neurologically impaired patients (Rothi et al., 1997). This test consists of 30 items presented verbally (Table 7-6). The patient uses the dominant arm if possible. Prior to testing, patients practice pantomiming such that they pretend they to hold the imagined tool and act on the imagined object. This rehearsal is important to discourage use of a body part as the imagined tool itself. Normal subjects may use a body part as tool but with instruction they correct their performance, while apraxic patients continue to do so even with the instruction (Raymer et al., 1997). Scoring for the *FAST-R* includes multiple error types based on content of the pantomime, timing and sequencing of the response, and spatial features (Table 7-7).

Constructional Apraxia

Constructional apraxia is a specific deficit in spatial–organizational performance (Benton & Tranel, 1993). Patients with constructional apraxia have difficulty with copying, drawing, and constructing designs in two and three dimensions. Constructional apraxia has been found to correlate with deficits of activities of daily living (Baum & Hall, 1981; Neistadt, 1993; Warren, 1981). It can be seen functionally as difficulty with such activities as setting a table, making a sandwich, and making a dress and with any mechanical activity in which parts are to be combined into a whole.

Constructional apraxia can be found in both RBD and LBD patients. Because of qualitative differences noted in the performance of RBD and LBD patients (Box 7-1), constructional apraxia in RBD is believed to be the result of visuospatial deficits, while that in LBD is thought to be caused by an executive or conceptual disorder (Benton, 1967; Piercy et al., 1960). It has often been found to be more frequent and more severe in RBD patients (Arrigoni & DeRenzi, 1964; Benton & Fogel, 1962; Piercy, et al., 1960; Warrington et al., 1966).

TABLE 7-7
Apraxia Error Types

Error Type	Description
Content errors	
Perseveration	Patient's response includes all or part of a previously produced pantomime.
Related	Pantomime is correctly produced but only related to that requested (e.g., playing the trombone instead of a bugle).
Unrelated	Pantomime is accurately produced but unrelated to request (e.g., playing the trombone for shaving).
Hand	Performs the action without use of a real or imagined tool (e.g., turning a screw with the fingers rather than an imaginary screwdriver).
Temporal	
Sequencing	Addition, deletion, or transposition of the elements of a sequence.
Timing	Any alteration in the timing or speed of a pantomime: abnormally increased, decreased, or irregular rate of production.
Occurrence	Any multiplication of characteristically single-cycle movements (e.g., unlocking a door) or reduction of a characteristically repetitive cycle (e.g., screwing in a screw) to a single event.
Spatial	
Amplitude	Any increase, decrease or irregularity of the characteristic movement.
Internal configuration	Any abnormality of the required finger/hand posture and its relationship to the target tool (e.g.; when pretending to brush the teeth, the hand may be closed tightly into a fist with no space allowed for the imagined toothbrush handle).
Body part as tool	Patient uses finger, hand, or arm as the imagined tool even when requested to pretend holding the object (e.g., Uses the finger to brush the teeth).
External configuration	Difficulties orienting the fingers/hand/arm to the object or in placing the object in space (e.g., brushing teeth with the hand so close to the mouth as to not allow room for the imagined toothbrush).
Movement	Any disturbance of the characteristic movement used when acting on an object (e.g., activates movement at incorrect joint—when pantomiming a screwdriver and rotation occurs at the shoulder rather than at the forearm).
Other	
Concretization	Patient performs pantomime not on an imagined object but instead on a real object not normally used in the task (e.g., instead of pretending to saw wood, pantomimes sawing on leg).
No response	
Unrecognizable	Response shares no temporal or spatial features of the target; it is unrecognizable.

Adapted from Rothi et al. (1997).

TABLE 7-8
Scoring for Drawing to Command

Shape	Instruction	Scoring
Clock	"Draw the face of a clock showing the numbers and the two hands."	0–3: one point each for approximately circular face, symmetry of number placement, and correctness of numbers
Daisy	"Draw a daisy."	0–2: one point each for general shape (center with petals around it) and symmetry of petal arrangement
Elephant	"Draw an elephant."	0–2: one point each for general shape (legs, trunk, head, body) and relative proportions correct
Cross	"You know what the Red Cross looks like? Draw an outline of it without taking your pencil off the paper."	0–2: one point each for basic configuration and ability to form all corners adequately with a continuous line
Cube	"Draw a cube in perspective, as it would look if you could see the top and two sides."	0–2: one point each for grossly correct attempt and correctness of perspective
House	"Draw a house in perspective, so you can see the roof and two sides."	0–2: one point each for grossly correct features of house and accuracy of perspective

Reprinted by permission from Goodglass, H., & Kaplan, E. (1972). *The Assessment of Aphasia and Related Disorders.* Philadelphia: Lea & Febiger.

There are two types of constructional activities used in assessment: graphic (e.g., copying line drawings and drawing to command) and assembly tasks (e.g., block and stick designs). Both types are included in an evaluation of constructional apraxia. The most common example of a graphic task is copying geometric shapes (from simple to complex) and drawing without a model (e.g., house, clock, flower). It is best to begin with a simple task (e.g., simple geometric figures, three-dimensional block design), as a more complex task involves a greater number of skills and becomes less specific (DeRenzi, 1997).

Goodglass and Kaplan (1972) describe a test of drawing to command. This test includes having the patient draw a clock, daisy, elephant, cross, cube, and house; scoring criteria are given in Table 7-8.

Assembly tasks include such activities as stick arrangement and three-dimensional block designs. Common errors on stick arrangement include selecting sticks of incorrect length; failing to reproduce parts of the model, especially lateral; making lines more oblique than the model indicates; tending to remove part of the model to make the copy; and crowding in (the patient's copy rests on top of or touches the model) (Critchley, 1966). Assembly tasks can be varied in numerous ways. For example, constructing from memory may be more difficult than copying from a model (representational or actual). Patients may be asked to choose the correct pieces from a large number of blocks and sticks versus providing them with the correct number and type of blocks and sticks, which structures the task and makes it simpler.

In general, these tasks are not standardized, and they rely on subjective judgment of the results. It is important to note the patient's method of completing the task; the patient's comments; any emotional display, hesitancy, indecision, and change of mind; and the type of errors made.

The *Lowenstein Occupational Therapy Cognitive Assessment* (*LOTCA*) was standardized on brain-injured adults. It contains a section on visuomotor organization (Katz et al., 1989) that contains block design, copying, drawing, and pegboard design (see Table 8-1).

Dressing Apraxia

Dressing apraxia refers to inability to dress oneself. It is usually due to RBD and secondary visuospatial disorganization. It is evaluated functionally by watching patients dress themselves. The underlying problem must be determined (e.g., visual deficits, unilateral neglect, apraxia, constructional apraxia), rather than evaluating dressing apraxia per se.

Summary Review Questions

1. What are the visual foundational skills and why should they be evaluated before higher-level visual perceptual skills?
2. A patient with brain injury does poorly on a test of figure ground. List at least four possible reasons.
3. Why is it important to assess contrast sensitivity?
4. Under what circumstances might you evaluate

visual foundation skills in a neurologically intact person?

5. Who are the eye care professionals and in what ways do occupational therapists interact with them? What information might you request, and what information might you be able to share?

6. Describe how you would differentiate between a visual field deficit and unilateral neglect in a stroke patient. Compare the assessment methods used to assess each of these problem areas.

7. Why is it important to screen vision as early as possible?

8. Your patient has LBD with resultant right hemiparesis and nonfluent aphasia. Why and how do you evaluate for apraxia?

Acknowledgment

Thanks to Liz Stuewe, MS, OTR for her input and assistance with preparation of the case study.

References

Arrigoni, G., & DeRenzi, E. (1964). Constructional apraxia and hemispheric locus of lesions. *Cortex, 1,* 170–197.

Baum, B., & Hall, K. M. (1981). Relationship between constructional praxis and dressing in the head-injured adult. *American Journal of Occupational Therapy, 35,* 438–442.

Benton, A. L. (1967). Constructional apraxia and the minor hemisphere. *Confinia Neurologica, 29,* 1–16.

Benton, A. L., & Fogel, M. L. (1962). Three-dimensional constructional praxis. *Archives of Neurology, 7,* 347–354.

Benton, A., & Tranel, D. (1993). Visuoperceptual, visuospatial, and visuoconstructional disorders. In K. M. Heilman & E. Valenstein (Eds.), *Clinical Neuropsychology* (3rd ed., pp. 165–213). New York: Oxford University.

Beschin, N., Cocchini, G., Sala, S. D., & Logie, R. H. (1997). What the eye perceives, the brain ignores: A case of pure unilateral representational neglect. *Cortex, 33,* 3–26.

Beschin, N., & Robertson, I. H. (1997). Personal versus extrapersonal neglect: A group study of their dissociation using a reliable clinical test. *Cortex, 33,* 379–384.

Bisiach, E., Geminiani, G., Berti, A. & Rusconi, M. L. (1990). Perceptual and premotor factors of unilateral neglect. *Neurology, 40,* 1278–1281.

Chatterjee, A., & Mennemeier, M. (1997). Diagnosis and treatment of spatial neglect. In T. E. Fineberg & M. J. Farah, *Behavioral Neurology and Neuropsychology* (pp. 597–612). New York: McGraw-Hill.

Coslett, H. B., Bowers, D., Fitzpatrick, E., Haws, B., & Heilman, K. M. (1990). Directional hypokinesia and hemispatial inattention in neglect. *Brain, 113,* 475–486.

Cowey, A., Small, M., & Ellis, S. (1994). Left visuo-spatial neglect can be worse in far than in near space. *Neuropsychologia, 32,* 1059–1066.

Crepeau, E. B. (1998). Activity analysis: A way of thinking about occupational performance. In M. E. Neistadt & E. B. Crepeau (Eds.), *Willard & Spackman's Occupational Therapy* (pp. 135–147). Philadelphia: Lippincott.

Critchley, M. (1966). *The parietal lobes.* New York: Hafner.

Dawson, D. R., & Tanner-Cohen, C. (1997). Visual scanning patterns in an adult Chinese population: Preliminary normative data. *Occupational Therapy Journal of Research, 17,* 264–279.

DeRenzi, E. (1997). Visuospatial and constructional disorders. In T. E. Feinberg & M. J. Farah (Eds.), *Behavioral Neurology and Neuropsychology* (pp. 297–307). New York: McGraw Hill.

Foundas, A. L., Macauley, B. L., Raymer, A. M., Maher, L. M., Heilman, K. M., & Rothi, L. J. G. (1995). Ecological implications of limb apraxia: Evidence from mealtime behavior. *Journal of the International Neuropsychology Society, 1,* 62–66.

Freidman, P. J. (1992). The *Star Cancellation Test* in acute stroke. *Clinical Rehabilitation, 6,* 23–30.

Giantusos, R. (1997). Vision rehabilitation following acquired brain injury. In M. Gentile (Ed.), *Functional Visual Behavior* (pp. 267–294). Bethesda, MD: American Occupational Therapy Association.

Goodglass, H., & Kaplan, E. (1972). *The Assessment of Aphasia and Related Disorders.* Philadelphia: Lea & Febiger.

Haaland, K. (1993, March). *Typology and assessment of individuals with limb apraxia.* Paper presented at the American Occupational Therapy Association's Neuroscience Institute conference: Treating Adults with Apraxia, Baltimore.

Haaland, K. Y., Harrington, D. L., & Yeo, R. (1987). The effects of task complexity on motor performance in left and right CVA patients. *Neuropsychologia, 25,* 783–794.

Haarmeier, T., & Thier, P. (1999). Impaired analysis of moving objects because of deficient smooth pursuit eye movements. *Brain, 122,* 1490–1505.

Halligan, P. W., & Marshall, J. C. (1998). Visuospatial neglect: The ultimate deconstruction? *Brain and Cognition, 37,* 419–438.

Heilman, K. M. & Rothi, L. J. G. (1993). Apraxia. In K. M. Heilman & E. Valenstein (Eds.), *Clinical Neuropsychology* (3rd. ed., pp. 141–163). New York: Oxford University.

Heilman, K. M., Rothi, L. J. G., & Watson, R. T. (1997). Apraxia. In S. C. Schachter & O. Devinsky (Eds.), *Behavioral Neurology and the Legacy of Norman Geschwind* (pp. 171–182). Philadelphia: Lippincott-Raven.

Heilman, K. M., & Watson, R. T. (1977). The neglect syndrome: A unilateral defect of the orienting response. In S. Hardned, R. W. Doty, L. Goldstein, J. Janynes, & G. Kean Thamer (Eds.), *Lateralization in the Nervous System* (pp. 285–302). New York: Academic.

Heilman, K. M., Watson, R. T., & Rothi, L. G. (1997). Disorders of skilled movements: Limb apraxia. In T. E. Fineberg & M. J. Farah (Eds.), *Behavioral Neurology and Neuropsychology* (pp. 227–235). New York: McGraw-Hill.

Heilman, K. M., Watson, R. T., & Valenstein, E. (1993). Neglect and related disorders. In K. M. Heilman & E. Valenstein (Eds.), *Clinical Neuropsychology* (3rd. ed., pp. 297–336). New York: Oxford University.

Heilman, K. M., Watson, R. T., & Valenstein, E. (1997). Neglect: Clinical and anatomic aspects. In T. E. Fineberg & M. J. Farah, *Behavioral Neurology and Neuropsychology* (pp. 309–317). New York: McGraw-Hill.

Helm-Estabrooks, N., & Albert, M. L. (1991). *Manual of aphasia therapy.* Austin, TX: Pro-ed.

Joseph, R. (1996). *Neuropsychiatry, Neuropsychology, and Clinical Neuroscience* (2nd ed.). Baltimore: Williams & Wilkins.

Kageyama, S., Imagase, M., Okubo, M., & Takayama, Y. (1994). Neglect in three dimensions. *American Journal of Occupational Therapy, 48,* 206–210.

Kartsounis, L. D., & Findley, L. J. (1994). Task specific visuospatial neglect related to density and salience of stimuli. *Cortex, 30,* 647–659.

Katz, N., Itzkovich, M., Averbach, S., & Elazar, B. (1989). Lowenstein Occupational Therapy Cognitive Assessment (LOTCA) battery for brain injured patients: Reliability and validity. *American Journal of Occupational Therapy, 43,* 184–192.

Kinsbourne, M. (1993). Orientation bias model of unilateral neglect: Evidence from attentional gradients within hemispace. In I. H. Robertson & J. C. Marshall (Eds.), *Unilateral Neglect: Clinical and Experimental Studies* (pp. 63–86). Hove, UK: Lawrence Erlbaum.

Ladavas, E., Carletti, M., & Gori, G. (1994). Automatic and voluntary orientating of attention in patients with visual neglect: Horizontal and vertical dimensions. *Neuropsychologia, 32,* 1195–1208.

Marchetti, C., & Della Sala, S. (1997). On crossed apraxia: A description of a right-handed apraxic patient with right supplementary motor area damage. *Cortex, 33,* 341–354.

Mattingley, J. B., Driver, J., Beschin, N., & Robertson, I. H. (1997). Attentional competition between modalities: Extinction between touch and vision after right hemisphere damage. *Neuropsychologia, 35,* 867–880.

Mennemeier, M., Vezey, E., Chatterjee, A., Rapcsak, S. Z., & Heilman, K. M. (1997). Contributions of the left and right cerebral hemispheres to line bisection. *Neuropsychologia, 35,* 703–715.

Mercier, L., Hebert, R., & Gauthier, L. (1995). Motor free visual perception test: Impact of vertical answer cards position on performance of adults with hemispatial visual neglect. *Occupational Therapy Journal of Research, 15,* 223–237.

Neistadt, M. E. (1993). The relationship between constructional and meal preparation skills. *Archives of Physical Medicine & Rehabilitation, 74,* 144–148.

Piercy, M., Hecaen, H., & Ajuriaguerra, J. (1960). Constructional apraxia associated with unilateral cerebral lesions: Left and right sided cases compared. *Brain, 83,* 225–242.

Poeck, K. (1985). Clues to the nature of disruptions to limb praxis. In E. A. Roy (Ed.), *Neuropsychological Studies of Apraxia and Related Disorders* (pp. 99–109). Amsterdam: Elsevier.

Posner, M. I., & Rafal, R. D. (1987). Cognitive theories of attention and the rehabilitation of attentional deficits. In M. J. Meier, A. L. Benton, & L. Diller (Eds.), *Neuropsychological Rehabilitation* (pp. 182–201). New York: Churchill Livingston.

Raymer, A. M., Maher, L. M., Foundas, A. L., Heilman, K. M., & Rothi, L. J. (1997). The significance of body part as tool errors in limb apraxia. *Brain and Cognition, 34,* 287–292.

Riddoch, M. J., & Humphreys, G. W. (1994). Towards an understanding of neglect. In M. J. Riddoch & G. W. Humphreys (Eds.), *Cognitive Neuropsychology and Cognitive Rehabilitation* (pp. 125–147). Hove, UK: Laurence Erlbaum.

Robertson, I. H., Manly, T., Beschin, N., Daini, R., Haeski-Deivick, H., Homberg, V., Jehkonen, M., Pizzamiglio, G., Shiel, A., & Weber, E. (1997). Auditory sustained attention is a marker of unilateral spatial neglect. *Neuropsychologia, 35,* 1527–1532.

Rothi, L. J. G., Raymer, A. M., & Heilman, K. M. (1997). Limb praxis assessment. In L. J. G Rothi & K. M. Heilman (Eds.), *Apraxia: The Neuropsychology of Action* (pp. 61–73). East Sussex, UK: Psychology.

Scheiman, M. (1997). *Understanding and Managing Vision Deficits: A Guide for Occupational Therapists.* Thorofare, NJ: Slack.

Scheiman, M. (1999, March). *Understanding and Managing Visual Deficits: Theory, Screening, Procedures, Intervention Techniques.* Conference of Vision Education Seminars, Jacksonville, FL.

Schenkenberg, T., Bradford, D. C., & Ajax, E. T. (1980). Line bisection and unilateral visual neglect in patients with neurologic impairment. *Neurology, 30,* 509–517.

Sea, M.-J. C., Henderson, A., & Cermak, S. A. (1993). Patterns of visual spatial inattention and their functional significance in stroke patients. *Archives of Physical Medicine & Rehabilitation, 74,* 355–360.

Simon, R. P., Aminoff, M. J., & Greenberg, D. A. (1999). *Clinical Neurology* (4th ed.). Stamford, CT: Appleton & Lange.

Stam, C. J., & Bakker, M. (1990). The prevalence of neglect: Superiority of neuropsychological over clinical methods of examination. *Clinical Neurology and Neurosurgery, 92,* 229–235.

Stone, S. P., Halligan, P. W., & Greenwood, R. J. (1993). The incidence of neglect phenomena and related disorders in patients with an acute right or left hemisphere stroke. *Age and Aging, 22,* 46–52.

Stone, S. P., Halligan, P. W., Marshall, J. C., & Greenwood, R. J. (1998). Unilateral neglect: A common but heterogeneous syndrome. *Neurology, 50,* 1902–1905.

Suderland, A., Bowers, M. P., Sluman, S. M., Wilcock, D. J., & Ardron, M. E. (1999). Impaired dexterity of the ipsilateral hand after stroke and the relationship to cognitive deficit. *Stroke, 30,* 949–955.

Tegner, R., & Levander, M. (1991). Through a looking glass: A new technique to demonstrate directional hypokinesia in unilateral neglect. *Brain, 114,* 1943–1951.

Titcomb, R. E., Okoye, R., & Schiff, S. (1997). Introduction to the dynamic process of vision. In M. Gentile (Ed.), *Functional Visual Behavior* (pp. 3–39). Bethesda MD: American Occupational Therapy Association.

Trobe, J. D., Acosta, P. C., Krischer, J. P., & Trick, G. L. (1981). Confrontation visual field techniques in the detection of anterior visual pathway lesions. *Annals of Neurology, 10,* 28–34.

Van Deusen, J. (1983). Normative data for ninety-three elderly persons in the Schenkenberg line bisection test. *Physical & Occupational Therapy in Geriatrics, 3,* 49–54.

Warren, M. (1981). Relationship of constructional apraxia and body scheme disorders to dressing performance in adult CVA. *American Journal of Occupational Therapy, 35,* 431–437.

Warren, M. (1993a). A hierarchical model for evaluation and treatment of visual perceptual dysfunction in adult acquired brain injury, part 1. *American Journal of Occupational Therapy, 47,* 42–54.

Warren, M. (1993b). A hierarchical model for evaluation and treatment of visual perceptual dysfunction in adult acquired brain injury, part 2. *American Journal of Occupational Therapy, 47,* 55–66.

Warren, M. (1996). *Brain Injury Vision Assessment Battery for Adults.* Lenexa, KS: visABILITIES Rehab.

Warren, M. (1999). *Evaluation and Treatment of Visual Perceptual Dysfunction in Adult Brain Injury, Part 1.* Conference of visABILITIES Rehab Services, Nashville, TN.

Warrington, E. K., James, M., & Kinsbourne, M. (1966). Drawing disability in relation to laterality of cerebral lesion. *Brain, 89,* 53–82.

Whyte, J., & DiPasquale, M. C. (1995). Assessment of vision and visual attention in minimally responsive brain injured patients. *Archives of Physical Medicine and Rehabilitation, 76,* 804–810.

Wilson, B., Cockburn, J., & Halligan, P. (1987). Development of a behavioral test of visuospatial neglect. *Archives of Physical Medicine & Rehabilitation, 68,* 98–102.

York, C. D., & Cermak, S. A. (1995). Visual perception and praxis in adults after stroke. *American Journal of Occupational Therapy, 49,* 543–550.

8

Assessing Abilities and Capacities: Cognition

Mary Vining Radomski

LEARNING OBJECTIVES

After studying this chapter, the reader will be able to do the following:

1. Describe specific cognitive capacities and abilities and analyze their influence on occupational function.
2. Select cognitive assessment methods and tools based on individual patients' characteristics and requirements.
3. Anticipate and describe factors that may confound performance during cognitive assessment.
4. Distinguish occupational therapy's contribution to multidisciplinary cognitive assessment from that of other rehabilitation disciplines.

*C*ognition refers to the integrated functions of the human mind that together result in thought and goal-directed action. Simply put by Diller (1993), "Cognition involves the acquisition, processing, and application of information in daily life" (p. 9). Cognition is at the core of an individual's essence or personhood. In fact, Schacter (1996) suggested that without the capacity to remember the past, humans lose a sense of self. Cognition not only influences what a person chooses to do (Bandura, 1986), it also dictates how an experience is remembered and interpreted. Cognition clearly drives the selection, performance, analysis, and learning of all human occupations, which is why this important dimension is reflected in the profession's uniform terminology (American Occupational Therapy Association, 1994) and the occupational science model of human subsystems (Clark et al., 1991).

GLOSSARY

Attention—The ability to deploy limited mental resources for purposes of concentration. Human activities have various attentional demands, including sustained attention (length of time), selective attention (competing stimuli), divided attention (multiple simultaneous stimuli), and alternating attention (shifts back and forth to various stimuli).

Cognition—The general term that reflects the mental enterprises related to absorbing information, thinking, and goal-directed action.

Concept formation—The ability to analyze relationships between objects and their properties (Sohlberg & Mateer, 1989).

Executive function—Metaprocess that enables a person to initiate, plan, self-monitor, and correct his or her approach to goal-directed tasks. Executive disorders often result from frontal lobe damage and are evidenced by problems with self-control, self-direction, and organization (Lezak, 1995).

Higher-order thinking abilities—Complex mental operations that include problem solving, reasoning, and concept formation. Thinking generally entails the manipulation of remembered information (Mayer, 1992) and depends on intact primary cognitive capacities (orientation, attention, and memory) (Sohlberg & Mateer, 1989).

Memory—The result of interactive cognitive systems that receive, code, store, and retrieve information.

Neuropsychological evaluation—A long battery of standardized tests for purposes of diagnosis, patient care and planning, rehabilitation evaluation, and research (Lezak, 1995). Typically, the examiner is a doctor of psychology with specialized training in cognitive processes and brain–behavior relationships.

Orientation—The awareness of self in relation to one's physical and temporal environment that depends upon reliable integration of attention, memory, and perception (Lezak, 1995). Impaired orientation is strongly suggestive of cerebral dysfunction (Lezak, 1995).

Problem solving—The multistage process consisting of identifying a problem, generating possible solutions, implementing a preferred solution, and evaluating the results. Everyday problem solving, however, does not always follow this logical sequence of steps.

Reasoning—The ability to draw inferences or conclusions from known or assumed facts.

Self-awareness—The capacity to objectively perceive the self (Prigatano & Schacter, 1991) and (with a reasonable degree of accuracy) to compare that conception to a pre-morbid standard.

In addition to its central role in occupational functioning, cognition also predicts rehabilitation outcome after injury and illness. MacNeill and Lichtenberg (1997) found that for geriatric inpatients, levels of cognitive function predicted ability to return home alone at discharge from rehabilitation. Sandstrom and Mokler (1999) also described cognitive function as a key outcome variable for persons with severe motor stroke, and Hanks et al. (1999) found that cognition predicted functional abilities and social integration 6 months after discharge from acute rehabilitation. Clearly, to identify and remove barriers to a patient's optimal occupational functioning and to anticipate rehabilitation outcomes, occupational therapists endeavor to understand the nature of patients' cognitive function as part of the assessment.

This chapter begins with descriptions of specific cognitive capacities and abilities and follows with a discussion of various influences on cognitive function. It reviews clinical reasoning considerations pertinent to cognitive assessment and describes specific methods and tools based on two complementary approaches to cognitive assessment.

Defining Cognitive Capacities and Abilities

Cognition consists of an interactive hierarchy (Ben-Yishay cited in Goldstein & Levin, 1987) that includes primary cognitive capacities (**orientation**, **attention**, and **memory**), **higher-level thinking abilities** (**reasoning**, **concept formation**, and **problem solving**), and metaprocesses (**executive functions** and **self-awareness**).

Primary Cognitive Capacities

The primary cognitive capacities of orientation, attention, and memory largely reflect the neuroanatomical and physiological integrity of the brain (Radomski,

1998). They are thought to be prerequisite to higher-level thinking abilities and to influence metaprocessing.

Changes in primary cognitive capacities are seen in many recipients of occupational therapy services. After a severe traumatic brain injury (TBI), many patients enter a confusional stage of recovery in which they are disoriented (Levin et al., 1979). Stroke and TBI often result in problems with attention, memory, and language (Capruso & Levin, 1992; Hochstenbach et al., 1998). Persons with chronic conditions such as multiple sclerosis (Foong et al., 1998), epilepsy (Giovagnoli et al., 1997), systemic lupus erythematosus (Denburg et al., 1997), and acquired immunodeficiency syndrome (AIDS) (Poutiainen et al., 1996) may also experience deterioration in attention and memory.

Orientation

Orientation refers to the awareness of self in relation to person, place, time, and circumstance (Sohlberg & Mateer, 1989). Orientation deficits are typically symptoms of brain dysfunction, with disorientation to time and place most common (Lezak, 1995).

Attention

Attention is the deployment of mental resources for concentration. Each person is thought to have a limited capacity for consciously attending to information—a hard-wired upper limit that dictates how many inputs can be simultaneously processed (Lezak, 1995). Let us examine four levels of attention in the context of preparing a meal.

1. *Sustained attention* is the capacity to maintain attentional performance over time (Lezak, 1995). To prepare a meal with several dishes, an individual must stay focused for the duration of the task.
2. *Selective attention* occurs when an individual concentrates on one set of stimuli while ignoring competing stimuli (Lezak, 1995), as when the cook ignores the noise from the television while measuring or counting ingredients.

3. *Divided attention* allows a person to respond to more than one task at a time—a more complex mental skill than sustained and selective attention (Sohlberg & Mateer, 1989). The cook browns the meat while talking with a family member.
4. *Alternating attention* is necessary as one flexibly shifts attention between multiple operations (Lezak, 1995). The cook interrupts meal preparation to answer the telephone and then quickly resumes setting the table while monitoring the status of food simmering on the stove.

Memory

Memory broadly refers to information storage and retrieval (Lezak, 1995). There are many conceptions of the way this process occurs (Baddeley, 1990; Lezak, 1995). Atkinson and Shiffrin's (1971) Information-Processing Model of memory highlights stages of acquiring and employing new knowledge and skills (Fig. 8-1). Box 8-1 outlines terms commonly used in the discussion of memory.

Sensory Registers

Information from the environment is briefly (milliseconds) held in registers (or stores) specific to the human senses (Lezak, 1995). This registration stage has been called the intake valve for determining what data from the environment are ultimately stored (Lezak, 1995). This phase is influenced by acuity of the senses (such as hearing and vision), affective set, and perception (Lezak, 1995).

Short-Term Memory

The short-term phase of information processing has many labels: immediate memory, short-term memory, working memory (Lezak, 1995). The term *working memory* connotes the effortful deployment of cognitive resources during this stage. In short, for input from sensory registers to proceed to storage in long-term memory, it must be the subject of deliberate concentra-

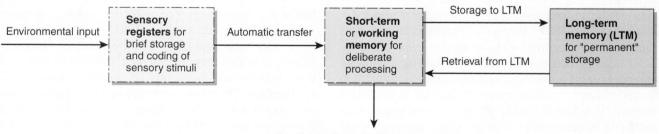

Figure 8-1 Human information processing model of memory. (Modified with permission from Atkinson, R. C., & Shiffrin, R. M. [1971]. The control of short-term memory. *Scientific American, 225,* 82–90.)

BOX 8-1
Memory Terms (Quintana, L., 1995)

Term	Definition
Memory	
Recent	Usually corresponds to long-term memory; includes memory hours to months post stimulus presentation
Remote	Very long term memory, as from childhood
Episodic	Memory of one's personal history (e.g., what you had for breakfast this morning)
Semantic	Personal knowledge of the world (e.g., that horses are big and ants are small)
Amnesia	
Retrograde	Loss of ability to recall events that occurred before the trauma
Anterograde	Decreased memory of events occurring post trauma
Postraumatic	Period following trauma during which the patient is confused and disoriented and seems to lack the ability to store and retrieve new information

---

tion in working memory for approximately 30 seconds (Lezak, 1995). Without this focused attention the memory trace decays and the memory is not retained (Lezak, 1995). Unlike long-term memory, which is thought to have an infinite capacity, working memory has a restricted holding capacity of seven plus or minus two chunks of information (Miller, 1956). In addition to its role in information processing, working memory is the seat of conscious thought used in concentration and problem solving (Baddeley, 1990). Based on electrochemical activity in the brain, working memory reflects the contribution of attention to the memory process (Lezak, 1995).

Long-Term Memory

Whereas data in working memory has a short shelf life, information in long-term memory can be stored for a lifetime (Lezak, 1995). When we remember information (an event that occurred an hour ago or a year ago), we have located and retrieved data from long-term memory and are holding it for conscious attention and thought in limited-capacity working memory. Storage in long-term memory is based on relatively permanent changes in brain cell structure (Glover et al., 1990), although there does not appear to be a single local storage site for stored memories (Lezak, 1995). Long-term memory is thought

to consist of two subsystems, declarative memory and procedural memory (Abreu, 1999). Declarative memory holds factual information, which is subdivided into episodic memory (knowledge of personal information and events) and semantic memory (knowledge of facts about the world) (Eysenck & Keane, 1990). Procedural memory holds information related to knowing how to do things; it allows us to learn and perform skilled motor actions (Eysenck & Keane, 1990).

Higher-Level Thinking Abilities

Higher-level thinking abilities are the result of complex and dynamic interactions between a number of brain structures united in functional systems (Hochstenbach, et al., 1998); they depend on intact primary cognitive capacities (Sohlberg & Mateer, 1989). After brain injury, people may have difficulty with reasoning and abstraction (Scherzer et al., 1993) and with sequencing and classification (Adamovich et al., 1985), all of which interfere with higher-level thought. Sohlberg and Mateer (1989) described three interrelated categories of higher-level thinking abilities: problem solving, reasoning, and concept formation.

Problem Solving

Most people use problem-solving skills hundreds of times a day. Problem solving occurs whenever the situation is different from a desired situation or goal and the person does not immediately know what series of actions to take (Bransford & Stein, 1984). In fact, at a basic level, all human responses that are not routine or habitual can be construed as problem solving (Radomski, 1998). Problem solving is usually conceptualized as the following multistage process:

- ► Identify the problem
- ► Define the problem
- ► Generate possible solutions and select one
- ► Implement the preferred solution
- ► Evaluate the outcome against the desired goal

However, everyday problem solving does not always follow this logical sequence. In his discussion of managerial problem solving, Wagner (1991) reported that high-level managers most often employ nonlinear problem solving in which they rely on tacit knowledge and base their actions and decisions on intuition rather than deliberation. Therefore, occupational therapists use the aforementioned sequence to organize their observations during assessment of problem solving rather than as a singular "right" sequence against which to judge effectiveness.

Reasoning

Reasoning entails drawing inferences or conclusions from known or assumed facts. It can make use of sequencing, classification, and deductive and inductive reasoning (Sohlberg & Mateer, 1989). Sequencing is ordering information properly (Sohlberg & Mateer, 1989), whereas classification requires grouping objects or ideas according to characteristics (Bruce, 1994). During deductive reasoning, a thinker uses general information to identify specific facts and principles (Bruce, 1994). For example, a patient who is doing a task observes the therapist signaling that a high degree of accuracy is required. The patient deduces from that general feedback that she should slow down and periodically check the work. During inductive reasoning, a thinker is given a set of examples and must create the general rule (Mayer, 1992). For example, a patient tells frequent anecdotes about her grandchildren and has numerous drawings and photos of them on the wall of her hospital room; the therapist uses inductive reasoning to conclude that the role of grandmother is important to this patient.

Concept Formation

Closely linked to reasoning, concept formation is the ability to analyze relationships between objects and their properties (Sohlberg & Mateer, 1989). Sohlberg and Mateer suggested that "forming a concept requires that an individual identify critical features of instances of that concept and also determine how those features interrelate" (p. 267). A person forms a concept when sorting a box of assorted kitchen tools, for example determining whether to organize them by function, size, or color). Thinking can be further qualified on a continuum of concrete to abstract (Mosey, 1993). Concrete thinking is characterized by the tendency to be bound to obvious stimulus properties and the inability to remove oneself from the immediate task (Sohlberg & Mateer, 1989). On the other end of the continuum, abstract thinking involves the ability to transcend the immediate situation, appreciate various aspects of the problem, and think symbolically (Sohlberg & Mateer). In the sorting example, a concrete thinker might choose to organize the kitchen tools by color, whereas the more abstract thinker might organize by common function.

Metaprocessing Abilities

Executive functions and self-awareness are metaprocesses that contribute initiation, planning, monitoring, reflection, and self-evaluation to cognitive function (Sternberg, 1990). Bewick et al. (1995) depicted these abilities as cognitive directors, as they facilitate the interplay of primary cognitive capacities and higher-level thinking in the execution of complex tasks.

The importance of executive functions and self-awareness to satisfying and productive role performance cannot be overstated. Impairments in executive functions are major factors associated with loss of social autonomy and inability to return to work long after TBI (Mazaux, et al., 1997). Decreased self-awareness after TBI prevents the survivor from recognizing the deficits that limit performance and diminishes motivation to participate in rehabilitation therapies. Interestingly, some family members view unawareness as a blessing in persons with dementia (Fleming et al., 1996), whereas for other caregivers, it is associated with higher levels of subjective distress (Seltzer et al., 1997).

Executive Functions

Intact executive functions are necessary for the successful performance of unstructured multistep occupational tasks and roles. Lezak (1995) described four components of executive functions: volition, planning, purposive action, and effective performance.

1. Volitional behavior is dictated by determining what one needs or wants and then formulating a goal or an intention to act (Lezak, 1995). It is influenced by self-awareness, as needs, wants, and goals are often moderated by people's understanding of their circumstances and ability to realize an objective (Lezak, 1995).
2. Planning is identifying and sequencing steps to move toward the goal or end point (Lezak, 1995).
3. Purposive action is "the translation of an intention or plan into productive, self-serving activity [requiring] the actor to initiate, maintain, switch and stop sequences of complex behavior in an orderly and integrated manner" (Lezak, 1995, p. 658).
4. Effective performance requires that an individual monitor and self-correct while regulating the intensity, speed, and strategies used during the task (Lezak, 1995).

Self-Awareness

Prigatano and Schacter (1991) suggested that self-awareness is the highest of all integrated activities of the brain. It is the ability to process information about the self and compare it to a longstanding self-evaluation (Dougherty & Radomski, 1993). Self-awareness has two primary dimensions: (1) appreciation of personal attributes, such as physical and cognitive strengths and weakness, and (2) initiation of compensatory strategies in response to known personal attributes. (In general, persons with TBI tend to be more aware of physical deficits than cognitive or emotional changes [Anderson & Tranel, 1989]).

Crosson et al. (1989) proposed a three-level self-awareness hierarchy consisting of intellectual awareness, emergent awareness, and anticipatory awareness:

1. Intellectual awareness is a person's ability to understand at some level that a particular function is impaired. Severe deficits in memory impede intellectual awareness because such awareness requires recall of the past.
2. Emergent awareness is the ability of a person to recognize a problem when it is actually happening.
3. Anticipatory awareness, which depends on the existence of intellectual and emergent awareness, is the ability to anticipate a challenge or problem resulting from physical or cognitive impairments. Metacognition—knowledge and regulation of one's own cognitive capacities and strategies (Toglia, 1998)—is closely linked to anticipatory awareness. For a person to begin taking notes in response to novel instructions (a metacognitive strategy), he or she must appreciate vulnerability from memory deficits and anticipate the challenge the activity represents (intellectual and anticipatory awareness).

Executive functions reciprocally influence self-awareness. Self-knowledge informs the selection of reasonable goals for a given undertaking and drives selection of strategies that best facilitate performance. Ongoing monitoring of task performance with adjustment of strategies and incorporation of feedback can in turn affect self-awareness, altering percepts of personal strengths and weaknesses.

Multiple-Determinant Model of Cognitive Function

The dissection of specific cognitive capacities and abilities for purposes of description belies the complexity of their interrelationships and redundancies. In actuality, an individual's cognitive state is dynamic, determined by many interacting variables: neurobiological, affective, experiential, social, and cultural influences, all of which are mediated by the task and environment. Changes in any of these domains improve or detract from a person's cognitive state and thereby his or her occupational functioning. To assess cognition and interpret findings, occupational therapists must understand how variables can affect performance during cognitive assessment. What follows is a brief summary of each influence, supported with specific examples from the literature.

Neurobiological Influence on Cognition

The neurobiological influence on cognition is best understood as foundational cognitive capacities resulting from dynamic neural networks (Hochstenbach et al., 1998). These neural networks represent innate cognitive strengths and weaknesses that are based on the integrity and composition of the brain (Hochstenbach et al., 1998). For example, in his theory of multiple intelligences, Gardner (1983) suggested a biological basis for at least seven specialized intelligences (linguistic, musical, logical–mathematical, spatial, bodily–kinesthetic, intrapersonal, and interpersonal) that human beings possess to greater or lesser extents. The neurobiological influence on cognition is most apparent following changes to the anatomy and physiology of the brain, as with injury and aging. Persons with stroke have local damage to brain tissue that often results in predictable and specific cognitive deficits, such as frontal lobe damage leading to executive dysfunction and temporal lobe damage affecting memory. Neurobiological changes that accompany aging also seem to affect thinking abilities and memory. Crystallized intelligence (well-practiced, overlearned skills and knowledge) is reportedly maintained or strengthened into the eighth decade of life, whereas fluid intelligence, which entails reasoning and problem solving for unfamiliar challenges, begins a slow decline in the sixth decade of life (Lezak, 1995). Small et al. (1999) found that healthy adults aged 70 and older demonstrated a decline in specific aspects of memory performance when compared with subjects 60 to 69 years old. They suggest that this profile of age-related memory decline is related to changes in the hippocampal formation (Small et al., 1999).

Changes or deterioration of other functions of the human body have secondary neurobiological influences on cognition. For example, visual–perceptual impairments alter the inputs into the memory process, limiting what a person can accurately remember. Medications can also have a neurobiological influence on cognition. Schagen et al. (1999) found that women who had adjuvant chemotherapy for operative primary breast cancer complained of more frequent memory and concentration problems and performed worse on neuropsychological tests than controls who received the same surgical and radiation therapy but did not receive systemic chemotherapy. Cognitive impairment was not explained by anxiety, depression, fatigue, or time since treatment.

Affective Influences on Cognition

Although it is clear that emotions affect cognition, the underlying mechanism is not known. Anxious people differ from others in several aspects of attentional functioning. Anxious people are more likely to attend to threat-related stimuli and use limited-capacity working memory for worry, self-concern, and other task-irrelevant distractions (Eysenck & Keane, 1990). Persons with depression also frequently complain about poor memory but often do not demonstrate memory deficits on neuropsychological testing (Lezak, 1995). Depressed individuals are thought to show passive disengagement with the environment in that their attentional focus is on internal concerns rather than environmental events (Eysenck & Keane, 1990). Depressed people also demonstrate a negative recall bias (a tendency to recall more negative information about themselves than others do) (Baddeley, 1990; Eysenck & Keane, 1990). Memory problems associated with depression seem to have a secondary effect on executive processes. Channon and Green (1999) found that otherwise healthy but depressed individuals performed worse than controls who were not depressed on three measures of executive function. They explained this difference as possibly related to alterations in neurotransmitter activities and/or distractions by dysfunctional negative thoughts that occupy limited-capacity working memory during problem solving and task performance.

Similarly, transient mental distractions can impair cognition. Pain and fatigue are thought to be irrelevant inputs that diminish the function of limited-capacity working memory by occupying attention that is therefore unavailable to incoming data (Denburg et al., 1997). Therefore, patients who are exhausted or in physical or emotional pain are unlikely to be able to demonstrate their cognitive capabilities during assessment, with or without neurobiological impairments.

Experiential, Social, and Cultural Influence on Cognition

Feuerstein (1980) hypothesized that experience and sociocultural background play superordinate roles in the development of cognitive capacities and habits. An Israeli psychologist–educator, Feuerstein became convinced that the large number of "retarded" adolescent immigrants after World War II lacked cognitive skills primarily because of poverty and socially deprived surroundings. Participants in his 2-year intervention program, which focused on acquisition of cognitive habits and strategies, demonstrated improvements in general intellectual aptitude, interpersonal conduct, self-sufficiency, and adaptation (Perkins, 1995). Belenky et al. (1986) suggested that culture and social institutions also influence gender differences in learning and thinking. They posited that women acquire a sense of knowing and sense of themselves as thinkers through methods and sequences different from those of men.

Finally, Prigatano et al. (1997) found that self-awareness after TBI is affected by culture. They suggested that because incompetence in personal care is a sign of disgrace in Japan, Japanese patients with TBI tended to overestimate their abilities in this realm. On the other hand, because Japanese generally view high estimations of social and interpersonal skills as impolite, Japanese patients with TBI tended to underestimate their abilities in this realm.

Task and Environment As Contextual Mediators of Cognition

People bring their neurobiological, emotional, experiential, social, and cultural predispositions to all information processing, but performance at a given moment is mediated by characteristics of the task and environmental contexts. In her Dynamic Interactional Model of Cognition, Toglia (1998) reviewed the contributions of task and environment to cognition. Task variables that influence cognition include complexity, arrangement, and movement demands (Toglia, 1998). Here is an example of task–cognition interplay. When a task is familiar, the thinker requires relatively little attention to recognize a problem type and determine a hypothesis and plan of action (Mayer, 1992). A familiar task or problem prompts the individual to retrieve a large number of interconnected units of knowledge, both related facts and previous solutions (Mayer, 1992). Tasks that optimally challenge an individual's cognitive capacities and abilities and engage his or her interest elicit an individual's peak cognitive performance (Csikszentmihalyi, 1990).

The environment similarly affects cognition. Contextual cues in the environment enhance recall of similar tasks or previously effective techniques or solutions. The stimulus–arousal properties of the environment also influence cognitive function. Lighting and noise can focus attention or, as is often the case for persons with brain injury, provide distractions that derail thinking.

In summary, cognition consists of specific but interrelated capacities and abilities that are influenced by neurobiological, affective, experiential–sociocultural variables, and task and environmental contexts. This discussion, although not exhaustive, highlights the complexity if not the mystery of cognitive function—an appreciation necessary for assessing cognitive capacities and abilities in occupational therapy. In judging the cognitive status of another person, teasing out performance confounders is as important as selecting and correctly administering the assessment tool. Whereas assigning and summing scores on standardized instruments requires the attentiveness of a trained technician, observing and interpreting performance during assessment requires the insight of a professional.

Case Example

ASSESSING COGNITION AFTER TRAUMATIC BRAIN INJURY

Patient Information

Mr. B. is a 26-year-old single man who sustained a traumatic brain injury as a result of a pedestrian–auto accident. Upon admission to the emergency room, he had a *Glasgow Coma Scale* score of 6, and records indicate that he was in coma for approximately 10 days. In addition to the brain injury, Mr. B. sustained fractures in both legs: tibia–fibula fracture on the right, fracture of the femur on the left. Mr. B. graduated from college with a degree in law enforcement and worked in a rural community as a police officer at the time of his injury. Mr. B. participated in inpatient rehabilitation for 3 weeks. Unable to return to his apartment because of concerns about safety, Mr. B. was discharged to his brother's home. Approximately 3 months post injury, Mr. B. was referred to outpatient occupational therapy to assess readiness for independent living.

The occupational therapist wanted to determine Mr. B.'s ability to assume self-maintenance roles and to identify cognitive deficits interfering with role and task performance. The therapist used the following tools: *Canadian Occupational Performance Measure (COPM)* to obtain information about the patient's perceived problems and priorities; *Kohlman Evaluation of Living Skills (KELS)*; *Cognitive Assessment of Minnesota (CAM)* to obtain a general picture of cognitive capabilities; and systematic observation of the patient's response to the presentation of homework.

Results

In an interview using the *COPM*, Mr. B. indicated that his ability to function independently was limited because of lower extremity fractures. He was dissatisfied with his inability to drive, the slowness with which he donned lower extremity clothing, his low stamina when walking outside, and lack of avocational outlets because of mobility limitations. When queried about known dependence on family members for taking medications and his lack of initiation of self-maintenance tasks, Mr. B. quickly dismissed these reports as awkwardness associated with being a guest in their home.

Mr. B. needed assistance to perform two activities in the money management component of the *KELS* (use of banking forms, payment of bills). He seemed capable of carrying out basic arithmetic operations but made transcription errors that he did not detect or correct on his own. In areas of self-care and safety and health, he demonstrated adequate awareness of and responses to personal and household hazards.

On the *CAM*, Mr. B.'s scores in recall and recognition, problem solving, and abstract thinking ranked as moderate to severe impairment. Performance ranked within normal limits for such domains as orientation, following directions, immedi-

ate memory, temporal awareness, auditory memory and sequencing, and simple math and money skills.

During each of his two outpatient evaluation sessions, the therapist gave Mr. B. oral instructions specific to three assignments to complete at home, all of which he agreed to do but did not make note of. He completed none of them. He seemed motivated throughout the assessment and did not appear distracted by pain or emotional distress during his sessions.

Analysis

The occupational therapist hypothesized that Mr. B. continued to have superficial awareness of his limitations, acknowledging physical but not cognitive changes. Mr. B.'s description of challenges coupled with his brother's report suggested that Mr. B. was physically capable of performing ADL and IADL but required prompting to initiate them. Problems with memory and lack of initiation were evident in Mr. B.'s performance of the *CAM* and his response to homework assignments. Inattention to detail seemed to explain his difficulties with money management on the *KELS*. Because of the structured nature of the assessment, the occupational therapist concluded that Mr. B.'s problem-solving ability was not adequately assessed and decided to create opportunities to observe strategy use, planning, and organization in the treatment plan.

Occupational Therapy Problem List

1. Decreased initiation of ADL and IADL
2. Decreased productivity due to poor stamina and limited repertoire of appropriate avocational outlets
3. Memory insufficiency and inadequate repertoire of memory compensation strategies
4. Decreased awareness of cognitive deficits interfering with compensatory strategy use

---

CLINICAL REASONING
in Occupational Therapy Practice

Effects of Environment on Cognitive Function

During his inpatient rehabilitation, Mr. B. was observed to have decreased attentional capacities, especially with complex tasks. How might this problem be evident during the occupational therapy ADL assessment? What factors in the environment might exaggerate these problems? What factors might minimize them?

The Process of Cognitive Assessment

Occupational therapists in clinical practice assess cognition for three primary reasons:

1. To establish a baseline against which to measure change
2. To inform intervention and discharge planning
3. To identify those who would benefit from more detailed **neuropsychological evaluation**

As previously discussed, many persons requiring the attention of medical and rehabilitation professionals have cognitive deficits that interfere with function. Cognitive changes can be temporary, relatively static, or progressive. Periodic assessment using standardized tools helps the rehabilitation team to interpret these cognitive changes and respond appropriately. Occupational therapists use findings to determine what problems to address and to select intervention strategies.

Occupational therapists exchange information about their findings with the family and other rehabilitation professionals so that the rehabilitation team together can create a comprehensive picture of the patient's function. For example, language is inextricably linked to almost every aspect of cognitive function. Occupational therapists review the results of speech and language assessment to understand the language capacities and abilities of a given patient and the influence of any impairment on cognitive assessment. Neuropsychology is informed by occupational therapists' observations of cognitive function in the context of daily life tasks and life roles. Neuropsychologists use a variety of standardized tests to diagnose localized deficits and differentiate between neurological and psychiatric symptoms. A full neuropsychological evaluation, which typically entails 2 to 8 hours of tests, guides decision making prior to major rehabilitation transitions (return to work, moving from supervised to independent living or vice versa) and establishes the permanence of cognitive impairments for legal purposes. Because neuropsychological evaluation is so expensive, occupational therapists often assess cognition on behalf of the team during acute rehabilitation, when cognitive capacities and abilities are in a period of rapid change.

Clinicians select the most appropriate cognitive assessment methods and tools based on the objectives of assessment and specific needs and characteristics of the patient. Occupational therapists use two complementary approaches to assessing cognition: (1) assessing function to make inferences about cognitive capacities and abilities and (2) assessing cognitive capacities and abilities to make inferences about function.

Methods and Tools for Assessing Function to Make Inferences About Cognition

Occupational therapists begin any new assessment by evaluating the patient's roles and performance in occupations (Moyers, 1999). Assessment of cognition is part of that process. Informal and formal functional assessments provide opportunities to make hypotheses about cognitive strengths and weaknesses, allowing the clinician to identify domains warranting further evaluation. For example, during an activities of daily living (ADL) or homemaking evaluation, occupational therapists observe attention to task by counting episodes of distractions, memory for instructions, and evidence of organization and planning. Of course, informal functional assessments of cognition are highly subjective, easily influenced by the clinician's definition of "normal" and his or her acumen in using the observable (behavior) to make inferences about internal cognitive processes. This method of cognitive assessment, however, is preferable for patients who cannot understand verbal or written instructions, as with communication deficits or speaking another language.

Three standardized functional assessments help clinicians simultaneously examine function and cognition: the *Arnadottir OT-ADL Neurobehavioral Evaluation (A-ONE)* (Arnadottir, 1990), the *Rabideau Kitchen Evaluation—Revised* (Neistadt, 1992), the *Kitchen Task Assessment* (Baum & Edwards, 1993), and its recent adaptation, the *Executive Function Performance Task* (in development by Baum & Edwards).

Arnadottir OT-ADL Neurobehavioral Evaluation

The *A-ONE* evaluates performance of ADL and examines the effect of neurobehavioral dysfunction on task performance. There are two parts of the instrument; part 2 is considered optional. During part 1, the occupational therapist observes the patient performing dressing, hygiene, transfer and mobility, feeding, and communication tasks and completes the *Functional Independence Scale* by assigning a numerical score (0–4) for each aspect of the various tasks. For example, a score is assigned to each of the activities of dressing (donning shirt, pants, socks, shoes; fastening clothing). While observing the patient's performance of each component, the therapist also rates the patient in terms of presence of neurobehavioral impairments, again using a 0 to 4 scale. For example, the patient is scored on each of the following possible neurobehavioral impairments specified for the task of dressing: motor apraxia, ideational apraxia, unilateral body neglect, somatoagnosia, spatial relations, unilateral spatial neglect, abnormal tone, perseveration, and organization and sequencing. The scores on the *Functional Independence* and *Neurobehavioral* scales are not additive but used to establish patterns of performance and impairment. Occupational therapists may use the results of part 1 to localize cerebral dysfunction based on functional performance (part 2). Part 1 of the *A-ONE*, which takes approximately 25 minutes to administer, was standardized on patients with cortical central nervous system dysfunction. Its author recommends that therapists attend a training seminar before using the tool (Arnadottir, 1990).

Rabideau Kitchen Evaluation—Revised

The *Rabideau Kitchen Evaluation—Revised* (*RKE-R*) requires that persons with brain injury synthesize an array of cognitive capacities and abilities in the context of preparing a simple meal, a cold sandwich with two fillings and a hot beverage. Each of the 40 component activities is rated on a 0 to 3 scale indicating level of assistance or cueing required, and the total time for completion is recorded. Neistadt (1994) recommended that therapists use scores on the *RKE-R* to determine where to begin with a treatment protocol designed to improve meal preparation skills but suggested that this test may not be sensitive enough to use with persons who have subtle cognitive or perceptual deficits (Neistadt, 1992).

Kitchen Task Assessment

The *Kitchen Task Assessment* (*KTA*) measures the cognitive support necessary for the patient to prepare cooked pudding. Specific neurobehavioral components, such as initiation, organization, and safety, are scored on a 0 to 3 scale, reflecting the degree of cueing or physical assistance required for that aspect of the task. This test was standardized on patients with Alzheimer's disease.

Executive Function Performance Task

Because of its insensitivity to improvement when used with brain injury patients, Baum and Edwards recently expanded the *KTA*, creating the *Executive Function Performance Task* (*EFPT*). The *EFPT* emphasizes the role of executive functions in examining what a person can do when attempting five tasks: washing hands, preparing oatmeal, using a telephone, taking medications, and paying bills. Each task is rated 0 to 5 based on the extent to which a person is able to initiate, plan, shift from step to step, and detect and correct errors. Similar to the *RKE-E* and *KTA*, scores reflect the amount of verbal or physical assistance required for successful completion.

Work Simulations

Work simulations are another method for assessing cognition through functional activity. Nadeau and Buckheit (1995) recommended a three-phase Work Simulation Model for outpatients with TBI as a means to observe executive functions. In the setup phase, after patients are provided with a workspace and scheduled work time, they make a list of supplies they need for the job. Before beginning the simulation phase, patients predict their performance on projects that are somewhat similar to work tasks they would have done before the injury. In the postsimulation phase, patients rate actual performance and compare self-ratings to that of the therapist. Dougherty and Radomski (1993) described a similar assessment of work behaviors in which following directions, accuracy, and vigilance are rated in the context of four tasks, balancing a checkbook and using a calculator, Yellow Pages, and transportation schedules.

Dynamic Investigative Approach

Finally, therapists can convert any task to an opportunity for cognitive assessment by using a dynamic investigative approach (Toglia, 1989). Therapists deliberately manipulate performance variables related to task, environment, strategies, and cueing to determine in what conditions the patient performs at his or her best (Dougherty & Radomski, 1993). *Dynamic Interactional Assessment* (*DIA*) (Toglia, 1998) is a formal example of a dynamic investigative approach. *DIA* consists of awareness questioning, cueing and task grading, and strategy investigation (Toglia, 1998). During awareness questioning, patients answer increasingly specific questions that tap their intellectual awareness of potential problems. They also predict their performance before beginning the assessment task. Graded verbal cues are offered as needed once the patient begins work, and parameters of the task are changed, if necessary, to buoy the patient's performance. During task performance, the therapist seeks to understand what strategies or approaches the patient uses by asking strategy questions. Toglia incorporates *DIA* into a number of the standardized assessment tools she developed, including the *Contextual Memory Test* (Toglia, 1993) and the *Toglia Category Assessment* (Toglia, 1994).

When using methods and tools for assessing function to make inferences about cognition, occupational therapists generally seek to determine what the patient can do given various supports and conditions. These less structured approaches to evaluation allow for observation of metaprocesses and qualitative aspects of performance that are not easily captured using more structured methods. Because of their foundation in function, such methods capitalize on the unique expertise of occupational therapists. However, Hajek et al. (1997) suggested that functional assessments may not be sufficient for identifying cognitive disability and that rehabilitation outcome would be better predicted if the results of functional assessment were coupled with a detailed assessment of specific cognitive capacities and abilities.

Methods and Tools for Assessing Cognitive Capacities and Abilities to Make Inferences About Function

Based on the results of assessing performance of tasks and activities, clinicians generate hypotheses as to what specific barriers or impairments interfere with a patient's optimal occupational function. Tools and methods that assess specific cognitive capacities and abilities are then used to verify these hypotheses and establish a baseline against which to measure improvement. Many instruments have demonstrated reliability and validity, and standardized scoring criteria greatly reduce therapist bias. However, assessments of specific cognitive capacities and abilities may be predicated on a serious theoretical fallacy, the notion that these constructs can be separated from one another. Based on the interrelatedness of various aspects of human cognition, one questions whether, for example, memory can be assessed apart from attention. Table 8-1 provides examples

---

TABLE 8-1

Selected Tools for Assessing Cognitive Capacities and Abilities to Make Inferences About Function

Cognitive Capacity or Ability	Test	Description
Orientation	*Galveston Orientation and Amnesia Test* (Levin et al., 1979)	A widely used measure of orientation to person, place, time, and memory for events preceding and following injury. 10 questions with weighted error points deducted from a total of 100 points Example: "What is your name?" (2 points deducted for errors); "On what date were you admitted to the hospital?" (5 points deducted for errors); "What is the year?" (10 points deducted for each year removed from correct one to maximum of 30) (Levin et al., 1979, p. 677).
	Test of Orientation for Rehabilitation Patients (Dietz et al., 1990)	Uses 46 open-ended questions to evaluate orientation to person and personal situation, place, time, schedule, temporal continuity. Can be adapted to a recognition format for patients with expressive language deficits.
	Orientation Log (Jackson et al., 1998)	Evaluates orientation to place, time, situation in terms of the cueing needed for correct responses. 10-item scale designed for repeated administration.
Attention (sustained)	Letter cancellation tests (Lezak, 1995)	Rows of letters or numbers randomly interspersed with target letters or numbers. The patient is instructed to cross out all targets, with performance scored in terms of missed targets (errors) and completion time. Visual scanning, activation, and inhibition are also required for successful performance.
Memory	*Rivermead Behavioral Memory Test* (Wilson et al., 1985)	Assesses memory skills necessary for everyday life, including remembering names, faces, routes, and appointments. Consists of 11 subtests and 4 parallel versions for retest. Takes approximately 30 minutes to administer. Makatura et al. (1999) found the *Rivermead* more accurate in classifying severity of memory impairment (with clinicians' observations providing the benchmark) than traditional measures of memory (*Luria Nebraska Neuropsychological Battery Memory Scale, Wechsler Memory Scale—Revised*).
	Contextual Memory Test (Toglia, 1993)	Evaluates awareness of memory capacity, recall, and strategy use by employing *Dynamic Interactional Assessment* methods (Toglia, 1998). After answering questions about his or her memory and predicting performance, the patient studies a picture card containing 20 items from a restaurant or morning hygiene scene. The patient attempts to recall the items immediately and again after 15–20 min, then answers reflective questions about strategy use.
Higher-level thinking abilities	*Toglia Category Test* (Toglia, 1994)	Evaluates concept formation and ability to switch conceptual sets and incorporates *Dynamic Interactional Assessment* (Toglia, 1998). Patient is given 18 plastic utensils (knife, spoon, fork) of 2 sizes and 3 colors and asked to sort so that items in one group are different from the others. The patient sorts twice more, with therapist providing cues as necessary. Patient's performance is analyzed in terms of responsiveness to cues and the extent to which awareness can be facilitated.

(continued)

TABLE 8-1

Selected Tools for Assessing Cognitive Capacities and Abilities to Make Inferences About Function *(Continued)*

Cognitive Capacity or Ability	Test	Description
Executive functions	*Tinkertoy Test* (Lezak, 1995)	Patient is provided with 50 specific Tinkertoy pieces and given 2 instructions: "Make whatever you want with these" and "You will have at least 5 minutes and as much more time as you wish to make something." In this unstructured activity, the patient's approach is observed and the final construction is assigned a numerical score based on its complexity and sophistication, including mobility and symmetry.
	Woodrow Wilson Rehabilitation Center Executive Functions Route-Finding Task (Sohlberg & Mateer, 1989)	Patient is asked to find an unfamiliar location within the rehabilitation or health care setting as efficiently as possible. The therapist accompanies and observes the patient but may not answer questions about how to get there. Performance is rated in a number of domains, including task understanding, incorporation of information seeking, retention of directions, and error detection and correction.
Screen of general cognitive function	*Modified Mini-Mental State Examination—Clock Drawing* (Suhr & Grace, 1999)	Teng and Chui (1987) expanded the *Mini-Mental State Examination* (Folstein et al., 1975) to tap a wider range of cognitive abilities and provide a wider range of scores (0–100 rather than 0–30). Suhr and Grace combined the *Modified Mini-Mental State Examination* with the clock drawing. They found that this combination was more sensitive than either test alone and better distinguished persons with cognitive impairment (right hemisphere stroke) from controls. Patients with right hemisphere stroke who did poorly on these tests had lower discharge *Functional Independence Measure* scores than patients with right hemisphere stroke who did well. Suhr and Grace used the methods of Watson et al. (1993) for scoring the clock drawing.
Microbatteries for multiple cognitive capacities and abilities	*Loewenstein Occupational Therapy Cognitive Assessment* (*LOTCA*) (Katz et al., 1989)	Developed in Israel and standardized on American and Israeli patients with stroke and traumatic brain injury (Cermak et al., 1995). Designed to detect cognitive impairment, establish a baseline, and identify patients needing detailed cognitive assessment. Consists of 20 subtests in four areas: orientation, perception, visuomotor operations, thinking operations. Does not pick up subtle cognitive deficiencies on persons with mild injuries. Administration takes approximately 30 min.
	Cognitive Assessment of Minnesota (Rustad et al., 1993)	Standardized for use with adult neurological patients. Consists of 17 subtests, including attention, memory, orientation, neglect, following directions, money and math skills, planning, abstract reasoning, and problem solving. Performance is reported in a profile format indicating presence or extent of impairment. Appropriate for persons at level IV or above on the *Rancho Los Amigos Scale of Cognitive Functioning*. Administration of the battery takes approximately 45 min.
	COGNISTAT (*Neurobehavioral Cognitive Status Examination*) (Kiernan et al., 1987)	Standardized for use with neurologically impaired adults. Provides separate scores for orientation, attention, language, construction, memory, calculation, similarities, and judgment. Administration of the battery takes approximately 15–30 min. Scores are presented in profile of performance in each domain (average, mild, moderate, severe impairment). Osman et al. (1992) found *COGNISTAT* sensitive to cognitive effects of stroke but it did not discriminate right- and left-sided strokes. Katz et al. (1997) found significantly different scores for healthy elderly people, neurosurgical patients, and persons with dementia. Katz et al. (1996) suggested that the *LOTCA* and *COGNISTAT* are complementary.

of various measures of specific cognitive capacities and abilities, including a cognitive screen and three microbatteries. A cognitive screen takes less than 15 minutes to administer and provides the clinician with a general sense of a patient's cognitive status but little information about what specific areas may be impaired. A microbattery may take up to 45 minutes to administer and consists of a number of subtests, typically associated with an array of cognitive capacities and abilities.

Self-Reports and Informant Reports of Cognition

A final method for understanding the influence of cognitive changes on daily life is to ask the patient and/or significant other about their perceptions of the problem. Table 8-2 has examples of standardized instruments. As with other evaluation methods, occupational therapists interpret these self-reports in the context of the myriad of variables affecting cognition and self-awareness. As opposed to an interview or casual conversation, administration of a report questionnaire permits quantitative rating of observed changes (Mackinnon & Mulligan, 1998). Many instruments reported in the literature, including the *Subjective Memory Questionnaire*, were standardized on "normal" subjects (Bennett-Levy & Powell, 1980). In general, self-reports of memory have a weak association with actual performance memory

tests; also, they are influenced by depression and anxiety (Giovagnoli et al., 1997). Informant reports from significant others, coupled with an objective screen for cognition, were found to be more effective in identifying dementia patients than either method used alone (Mackinnon & Mulligan, 1998). Informed interpretation is critical. Mackinnon and Mulligan suggest that informant reports may also be influenced by noncognitive factors, such as affective state of the patient and informant, personality of the patient, and quality of the relationship between the informant and the patient.

Summary Review Questions

1. Analyze bill paying and grocery shopping in terms of the specific cognitive capacities and abilities required.
2. Compare the advantages and disadvantages of the two approaches to cognitive assessment described in this chapter.
3. Describe each variable that influences a person's ability to think. How would you expect these variables to affect cognitive assessment of an elderly illiterate patient? How would you expect these

TABLE 8-2
Informant Tools for Assessing Influence of Cognitive Changes on Daily Life

Test	Description
Patient Competency Rating Scale (Prigatano et al., 1986)	Designed for persons with traumatic brain injury.
	The patient is asked to answer 30 questions related to everyday tasks, rating how easy or difficult each is (can't do, very difficult, some difficulty, fairly easy, can do with ease). A person familiar with the patient's abilities (family member or rehabilitation staff) also rates the patient's proficiency with the 30 tasks. The magnitude of differences between self-ratings and that of relative or staff quantifies the patient's tendency to minimize deficits. Examples: "How much problem do I have preparing my own meals?" "How much problem do I have keeping appointments on time?" "How much problem do I have controlling my temper when something upsets me?" (Prigatano et al., 1986, pp. 148, 150).
Self-Awareness of Deficits Interview (Fleming et al., 1996)	Designed to obtain both qualitative and quantitative data on status of self-awareness.
	The patient is asked about self-awareness of deficits, self-awareness of functional limitations because of deficits, and ability to set realistic goals. The therapist assigns a score (0–3, with 0 representing full awareness) in each realm.
	To assign scores, the therapist must be familiar with the patient's level of functioning. Example of self-awareness of deficits questions: "Are you any different now compared to what you were like before your accident? In what way?" "Do you feel anything about you or your abilities has changed?" "Do people who know you well notice anything is different about you since the accident?" (Strong et al., 1996, p. 14).
Questionnaire of Memory Efficiency (Giovagnoli et al., 1997)	A 28-item self-report with questions pertaining to episodic memory, prospective memory, use of memory, and awareness of memory.
	Uses a 5-point Likert scale with scores ranging from 28–140 (higher points reflecting subjective impression of better memory)
	Giovagnoli et al. found that for persons with epilepsy, subjective perception of memory failure correlated with scores on measures of memory, anxiety, and depression.

variables to affect cognitive assessment of a college student?

4. Explain the occupational therapist's contribution to the rehabilitation team in the realm of cognitive assessment. Specifically, outline the ways in which occupational therapy complements the assessments of other professionals and the unique elements of occupational therapy.

Acknowledgment

I gratefully acknowledge Carolyn Baum, PhD, OTR/C, FAOTA for her helpful suggestions to an earlier draft of this chapter.

References

Abreu, B. C. (1999). Evaluation and intervention with memory and learning impairments. In C. Unsworth (Ed.), *Cognitive and Perceptual Dysfunction* (pp. 163–207). Philadelphia: Davis.

Adamovich, B. B., Henderson, J. A., & Auerbach, S. (1985). *Cognitive Rehabilitation of Closed Head Injured Patients*. San Diego: College-Hill.

American Occupational Therapy Association (1994). Uniform terminology for occupational therapy (3rd ed.). *American Journal of Occupational Therapy, 48*, 1047–1054.

Anderson, S. W., & Tranel, D. (1989). Awareness of disease states following cerebral infarction, dementia, head trauma: A standardized assessment. *Clinical Neuropsychologist, 3*, 327–339.

Arnadottir, A. (1990). *The Brain and Behavior: Assessing Cortical Dysfunction Through Activities of Daily Living*. St. Louis: Mosby.

Atkinson, R. C., & Shiffrin, R. M. (1971). The control of short-term memory. *Scientific American, 225*, 82–90.

Baddeley, A. (1990). *Human Memory: Theory and Practice*. Boston: Allyn & Bacon.

Bandura, A. (1986). *Social Foundations of Thought and Action: A Social Cognitive Theory*. Englewood Cliffs, NJ: Prentice-Hall.

Baum, C., & Edwards, D. F. (1993). Cognitive performance in senile dementia of the Alzheimer's type: The Kitchen Task Assessment. *American Journal of Occupational Therapy, 47*, 431–436.

Belenky, M. F., Clinchy, B. M., Goldberger, N. R., & Tarule, J. M. (1986). *Women's Ways of Knowing: The Development of Self, Voice, and Mind*. New York: Basic Books.

Bennett-Levy, J., & Powell, G. E. (1980). The Subjective Memory Questionnaire (SMQ). An investigation into the self-reporting of "real-life" memory skills. *British Journal of Social and Clinical Psychology, 19*, 177–188.

Bewick, K. C., Raymond, M. J., Malia, K. B., & Bennett, T. L. (1995). Metacognition as the ultimate executive: Techniques and tasks to facilitate executive functions. *NeuroRehabilitation, 5*, 367–375.

Bransford, J. D., & Stein, B. S. (1984). *The IDEAL Problem Solver: A Guide for Improving Thinking, Learning, and Creativity*. New York: Freeman.

Bruce, M. A. G. (1994). Cognitive rehabilitation: Intelligence, insight, and knowledge. In C. B. Royeen (Ed.), *AOTA Self-Study Series: Cognitive Rehabilitation*. Rockville, MD: American Occupational Therapy Association.

Capruso, D. X., & Levin, H. S. (1992). Cognitive impairment following closed head injury. *Neurologic Clinics, 10*, 879–893.

Cermak, S. A., Katz, N., McGuire, E., Greenbaum, S., Peralta, C., & Maser-Flanagan, V. (1995). Performance of Americans and Israe-lis with cerebrovascular accidents on the Loewenstein Occupational Therapy Cognitive Assessment (LOTCA). *American Journal of Occupational Therapy, 49*, 500–506.

Channon, S., & Green, P. S. S. (1999). Executive function in depression: The role of performance strategies in aiding depressed and non-depressed participants. *Journal of Neurology, Neurosurgery, and Psychiatry (London), 66*, 162-171.

Clark, F. A., Parham, D., Carlson, M. E., Frank, F., Jackson, J., Pierce, D., Wolfe, R. J., & Zemke, R. (1991). Occupational science: Academic innovation in the service of occupational therapy's future. *American Journal of Occupational Therapy, 45*, 300–310.

Crosson, B., Barco, P. P., Velozo, C. A., Bolesta, M. M., Cooper, P. V., Werts, D., & Brobeck, T. C. (1989). Awareness and compensation in postacute head injury rehabilitation. *Journal of Head Trauma Rehabilitation, 4*, 46–54.

Csikszentmihalyi, M. (1990). *Flow: The Psychology of Optimal Experience*. New York: Harper Collins.

Denburg, S. D., Carbotte, R. M., & Denburg, J. A. (1997). Cognition and mood in systemic lupus erythematosus. *Annals of the New York Academy of Sciences, 823*, 44–59.

Dietz, J. C., Tovar, V. S., & Beeman, C. (1990). The test of orientation for rehabilitation patients: Adults inter-rater reliability. *American Journal of Occupational Therapy, 44*, 783–790.

Diller, L. (1993). Introduction to cognitive rehabilitation. In C. Royeen (Ed.). *AOTA Self-Study Series: Cognitive Rehabilitation*. Rockville, MD: American Occupational Therapy Association.

Dougherty, P. M., & Radomski, M. V. (1993). *The Cognitive Rehabilitation Workbook*. Gaithersburg, MD: Aspen.

Eysenck, M. W., & Keane, M. T. (1990). *Cognitive Psychology: A Student's Handbook*. London: Lawrence Erlbaum.

Feuerstein, R. (1980). *Instrumental Enrichment: An Intervention Program for Cognitive Modifiability*. Baltimore: University Park.

Fleming, J. M., Strong, J., & Ashton, R. (1996). Self-awareness of deficits in adults with traumatic brain injury: How best to measure? *Brain Injury, 10*, 1–15.

Folstein, M. F., Folstein, S. E., & McHugh, P. R. (1975). "Mini-Mental State": A practical method for grading cognitive state of patients for the clinician. *Journal of Psychiatric Research, 12*, 189–198.

Foong, J., Rozewicz, L., Quaghebeur, G., Thompson, A. J., Miller, D. H., & Ron, M. A. (1998). Neuropsychological deficits in multiple sclerosis after acute relapse. *Journal of Neurology, Neurosurgery, and Psychiatry (London), 64*, 529–532.

Gardner, H. (1983). *Frames of Mind: The Theory of Multiple Intelligences*. New York: Basic Books.

Giovagnoli, A. R., Mascheroni, S., & Avanzini, G. (1997). Self-reporting of everyday memory in patients with epilepsy: Relation to neuropsychological, clinical, pathological and treatment factors. *Epilepsy Research, 28*, 119–128.

Glover, J. A., Ronning, R. R., & Bruning, R. H. (1990). *Cognitive Psychology for Teachers*. New York: Macmillan.

Goldstein, F. C., & Levin, H. S. (1987). Disorders of reasoning and problem-solving ability. In M. J. Meier, A. L. Benton, & L. Diller (Eds.), *Neuropsychological Rehabilitation* (pp. 327–354). New York: Guilford.

Hanks, R. A., Rapport, L. J., Millis, S. R., & Deshpande, S. A. (1999). Measures of executive functioning as predictors of functional ability and social integration in a rehabilitation sample. *Archives of Physical Medicine and Rehabilitation, 80*, 1030–1037.

Hajek, V. E., Gagnon, S., & Ruderman, J. E. (1997). Cognitive and functional assessments of stroke patients: An analysis of their relation. *Archives of Physical Medicine and Rehabilitation, 78*, 1331–1337.

Hochstenbach, J., Mulder, T., van Limbeek, J., Donders, R., & Schoonderwaldt, H. (1998). Cognitive decline following stroke: A comprehensive study of cognitive decline following stroke. *Journal of Clinical and Experimental Neuropsychology, 20*, 503–517.

Jackson, W. T., Novack, T. A., & Dowler, R. N. (1998). Effective serial measurement of cognitive orientation in rehabilitation: The Orientation Log. *Archives of Physical Medicine and Rehabilitation, 79*, 718–720.

Katz, N., Itzkovich, M., Averbuch, S., & Elazar, B. (1989). Loewenstein Occupational Therapy Cognitive Assessment (LOTCA) battery for brain-injured patients: Reliability and validity. *American Journal of Occupational Therapy, 43*, 184–192.

Katz, N., Elazar, B., & Itzkovich, M. (1996). Validity of the Neurobehavioral Cognitive Status Examination (COGNISTAT) in assessing patients post CVA and healthy elderly in Israel. *Israel Journal of Occupational Therapy, 5*, E185–E198.

Katz, N., Hartman-Maeir, A., Weiss, P., & Armon, N. (1997). Comparison of cognitive status profiles of healthy elderly persons with dementia and neurosurgical patients using the neurobehavioral cognitive status examination. *NeuroRehabilitation, 9*, 179–186.

Kiernan, R. J., Mueller, J., Langston, J. W., & Van Dyke, C. (1987). The Neurobehavioral Cognitive Status Examination: A brief but differentiated approach to cognitive assessment. *Annals of Internal Medicine, 107*, 481–485.

Levin, H. S., O'Donnell, V. M., & Grossman, R. G. (1979). The Galveston Orientation and Amnesia Test. *Journal of Nervous and Mental Disease, 167*, 675–684.

Lezak, M. D. (1995). *Neuropsychological Assessment* (3rd ed.). New York: Oxford University.

Mackinnon, A., & Mulligan, R. (1998). Combining cognitive testing and informant report to increase accuracy in screening for dementia. *American Journal of Psychiatry, 155*, 1529–1535.

MacNeill, S. E., & Lichtenberg, P. A. (1997). Home alone: The role of cognition in return to independent living. *Archives of Physical Medicine and Rehabilitation, 78*, 755–758.

Makatura, T. J., Lam, C. S., Leahy, B. J., Castillo, M. T., & Kalpakjian, C. Z. (1999). Standardized memory tests and the appraisal of everyday memory. *Brain Injury, 13*, 355–367.

Mazaux, J. M., Masson, F., Levin, H. S., Alaoui, P., Maurette, P., & Barat, M. (1997). Long-term neuropsychological outcome and loss of social autonomy after traumatic brain injury. *Archives of Physical Medicine and Rehabilitation, 78*, 1316–1320.

Mayer, R. E. (1992). *Thinking, Problem Solving, Cognition.* New York: Freeman.

Miller, G. A. (1956). The magical number seven, plus or minus two: some limits on our capacity for processing information. *Psychological Review, 63*, 81–97.

Mosey, A. C. (1993). Working taxonomies. In C. Royeen (Ed.), *AOTA Self Study Series: Cognitive Rehabilitation* (pp. 23–35). Rockville, MD: American Occupational Therapy Association, Inc.

Moyers, P. A. (1999). The guide to occupational therapy practice. *American Journal of Occupational Therapy, 53*, 247–322.

Nadeau, B., & Buckheit, C. (1995). Work simulation as a diagnostic tool in the rehabilitation setting. *Occupational Therapy in Health Care, 9*, 37–44.

Neistadt, M. E. (1992). The Rabideau Kitchen Evaluation—Revised: An assessment of meal preparation skill. *Occupational Therapy Journal of Research, 12*, 242–253.

Neistadt, M. E. (1994). A meal preparation treatment protocol for adults with brain injury. *American Journal of Occupational Therapy, 48*, 431–438.

Osmon, D. C., Smet, I. C., Winegarden, B., & Gandhavadi, B. (1992). Neurobehavioral Cognitive Status Examination: Its use with unilateral stroke patients in a rehabilitation setting. *Archives of Physical Medicine and Rehabilitation, 73*, 414–418.

Perkins, D. (1995*). Outsmarting IQ.* New York: Free Press.

Poutiainen, E., Elovaara, I., Raininko, R., Vilkki, J., Lahdevirta, J., & Iivanainen, M. (1996). Cognitive decline in patients with symptomatic HIV-1 infection: No decline in asymptomatic infection. *Acta Neurologica Scandinavica, 93*, 421–427.

Prigatano, G. P., Fordyce, D. J., Zeiner, H. K., Rouche, J. R., Pepping, M., & Wood, B. C. (1986). *Neuropsychological Rehabilitation After Brain Injury.* Baltimore: John Hopkins University.

Prigatano, G. P., & Schacter, D. L. (1991). *Awareness of Deficit After Brain Injury: Clinical and Theoretical Issues.* New York: Oxford University.

Prigatano, G. P., Ogano, M., & Amakusa, B. (1997). A cross-cultural study on impaired self-awareness in Japanese patients with brain dysfunction. *Neuropsychiatry, Neuropsychology, and Behavioral Neurology, 10*, 135–143.

Radomski, M. V. (1998). Problem-solving deficits: Using a multidimensional definition to select a treatment approach. *Physical Disabilities Special Interest Section Quarterly, 21*, 1–4.

Rustad, R. A., DeGroot, T. L., Jungkunz, M. L., Freeberg, K. S., Borowick, L. G., & Wanttie, A. M. (1993). *The Cognitive Assessment of Minnesota.* Tucson: Therapy Skill Builders.

Sandstrom, R., & Mokler, P. J. (1999). Cognitive function and key rehabilitation outcomes: Understanding the structure of human disability after sever motor stroke. *Journal of Rehabilitation Outcomes, 3*, 22–26.

Schacter, D. L (1996). *Searching for Memory: The Brain, the Mind, and the Past.* New York: Basic Books.

Schagen, S. B., van Dam, F. S. A. M., Muller, M. J., Boogerd, W., Lindeboom, J., & Bruning, P. F. (1999). Cognitive deficits after postoperative adjuvant chemotherapy for breast carcinoma. *Cancer, 85*, 640–650.

Scherzer, B. P., Charbonneau, S., Solomon, C. R., & Lepore, F. (1993). Abstract thinking following severe traumatic brain injury. *Brain Injury, 7*, 411–423.

Seltzer, B., Vasterling, J. J., Yoder, J., Thompson, K. A. (1997). Awareness of deficit in Alzheimer's disease: Relation to caregiver burden. *The Gerontologist, 37*, 20–24.

Small, S. A., Stern, Y., Tang, M., Mayeux, R. (1999). Selective decline in memory function among healthy elderly. *Neurology, 52*, 1392–1396.

Sohlberg, M. M., & Mateer, C. A. (1989). *Introduction to Cognitive Rehabilitation Theory and Practice.* New York: Guilford.

Sternberg, R. J. (1990). *Metaphors of Mind: Conceptions of the Nature of Intelligence.* New York: Cambridge University.

Suhr, J. A. & Grace, J. (1999). Brief cognitive screening of right hemisphere stroke: Relation to functional outcome. *Archives of Physical Medicine and Rehabilitation, 80*, 773–776.

Teng, E. L., & Chui, H. (1987). The Modified Mini-Mental State (3MS) Examination. *Journal of Clinical Psychiatry, 48*, 314–318.

Toglia, J. P. (1989). Approaches to cognitive assessment of the brain-injured adult. *Occupational Therapy Practice, 1*, 36–55.

Toglia, J. P. (1993). *The Contextual Memory Test.* Tucson: Therapy Skill Builders.

Toglia, J. P. (1994). *Dynamic Assessment of Categorization Skills: The Toglia Category Assessment.* Pequannock, NJ: Maddak.

Toglia, J. P. (1998). A dynamic interactional model to cognitive rehabilitation. In N. Katz (Ed.), *Cognition and Occupation In Rehabilitation.* Bethesda, MD: American Occupational Therapy Association.

Wagner, R. K. (1991). Managerial problem solving. In R. J. Sternberg & P.A. Frensch (Eds.), *Complex Problem Solving: Principles and Mechanisms* (pp. 159—183). Hillsdale, NJ: Lawrence Erlbaum.

Watson, Y. I., Arfken, C. L., & Birge, S. J. (1993). Clock completion: An objective screening test for dementia. *Journal of the American Geriatric Society, 41*, 1235–1240.

Wilson, B. A., Cockburn, J., & Baddeley, A. (1985). *The Rivermead Behavioral Memory Test.* Reading, UK: Thames Valley Test; Gaylord, MI: National Rehabilitation Services.

9

Assessing Context: Personal, Social, and Cultural

Mary Vining Radomski

LEARNING OBJECTIVES

After studying this chapter, the reader will begin to do the following:

1. Describe the components of personal, social, and cultural context that influence occupational therapy assessment and guide treatment planning.
2. Employ methods for quantifying the influence of various contextual factors on performance.
3. Recognize the role of contextual factors in the development of conditional reasoning in clinical practice.
4. Examine his or her own contextual fabric—the personal, social, and cultural factors that shape the therapist's everyday experiences.

Much as a phrase, punch line, or couplet can be understood only in the larger **context** of a story, joke, or poem, a patient's performance during occupational therapy assessment can be interpreted only in light of the broader context of his or her life and background. For example, lack of eye contact during an initial interview can easily be misinterpreted as lack of interest or motivation unless the therapist appreciates the contribution of cultural background: that avoiding eye contact is a way of showing respect in some cultures, including the Vietnamese culture (Farrales, 1996). Difficulty selecting clothing during a dressing assessment may be erroneously attributed to a patient's poor decision-making skills unless the therapist appreciates the contribution of social role experiences, that for 50 years, the patient's wife set out his clothing each morning.

GLOSSARY

Context—The whole situation, background, or environment that is relevant to a particular event or personality (Webster's New World Dictionary, 1994).

Culture—The norms, values, and behavior patterns that serve as guidelines for people's interactions with others and their environments (Krefting, 1991).

Cultural context—Stable and dynamic norms, values, and behaviors associated with the community or societal environments in which occupational functioning occurs.

Ethnicity—Membership by virtue solely of one's birth in a racial, religious, national, or linguistic group (McGruder, 1998). In and of itself, ethnicity does not predict cultural identity.

Personal context—A person's internal environment, derived from stable and dynamic factors such as sex, age, mood, cultural identity.

Social context—The social environment consisting of stable and dynamic factors such as premorbid roles, social network, support resources.

Social network—An interactive web of people who provide each other with helpfulness and protection. Social networks typically vary in terms of reciprocity, complexity, intensity, and density (Heaney & Israel, 1997).

Social support—The aid and assistance (emotional, instrumental, information, appraisal) exchanged through a social network (Heaney & Israel, 1997).

Spirituality—Beliefs and practices that give a person transcendent meaning in life (Puchalski, 1996).

The term *context* refers to the whole situation, background, or environment that is relevant to a particular event or personality; it has its roots in the Latin word *contexere*, to weave together (Webster's New World Dictionary, 1994). Occupational therapists appreciate that a person's function at any moment is shaped by a tapestry of contextual factors, not solely his or her capacities, acquired skills, and abilities. Without deliberate attention to these personal, social, cultural, and physical mediators of performance, therapists may misunderstand what they observe during assessment and risk assigning erroneous labels of dysfunction.

This chapter describes the personal, social, and cultural contextual factors that help or hinder performance during occupational therapy assessment. (Chapter 10 focuses on assessing contextual factors associated with the built or physical environment.) After summarizing the role of context in human functioning, this chapter discusses specific examples of personal, social, and cultural context in terms of their potential for influencing occupational therapy assessment and treatment. Using these examples, readers are encouraged to reflect on other contextual factors not discussed herein. The role of context in occupational function cannot be exhaustively explored in one chapter; whole texts and careers have been devoted to each of these complex constructs. This overview, however, has one superordinate aim: to inspire therapists to try to interpret patients' performance in the broader context of their background, changing circumstances, and envisioned futures.

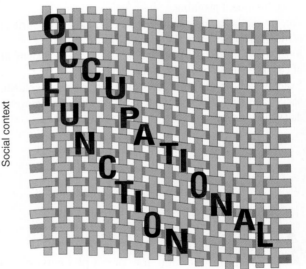

Figure 9-1 Interwoven tapestry of personal, social, cultural, and physical contextual factors.

Context and Occupational Function

Occupational function is always embedded in context, with physical, cultural, social, and personal factors shaping its form (Nelson, 1988). Figure 9-1 depicts the interweaving of personal, social, cultural, and physical context that creates the parameters of a given occupational experience. Consider how minor changes in any dimension change the tapestry: a middle-aged homemaker preparing eggs and toast for her children before they leave for school versus a middle-aged homemaker preparing the same breakfast for her therapist as part of a rehabilitation assessment.

The important role of context in occupational function is described by a number of models and frameworks from occupational therapy, rehabilitation, and health fields. Each of the models or frameworks summarized in Table 9-1 emphasizes the dynamic relationship between a person, his or her cultural, social, and physical contexts and the continuum of function to disability relative to chosen roles and tasks. In fact, two of these models downplay the contribution of physical impairments and bodily dysfunctions and emphasize the contribution of contextual factors to function and disability in society (Institute of Medicine, 1997; World Health Organization [WHO], 1999).

The aforementioned models universally elevate the role of context in the explanation of human functioning and disablement but use slightly different terminology. In this chapter, contextual factors are presumed to be peripheral or unrelated to patients' primary diagnoses or disabling conditions (WHO, 1999) but central to the broad realms within which people carry out their lives.

► **Personal context** is an individual's internal environment derived from his or her gender, values, beliefs, cultural background, or state of mind.
► **Social context** refers to factors in the human environment (roles, resources, and structure) that enable or deter the person's occupational function.
► **Cultural context** is the norms, values, and behaviors related to the community or society in which the occupational function occurs.

The convenience of describing personal, social, and cultural contextual factors as separate and distinct

---

TABLE 9-1

Models and Frameworks That Specifically Include Context As an Element in Human Function

Models and Frameworks	Synopsis of Role of Context in Occupation and/or Human Function
Ecology of Human Performance (Dunn et al., 1994)	The interaction between a person and the environment affects behavior and performance. Human performance can be understood only through the lens of context, which includes temporal (age, development, health status), physical, cultural, and social features that are external to a person. In essence, the interrelations between person and context determine which tasks fall within the individual's performance range.
Person–Environment–Occupation Model of Occupational Performance (Law et al., 1996)	Occupational function is the result of the transactive relations "between people, their occupations and roles, and the environments in which they live, work, and play" (p. 9). This model emphasizes the interdependence of person and environment (defined as contexts and situations outside the individual, such as cultural, socioeconomic, institutional, and social considerations). It also recognizes the temporal, or changing, nature of person, environment, occupational characteristics, and their interrelationships.
Enabling–Disabling Process (Institute of Medicine, 1997)	The relationships between a person's physical conditions and the environment (rather than levels of disease, impairment, or functional limitations) determines the ability to function. Environment is defined broadly to include the physical or built environment, psychological and social environments (including influences of culture, family, community, and political climate) and intrapersonal environment (such as one's thoughts, beliefs, and expectations).
Occupational Therapy Intervention Process Model (Fisher, 1998)	Occupational performance is a "transaction between the person and the environment as he or she enacts a task" (p. 514). Therapists must be aware of the client's performance context (composed of temporal, environmental, cultural, societal, social, role, motivational, capacity, and task dimensions) to understand, evaluate, and interpret a person's occupational performance.
ICIDH-2 (WHO, 1999)	"Functioning and disability are conceived as a dynamic interaction between health conditions and contextual factors" (p. 12). Context includes personal and environmental factors. Personal factors are internal influences of functioning that are not part of a health condition or functional state such as gender, age, social background, character, and coping styles. Environmental factors, external influences on functioning, include features of the physical, social, attitudinal world.

Context	Stable ← ———————————————————————————————— → Dynamic		
Personal (influence of the individual's internal variables on occupational function)	• Age*		
	• Gender identity		
		• Values and preferences	
		• Spirituality and meaning systems*	
	• Coping style (including substance use)*		
		• Comorbidities	
	• Cultural identity*		
	• Educational background (See Box 9-1 for assessing literacy)*		
			• Fatigue
			• Pain*
			• Mood*
		• Place in adaptation continuum	
Social (influence of individual's social structure and experience on occupational function)	• Socioeconomic status/social class		
	• Social network (nature and extent)*		
	• Social role expectations (See Law, Chapter 3)		
		• Significant others' adjustment to disability*	
		• Norms, values, behaviors of patient–therapist social interactions*	
Cultural (influence of norms, values, behaviors expected of the individuals living in a particular country or community)	• Norms, values, behavior of broader community*		

* These factors are discussed in this chapter

Figure 9-2 Examples of interrelated personal, social, and cultural contextual factors.

entities belies their complexity, interrelatedness, and interactive influences (Fig. 9-2). Krefting (1991) described the pervasive influence of **culture** on community, families (norms, values, and behaviors of a familial social group), and individuals (such as distinc-tive food preferences, humor, definition of personal space—in this chapter considered to be a part of personal context). Likewise, personal context may influence social and cultural context. For example, a person's spiritual beliefs often shape his or her social network, preferred roles, and definitions of acceptable behavior.

Personal, social, and cultural contextual factors can be examined on a continuum of highly stable to highly dynamic. The relatively stable factors, such as age, gender identity, and premorbid coping style tend to pervade most tasks and situations and are not easily changed in therapy. For example, a patient's educational background may affect how the therapist provides home instruction but is unlikely to be a focus of intervention (Box 9-1). On the other hand, the more dynamic contextual factors are transient and situational, more responsive to environment, task, and therapy than stable contextual factors. The headache that interferes with an individual's concentration today will likely be better tomorrow. The spouse's ability to use resources and encourage his or her loved one's independence change as both patient and spouse adapt to the sequelae of stroke.

Importance of Personal, Social, and Cultural Context to Assessment

Personal, social, and cultural context influence occupational therapy assessment and treatment in at least three ways. First, contextual factors mediate (help or hinder) performance on traditional occupational therapy assessments, skewing the results and muddying their interpretation. For example, Mr. J.'s difficulty attending to instructions during a homemaking assessment might be interpreted as solely a cognitive impairment related to his right cerebrovascular accident if the therapist did not know he was awake much of the previous night as nurses addressed his roommate's deteriorating medical condition. Second, contextual factors may be facilitators or barriers to function and therefore targets of occupational therapy intervention. Consider the influence of social context on occupational therapy goals. Despite adequate strength and technical skills, Mrs. S. remains dependent in lower extremity dressing after her total hip replacement because her husband, fearful that she may overexert, insists on assisting with dressing. The home health therapist, who brings his or her own biases regarding the goal of independence, ultimately collaborates with Mr. and Mrs. S. regarding their expectations of therapy. Should they choose to work toward complete independence in self-care, the therapist helps Mr. S. become comfortable with Mrs. S. dressing herself and helps Mrs. S. improve her skills. Finally, throughout the assessment, occupational therapists trawl for glimpses of what patients find meaningful—lures to hook them into therapy. Each dimension of context holds such possibilities as goals are set and treatment is planned.

Conditional Reasoning

Awareness of interwoven contextual factors is a foundation for what Mattingly and Fleming (1994) describe as conditional reasoning: viewing the patient as a complex composite of premorbid characteristics and preferences, condition-specific limitations, and future potentialities.

"Therapists try to understand what is meaningful to the patients, and to their perceptions of themselves and others in the physical and social contexts in which they experience their lives. In order to do this therapists need an ability to imagine the clients, both as they were before the illness, and as they could be in the future. They also need to be able to enlist the patients in imagining a possible future for themselves" (Mattingly & Fleming, 1994, p. 197).

Conditional reasoning enables the therapist to appreciate the wholeness of the patient and his or her situation. While it is more often employed by experienced therapists than novices (Mattingly & Fleming), one may presume that desire to learn may expedite the acquisition of this mind-set.

Looking in the Mirror: Therapist as Contextually Influenced Being

Appreciation for the influence of personal, social, and cultural context requires that therapists acquire a complex combination of knowledge, attitudes, and skills. The goal is to shift from viewing how a patient can fit into the therapist's world to examining how the therapist can understand and fit into the patient's world (St. Clair & McKenry, 1999). To accomplish this shift, therapists must acknowledge and inventory the personal, social, and cultural factors that influence their own function. As I become aware of my own beliefs and biases, social background, and culturally based expectations, I will be able to appreciate their influence on collaborations with patients and coworkers.

In summary, clinicians need not obsess about correctly labeling or pigeonholing each and every contextual factor. Rather, therapists aim to tease out various contributions to patients' performance during assessment so as to inform treatment planning by asking whether this patient's present performance is influenced by the following:

▶ Personal, social, or cultural factors that obscure identification of strengths or weaknesses in occupational function
▶ Longstanding personal, social, or cultural factors that are unlikely to change as a result of therapy

BOX 9-1
PROCEDURES FOR PRACTICE

Assessing Literacy

Occupational therapists use written materials in assessment and treatment. Patients with low literacy may try to hide their difficulties with reading, compromising the assessment and the value of written home instructions (Parikh et al., 1996). Use of a reading screen allows the clinician to identify patients who need simplified, audiotaped, or pictorial education materials for patients.

The *Rapid Estimate of Adult Literacy in Medicine* (*REALM*) (Murphy et al., 1993) is a reading recognition test that takes 2 to 3 minutes to administer and score. It contains three columns of health-related words of increasing difficulty, 66 words in all. The patient is asked to start at the top of list 1 and read the words aloud until he or she completes the three lists or is unable to read additional words. The patient is allowed 5 seconds to pronounce each word. The clinician takes note of all words pronounced correctly; this number becomes the raw score that is converted to grade range estimates. Murphy et al. suggested that patients who score below the 9th grade level need adapted education materials.

Rapid Estimate of Adult Literacy in Medicine (REALM)©

Reading level _____

Patient name/subject # _____ Date of birth _____ Grade completed _____

Date _____ Clinic _____ Examiner _____

List 1		List 2		List 3	
fat	_____	fatigue	_____	allergic	_____
flu	_____	pelvic	_____	menstrual	_____
pill	_____	jaundice	_____	testicle	_____
dose	_____	infection	_____	colitis	_____
eye	_____	exercise	_____	emergency	_____
stress	_____	behavior	_____	medication	_____
smear	_____	prescription	_____	occupation	_____
nerves	_____	notify	_____	sexually	_____
germs	_____	gallbladder	_____	alcoholism	_____
meals	_____	calories	_____	irritation	_____
disease	_____	depression	_____	constipation	_____
cancer	_____	miscarriage	_____	gonorrhea	_____
caffeine	_____	pregnancy	_____	inflammatory	_____
attack	_____	arthritis	_____	diabetes	_____
kidney	_____	nutrition	_____	hepatitis	_____
hormones	_____	menopause	_____	antibiotics	_____
herpes	_____	appendix	_____	diagnosis	_____
seizure	_____	abnormal	_____	potassium	_____
bowel	_____	syphilis	_____	anemia	_____
asthma	_____	hemorrhoids	_____	obesity	_____
rectal	_____	nausea	_____	osteoporosis	_____
incest	_____	directed	_____	impetigo	_____

Score

List 1 _____
List 2 _____
List 3 _____
Raw
score _____

Note: While the set of words used in REALM is copyrighted, its authors are placing the test in the public domain to encourage its use by physicians and reading specialists. Plastic laminated copies of the word list and examiner copies with instructions are available from Peggy Murphy, Department of Internal Medicine, LSUMC-S, PO Box 33932, Shreveport, LA 71130-3932, USA. Telephone: (318) 674-5813.

(continued)

BOX 9-1
PROCEDURES FOR PRACTICE

Assessing Literacy (Continued)

REALM grade estimate	
Raw Score	Estimated Grade Range and Practical Meaning
0-18	**Third grade and below** These patients may not be able to read most educational materials and probably cannot even understand simple prescription labels. Repeated oral instructions will be needed to enhance compliance; the doctor cannot simply write a prescription or give standard levels of instruction and expect compliance. Materials, including simple video and audio tapes, may be helpful if a health care worker is present during their use and is available to answer questions. Repeated oral instructions will be the key to establishing long-term compliance.
19-44	**Fourth to sixth grade** Tremendous potential for improvement exists in this group. They should respond well to direct instruction by health care providers and should be able to read and comprehend materials written on elementary school levels. Appropriately written materials may still require one-on-one counseling for adequate understanding.
45-60	**Seventh to eighth grade** These patients will certainly benefit from appropriately written materials, but material (both oral and written) should not be too simple (e.g., first grade) or too complex. Material written for a fourth- to sixth-grade level may be appropriate.
61-66	**Ninth grade and above** These readers can understand much high school level material presented to them; therefore, current educational brochures may be effective. These individuals should also be able to converse with their physicians about matters of lifestyle.

▶ Personal, social, or cultural factors that are transient or situational; factors that may be affected by occupational therapy intervention

▶ The therapist's personal, social, or cultural contextual factors

Personal Context

"Life is suddenly reduced to a one dimension picture, known as physical function, and continually referred to as 'outcome.' The typical outcome process ignores . . . emotional and interpersonal needs and skills. Within those parameters lies the answer to true recovery . . . I refuse to have an 'outcome.' I do have a *life!*"
(Cannon, 1994, p. 3)

Personal context refers to the intrapersonal environment that shapes an individual's experience. These factors play a role in determining the patient's unique response to the onset of illness or impairment and contribute to the patient's ability to adapt (National Center for Medical Rehabilitation and Research, 1993). Some aspects of a person's internal environment, such as age and longstanding beliefs, are stable; others, such as pain, mood, and adaptation to illness or injury (see Chapter 35), may be constantly in flux.

Personal Demographics: Age

A person's age influences his or her occupational functioning in three primary ways: (1) age-related changes in capacities and abilities; (2) developmental shifts in goals, values, and priorities; and (3) the individual's generation-based worldview.

Table 9-2 summarizes typical changes in capacities and abilities associated with normal aging. In tandem with physiological changes in capacities, Royeen (1995) hypothesized that people undergo "occupational shifts" (p. 11) during the life cycle that lead to major changes in patterns of activity. She posited that early adulthood is characterized by establishing worker roles while realigning social roles to adjust to marriage and parenthood. In middle adulthood, people maintain work and leisure roles but may undergo sudden occupational shifts related to caregiving roles of parents, children, and grandchildren. During maturity (45 years to retirement), people continue their work and leisure roles, but occupational shifts arise from death of family members, loss of provider status, and adjustments in life goals. Persons in old age must adjust to changes in role performance commensurate with deterioration of physical and mental capacities.

TABLE 9-2
Age-Related Changes in Physical and Cognitive Capacities and Abilities

Age Group	Physical Development	Cognitive Development
20s	▶ Fully developed body shape and proportions except weight and body mass, which fluctuate throughout life ▶ Peak muscle strength ▶ Fully mature reproductive systems, with both sexes subject to involuntary cyclic alterations in sex hormone production	▶ Peak brain cell development, although the final number of neurons and supportive cells is determined by the end of the first year of life ▶ Memory capacity peaks with the brain's greatest mass
30s and 40s	▶ Gradual slowing of body functions (dependent on diet, exercise, stress, genetic predisposition, any disease) ▶ Without regular exercise, gradual loss of muscle mass and strength and bone mass and density ▶ Decreasing elasticity in cardiorespiratory system resulting in gradually decreasing respiratory capacity and increasing blood pressure ▶ Beginnings of hearing loss (first limited to high pitches) ▶ Beginnings of presbyopia, which necessitates reading glasses or bifocals	▶ Gradual shrinkage of brain cells around age 30, but because of the vast number of unused brain cells, these changes do not affect function ▶ Continued gradual brain shrinkage but increasing life experiences result in high mental acumen
50s and 60s	▶ Physical changes continue, faster and to a greater extent ▶ Fewer calories are required, necessitating changes in intake and/or activities to maintain weight ▶ Changes in amounts and patterns of hormone production affecting metabolism, energy, sexuality, reproduction	▶ Continued brain shrinkage offset by reservoir of life experience, wisdom, judgment
70s and older	▶ Loss of vestibular function in inner ears resulting in decreased balance ▶ Steady deterioration of vision and hearing ▶ Loss of cartilage and connective tissue leading to decreased range of motion, pain, postural changes ▶ Reduced appetite due to inactive taste buds and changes in digestion ▶ Changes in metabolism making adaptation to changing temperatures more difficult	▶ Decreasing memory capacity ▶ Decreasing abilities in abstract reasoning and novel problem solving ▶ Enriched perspectives based on lifelong learning and integrated experiences

Adapted with permission from Freiberg, K. L. (1987). *Human Development: A Life-Span Approach* (3rd ed.). Boston: Jones & Bartlett.

Finally, Strauss and Howe (1991) suggested that a person's age location in history influences his or her personality and beliefs. They characterized the attributes of four contemporary generational groups in the United States:

▶ G. I. elders (born 1901–1924) strive for public harmony and cooperative social discipline and subscribe to a philosophy that optimism and hard work guarantee goal achievement.
▶ Silent midlifers (born 1925–1942) appreciate a variety of mind-sets, virtues, and flaws and subscribe to a philosophy that promotes compromise and consensus as means to happy endings.
▶ Boomer adults (born 1943–1960) appreciate their own opinions and perspectives as morally correct

and subscribe to a philosophy suggesting that adherence to moral ideals leads to satisfying experience.
▶ 13ER youths (born 1961–1981) appreciate the need for personal determinism and subscribe to a philosophy that elevates the acquisition of money to personal survival in response to perceived uncertainties in their economic future.

Of course, generalizations about patterns of aging may or may not apply to specific individuals. Human function over time is influenced by an array of factors, such as lifetime habits related to diet and exercise, stress, genetic predispositions, and sociocultural background (Freiberg, 1987). However, catastrophic loss of function, as with illness or disability, takes place against a backdrop of other age-related changes, developmental tasks, and worldviews. For example, a person's adaptation to a spinal cord injury may occur as he or she is also adapting to a new marriage or career. An elderly patient's efforts to relearn motor skills and standing balance may be complicated by declines in capacities associated with age and beliefs that if a person works hard enough, he or she will always achieve goals.

Coping Strategies and Beliefs

Premorbid coping styles and long-term spiritual beliefs and meaning systems influence peoples' reactions to catastrophic injury and chronic illness.

Coping Style

The ways that people typically face stressful circumstances affect whether they seek health-related services and the extent to which they follow professionals' advice (Lerman & Glanz, 1997). Coping styles are relatively stable characteristics of a person and are thought to mediate the effects of stress on function (Lerman & Glanz, 1997). (Box 9-2 describes assessment of substance use, a maladaptive coping style.)

Lerman and Glanz (1997) summarized two aspects of coping. Consider how each of them contributes to or derails occupational therapy assessment and treatment when they are part of the patient or therapist's longstanding coping style.

► Optimism is the tendency to have positive rather than negative expectations for outcomes. Optimism is associated with relatively few physical symptoms during stress, and it predicts psychological adjustment. Optimists tend to use active coping strategies, such as planning, problem solving, and acceptance rather than avoidance.

► Locus of control is a general belief about one's ability to control relevant life circumstances and events. People with an internal locus of control are likely to take responsibility for change, while those with an external locus of control tend to expect other people or factors ultimately to determine a particular outcome. The assumption that one can affect one's circumstances leads to active coping and goal-directed activity that influence outcome.

Spirituality

Puchalski (1996) defines **spirituality** as beliefs and practices that give a person transcendent meaning in life. These beliefs may be expressed as a religious faith or directed toward nature, family, or community. According to Cox and Waller (1991), spirituality helps people make sense of confusion and find meaning in daily living. It reflects a person's overriding system of meaning that influences use of time, choice of actions, and

perceptions of purpose. As such, spirituality is central to a person's occupational function (Christiansen, 1997). In a survey of 270 registered occupational therapists in the United States, 84% of the respondents viewed spirituality as an important dimension of health and rehabilitation, but fewer than 40% of the respondents thought their patients' spiritual needs were within their scope of practice (Engquist et al., 1997).

The onset of illness, ongoing disability, and suffering force patient and therapist alike to confront their own spirituality and meaning systems. Based on their study of 216 inpatients with a variety of illnesses and disabilities, Riley et al. (1998) suggested three classes of spiritual well-being. Persons in the religious cluster derived satisfaction from a relationship with God or a higher

BOX 9-2
PROCEDURES FOR PRACTICE

Assessing Possible Substance Abuse

Alcohol use is a risk factor for spinal cord and brain injury (Kolakowsky-Hayner et al., 1999). Kolakowsky-Hayner et al. found alarmingly high rates of preinjury heavy drinking among patients who were treated in a level I trauma center and subsequently in rehabilitation (57% of patients admitted with spinal cord injury, 42% of patients admitted with traumatic brain injury). Preinjury substance abuse has been associated with worse rehabilitation outcomes (Kelly et al., 1997; Moyers & Stoffel, 1999) and predicts postinjury substance abuse (Kolakowsky-Hayner et al.). Despite the implications for rehabilitation, health care providers are often reluctant to ask patients about substance use because of time constraints, lack of knowledge, and reluctance to intervene (Taj et al., 1998).

An occupational therapist who suspects that a patient is a substance abuser has an ethical obligation (Moyers & Stoffel) to perform a screening test and, if indicated, refer the patient for further assessment and intervention. Here are two screening methods.

1. Ask a pointed question. Taj et al. were able to identify 74% of at-risk or problem drinkers when physicians incorporated a simple question into their routine examinations ("On any single occasion during the past 3 months, have you had more than 5 drinks containing alcohol?"). They presented the alcohol screening question between two other general health questions ("In the past 3 months, have you used tobacco?" and "Do you regularly wear your seat belt when riding in the car?," p. 329).
2. Use a mnemonic when interviewing patients about suspected alcohol abuse. The *CAGE Questionnaire* (Ewing, 1984) asks 4 questions related to patients' perceptions of need to **cut** down, **annoyance** with criticism, **guilt** about drinking, and need for a drink as an **eye-opener** first thing in the morning. Soderstrom et al. (1997) found CAGE to be an efficient screening test to detect alcohol dependence of patients admitted to a trauma center.

power and tended to believe that they would be fine despite their illness or condition. They generally described their relationship with God as close, meaningful, and loving and had a more positive view of their future than other groups. People in the existential cluster derived satisfaction from a sense of purpose and their deep connection to others and the environment. This group reportedly had the highest levels of physical, social, emotional, and mental functioning. Finally, people in the nonspiritual cluster had significantly less social, physical, and emotional well-being than the other groups, and their sense of health and vitality was significantly poorer. Riley et al. suggested that knowledge of a patient's spiritual beliefs informs treatment planning and intervention and "is clearly too important a variable to be neglected in the rehabilitation process" (p. 263). Box 9-3 suggests ways to discuss coping, spiritual belief, and meaning systems with patients.

Cultural Background and Identity

Culture provides guidelines for peoples' interactions with others and their environments (Krefting,1991). Socialization teaches these guidelines for values, beliefs, and behavior patterns. Culture is not biologically inherited nor determined by geography or ethnicity (Krefting). **Ethnicity** is defined as "membership, conveyed by birth, in a racial, religious, national, or linguistic group" (McGruder, 1998, p. 55). While ethnicity may have implications in economic, social, and political realms, it contributes little to a therapist's appreciation of a patient's personal context. Because there is as much variation within ethnic groups as between them (McGruder), a person's ethnic background is not a reliable gauge of his or her cultural identity.

The influence of culture on a person's experience is hard to state precisely. While cultural rules are learned, they are also graded, flexible, task- and environment-

BOX 9-3
PROCEDURES FOR PRACTICE

Assessing Patients' Coping, Spiritual Beliefs, and Meaning Systems

People typically share personal information with those they trust. Therefore, to explore patients' beliefs and meaning systems, therapists invest in establishing therapeutic rapport (see Chapter 13). Without the rapport that comes with time and consistency of care providers, patients may perceive questions about their spirituality, for example, as intrusive or offensive. Therapists who are aware of their own coping strategies and belief systems will be best able to comfortably discuss these issues with their patients.

In general, discussions of these very personal and potentially sensitive matters begin at a superficial level and progress to deeper, more personal levels as dictated by the patient and therapist's comfort with each other and the subject matter. Here are examples of this progression.

► Ask the patient to provide an hour-by-hour account of a typical day prior to the injury or onset of illness (Radomski, 1995). How a person is used to spending his or her time richly defines his or her valued activities and priorities.
► Take a brief life history, asking the patient to give you an overview of his or her life course, including past goals and obstacles (Kleinman, 1988). People often use stories or narratives to make connections and meaning attributions between a series of life events (Mattingly, 1991).
► Ask the patient about his or her explanatory model of the illness or disability. Kleinman suggested that faced with illness, disability, or suffering, people attempt to construct models to explain the whys of their experiences. They make attributions about causation and outcome that are more likely to be based on personal beliefs and

culture than on facts or medical information. For example, patients may feel responsible for permanent impairments because they didn't try hard enough in rehabilitation to overcome them (Luborsky, 1997). If the person views onset of illness or disability as God's punishment for a past sin or mistake, he or she may not feel empowered to invest in rehabilitation efforts. Only as patients' explanatory models are acknowledged may they be negotiated with the therapist or health care team (Kleinman).

► Cox and Waller (1991, p. 86) suggested that clinicians ask patients about past experiences in which their coping skills were taxed:
1. When you're discouraged and feeling despondent, what keeps you going?
2. Where have you found strength in the past?
3. What have you done in the past when you've lost someone or something important?
4. What do you think the message in this is for you?
► Puchalski (1996) recommended an acronym for aspects of a spiritual assessment (F, Faith; I, Importance and influence; C, Community; A, Address).
F. What things do you believe in that give meaning to your life?
I. How have your beliefs influenced your behavior during this illness? What roles do your beliefs play in regaining your health?
C. Are you a part of a spiritual or religious community? Is this a support to you and how?
A. How would you like me, your health care provider, to address these issues in your health care?

specific, and often self-selected. For example, the degree to which immigrants have assimilated the customs and patterns of behavior of their new country or region is determined by how recently they emigrated, the primary language spoken at home, and the amount of contact with their homeland (Krefting, 1991). People adopt the culture of specific subgroups and environments; the expectations for behavior of a clinician in an occupational therapy clinic are different from expectations for brokers working at the New York Stock Exchange. The dynamic influence of culture on human experience requires that clinicians resist attempts to characterize or stereotype patients based on ethnic or geographical background. Rather, occupational therapists attempt to recognize and then step outside of their own cultural backgrounds and biases to appreciate and accept the culturally based customs, values, and beliefs of each patient.

Lipson (1996) characterized culturally competent care as sensitive to "issues related to culture, race, gender, sexual orientation, social class, and economic situation" (p. 1). Culturally competent occupational therapists address the contribution of culture to occupational function in two ways: (1) seeking information about the cultural identity of each patient (Box 9-4); and (2) selecting and interpreting performance on standardized tests based on this knowledge.

Many occupational therapy evaluation tools are based on norms developed for a white middle-class population (Krefting, 1991; Paul, 1995). Culturally competent clinicians assess the cultural validity of their standardized assessment tools (Krefting) and select criterion-referenced and norm-referenced tests appropriate for the person's background (Paul). Paul described the challenges of devising culturally unbiased tests that include only items that reflect knowledge, experiences, and skills common to all cultures. He recommended the use of culture-specific evaluation tools, which include items relevant to a specific cultural group, when available. Practically speaking, it is impossible to locate culture-specific tools for all of the diverse cultural groups in North America. Therefore, therapists must make every effort to attempt to understand a patient's individual cultural background before interpreting performance on the most appropriate standardized tests.

Pain

Pain, acute and chronic, interferes with occupational function and quality of life for many people receiving occupational therapy services. People with spinal cord injury who use manual wheelchairs report upper extremity pain, with most severe pain while pushing the

BOX 9-4
PROCEDURES FOR PRACTICE
Cultural Assessment

Experts advise against using cultural cookbooks to gain insights about culturally based habits and behaviors of various ethnic groups, as they can lead to stereotyping individual patients (Krefting, 1991; Lipson, 1996). Instead, therapists consider the unique influence of culture on each individual's experience (Krefting).

Lipson (p. 3) suggested the following questions as key elements of a cultural assessment of any patient. Occupational therapists may get the answers to these questions in the medical record or talk directly with patients or loved ones.

- Where was the patient born? If an immigrant, how long has the patient lived in this country?
- What is the patient's ethnic affiliation and how strong is the patient's ethnic identity?
- Who are the patient's major support people, family members or friends? Does the patient live in an ethnic community?
- What are the primary and secondary languages and the speaking and reading ability?
- How would you characterize the nonverbal communication style?
- What is the patient's religion, its importance in daily life, and current practices?
- What are the patient's food preferences and prohibitions?
- What is the patient's economic situation, and is the income adequate to meet the needs of the patient and family?
- What are the health and illness beliefs and practices?
- What are the customs and beliefs around such transitions as birth, illness, and death?

wheelchair up an incline and during sleep (Curtis et al., 1999). Dalyan et al. (1999) found that upper extremity pain was associated with lower employment rates and greater disability for outpatients with spinal cord injury. Many stroke patients have upper extremity pain as well, typically beginning 2 weeks post onset of stroke (Chantraine et al., 1999). Finally, pain is a common problem for adults with cerebral palsy, with fatigue, stress, depression, overexertion, and weather changes reportedly making pain worse (Schwartz et al., 1999). In addition to its contribution to disability and to decreased quality of life, pain is linked to depression (Dalyan et al.) and inefficiencies in information processing (Luoto et al., 1999).

The patient's pain should be measured when it is both a barrier to occupational function and a target of intervention. Million et al. (1982) described two categories of pain assessment techniques: (1) those that assess the patient's subjective experience with pain and limitations in activities and (2) those that quantify physical signs, such as moving during a physical examination and biochemical changes during activity. Beyond observing function and behavior, the former methods seem most appropriate for occupational therapists.

Pain is a highly personal experience; an individual's pain in the present is influenced by his or her recollections of past pain, expectations of pain, and perceptions regarding its cause (Smith et al., 1998). Two commonly used subjective measures of pain are described: the *Visual Analogue Scale* (*VAS*) (Huskisson, 1974; Million et al., 1982) and the *McGill Pain Questionnaire* (*MPQ*) (Melzack, 1975).

Visual Analogue Scale

The *VAS* is a self-administered measure of pain intensity. Patients are asked to indicate the severity of their pain by marking a point on a 10-cm line on which the end points are labeled "Pain as bad as it could be" or "No pain" (Huskisson, 1974). The rating is converted to a score by measuring the distance of the mark from the origin of the scale. Million et al. (1982) suggested that asking patients to provide one global rating of pain demands that they provide a singular estimate of their pain experience across time and situation, when in reality, pain varies with time and activity. Therefore, they developed 15 questions related to severity of pain associated with various activities, each accompanied by a *VAS*. Each question is answered as the patient marks the *VAS* based on the continuum of symptoms or limitations. The ends of each scale are described with extreme answers to the question. Here are two examples:

Does your back pain interfere with your freedom to walk? (Complete freedom to walk—completely unable to walk)

To what extent does your pain interfere with your work? (No interference at all—totally incapable of work) (Million et al., pp. 211–212).

McGill Pain Questionnaire

The *MPQ* is widely used to measure pain and response to pain interventions (Melzack, 1975, 1987). People indicate which words best describe the characteristics of their pain. These word lists represent three major categories of the pain experience (sensory, affective, evaluative). For example, the patient is asked to indicate which, if any, of the following words describes his or her present pain (sensory): pinching, pressing, gnawing, cramping, crushing. The patient receives a numerical score based on the rank value of words selected and the total number of words chosen. The *MPQ* also incorporates an index of pain intensity; it takes approximately 15 minutes to complete. Melzack

developed a shorter version (*SF-MPQ*) that takes 2 to 5 minutes to complete. The short form consists of 15 word descriptors (sensory and affective) and the *Present Pain Index* and a *VAS* to indicate the overall intensity of the pain.

Mood

Many people who receive occupational therapy services have mood disorders, such as depression and anxiety (Arruda et al., 1999). Paolucci et al. (1999) found that 27.4% of rehabilitation inpatients with stroke were depressed, and while not linked to site or side of cerebral lesion, depression was associated with poorer rehabilitation outcomes. Persons with spinal cord injury, traumatic brain injury (Kreuter et al., 1998), and Parkinson's disease (Meara et al., 1999) tend to be more depressed than the general population. Early identification and treatment of mood disorders is important, as depression and anxiety appear to interfere with attention and concentration during assessment (Eysenck & Keane, 1990) and negatively influence outcome of intervention (Paolucci et al.). While occupational therapists do not diagnose mood disorders, they have numerous opportunities to observe behavior. According to Scherer and Cushman (1997), certain patterns of behavior may indicate psychological distress and warrant referral to a psychologist or psychiatrist for further assessment and treatment.

Depression

While people feeling transitory sadness and discouragement or normal grief may display signs that are similar to those of depression, they differ in terms of persistence of symptoms and their effect on self-esteem (Gorman et al., 1989). That is, sadness and normal grief resolve with time and generally do not lead to lowered self-esteem, as suggested by the following signs of possible clinical depression (Gorman et al.; Scherer & Cushman, 1997):

► Significant declines in functioning lasting 2 weeks or more
► Feelings of worthlessness, inadequacy, self-doubt
► Diminished interest in virtually all activities, even formerly enjoyable activities
► Depressed or irritable mood most of the time
► Vegetative disturbances: lethargy; insomnia or excessive sleep; change of appetite with weight change of more than 5%; periods of excessive activity or slowness almost every day
► Very poor concentration
► Withdrawal from social interaction
► Recurrent thoughts of death or suicide

TABLE 9-3
Commonly Used Standardized Screens of Mood Disorders

Test	Description
Self-Rating Depression Scale (Zung et al., 1965)	▶ Self-administered tool designed to document symptoms and changes in the patient's clinical course ▶ Consists of 20 statements, 10 worded positively ("Morning is when I feel the best," p. 510) and 10 worded negatively ("I feel downhearted and blue," p. 510). The patient checks the statement that most accurately reflects his or her state of mind at that moment ("A little of the time," "Some of the time," "Good part of the time," "Most of the time," p. 510).
Center for Epidemiologic Studies Depression Scale (CES-D Scale) (Radloff, 1977)	▶ Self-administered questionnaire designed to detect depression in the general population ▶ The person rates 20 statements, such as "I was bothered by things that usually don't bother me" (p. 387), based on how often he or she has felt this way during the past week. ▶ Range of scores is 0–60, with the higher scores indicating more symptoms.
Hospital Anxiety and Depression Scale (Zigmond & Snaith, 1983)	▶ Self-administered questionnaire designed to detect depression and anxiety in a hospital medical outpatient clinic. ▶ Consists of 16 questions, 8 related to depression ("Do you take as much interest in things as you used to?" p. 362) and 8 related to anxiety ("Do you ever feel tensed up?" p. 362).

Anxiety

Anxiety is defined as a "subjectively painful warning of impending danger, real or imagined, that motivates the individual to take corrective action to relieve the unpleasant feelings and is experienced both psychologically and physiologically" (Gorman et al., 1989, p. 51). Anxiety is different from fear. Anxiety is characterized by a diffuse feeling of dread, whereas fear is a reaction to a specific temporary external danger (Gorman et al.). Here are some signs of possible anxiety disorder (Gorman et al.; Scherer & Cushman, 1997) that may prompt referral to a psychiatrist or psychologist:

▶ Panic attack—choking feeling, nausea, dizziness, palpitations or chest pain, fear of dying or losing control

▶ Distorted, unrealistic fears or perceptions of a situation or object

▶ Disruption of normal routines or daily activities associated with irrational fears

Occupational therapists may also use standardized screens to identify patients in need of psychological or psychiatric services. Table 9-3 describes some frequently used standardized screens, each of which takes 10 to 20 minutes to self-administer.

Social Context

"In the acute stages of an illness, it's easy to be a good friend—exhausting but rewarding to nurse a loved one back to health. But her health never returned and chronic care takes tenacious strength when you're also battling grief. I often feel unequal to the challenge."

(Osborne, 1998, p. 46)

Social context, including the person's social resources, roles, and preferences, influences occupational pursuits and satisfaction. For example, some people select tasks and activities that put them in contact with a social network; others select occupations that allow them to avoid social interaction, as in the case of individual preferences for hobbies or careers. Social networks may facilitate an individual's chosen occupations through emotional support, assistance, or instruction; unfortunately, some social relationships interfere with a person's optimal function. Only as occupational therapists are aware of the social context in which occupational function occurs can they orchestrate intervention that will outlive their own involvement in a patient's recovery and adaptation.

Social Network and Support

The characteristics of a person's social network are relatively stable social contextual factors that influence his or her identity, opportunities, and function. Langford et al. (1997) suggested that a **social network** is an interactive web of people who provide each other with help and protection; that is, they give and receive **social support**. Social networks vary in terms of the following characteristics: reciprocity (extent to which resources and support are both given and received); intensity (extent to which social relationships offer emotional closeness); complexity (extent to which social relationships serve many functions); and density (extent to which network members know and interact with each other) (Heaney & Israel, 1997).

Social support is defined as aid and assistance exchanged through social relationships and interactions

Case Example

ASSESSING PERSONAL, SOCIAL, CULTURAL CONTEXT DURING OCCUPATIONAL THERAPY ASSESSMENT

Patient Information

Mrs. N., a 30-year-old wife and mother of three young children, was referred to outpatient occupational therapy for assessment and treatment approximately 6 months after a suspected brain injury. She was injured when a shelf at a convenience store broke and its contents fell on her head. After the accident, Mrs. N. frequently complained of headaches, fatigue, and dizziness accompanied by dramatic decrease in her activity level and was observed to be forgetful, even unsafe (e.g., leaving stove burners turned on, losing tracking of her children, forgetting to take medication). With a high school education, Mrs. N. worked full time as a teaching assistant at a day care center but was unable to return to work following her injury. As a recent immigrant from Saudi Arabia, Mrs. N. spoke very little English. (She spoke and wrote in Arabic.) The consulting neuropsychologist opted not to perform a battery of standardized cognitive assessments because of concerns about communication, cultural biases of the tests themselves, and possible religious discomfort associated with spending hours of assessment time with the neuropsychologist, a man. Therefore, assessment and observations in occupational therapy were particularly important in establishing her rehabilitation needs.

Description of Assessment

Mrs. N. appeared to doze in the waiting room prior to her initial occupational therapy session. She was cooperative and soft-spoken; she was able to respond in English to approximately 30% of the questions. She stayed awake for most of each of the three 1-hour assessment sessions. Mr. N., also a native of Saudi Arabia, served as translator but often dominated interactions with details of his own stress related to his wife's status. He appeared to be on the verge of tears on at least two occasions as he described his inability to work full time because of his wife's need for supervision, assistance, and transportation to medical appointments.

Patient's and Husband's Report of Abilities and Limitations

Through her husband, Mrs. N. indicated that she was primarily concerned about her memory and endurance and that her ultimate goals were to completely resume her roles as mother, homemaker, and worker. (At the time of her assessment, Mr. N. prepared all of the family meals and their oldest daughter, aged 9, did most of the household chores.) Through her husband, Mrs. N. indicated that she had very little activity or routine in her day. She woke anywhere between 8:00 A.M. and noon. After rising, she sat for approximately half an hour, avoiding movement so as to avoid dizziness. She did not prepare meals for herself, eating only a cookie with tea instead of breakfast or lunch. She typically spent her afternoons napping, sitting alone at the window, or watching television. She fell asleep at approximately 9:00 P.M., but her husband reported that he regularly found her crying in the middle of the night. Her inactivity contrasted dramatically with reports of her premorbid status: working full time, attending language and driving classes, managing all household tasks, caring for her children, socializing with friends. With the patient's permission, the therapist also contacted Mrs. N.'s American-born, English-speaking sister-in-law, who confirmed the dramatic decline in Mrs. N.'s activity level and abilities, Mr. N.'s understandable stress given these changes, and her own willingness to serve as a resource.

Observations of Cognitive Function

Mrs. N. performed the *Contextual Memory Test* (Toglia, 1993), a test of immediate and delayed recall of 20 pictures associated with morning hygiene. Her performance on this test suggested moderate memory deficits but adequate awareness of these limitations (though the veracity of these findings was questioned, as all responses were reported through her husband). Her husband translated instructions to a 10-step task to which she jotted notes. After a 25-minute delay and interference activities, she was able to use her own notes to carry out the task with 70% accuracy. She appeared to make errors because she did not carefully review her notes and approached two steps with what appeared to be a hasty and impulsive manner.

Observations of Performance of Functional Tasks

The therapist requested that Mrs. N. select a familiar stove-top meal to prepare in occupational therapy and asked her to bring necessary supplies and ingredients to one of her assessment sessions. Mr. N. reportedly reminded Mrs. N. to do so. As instructed by the therapist, Mrs. N. made an obvious effort to remember to turn off the stove burner once she finished preparing her dish. She sat next to the stove throughout the task, but having removed the pan from the stove to serve the food, she did not return to turn off the burner (which was left on for 5 minutes, until the therapist turned it off). She appeared well organized in her approach to the task, removing all ingredients and supplies from the cupboard ahead of time and cleaning up as she proceeded. Despite these efforts, she forgot to add one of the ingredients she had set out on the table and asked the therapist whether she had added another.

Mrs. N. frequently requested rest during occupational therapy sessions that entailed physical activity. She generally tolerated approximately 5 minutes of standing or walking before requesting to sit and rest because of fatigue and dizziness. During one of the three sessions, Mrs. N. complained of headache and intermittently rested her head on the table.

Analysis of Results

Mrs. N.'s performance of functional tasks in occupational therapy seemed consistent with the kinds of problems reported at home by Mrs. N., her husband, and her sister-in-law. Specifically, Mrs. N.'s performance on pencil-and-paper and kitchen tasks were marked by forgetfulness, absent-mindedness, and poor endurance. Furthermore, given her dramatic decline in activity, reports of frequent crying and decreased appetite, the therapist was concerned about depression. Given his own stress, the therapist questioned whether Mr. N. would be able to maintain all of the roles he had assumed since his wife's injury.

Descriptions of Mrs. N.'s premorbid activities and her self-reports of long-term goals contrasted with the therapist's assumptions about Muslim women from the Middle East. Prior to meeting Mrs. N., the therapist expected that Mrs. N.'s narrow sphere of activities would center exclusively on her home and children. Mrs. N.'s premorbid engagement in work outside of her home and language and driving lessons and her goals to return to these roles exemplify the importance of attempting to understand each patient as an individual rather than drawing conclusions based on cultural or ethnic stereotypes. (Concerns about Mrs. N.'s potential for discomfort with unfamiliar men health care workers was, however, confirmed later, when the hospital sent a male interpreter to an occupational therapy session.)

Occupational Therapy Recommendations

The following recommendations were suggested as prerequisite to commencing occupational therapy treatment:

1. Referral to a woman psychologist for further evaluation and treatment of possible mood disorder.
2. Referral to a neurologist specializing in balance disorders (she had never had this complaint exhaustively evaluated).

3. Scheduling of a family conference with Mrs. N.'s sister-in-law, brother-in-law, and attorney to make arrangements to assist Mr. N. at home, enabling him to put in more hours at work.
4. Request of the hospital patient representative to provide a translator for future occupational therapy sessions so as to provide Mr. N. with more time for other activities.
5. Participation in an occupational therapy home safety evaluation.

Occupational Therapy Problem List

1. Decreased memory and concentration capabilities and inadequate strategies to compensate for these problems.
2. Deconditioning associated with prolonged inactivity complicated by poor nutrition.
3. Lack of structure or routine for daily activities and inability to judge independently which tasks were within her competence level.

CLINICAL REASONING
in OT Practice

Adapting Assessment to Contextual Factors

The occupational therapist working with Mrs. N. used only one standardized assessment tool because of concerns related to language barriers and cultural biases. How might the assessment have been different if Mrs. N. had presented the same symptoms and complaints but was born in Pittsburgh and spoke English all of her life?

(Heaney & Israel, 1997). There are four types of social support: (1) emotional (expressions of empathy, love, trust, and caring); (2) instrumental (tangible aid and service); (3) information (including advice and suggestions); (4) appraisal (feedback and affirmation) (Heaney & Israel).

During the assessment, occupational therapists first try to identify the composition and characteristics of the patient's social network: who these individuals are and the nature of their relationships. Occupational therapists must step outside of their own biases and expectations to appreciate that patients' social networks take many forms, including traditional nuclear families, same-sex partners, friendships, and acquaintances. Such biases remain prevalent, insidious, and hurtful. For example,

Jackson (2000) described many occupational therapy clinics as noninclusive environments in which a heterosexist perspective pervades conversations, humor, and assumptions.

Second, therapists attempt to determine the types of support that individuals in the social network are willing and able to provide. For example, longstanding intimate ties typically provide emotional support and long-term assistance, while neighbors and friends most often provide short-term instrumental and informational support (Heaney & Israel, 1997). Key players in the social network assume as much or as little responsibility as they are able, and the patient–family unit become the primary recipient of occupational therapy services (Brown et al., 1997). Therapists can learn a lot about patients' social network and resources by simply talking with them. However, interpretation may be confounded by therapists' personal perceptions of what constitutes adequate social support. An alternative method of assessing a patient's social network and resources is the *Norbeck Social Support Questionnaire* (Norbeck et al., 1981). It is a standardized, self-administered questionnaire consisting of 9 items and taking about 10 minutes to complete. Patients list individuals in their personal network and specify the nature of these relationships. Patients then indicate the extent to which each person listed provides emotional, appraisal, and instrumental support.

Finally, occupational therapists appreciate that some social relationships are harmful to patients. Accredited hospitals and rehabilitation facilities are mandated to have policies in place to respond to patients considered to be vulnerable adults or potential victims of intimate partner violence (Joint Commission on Accreditation of Healthcare Organizations, 1999). Therapists must familiarize themselves with employers' policies and procedures that describe how to report, document, and respond to cases of suspected maltreatment. For example, at Mercy and Unity Hospitals in suburban Minneapolis, physical and occupational therapists are expected to screen all outpatients for family violence (Fig. 9-3) (J. L. Miller, personal communication, January 10, 2000).

Caregiver Adaptation: A Dynamic Social Factor

Longstanding intimate ties in the patient's social network (hereafter also referred to as family) are critical to patients' ability to adapt to chronic illness and disability. Brown et al. (1997) suggested that families influence outcome of services because they provide a context for individual change and because they represent continuity in patients' lives. However, the ability of significant others to provide needed support is dictated in part by their own emotional and physical health and place in the adaptation process. Many relatives of persons with traumatic brain injury (Webster et al., 1999) and Alzheimer's disease (Pruchno & Potashnik, 1989), for example, experience significant levels of subjective burden and mood disorders as well as role changes in work, leisure, and social life (Frosch et al., 1997). To contribute to patients' long-term quality of life, occupational therapists assess family members' adaptation needs on an ongoing basis.

All of the personal, social, and cultural contextual factors described in Figure 9-2 can be applied to the significant other's occupational functioning as caregiver. That is, a spouse's ability to learn and apply new techniques and strategies is affected by his or her own

health concerns and distractions, age and generation, sex, mood, cultural background, makeup of the social network, and culture of the community. Furthermore, caregivers goals and perceptions of need from health providers change as they adapt to the patient's illness or injury.

Corbin and Strauss (1988) described the work of adapting to chronic disability over time as "a set of tasks performed by an individual or couple, alone or in conjunction with others, to carry out a plan of action designed to manage one or more aspects of the illness" (p. 9). This work consists of not only adjustments to self-maintenance tasks and roles but also the work involved in redefining one's identity. Corbin and Strauss used the term *illness trajectory* to refer to the sequence of physiological changes associated with an illness, injury, or disorder and the adaptive work demanded of a patient and family that accompanies each phase. They further suggested that most trajectories have five types of phases, distinctly ordered according to various diagnoses and individual courses: acute, comeback, stable, unstable, and downward.

▶ Acute phase—The patient requires immediate medical attention and focuses on physiological stabilization and recovery. Patient and family may wonder how life will change because of the illness, injury, or disorder.

▶ Comeback phase—The patient is in the midst of physical and emotional recovery and focuses on getting physically well and regaining functional abilities. Patient and family may ask questions such as these: Will I (he or she) come back? How long will it take before I (he or she) peak? "In the comeback trajectory, the present is seen as overbearing, and the future is put on hold while one awaits answers to the foregoing questions" (Corbin and Strauss, 1988, p. 46).

▶ Stable phase—The patient undergoes very few changes in course of illness or functional abilities, as in the remission phase of multiple sclerosis or permanent spinal cord injury. Patient and family focus on maintaining stable health while wondering how long the phase will last and what can be done to extend it.

▶ Unstable phase—The patient has periodic but erratic downturns in function or exacerbations of illness (as might come, for example, with bladder infection). Unstable phases hamper normal living, and people in this phase ask questions like these: How long until we get this under control? How much longer can I (or we) go on like this?

▶ Downward phase—The patient slowly or rapidly loses health and function. With increasing

Family Violence Screening and Response Tool

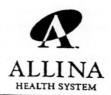

ALLINA HEALTH SYSTEM

What to do: RADAR mnemonic *

Routinely ask. Inquiring about family violence can be an intervention. You're signaling that violence is inappropriate; you may be helping to end the isolation.
Affirm and support patients who acknowledge abuse.
Document objective findings; patient statements in quotes.
Address your patient's safety.
Refer the patient to people skilled in family violence and safety planning.

When do you screen?

➤ Patient must always be alone. The exception is with infants or nonverbal toddlers.
➤ Screen all adults—both males and females.

When do you introduce the screening?

An introductory statement will lead you into asking the screening questions. This statement gives the patient the following messages:

➤ Violence in the home is a major health care issue;
➤ I care about you;
➤ All patients are asked these questions; and
➤ This is a safe place.

STATE: *We at (name clinic/hospital) are concerned about the violence that is impacting the health of many of our patients, so we routinely ask everyone the following confidential questions.*

Screening Questions

➤ Have you ever been hit, kicked, pushed, or otherwise hurt or mistreated by someone important to you?
➤ Is someone important to you yelling at you, threatening you, or otherwise trying to control your life?

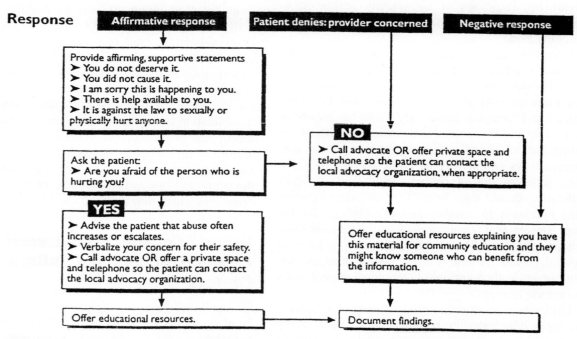

* Alpert, E.J. (1999). *Partner Violence: A Guide for Physicians and Other Health Care Professionals (3rd Edition) – Use Your "RADAR".* Waltham, MA: Massachusetts Medical Society.

Figure 9-3 Family Violence Screening and Response Tool (Reprinted with permission from Allina Health System, Minnetonka, MN 55343.)

incapacity, the patient and family view the present as temporary and the future as unknown. They are concerned with questions such as these: How fast and how far? When will it end? What can we do to slow it down?

While there are no standardized methods for determining a person's phase in an illness trajectory, sensitivity to each person's changing path in this journey is prerequisite to creating a treatment plan that meshes with patient and family real-time needs and priorities. A family-centered approach allows the therapist to capitalize on the family's priorities and contributions to the patient's recovery and adaptation. This mind-set, however, requires that therapists "follow the family's lead rather than impose professional decisions," (Brown et al., 1997, p. 598).

Patient–Therapist Social Interactions

Occupational therapy assessment is not a neutral process (Luborsky, 1997). Gans (1998) suggests, "Part of the way the patient behaves with you is a function of the way you are with the patient. This effect may comprise 75%, 25%, or 2% of what goes on between you and the patient, but it is there" (p. 4). Social convention and cultural norms organize the patient's self-report of problems and symptoms and the therapist's response to these concerns (Luborsky, 1997). The therapist is endowed with power to shape the interaction by selecting certain questions and omitting others (Luborsky, 1995), to judge or evaluate the responses of the patient, and even to determine whose expectations and "reality" are correct (Abberley, 1995).

Occupational therapists monitor the extent to which their own needs infiltrate social interactions with patients. Perhaps to meet self-imposed expectations around outcome, Abberley (1995) suggested that some occupational therapists unwittingly define the patient as the problem and themselves as the solution, with failure of intervention always attributed to the patient and success always credited to the clinician's efforts. Gans (1998) believes that a primary source of clinician gratification should stem from "the privilege of participating intimately in another person's life" (p. 5). He further suggests that when the work no longer feels like a privilege, one should try to figure out why (volume of caseload, private life that is distracting or burdensome, burnt out, ethically questionable employer expectations that corrode integrity).

Clinicians also examine their expectations of their own supportive roles in patients' lives. They recognize that professional helpers are typically not able to provide support over long periods. They realize that professional–lay relationships are not characterized by reciprocity typical of social networks and often entail invisible but palpable power differentials that interfere with the provision of genuine emotional support (Heaney & Israel, 1997). In essence, they realize that as professionals, they should not attempt to assume a long-term role in the social network but rather work with the patient and family to create permanent social links that meet their needs.

Cultural Context of the Larger Society and Community

"I used to dream about being in a world where being disabled was no big deal, where no one considered it a tragedy. No one thought you were inspiring or felt sorry for you . . . . I imagined what a relief it would be to be seen every day as perfectly ordinary."
(Tollifson, 1997, p. 105)

The dominant culture influences the ease with which a person with disabilities feels accepted and integrated into the community. Luborsky (1994) suggested that culturally based requirements for status of full adult person in Europe and North America, such as self-sufficiency, activity, and upright posture, are often at odds with full participation for persons with disabilities. Adapted equipment may be rejected because of its appearance and acceptability in public rather than its functional value (Luborsky, 1994, 1997). Patients and family may respond to embarrassment or guilt over disability by attempting to keep the disability private and denying help from friends or neighbors (Armstrong & Fitzgerald, 1996). Loss of social status is further compounded when insidious cultural beliefs hold persons with disabilities responsible for their impairments. "At a deep level there is a bias that either they are culpable for the cause of the impairment, or for not working harder at rehabilitation to be able to 'overcome' the odds regardless of how realistic that is" (Luborsky, 1994, p. 251). As abhorrent and illogical as such notions are, patients, families, and occupational therapists are not immune to the subtle but pervasive influences of the sociocultural context in which they live.

General Comments on Assessing Personal, Social, and Cultural Context

Occupational therapists struggle to balance their preeminent concerns for service to patients with very real demands for efficiency and productivity. Clinicians typically devote 30 minutes to 3 hours assessing each patient; the short lengths of stay in acute settings allow less time; inpatient rehabilitation settings (with possibly longer stays) allow somewhat more. How does one have time to assess the web of personal, social, and cultural contextual factors on top of all pertinent areas of occupational function (roles, tasks, activities, abilities and skills, and capacities)? Here are some general guidelines:

▶ Review the assessments of other professionals. Many patients who are referred to occupational therapy are also assessed by social workers, psychologists, speech–language pathologists, physical therapists, physicians, therapeutic recreation specialists, chaplains, and/or nurses. Reviewing the assessments of team members greatly adds to the occupational therapist's ability to understand a patient's personal, social, and cultural context without using limited assessment time to do so.

▶ Use specific tools (many discussed in this chapter) to measure contextual factors that appear to bias or confound performance during assessment or that are expected to be targets of occupational therapy intervention (to establish a baseline).

▶ Take advantage of informal conversations with patients. Luborsky (1997) pointed out the value of attending to patients' informal remarks made during structured assessments. He described how a patient's comments during transitions between various standardized tools provide insights not captured by the tools themselves. He further stated that patients' informal remarks "can be essential to gaining an understanding of the way subjects make sense of the assessment; to providing us with important information on the validity of the assessment tool; and to identifying important areas for clinical intervention" (p. 12).

It is advisable to use each and every moment with patients to try to understand who they are, where they come from, and how they are interpreting their experience in therapy. Gans (1988) links this investment to patient outcome: "our ongoing, relentless determination to understand the uniqueness of each patient is what the patient, to the degree he or she can, experiences as love . . . [and] patients who feel cared about and valued make the most gains in therapy" (p. 5). It is unrealistic to expect therapists to unravel the mysteries of a patient's contextual fabric during an arbitrarily defined assessment period. The richness of conversations that relate to personal, social, and cultural context grows as the therapeutic relationship deepens and continues to inform the treatment process.

Summary Review Questions

1. Consider your morning self-care routine—the activities you performed today to get ready to leave for school or work. List the personal, social, and contextual factors that influenced your performance. If someone who did not know you judged your performance, what aspects might they consider unusual? What aspects might he or she consider normal for someone of your age and background?
2. Review Table 9-2 and write a paragraph describing the possible influences on occupational functioning of one of the contextual factors not discussed in this chapter. For example, how might social class or gender help or hinder performance?
3. Outline circumstances in which you would use standardized instruments to assess contextual factors and those in which you would use more informal methods.
4. Make a private list of your own biases. What assumptions do you have about people who are different from you in terms of age, sex, cultural and educational background, sexual orientation, and abilities (physical, cognitive, emotional)? List the steps you can take to debunk these biases and measures to minimize their effects during interactions with patients.
5. Observe the interactions of another clinician and patient during assessment. What if any comments made by the therapist could be attributed to his or her personal, social, and cultural context? What comments made by the patient could be attributed to his or her personal, social, and cultural context?

Acknowledgments

I thank Jo Solet, PhD, OTR, and Cathy Lysack, PhD, OTC, for helpful suggestions on an earlier version of this chapter. I also appreciate Cathy's willingness to share the readings for her course at Wayne State University on Culture and Disability.

References

Abberley, P. (1995). Disabling ideology in health and welfare: The case of occupational therapy. *Disability & Society, 10,* 221–232.

Armstrong, M. J., & Fitzgerald, M. H. (1996). Culture and disability studies: An anthropological perspective. *Rehabilitation Education, 10,* 247–304.

Arruda, J. E., Stern, R. A., & Sommerville, B. A. (1999). Measurement of mood states in stroke patients: Validation of the Visual Analog Mood Scale. *Archives of Physical Medicine and Rehabilitation, 80,* 676–680.

Brown, S. M., Humphry, R., & Taylor, E. (1997). A model of the nature of family-therapist relationships: Implications for education. *American Journal of Occupational Therapy, 51,* 597–603.

Cannon, P. (1994). If I live, does the injury take my life? *Viewpoints: Issues in Brain Injury Rehabilitation, 26,* 3–4.

Chantraine, A., Baribeault, A., Uebelhart, D., & Gremion, G. (1999). Shoulder pain and dysfunction in hemiplegia: Effects of functional electrical stimulation. *Archives of Physical Medicine and Rehabilitation, 80,* 328–331.

Christiansen, C. (1997). Acknowledging a spiritual dimension in occupational therapy practice. *American Journal of Occupational Therapy, 51,* 169–172.

Corbin, J. M., & Strauss, A. (1988). *Unending Work and Care: Managing Chronic Illness at Home.* San Francisco: Jossey-Bass.

Cox, B. J., & Waller, L. L. (1991). *Bridging the Communication Gap with the Elderly.* Chicago: American Hospital.

Curtis, K. A., Drysdale, G. A., Lanza, D., Kolber, M., Vitolo, R. S., & West, R. (1999). Shoulder pain in wheelchair users with tetraplegia and paraplegia. *Archives of Physical Medicine and Rehabilitation, 80,* 453–457.

Dalyan, M., Cardenas, D. D., & Gerard, B. (1999). Upper extremity pain after spinal cord injury. *Spinal Cord, 37,* 191–195.

Dunn, W., Brown, C., & McGuigan, A. (1994). The ecology of human performance: A framework for considering the effect of context. *American Journal of Occupational Therapy, 48,* 595–607.

Engquist, D. E., Short-DeGraff, M., Gliner, J., & Oltjenbruns, K. (1997). Occupational therapists' beliefs and practices with regard to spirituality and therapy. *American Journal of Occupational Therapy, 51,* 173–180.

Ewing, J. A. (1984). Detecting alcoholism: The CAGE questionnaire. *Journal of the American Medical Association, 252,* 1905–1907.

Eysenck, M. W., & Keane, M. T. (1990). *Cognitive Psychology: A Student's Handbook.* London: Lawrence Erlbaum.

Farrales, S. (1996). Vietnamese. In J. G. Lipson, S. L. Dibble, & P. A. Minarik (Eds.), *Culture & Nursing Care: A Pocket Guide* (pp. 280–290). San Francisco: UCSF Nursing.

Fisher, A. G. (1998). Uniting practice and theory in an occupational framework. *American Journal of Occupational Therapy, 52,* 509–521.

Freiberg, K. L. (1987). *Human Development: A Life-Span Approach* (3rd Ed.). Boston: Jones & Bartlett.

Frosch, S., Gruber, A., Jones, C., Myers, S., Noel, E., Westerlund, A., & Zavisin, T. (1997). The long term effects of traumatic brain injury on the roles of caregivers. *Brain Injury, 11,* 891–906.

Gans, J. S. (1998). Enhancing the therapeutic value of talking with patients in the rehabilitation setting. *Rehabilitation Outlook,* Summer, 4–5.

Gorman, L. M., Sultman, D., & Luna-Raines, M. (1989). *Psychosocial Nursing Handbook for the Nonpsychiatric Nurse.* Baltimore: Williams & Wilkins.

Heaney, C. A., & Israel, B. A. (1997). Social networks and social support. In K. Glanz, F. M. Lewis, & B. K. Rimer (Eds.), *Health Behavior and Health Education* (pp. 179–205). San Francisco: Jossey-Bass.

Huskisson, E. C. (1974). Measurement of pain. *Lancet, 2,* 1127–1131.

Institute of Medicine (1997). *Enabling America.* E. N. Brandt & A. M. Pope (Eds.). Washington: National Academy.

Jackson, J. (2000). Understanding the experience of noninclusive occupational therapy clinics: Lesbians' perspectives. *American Journal of Occupational Therapy, 54,* 26–35.

Joint Commission on Accreditation of Healthcare Organizations (1999). *Comprehensive Accreditation Manual for Hospitals.* Oakbrook Terrace, IL: Author.

Kelly, M. P., Johnson, C. A., Knoller, N., Drubach, D. A., & Winslow, M. M. (1997). Substance abuse, traumatic brain injury, and neuropsychological outcome. *Brain Injury, 11,* 391–402.

Kleinman, A. (1988). *The Illness Narratives: Suffering, Healing, and the Human Condition.* New York: Basic Books.

Kolakowsky-Hayner, S. A., Gourley, E. V., Kreutzer, J. S., Marwitz, J. H., Cifu, D. X., & McKinley, W. O. (1999). Pre-injury substance abuse among persons with brain injury and spinal cord injury. *Brain Injury, 13,* 571–581.

Krefting, L. (1991). The culture concept in the everyday practice of occupational and physical therapy. *Physical and Occupational Therapy in Practice 11* (4), 1–16.

Kreuter, M., Sullivan, M., Dahllof, A. G., & Siosteen, A. (1999). Partner relationships, functioning, mood and global quality of life in persons with spinal cord injury and traumatic brain injury. *Spinal Cord, 36,* 252–261.

Langford, C. P. H., Bowsher, J., Maloney, J. P., & Lillis, P. (1997). Social support: A conceptual analysis. *Journal of Advanced Nursing, 25,* 95–100.

Law, M., Cooper, B., Strong, S., Stewart, D., Rigby, P., & Letts, L. (1996). The person-environment-occupation model: A transactive approach to occupational performance. *Canadian Journal of Occupational Therapy, 63,* 9–23.

Lerman, C., & Glanz, K. (1997). Stress, coping, and health behavior. In K. Glanz, F. M. Lewis, B. K. Rimer (Eds.), *Health Behavior and Health Education* (pp. 113–138). San Francisco: Jossey-Bass.

Lipson, J. G. (1996). Culturally competent nursing care. In J. G. Lipson, S. L. Dibble, P. A. Minarik (Eds.), *Culture & Nursing Care: A Pocket Guide* (pp. 1–10). San Francisco: UCSF Nursing.

Luborsky, M. R. (1994). The cultural adversity of physical disability: Erosion of full adult personhood. *Journal of Aging Studies, 8,* 239–253.

Luborsky, M. R. (1995). The process of self-report of impairment in clinical research. *Social Science Medicine, 40,* 1447–1459.

Luborsky, M. (1997). Attuning assessment to the client: Recent advances in theory and methodology. *Generations, 21* (1), 10–15.

Luoto, S., Taimela, S., Hurri, H., & Alaranta, H. (1999). Mechanisms explaining the association between low back trouble and deficits in information processing. *Spine, 24,* 255–261.

Mattingly, C. (1991). The narrative nature of clinical reasoning. *American Journal of Occupational Therapy, 45,* 998–1005.

Mattingly, C., & Fleming, M. H. (1994). *Clinical Reasoning.* Philadelphia: Davis.

McGruder, J. (1998). Culture and other forms of human diversity in occupational therapy. In M. E. Neistadt & E. B. Crepeau (Eds.), *Willard and Spackman's Occupational Therapy* (9th ed.). Philadelphia: Lippincott.

Meara, J., Michelmore, E., & Hobson, P. (1999). Use of the GDS-15 geriatric depression scale as a screening instrument for depressive symptomatology in patients with Parkinson's disease and their carers in the community. *Age & Ageing, 28,* 35–38.

Melzack, R. (1975). The *McGill Pain Questionnaire*: Major properties and scoring methods. *Pain, 1,* 277–299.

Melzack, R. (1987). The short-form McGill Questionnaire. *Pain, 30,* 191–197.

Million, R., Hall, W., Nilsen, K. H., Baker, R. D., & Jayson, M. I. V. (1982). Assessment of the progress of the back pain patient. *Spine, 7,* 204–212.

Moyers, P. A., & Stoffel, V. C. (1999). Alcohol dependence in a client with a work-related injury. *American Journal of Occupational Therapy, 53,* 640–645.

Murphy, P. W., Davis, T. C., Long, S. W., Jackson, R. H., & Decker, B. C. (1993). *Rapid Estimates of Adult Literacy in Medicine* (REALM): A quick reading test for patients. *Journal of Reading, 37,* 124–130.

National Center for Medical Rehabilitation Research (1993). Research plan for the National Center for Medical Rehabilitation Research (NIH Publication 93-3509). Bethesda: MD: Author.

Nelson, D. L. (1988). Occupation: Form and performance. *American Journal of Occupational Therapy, 42,* 633–641.

Norbeck, J. S., Lindsey, A. M., & Carrieri, V. L. (1981). The development of an instrument to measure social support. *Nursing Research, 30,* 262–269.

Osborne, C. L. (1998). *Over My Head.* Kansas City, MO: Andrews McMeel.

Paolucci, S., Antonucci, G., Pratesi, L., Traballesi, M., Grasso, M. G., & Lubich, S. (1999). Post stroke depression and its role in rehabilitation of inpatients. *Archives of Physical Medicine and Rehabilitation, 80,* 985–990.

Parikh, N. S., Parker, R. M., Nurss, J. R., Baker, D. W., & Williams, M. V. (1996). Shame and health literacy: The unspoken connection. *Patient Education and Counseling, 27,* 33–39.

Paul, S. (1995). Culture and its influence on occupational therapy evaluation. *Canadian Journal of Occupational Therapy, 62,* 154–161.

Pruchno, R. A., & Potashnik, S. L. (1989). Caregiving spouses: Physical and mental health in perspective. *Journal of the American Geriatrics Society, 37,* 697–705.

Puchalski, C. M. (1996). F.I.C.A.: A Spiritual Assessment. National Institute for Healthcare Research. Available at http://www.nihr.org/education/fica.html. Accessed March 13, 2000.

Radloff, L. S. (1977). *The CES-D Scale:* A self-report depression scale for research in the general population. *Applied Psychological Measurement, 1,* 385–401.

Radomski, M. V. (1995). There is more to life than putting on your pants. *American Journal of Occupational Therapy, 49,* 487–490.

Riley, B. B., Perna, R., Tate, D. G., Forchheimer, M., Anderson, C., & Luera, G. (1998). Types of spiritual well-being among persons with chronic illness: Their relation to various forms of quality of life. *Archives of Physical Medicine and Rehabilitation, 79,* 258–264.

Royeen, C. B. (1995). The human life cycle: Paradigmatic shifts in occupation. In C. B. Royeen (Ed.), *The Practice of the Future: Putting Occupation Back into Therapy.* Bethesda, MD: American Occupational Therapy Association.

Scherer, M. J., & Cushman, L. A. (1997). A functional approach to psychological and psychosocial factors and their assessment in rehabilitation. In S. S. Dittmar & G. E. Gresham (Eds.), *Functional Assessment and Outcome Measures for the Rehabilitation Health Professional* (pp. 57–67). Gaithersburg, MD: Aspen.

Schwartz, L., Engel, J. M., & Jensen, M. P. (1999). Pain in persons with cerebral palsy. *Archives of Physical Medicine and Rehabilitation, 80,* 1243–1246.

Smith, W. B., Gracely, R. H., & Safer, M. A. (1998). The meaning of pain: Cancer patients' rating and recall of pain intensity and affect. *Pain, 78,* 123–129.

Soderstrom, C. A., Smith, G. S., Kufera, J., Dischinger, P. C., Hebel, J. R., McDuff, D. R., Gorelick, D. A., Ho, S. M., Kerns, T. J., & Read, K. M. (1997). The accuracy of CAGE, the Brief Michigan Alcoholism Screening Test, the Alcohol Use Disorders Identification Test in screening trauma center patients for alcoholism. *The Journal of Trauma: Injury, Infection, and Critical Care, 43,* 962–969.

St. Clair, A., & McKenry, L. (1999). Preparing culturally competent practitioners. *Journal of Nursing Education, 38,* 228–234.

Strauss, W., & Howe, N. (1991). *Generations.* New York: William Morrow.

Taj, N., Devera-Sales, A., & Vinson, D. C. (1998). Screening for problem drinking: Does a single question work? *Journal of Family Practice, 46,* 328–335.

Toglia, J. P. (1993). *The Contextual Memory Test.* Tucson: Therapy Skill Builders.

Tollison, J. (1997). Imperfection is a beautiful thing: On disability and meditation. In K. Fries (Ed.), *Staring Back: The Disability Experience From the Inside Out.* New York: Penguin Putnam.

Webster's New World Dictionary of American English (3rd college ed). (1994). New York: Prentice Hall.

Webster, G., Daisley, A., & King, N. (1999). Relationship and family breakdown following acquired brain injury: The role of the rehabilitation team. *Brain Injury, 13,* 593–603.

World Health Organization (1999). *ICIHD-2: International Classification of Impairments, Activities, and Participation (Beta-2 draft for field trials).* Geneva: Author.

Zigmond, A. S., & Snaith, R. P. (1982). The Hospital Anxiety and Depression Scale. *Acta Psychiatrica Scandinavia, 67,* 361–370.

Zung, W. W. K., Richards, C. B., & Short, M. J. (1965). Self-rating Depression Scale in an outpatient clinic. *Archives of General Psychiatry, 13,* 508–515.

10
Assessing Context: Home, Community, and Workplace Access

Barbara Acheson Cooper, Patricia Rigby, Lori Letts, Debra Stewart, Susan Strong, and Mary Law

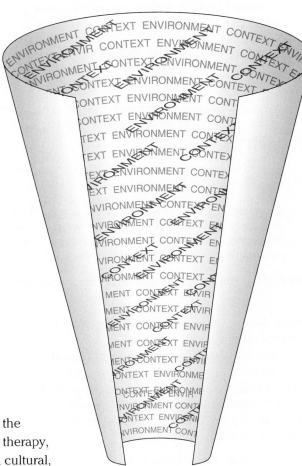

LEARNING OBJECTIVES

After studying this chapter, the reader will be able to do the following:

1. Identify the roles and responsibilities of the occupational therapist in the evaluation of access to physical environments.
2. Identify factors that act as environmental barriers and supports to occupational performance.
3. Identify assessment instruments appropriate for use in evaluating access to home, community and workplace.
4. Identify the properties that make access assessment tools useful in clinical practice.
5. Identify how legislation and building standards influence the degree of access to the physical environment available for people with disabilities.

*T*he environment influences human behavior and provides the context within which all roles are performed. In occupational therapy, the environment is broadly defined as having physical, social, cultural, organizational, and institutional dimensions. These dimensions interact with each other and are difficult to tease apart; that is, they are said to be **transactive** (Law et al., 1996).

A number of occupational therapy theories specifically address the issue of environmental influences on occupational functioning (e.g., Dunn et al., 1994; Law et al., 1996). These vary slightly in terminology and approach, but all agree on the importance of environmental considerations in the practice of occupational therapy. Central to these theories is the notion that **environmental barriers** to occupational performance for people with disabilities can be modified or eliminated more easily than most other negative influences. Also, the theories all emphasize that

GLOSSARY

Accessibility—The ease with which the physical environment may be reached, entered, and used by all individuals.

Accommodation—Any changes in the environment or the way in which an activity or task is customarily performed that enables a person with a disability to enjoy equal opportunity.

Barrier-free design—Design features of the built environment that remove physical barriers to full and equal accessibility for all persons with disabilities.

Environmental barrier—Any component of the environment that impedes a person's ability to attain optimal occupational functioning.

Environmental support—Any component of the environment that encourages, facilitates, or provides assistance to allow a person to achieve optimal occupational function.

Person–environment fit—The degree to which an environment matches the functional, social, and psychological needs of an individual.

Physical environment—The built or natural context within which all occupational functioning occurs.

Reasonable accommodation—The steps required to ensure that no person with a disability is excluded from or denied services, segregated, or otherwise treated differently from the general population because of the absence of auxiliary aids or services.

Reliability—The extent to which the results of an assessment are reproducible or give the same results on different days (test–retest reliability) or by different observers (interrater reliability). The level of reliability is excellent when the correlation coefficient (r), or intraclass correlation, is above .80, is adequate when it is between .60 and .79, and is poor when it is less than .60 (Gowland et al., 1991).

Standardization—The process of making an assessment available in a manual with standard procedures for testing, scoring, and interpreting the results. Environmental assessments do not usually undergo a normative process because of the variability in environments, yet many are based on standards developed by the ANSI, government building codes, and interpretations of the ADA.

Transactive—Integrated, codependent (of a relationship).

Universal design—Design features of the built environment that enhance optimal function and convenience for all individuals, regardless of their ability.

Validity—The extent to which the assessment measures what it is intended to measure. Content validity is most relevant to environmental assessments and is considered excellent for evaluative purposes when the assessment tool includes items that have the potential to change (e.g., physical barriers and supports). Items selected for an assessment should be the result of a thorough review of the literature on the topic and consultation from experts in the area of study, including the input of people with physical disabilities (Gowland et al., 1991).

---

environmental supports promote optimal occupational performance.

The congruence between a person and the environment is the **person–environment (P/E) fit**. Occupational therapists are frequently called upon to determine the fit between people with disabilities and the various environments in which they operate. In this capacity, the therapist's role is as follows:

► To identify and evaluate barriers that may challenge the competency and ability of individuals to carry out their chosen activities and roles
► To identify and evaluate supports that facilitate occupational functioning
► To develop strategies to eliminate or ameliorate barriers
► To foster supports

This chapter focuses on the assessment of the **physical environment**, specifically ways to evaluate the physical attributes of the environment when assessing the context in which occupational functioning occurs. The assessment measures selected are those that we consider the best available and that reflect the transactive nature of the relationship between people and the physical environments in which they live and work.

Evaluation of the Physical Environment

The physical environment provides the context for human activity. Consequently, an assessment of its attributes should be augmented with information about those who will use the environment and the functions they will carry out there. In the practice of occupational therapy, it is important to begin this process with the person.

Client-Centered Approach

The client is central to all occupational therapy services (Canadian Association of Occupational Therapists, 1997; Trombly, 1995). The client–therapist interaction begins with an interview to determine what roles and occupations the client previously had and what the client wants or is expected to be able to do. The client's perspective on the importance of these activities and current level of performance are thereby determined. This can be done informally or using an assessment such as the *Canadian Occupational Performance Measure (COPM)* (Law et al., 1994). The occupational therapist also ascertains the client's competence and the contexts within which these activities and roles will be carried out. For example, a therapist could be asked to determine the degree of disability that will be experienced by a hospitalized client currently using a wheelchair to move through wide doorways and corridors in the hospital, when faced with negotiating narrow doors and hallways at home after discharge.

Clients' Roles

The roles carried out by clients consist of self-maintenance, self-enhancement, and self-advancement activities. Each individual ascribes different meaning and value to his or her roles. Specific features of the environment support or hinder the fulfillment of valued roles within the home, community, and workplace.

Environmental Barriers and Supports

The occupational therapist must be able to identify the key environmental barriers and supports that influence the occupational functioning of clients. In clinical practice, barriers and supports are broadly defined. However, this chapter discusses only physical barriers and supports; other contextual barriers and supports are described in Chapter 9.

Physical barriers are characteristics of the built or natural environment that prevent or impede a person with a disability from completing role activities. For example, consider the challenge that stairs or rocky paths impose on a person using a wheelchair. These barriers can be removed or reduced by adding supports such as elevators or ramps to replace stairs and a ramped bridge across the rocks to allow access for a wheelchair.

Access that is discriminatory or inconvenient, such as when persons with physical disabilities must use freight elevators or ramped entrances at the back of buildings, is no longer considered a viable solution to eliminating access barriers. Improved **accessibility** through the use of **universal design** and **barrier-free design** is preferred. These two terms are similar but not synonymous. Universal design refers to features of the built environment that enhance optimal function and convenience for everyone, regardless of ability. Barrier-free design refers to features of the built environment

that remove physical barriers to allow full and equal accessibility for all persons with disabilities. Universal design can encompasses barrier-free design, but the converse is not necessarily true. For this reason, it is preferable to promote the use of universal design (see Resources).

Influences on Environmental Accessibility

Various societal and cultural attitudes influence the degree to which the physical environment is made accessible to people with disabilities. Occupational therapy practice standards also reflect these global views. These influences manifest as national and state or provincial legislation, building standards, and professional practice requirements.

Legislation

A number of recent laws address the restrictions that environmental barriers impose on people with disabilities. The most significant of these, the Americans with Disabilities Act (ADA) (1990), is a civil rights law designed to increase the integration and successful community living of people with disabilities in American society. Comprehensive civil rights protection is focused on five areas:

▶ Employment
▶ Public accommodations (i.e., places frequented by the general public)
▶ State and local government
▶ Public transportation
▶ Telecommunications

For example, the ADA mandates that a qualified person with a disability cannot be discriminated against when seeking or participating in employment. The intent of the law is to create equal opportunity and equal access to public environments, services, and transportation for persons with disabilities. The ADA is a dynamic legal document that focuses on achieving integration and independent living for people with disabilities through societal change.

The key phrase in the ADA is the obligation of society to provide **reasonable accommodation** to ensure that public services, facilities, transportation, employment, accommodations, and telecommunications are accessible. Reasonable accommodation is defined by federal law; legal parameters are developed through challenge on a case-by-case basis.

Titles II and III of the ADA detail the steps to be taken by state and local government services, programs, and facilities to comply with and implement the requirements of the ADA. They address the public accommodations required and the availability of these resources;

modifications to policies, practices, and procedures; the removal of barriers; and alternative forms of services, such as paratransit services when mainline public facilities are unavailable. In time these regulations are expected to eliminate the social barriers against people with disabilities (Kalscheur, 1991). See Resources for further information on the ADA.

Although the ADA does not mandate professional involvement in achievement of the criteria it sets forth, occupational therapists, skilled in occupational analysis, environmental assessment and determining P/E fit, are well suited to assist with meeting the requirements of the ADA. A number of guides are available to facilitate compliance with the ADA (see Resources).

Building Standards

The American National Standards Institute (ANSI) (1998) outlines design specifications that must be met to allow accessibility of buildings by people with disabilities. Examples of these standards of barrier-free design include the provision of ramps, wide doorways, and grab bars. Some examples from the ANSI document are provided to show the type of standards and specifications it addresses (Figs. 10-1 and 10-2). The ANSI document is essential for occupational therapists who are

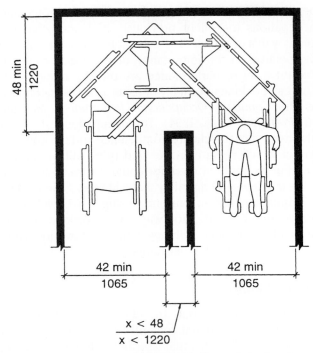

Figure 10-2 Clear width at turn. (Reprinted with permission from International Code Council, Inc., Falls Church, Va. ICC/ANSI A117.1-1998.)

planning and adapting environments for maximum accessibility.

Other standards have been developed for specific environments, such as the workplace. For example, the National Institute of Occupational Safety and Health (NIOSH) publishes criteria directed at reducing the rate of workplace injuries (Aja, 1995). Occupational therapists who work in these environments must become familiar with the standards and guidelines relevant to their area of practice.

Professional Practice Requirements

The practice of occupational therapy is also guided by professional regulations. Standards of practice, core competencies, and functions expected of therapists are developed at the national and state or provincial levels to provide performance evaluation criteria. These guidelines are usually generic, applying to all therapists, regardless of the area, setting, or focus of practice. Entry-level requirements for occupational therapists are established by councils of accreditation for university programs. These include the curriculum content, which must be addressed by every academic program (American Occupational Therapy Association, 1998). Knowledge of and ability to perform assessments of context and environment are considered to be core competencies and functions of practice for all occupational therapists (American Occupational Therapy Association, 1995; Canadian Association of Occupational Therapists, 1996; Moyers, 1999).

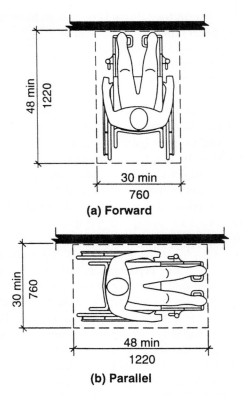

Figure 10-1 Position of clear floor or ground. (Reprinted with permission from International Code Council, Inc., Falls Church, Va. ICC/ANSI A117.1-1998.)

Assessments of Person–Environment Fit

Ideally, instruments used to assess P/E fit should consider qualities of the person and the environment as well as the activities that take place there. The P/E relationship is dynamic, complex, and interwoven and therefore more difficult to measure than interactions that can be understood by assessing discrete components. The following assessments have been selected for their ability to reflect this transactive relationship.

Assessments Rated by Authors

Through a literature review and consultation, we identified instruments used to measure access to the physical environment. These were evaluated and rated as excellent, adequate, or poor according to guidelines developed by Gowland et al. (1991). Instruments rated as excellent or adequate have been listed along with their sources. The measures have been categorized by setting:

those suitable for assessing homes (Table 10-1), the community (Table 10-2), and the workplace (Table 10-3). The tables also include some unique measures that have good content validity and clinical utility but for which formal studies of psychometric properties are unavailable or incomplete. These measures are identified in the tables with an asterisk, and some are discussed in the section on universal assessments. The rating process addressed the following factors:

▶ Intended use of the assessment instrument
▶ Focus (e.g., location, factors)
▶ Clinical utility (e.g., time to administer, cost, convenience, usefulness, training required)
▶ **Standardization** (e.g., published information on **reliability** and **validity** of the measure; availability of a manual).

Forms and detailed information on the process can be downloaded from the Internet (see Resources). An example of a completed assessment is also provided in Box 10-1 to illustrate the review process.

TABLE 10-1
Assessments of Access to Home

Assessment	Source
Accessibility Checklist (Goltsman et al., 1992)	M.I.G. Communications, 1802 Fifth Ave., Berkeley, CA 94710
Assessment Tool (Maltais et al., 1998)	Canada Mortgage and Housing Corporation, National Office, 700 Montreal Rd., Ottawa, ON, Canada K1A 0P7. Web: www.cmhc-schl.gc.ca
*EASE3 (Lifease, 1998)	Margaret Christiansen, 615-636-6869
*Enabler (Steinfeld et al., 1979)	HUD User, P.O. Box 6091, Germantown, MD 20850
Enviro-FIM, Usability Rating Scale (Steinfeld & Danford, 1997)	Dr. E. Steinfeld, Department of Architecture, 382 Hayes Hall, 3435 Main St., Buffalo, NY 14214
Home Modifications Workbook (Adaptive Environments Center, 1988)	Web: www.adaptenv.org
Home Observation for Measurement of the Environment (Revised Edition) (*HOME Inventory*) (Caldwell & Bradley, 1984)	Center for Child Development and Education. University of Arkansas at Little Rock, 33rd and University Ave., Little Rock AR 72204
Housing Enabler (OT) (Iwarsson & Isacsson, 1996)	*Enabler*. Manual and assessment form. Swedish revised occupational therapy version. Available in English from Dr. S. Iwarsson, Lund University, Sweden. Fax: +46-46-222-1959
Multiphasic Environmental Assessment Procedure (*MEAP*):	*Evaluating Residential Facilities: the Multiphasic Environmental Assessment Procedure*. Thousand Oaks, CA: Sage. Fax: 415-852-3420.
Physical Architectural Features Checklist	Moos & Lemke, 1996
POE	Cooper, Ahrentzen, & Hasselkus, 1991
Safety Assessment of Function and the Environment for Rehabilitation (*SAFER*) Tool (Oliver et al., 1993)	Community Occupational Therapists and Associates, 199. 3101 Bathurst St., Toronto, ON M6A 2A6. Telephone: 416-785-8797
The Source Book (Kelly & Snell, 1989)	Barrier-Free Design Consultants, 31 Biggar Ave., Toronto, ON, Canada M6H 2N5. Telephone 416-223-4217; fax 416-223-7049
Westmead Home Safety Assessment (*WeHSA*) (Clemson, 1997)	Co-ordinates Publications, P.O. Box 59, West Brunswick, Victoria 3055, Australia

*Unique instrument of measure with incomplete psychometric validation.

TABLE 10-2
Assessments of Access to Community

Assessment	Source
ADA Accessibility Guidelines for Buildings and Facilities	U.S. Architectural and Transportation Barriers Compliance Board, 1111 18th St., N.W., Suite 501, Washington, D.C. 20036-3894; Telephone: 202-272-5434
Community Mobility Assessment	Kelly Brewer, Bloorview MacMillan Centre, 350 Rumsey Rd., Toronto, ON, Canada M4G 1R8. Telephone 416-424-3855 ext. 3493; email vwright@bloorviewmacmillan.on.ca
Enabler (Steinfeld et al., 1979)	HUD User P.O. Box 6091, Germantown, MD 20850
Enviro-FIM and *Usability Rating Scale* (Steinfeld & Danford, 1997)	Dr. E. Steinfeld, Department of Architecture, 382 Hayes Hall, 3435 Main St., Buffalo, NY 14214
The Travel Enabler (OT) (Iwarsson & Isacsson, 1996)	*The Enabler.* Manual and assessment form. Swedish revised occupational therapy version. Available in English from Dr. S. Iwarsson, Lund University, Sweden. Fax: 001-46-46-222-1959 email: Luc.Noreau@pht.ulaval.ca
Measuring the Quality of the Environment (*MQE*) (Fougerollas et al., 1997)	
Multilevel Assessment Instrument (*MAI*) (Lawton et al., 1982)	Philadelphia Geriatric Center, 5301 Old York Rd., Philadelphia, PA 19141, 215-455-6162
Multiphasic Environmental Assessment Procedure (*MEAP*):	Evaluating residential facilities: the Multiphasic Environmental Assessment Procedure. Thousand Oaks, CA: Sage.
Physical Architectural Features Checklist	(Moos & Lemke, 1996)
POE	Cooper, Ahrentzen, & Hasselkus, 1991
Readily Achievable Checklist (Cronburg, Barnett, & Goldman, 1993)	Cronburg et al., 1993. CAT Adaptive Environments Center, 374 Congress Street, Suite 301, Boston, MA 02210. Telephone: 617-695-1225

*Unique instrument of measure with incomplete psychometric validation.

TABLE 10-3
Assessments of Access to Workplace

Assessment	Source
Americans with Disabilities Act Work-Site Assessment (Jacobs & Bettencourt, 1999)	Appendix B. *Ergonomics for Therapists.* (2nd ed., pp. 345–354). Boston: Butterworth-Heinemann.
Enabler (Steinfeld et al., 1979)	HUD User, P.O. Box 6091, Germantown, MD 20850
Job Analysis During Employer Site Visit (Jacobs & Bettencourt, 1999)	Appendix C
Life Stressors and Social Resources Inventory—Adult Form (*LISRES*-A) (Moos, 1995)	Psychological Assessment Resources Inc., P.O. Box 998, Odessa, FL, 800-311-TEST (800-311-8378)
POE	Cooper, Ahrentzen, & Hasselkus, 1991
Work Environment Impact Scale (*WEIS*) (Corner, Kielhofner, & Lin, 1997)	Moore-Corner et al., 1998. Model of Human Occupational Clearinghouse, University of Illinois at Chicago.
Work Environment Scale (*WES*), 3rd ed. (Moos, 1993)	Consulting Psychologists Press, 3803 E. Bayshore Rd., Palo Alto, CA 94303

*Unique instrument of measure with incomplete psychometric validation.

Universal Assessments

Universal assessments are those that can be used to evaluate the environmental needs of any group using all sizes and types of settings. They usually do not require specific skills or knowledge of terminology to administer. Such measures are particularly useful when multidisciplinary teams are involved.

The Enabler

A useful universal assessment, the *Enabler* provides a multiprofessional approach to conceptualizing disability and a mechanism for identifying problems of access to the physical environment (Steinfeld et al., 1979). The 13 matrices of the tool describe all possible access conditions and rank the difficulty of access that individuals with a variety of disabilities may encounter (see Fig. 10-3). The P/E concepts emphasized are safety, accessibility, mobility, and performance. This well-developed measure was the byproduct of an extensive literature review and work conducted by Steinfeld et al. (1979) to develop barrier-free design standards for the U.S. Department of Housing and Urban Development; however, it has never undergone extensive psychometric testing (Cooper, Cohen & Hasselkus, 1991). The *Enabler* has recently been modified for use as a specific occupational therapy home access measure (Iwarsson & Isaacson, 1996). This version, the *Housing*

Enabler, has been tested repeatedly in Sweden and found to be psychometrically sound and clinically useful, although usefulness may be somewhat limited in North America by the need for therapists to be trained by Iwarsson in the use of the instrument (Cooper et al., 2001).

Postoccupancy Evaluation

Postoccupancy evaluation (POE) is a term used by architects, social scientists, and others working in environment and behavior to describe a generic, comprehensive, and systematic approach to assessing any physical environment to determine P/E fit (Cooper, Ahrentzen, & Hasselkus, 1991). It is, therefore, a process model rather than a specific assessment. A POE may be simple (individual home), somewhat complex (nursing home), or highly complex (school system or several hospitals). A POE uses a variety of instruments and strategies to gather data on the environment and user needs. The reliability and validity of the results depend on whether the total battery (e.g., Moos & Lemke, 1996) or components of the battery have undergone such testing.

Current practice calls on occupational therapists to administer simple POEs (e.g., home accessibility evaluations). As occupational therapy practice expands further into community issues, therapists will likely be called on to conduct broader and more extensive environmental

---

BOX 10-1
Example of an Evaluation of a Measurement

Name	*Enviro-FIM* and *Usability Rating Scale (URS)* (Steinfeld & Danford, 1997)
Type	Home and community
Availability	Dr. E. Steinfeld, Department of Architecture, 382 Hayes Hall, 3435 Main Street, Buffalo, NY 14214
Purpose	Measures the influence of architectural design on functional performance of people with disabilities (personal care, mobility, accessibility of indoor architecture, self-management)
Focus	Uses format of modified *International Classification of Impairment Disability and Handicap* (Fougerollas et al., 1997)
Clinical utility	Requires therapist to observe client completing five specific ADL tasks involving access to physical environment and to complete a decision tree for these. The client rates his or her performance on each task. Time to complete assessment depends on the time the client needs to complete the tasks. Scale construction (ordinal) is excellent and based on widely used measures of functional ability used in rehabilitation. Cost is still to be determined.
Standardization	Reliability: one study completed with the *Enviro-FIM* with excellent ICC observer scores; one study completed with each tool indicating high levels of test–retest agreement. Validity: extensive testing indicates excellent content validity for the *Enviro-FIM*. One study completed for each tool on construct validity (adequate). These reveal that the *Enviro-FIM* scores measure the influence of design on performance and the *URS* can discriminate between ease and difficulty of access and between user groups. Manual is under development.
Rating	Adequate to excellent. The *Enviro-FIM* and *URS* have shown strong psychometric properties with initial testing. They show promise of good clinical utility when used in conjunction with the *FIM* (Uniform Data Systems, 1993) to assess the effect of architecture on the function of people with disabilities.

For additional information on the assessment of many of the other measures listed in this chapter see Cooper et al. (2001).

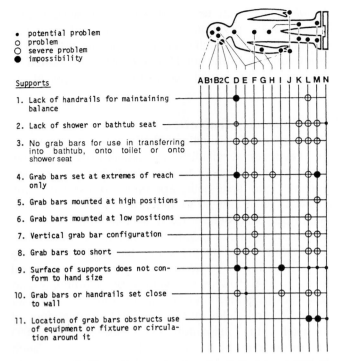

- • potential problem
- ○ problem
- ⊘ severe problem
- ● impossibility

Supports

1. Lack of handrails for maintaining balance
2. Lack of shower or bathtub seat
3. No grab bars for use in transferring into bathtub, onto toilet or onto shower seat
4. Grab bars set at extremes of reach only
5. Grab bars mounted at high positions
6. Grab bars mounted at low positions
7. Vertical grab bar configuration
8. Grab bars too short
9. Surface of supports does not conform to hand size
10. Grab bars or handrails set close to wall
11. Location of grab bars obstructs use of equipment or fixture or circulation around it

Figure 10-3 *Enabler* problem matrix using a hypothetical case. A, difficulty interpreting information; B1, severe loss of sight; B2, complete loss of sight; C, severe loss of hearing; D, prevalence of poor balance; E, incoordination; F, limitations of stamina; G, difficulty moving head; H, difficulty reaching with arms; I, difficulty in handling and fingering; J, loss of upper extremity skills; K, difficulty bending, kneeling, and so on; L, reliance on walking aids; M, inability to use lower extremities; N, extremes of size and weight. (Reprinted from Steinfeld, E., Schroeder, S., Duncan, J., Faste, R., Chollet, D., Bishop, M., Wirth, P., & Cardell, P. [1979]. *Access to the Built Environment: A Review of the Literature* [HUD #660]. Washington: U.S. Government Printing Office.)

assessments of this type as part of multidisciplinary teams.

Computerized Assessments

EASE3 (Lifease, 1999) consists of a computerized notebook that responds to assessment information on clients and their home environment. The program, which is updated regularly, offers options for measurement and modifications, usually in the form of assistive devices. Preliminary psychometric work is under way.

Assessment of Access to Home

A home assessment completed by an occupational therapist can be pivotal in the rehabilitation program of a client with a disability and critical to injury prevention for the elderly (Head & Patterson, 1997; Rogers et al., 1997). The occupational therapist evaluates home accessibility, safety, and housing options to match the individual's abilities and needs with the environmental

demands of the home. Park et al. (1994) advise that assessment should take place in the client's home, as this improves accuracy and provides the occupational therapist with a greater understanding of the client's situation.

Standardized home assessments are available for the occupational therapist to use with clients and families to identify occupational performance problems in the home. Table 10-1 lists the home assessments we selected on the basis of their psychometric properties and tells where to obtain them. The assessments vary slightly in focus and should be chosen to suit the client's requirements. The *Assessment Tool* (Canada Mortgage and Housing Corporation, 1989), the *Home Modification Workbook* (Adaptive Home Environments Center, 1988), the *Source Book* (Kelly & Snell, 1989) and EASE3 (Lifease, 1999) are four measures that address environmental factors in relation to clients' needs and ability. Figure 10-4 provides an example from the *Source Book*. It illustrates the process using information from the case study presented in this chapter.

Housing options can also be reviewed to determine the best fit for clients with disabilities. Options are numerous, and most communities have innovative, barrier-free housing with access to attendant care and other support services, meals, and recreation. Many seniors and persons with severe physical disabilities choose to live in these housing projects, since they can more easily achieve independence within a supportive system. Transitional housing programs also assist clients to develop independent living skills and to develop knowledge of resources. The occupational therapist can use assessment tools such as the *Housing Enabler* (Iwarsson & Isacsson, 1996) and the *Assessment Tool* (Canada Mortgage and Housing Corporation, 1989) to determine clients' needs and ensure that accessibility is achieved.

The ADA does not apply to housing, but the Fair Housing Act Amendments (FHAA) (1995) provide accessibility standards for rental facilities, such as apartment buildings. The FHAA does not fully remove barriers to accessibility but has increased the housing options for persons with physical disabilities (Mace, 1998). Occupational therapists conducting an environmental assessment of an apartment must also remember to evaluate building access, parking, halls, facilities, and fire routes. The *Accessibility Checklist* (Goltsman et al., 1992) can be used to accomplish this.

Assessment of Access to Community

Occupational therapists have not been extensively involved in changing environments to facilitate their clients' abilities to engage in roles within their communities. However, this is clearly within their scope of practice and is becoming more widespread. For example, occupational therapists have a role to educate and empower clients about their civil rights as defined by such legislation as the ADA (McClain et al., 1999). This may be particularly important for achieving community participation and the realization of self-enhancement roles. Title III of the ADA guarantees access to the community and requires the implementation of reasonable accommodations to accomplish this (U.S. Department of Justice, 1991). Occupational therapists can assume consultation or advocacy roles with groups seeking to make educational, cultural, commercial, and religious facilities accessible.

Persons with disabilities may not be aware that community businesses and services must be made accessible to them (McClain, et al., 1999). For example, those with disabilities should have access to shopping for basic needs and to public washrooms when visiting public places. The *Assessment Tool* (Canada Mortgage and Housing Corporation, 1989) and *Accessibility Checklist* (Goltsman et al., 1992) shown in Figures 10-5 and 10-6, are instruments that can be used to evaluate the accessibility of these services.

The transportation needs of persons with disabilities should not be overlooked. Useful information about standards and devices for vehicular transportation for persons with physical disabilities can be sought from the U.S. Department of Transportation and the National Highway Traffic Safety Administration (see Resources). Commercial transportation companies, such as airlines, buses, and trains, must also comply with accessibility standards and make reasonable accommodations according to the ADA.

Text continued on p. 249.

Figure 10-4 Case example of home assessment. (Reprinted with permission from Kelly, C., & Snell, K. [1989]. *The Source Book: Architectural Guidelines for Barrier-Free Design.* Toronto: Barrier-Free Design Centre.)

(continued)

PART II: Description of Activities

Please check the box that best describes how you would normally do the activity.

This section asks questions about how you do certain activities in specific rooms in your home. Please tell us as much as you can about your abilities, and the problems or solutions you have come up with in your house.

1. The Site

I can:	Does not apply	Can manage alone	Can manage with equipment (wheelchair, reacher, etc.)	Can manage with someone helping	Cannot manage at all
Move around outside the house				✓	
Manage curbs				✓	
Manage rough ground				✓	
Manage slopes				✓	
Manage ice/snow				✓	
Carry things outdoors				✓	
Get into and out of a car				✓	
Load and unload things into and out of a car				✓	
Use a bus, or special transportation service			✓		
Drive a car					✓

Do you have any special outdoor interests or hobbies?

Going to the store for groceries and personal items such as toiletries. Playing bridge weekly with friends; visiting with friends and family.

Do you have any special needs when going out of doors? (ie. Sensitive to sun)

Does not feel safe nor capable of getting around community without someone to assist her.

Do you use a scooter or wheelchair when you are outside? Please describe.

Uses manual wheelchair, which she can propel herself for short distances; typically someone pushes her.

What are the biggest problems to you when you are outside, or in your yard?

Carrying items while propelling w/c; getting in + out of car

2. Front and Back Door

I can:

	Does not apply	Can manage alone	Can manage with equipment (wheelchair, reacher, etc.)	Can manage with someone helping	Cannot manage at all
Climb up stairs	✓				
Go down stairs	✓				
Go up a ramp				✓	
Go down a ramp				✓	
Use a hand rail			✓		
Open and go through a door		✓			
Use a key		✓			
Use the door lock		✓			
Use the door knob		✓			
Use lever handles		✓			
Reach and use the mailbox				✓	
Walk, (wheel) over the lip at the door				✓	

What are the biggest problems you now have when going in and/or out of your house.

Propelling w/c or walk with quad cane over sloped surfaces (e.g. ramp) and over raised lip at entrance ways.

3. Hallways and Inside Doors

I can:

	Does not apply	Can manage alone	Can manage with equipment (wheelchair, reacher, etc.)	Can manage with someone helping	Cannot manage at all
Manage carpeted areas			✓		
Manage hallways			✓		
Open and go through doors to rooms		✓			
Manage door knobs		✓			
Manage lever handles		✓			

When I move from room to room I use a:

✓ cane ☐ crutches ☐ artificial limb ☐ manual/electric wheelchair

☐ power scooter ☐ other

What are the biggest problems you now have when going from room to room in your house?

Fear that she may slip when walking over scatter rugs in hallways and living room

4. Stairs

I can:

	Does not apply	Can manage alone	Can manage with equipment (wheelchair, reacher, etc.)	Can manage with someone helping	Cannot manage at all
Climb up stairs				✓	
Go down stairs				✓	
Use a handrail				✓	
Use elevator controls		✓			
Use a lift device	✓				

Is going from one level up or down to another level of your house very important to you? How do you manage going up or down?

Must use elevator within apartment building to get to and from apartment. Apartment is on one level.

What are the biggest problems you now have when going from one level to another in your house?

Rarely uses stairs in apartment building. Would need to use stairs in the event of fire.

Figure 10-4 *(Continued).*

5. Bathroom

I can:	Does not apply	Can manage alone	Can manage with equipment (wheelchair, reacher, etc.)	Can manage with someone helping	Cannot manage at all
Turn the lights on and off	☐	☑	☐	☐	☐
Use the electrical outlets	☐	☑	☐	☐	☐
Use the cabinets and closets	☐	☐	☐	☑	☐
See myself in the mirror	☐	☑	☐	☐	☐
Wash hands and face and brush my teeth	☐	☐	☑	☐	☐
Use taps	☐	☑	☐	☐	☐
Use the sink	☐	☑	☐	☐	☐
Get on the toilet	☐	☐	☑	☐	☐
Get off the toilet	☐	☐	☑	☐	☐
Manage conventional toileting	☐	☐	☑	☐	☐
Reach the toilet paper	☐	☐	☑	☐	☐
Use grab bars	☐	☐	☑	☐	☐
Get into the bath tub	☐	☐	☐	☑	☐
Get out of the bath tub	☐	☐	☐	☑	☐
Take a bath	☐	☐	☐	☑	☐
Get into the shower	☐	☐	☐	☑	☐
Get out of the shower	☐	☐	☐	☑	☐
Take a shower	☐	☐	☐	☑	☐
Use taps	☐	☐	☐	☑	☐
Dry off after a bath/shower	☐	☐	☐	☑	☐
Get dressed after a bath/shower	☐	☐	☐	☑	☐

Do you have any special needs or procedures in the bathroom?

Attendant or husband assist with bathing; grab bars and bath bench have been installed.

What are the biggest problems you now have when using the bathroom in your house?

Balance during performance of bathroom tasks and fear of falling during tub or shower transfers.

6. Kitchen

I can:	Does not apply	Can manage alone	Can manage with equipment (wheelchair, reacher, etc.)	Can manage with someone helping	Cannot manage at all
Turn the lights on and off	☐	☑	☐	☐	☐
Use the electrical outlets	☐	☑	☐	☐	☐
Reach the garbage	☐	☑	☐	☐	☐
Move around in the kitchen	☐	☐	☑	☐	☐
Take food out of the fridge	☐	☐	☐	☑	☐
Take food out of the freezer	☐	☐	☐	☑	☐
Take things out of the cupboards	☐	☐	☐	☑	☐
Wipe the counters	☐	☐	☐	☑	☐
Wash dishes	☐	☐	☐	☑	☐
Use the dishwasher	☐	☐	☐	☑	☐
Clean the floor	☐	☐	☐	☑	☐

Figure 10-4 *(Continued).*

6. Kitchen (cont'd)

I can:

	Does not apply	Can manage alone	Can manage with equipment (wheelchair, reacher, etc.)	Can manage with someone helping	Cannot manage at all
Open cans, bottles, boxes	☐	☐	☑	☐	☐
Mix ingredients in a bowl	☐	☐	☑	☐	☐
Fill pot with water	☐	☐	☐	☑	☐
Place pot on stove	☐	☐	☐	☑	☐
Turn stove on and off	☐	☐	☑	☐	☐
Use a microwave	☐	☐	☐	☑	☐
Open and close oven door	☐	☑	☐	☐	☐
Put pan in oven	☐	☐	☐	☑	☐
Pour hot water from a pot	☐	☐	☐	☑	☐
Cook on stove top	☐	☐	☐	☑	☐
Use range fan	☐	☑	☐	☐	☐
Set the table	☐	☐	☐	☑	☐
Eat in the kitchen	☐	☐	☑	☐	☐
Eat in the dining room	☐	☐	☑	☐	☐
Prepare a meal	☐	☐	☐	☑	☐
Prepare a snack	☐	☐	☑	☐	☐
Feed myself	☐	☑	☐	☐	☐

Do you have any special needs in the kitchen?

Cannot reach back of 2nd shelf nor lower shelves — need to re-arrange kitchen to enable easier access to items used daily

Is using the kitchen very important to you?

Meal preparation has been an important occupation throughout life to fulfill self-maintenance and self-enhancement roles

What are the biggest problems you now have when using the kitchen in your house?

Cannot safely reach for and access items from many cupboards and fridge without help. Cannot stand safely at counter to prepare meals.

7. Living Room or Family Room

I can:

	Does not apply	Can manage alone	Can manage with equipment (wheelchair, reacher, etc.)	Can manage with someone helping	Cannot manage at all
Get into the living room	☐	☐	☑	☐	☐
Use the T.V. controls	☐	☑	☐	☐	☐
Use the radio/stereo controls	☐	☑	☐	☐	☐
Use the telephone	☐	☐	☐	☑	☐
Turn the lights on and off	☐	☑	☐	☐	☐
Move around in the living room	☐	☐	☑	☐	☐
Use the living room chairs	☐	☑	☐	☐	☐

What are the biggest problems you now have when using the living room or family room in your house?

Fear of tripping or slipping on scatter rugs. Getting up and down from couch; accessing the phone as it is not placed near chair that Mrs. P. typically used.

Figure 10-4 *(Continued).*

8. Bedroom

I can:	Does not apply	Can manage alone	Can manage with equipment (wheelchair, reacher, etc.)	Can manage with someone helping	Cannot manage at all
Turn lights on and off	☐	☑	☐	☐	☐
Use electrical outlets	☐	☐	☐	☑	☐
Open and close windows	☐	☑	☐	☐	☐
Pull drapes open and closed	☐	☑	☐	☐	☐
Get into my bedroom	☐	☐	☑	☐	☐
Reach clothes in closet	☐	☐	☐	☑	☐
Open drawers	☐	☐	☐	☑	☐
Dress myself	☐	☐	☐	☑	☐
Undress myself	☐	☐	☐	☑	☐
Get into bed	☐	☐	☑	☐	☐
Get out of bed	☐	☐	☑	☐	☐
Get into the other bedrooms in the house	☐	☐	☐	☑	☐

What are the biggest problems you now have when using your bedroom?

The bedroom is small with a lot of furniture and limited space to manuver using cane. Cannot reach clothes or other items from closet.

9. Laundry

I can:	Does not apply	Can manage alone	Can manage with equipment (wheelchair, reacher, etc.)	Can manage with someone helping	Cannot manage at all
Get into the laundry room	☐	☐	☑	☐	☐
Turn the lights on and off	☐	☑	☐	☐	☐
Use the electrical outlets	☑	☐	☐	☐	☐
Reach the closets and cupboards	☐	☐	☐	☑	☐
Use the washer and dryer controls	☐	☑	☐	☐	☐
Put the laundry in the machine	☐	☐	☐	☑	☐
Take the laundry out of the machine	☐	☐	☐	☑	☐
Reach the taps	☐	☐	☐	☑	☐
Do hand laundry	☐	☐	☐	☑	☐
Do the ironing	☐	☐	☐	☑	☐

What are the biggest problems you now have when doing the laundry?

Cannot carry loads of laundry to + from laundry room, which is down hall from apartment. Cannot maintain safe standing balance while doing bi manual tasks such as ironing

Figure 10-4 *(Continued).*

Do you purchase/store groceries?
☐ No   ☐ Yes   ☐ N.A.

		Recommendations	
Functional Limitations	Home Checklist	Housing	Other
☐ Poor tolerance ☐ Muscle weakness ☐ Poor balance ☐ Reduced mobility ☐ Wheelchair dependent ☐ Poor vision	☐ Adequate/usable re-frigerator and cup-board storage space for storing items ☐ Sufficient food supply to last until next shop-ping day ☐ Bulletin board near storage for list	☐ Adequate cold storage space for 1 week (or more) of supplies ☐ Increase storage space (add pantry, shelves, baskets, etc.)	☐ Walking aids (walker with basket) ☐ Shopping cart ☐ Meals on Wheels ☐ List of local stores that deliver ☐ List of local stores that take tele-phone orders ☐ Emergency pack ☐ Escort to store ☐ Assistance

Figure 10-5 Assessing the functional ability to purchase and/or go to the store for groceries. (Reprinted with permission from Canada Mortgage and Housing Corporation [1989]. *The Assessment Tool.*)

Complies	Does Not Comply	Actual Measure	Space around Toilet
☐	☐	____	1. Clear space from the side of the toilet to the sink is 28 inches minimum. or Clear space from one side of the toilet to the wall is 32 inches.
☐	☐	____	2. Clear space from the other wall to the center of the toilet is 18 inches.
☐	☐	____	3. Clear space in front of the toilet is 48 inches minimum.
☐	☐	____	4. Toilet seat height is 17 to 19 inches. (Note height of lifts if pro-vided: ____.)
☐	☐	____	5. Flush controls are located on wide side of the toilet and 44 inches maxi-mum above floor.
☐	☐	____	6. Toilet paper turns freely, is 12 inches maximum in front of the toilet, and is 40 inches maximum high.
☐	☐	____	7. Seat cover dispenser is 40 inches maximum above the floor.
			8. Grab Bars
☐	☐	____	a. Bars are mounted 33 inches above the floor, parallel to the floor sur-face (36 inches rear grab bar height acceptable if tank-type toilet).
☐	☐	____	b. Rear grab bar is 36 inches minimum long.
☐	☐	____	c. Side grab bar is 42 inches minimum long.
☐	☐	____	d. Side grab bars are positioned so the front end is 24 inches minimum in front of the toilet.
☐	☐	____	e. Diameter of bars is 1¼ to 1½ inches. or Bars provide an equivalent gripping surface with a ⅛-inch minimum edge radius.
☐	☐	____	f. Space between the wall and the grab bar is 1½ inches.
☐	☐		g. Grab bars do not rotate in fittings.
☐	☐		h. Grab bars have rounded and nonabrasive surfaces.
☐	☐		i. Grab bars will withstand 250-pound load.

Figure 10-6 Assessment of single-user restroom. (Reprinted with permission from Goltsman, S. M., Gilbert, T. A., & Wohlford. S. D. [1992]. *The Accessibility Checklist: An Evaluating System for Buildings and Outdoor Settings.* Berkeley: MIG Communications.)

The occupational therapist can assess community structures with tools such as the *Readily Achievable Checklist* (Cronburg et al., 1993) and the *Enviro-FIM* and *Usability Rating Scale* (Steinfeld & Danforth, 1997) to determine whether they meet accessibility standards. The guidelines set forth in *Achieving Physical and Communication Accessibility* (Adaptive Environments Center, 1995) also suggest ways to make reasonable accommodations in community structures. An instrument for assessing accessibility of urban public transport is under development in Sweden by occupational therapist Susanne Iwarsson and her colleagues. This too is based on the *Enabler* (Steinfeld et al., 1979); it is called the *Travel Chain Enabler*. A full list of these assessment instruments and their sources is provided in Table 10-2.

Assessment of Access to Workplace

Occupational therapists play an important part in enabling clients to fulfill self-advancement roles (Jacobs & Bettencourt, 1999) by assisting them to seek work or return to work. The ADA strongly supports the occupational therapist's efforts to reduce barriers in the workplace and to recommend methods of reasonable accommodation to support workers with physical disabilities (Jacobs & Bettencourt). Occupational therapy interventions in the workplace focus mainly on ergonomics (Jacobs & Bettencourt), the functional aspects of work assessment, and environmental assessments to determine barriers to accessibility (Velozo, 1993).

BOX 10-3
PROCEDURES FOR PRACTICE

Supplies and Materials Required for Site Visit

- Paper, pens, pencils
- Clipboard
- Measuring tape
- Stopwatch
- Force gauge dynamometer
- Videotape recorder, tapes, log
- Instant camera, film, batteries
- Job description and duties list
- Charts, assessment forms to record findings
- List of evaluation activities and questions

CLINICAL REASONING
in Occupational Therapy Practice

Professional Issues to Consider When Making a Work Site Assessment

During a site visit, the occupational therapist observed department store clerks performing a full range of duties. What environmental factors should be noted and evaluated? In particular, consider transportation, access to the building, offices, and public areas, workstations and work areas, and the essential tasks of the job. What methods should be used to collect data? What additional sources of information could be sought and considered to determine the degree of P/E fit present?

BOX 10-2
PROCEDURES FOR PRACTICE

Preparing for a Site Visit

The occupational therapist is asked to perform a work site assessment to determine the risk factors contributing to an unusually high number of cumulative trauma disorders impeding productivity (Meuller, 1990).
Background Information to Be Gathered in Advance

- Description of job (e.g., duties, activities, temporal patterns, risks)
- Workstation (e.g., structure, ambiance)
- Work site (e.g., location, access, physical layout, transportation)
- Workers' perspective (e.g., expectations, issues)
- Employer or supervisor's perspective (e.g., expectations, issues)
- Occupational therapist's capabilities and limitations (e.g., experience, resources)
- Relevant legislation

Accessibility can be assessed using a tool such as the *Readily Achievable Checklist* (Cronburg et al., 1993) to determine access to parking, entranceways, toilets, cafeterias, and other necessary areas of the building. Tools such as the *ADA Work-Site Assessment* (Jacobs & Bettencourt, 1999) and the *Accessibility Checklist* (Goltsman et al., 1992) help the occupational therapist focus on physical barriers that prevent the worker from fulfilling the requirements of the job. Strategies such as workstation modifications and assistive technologies can be implemented to reduce performance barriers. A POE can be developed for large-scale projects. An expanded list of assessment measures and their source is provided in Table 10-3. Boxes 10-2 and 10-3 outline ways to prepare in for a work-site visit. The Clinical Reasoning box above presents issues around P/E fit and client activities that an occupational therapist would consider when making a workplace assessment.

Case Example

HOME VISIT

Client Information

Mrs. P. is a 75-year-old woman who ago sustained a right-sided cerebrovascular accident (CVA) 2 months with resultant left-sided hemiparesis. She was recently discharged from the rehabilitation center to an apartment that she shares with her husband. At the time of discharge, she required help with grooming, bathing, dressing, toileting, and bath transfers. Mrs. P.'s total *FIM* (Uniform Data System, 1993) score was 99 (Fig. 10-7). She can walk short distances using a quad cane and uses a wheelchair for community mobility. Mrs. P. has poor motor return in the left upper extremity, and because she is right dominant, now does most manual tasks with her right hand. Mr. P. and their daughter have been doing the housekeeping and most of the meal preparation. Recently, Mr. P. hired an attendant to work a few hours a day to assist with Mrs. P.'s personal care and to help with the housekeeping. The home health occupational therapist assessed the home. She also used the *COPM* (Law et al., 1994) to help Mrs. P. to establish priorities in bathing, using the toilet, meal preparation, laundry, and housekeeping, as goals for intervention. Mrs. P. notes that she doesn't like her husband to help with housekeeping and meal preparation. She has always looked after him, has always completed the household tasks, and does not like these changes in roles. These responsibilities have fulfilled both self-achievement and self-maintenance roles for Mrs. P. throughout her married life.

Description of Assessments

The *Home Assessment* (Kelly & Snell, 1989) was used to assess Mrs. P.'s occupational performance at home. This tool allowed the therapist to ask Mrs. P. how she performs specific tasks throughout all parts of her home and whether she has difficulties with access to certain areas, including entrance-ways, hallways, kitchen, and bathroom. Mrs. P. was also asked to identify her specific needs and main functional problems for every room of her apartment. Figure 10-4 shows the results of this assessment. Data were summarized for final conclusions and recommendations.

Results

The *Home Assessment* helped the occupational therapist to identify a number of problem areas in Mrs. P.'s apartment and access to the immediate community from her apartment. These were contributing to her difficulties with occupational functioning, as reported on the *COPM* and *FIM*. Mrs. P. needs help getting in and out of her apartment and can use a wheelchair successfully with some assistance of her husband. She goes on outings with her husband but still has not gone shopping for groceries or visited her friends. She can manage the elevator to her apartment and the doors and locks at the entrances to the building and apartment. In her apartment, Mrs. P. requires a considerable amount of help with her daily occupations. She wants help from the occupational therapist to determine strategies to make her more independent. Even though grab bars for the toilet and bath and a bath bench were installed prior to Mrs. P.'s discharge home, she continues to feel anxious about transfers because of slippery surfaces. The kitchen is poorly organized for the management of tasks with one hand, and Mrs. P. does not have a work surface where she can sit to prepare meals safely and efficiently. The bedroom is crowded and cluttered, and it is difficult for her to get what she needs. There are other obstacles to mobility throughout the apartment, such as side tables and scatter rugs in traveling zones. The laundry room is down the hall outside her apartment. She cannot do the laundry without a considerable amount of help.

Analysis of Results

The results of the home assessment confirmed problems identified by the *FIM* and *COPM* and added new information about personal and environmental factors that also contributed to Mrs. P.'s functional difficulties. This was used to formulate a more specific problem list and intervention plan.

Occupational Therapy Problem List

The following issues were identified:

► Decreased independence in self-care, particularly in bathing and toileting
► Decreased independence in instrumental activities of daily living at home, particularly in meal preparation, laundry, and housekeeping
► Physical barriers to independence identified in the kitchen and bathroom
► Limited funds available for assistive devices and home modifications
► Reluctance to modify the home and install assistive devices

Occupational Performance: Strengths and Weaknesses

Mrs. P. was highly motivated to gain more independence at home. She and her husband are both anxious to have her assume her previous roles at home and have expressed willingness to consider environmental adaptations. Although Mrs. P. does not want a lot of devices around the apartment, she sees that the suggested modifications for the kitchen and bathroom (grab bars and a bath bench) are necessary for her occupational functioning.

The therapist will help Mrs. P. establish functional goals. In particular, she wants to regain her ability to prepare meals. The therapist will have to consider the issues raised in the Clinical Reasoning Box. Having done so, she will recommend a number of modifications and assistive devices to improve Mrs. P.'s overall independence within her home. Their effect will be evaluated periodically. The cost of devices and modifications to the home should also be considered. Mr. P. has expressed an interest in comparison shopping for the assistive devices and has asked their son to make the home modifications where possible. EASE3 (Lifease,1998) can be used for these purposes.

CLINICAL REASONING
in Occupational Therapy Practice

Effects of the Physical Environment on Performance of Meal Preparation

Mrs. P. is a 75-year-old woman with left-sided hemiplegia who can walk short distances using a cane. Considering the occupational therapist's assessment findings, what would a therapist expect to observe if Mrs. P. tried to make a light meal in her apartment kitchen? What environmental factors might help or hinder her performance? How might family members help or hinder the process? What environmental modifications would you suggest to facilitate her task?

FIM™ instrument

	LEVELS		NO HELPER / HELPER
	7 Complete Independence (Timely, Safely) 6 Modified Independence (Device)		**NO HELPER**
	Modified Dependence 5 Supervision (Subject = 100%+) 4 Minimal Assist (Subject = 75%+) 3 Moderate Assist (Subject = 50%+) **Complete Dependence** 2 Maximal Assist (Subject =25%+) 1 Total Assist (Subject = less than 25%)		**HELPER**

	ADMISSION	DISCHARGE	FOLLOW-UP
Self-Care			N/A
A. Eating	5	6	
B Grooming	3	4	
C. Bathing	2	3	
D. Dressing - Upper Body	3	4	
E. Dressing - Lower Body	2	4	
F. Toileting	4	5	
Sphincter Control			
G. Bladder Management	5	7	
H. Bowel Management	5	7	
Transfers			
I. Bed, Chair, Wheelchair	3	6	
J. Toilet	3	6	
K. Tub, Shower	1	4	
Locomotion			
L. Walk/Wheelchair	2 W	6 B	W Walk C Wheelchair B Both
M. Stairs	2	5	
Motor Subtotal Score	40	67	
Communication			
N. Comprehension	7 B	7 B	A Auditory V Visual B Both
O. Expression	7 B	7 B	V Vocal N Nonvocal B Both
Social Cognition			
P. Social Interaction	7	7	
Q. Problem Solving	4	5	
R. Memory	5	6	
Cognitive Subtotal Score	30	32	
TOTAL FIM Score	70	99	

NOTE: Leave no blanks. Enter 1 if patient not testable due to risk

Figure 10-7 Case example of FIM™ assessment. (Reprinted with permission from Uniform Data System for Medical Rehabilitation, Buffalo, NY [1993].)

Looking Ahead

Many occupational therapists rely mainly on experience, observation, and interviews when called on to evaluate the environment. While these strategies are necessary components of good practice, they cannot stand alone. The use of well-validated, standardized instruments is also necessary. Information on the reliability and validity of measures changes constantly and may not be easily available to the busy practitioner. It is reasonable to suggest that in the future, summaries of data should be readily available for clinicians on computer programs or the Internet. These will greatly facilitate the selection of appropriate and well-tested measures.

Summary Review Questions

1. Why would an occupational therapist assess the physical environment?
2. List seven examples of environmental barriers that a person with mobility impairment might encounter when returning to work.
3. List seven examples of environmental supports that would allow a senior with arthritis to continue to live at home.
4. How can you be sure that an assessment provides you with information you can trust?
5. What should you look for in an assessment tool to ensure that your results will be consistent with those of another occupational therapist using the same assessment?
6. What factors contribute to clinical utility of an assessment instrument?
7. What assessments would you use to evaluate whether a client with a spinal cord injury can live independently in the community?
8. As an occupational therapist consultant to an assisted-living facility, what assistance could you offer the facility's administration regarding their plans to renovate the building?
9. What are some reasonable accommodations mandated by the ADA with which occupational therapists should be familiar?

Resources

Universal Design Resource Notebook

To inquire or order call Adaptive Environments · 617-695-1225
http//www.adaptenv.org/publist.htm

The ADA Core Curriculum

This is a comprehensive set of presentation materials covering every title of the ADA. Available through Adaptive Environments ($425).

Revised 2/96. For training on the core curriculum contact the Disability and Technical Assistance Centers at 800-949- 4ADA.

ADA Compliance Guides

For example, see those addressed by the Adaptive Environments Center (1992), Bartels & Easry (1992), and Texas Governor's Committee for Disabled Persons, 1992.

Website: Critical Review Process and Form

CanChild, McMaster University, Hamilton, ON
Form: www.fhs.mcmaster.ca/canchild/publications/measrate.pdf
Guideline: www.fhs.mcmaster.ca/canchild/publications/measguid.pdf

Transportation Websites

For additional information see U.S. Department of Transportation (http://www.dot.gov), 202-366-4000; National Highway Traffic Safety Administration (http://www.nhtsa.dot.gov/)

References

Adaptive Environments Center. (1988). *Home Modification Workbook.* Boston: Author.

Adaptive Environments Center (1992). *The Americans With Disabilities Act Checklist for Readily Achievable Barrier Removal.* Washington: National Institute on Disability and Rehabilitation Research.

Adaptive Environments Center (1993). *Readily Achievable Checklist: A Survey for Accessibility* (rev. ed.). Boston: Author.

Adaptive Environments Center (1995). *Achieving Physical and Communication Accessibility.* Boston: Author.

Aja, D. (1995). Revised NIOSH equation for the design and evaluation of manual lifting tasks. In K. Jacobs & C. M. Bettencourt (Eds.). *Ergonomics for Therapists* (pp.115–136). Newton, MA: Butterworth-Heinemann.

Americans With Disabilities Act. (1990). *Public Law 101–336, 42* U.S.C. 12101.

American National Standards Institute (1998). *Accessible and Usable Buildings and Facilities.* New York: ANSI. ICC A117.1.

American Occupational Therapy Association (1995). *Developing, Maintaining, and Updating Competency in Occupational Therapy: A Guide to Self-Appraisal.* Bethesda, MA: Author.

American Occupational Therapy Association (1998). *Standards for an Accredited Educational Program for the Occupational Therapist.* Adopted by the Accreditation Council for Occupational Therapy Education. Bethesda, MD: Author.

Bartels, E. C. & Easry, N. F. (1992). *Americans With Disabilities Act: Examples of Reasonable Accommodation.* Boston: Massachusetts Rehabilitation Commission, Legal Department.

Caldwell, B. M., & Bradley, R. H. (1988). Using the HOME inventory to assess family environment. *Pediatric Nursing, 14,* 97–102.

Canadian Association of Occupational Therapists (1996). Profile of Occupational Therapy Practice in Canada. *Canadian Journal of Occupational Therapy, 63, 2,* 79–95.

Canadian Association of Occupational Therapists (1997). Enabling occupation: An occupational therapy perspective. Ottawa: Author.

Canada Mortgage and Housing Corporation (1989). *Maintaining Seniors' Independence: A Guide to Home Adaptations.* Ottawa: Author.

Clemson, L. (1997). *Home Fall Hazards: A Guide to Identifying Fall hazards in the Homes of Elderly People and an Accompaniment to the Assessment Tool,* The Westmead Home Safety Assessment. West Brunswick, Australia: Coordinates.

Cooper, B. A., Cohen, U., & Hasselkus, B. R. (1991). Barrier-free design: A review and critique of the occupational therapy perspective. *American Journal of Occupational Therapy, 45,* 344–350.

Cooper, B. A., Ahrentzen, S., & Hasselkus, B. R. (1991). Post-occupancy evaluation: An environment-behaviour technique for assessing the built environment. *Canadian Journal of Occupational Therapy, 58*, 181–188.

Cooper, B., Letts, L., Rigby, P., Stewart, D., & Strong, S. (2001). Measuring environmental factors. In M. Law, C. Baum, & W. Dunn (Eds.). *Measuring Occupational Performance*, pp. 229–256. Thorofare, NJ: Slack.

Corner, R., Kielhofner, G., & Lin, F.-L. (1997). Construct validity of a work environment impact scale. *Work, 9*, 21–34.

Cronburg, J., Barnett, J., & Goldman, N. (1993). *Readily Achievable Checklist: A Survey for Accessibility.* Boston: Adaptive Environments Center.

Dunn, W., Brown, C., & McGuigan, A. (1994). The ecology of human performance: A framework for considering the effect of context. *American Journal of Occupational Therapy, 48*, 595–607.

Fair Housing Act Amendments. (1995). 42 U.S.C. Sec. 3601.

Fougerollas, P., Noreau, L., & St. Michael, G. (1997). User guide: The Assessment of Life Habits (LIFE-H2.1) and Measurement of the Quality of the Environment (MQE). *ICIDH and Environmental Factors Network, 9*, 6–19.

Goltsman, S. M., Gilbert, T. A., & Wohlford, S. D. (1992). *The Accessibility Checklist: An Evaluating System for Buildings and Outdoor Settings.* Berkeley: M. I. G. Communications.

Gowland, C., King, G., King, S., Law, M., Letts, L., Mackinnon, L., Rosenbaum, P., & Russell, D. (1991). *Review of selected measures in neurodevelopmental rehabilitation research. Report 91–2.* McMaster University, Hamilton, Ont.: Neurodevelopmental Clinical Research Unit (Now called Can Child).

Head, J., & Patterson, V. (1997). Performance context and its role in treatment planning. *American Journal of Occupational Therapy, 51*, 453–457.

Iwarsson, S., & Isacsson, A. (1996). Development of a novel instrument for occupational therapy assessment of the physical environment in the home: a methodologic study on "The Enabler." *Occupational Therapy Journal of Research, 16*, 40, 227–244.

Jacobs, K., & Bettencourt, C. M. (Eds.). (1999). *Ergonomics for Therapists.* Newton, MA: Butterworth-Heinemann.

Kalscheur, J. A. (1991). Benefits of the Americans with Disabilities Act of 1990 for children and adolescents with disabilities. *American Journal of Occupational Therapy, 46*, 419–426.

Kelly, C., & Snell, K. (1989). *The Source Book: Architectural Guidelines for Barrier-Free Design.* Toronto: Barrier-Free Design Centre.

Law, M., Baptiste, S., Carswell, A., McColl, M. A., Polatajko, H., & Pollack, N. (1994). *Canadian Occupational Performance Measure* (2nd ed.). Toronto: CAOT.

Law, M., Cooper, B., Strong, S., Stewart, D., Rigby, P., & Letts, L. (1996). The Person-Environment-Occupation Model: A transactive approach to occupational performance. *Canadian Journal of Occupational Therapy, 63* (1), 9–23.

Lawton, M. P., Moss, M., Fulcomer, M., & Kleban, M. H. (1982). A research and service oriented Multilevel Assessment Instrument. *Journal of Gerontology, 37*, 91–99.

Lifease (1999). Ease 3.0 software. St. Paul, MN: Author.

Mace, R. L. (1998). Universal design in housing. *Assistive Technology, 10*, 21–28.

Maltais, D., Trickey, F., & Robitaille, Y. (1988). Élaboration d'une grille d'analyse du logement des personnes agées en perte d'autonomie physique. Ottawa: Canada Mortgage and Housing Corporation.

McClain, L., Cram, A., Wood, J., & Taylor, M. (1999). Wheelchair accessibility: Living the experience in the community. *Occupational Therapy Journal of Research, 18*, 25–43.

Moore-Corner, R. A., Keilhofner, G., & Olsen, L. (1998). *Model of Human Occupation.* Chicago: Clearinghouse, University of Illinois.

Moos, R. (1993). *The Work Environment Scale: An Annotated Bibliography.* Palo Alto, CA: Department of Veterans Affairs and Stanford University Medical Center, Center for Health Education.

Moos, R. (1994). *Work Environment Scale Manual.* (3rd ed.). Palo Alto, CA: Consulting Psychologists Press, Inc.

Moos, R. H. (1995). Development and applications of new measures of life stressors, social resources, and coping responses. *European Journal of Psychological Assessment, 11*, 1–13.

Moos, R. H., & Lemke, S. (1996). *Evaluating Residential Facilities: The Multiphasic Environmental Assessment Procedure.* Thousand Oaks, CA: Sage.

Moyers, P. A. (1999). The Guide to Occupational Therapy Practice. *American Journal of Occupational Therapy, 53*, 3, 247–320 (special edition).

Mueller, J. (1990). *The Workplace Workbook: An Illustrated Guide to Job Accommodation and Assistive Technology.* Washington: Dole Foundation.

Oliver, R., Blathwayt, J., Brackley, C., & Tamaki, T. (1993). Development of the Safety Assessment of Function and Environment for Rehabilitation (SAFER) Tool. *Canadian Journal of Occupational Therapy, 60*, 78–82.

Park, S., Fisher, A. G., & Velozo, C. A. (1994). Using the Assessment of Motor and Process Skills to compare occupational performance between clinic and home settings. *American Journal of Occupational Therapy, 48*, 697–709.

Rogers, J. C., Holm, M. B., & Stone, R. G. (1994). Evaluation of daily living tasks. The home care advantage. *American Journal of Occupational Therapy, 51*, 410–422.

Steinfeld, E., Schroeder, S., Duncan, J., Faste, R., Chollet, D., Bishop, M., Wirth, P., & Cardell, P. (1979). *Access to the built environment: A review of the literature (HUD #660).* Washington, DC: U.S. Government Printing Office.

Steinfeld, E., & Danford, G. S. (1997). Environment as a mediating factor in functional assessment. In S. Dittmar and G. Gresham (Eds). *Functional assessment and outcome measures for rehabilitation health professionals,* (pp. 37–56). Gaithersburg, MD: Aspen.

Texas Governor's Committee for Disabled Persons (1992). *ADA Self-evaluation Guide.* Houston, TX: Author.

Trombly, C. (1995). Occupation: Purposefulness and meaningfulness as therapeutic mechanisms. *American Journal of Occupational Therapy, 49*, 960–972.

Uniform Data Systems. (1993). *Guide for the Uniform Data Set for medical rehabilitation.* Buffalo, NY: University of Buffalo Foundation.

U.S. Department of Justice, (1991, July 26). Nondiscrimination on the basis of disability by public accommodations and in commercial facilities; Final Rule (DOJ 28CFR Part 36; No 1531-1591), Federal Register 35544-35691.

Velozo, C. A. (1993). Work evaluations: Critique of the state of art of functional assessment of work. *American Journal of Occupational Therapy, 47*, 203–208.

11
Occupation

Catherine A. Trombly

LEARNING OBJECTIVES

After studying this chapter, the reader will be able to do the following:

1. Describe how occupation is used as a therapeutic mechanism to regain key tasks and activities for roles important to the person or to remediate impaired abilities and capacities.
2. Analyze occupations to determine their value for remediation of impaired abilities and capacities.
3. Analyze occupations to determine whether they are within the capabilities of a particular person.
4. Select occupation-as-means to achieve particular goals.
5. Grade occupations to challenge the person's abilities to improve performance.
6. Adapt occupations to increase their therapeutic value or to bring them within the capability of a person.

*O*ccupation is the unique medium of occupational therapy (National Society for the Promotion of Occupational Therapy, 1917; Reilly, 1962). Long before there was scientific evidence, occupational therapists believed that occupation maintained or restored health. Evidence is beginning to accrue to support that belief. There is even evidence that social and productive activities (occupations) are independently associated with survival. This was found in a study that followed 2,761 men and women in one U. S. city over 13 years. The researchers controlled all other variables that could possibly explain the survival rate and found that social activities, defined as going to church, cinema, and restaurants; taking trips; playing cards and other games; and participating in social groups and productive activities, defined as gardening, preparing meals, and shopping, conferred survival advantages equivalent to those of fitness activities. They concluded that social and productive activities exert an independent protective effect not due exclusively to the associated physical activity (Glass et al., 1999).

GLOSSARY

Activity analysis—A process by which properties inherent in a given activity, task, or occupation may be gauged for their ability to elicit individual motivation and to fulfill patient's needs in occupational performance and performance components (Llorens, 1993).

Closed task—A closed task involves the least interaction with environment (Gentile, 1987). A closed task is one in which the task demands remain constant and for which habits can develop so that little conscious control is required once learned.

Constraints—Limitations imposed on purposeful movement or the completion of occupational performance. Extrinsic constraints include the physical and sociocultural environment and task demands. Intrinsic constraints include biomechanical and neuromuscular aspects of a person's body, as well as other personal contextual factors (Newell, 1986).

Dynamical systems theory of motor control—A theory of movement organization that originated from dynamical (nonlinear) systems theory developed from the study of chaotic systems. It proposes that the order and pattern of movement to accomplish a goal emerges from the interaction of multiple, nonhierarchical subsystems, such as biomechanical and neuromuscular constraints (coordinative structures), environmental constraints (context), and task constraints (demand) (Kamm et al., 1990; Newell, 1986). See Chapters 5, 21, and 22.

Electromyographic—Pertaining to recording the electrical activity produced by a contracting muscle. When a muscle is at rest, no electrical activity is recorded. As the muscle contracts, the electrical activity increases proportionately.

Kinematic—Spatial and temporal description of movement measured by optoelectric or videographic instruments. Velocity and acceleration are mathematically derived from positional data and from their plots allow detection of strategies for the organization of movement (Georgopoulos, 1986; Jeannerod, 1988).

MET (metabolic equivalent)—The amount of energy consumed when a person is at rest in a semireclined position and with the extremities supported. That amount is 3.5 mL of oxygen per minute per kilogram of body weight. Activities can be rated according to energy expenditure in terms of multiples of METs.

Open task—Task with most interaction between the performer and environment (Gentile, 1987). An open task is one for which the environment and/or objects may vary during performance and between trials. Open tasks require attention and vigilance.

Phase planes—Graphs of movement, with velocity of the end point on the ordinate and displacement on the abscissa. Movements using the same motor plan produce replicable phase planes, but movements using different plans produce unique phase planes.

Purposeful activity—Goal-directed behaviors or tasks that combine to constitute occupations (American Occupational Therapy Association, 1997).

Task analysis—Similar to activity analysis; term used primarily in relation to work assessment (ergonomics). Analysis of the dynamic relationship between the person and his or her everyday occupations and environments (Watson, 1997).

Task demands—The context (e.g., objects, surroundings, ritual) that evokes certain maneuvers required to accomplish the goal of the task.

To use occupation therapeutically, therapists design experiences that translate therapeutic principles into concrete activities and tasks that promote behavior away from dysfunction toward function (Cynkin & Robinson, 1990). The patient changes as a result of engaging in the occupation (Darnell & Heater, 1994; Nelson, 1988).

Although all occupational therapists agree that they use occupation or activity as the therapeutic medium, there is no consensus on the definition of occupation. The most widely accepted definition seems to be that occupations are "chunks of culturally and personally meaningful activity in which humans engage that can be named in the lexicon of the culture" (Clark et al., 1991, p. 301). These are the ordinary and familiar things that people do every day (e.g., dress, garden, do puzzles).

Therapeutic occupation, a special type of occupation, is further defined as "meaningful purposeful occupation performance leading to accurate assessment, positive adaptation, and successful compensation" (Nelson, 1996, p. 780) or activities in which the patient actively participates, identifies as purposeful and meaningful, uses real objects in natural environments, and focuses on remediation of impairments (Fisher, 1998).

The terms *occupation* and **purposeful activity** are used interchangeably by most therapists. However, the American Occupational Therapy Association (1997) distinguished between the two in this way: occupation is active participation in self-maintenance, work, leisure, and play, and purposeful activity is goal-directed behaviors or tasks that constitute occupations. The term *occupation* applies to the integration of the person's abilities,

BOX 11-1
Therapeutic Characteristics and Effects of Occupation-As-Means and Occupation-As-End

	Occupation-As-Means	Occupation-As-End
Purposefulness	Organizes abilities and capacities, e.g., movement, cognition, perception	Organizes capacities and abilities into activities, tasks, roles
Meaningfulness	Motivates engagement in therapeutic occupation	Motivates engagement in activities, tasks, life roles
Effect	Occupation, through task demand, remediates capacities and abilities	Occupation, through adaptation or education, restores activities and tasks of life roles

motivations, goals, and the environment to enable role performance. Purposeful activity is circumscribed; it demands particular responses within particular contexts and is used to facilitate change in impairments and functional limitations. In this text, occupation-as-end is equated to *occupation* and occupation-as-means to *purposeful activity*.

Occupational therapists traditionally help people achieve satisfying occupational lives in several ways. One way is to adapt the environment or tools and teach the person how to use these contextual adaptations or other adapted methods to accomplish activities and tasks of daily life (Moyers, 1999). In this case, occupation is both the treatment and the end goal. The second way is to remediate impaired capacities and abilities that prevent successful performance of activities and tasks required of a patient's roles (Moyers, 1999). In this case, occupation is the means to remediate impairments.

This chapter defines occupation-as-end and occupation-as-means (Box 11-1). It describes how occupational therapists use occupation to remediate impaired abilities and capacities or to enable a person to continue or regain important roles.

Occupation-As-End

Occupation-as-end refers to complex activities and tasks that comprise roles. Learning the occupation is the goal. Occupation-as-end is equivalent to the higher levels of the International Classification of Functioning, Disability and Health (ICIDH-2): activities and participation (see Chapter 1). At these levels the person has a functional goal and tries to accomplish it using what abilities and capacities he or she has. Occupation-as-end may remediate impairments, but this benefit is serendipitous and the occupation is not chosen for that purpose. Occupation-as-end achieves its therapeutic effect from the qualities of purposefulness and meaningfulness. Purposefulness is hypothesized to organize behavior and meaningfulness is hypothesized to motivate performance (Trombly, 1995).

Purposefulness

Occupation-as-end is purposeful by virtue of its focus on accomplishing activities and tasks. Purposeful occupation-as-end organizes a person's behavior, day, and life (Kielhofner, 1995; Meyer, 1922, 1977; Slagle, 1914; Yerxa & Baum, 1986; Yerxa & Locker, 1990). Early occupational workers, as they were called, imposed purposeful occupation on people who could not choose it for themselves, and those people could then act in healthier ways (Slagle).

Evidence That Occupation-As-End Organizes Time and Life

Time use studies indicate that people who are mentally able to envision goals fill their time with activities and tasks (Grady, 1992). The studies also indicate that this distribution is affected by age (McKinnon, 1992) and disability (Pentland et al., 1999; Yerxa & Baum, 1986; Yerxa & Locker, 1990). For example, Yerxa and Baum found the number of hours that community-living spinal cord–injured subjects devoted to particular occupations differed significantly from that of their nondisabled friends. The spinal cord–injured subjects worked fewer hours and devoted more hours to "other" activities, such as shopping, going to church, eating, and watching television. Pentland et al. found a similar pattern of time use. They found a significant difference between how 312 men with spinal cord injury and 3,617 able-bodied men in Canada used their time. The men with spinal cord injury spent an average of 7.2 hours in leisure activities, mostly television, versus 6 hours for the able-bodied; 4.4 versus 7.7 hours in productivity; and 3.7 versus 2.3 hours in personal care. The men with spinal cord injury rated their satisfaction with their daily routines as mediocre.

There are no studies on how occupational therapists use occupation-as-end to organize people's lives. There is some anecdotal evidence that occupation-as-end does organize people's lives. For example, an occupational therapist and a patient reported on how the patient reorganized her own life after traumatic brain injury using a synergistic mix of occupation and narration (Price-Lackey & Cashman, 1996).

Meaningfulness

Occupation-as-end is not only purposeful but also meaningful, since it is the performance of activities or tasks that a person sees as important. Only meaningful occupation remains in a person's life repertoire. Meaningfulness as a therapeutic aspect of occupation derives from our belief in the mind–body connection. The actions of the body are guided by the meaning ascribed to them by the mind (Bruner, 1990). Meaningfulness has an overarching quality when discussing activities and tasks of self-maintenance, self-advancement, and self-enhancement roles that are valued over the years and contribute to the definition of a person's life. Meaningfulness of occupation-as-end is based on a person's values acquired from family and cultural experiences. Meaningfulness also springs from a person's sense of the importance of participating in certain occupations or performing in a particular manner, from the person's estimate of his or her reward in terms of success or pleasure, and possibly from a threat of bad consequences if the occupation is not engaged in.

Meaning is individual (Bruner, 1990), and while the occupational therapist can guess what may be meaningful to the patient based on the person's life history, the therapist must verify with each patient that the particular occupation *is* meaningful to that person *now* and verify that the person sees value in relearning it. The therapist cannot substitute his or her own values in selecting appropriate occupational goals for the patient.

Evidence That Occupation-As-End Motivates Participation

No studies in occupational therapy have tested the hypothesis that meaningful occupation-as-end motivates behavior. Related studies indicate that life satisfaction is at least partially defined in terms of competent role performance. One can extrapolate from that that if a particular role is satisfying, one would be motivated to do the tasks associated with that role. For example, in the study by Yerxa and Baum (1986) of 15 spinal cord–injured subjects and their 12 nondisabled friends, a significant moderate correlation, $r = .44$, was found between satisfaction with performance in home management and overall life satisfaction. A slightly higher correlation, $r = .62$, was found between community skills and overall life satisfaction. Smith et al. (1986) studied 60 persons with a mean age of 78 years to determine the relationship between engagement in daily occupations and life satisfaction. They found that subjects in the high-satisfaction category engaged in work and recreation significantly more and in activities of daily living and rest significantly less than those in the low-satisfaction category.

Evidence That Occupation-As-End Restores Self-Maintenance, Self-Enhancement, and Self-Advancement Roles

The evidence of the effectiveness of occupation-as-end to restore life roles is sparse. The anecdote of the person who reorganized her own life after traumatic brain injury, as told by Price-Lackey and Cashman (1996), attests to the power of occupation-as-end with or without occupational therapists to guide it. Another study reported successful resumption of role performance in 17 randomly selected chronically disabled community-living elders after receiving home-based occupational therapy (Levine & Gitlin, 1993). As a result of the program, participants engaged in a greater range of tasks, such as wine making, visiting relatives, attending church, and cleaning, than they did before the intervention. They became more engaged in life, as shown by their volunteerism and increased social activities.

Implementation of Occupation-As-End in Therapy

Occupation-as-end is implemented by teaching the activity or task directly, using whatever abilities the patient has, or by providing whatever adaptations are necessary. Because occupation occurs within a person–task–environment interaction, change in any one of these variables may result in successful performance. Implementation of occupation-as-end, however, focuses on the task demands and/or the environment. Therapeutic principles for this approach derive from cognitive information processing and learning theories. It is the rehabilitative approach (Trombly & Scott, 1977). In this approach, occupations are analyzed to ensure that they are within the capabilities of the patient, but they are not used to bring about change in these capabilities per se. The patient learns, with the help of the therapist as teacher and adaptor, of the task demands and context. In the therapeutic encounter, the therapist

▶ Organizes the subtasks to be learned so the person will succeed
▶ Provides clear instructions
▶ Provides feedback to promote successful outcome
▶ Structures the practice to ensure improved performance and learning
▶ Makes adaptations as necessary

Occupation-As-Means

Occupation-as-means is the use of occupation as a treatment to improve the person's impaired capacities and abilities to enable eventual occupational functioning. Occupation-as-means refers to occupation acting as the therapeutic change agent. Various arts, crafts, games, sports, exercise routines, and daily activities that are systematically selected and tailored to each individual are used as occupation-as-means (Cynkin & Robinson, 1990).

Occupation-as-means is therapeutic when the activity has a purpose or goal that makes a challenging demand yet has a prospect for success. Furthermore, if it has meaning and relevance to the individual who is to change, it motivates the will to learn and improve (Cynkin & Robinson, 1990). The therapeutic aspects of occupation used as a means to change impairments, then, are purposefulness and meaningfulness.

Purposefulness

Therapeutic use of occupation-as-means was based on the assumption that the activity held within itself a healing property that would change organic or behavioral impairments. One mechanism of that change is purposefulness. Because the central nervous system (CNS) is organized to accomplish goals (Granit, 1977), the goal or purpose seems to organize the most efficient response, given the constraints of person and context.

Evidence That Occupation-As-Means Organizes Responses

Evidence concerning the organization of movement can be gained using instruments designed to track the spatial–temporal aspects of movement. Movement organization can be detected from the shape of the velocity profile (Georgopoulos, 1986; Kamm et al., 1990). Different velocity profiles, which indicate differences in movement organization and CNS control, emerge for particular goals (Jeannerod, 1988; Nelson, 1983) (Fig 11-1).

In 1987, Marteniuk et al. demonstrated for the first time the effect of goal on the organization of movement as detected from velocity profiles. They found that five university students organized movement differently when they reached for the same object for different purposes. One goal was to pick up a 4-cm disk and place it in a slot. The other goal was to pick up the disk and throw it into a basket. They measured the reach to the disk. The distance and biomechanical demands were exactly the same under both conditions. Only intent after reach was different. The two purposes produced different velocity profiles for reaching to the disk, indicating different movement organizations.

Goal is generated from the patient's own intention, from the therapist's directions (Fisk & Goodale, 1989), or from the context, including what objects are available, the relevance of the objects, and what the objects afford the person in terms of action. We are familiar with generation of goals by the person and by the therapist, but contextual indication of goal may be unfamiliar, so studies concerning this will be reviewed.

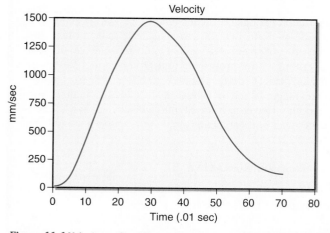
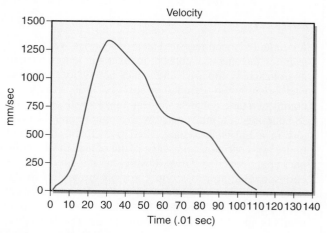

Figure 11-1 Velocity profiles. The profile on the left is symmetrical and bell-shaped, which is commonly seen in planned reach to a stationary, large target. The peak of the velocity profile (end of the acceleration phase) occurs between 33% and 50% of the reach. The profile on the right is left-shifted, which is commonly seen in guided reach to a small target. The peak velocity occurs early in the reach, and the deceleration phase is extended as the person guides the hand to the target.

Mathiowetz and Wade (1995) tested whether the same motor organization was elicited when 20 subjects with multiple sclerosis performed functional tasks in natural, impoverished, partial, and simulated conditions. In the natural condition the subjects actually ate applesauce from a dish with a spoon; in the impoverished condition they pretended to eat applesauce, with no applesauce, spoon, or dish; in the partial condition they pretended to eat applesauce using a dish and spoon but no applesauce; in the simulated condition they did the feeding subtest of the *Jebsen-Taylor Hand Function Test*, which has the subject pick up kidney beans with a spoon and transfer them to a can. The different contexts transmitted the idea of different goals to the subjects. Because subjects produced unique spatial–temporal maps (**phase planes**) in each context, the researchers concluded that subjects perceived each as an unique activity having a different goal.

Wu et al. (1994) investigated whether actually reaching for a pencil to write one's name, reaching the same distance for an imagined pencil, or reaching forward in a biomechanically similar way would produce different outcomes in terms of the organization of movement. In the sample of 37 normal college-aged subjects, reaching for an actual pencil elicited a significantly different and more efficient organization of movement than reaching for a pretend pencil or exercise. The reach to the actual pencil was faster, straighter, and more planned, and it used less force than in the other two conditions.

Trombly and Wu (1999) examined, in two conditions, the movement organization of 14 persons who had had a stroke. The conditions were goal object present and goal object absent (rote exercise). In the goal object–present condition, participants were asked to reach forward to take a piece of food off the plate and bring it to the mouth. In the goal object–absent condition, they were asked to reach forward to the same place but without the food goal. Although the two conditions were biomechanically equivalent, the reach was smoother, faster, more forceful, and more planned when the goal-object was present than when it was absent.

These findings have been verified in other studies (Ma et al., 1999; Wu et al., 1998, 2000). At least in terms of motor responses, then, purposiveness, as transmitted by context, does appear to organize behavior. Of course much more study is required to verify this and confirm it to be true for other performance components.

Meaningfulness

Meaningfulness is not only a psychological term but also a mechanism of change. In a positron emission tomography (PET) study, Decety et al. (1997) discovered that brain activation differed with the meaning of an action

---

RESEARCH NOTE

A Kinematic Study of Contextual Effects on Reaching Performance in Persons With and Without Stroke: Influences of Object Availability

Wu, C., Trombly, C. A., Lin, K., & Tickle-Degnen, L. (2000). *Archives of Physical Medicine and Rehabilitation, 81, 95–101*

ABSTRACT

A counterbalanced repeated-measures design was used to examine the effects of context on reaching performance in neurologically impaired and intact populations. Context was varied by the presence or absence of objects used to complete a task. Subjects were 14 persons with stroke and 25 neurologically intact persons. In a motor control laboratory in a university setting, each participant was tested under two conditions: presence of the object, in which the participant reached forward with the impaired arm or corresponding arm to scoop coins off the table into the other hand; and absence of the object, in which the participant reached forward to a place where the coins would be placed if the object were present. The dependent variables were kinematic variables of movement time, total displacement, peak velocity, percentage of reach where peak velocity occurs, and movement units derived from acceleration data for the reaching part of the activity. The condition of object present elicited significantly better ($p < .0055$) performance of reaching movements than the condition of object absent. Better performance was defined as faster (shorter movement time), more direct (less total displacement), more planned and less guided (greater percentage of reach where peak velocity occurs), and smoother (fewer movement units). Peak velocity (forcefulness) was not significantly different between conditions ($p = .2791$).

APPLICATION TO PRACTICE

▶ Occupation provides significant performance advantage over rote exercise.
▶ Tasks that use real objects elicit improved organization of movement.
▶ Treatment in simulated contexts using simulated objects and simulated goals may not help a patient learn occupational performance for real life.

regardless of subjects' strategies. Meaningful actions strongly engaged the frontal and temporal regions of the left hemisphere, while meaningless action activated mainly the right occipitoparietal areas.

Meaningfulness in the sense of occupation-as-means has an immediate aspect. Choice to participate in an activity at the moment is based on immediate motivation that is guided by currently perceived needs, feelings, and desires that may or may not be related to life goals. The meaningful aspect of occupation-as-means may be the emotional value that an interesting and creative experience offers the patient (Ayres, 1958). Or meaningfulness may stem from familiarity with the occupation or its power to arouse positive associations or the likelihood that completion of it will elicit approval from others who are respected and admired or its value in learning a prized skill or its potential to contribute to recovery (Cynkin & Robinson, 1990; Grady, 1992).

Although we often count on meaning to emanate from the activity, there is no inherent meaningful quality in a particular occupation. Meaningfulness is individual. "Meaning is rooted in the occupation's intrinsic value *to the person* [emphasis added]" (Grady, 1992, p. 1063). The importance of meaningfulness to therapists is that we believe it motivates the patient to engage in the therapy longer with the expectation that that will increase the therapeutic benefit. Although the therapist may determine what seems to be the ideal therapeutic occupation to accomplish a particular goal, it would be inappropriate to assign that activity to the patient. Meaningfulness should be developed through an exchange between therapist and patient to unmask or construct the meaning of the activity within the context of the patient's culture, life experiences, disability, and present needs (Kielhofner, 1994). In therapy, the patient should be allowed to choose an occupation from several that can be similarly effective. Being able to choose the occupation makes it more likely that the patient will be committed to doing it for therapeutic purposes.

Evidence That Occupation-As-Means Motivates Participation

Meaningfulness is expressed in occupational therapy research in four ways: (1) provide enjoyment; (2) offer a choice; (3) make an end product to keep; and (4) enhance the context or make the context more applicable to the person's life. The response, *motivation*, is expressed as the number of repetitions or length of time engaged in the occupation or the effort expended.

Fun or Enjoyment

Fun is immediately motivating. Several studies confirm that fun or enjoyment derived from play motivates attempts to perform an action or prolongs engagement in an action. King (1993) treated 146 patients in a hand clinic using either a computer game that required the person to pinch or grasp to play the game or by using pinch or grip strengthening devices. Both treatments lasted 3 minutes. Those who participated in the game did significantly more repetitions (237.2 grips, 240.5 pinches) than those who did the exercise without the game (170.7 grips, 203.2 pinches). Hoppes (1997) studied 10 elderly women who were unable to maintain a functional standing position. They alternatively played a game of their choice or did other chosen, nonplayful, activities, such as reading, conversing, or folding towels, all while standing at a raised table. Although the difference in standing tolerance was only a minute and a half, it was significantly greater for playing the game (386.5 seconds) than for the other activities (294.3 seconds).

Choice

Provision of a choice presumably creates emotional value because the person is likely to choose an activity that is interesting and creative and/or arouses positive associations from the past. Zimmerer-Branum and Nelson (1995) gave 52 elderly nursing home residents a choice between a simulated basketball game chosen to encourage shoulder flexion and rote shoulder flexion exercises. After trying both, 69% chose the game for the actual treatment session. LaMore and Nelson (1993) found a significant increase in repetitions when 22 adult subjects with mental disabilities were given a limited choice of which ceramic object to paint (26 repetitions) as compared to being told to paint a particular one (17 repetitions).

Keeping an End Product

Presumably letting the patient make a product that he or she can keep motivates by arousing positive emotions and through the potential of gaining approval from others. Murphy et al. (1999) found that 50 college-aged subjects worked significantly longer on a craft project of their choice when they could keep the product (21.2 minutes) than when they could not (16.9 minutes). However, this was true for only two of the four activities from which the subjects could choose, and only 80% of the subjects reported being interested in keeping the end product. So it is not safe to assume that offering an opportunity to keep an end product is motivational. One must ask.

Enriched Context

Enriched or natural contexts motivate through the positive emotions associated with familiarity and arousal of positive associations with one's home, culture, or previous life. Lang et al. (1992) tested the responses of 15 elderly nursing home residents under three conditions:

kicking a red balloon, kicking a described imagined balloon, and exercise in which they kicked as demonstrated. A significantly greater number of repetitions was associated with really kicking the balloon (54) versus in the imagery or exercise conditions (26 and 18, respectively). This study was later replicated by DeKuiper et al. (1993) with similar results.

A number of other researchers demonstrated significantly greater numbers of repetitions or duration of performance under enhanced context conditions (Bloch et al., 1989; Kircher, 1984; Miller & Nelson, 1987; Steinbeck, 1986; Thomas et al., 1999; Yoder et al., 1989).

Meaningfulness, as operationalized by fun and enjoyment, enhanced context, and possibly choice, appears to motivate continued performance. However, more research is needed on these as well as on the effects of familiarity of context on motivation.

Evidence That Occupation-As-Means Remediates Impairments

Occupational therapists believe that a person develops cognitive, perceptual, psychosocial, and motor skills through engagement in activity of interest and purpose, but this assumption has hardly been researched (Ramsbey, 1993; Trombly & Ma, 2000). A few studies of the effects of occupation-as-means on persons with diagnosed physical impairments are reported here.

Van der Weel et al. (1991) tested 9 children of normal intelligence aged 3 to 7 years who were diagnosed with right hemiparesis. They measured the children's range of supination and pronation when moving a drumstick back and forth in the frontal plane with the instruction to "move as far as you can." The children previously had experienced full range of movement passively. Range was also measured when the children were told to use the same drumstick to "bang the drums," which were placed to require full range of motion (ROM). Movement range was significantly greater for the task of banging the drums (> 93°) than for the exercise task (< 67°), which had a vague goal and probably was less fun.

Another group of researchers tested the effect of occupation-as-means on active range of shoulder motion of 20 brain-injured adults (Sietsema et al., 1993). In one condition, each subject reached to a point 3 inches above the center of a table placed to require full forward reach. In the other condition, each reached the same distance to play the Simon computer-controlled game of flashing lights and sounds. Overall active motion was significantly greater as a result of the Simon game (71.6 cm) than simply reaching to the center of the table (59.4 cm).

Nelson et al. (1996) briefly treated 26 elderly women who had had a stroke to decrease pronator spasticity and

to increase supination ROM. All participants engaged in a bilaterally assisted supination exercise. Half did so in the context of a dice game that required them to supinate to dump out the dice for a score. Those who participated in the game demonstrated significantly greater handle rotation [supination] (95.3°) than those who participated in rote exercise (81.9°).

Implementation of Occupation-As-Means in Therapy

Therapist and patient select occupations that are meaningful to the patient. The therapist analyzes the chosen occupation to determine that it demands particular responses from the person and that the responses demanded are slightly more challenging than what the person can easily produce. The therapist provides the opportunity to engage in the potentially therapeutic occupation (Meyer, 1922, 1977), and as the person makes the effort and succeeds, the particular impairment the occupation-as-means was chosen to remediate is reduced. The processes involved in using occupation therapeutically are analysis, selection and gradation, and adaptation. Guidelines for these processes are presented next.

Analysis

Activity analysis, or **task analysis**, is one of the key process skills of occupational therapists. Occupational therapists analyze an activity because they want to know (1) whether the patient, given certain abilities, can be expected to do the activity and (2) whether the activity can challenge latent abilities or capacities and thereby improve these.

Activity analysis developed from industrial time-and-motion study methods. Military occupational therapists applied these methods to rehabilitation of injured soldiers during World War I (Creighton, 1992) at the suggestion of Gilbreth and Gilbreth (1920), industrial engineers who observed injured soldiers in military hospitals. Gilbreth (1911) listed these steps for analyzing a task: "(1) Reduce . . . practice to writing; (2) enumerate motions used; (3) enumerate variables which affect each motion" (p. 5). Variables considered were characteristics of the worker, the surroundings, and the motion. This method has been used by occupational therapists for many years when focusing the analysis on the activity. More dynamic forms of occupational analyses that focus on the performance of the patient are developing. Some are Performance Analysis (Fisher, 1998), Ecological Task Analysis (Burton & Davis, 1996; Davis & Burton, 1991), and Dynamic Performance Analysis (Polatjko et al., 2000). The dynamical observational methods require skill based on practice. The activity-focused analysis is presented in this chapter because it demonstrates the process to the inexperienced activity analyst.

Both activity and performance analyses entail unnesting the component tasks and activities that constitute the occupation and determining what abilities, skills, and capacities are needed to do the specified activity or that may improve if the person does the activity (Mayer et al., 1986; Trombly, 1995).

Analyzing for component abilities and capacities presupposes that activities have reliably identifiable inherent therapeutic aspects. This belief is stated in a position paper of the American Occupational Therapy Association (1995): "Whether physical or mental in nature, the behaviors necessary for completion of tasks in daily occupations can be analyzed according to specific components related to moving, perceiving, thinking, and feeling" (p. 1015). Although the concept that tasks, activities, and occupation components possess inherent factors (Llorens, 1986) still serves as the basis for activity analysis, a survey of 120 experienced therapists indicated that there was limited consensus on the sensorimotor, cognitive-perceptual, or psychosocial components inherent to particular activities (Tsai, 1994). Neistadt et al. (1993) also reported discrepancies among therapists in identifying components of common activities. Much research on activity analysis and the inherent qualities of activities is necessary.

Activity-Focused Analysis

Using an analytical approach, the therapist examines an activity to determine its components and the level of capability demanded. The outcome can be used to select activities for remediation or to match a particular person's skills with the demands of the task. A person feels best when engaging in activity if his or her skills match the situational challenges posed by the activity and the challenge of the activity matches the person's skills—called "flow" by Csikszentmihalyi (1990).

All analyses should occur within some conceptual framework to give it direction, coherence, and meaning (Mosey, 1981). For example, planting a tulip bulb in a plant pot can be analyzed from various frames of reference. The biomechanical approach prompts the therapist to examine the physical aspects, such as grasp and ROM, whereas the cognitive-perceptual approach examines the activity according to its cognitive or perceptual demands. The Model of Human Occupation might focus the therapist's attention on how this planting activity may meet the patient's nurturing needs and values.

Whereas biomechanical analysis examines joint ROM and muscle contraction used to carry out the activity, contemporary thinking about human movement based on **electromyographic** (EMG) and **kinematic** research indicates that this may not be wholly valid because of individual differences in muscle action and differences in movement strategies secondary to learning, maturation, and perception of goal (Trombly & Quintana, 1983). Each person's CNS plans movement to accomplish the goal with the resources the person has. Reaching for a glass of milk on the table may or may not activate the anterior deltoid. If that muscle is weak, the patient may accomplish the goal by substituting other muscles or strategies, such as turning sidewise to the table to make use of the stronger middle deltoid to reach the glass. The substitutions listed in the muscle testing section of Chapter 4 are common ways people accomplish the movement goal when the prime mover is weak. The idea that doing a certain activity will always exercise a certain weak muscle may be naive. If it is essential that a particular muscle of a particular patient be contracting to a certain level of activity, as may be the case in tendon transfer rehabilitation, it is best to monitor the muscle directly using EMG biofeedback while the patient does the activity (Trombly & Cole, 1979; Trombly & Quintana, 1983).

However, on average, certain motions and muscle actions are more probable than others, and therefore an analysis can be based on this if the therapist realizes that actual performance of a particular patient must be verified and not assumed. Because understanding of human movement is in too early a stage of development to support a better method of activity analyses, by default the traditional biomechanical activity analysis is described here (Boxes 11-2 and 11-3).

The therapist begins the biomechanical analysis by stating the goal (purpose) and by establishing the task demands, that is, the exact placement of the selected tools and equipment in relation to the patient, the speed at which the activity is to be accomplished, the complexity of the task, and the context in which it will be carried out. Changes in any of these variables change the task demands and require a different analysis. The prerequisite abilities and capacities for accomplishing the whole activity are identified. If these prerequisite abilities are lacking, the way the activity is to be done would have to be modified (e.g., if the patient is blind) if the goal was the focus (occupation-as-end). Alternatively, a different activity would be chosen if the exercise was the focus (occupation-as-means).

The steps of an activity are identified. For example, the steps of vacuuming the carpet while standing are listed under No. 4 in Box 11-3. The potential repetitions of each motion are noted. Only the 4th step, pushing the vacuum cleaner back and forth, would be analyzed further because it is the repetitive, therapeutic aspect of this activity. The other steps occur too infrequently to be

BOX 11-2
PROCEDURES FOR PRACTICE

Activity-Focused Analysis

1. Name the activity goal.
2. Describe the task demands:
   ▶ Task constraints: How are the person and materials positioned, especially in relation to one another?
   ▶ Task constraints: What utensils/tools/materials are normally used to do this activity?
   ▶ Environmental constraints: Where is this activity usually carried out?
   ▶ Contextual constraints: Does this activity or the way it is carried out hold particular meaning for certain cultures or social roles?
3. What capacities and abilities are prerequisite to successful accomplishment of this activity?
4. List the steps of the activity.
5. Describe the biomechanical internal constraints for the most therapeutic or repetitive step.

Motions	ROM	Primary Muscles	Gravity Assists, Resists, No Effect	Minimal Strength Required	Type of Contraction

6. What must be stabilized to enable doing this activity, and how will that stabilization be provided?
7. For which ages is this activity appropriate?
8. What is the estimated MET level of this activity?
9. What precautions must be considered when using this activity in therapy?
10. For which short-term goal or goals is this activity appropriate?
11. How can this activity be graded to improve the following:
    ▶ Strength
    ▶ Active ROM
    ▶ Passive ROM
    ▶ Endurance
    ▶ Coordination and dexterity
    ▶ Edema
    ▶ Perceptual abilities
    ▶ Cognitive skills

therapeutic. Each repetitive step is subdivided into motions. For example, pushing the vacuum back and forth involves shoulder flexion with elbow extension, shoulder extension with elbow flexion, and trunk flexion and extension, although trunk movement may be eliminated, depending on how the person moves in relation to the machine. Wrist stabilization (cocontraction) in extension and cylindrical grasp are also "motions" associated with vacuuming.

The range of each motion is estimated by observing another person or doing the activity oneself. Each motion is further analyzed to determine which muscle or muscles are likely responsible, based on anatomical, kinesiological, and electromyographic knowledge. Examining the effect of gravity allows estimation of the minimal strength necessary to do the motion. The kind of

contraction demanded for each muscle group in each motion is established by definition.

Activities selected to restore motor function must also take into account the person's cognitive and perceptual abilities, emotional status, cultural background, and interests. Some cognitive aspects of the activity to be considered include the number and complexity of the steps involved in doing the activity, the requirements for organization and sequencing of the steps or stimuli, and the amount of concentration and memory required. Some perceptual factors to be considered are whether the activity requires the patient to distinguish figure from ground, determine position in space, construct a two- or three-dimensional object, or follow verbal or spatial directions. Other cognitive-perceptual considerations are found in Chapters 28

BOX 11-3
PROCEDURES FOR PRACTICE

An Activity-Focused Analysis

1. Name the goal: Vacuuming the hallway carpet using a light-weight vacuum with a 25-foot cord.
2. Describe the task demands:
   ▶ Task constraints: How are the person and materials positioned, especially in relation to one another?
      ▶ The vacuum cleaner is in a closet next to the area to be cleaned.
      ▶ The electrical plug is halfway between the two ends of the hallway, 5 inches from the floor.
      ▶ When vacuuming, the person will be directly behind the machine.
   ▶ Task constraints: What utensils, tools, and materials are normally used to do this activity?
      ▶ A lightweight vacuum cleaner
   ▶ Environmental constraints: Where is this activity usually carried out?
      ▶ The hallway is 30 feet long and 3 feet wide.
      ▶ No furniture is in the way.
      ▶ The carpet is a flat pile.
   ▶ Contextual constraints: Does this activity or how it is carried out hold particular meaning for certain cultures or social roles?
      ▶ The person takes pride in a clean, well-vacuumed home.
      ▶ The person is not willing to switch to a lighter, unmotorized carpet sweeper because of the feeling that it doesn't do a proper job.

3. What capacities and abilities are prerequisite to successful accomplishment of this activity?
   ▶ Standing balance
   ▶ Ability to bend over and straighten up
   ▶ Ability to grasp
   ▶ Ability to walk forward and backward on carpeting
   ▶ Ability to move dominant arm against gravity and moderate resistance
   ▶ Vision[1]
4. List the steps.
   1. Get the vacuum cleaner from the closet.
   2. Unwind the cord.
   3. Plug cord into wall socket and turn vacuum cleaner on.
   4. Push the vacuum cleaner back and forth.
   5. Unplug it and wind the cord.
   6. Return the vacuum cleaner to the closet.

5. Describe the biomechanical internal constraints for pushing the vacuum back and forth (step # 4).

Motions	ROM (degrees), Distances	Primary Muscles	Gravity Assists, Resists, No Effect	Minimal Strength Required	Type of Contraction
Shoulder flexion	0–75	Anterior deltoid, coracobrachialis, pectoralis major	Resists	4– to 4	Concentric
Elbow extension	90–0	Triceps	Assists	4– to 4	Concentric
Scapular protraction	1.5 in	Serratus anterior	No effect	4– to 4	Concentric
Shoulder extension	0–45	Posterior deltoid Latissimus dorsi Teres major	Assists No effect Resists	4– to 4	Concentric
Elbow flexion	90–120	Biceps, brachialis	Resists	4– to 4	Concentric
Scapular retraction	1.5 in	Middle trapezius	No effect	4– to 4	Concentric
Cylindrical grasp		Finger flexors, finger extensors, interossei	No effect	4– to 4	Isometric
Wrist stabilize		All wrist muscles	No effect	4– to 4	Isometric
Trunk flexion	0–30	Back extensors	Assists	3+ to 4–	Eccentric
Trunk extension	30–0	Back extensors	Resists	4– to 4	Concentric

(continued)

BOX 11-3
PROCEDURES FOR PRACTICE

An Activity-Focused Analysis (Continued)

6. What must be stabilized to enable doing this activity and how will that stabilization be provided?
   ▸ Nothing
7. For which ages is this activity appropriate?
   ▸ 18+ years primarily
   ▸ 10–17 years secondarily
8. What is the estimated MET level of this activity?
   ▸ 2–3 METs
9. What precautions must be considered when using this activity in therapy?
   ▸ If standing balance and bending over are not well developed, the patient must be guarded.
   ▸ Patient who is apt to lose balance walking on carpet must be guarded.
   ▸ Patient who has low back pain must be taught to do the activity without bending forward.
   ▸ Patient with low endurance needs to rest periodically.
10. For which short-term goal or goals is this activity appropriate?
    ▸ Strengthening of upper extremity musculature
    ▸ Developing dynamic standing balance
    ▸ Improving grip strength
    ▸ Improving central and peripheral endurance
    ▸ Learning proper back mechanics

11. How can this activity be graded to improve the following?
    ▸ Strength
      ▸ Heavier vacuum cleaner
      ▸ Thicker carpet
    ▸ Active ROM
      ▸ At limit
    ▸ Passive ROM
      ▸ Not applicable
    ▸ Endurance
      ▸ Increase amount of carpeting vacuumed before resting
    ▸ Coordination, dexterity
      ▸ Place furniture in the area so patient has to change directions of the vacuum to go around the obstacles
    ▸ Edema
      ▸ Not applicable
    ▸ Improve perceptual abilities (examples)
      ▸ Change the color of the "dirt" on the carpet, e.g., spread bits to be vacuumed either in contrasting colors or closer to the color of the carpet (figure ground)
      ▸ Put objects in the way for the person to figure out how to move around them (spatial relations)
    ▸ Improve cognitive skills
      ▸ Not applicable

¹The blind person needs to use adaptive methods for knowing which sections of the carpet have been cleaned and which have not.

and 29. Some psychosocial aspects of an activity that may be important to patients include whether the activity must be done alone or in a group, the length of time required to complete the activity, whether fine detailed work or large expansive movements are involved, how easily errors can be corrected, the view of the activity from the person's particular cultural and social background, and the likelihood of producing a satisfying outcome.

Other methods of analysis of activities have been published. Gentile (1987) has provided a detailed taxonomy of task analysis to be used for evaluation and selection of functionally relevant activities. The taxonomy is related to the learning of motor tasks. Her taxonomy is briefly described here; however, see the original material for a complete description and rationale. The taxonomy consists of 16 categories consisting of movement types and environmental regulatory **constraints**. The dimensions are presented separately in Box 11-4 for the sake of clarity, but they are meant to be combined. The easiest tasks are repetitive ones done in a stationary environment with the body in a stable position, such as sitting and brushing one's hair. Tasks are graded by changing one at a time the various parameters (environmental regulatory conditions, differences in performance between trials, body orientation, manipulation demands). The most demanding tasks are those done in an environment that changes with the performance, requirements that change between trials, with the body in motion while manipulating an object, such as playing basketball. Neistadt et al. (1993) published a model for analyzing activities in relation to cognitive and perceptual demands. Watson (1997) published a useful form based on the American Occupational Therapy Association uniform terminology.

Some activity analyses have been published: Hi-Q game (Neistadt et al., 1993); macramé (Chandani & Hill, 1990); planting a small garden (Nelson, 1988); using a computer for skill development, education, and prevocational training (Okoye, 1993); hand activities (Trombly & Cole, 1979); and bilateral inclined sanding (Spaulding & Robinson, 1984).

Performance-Focused Analyses

Using an analytic approach, the therapist observes the patient's performance of role-related occupations. Figure 11-2 and Box 11-5 depict analysis of role performance using the Occupational Functioning Model as the basis (Trombly, 1993). The first step is to determine whether the person is accomplishing the role as he or she wants, needs, or expects to do. If not, the patient identifies the tasks and activities within the role that are not being accomplished to criterion. Observing the person attempt these gives the therapist clues about which abilities and capacities may need further evaluation and treatment. This is the assessment described in Chapter 1. It is similar to the Dynamic Performance Analysis (DPA) proposed by Polatajko et al. (2000). The DPA is described as a performance-based dynamic iterative process of analysis that is carried out as the client performs an occupation. The steps are (1) establish whole-task performer prerequisites (motivation & knowledge of the task), (2) analyze observed performance to identify where the patient demonstrates perfor-

mance difficulties, and (3) establish the source of the difficulties within the relationship between client abilities and the environmental or occupational supports or demands.

The Performance Analysis proposed by Fisher (1998) involves observational evaluation of the "transaction between the client and the environment as the client performs a task that is familiar, meaningful, purposeful and relevant" (p. 517). To do this Fisher uses a standardized performance analysis, the *AMPS* (*Assessment of Motor and Process Skills*) (Fisher, 1997), although it can also be done by informal observation. The quality of performance, not the person's underlying capacities, is graded, although these are considered when interpreting the outcome and planning treatment.

The Ecological Task Analysis (ETA) is based on ideas of the dynamical systems theory of movement and Gibson's (1977) theory of affordances (Burton & Davis, 1996; Davis and Burton, 1991). This analysis examines the interacting constraints (limitations and enablers) of performer, environment, and task as the occupation is undertaken. The ETA is based on the premise that there

---

BOX 11-4
Examples of Tasks Described According to the Taxonomy of Gentile

Environmental Regulatory Dimension

Environmental Regulatory Conditions During Performance	No Differences in Performance Between Trials	Differences in Performance Between Trials
Stationary: the objects, people, and/or apparatus do not move	**Closed tasks** Climbing stairs at home Brushing teeth Unlocking the front door Turning on the bedroom light	Tasks in which objects are different but stationary during performance Walking on different surfaces Drinking from mugs, glasses, cups Putting on shirt, sweater
Motion: the objects, people, and/or apparatus move	Tasks in which objects move consistently over repeated encounters Stepping onto an escalator Lifting luggage from the conveyer belt at the airport Moving through a revolving door	**Open Tasks** Propelling a wheelchair down a crowded hall Catching a ball Carrying a wiggling child

Movement Type Dimension

Body Orientation	No Manipulation	Manipulation
Stability: body is positioned in one place	Body Stability Sit Stand Lean on table	Body stability plus manipulation Hold object while standing Reach for hairbrush while sitting Keyboard sitting at computer
Transport: body is moving through space	Body Transport Walk Run Propel wheelchair	Body transport plus manipulation Run to catch a ball Drive an automobile Dial phone while walking

Adapted with permission from Gentile, A. M., Higgins, J. R., Miller, E. A., & Rosen, B. (1975). Structure of motor tasks. In *Mouvement Actes du 7e Symposium Canadien en Appentissage Psycho-motor et Psychologie du Sport* (pp. 11–28). Quebec (out of print). Also printed in Gentile, A. (1987). Skill acquisition: Action, movement and neuromotor processes. In J. H. Carr, R. B. Shepherd, J. Gordon, A. M. Gentile, & J. M. Held (Eds.), *Movement Science: Foundations for Physical Therapy in Rehabilitation* (pp. 93–154). Rockville, MD: Aspen Systems.

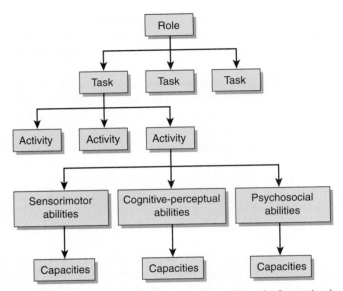

Figure 11-2 Performance-focused analysis according to the Occupational Performance Model. One role is composed of several tasks. Each task consists of several activities. Each activity depends on varying degrees of sensorimotor, cognitive-perceptual and psychosocial abilities. Those abilities depend on supporting capacities. The performance-focused analysis examines these from the top down by observing the patient. When the patient has difficulty performing, the therapist examines the next lower levels and/or the environment as possible constraints to the performance.

are many solutions to a particular task, determined by the unique interaction of performer and environment with the goal or intent of the action. The steps are as follows: (1) The therapist selects and establishes the task goal, structures the physical and social environments, and provides verbal and other cues to allow for an understanding of the task goal. (2) The patient practices the task, the therapist allowing the patient to choose movement solutions. (3) The therapist manipulates the performer, environment, or task variables to find the optimal performance. The therapist identifies specific contexts in which the person can always (sometimes, never) accomplish the task and discovers by perturbation (e.g., increase speed or force) the importance of performer or environmental variables on the performance of the task or movement. (4) The therapist provides direct instructions of other possibilities of movement solutions. See Chapter 21 for application of this analysis and teaching process.

Selection and Gradation

The therapist skilled in activity analysis can match the patient's abilities with activities the patient needs or wants to do. The therapist who is skilled in activity analysis can also easily select the most appropriate

activity for remediation from those that are available and that interest the patient. Activities that meet each goal of the patient's program are considered.

Selection of Occupation-As-End

Occupations-as-end are activities and tasks that constitute the patient's life roles. The patient and therapist identify key tasks and activities that would enable the patient to engage in the role. The therapist matches the particular patient's capabilities to the demand level of each activity. If the patient wants these activities to be part of his or her life, the comparison between task demands, usual environment, and the patient's capabilities determines whether the patient will be able to do the activity independently, with adaptation, or not at all. The patient may be taught new methods of accomplishing particular activities. For example, after having a stroke that causes paresis of one upper limb, a patient can learn a new method of putting on a shirt that requires only one hand. Or the environment in which a favorite activity was accomplished can be modified to allow engagement. For example, a gardener who undergoes bilateral lower extremity amputation because of diabetes can continue to garden from a wheelchair if the beds are raised. See Chapters 30 to 34 for ways to compensate for particular disabilities to enable role performance. For

BOX 11-5
PROCEDURES FOR PRACTICE

Performance-Focused Analysis According to the Occupational Performance Model

1. Name the role.
2. List the tasks the person identifies as important to this role.
3. List the activities the person identifies as part of one of the tasks.
4. Observe the person performing one of the activities.
5. If the person is able to perform the activity, observe another of the activities. When the person is unable to do an activity, one of two directions can be taken:
   ▶ Teach the person adapted methods to accomplish the activity
   ▶ Remediate impaired abilities and capacities
6. If remediation is chosen, analyze what abilities are limited.
7. After deciding on particular ability limitations, measure those abilities to confirm the limitation.
8. If the ability is actually limited, analyze what capacities are resulting in that limitation.
9. Measure those capacities. Treat when verified.

further study, do the assignment in the Clinical Reasoning Box below.

Selection of Occupation-As-Means

An activity that is to be used to restore one or more abilities or capacities must challenge the patient's level of ability so that through effort and/or practice the patient improves (Box 11-6). Some specific characteristics for the goals commonly addressed by occupational therapists who treat persons with physical disabilities are listed here and in Box 11-7. The dimensions along which the activity is to be graded are also listed; when more than one dimension is listed, the therapist should be careful to grade the changes one dimension at a time so that the patient has more of a chance at success. The best activity for remediation is one that intrinsically demands the exact response that has been determined to need improvement and that allows incremental gradations starting where the patient can be successful (Box 11-6). Contrived methods of doing an ordinary activity to make it therapeutic may diminish the value of the activity in the eyes of the patient. Contrived methods also require the patient constantly to focus directly on the process rather than the goal of the activity, undermining the therapeutic mechanisms.

To Retrain Sensory Awareness and/or Discrimination

The activity must provide components that offer a variety of textures, shapes, and sizes, graded from large, distinct, common shapes to small, less common shapes with less distinct differences between them. The texture of the various objects should be graded from diverse coarse materials to similar smooth materials. The patient and the therapist must also involve themselves in a teaching–relearning interactive experience in which the characteristics of the objects are discussed and correct identification by touch rewarded.

BOX 11-6
Characteristics of Therapeutic Occupation

Generally, activities should

- ► Have the necessary inherent characteristics to evoke the desired response
- ► Allow gradation of response to progress the patient to the next higher level of function
- ► Be within the patient's capabilities
- ► Be meaningful to the person
- ► Be as repetitive as required to evoke the therapeutic benefit

---

CLINICAL REASONING
in OT Practice

Occupation-As-End

Review the case examples in other chapters in this book. What examples of occupation-as-end do you find? Select three. What purpose was each designed to accomplish? What was the evidence in the case report that the behavior became better organized? What meaning did each hold for the patients? What was the evidence that the patient was motivated because of the occupation?

Occupation-as-End	Purpose	Behavior Organized?	Meaning	Motivated?
1.				
2.				
3.				

BOX 11-7
PROCEDURES FOR PRACTICE

Selecting and Grading a Therapeutic Occupation-As-Means

Remediation Goal	Key Factors of the Activity
To retrain sensory awareness or discrimination	Offer various textures, sizes, shapes. Grade from diverse, coarse, large to similar, smooth, small.
To decrease hypersensitivity	Offer various textures and degrees of hardness or softness. Grade from acceptable to barely tolerable.
To reacquire skilled voluntary movement	Be goal-directed, require sought-after response, allow feedback. Grade from simple movements to complex movements.
To improve coordination and dexterity	Require ROM the patient can control. Grade from slow, gross movement involving limited number of joints to fast, precise movement involving a greater number of joints.
To increase passive ROM	Provide controlled stretch or traction. Grade from lesser to greater ROM.
To increase strength	Require movement or holding against resistance or slow to fast movement. Grade from lesser to greater resistance or from slow to fast movement.
To improve cardiopulmonary endurance	Rated at the patient's current MET level. Grade by increasing duration, frequency, then intensity (METs).
To improve muscular endurance	Require movement or holding against 50% or less of maximal strength. Grade by increasing repetitions or duration.
To decrease edema	Allow use of the extremity in an elevated position and require isotonic contraction.
To improve problem solving	Require performance at outside edge of patient's current skill. Grade from simple (one step) to complex (multiple steps), from concrete to abstract.

To Decrease Hypersensitivity

The activity should involve objects or media whose textures can be graded from one that the patient perceives to be least noxious to textures perceived to be tolerably noxious. Another plan grades textures and objects from soft to hard to rough and the contact with the objects from touching them to rubbing them to tapping them.

To Relearn Skilled Voluntary Movement

Organization of voluntary movement depends both on the unique problem or goal and the constraints operating at a given time (Newell, 1986). The activity must have a clear goal or purpose, demand the sought-after movement or movements, and offer opportunity to self-monitor success (feedback). The context and task constraints should support natural responses. Grading should provide increasingly more difficult motor challenges (e.g., moving the body in various directions, moving the limbs in various directions, isolated movement of particular joints, faster movement, or more accurate movement in more challenging contexts).

Sensorimotor learning requires practice, so opportunities for vast amounts of varied practice should be provided. The activity may provide an opportunity for practice simply through the accomplishment of the intended goal. For example, weaving requires multiple passes of the shuttle to produce the desired product and offers good practice of bilateral horizontal abduction and adduction. For other activities the goal may be achieved quickly, so practice is sought through repetition of the whole action, as with ironing, polishing the silverware, throwing a ball, and other activities of daily living. Variable practice promotes learning. Unvaried (blocked) practice improves performance within a session but does not improve long-term learning. Blocked practice is used to begin to develop a new movement or skill (see Chapter 12).

To Increase Coordination and Dexterity

The activity should allow as much ROM as the patient can control and allow grading from slow, gross motions to precise, fast movements involving greater ROM or action at more joints. At first, if you are grading along the continuum of increasing speed, expect accuracy to suffer. A speed–accuracy trade-off is basic to the organization of the CNS (Fitts, 1954).

To Increase Active ROM

The activity must require that the part of the body being treated move to its limit repeatedly and be graded, naturally or through adaptations, to demand greater amounts of movement as the patient's limit changes.

To Increase Passive ROM, or Elongate Soft Tissue Contracture

The activity must provide controlled stretch or traction to the part being treated and held at the end of range for several seconds. ***Stretch should be slow and gentle to avoid tearing the tissue.*** Grade from lesser to greater ROM.

To Increase Strength

Stress to muscle tissue increases strength. Stress can be graded by increasing the velocity and/or resistance needed to complete the activity or, for very weak muscles, by increasing the number of repetitions of an isotonic contraction or the amount of time an isometric contraction is held.

To Increase Cardiopulmonary Endurance

The metabolic demand of the activity (**MET** level) should match the patient's status. The demand can be graded by increasing the duration a task is done, by increasing the frequency of doing the task, by changing the muscles used in the task (smaller muscles increase metabolic demand), or by increasing the intensity (METs). The metabolic intensities (METs) of some activities have been measured and are listed in Chapters 4 and 47.

To Increase Muscular Endurance

The activity must be repetitious over a controlled number of times or period. Resistance should be held to 50% or less of maximal strength.

To Decrease Edema

The activity should entail repetitive isotonic contractions of the muscles in the edematous part. An activity that requires repeated movement of the extremity into an elevated position helps to drain the fluid out of the extremity.

To Improve Perceptual Impairments or Problem-Solving Strategies

The activity should involve varied practice of information processing or perceptual processing at the outside edge of the person's capability. For example, if the person has impaired figure–ground skill, practice may start with detecting one figure from a plain background and progress through finding multiple figures on a plain background or finding one figure in more complex backgrounds until the person has developed the level of functional ability he or she requires (e.g., able to find the scissors in a kitchen "junk" drawer). Gradation is along a continuum of increasing complexity (more stimuli).

If the person has impaired problem-solving skill, practice may start with concrete problems involving objects that the person can see and touch, such as the problem of getting soup out of a can, with can, manual can opener, and electrical can opener at hand. The patient figures out that he or she must open the can to get the soup, selects a can opener, and figures out through exploration how to use the can opener. Therapy may proceed to a higher level of abstraction by asking the person to figure out how many pills he or she needs for

the week if he or she should take one (or two, or more) pill(s) every day. The pill bottle, calendar, and weekly pill minder container are present. The patient may solve the problem in one of several ways: using arithmetic (unlikely, since the patient is in treatment for cognitive deficits); using a calendar, taking out the pill or pills for each day and lining them up on the calendar and counting them; or putting a pill in each compartment of the pill minder and then counting them.

Gradation is along a continuum of concrete to abstract and few objects or ideas to multiple objects or ideas. See Chapters 28 and 29 for suggestions for particular impairments. To reinforce learning, do the assignment in the Clinical Reasoning Box on the next page.

Adaptation

Activity adaptation is the process of modifying a familiar activity of daily living, craft, game, sport, or other occupation to accomplish a therapeutic goal (Box 11-8). Although we may like to think that occupational therapists devised this process, actually Gilbreth did in the early 1900s (Creighton, 1992, 1993). He proposed adapting activity to suit the anatomy of workers to make work more efficient (Gilbreth, 1911).

There are three reasons to adapt an activity in the treatment of the physically disabled. One is to modify the activity to make it therapeutic when ordinarily it would not be so. Many examples of this can be seen in occupational therapy clinics. For example, in wall checkers, the board is mounted on the wall and has pegs at each square to hold the enlarged checkers (Fig. 11-3).

The second reason for adaptation is to graduate the exercise offered by the activity along therapeutic continua to accomplish goals. Grading of activity for this purpose is an original principle of occupational therapy (Creighton, 1993). For example, to increase coordination, the activity must be graded along a continuum from gross, coarse movement to fine, accurate movement.

BOX 11-8
Characteristics of a Good Adaptation

► Accomplishes the specific goal
► Does not encourage or require odd movements or postures
► Is soundly constructed and not dangerous to the patient
► Intrinsically demands a certain response that the patient does not have to concentrate on
► Does not demean the patient; some contrived adaptations seem ridiculous to the patient and so are embarrassing

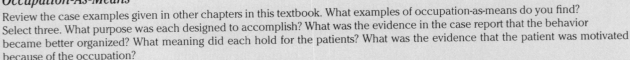

CLINICAL REASONING
in OT Practice

Occupation-As-Means

Review the case examples given in other chapters in this textbook. What examples of occupation-as-means do you find? Select three. What purpose was each designed to accomplish? What was the evidence in the case report that the behavior became better organized? What meaning did each hold for the patients? What was the evidence that the patient was motivated because of the occupation?

Occupation-as-Means	Purpose	Behavior Organized?	Meaning	Motivated?
1.				
2.				
3.				

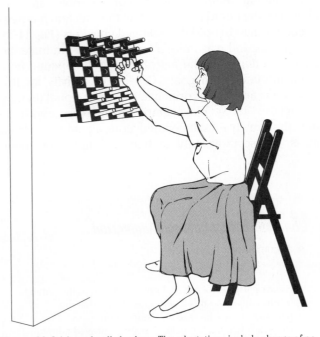

Figure 11-3 Adapted wall checkers. The adaptations include change of position (mounted on wall), size of object (checker), and methods of doing the activity (lift checker off dowels rather than push it).

Checkers and other board games lend themselves easily to such gradations; the board and pieces can be changed from large to small so that the checker aficionado can continue a favorite game while continuing to benefit therapeutically.

The third reason for adapting activities is to enable a person with physical impairments to do an activity or task he or she would be unable to do otherwise. For example, a vehicle can be adapted so that a person with weak upper extremities can drive. Chapters 30 to 34 describe various adaptations for achieving activities and tasks of important roles despite various impairments.

As with all therapeutic techniques, it is vital for the patient to understand the reason that an activity is adapted (Peloquin, 1988). Ways to modify activities are described here and summarized in the Clinical Reasoning box on the following page.

Positioning the Task Relative to the Person

The position of the person relative to the work to be done dictates the movement demanded by the activity and therefore which muscle groups are likely to be used (McGrain & Hague, 1987). Adaptation by positioning

CLINICAL REASONING
in OT Practice

Adapting Occupation for Therapeutic Purpose

Adaptation	Therapeutic Purpose
Positioning the task relative to the person	Increase ROM Specify muscles, motions Enable person to do the task
Arranging objects in relation to others	Improve perceptual responses Require specific movements Decrease energy expenditure
Changing lever arms	Increase strength Reduce strength needed Prevent injuries
Changing materials or texture of materials	Increase strength Increase coordination Challenge sensory system
Changing level of difficulty	Increase cognition Increase perception Increase motor planning Enable person to do the task
Changing the size or shape of objects	Improve dexterity Enable activities, such as feeding, with enlarged handles on utensils Increase strength Increase ROM
Changing color contrast between objects	Improve figure–ground discrimination Enable performance by those with low vision
Changing method of doing the activity	Enable person to do the task Increase strength Increase ROM Increase coordination, dexterity Increase cognitive-perceptual demands
Modifying tool	Enable the person to do the task Prevent deformity Prevent cumulative trauma disorders
Add weights	Increase strength Reduce incoordinated movements Provide PROM
Add springs or rubber bands	Increase strength Reduce incoordinated movements Provide PROM Assist weak muscles

can be made more or less resistive by changing the incline of the surface. For example, if the surface is inclined down and away from the patient, resistance is given to shoulder extension and elbow flexion. If the incline is up and toward the patient, resistance is given to shoulder flexion and elbow extension.

The standard horizontal work surface itself can be raised or lowered to make demands on certain muscle groups or to alter the effect of gravity. For example, a table raised to axilla height allows flexion and extension of the elbow on a gravity-eliminated plane and may enable a person with grade 3+ muscles to eat independently.

Placing items such as nails, mosaic tiles, pieces of yarn, beads, darts, bean bags, and paint brushes in various locations changes the motion required to reach them when performing the activity in an otherwise standard manner. Placement may be high enough to encourage shoulder flexion or abduction; lateral to encourage shoulder rotation, trunk rotation, or horizontal motion; or low to encourage trunk flexion or lateral trunk flexion. All of the placements would encourage improvement in dynamic balance.

Arrangement of Objects Relative to Each Other

To grade an activity for increasing perceptual skills (e. g., figure–ground, unilateral neglect), the arrangement of objects to be used, the printing on a page, and so on can

refers to changes in incline of work surface, height of work surface, or placement of pieces to be added to the project (Figs. 11-4 to 11-8).

Activities that are usually done on a flat surface, such as finger painting, board games, and sanding wood

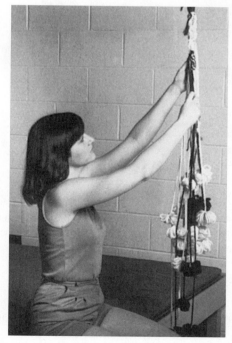

Figure 11-4 Macramé repositioned to require shoulder flexion.

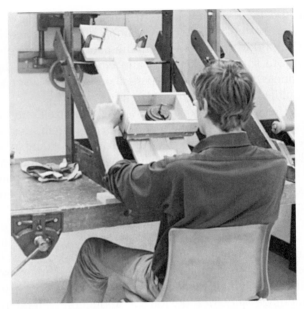

Figure 11-5 Wood repositioned to require shoulder flexion and elbow extension. Sander is adapted to require bilateral usage and can be weighted to adjust resistance.

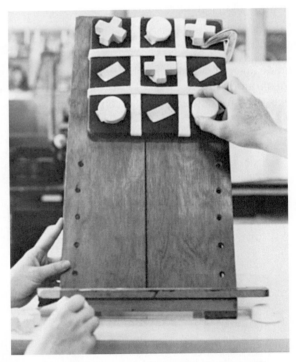

Figure 11-6 Adapted tic-tac-toe repositioned to require shoulder motions and size changed to accommodate poor coordination. The pieces are held in place with Velcro.

hand, while placement on the left encourages use of the left hand. Placement of ingredients on a kitchen counter across the room from the mixing bowl encourages walking in the kitchen that would not occur if all were

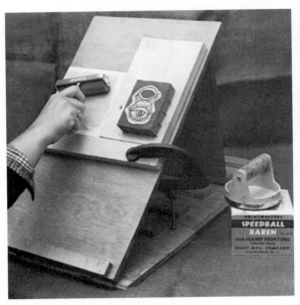

Figure 11-7 Block printing repositioned. Nails below and to the right of the block hold it in place. Height can be changed by moving the board that is held by a C-clamp to the incline board.

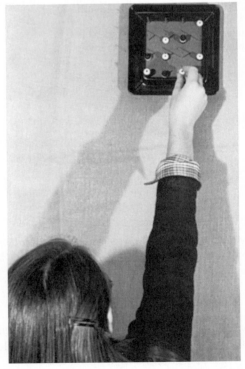

Figure 11-8 Score Four game mounted on the wall to require shoulder flexion and elbow extension.

be graded from sparse to dense (i.e., fewer objects or words with space between versus many objects or words with no space between). Putting game pieces on the right side of the game board encourages use of that

together. On the other hand, placing all objects needed for a task together reduces the energy required to do the task.

Changing Length of Lever Arm

The amount of work a muscle or muscle group is doing depends on the resistance. Resistance is determined by the pull of gravity on the limb and the implements the patient is using, which together act as the resistance lever arm. The effect of a given amount of resistance can be altered by lengthening or shortening the resistance lever arm. The longer the resistance arm, the greater the force required to counterbalance it. The lever arm can be lengthened or shortened by changing the location of the resistance on the limb; for example, applying a weight at the end of the humerus rather than at the wrist reduces the amount of force that the shoulder flexors must generate to lift the weight. The lever arm can also be altered by shortening or lengthening the limb; for example, flexing the knee, which shortens the limb, offers less resistance to hip extension than if the knee were extended. Another example is carrying an object close to the body, which requires less activity of back muscles than if the object is carried at arm's length. Use of a reacher to pick up an object involves more resistance and therefore more muscle output than if the object is picked up directly. Use of a large paintbrush to paint a mural on the wall increases the resistance over using finger paint.

On the other hand, increasing the length of the force lever arm decreases the muscle output needed to accomplish a task. For example, in Figure 11-9, if the clothespin were adapted to have longer handles, less pinch force would be required to open it the same distance.

Attention to lengths of lever arms is important not only in adapting an activity to make it more therapeutic but also in adapting utensils and tools used in daily life tasks to enable weak persons to use them. Furthermore, this idea guides workers in methods of lifting and handling on their jobs to avoid musculoskeletal injuries. See illustrations of lever arms in Chapter 20.

Change of Materials or Texture of Materials

Gradation along the strengthening continuum may be accomplished by selection of material by type and also by variations of texture or density to change resistance. Resistance can be changed, for example, by starting a cutting project with tissue paper and then progressing to heavier materials, such as construction paper, cloth, and leather. Metal tooling can be graded for resistance by choosing materials in grades from thin aluminum to

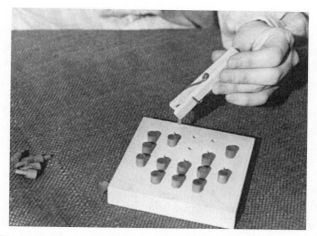

Figure 11-9 Game played using a clothespin to move the pieces to strengthen pinch.

thick copper. Sandpaper is graded from extra fine to coarse, and resistance increases as the grade coarsens. Mixing can be graded from making gelatin dessert to scrambled eggs to biscuit batter and so on. If materials are graded in the opposite direction, that is, from heavy to light, the activity demands increased coordination from the patient. Weaving may begin using rug roving and be graded toward fine linen threads as the patient progresses in coordination.

Cutaneous stimulation changes with the amount of texture of objects or surfaces. By making balls from yarn or terry toweling, carpeting the surfaces the person works on, padding handles with textured material, and so on, the therapist adapts the activity to increase sensory stimulation.

Change in Level of Difficulty

Patterns for craft activities, game rules, extent of task (e.g., prepare instant coffee versus espresso), and level of creativity can be downgraded to enable the patient to succeed or upgraded to demand performance at higher levels. Changing the difficulty entails changing the number of pieces or the ideas that must be manipulated, changing the problem-solving level from concrete reasoning to abstract reasoning, changing the directions from specific to general, and so on. For example, a patient with traumatic brain injury may be unable to pay the bills if the top of the desk is littered with bills and papers but may be able to manage if one bill is taken out at a time.

Change the Size or Shape of Objects

Playing pieces of board games can vary in size and shape (Figs. 11-3 and 11-6) and can therefore offer a therapeutic benefit that the standard objects would not. For example, checkers, which are usually flat pieces approximately 2.5 cm in diameter, can be cylinders, squares, cubes, or spheres and can range in size from tiny to as large as a person's grasp permits.

Reducing the size or changing the shape of the pieces being worked on facilitates the goals of increased dexterity and fine coordination. Therapists creatively change sizes of craft materials (e.g., weaving thread, tiles, paint-by-number guidelines, and ceramic pieces) and recreational materials (e.g., puzzle pieces, chess pieces, and target games) to increase coordination. Tools and utensils can be adapted by changing the size or shape of their handles or adding handles to tools that do not normally have them. In a study of 30 healthy young women, changing the size of the handle on a cup significantly influenced the number of fingers placed through the handle, regardless of cup size or weight, indicating that patients with weak grasps may be able to use a cup with a longer handle that accommodates more fingers and provides leverage (Fuller & Trombly, 1997).

The actual size of the tool can be chosen to offer more or less resistance. For example, saws range in size from small coping saws and hacksaws to large cross-cut and rip saws. Resistance of saws can also be graded by the number of teeth per inch on the blade; the fewer the teeth, the greater the resistance. Woodworking planes vary in size, and the amount of exposed blade can be

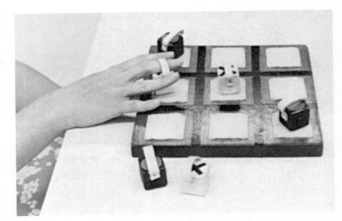

Figure 11-11 Adapted tic-tac-toe to exercise finger extensors; Velcro holds pieces, requiring force to lift them.

adjusted to provide resistance. Size of scissors, screwdrivers, stirring spoons, and other tools and utensils can also be varied.

Change of Color of Multiple Objects

Neistadt et al. (1993) suggested grading challenge to figure–ground ability by changing game objects from contrasting colors to increasingly similar colors.

Change of Method of Doing the Activity

Bowling, basketball, and many other sports can be done seated instead of standing. Change of rules adapts some sports, such as track and field events, to certain requirements of the physically impaired. Sewing and needlework, normally bilateral activities, can be made unilateral by adaptations that hold the material steady for the working hand (Fig. 11-10). Holes can be punched in leather or packs of paper with a drill press in lieu of regular leather or paper punches. Block printing can be done in a hand- or foot-operated printing press rather than in a block printing press. Instead of rolling over on a therapy mat, rolling can be done in bed for more functional relevance.

Change of method is used both for exercise, that is, occupation-as-means, (Figs. 11-9 and 11-11) and for compensation, that is, occupation-as-end (Figs. 11-12 and 11-13). Such compensatory adaptation allows performance of an activity that would otherwise be impossible because of the person's disability.

There is ample evidence, however, that performance in simulated contexts using simulated objects is poorer than performance in natural contexts with actual objects (Dunn, 1993; Flinn, 1999; Ma et al., 1999; Mathiowetz & Wade, 1995; Trombly & Wu, 1999; Wu

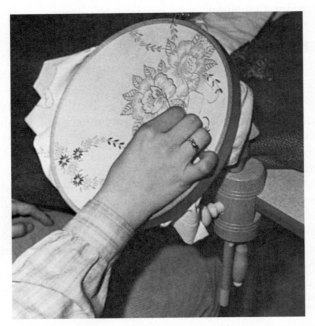

Figure 11-10 Embroidery adapted with use of a hoop that fastens to the table; requires only one hand.

et al., 1998, 2000). Some rehabilitation centers, heeding these research findings, now have simulated real environments to allow patients to practice in realistic contexts (Fig. 11-14).

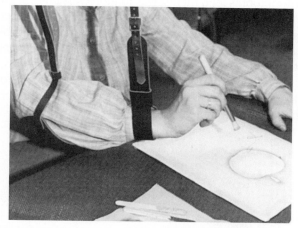

Figure 11-12 Stenciling is made possible by use of a suspension sling. Wrist extensors get exercise.

Use of Modified or Supplemental Tools and Utensils

Using tools when normally none are used or modifying tools or utensils enables a person to accomplish activities and tasks that he or she would not be able to do otherwise. For example, toast can be retrieved from a toaster by use of a wooden spring clothespin when sensory precautions are in effect (Fig. 11-15). Angling the handles on carving knives allows a person with rheumatoid arthritis to cut meat or vegetables without putting deforming forces on the wrist and fingers. Changing keyboard or mouse designs can prevent carpal tunnel syndrome.

Adding Weights

The addition of weights adapts an activity to meet such goals as increase of strength, promotion of co-contraction, and increase of passive ROM by stretch. Some nonresistive activities can be made resistive by adding weights to the apparatus directly or by use

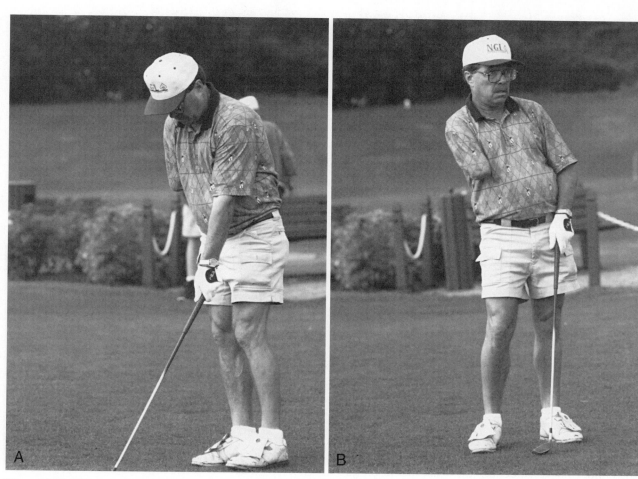

Figure 11-13 Golf is made possible for a person with the use of only one side of the body by changing the method of swinging the club. **B.** Watching the ball land. (Photographs by Jim Hanson.)

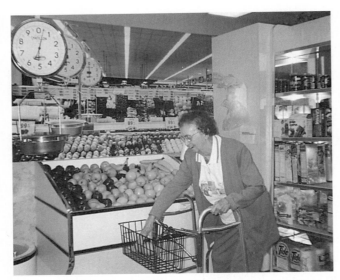

Figure 11-14 "Shopping" at Independence Square Market, a simulated "real" environment to promote best performance in preparation to return to the community. (Photo by Mary Vining Radomski.)

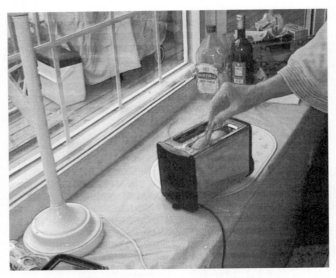

Figure 11-15 Retrieving toast with a spring clothespin.

the patient, as with weighted cuffs, (Fig. 11-16) or by pulley line attachments. With a weighted wrist cuff, leather lacing can be resistive to external rotation and elbow flexion.

Resistance can be changed on all looms; however, the floor looms lend themselves to more versatility in the application of the resistance. Weights can be added directly to the harnesses, treadles, or beater or can be added indirectly to the beater by the use of a pulley system (Fig. 11-17). Tools also are weights, and they can be selected or adjusted to offer graded resistance; for instance, hammers range from lightweight tack hammers to heavy claw hammers.

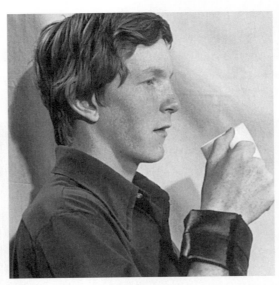

Figure 11-16 Weight cuff used to damp intention tremor or other uncoordinated movements or to add resistance to an action that is not normally resistive.

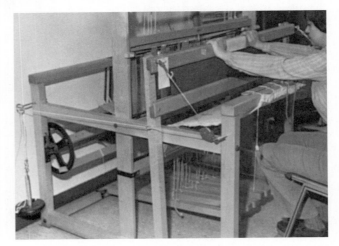

Figure 11-17 Floor loom adapted with weights and pulleys to resist elbow extension.

of pulleys, while others may be made resistive by adding weights to the person. For example, to resist shoulder extension and elbow flexion, weights can be suspended from pulleys attached across from the person on a flat or inclined surface, with the weight lines running from each handle of a bilateral sanding block. The line of pull can be reversed to resist shoulder flexion and elbow extension by attaching the pulleys behind the person. As another example, braid weaving can be made resistive to shoulder flexion by means of weights and pulleys attached over the back of the patient's chair, with the lines running to a cuff fastened around the humerus. Weights can be attached directly to

Adding Springs or Rubber Band

Springs and rubber bands are means of adapting activity to increase strength through resistance, to assist a weak muscle, or to stretch muscle and other soft tissue to increase passive ROM. When offering resistance, the spring or rubber band is positioned so that its pull is opposite to the pull of motion of the target muscle group, whereas if used for assistance, they are set to pull in the same direction as the contracting muscle group. Springs and rubber bands applied for the purpose of stretching are placed so the pull is against the tissue to be stretched.

Springs of graduated tensions may be applied directly to the equipment. A beater of a floor loom can be made resistive to elbow extension or flexion by attaching springs either from the breast beam to the beater to resist elbow extension or from the beater to the castle (the center upright of the loom) to resist elbow flexion. Rubber bands can be added to smaller pieces of equipment and can be graded from thin and light tension to thick and heavy tension. For example, a rubber band can be wrapped around the pincer end of a spring-type clothespin to add resistance when it is used in games involving picking up small pieces (Fig. 11-9).

When rubber bands or springs are used to create a force of resistance in one direction, the return motion can involve passive stretch of the same muscle group during motion in the opposite direction, unless the person does an eccentric contraction of the resisted muscles to prevent the stretching pull. For example, if a spring is attached to a loom's beater to resist elbow flexion when the beater is pulled toward the person, on the return motion the spring will pull into extension, stretching the flexors unless the patient eccentrically contracts the flexors. Eccentric contraction would be desired, as it also exercises the weak flexors.

Summary Review Questions

1. Define occupation-as-end.
2. Define occupation-as-means.
3. What are the general characteristics required of an activity to be used to treat motor impairments?
4. How does analysis relate to selection of an occupation or activity?
5. How do goals and treatment principles relate to selection of occupation-as-means? Occupation-as-end?
6. What are two reasons for adapting an occupation used as means? Occupation-as-end?
7. What are the five characteristics of good adaptations?

8. What therapeutic goals can be accomplished by the following?
   ▶ Changing the position of the task relative to the person
   ▶ Adding weights to tools or game pieces
   ▶ Adding springs or rubber bands to craft equipment or tools
   ▶ Changing the length of lever arms of tools, equipment, or the limb itself
   ▶ Changing the material to be used in a project
   ▶ Changing the method of doing an activity

Acknowledgments

I thank my former students Janice Ferguson, Julie Pope, Natalia Ramsbey, Pei-Luen Tsai, Ellen Rosenberg, Yvonne Fuller, Dr. Susan Murphy, Dr. Pimjai Sudsawad, Dr. Steven Cope, Dr. Ching-Yi Wu, Dr. Hui-Ing Ma, and Dr. Susan Fasoli for their assistance and conversations about occupation.

References

American Occupational Therapy Association (1995). Position paper: Occupation. *American Journal of Occupational Therapy, 49,* 1015–1018.

American Occupational Therapy Association (1997). Statement: Fundamental concepts of occupational therapy: Occupation, purposeful activity, and function. *American Journal of Occupational Therapy, 51,* 864–866.

Ayres, A. J. (1958). Basic concepts of clinical practice in physical disabilities. *American Journal of Occupational Therapy, 12,* 300–302, 311.

Bloch, M. W., Smith, D. A., & Nelson, D. L. (1989). Heart rate, activity, duration, and affect in added-purpose versus single-purpose jumping activities. *American Journal of Occupational Therapy, 43,* 25–30.

Bruner, J. (1990). *Acts of meaning.* Cambridge, MA: Harvard University.

Burton, A. W., & Davis, W. E. (1996). Ecological task analysis: Utilizing intrinsic measures in research and practice. *Human Movement Science, 15,* 285–314.

Chandani, A., & Hill, C. (1990). What really is therapeutic activity? *British Journal of Occupational Therapy, 53,* 15–18.

Clark, F., Parham, D., Carlson, M. E., Frank, G., Jackson, J. Pierce, D., Wolfe, R. J., & Zemke, R. (1991). Occupational science: Academic innovation in the service of occupational therapy's future. *American Journal of Occupational Therapy, 45,* 300–310.

Creighton, C. (1992). The origin and evolution of activity analysis. *American Journal of Occupational Therapy, 46,* 45–48.

Creighton, C. (1993). Looking back: Graded activity: Legacy of the sanatorium. *American Journal of Occupational Therapy, 47,* 745–748.

Csikszentmihalyi, M. (1990). *Flow: The Psychology of Optimal Experience.* New York: Harper & Row.

Cynkin, S., & Robinson, A. M. (1990). *Occupational Therapy and Activities Health: Toward Health Through Activities.* Boston: Little, Brown.

Darnell, J. L., & Heater, S. L. (1994). The issue is: Occupational therapist or activity therapist: Which do you choose to be? *American Journal of Occupational Therapy, 48,* 467–486.

Davis, W. E., & Burton, A. W. (1991). Ecological task analysis: Translating movement behavior theory into practice. *Adapted Physical Activity Quarterly, 8,* 154–177.

Decety, J., Grezes, J., Costes, N., Perani, D., Jeannerod, M., Procyk, E., Grassi, F., & Fazio, F. (1997). Brain activity during observation of actions: Influence of action content and subject's strategy. *Brain, 120* (Pt 10), 1763–1777.

DeKuiper, W. P., Nelson, D. L., & White, B. E. (1993). Materials-based occupation versus imagery-based occupation versus rote exercise: A replication and extension. *Occupational Therapy Journal of Research, 13,* 183–197.

Dunn, W. (1993). The issue is: Measurement of function: Actions for the future. *American Journal of Occupational Therapy, 47,* 357–359.

Fisher, A. G. (1997). *Assessment of Motor and Process Skills* (2nd ed.). Fort Collins, CO: Three Star.

Fisher, A. G. (1998). Uniting practice and theory in an occupational framework. *American Journal of Occupational Therapy, 52,* 509–521.

Fisk, J. D., & Goodale, M. A. (1989). The effects of instructions to subjects on the programming of visually directed reaching movements. *Journal of Motor Behavior, 21,* 5–19.

Fitts, P. M. (1954). The information capacity of the human motor system in controlling the amplitude of movement. *Journal of Experimental Psychology, 47,* 381–391.

Flinn, N. A. (1999). Clinical interpretation of "Effect of rehabilitation tasks on organization of movement after stroke." *American Journal of Occupational Therapy, 53,* 345–347.

Fuller, Y., & Trombly, C. A. (1997). Effect of object characteristics on female grasp patterns. *American Journal of Occupational Therapy, 51,* 481–487.

Gentile, A. M., Higgins, J. R., Miller, E. A., & Rosen, B. (1975). Structure of motor tasks. In *Mouvement Actes du 7e Symposium Canadien en Appentissage Psycho-motor et Psychologie du Sport* (pp. 11–28). Quebec (out of print).

Gentile, A. (1987). Skill acquisition: Action, movement and neuromotor processes. In J. H. Carr, R. B. Shepherd, J. Gordon, A. M. Gentile, & J. M. Held (Eds.), *Movement Science: Foundations for Physical Therapy in Rehabilitation* (pp. 93–154). Rockville, MD: Aspen Systems.

Georgopoulos, A. P. (1986). On reaching. *Annual Review of Neurosciences, 9,* 147–170.

Gibson, J. J. (1977). The theory of affordances. In R. E. Shaw & J. Bransford (Eds.), *Perceiving, Acting, and Knowing: Toward an Ecological Psychology* (pp. 67–82). Hillsdale, NJ: Lawrence Erlbaum.

Gilbreth, F. B. (1911). *Motion Study.* New York: Van Nostrand.

Gilbreth, F. B., & Gilbreth, L. M. (1920). *Motion Study for the Handicapped.* London: Routledge.

Glass, T. A., Mendes de Leon, C., Marottoli, R. A., & Berkman, L. F. (1999). Population based study of social and productive activities as predictors of survival among elderly Americans. *British Journal of Medicine, 319,* 478–483.

Grady, A. P. (1992). Nationally speaking: Occupation as vision. *American Journal of Occupational Therapy, 46,* 1062–1065.

Granit, R. (1977). *The Purposive Brain.* Cambridge, MA: MIT.

Hoppes, S. (1997). Can play increase standing tolerance? A pilot study. *Physical & Occupational Therapy in Geriatrics, 15,* 65–73.

Jeannerod, M. (1988). *The Neural and Behavioral Organization of Goal-Directed Movements.* Oxford, UK: Clarendon.

Kamm, K., Thelen, E., & Jensen, J. L. (1990). A dynamical systems approach to motor development. *Physical Therapy, 70,* 763–775.

Kielhofner, G. (1994). *Knowledge and Practice in Occupational Therapy.* Philadelphia: Davis.

Kielhofner, G. (Ed.). (1995). *A Model of Human Occupation: Theory and Application* (2nd ed.). Baltimore: Williams & Wilkins.

King, T. I. (1993). Hand strengthening with a computer for purposeful activity. *American Journal of Occupational Therapy, 47,* 635–637.

Kircher, M. A. (1984). Motivation as a factor of perceived exertion in purposeful versus nonpurposeful activity. *American Journal of Occupational Therapy, 38,* 165–170.

LaMore, K. L., & Nelson, D. L. (1993). The effects of options on performance of an art project in adults with mental disabilities. *American Journal of Occupational Therapy, 47*(5), 397–401.

Lang, E. M., Nelson, D. L., & Bush, M. A. (1992). Comparison of performance in materials-based occupation, imagery-based occupation, and rote exercise in nursing home residents. *American Journal of Occupational Therapy, 46,* 607–611.

Levine, R. E., & Gitlin, L. N. (1993). A model to promote activity competence in elders. *American Journal of Occupational Therapy, 47,* 147–153.

Llorens, L. A. (1986). Activity analysis: Agreement among factors in a sensory processing model. *American Journal of Occupational Therapy, 40,* 103–110.

Llorens, L. A. (1993). Activity analysis: Agreement between participants and observers on perceived factors in occupation components. *Occupational Therapy Journal of Research, 13,* 198–211.

Ma, H., Trombly, C. A., & Robinson-Podolski, C. (1999). The effect of context on skill acquisition and transfer. *American Journal of Occupational Therapy, 53,* 138–144.

Marteniuk, R. G., MacKenzie, C. L., Jeannerod, M., Athenes, S., & Dugas, C. (1987). Constraints on human arm movement trajectories. *Canadian Journal of Psychology, 41,* 365–378.

Mathiowetz, V., & Wade, M. G. (1995). Task constraints and functional motor performance of individuals with and without multiple sclerosis. *Ecological Psychology, 7,* 99–123.

Mayer, N. H., Keating, D. J., & Rapp, D. (1986). Skills, routines, and activity patterns of daily living: A functional nested approach. In B. Uzzell & Y. Gross (Eds.), *Clinical Neuropsychology of Intervention* (pp. 205–222). Boston: Martinus Nijhoff.

McGrain, P., & Hague, M. A. (1987). An electromyographic study of the middle deltoid and middle trapezius muscles during warping. *Occupational Therapy Journal of Research, 7,* 225–233.

McKinnon, A. L. (1992). Time use for self care, productivity, and leisure among elderly Canadians. *Canadian Journal of Occupational Therapy, 59,* 102–110.

Meyer, A. (1922, 1977). The philosophy of occupational therapy. *Archives of Occupational Therapy, 1,* 1-10; *American Journal of Occupational Therapy, 31,* 639–642.

Miller, L., & Nelson, D. L. (1987). Dual-purpose activity versus single-purpose activity in terms of duration of task, exertion level, and affect. *Occupational Therapy in Mental Health, 1,* 55–67.

Mosey, A. C. (1981). *Occupational Therapy: Configuration of a Profession.* New York: Raven.

Moyers, P. A. (1999). The guide to occupational therapy practice. *American Journal of Occupational Therapy, 53,* 247–322.

Murphy, S., Trombly, C. A., Tickle-Degnen, L., & Jacobs, K. (1999). The effect of keeping as end-product on intrinsic motivation. *American Journal of Occupational Therapy, 53,* 153–158.

National Society for the Promotion of Occupational Therapy. (1917). *Constitution of the National Society for the Promotion of Occupational Therapy.* Baltimore: Sheppard Hospital.

Neistadt, M. E., McAuley, D., Zecha, D., & Shannon, R. (1993). An analysis of a board game as a treatment activity. *American Journal of Occupational Therapy, 47,* 154–160.

Nelson, W. L. (1983). Physical principles for economies of skilled movements. *Biological Cybernetics, 46*, 135–147.

Nelson, D. L. (1988). Occupation: Form and performance. *American Journal of Occupational Therapy, 42*, 633–641.

Nelson, D. L. (1996). Therapeutic occupation: A definition. *American Journal of Occupational Therapy, 50*, 775–782.

Nelson, D. L., Konosky, K., Fleharty, K., Webb, R., Newer, K., Hazboun, V. P., Fontane, C., & Licht, B. C. (1996). The effects of an occupationally embedded exercise on bilaterally assisted supination in persons with hemiplegia. *American Journal of Occupational Therapy, 50*, 639–646.

Newell, K. M. (1986). Constraints on the development of coordination. In M. G. Wade & H. T. A. Whiting (Eds.), *Motor Development in Children: Aspects of Coordination and Control* (pp. 341–360). Boston: Martinus Nijhoff.

Okoye, R. L. (1993). Computer applications in occupational therapy. In H. L. Hopkins & H. D. Smith (Eds.), *Willard and Spackman's Occupational Therapy* (8th ed., pp. 341–353). Philadelphia: Lippincott.

Peloquin, S. M. (1988). Linking purpose to procedure during interactions with patients. *American Journal of Occupational Therapy, 42*, 775–781.

Pentland, W., Harvey, A. S., Smith, T., & Walker, J. (1999). The impact of spinal cord injury on men's time use. *Spinal Cord, 37*, 786–792.

Polatajko, H. J., Mandich, A., & Martini, R. (2000). Dynamic performance analysis: A framework for understanding occupational performance. *American Journal of Occupational Therapy, 54*, 65–72.

Price-Lackey, P., & Cashman, J. (1996). Jenny's story: Reinventing oneself through occupation and narrative configuration. *American Journal of Occupational Therapy, 50*, 306–314.

Ramsbey, N. (1993). Is purposeful activity effective in remediating physical impairments and/or restoring function? *Journal of Occupational Therapy Students, 7*, 7–14.

Reilly, M. (1962). Occupation can be one of the great ideas of 20th century medicine. *American Journal of Occupational Therapy, 16*, 1–9.

Sietsema, J. M., Nelson, D. L., Mulder, R. M., Mervau-Scheidel, D., & White, B. E. (1993). The use of a game to promote arm reach in persons with traumatic brain injury. *American Journal of Occupational Therapy, 47*, 19–24.

Slagle, E. C. (1914). History of the development of occupation for the insane. *Maryland Psychiatric Quarterly, 4*(1), 14–20.

Smith, N. R., Kielhofner, G., & Watts, J. H. (1986). The relationships between volition, activity pattern, and life satisfaction in the elderly. *American Journal of Occupational Therapy, 40*, 278–283.

Spaulding, S. J., & Robinson, K. L. (1984). Electromyographic study of the upper extremity during bilateral sanding: Unresisted and resisted conditions. *American Journal of Occupational Therapy, 38*, 258–262.

Steinbeck, T. M. (1986). Purposeful activity and performance. *American Journal of Occupational Therapy, 40*, 529–534.

Thomas, J. J., Vander Wyk, S., & Boyer, J. (1999). Contrasting occupational forms: Effects on performance and affect in patients undergoing Phase II cardiac rehabilitation. The *Occupational Therapy Journal of Research, 19*, 187–202.

Trombly, C. A. (1993). The issue is: Anticipating the future: Assessment of occupational function. *American Journal of Occupational Therapy, 47*, 253–257.

Trombly, C. A. (1995). Occupation: Purposefulness and meaningfulness as therapeutic mechanisms. *American Journal of Occupational Therapy, 49*, 960–972.

Trombly, C. A., & Cole, J. M. (1979). Electromyographic study of four hand muscles during selected activities. *American Journal of Occupational Therapy, 33*, 440–449.

Trombly, C. A., & Ma, H. (2000). *Evidence Based Literature Review on Occupational Therapy and Stroke*. Bethesda, MD: American Occupational Therapy Association.

Trombly, C. A., & Quintana, L. A. (1983). Activity analysis: Electromyographic and electrogoniometric verification. *Occupational Therapy Journal of Research, 3*, 104–120.

Trombly, C. A., & Scott, A. D. (1977). *Occupational therapy for physical dysfunction*. Baltimore: Williams & Wilkins.

Trombly, C. A., & Wu, C. (1999). Effect of rehabilitation tasks on organization of movement after stroke. *American Journal of Occupational Therapy, 53*, 333–344.

Tsai, P.-L. (1994). *Activity analysis and activity selection among occupational therapists: A survey*. Unpublished Master's thesis, Boston University.

van der Weel, F. R., van der Meer, A. L. H., & Lee D. N. (1991). Effect of task on movement control in cerebral palsy: Implications for assessment and therapy. *Developmental Medicine and Child Neurology, 33*, 419–426.

Watson, D. E. (1997). *Task Analysis: An Occupational Performance Approach*. Bethesda, MD: American Occupational Therapy Association.

Wu, C., Trombly, C. A., & Lin, K. (1994). The relationship between occupational form and occupational performance: A kinematic prospective. *American Journal of Occupational Therapy, 48*, 679–687.

Wu, C., Trombly, C. A., Lin, K., & Tickle-Degnen, L. (1998). Effects of object affordances on reaching performance in persons with and without cerebrovascular accident. *American Journal of Occupational Therapy, 52*, 447–456.

Wu, C., Trombly, C. A., Lin, K., & Tickle-Degnen, L. (2000). A kinematic study of contextual effects on reaching performance in persons with and without stroke: Influences of object availability. *Archives of Physical Medicine and Rehabilitation, 81*, 95–101.

Yerxa, E. J., & Baum, S. (1986). Engagement in daily occupations and life satisfaction among people with spinal cord injuries. *Occupational Therapy Journal of Research, 6*, 271–283.

Yerxa, E. J., & Locker, S. (1990). Quality of time use by adults with spinal cord injuries. *American Journal of Occupational Therapy, 44*, 318–326.

Yoder, R. M., Nelson, D. L., & Smith, D. A. (1989). Added-purpose versus rote exercise in female nursing home residents. *American Journal of Occupational Therapy, 43*, 581–586.

Zimmerer-Branum, S., & Nelson, D. L. (1995). Occupationally embedded exercise versus rote exercise: A choice between occupational forms by elderly nursing home residents. *American Journal of Occupational Therapy, 49*, 397–402.

12

Learning

Nancy Ann Flinn and Mary Vining Radomski

LEARNING OBJECTIVES

After studying this chapter, the reader will be able to do the following:

1. Differentiate between patient performance and patient learning.
2. Outline clinical considerations necessary for planning patient-specific teaching.
3. Explain the roles of context, feedback, and practice in the acquisition of both task-specific skills and general strategies.
4. List phases of teaching patients and describe the advantages and disadvantages of various teaching technologies.

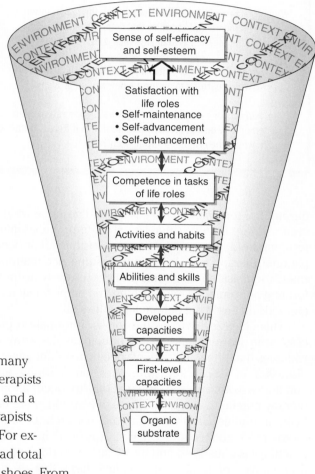

*L*earning is a primary therapeutic mechanism underlying many if not all occupational therapy interventions. Occupational therapists teach patients to use adaptive equipment, new ways to move, and a variety of compensatory skills and strategies. As teachers, therapists must determine whether and when learning has taken place. For example, after a 30-minute dressing session, a patient who has had total knee replacement surgery is able to don his pants, socks, and shoes. From a traditional learning perspective, the patient's performance at the end of the session reflects the extent to which he or she has learned the desired skill or strategy. However, what if a nurse later reports that the patient is unable to carry out the activities he demonstrated proficiency with the day before? One can easily deduce that while within-session performance was buoyed by cues and practice, true learning did not occur.

Schmidt's (1988) contemporary definition of motor learning allows us to differentiate learning from within-session **performance**. According to Schmidt (1988), "Motor learning is a set of processes associated with practice or experience leading to relatively permanent changes in the capability for responding" (p. 346). Based on this definition of learning, we would expect the knee replacement patient to demonstrate similar levels of proficiency after the occupational therapy session as during. The term *performance* is used to describe what is seen during training, that is, short-term capabilities resulting from instruction, cues, or assistance. For occupational therapy to help patients resume occupational roles, therapists must understand the process of transforming performance into learning and employ teaching methods that help the patient learn the skills.

This chapter discusses the role of information processing in learning and then summarizes the array of variables that affect the patient-specific teaching plan. It discusses in detail key influences on learning and concludes with specific applications to occupational therapy practice. As regards issues of learning, there has been a traditional division in the research between motor tasks and cognitive tasks. However, in clinical practice it is unusual to find motor tasks that do not have a cognitive component or cognitive tasks that do not have a motor component. Therefore, because this distinction does not translate well into practice and because principles in the two areas are similar, they will be reviewed together in this chapter.

Human Information Processing Model of Learning

Learning is inextricably linked to memory, specifically the **encoding** and **retrieval** of information. As explained in Chapter 8, people hold environmental stimuli very briefly in a series of short-term sensory stores before transferring it to limited-capacity working memory (Atkinson & Shiffrin, 1971). In working memory, also called short-term memory, people may use control processes to encode information for storage in long-term memory (Schneider & Shiffrin, 1977). These control processes include but are not limited to rehearsal, coding, and imaging (Atkinson & Shiffrin). Rehearsal is rote repetition of information, whereas coding entails linking the new information to something already meaningful. Imaging transforms verbal information to visual images that are stored in memory. Craik and Tulving (1975) found that the durability of the memory trace is a function of depth of processing. That is, deep processing, as in the time-consuming process of linking new information to personally relevant old knowledge, results in better retention than shallow processing, such as rote rehearsal. If the learner does not use some form of conscious control, the memory trace quickly fades from working memory and cannot be recovered or stored (Atkinson & Shiffrin). From the standpoint of human information processing, learning is the transfer of information from short-term or working memory to long-term memory (Shiffrin & Schneider, 1977).

Controlled Versus Automatic Information Processing

Consider the attentional resources required of you the first time you drove a car compared with the attention required for the same task now. After years of experience, the car seems to drive itself, freeing the driver to concentrate on plans for the day or talk to a passenger. This example typifies the difference between controlled and automatic processing.

Controlled Processing

A controlled process is technically a temporary activation of a series or sequence of elements in long-term memory under the control and attention of the thinker (Schneider & Shiffrin, 1977). For example, the new driver must actively recall specific rules and instructions and direct his or her attention to each motor sequence of the task. Controlled processing is limited by the capacity of working memory and therefore effortful but flexible in handling novel situations. When learning a new task or skill that requires effortful concentration, people employ controlled processing. Because of this, patients learning new skills or behaviors can process only a limited number of inputs (instructions, cues, environmental distractions) at a time.

Automatic Processing

With enough controlled processing, a task requires less and less concentration to carry out (Shiffrin & Schneider, 1977). That is, the task becomes increasingly automatic, as in the example of the proficient driver. Automatic processing occurs when specific contextual stimuli internal or external to the person trigger the activation of a specific learned sequence in long-term memory (Schneider & Shiffrin, 1977). Given enough repetition, the individual performs the skill or task in a consistent manner with little or no attention. Sternberg (1986) suggested that development of a full level of automatization requires at least 200 trials of a task but that automatization begins in as few as 10 trials, so long as those trials involve consistency. With fully automatic

---

BOX 12-1
Definition of Error-Free Learning

Wilson and Evans (1996) propose error-free learning methods for persons with severe memory impairments. They suggest that these individuals have difficulty remembering what they learned if they made errors during the training process. Error-free learning is based on implicit learning in that learners are helped to do it right each time the new skill is performed by introducing and then fading preemptive cues and/or assistance. Guessing and trial-and-error are avoided, and because training generally occurs in the context in which the new skills will be used, expectations of transfer are minimized.

BOX 12-2
Definitions of Implicit and Explicit Learning

With any new task, subjects learn through several processing methods. These methods are supported by separate brain structures and have very different characteristics:

Explicit Learning
The conscious learning of the rules of the task, often called declarative learning. This type of learning includes conscious recollections about facts and events. It can be facilitated by a therapist through direct instruction about key environmental features, task-relevant feedback, and cues regarding movement organization (Reber & Squire, 1994). Explicit learning is more flexible than implicit learning and has been shown to generalize more easily, probably because it is not as context dependent as implicit learning (Squire, 1994).

Implicit Learning
Learning how to do a task, is similar to procedural learning. This includes motor skill learning, perceptual and cognitive skills, habits, and simple forms of conditioning (Reber & Squire, 1994). Much of the learning of a motor task is thought to be implicit, including the dynamics of force production in the task, the interaction of active and passive components of the multiple joints involved in the task. Implicit learning, because it does not occur at a conscious level, is facilitated through structuring the environment to create opportunities for appropriate practice of the task (Gentile, 1998). Implicit learning is more robust than explicit learning and retains its strength even when the explicit knowledge about a task has decayed (Lee & Vakoch, 1996). For example, an individual may be unable to describe how to cook a familiar dish but able to cook the dish without any difficulty.

---

skills, people cannot stop themselves from performing the overlearned sequence unless control processes are employed to override it. Box 12-1 discusses implications related to helping patients with memory impairment to reacquire skills.

According to Giles (1998), overlearning is practice of a skill or strategy well beyond demonstration of learning or proficiency; it increases the likelihood that the skill or strategy will become automatic. These automatic skills and strategies become the easiest behaviors to initiate from an array of possible behaviors (Giles, 1998), minimizing demands on attention and decision making. Habits are examples of automatic motor sequences that according to Kielhofner et al. (1982), organize a person's tasks, space, and time. Characteristic of automatic skills and strategies, habits are responsive to the environmental conditions under which they are learned and develop with repetition (Kielhofner et al., 1982). Occupational therapists often help patients resume or relearn self-maintenance tasks that once were automatic. Box 12-2 has examples of other ways in which information can be learned.

Implications of the Information Processing Memory Model

Attention and memory play an important role in many aspects of learning. Therefore, occupational therapists assess these domains before they try to teach patients skills or strategies. Sensitivity to distractions, such as pain, fatigue, and noise, allows therapists to optimize the likelihood that patients will use limited-capacity cognitive resources to hold and ultimately store stimuli related to the new skills or strategies. Therapists also facilitate memory storage and retrieval by helping patients use effective control processes, such as linking the new information to something they already know. Finally, therapists recognize that for many skills, the learning end point is not proficiency but automaticity. Therapists ultimately enable their patients to carry out these tasks with accuracy and ease if they encourage consistency in performance (consistent environment, consistent sequence of steps).

Clinical Considerations in Teaching Patients

In advance of every teaching intervention, occupational therapists make deliberate decisions regarding appropriate teaching methods. These decisions are based on the characteristics of the patient, anticipated length of intervention, desired learning outcome (specific task versus general strategy), and expectations for transfer and generalization.

Patients' Characteristics

A patient's learning potential is determined by many factors. Variables affecting cognitive status (reviewed in Chapter 8) are critical contributors to learning potential. They include neurobiological, affective, experiential, and sociocultural influences. In brief, the *neurobiological influences* on cognitive function are largely associated with the physiological and anatomical integrity of a person's brain. *Affective influences* may interfere with learning because depression and anxiety, for example, distract a person from attending to new information and storing that information in memory. Therapists consider other personal affective influences with similar effects on learning, such as motivation to improve function and pain and fatigue. (Chapter 9 discusses assessing these aspects of personal context.) Finally, each individual brings his or her *experiential sociocultural* background to the lesson. Literacy is one important dimension of the experiential sociocultural influence on learning, with many implications regarding teaching methods. (Again, see Chapter 9 regarding assessing literacy.) Furthermore,

Neistadt (1995) suggested that occupational therapists attempt to answer four questions regarding patients' learning capacities during the course of their traditional evaluation. These questions include the following:

1. What modes of input (visual, auditory, tactile) can this patient process most easily?
2. What approaches to tasks (outputs or behaviors) are still available to this patient?
3. What tasks remain meaningful or are most likely to facilitate learning for this patient?
4. How well is this patient able to transfer learning, that is, apply specific skills to a variety of tasks under a variety of circumstances?

Anticipated Length of Treatment

Occupational therapists also consider how many teaching sessions are likely to be available. Typically this is dictated by expected length of stay at the hospital, rehabilitation center, or nursing facility, insurance coverage of rehabilitation services, acuteness of medical condition, and learning potential of the patient. Awareness of time constraints for teaching allows the clinician to anticipate what stage of learning the patient will attain by the completion of treatment. Discharge planning then incorporates recommendations for continuing and extending the learning that began in treatment.

Stages of Learning

Poole (1995) summarized Fitts and Posner's (1967) three sequential stages of learning, cognitive, associative, and autonomous. During the cognitive stage, the patient tries to understand the requirements of the task. The patient uses conscious control to acquire the new skill or strategy: thinking through or verbalizing the steps, attending to visual and verbal feedback from the therapist, and determining what cues to heed.

In the associative stage, the patient has determined the most effective way of doing the task and begins to make refinements in performance. The learner relies less on vision and verbal feedback and begins to use internal feedback mechanisms. During this stage, practice takes on primary importance; this important dimension of learning is discussed in more detail later in this chapter.

During the autonomous stage the new skill or strategy becomes increasingly automatic or habitual. The patient can accurately perform most of the skill or strategy without thinking about it and is less subject to interference from other activities or environmental distractions.

Desired Learning Outcomes: Task-Specific Skills Versus General Strategy Related to Expectations for Transfer and Generalization

Recipients of occupational therapy services have a variety of learning needs. Two categories of learning end points include acquisition of task-specific skills and acquisition of general strategies. Therapists deliberately determine the patient-specific learning end point, as it dictates teaching methods, length of treatment, and expectations for transfer and generalization.

Task-Specific Skills and Transfer of Training

After a stroke, many patients receive occupational therapy services to learn task-specific skills such as how to dress themselves using only one hand. Acquired skills are expected to enhance function solely within the training tasks. For example, a patient who receives home-based treatment may learn techniques specific to donning her housecoat and slippers (her usual attire) at the side of her bed, which rests on shag carpeting. Teaching in this situation (within the environment and context that the skill will be used) is task specific. The learning process is embedded in the performance environment, with surroundings and objects becoming cues. The therapist does not expect the patient to apply skills learned in this sequence to a whole host of new tasks, and therefore, training time is minimized. Typically the therapist hopes that given enough consistent repetition, the routine will be carried out automatically.

However, occupational therapy intervention, such as activities of daily living (ADL) training, typically begins while the patient is hospitalized. Patients often learn one-handed dressing techniques from hospital beds in rooms with very different characteristics from those of their homes. For the intervention to improve the patient's level of independence after discharge, the therapist must train to transfer. That is, therapists employ teaching techniques that optimize patients' chances of being able to apply the task-specific dressing skills learned at the hospital when they get home.

Transfer of learning refers to a person's ability to carry out the same task in a different environment. According to Toglia (1991), transfer is not an all-or-none phenomenon. She described four levels of transfer, near, immediate, far, and very far, based on the number of differences in the surface characteristics between the learning and real-life environments. In general, near transfer requires the person to apply the same skill in very similar circumstances, whereas far transfer implies greater differences in application environment (Perkins, 1995). Transfer is associated with perceptual similarities of tasks, not similarities in underlying principles (Perkins). Therefore, transfer places minimal demands

on metaprocessing abilities (see Chapter 8) and requires less training time than generalization of newly learned strategies (Saloman & Perkins, 1989).

Strategies and Generalization of Learning

Whereas acquisition of task-specific skills involves learning targeted behavioral sequences, the acquisition of strategies entails learning rules or principles that can be broadly applied. For example, many therapists expect persons with stroke to learn this general strategy: dress the weak side first and undress the weak side last. This rule or principle enables patients to don and doff sweatshirts, dress shirts, slacks, and outwear, but it presumes **generalization** of learning.

Generalization occurs when the person is able to apply the newly learned strategy to a new task in a new environment. For example, the patient who demonstrates the ability to get dressed one-handed in the hospital can use the same strategies to put on a raincoat at home. Generalization, as it is here defined, depends on the learner's mindful abstraction of a principle and is based on conceptual similarities between the learning task and environment and the real-world application (Perkins, 1995). Generalization of learning places greater demands on patients' metaprocessing abilities (Saloman & Perkins, 1989). In fact, the more abstract the strategy, the more difficult it is to learn (Kirby, 1984). (It is easier for a patient to learn to dress the weak extremity before the strong one than to learn to use a higher-order problem-solving strategy.)

Fundamentals of the Teaching–Learning Process

Clearly, the value of occupational therapy intervention will largely be judged by the extent to which new skills and strategies are carried out in patients' real-life environments. Therapists interested in helping patients achieve transfer and generalization objectives incorporate research findings about critical constructs in teaching–learning theory. These constructs relate to the therapeutic use of context, **feedback**, and **practice**.

Therapeutic Use of Context

Many conceptions of context as a facilitator or barrier to function can be found in the occupational therapy and rehabilitation literature (American Occupational Therapy Association, 1994; Dunn et al., 1994; Fisher, 1998; World Health Organization, 1997) (see Chapters 9 and 10). Fisher (1998) broadly defined context to include the following dimensions: temporal, environmental, cultural, societal, social, role, motivational, capacity, and task. We now briefly discuss the influence of task and environmental context on learning.

Role of Context in Learning

Research indicates that task context has a stronger influence on motor performance than previously believed and must be carefully manipulated in treatment. Wu et al. (1994) demonstrated that college students elicited smoother and faster arm movements when using real objects in movement tasks. Students were asked to perform three movements: picking up a pencil and preparing to write their name (materials-based task), pretend picking up a pencil and prepare to write their name (imagery-based task), and moving the arm forward to a target (exercise task). Students performed the three tasks differently, with the material-based task eliciting the smoothest and fastest movements.

The finding that the use of real objects elicits different movements than imagery-based tasks or rote exercise has also been demonstrated by persons with disabilities such as cerebral palsy, stroke, and multiple sclerosis (Mathiowetz & Wade, 1995; Trombly & Wu, 1999; van der Weel et al., 1991). Mathiowetz & Wade (1995) demonstrated that both subjects with multiple sclerosis and those without benefited from context provided by real objects. Subjects were asked to eat applesauce, with a spoon, bowl and applesauce available (materials-based task); pretend to eat applesauce, with a spoon and bowl available (partial-support task); and pretend to eat applesauce without a spoon or bowl (imagery-based task). Again, the movement patterns in the three conditions were significantly different. Trombly and Wu (1999) demonstrated that subjects who had strokes benefited from having objects to reach to rather than just reaching for a point in space. These findings support occupational therapy approaches that emphasize the significance of real-life tasks in optimizing function (Mathiowetz & Haugen, 1994). (See Chapters 5 and 21 for more about this approach.)

Environmental context is equally important to cognitive learning. In a classic study by Godden and Baddeley (1975) scuba divers who learned lists of words while underwater recalled them better underwater than on dry land, while divers who learned the lists on dry land recalled them better in that setting. These and previous findings are likely explained by two important principles: encoding specificity and contextual interference.

Encoding Specificity

The principle of encoding specificity suggests that events are stored in memory in such a way as to be inseparable from their contexts (Tulving & Thompson, 1973). That is, people encode features of the learning task and environment along with the newly acquired skill or strategy. Encoding specificity limits transfer and generalization because new tasks and environments do not have the same cueing properties as those present during original learning, making retrieval from long-term memory more difficult. For example, imagine that a therapist works with a patient on the same grasp and release task every day; even the work space is consistent. The patient improves performance on the task, but because the information about control of grasp and release is stored along with the context of the practice task and environment, he or she may not be able to elicit these skills during ADL.

Contextual Interference

One way to mitigate the influence of encoding specificity on learning is to employ high **contextual interference** training (Battig, 1978). Low contextual interference occurs when the context and training task are invariant, forcing the learner to perform the same task repetitively in a consistent environment, as in the previous example. On the other hand, high contextual interference occurs when the task and environment keep changing throughout the learning process. This principle asserts that task and environmental variation force people to use multiple and varied information processing strategies, which makes retrieval easier. Contextual interference forces elaborate processing strategies, and transfer is facilitated.

Put another way, high contextual interference is a barrier to rote responding because it introduces problem-solving demands with each change of the context (Lee et al., 1991). Had the therapist from the previous example provided a variety of grasp and release activities in a variety of settings, the patient would have used more complex processing strategies during the learning process. Information about many similar grasp and release movements would be stored in memory along with a variety of environments and objects. As a result, the patient would be more likely to use the newly learned skills to solve problems within the inevitable variety of the real world. Therefore, to facilitate transfer of task-specific skills and generalization of newly learned strategies, therapists deliberately vary the learning tasks and environments.

Therapeutic Use of Feedback

Feedback also can enhance or interfere with learning. Occupational therapists understand the functions of feedback and deliberately select the types and schedules of feedback in designing a patient's learning experience. Box 12-3 discusses videotaped feedback.

Teaching Technologies: Videotape Feedback

Much investigation into the use of videotape for feedback to improve learning has been done (Brotherton et al., 1988; Morgan & Salzberg, 1992; Tham & Tegner, 1997). It has been applied to a broad variety of situations and a large number of patient populations. These studies have consistently demonstrated that videotape feedback can improve a patient's awareness of his or her performance. However, researchers have also found that simply showing a videotape of performance does not lead to improvements. Effective feedback must be structured by the clinician to focus the attention of the patient on pertinent actions and events. The advantage of videotape feedback is that the therapist can stop the tape at critical points, focus attention on specific features, and ask the subject to analyze and suggest appropriate changes. For example, in an investigation of the effectiveness of videotape feedback in the treatment of neglect syndrome, patients were videotaped performing a simulated cooking task that involved arranging pastries on a baking tray (Tham & Tegner, 1997). Therapists showed the subjects structured videotapes of their performance and provided feedback during the viewing. Subjects improved on follow-up on this test, but no generalization was noted.

Videotape has also been used to assist with social skills training of patients with brain injuries and severe mental retardation (Brotherton et al., 1988; Morgan & Salzberg, 1992). In both cases, the videotape feedback was used to help patients identify problematic behaviors which was followed by rehearsal of appropriate behaviors. Again, in these cases, the therapist structured viewing of the videotape, with identification of the problems and the appropriate behaviors as part of an ongoing dialogue. Rehearsal of appropriate responses was also part of the training program.

As these studies show, the use of videotaped feedback can assist in the teaching process, but it must be used in a structured and purposeful way. Showing patients specific sections of tape, pointing out relevant details, and asking patients to describe their behavior and solve problems are all effective ways to use videotape. Furthermore, if reasonable for the specific task, rehearsal of appropriate responses provides patients with a repertoire of appropriate behaviors.

Functions of Feedback

Feedback regarding performance has several functions (Salmoni et al., 1984). It has a temporary motivating or energizing effect and a guidance effect that informs the subject how to correct an error on the next trial. However, feedback can permanently impair motor learning if provided beyond the point that the person has a rough idea of the desired motion.

Types of Feedback

To help patients learn and sustain skills and strategies, therapists initially provide extrinsic feedback on performance but ultimately facilitate the development of intrinsic feedback.

Extrinsic Feedback: Knowledge of Results and Knowledge of Performance

Therapists typically provide feedback about performance in verbal form. Extrinsic, or external, information presented after the task is complete is called **knowledge of results**. This feedback allows subjects to alter or adapt their responses or behaviors on subsequent trials. Knowledge of results provides information about outcome, such as "You got your shirt on" or "You took the cap off that jar." A second type of feedback, **knowledge of performance**, is related to qualitative descriptions of a performance, such as "You shifted your weight too far to the left" or "You bent your elbow." This information directs patients' attention not to outcome but to components of movement that they need to change or attend to. This type of feedback duplicates information patients already have available through intrinsic feedback but on which they may not be focusing.

Other external information provided to patients during practice falls into the category of encouragement. It is important that patients and therapists not confuse encouragement ("Keep going") with feedback ("You're doing great"), especially if the latter is not true, as incorrect feedback is highly detrimental to learning (Buekers et al., 1992).

Intrinsic Feedback

Intrinsic feedback, or internal feedback, is information that patients receive through their own senses, such as seeing an egg break as it hits the floor after dropping it or feeling the pain of hitting the ground after an unsuccessful transfer. While this information is readily available to patients, they may need cueing to focus on the most important components of a skill or strategy, such as learning to use vision when moving an anesthetic limb. Intervention that incorporates self-monitoring and self-estimation (task difficulty, completion time, accuracy score, amount of cueing or assistance needed) enables patients to create mechanisms for self-generated feedback (Cicerone & Giacino, 1992; Toglia,1998), lessening dependence on therapists for successful performance.

Feedback Schedules

The frequency and content of feedback are critical to the learning process and must be considered when a teaching situation is planned.

Immediate and Summary Feedback

The frequency and rate at which feedback is given can profoundly influence the acquisition and retention of task-specific skills and strategies. For example, Lavery (1962) wanted to know which schedule of feedback best facilitated learning: immediate feedback provided after each trial was completed, also referred to as constant feedback; summary feedback provided after a number of trials were completed; or both. Lavery found that subjects who received immediate or combined feedback improved their performance of the task more quickly during the acquisition phase than the group receiving only summary feedback. However, when tested for retention of the task 4, 37, and 93 days post training, the subjects who received only summary feedback did significantly better than those who received either immediate feedback or both types.

Lavery hypothesized that people who received immediate feedback came to rely on it when performing the task and those that received only summary feedback were forced to analyze their own movements. The subjects who received both immediate and summary feedback did just as poorly as those who received only immediate feedback, suggesting that the immediate feedback interfered with the processing of the summary feedback. Beyond its implications about the schedule of feedback, these findings support the idea that performance during the training phase does not reflect actual learning of the skill.

Faded Feedback

Therapists are often concerned that providing only summary feedback after a series of trials will not help their patients understand tasks that are complex or new. Winstein and Schmidt (1990) evaluated the effectiveness of feedback given at 50% and 100% of trials on the learning of a task by college students. The 50% feedback was faded, with the feedback given on every trial initially and then decreased to no feedback at the end of training. On average, feedback was provided on half the trials. They found a slight advantage for the 100% feedback group during acquisition of the skill, but there were significant differences during the retention phase, which is the true test of learning. The group that received faded feedback performed significantly better than the immediate feedback group on the retention trials, at 10 minutes and 2 days, with the effect at 2 days more noticeable. Remember that from the standpoint of encoding specificity, subjects who received no feedback at the end of the acquisition phase were performing the task in exactly the same way as they did during the retention phase. Also, these findings point out an important irony: factors that degrade performance during acquisition may improve learning.

Bandwidth Feedback

With bandwidth feedback, an acceptable range of performance is defined, and the subject receives feedback only when performance is outside of that range. As the subject's performance improves, feedback is provided less frequently. The research note on the next page further discusses this point (Goodwin & Meeuwsen, 1995).

Therapeutic Use of Practice

In addition to planning feedback, the design of a treatment session must include a plan for practicing the material.

Blocked Versus Random Practice

As discussed earlier, traditional models of learning did not distinguish between learning and performance. These models also promoted blocked forms of practice, such as drill, as the most efficient schedule for learning a task. Using a blocked format, the same skill or strategy is practiced over a number of repetitions, after which the next skill or strategy is rehearsed. As such, blocked practice is a form of practice with low contextual interference.

Shea and Morgan (1979) studied whether increasing the contextual interference by random practice during skill acquisition leads to improved retention and transfer of motor skills. Their experiments entailed knocking over wooden barriers with a tennis ball held in the hand. In brief, they found that blocked practice provided low contextual interference, whereas random practice provided high contextual interference, requiring subjects to formulate a new movement plan for each trial. Subjects who practiced with high contextual interference demonstrated better retention and transfer than those who used blocked practice. This study demonstrated two important findings: (1) Performance during acquisition of a skill does not necessarily relate to later learning. (2) Conditions that may improve performance during acquisition do not necessarily create better learning. In fact, structuring training to improve performance during practice by using blocked practice schedules is actually detrimental to learning.

The advantage of random practice over blocked practice was also demonstrated for patients with hemiplegia (Hanlon, 1996). Patients practiced a multistep functional activity that consisted of reaching for a cupboard door, opening it, picking up a coffee cup by the handle, transferring it to a counter, and releasing the handle. The subjects practiced these steps in either a blocked or a random pattern. The random pattern group performed significantly better than either the blocked or control group on both 2-day and 7-day retention trials.

RESEARCH NOTE

Using Bandwidth Knowledge of Results to Alter Relative Frequencies During Motor Skills Acquisition

Goodwin, J. E., & Meeuwesen, H. J. (1995). *Research Quarterly for Exercise and Sport, 66, 99–104*

ABSTRACT

Goodwin and Meeuwsen (1995) examined the effect of using bandwidth feedback on a golfing task. Subjects were assigned to four groups. The first group received feedback on every trial that did not hit the hole, whereas the second group received feedback on every trial that the ball was more than 18 inches from the hole. The third group was given feedback on a shrinking bandwidth schedule, tolerating increasingly smaller errors (initially if the ball missed the hole by 27 inches, then 18 inches, 9 inches, then 0 inches). The fourth group received feedback on an expanding schedule, tolerating increasingly larger errors, starting with 0 inches, then 9 inches, 18 inches 27 inches and finally 36 inches. Interestingly, the groups that received the least feedback (i.e., the group that got feedback only when the ball was more than 18 inches from the hole and the expanding [fourth] group) performed the best during the retention phase. The third (shrinking) group performed similarly to the group that received feedback whenever the ball did not hit the hole. These findings led the authors to suggest that receiving high frequencies of feedback at the end of the acquisition phase increases the subject's dependence on that feedback and is as detrimental to learning as providing high frequencies of feedback throughout the acquisition phase.

IMPLICATIONS FOR PRACTICE

▶ Frequent indiscriminate feedback seems detrimental to learning. Therefore, therapists must monitor the timing and frequency of comments to patients as they learn new skills and strategies.

▶ When it comes to feedback, it appears that less is more. Patients who receive less feedback may increasingly rely on intrinsic feedback and be more likely to retain the new skill or strategy than persons who get a lot of feedback when they make errors. Therapists should provide opportunities for patients to determine when and why they have made errors.

Part–Whole Practice

Therapists also decide whether patients practice the whole task or components of a task (referred to as part–whole training). Mané et al. (1989) manipulated two dimensions of practice: whole versus part task and speed of performance. Subjects learned to play a goal-directed computer game. The part–whole study examined the extent to which practicing part of a critical component of the task improved performance of the whole game. In this study, subjects who practiced a critical skill extracted from the game did improve performance on the overall game. However, changing the speed of practice was met with varying success. Practice at the slowest speed fundamentally changed the demands of the task, leading to poor transfer of skills to the task at original speeds. On the other hand, slight slowing of task speed during training did enhance learning.

Winstein et al. (1989) examined the effect of part-task practice with gait training. One group of patients with hemiplegia received traditional physical therapy gait training. The second group received traditional physical therapy and specific training in standing balance symmetry (proposed as a reasonable critical component of symmetrical gait). After several weeks of training, the group that had practiced symmetry in standing showed improvement in that component of the activity, but there was no carryover to the whole task of gait. There was no significant difference in gait symmetry between the two groups.

These findings demonstrate that although part–whole training may work in some situations, such as the computer game, it is not successful in all situations. Furthermore, therapists may not be able to identify the specific critical components that would improve overall learning. It will require much more research to identify the components that will transfer to the whole task before part-task training can be the preferred method. Winstein et al. (1989) suggested that tasks that are continuous and cannot be easily separated into component parts may not be appropriate for part training. Examples of this type of movement include walking or driving a car—tasks that require many adjustments with components that occur simultaneously and cannot be easily separated.

Making Personal Change

Employing a newly learned skill or strategy is fundamentally a personal change. Using a new skill or strategy in daily life depends not only on recall, transfer, or generalization but also on learners' beliefs about their competence and their stage in the change process.

Bandura (1977) posited that people's beliefs about their ability to handle a new situation largely determine

Case Example

TREATMENT IN THE HOME OF A CLIENT WITH MOTOR AND PERCEPTUAL DEFICITS

Patient Information

Mr. O. was a 69-year-old married man seen by occupational therapy in home care 1 month post stroke. He had received therapy in both the acute hospital and in a rehabilitation unit. When he was interviewed at home, he identified working as the head of an advertising agency, golfing, driving, and being independent at home as roles that he wanted to resume. He indicated that his goals for therapy included being safe and independent for short periods, able to walk and drive independently, and independent in self-care, light meal preparation, and going to the bathroom. He also wanted to use his involved left arm like he did before. He viewed these skills and tasks as prerequisite to resumption of his identified roles.

Assessment Results

The client was assessed at home, with the following results:

▶ ADL—Mr. O. was able to dress with minimal assistance and cues but needed maximal assistance in toileting, bathing, and meal preparation.

▶ Upper extremity function—He did not use his left arm in any functional activities, although he did have active movement and strength of muscle grades 3 to 4 throughout. He had difficulty using the available motion in tasks requiring movement at more than one joint.

▶ Walking and mobility—He was able to stand with moderate assistance but was unable to propel his wheelchair in the house. He walked with moderate assistance and a wide-based quad cane.

▶ IADL—Driving was not evaluated. Because of his need for assistance in standing, golf was not evaluated initially.

▶ Component evaluations—Problems in performance were related to severe left neglect, which the patient strongly denied. He knew adapted dressing techniques but needed cues regarding neglect of his left arm. There were also environmental barriers to using the wheelchair, and adaptive equipment was needed for the bathroom.

▶ Patient's safety—This was also a concern because of his deficits in awareness. He fell several times in the hospital and had been labeled impulsive. However, conversation with the patient revealed that the problem was not so much impulsivity as awareness. As he put it, "I forget that my leg and arm don't work when I stand up, but remember as I'm falling."

Recommendations

Home-based occupational therapy was recommended for four times a week for 3 weeks, then two or three times a week for 3 weeks, followed by transition to outpatient OT. Short-term goals for home care (3 weeks) were identified as (1) minimal assistance in toileting and clothing adjustment, (2) independence in using the wheelchair at home, (3) independence in light meal preparation, (4) standby assistance with showering, and (5) safe and independent for short periods during the day (1–2 hours).

Treatment

The first week of therapy focused on environmental adaptations so that Mr. O. could move about the house in his wheelchair. Also, a raised tub seat, raised toilet seat, and grab bars were installed in the bathroom to increase safety and decrease his dependence on his wife. Because of his denial of and refusal to address left neglect, this was not an initial focus of treatment. Attempts to increase his awareness of neglect were integrated into almost all contacts. He did make some improvements in compensation for the left neglect, specifically as it related to wheelchair propulsion and toileting.

During the second week of home care, the patient attempted to walk without assistance and fell. He received a large gash to his face and ear and spent the night in the emergency room. When the occupational therapist arrived the next day, he announced that this "left neglect thing" might be more of a problem than he had thought and that he was now willing to work on it. A number of functional tasks were practiced, including playing cards and doing crossword puzzles, activities he had previously enjoyed. Over the next 2 weeks, he became more aware of his left visual space, compensating spontaneously in most simple activities around the house and becoming much safer at home.

During this same 2-week period, he continued to make gains in gait and all ADL. Improvements in both strength and compensation for neglect allowed him to go to the bathroom and transfer into and out of the bathtub with minimal assistance. However, he continued to need constant cueing to incorporate his left arm into most activities. When cued to use his arm, he insisted that it had been involved with the activity or that he always did that task with only his right arm.

Feedback

In an attempt to increase his awareness of the use of the left arm, video feedback was employed during a golfing task. The client tried putting several times, and these attempts were videotaped. The client consistently neglected his left hand but insisted that he was using it. Following the unsuccessful cues, four more putts were taped. Mr. O. was then shown the videotape as a form of summary feedback. He was surprised by his lack of use of his arm and hand and identified that as part of the cause of his poor performance. Following the viewing of the tape, he putted some more. The client consistently incorporated his left arm into the task, and his performance improved. Most surprisingly, this awareness transferred to other activities, increasing his safety and efficiency in a variety of tasks, including transfers, walking, meal preparation, and emptying the dishwasher.

Revised Goals

Following the first 3 weeks of treatment, new goals for therapy were set. They included (1) independence in light meal preparation, (2) independence in toileting, (3) standby assistance for transfers in and out of shower, and (4) safe and independent for short periods (1–2 hours).

CLINICAL REASONING
in OT Practice

Differentiating Between the Acquisition of Skills Versus Strategies

Mr. O.'s assessment suggested a number of learning needs related to his self-identified goals. List learning needs characterized as task-specific skills. List learning needs that are best characterized as general strategies. Compare Mr. O.'s learning processes for the task-specific skills and general strategies in terms of speed and ease of acquisition and teaching methods.

Training for Transfer and Generalization

Mr. O.'s treatment took place in his home in the context of his everyday activities. Describe how encoding specificity contributed to the acquisition of skills and strategies in this setting. Imagine that Mr. O. works toward similar goals while a patient on a rehabilitation unit. In what ways should his treatment program change to optimize the likelihood of transfer and generalization of skills and strategies?

---

whether they attempt the new task and their ultimate performance. Self-percepts of efficacy (self-perceptions of competence) predict success with a wide range of acquired health behaviors, including smoking cessation (Stewart et al., 1994), exercise maintenance (McAuley, 1993), and medication compliance (DeGeest et al., 1994). Bandura (1977) demonstrated that people make judgments about their competence (self-efficacy) by thinking about past accomplishments, vicarious experience (observing similar others), verbal persuasion, and emotional arousal, such as anxiety. Because self-percepts of competence seem to explain the discrepancy between what people can do and what they actually do (Bandura, 1981), occupational therapists actively create opportunities for patients to demonstrate to themselves that they are indeed competent with the new skill or strategy.

Many patients served by occupational therapists have had sudden onset of changes in physical functioning. Persons who are insulated from ramifications of these changes (perhaps have been hospitalized continuously since onset) may not fully appreciate the need for the skills and strategies therapists are attempting to teach them. The Stages of Change Model (Prochaska & DiClemente, 1982) helps therapists target their teaching–learning intervention to address the learning predispositions of the patient and family.

This model identifies four stages of change: contemplation, determination, action, and maintenance. During the first stage, patients become aware of the problem or concern; in the determination stage, they resolve to do something about it; during the action stage, patients work to address the problem or issue; and patients must still put forth some degree of effort to sustain the desired skill or behavior during the maintenance stage. The researchers suggested that verbal intervention strategies are most appropriate during the first two stages (pointing out the problem, discussing possible approaches), whereas action-oriented behavioral interventions are most helpful during the last two stages. Essentially, for example, before a patient routinely employs strategies for scanning the left visual field, he or she must believe that parts of the environment are missing or that personal safety is in jeopardy. Merely elucidating the problem is not enough. Once convinced and motivated, the patient is taught specifically how to handle the problem.

Occupational Therapist As Teacher

The extent to which occupational therapy contributes to a patient's resumption of roles depends to a large extent on the effectiveness of the therapist as a teacher. Principles of teaching parallel therapy: assessment, goal setting, intervention, and evaluation (Redman, 1997).

While this process rarely follows a predictable, orderly sequence, these steps serve as a checklist to ensure that therapists consider variables affecting the outcome of their teaching efforts (Redman, 1997).

Assess Learning Needs and Readiness

Before teaching begins, therapists complete a traditional occupational therapy assessment so as to understand the patient's occupational needs, priorities, capacities, skills, and competencies. Therapists attempt to identify barriers to learning, such as low literacy; distracters, such as pain and fatigue; lack of human or financial support; awareness of problem areas; and incongruous values between patient and therapist (Vanetzian, 1997). Dynamic assessment provides information about the circumstances (task, environment, strategies, cueing) in which the patient is best able to learn (Toglia, 1989) (see Chapter 8). Therefore, the therapist determines who will be the subject or subjects of the teaching—the patient, family member (if the patient seems unlikely to retain the information), or both.

Set Patient-Specific Learning Goals

Therapists use the results of their assessments and estimates of the treatment time available to set learning and cognitive objectives for each patient (Fig. 12-1). Therapists plan treatment around transfer and generalization goals by identifying reinforcements in the natural environment and incorporating into the treatment stimuli common to both training and real-world environments (Sohlberg & Raskin, 1996). If the intervention ultimately is to change an existing routine, skill, or strategy, the therapist attempts to determine where in the process of change the learner is. For example, a patient with little or no awareness of a memory problem is likely to have minimal interest in learning to use compensatory

memory techniques. Therefore, the therapist sets goals that move the patient toward the contemplative stage of change by allowing him or her to take the consequences of forgetting. Finally, therapists merely recommend learning goals. Goals that direct teaching–learning efforts are set in collaboration with patients and their families.

Create Learning Opportunities Throughout Treatment

Therapists deliberately use context, feedback, and practice to help patients meet learning goals (Box 12-4). They

BOX 12-4
PROCEDURES FOR PRACTICE

Therapeutic Use of Context, Feedback, and Practice to Promote Transfer and Generalization

▶ Vary the training environmental context to achieve transfer; vary training tasks and environments to achieve generalization of new strategies.
▶ Provide extrinsic feedback just until the learner understands the desired movement, skill, or strategy. Use cueing and the patient's own performance prediction and analysis to help the learner increasingly rely on intrinsic feedback.
▶ Provide summary feedback when possible. Tolerate a slower or longer acquisition phase of learning, appreciating the later benefits in terms of retention, transfer, and generalization.
▶ Fade therapist feedback and cues so that these elements of training do not get encoded with the new skill or strategy so that they are required for recall.
▶ Attempt to teach movement, skills, and strategies within whole tasks. Address components or subskills only when they are critical to whole task performance.

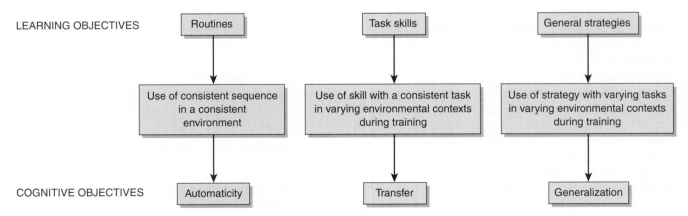

Figure 12-1 Teaching objectives in occupational therapy.

Low literacy affects comprehension and use of health-related written materials for many adults (Davis et al., 1998). Citing the results of the *National Adult Literacy Survey* (1993), Davis et al. (1998) reported that 21% of adults are functionally illiterate and another 27% have marginal literacy skills. Problems with literacy pervade all socioeconomic and ethnic groups (Thomas, 1999). People with low literacy tend to be ashamed of their difficulties with reading and reluctant to admit the problem, even to family members (Parikh et al., 1996). Thomas offered the following suggestions for addressing this issue in occupational therapy:

- ▶ Incorporate a brief evaluation of literacy into the occupational therapy assessment process (see Chapter 9 for a discussion of REALM).
- ▶ Limit the quantity of information to the most important messages. Collaborate with the patient, family, and other team members to establish priorities.
- ▶ Reduce the reading level of printed materials by using one- or two-syllable words, shortening sentences to 10 to 15 words, and targeting materials to the fifth or sixth grade reading level.
- ▶ Make sure text and graphics are well organized. Davis et al. (1998) found both preference for and improved comprehension with a question-and-answer list format over a paragraph format for text.
- ▶ Use materials that are racially and culturally sensitive. As recommended by Thomas (1999), "make sure that patients can 'see themselves' in materials provided."

try to enhance motivation and recall by linking new skills or strategies with patients' specific interests, knowledge, and abilities. Effective teachers also make an effort to overcome barriers to learning. They select the optimal time of day and environment for teaching, change their schedules occasionally to adapt to family needs, and use written materials that are well organized and easy to read (Box 12-5). Finally, to achieve transfer and generalization goals, therapists use the continuum of care to reinforce long-term learning. Often this means teaching family members how to extend the learning process and providing copies of the discharge instructions to other providers, such as the home health occupational therapist, vocational specialist, and nurse case manager.

Evaluate Achievement of Learning Goals

Effective teachers routinely assess patients' progress toward learning goals, typically by changing the training

task or environment and evaluating carryover. Family members perform return demonstrations of new techniques, such as transfers. Based on performance or other changes in learning status, therapists adjust learning goals throughout the intervention.

Summary Review Questions

1. List the types of practice patterns and discuss the advantages and disadvantages of each.
2. Design two ADL training sessions, one for learning a specific task and the second for learning a general strategy.
3. Discuss the different feedback schedules and compare their advantages and disadvantages.
4. Identify Fitts and Posner's three stages of learning. Describe the characteristics of performance that you might see as patients learn to use a piece of adaptive equipment.
5. List characteristics of practice mostly likely to facilitate transfer and generalization of practice.
6. Describe the influences on the learning readiness of a family caregiver. What will you do to optimize the learning process in response to these influences?

References

American Occupational Therapy Association (1994). Uniform terminology for occupational therapy (3rd ed.). *American Journal of Occupational Therapy, 48,* 1047–1054.

Atkinson, R. C., & Shiffrin, R. M. (1971). The control of short-term memory. *Scientific American, 225,* 82–90.

Bandura, A. (1977). Self-efficacy: Toward a unifying theory of behavior change. *Psychological Review, 84,* 191–215.

Bandura, A. (1982). Self-efficacy mechanism in human agency. *American Psychologist, 37,* 122–147.

Battig, W. F. (1978). The flexibility of the human memory. In L. S. Cermak, & F. I. M. Craik (Eds.), *Levels of Processing and Human Memory* (pp. 23–44). Hillsdale, NJ: Erlbaum.

Brotherton, F. A., Thomas, L. L., Wisotzek, I. E., & Milan, M. A. (1988). Social skills training in the rehabilitation of patients with traumatic closed head injury. *Archives of Physical Medicine and Rehabilitation, 69,* 827–832.

Buekers, M. J. A., Magill, R. A., & Hall, K. G. (1992). The effect of erroneous knowledge of results on skill acquisition when augmented information is redundant. *Quarterly Journal of Experimental Psychology, 44* (1), 105–117.

Cicerone, K. D., & Giacino, J. T. (1992). Remediation of executive function deficits after traumatic brain injury. *NeuroRehabilitation, 2,* 12–22.

Craik, F. I. M., & Tulving, E. (1975). Depth of processing and retention of words in episodic memory. *Journal of Experimental Psychology: General, 104,* 268–294.

Davis, T. C., Fredrickson, D. D., Arnold, C., Murphy, P. W., Herbst, M., & Bocchini, J. A. (1998). A polio immunization pamphlet with increased appeal and simplified language does not improve comprehension to an acceptable level. *Patient Education and Counseling, 33*, 25–37.

DeGeest, S., Abraham, I., Gemoets, H., & Evers, G. (1994). Development of the long-term medication behavior self-efficacy scale: Qualitative study for item development. *Journal of Advanced Nursing, 19*, 233–238.

Dunn, W., Brown, C., & McGuigan, A. (1994). The ecology of human performance: A framework for considering the effect of context. *American Journal of Occupational Therapy, 48*, 595–607.

Eysenck, M. W., & Keane, M. T. (1990). *Cognitive Psychology: The Student's Handbook*. East Sussex, UK: Lawrence Erlbaum.

Fisher, A. G. (1998). Uniting practice and theory in an occupational framework. *American Journal of Occupational Therapy, 52*, 509–521.

Fitts P. M., & Posner, M. I. (1967). *Human Performance*. Belmont, CA: Brooks/Cole.

Gentile, A. M. (1998). Implicit and explicit processes during acquisition of functional skills. *Scandinavian Journal of Occupational Therapy, 5*, 7–16.

Giles, G. M. (1998). A neurofunctional approach to rehabilitation following severe brain injury. In N. Katz (Ed.), *Cognition and Occupation in Rehabilitation*. Bethesda, MD: American Occupational Therapy Association.

Godden, D. R., & Baddeley, A. D. (1975). Context-dependent memory in two natural environments: On land and underwater. *British Journal of Psychology, 66*, 325–331.

Goodwin, J. E. & Meeuwsen, H. J. (1995). Using bandwidth knowledge of results to alter relative frequencies during motor skills acquisition. *Research Quarterly for Exercise and Sport, 66* (2), 99–104.

Hanlon, R. E. (1996). Motor learning following unilateral stroke. *Archives of Physical Medicine and Rehabilitation, 77*, 811–815.

Kielhofner, G., Barris, R., & Watts, J. H. (1982). Habits and habit dysfunction: A clinical perspective for psychosocial occupational therapy. *Occupational Therapy in Mental Health, 2*, 1–21.

Kirby, J. R. (1984). Educational roles of cognitive plans and strategies. In J. R. Kirby (Ed.), *Cognitive Strategies and Educational Performance* (pp. 51–88). Orlando, FL: Academic.

Lavery, J. J. (1962). Retention of simple motor skills as a function of type of knowledge of results. *Canadian Journal of Psychology, 16* (4), 300–311.

Lee, T. D., Swanson, L. R., & Hall, A. L. (1991). What is repeated in a repetition? Effects of practice conditions on motor skill acquisition. *Physical Therapy, 71*, 150–156.

Lee, Y., & Vakoch, D. A., (1996). Transfer and retention of implicit and explicit learning. *British Journal of Psychology, 87*, 637–651.

Mané, A. M., Adams, J. A., & Donchin, E. (1989). Adaptive and part–whole training in the acquisition of a complex perceptual-motor skill. *Acta Psychologica, 71*, 179–196.

Mathiowetz, V., & Haugen, J. B. (1994). Motor behavior research: Implications for therapeutic approaches to central nervous system dysfunction. *American Journal of Occupational Therapy, 48*, 733–745.

Mathiowetz, V., & Wade, M. G. (1995). Task constraints and functional motor performance of individuals with and without multiple sclerosis. *Ecological Psychology, 7* (2), 99–123.

McAuley, E. (1993). Self-efficacy and the maintenance of exercise participation in older adults. *Journal of Behavioral Medicine, 16*, 103–113.

Morgan, R. L., & Salzberg, C. L. (1992). Effects of video-assisted training on employment-related social skills of adults with severe mental retardation. *Journal of Applied Behavioral Analysis, 25*, 365–383.

Neistadt, M. E. (1995). Assessing learning capabilities during cognitive and perceptual evaluations for adults with traumatic brain injury. *Occupational Therapy in Health Care, 9*, 3–16.

Parikh, N. S., Parker, R. M., Nurss, J. R., Baker, D. W., & Williams, M. V. (1996). Shame and health literacy: The unspoken connection. *Patient Education and Counseling, 27*, 33–39.

Perkins, D. (1995). *Outsmarting IQ: The emerging science of learnable intelligence*. New York: Free Press.

Poole, J. L. (1995). Learning. In C. A. Trombly (Ed.), *Occupational Therapy for Physical Dysfunction* (pp. 265–276). Baltimore: Williams & Wilkins.

Prochaska, J. O., & DiClemente, C. C. (1982). Transtheoretical therapy: Toward a more integrative model of change. *Psychotherapy: Theory, Research and Practice, 19*, 276–288.

Reber P. J., & Squire, L. R. (1994). Parallel brain systems for learning with and without awareness. *Learning and Memory 1*, 217–229.

Redman, B. K. (1997). *The Practice of Patient Education*. St. Louis, MO: Mosby.

Salmoni, A. W., Schmidt R. A., & Walter, C. B. (1984). Knowledge of results and motor learning: A review and critical reappraisal. *Psychological Bulletin, 95*, 355–386.

Saloman, G., & Perkins, D. N. (1989). Rocky roads to transfer: Rethinking mechanisms of a neglected phenomenon. *Educational Psychologist, 24*, 113–142.

Schmidt, R. A. (1988). *Motor Control and Learning: A Behavioral Emphasis* (2nd ed.) Champaign, IL: Human Kinetics.

Schneider, W., & Shiffrin, R. M. (1977). Controlled and automatic human information processing: I. Detection, search, and attention. *Psychological Review, 84*, 1–66.

Shea, J. B., & Morgan, R. L. (1979). Contextual interference effects on the acquisition, retention and transfer of a motor skill. *Journal of Experimental Psychology: Human Learning and Memory, 5*, 179–187.

Shiffrin, R. M., & Schneider, W. (1977). Controlled and automatic human information processing: II. Perceptual learning, automatic attending, and a general theory. *Psychological Review, 84*, 127–190.

Sohlberg, M. M., & Raskin, S. A. (1996). Principles of generalization applied to attention and memory interventions. *Journal of Head Trauma Rehabilitation, 11*, 65–78.

Squire, L. R. (1994). Declarative and nondeclarative memory: Multiple brain systems support learning and memory. In D. Schacter & E. Tulving (Eds.), *Memory Systems 1994* (pp. 203–231). Cambridge, MA: MIT.

Sternberg, R. J. (1986). *Intelligence Applied: Understanding and Increasing Your Intellectual Skills*. New York: Harcourt Brace Jovanovich.

Stewart, K., Borland, R., & McMurray, N. (1994). Self-efficacy, health locus of control, and smoking cessation. *Addictive Behaviors, 19*, 1–12.

Tham, K., & Tegner, R. (1997). Video feedback in the rehabilitation of patients with unilateral neglect. *Archives of Physical Medicine and Rehabilitation, 78*, 410–413.

Thomas, J. J. (1999). Enhancing patient education: Addressing the issue of literacy. *Physical Disabilities Special Interest Section Quarterly, 22*, 3–4.

Toglia, J. P. (1989). Approaches to cognitive assessment of the brain-injured adult. *Occupational Therapy Practice, 1*, 36–55.

Toglia, J. P. (1991). Generalization of treatment: A multicontext approach to cognitive perceptual impairment in adults with brain injury. *American Journal of Occupational Therapy, 45*, 505–516.

Toglia, J. P. (1998). A dynamic interactional model to cognitive rehabilitation. In N. Katz (Ed.), *Cognition and Occupation in Rehabilitation*. Bethesda, MD: American Occupational Therapy Association.

Trombly, C. A., & Wu, C. (1999). Effect of rehabilitation tasks on organization of movement after stroke. *American Journal of Occupational Therapy. 53*, 333–344.

Tulving, E., & Thompson, D. (1973). Encoding specificity and retrieval processes in episodic memory. *Psychological Review, 80,* 352–373.

van der Weel, F. R., van der Meer, A. L. H., & Lee, D. N., (1991). Effect of task on movement control in cerebral palsy: Implications for assessment and therapy. *Developmental Medicine and Child Neurology. 33,* 419–426.

Vanetzian, E. (1997). Learning readiness for patient teaching in stroke rehabilitation. *Journal of Advanced Nursing, 26,* 589–594.

Wilson, B. A., & Evans, J. J. (1996). Error-free learning in the rehabilitation of people with memory impairments. *Journal of Head Trauma Rehabilitation, 11,* 54–64.

Winstein, C. J., Gardner, E. R., McNeal, D. R., Barto, P. S., & Nicholson, D. E. (1989). Standing balance training: Effect on balance and locomotion in hemiparetic patients. *Archives of Physical Medicine and Rehabilitation. 70,* 755–762.

Winstein, C. J., & Schmidt, R. A. (1990). Reduced frequency of knowledge of results enhances motor skill learning. *Journal of Experimental Psychology: Learning, Memory, and Cognition, 16,* 677–691.

World Health Organization (1997). *ICIHD-2: International Classification of Impairments, Activities, and Participation (Beta-1 draft for field trials)*. Geneva: Author.

Wu, C., Trombly, C. A., & Lin, K. (1994). The relationship between occupational form and occupational performance: A kinematic perspective. *American Journal of Occupational Therapy, 48,* 679–687.

13
Therapeutic Rapport

Linda Tickle-Degnen

LEARNING OBJECTIVES

After studying this chapter, the reader will be able to do the following:

1. Define high therapeutic rapport.
2. Describe how rapport influences intervention and the client's occupational functioning.
3. Describe how collaboration between therapist and client contributes to achieving high therapeutic rapport.
4. Select methods to enhance rapport with a client.
5. Identify therapists' and clients' attributes that can influence the development of rapport.
6. Apply knowledge of ethics of practice to the therapeutic relationship.

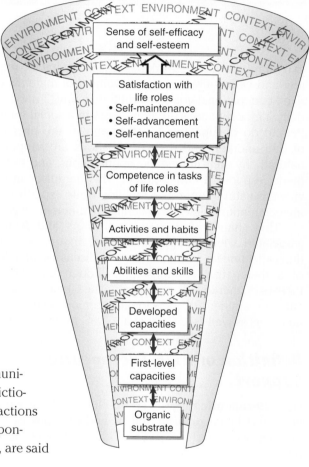

*T*he origins of the term *rapport* reflect an emphasis on communication and connection between individuals (Oxford English Dictionary, 1971). Individuals who are finely tuned to one another's actions and ideas so that they respond to one another "immediately, spontaneously, and sympathetically" (Park & Burgess, 1924, p. 893), are said to be in rapport with one another.

Although rapport can occur in any social situation, the type of rapport developed in occupational therapy has its own special characteristics. Rapport is one mechanism, or means, by which a client achieves positive therapeutic outcomes; in the case of occupational therapy, this means confident and competent occupational functioning. It involves the interpersonal influences arising between client and therapist that can support the client's desire to try occupational therapy, maintain continued involvement in therapy despite the need for considerable effort and courage, and participate with the therapist in constructing a new vision of life possibilities that project into the client's occupational future (Mattingly & Fleming, 1994).

A client who shares a high rapport with the therapist at the point of assessment may want to try therapy simply because of an initial liking of the therapist; once in the midst of therapy, he or she may

GLOSSARY

Mutuality—Interaction between the client and therapist in which they influence one another.

Nonverbal communication—The process of interpreting another's nonverbal behavior and expressing one's own thoughts and emotions through nonverbal behavior. Nonverbal behavior includes positions and movements of the face and body and qualities of the voice, such as vocal tone, intensity, and speed.

Therapeutic rapport—The qualities of experience and behavior between client and therapist that affect the client's performance and involvement in therapy.

Verbal communication—Interpreting another's words and expressing one's own thoughts and emotions through words.

Working alliance—Working together to achieve agreed-upon goals.

carry through with the work because of having a competent and caring ally in the achievement of mutually derived occupational goals. In addition, many, if not most, daily life occupations are conducted in a social milieu. People do occupations together and in the presence of one another, and their occupations are supported naturally by their immediate, spontaneous, and sympathetic responses to one another. The therapist can provide this natural supportive function while expertly guiding occupation-as-means to achieving therapeutic goals.

This chapter defines the behaviors and feelings associated with therapeutic rapport, describes conditions affecting its development, and discusses the ethics of a therapeutic relationship. Although this chapter focuses on therapeutic rapport with the client, its content can be applied to developing rapport with family members as well (see Clark et al., 1995, for more detail).

Definition of High Therapeutic Rapport

High **therapeutic rapport** (Box 13-1) entails the experience and behavior of the client and therapist as they interact with each other and the outcome of the interaction for the client:

1. It is an optimal, interpersonal *experience* for both the client and the therapist that requires concentration, masterful communication, and enjoyment (Csikszentmihalyi, 1990).
2. It occurs with *behavior* that reflects high levels of mutual attentiveness, interpersonal coordination, and mutual positivity (Tickle-Degnen & Rosenthal, 1990, 1992).
3. It has a *beneficial effect* on the client's performance and follow-through with intervention plans (Feinberg, 1992; Hall et al., 1995; Porszt-Miron et al., 1988).

BOX 13-1
A Definition of High Therapeutic Rapport

Qualities of Experience

Concentration	The client and therapist experience a deep and effortless concentration on the interaction. Distractions, worries, and self-concern disappear.
Masterful communication	They are challenged by the interaction yet feel skillful in meeting the challenge. The goals of the interaction are experienced as clear and shared by both. Each understands immediately how well these goals are being met.
Enjoyment	They experience the interaction with deep satisfaction.

Qualities of Verbal and Nonverbal Behavior

Attentiveness	The client and therapist demonstrate verbally and nonverbally that their attention is focused on the other.
Interpersonal coordination	They demonstrate a highly tuned responsiveness to each other such that behavior and emotional expression are highly coordinated between the two.
Positivity	They demonstrate verbally and nonverbally that their feelings are positive towards one another and the interaction.

Beneficial Effects for the Patient

Enhanced client performance	Qualities of the client-therapist interaction are beneficial if they improve client performance during evaluation and intervention.
Client follow-through with therapeutic activities	Qualities of the client-therapist interaction are beneficial if they support clients' continued involvement in activities that enable them to make progress toward their goals.

Mutuality and Therapeutic Rapport

Mutuality in the relationship between client and therapist is relatively new in the espoused philosophy of occupational therapy. In the first half of the 20th century, occupational therapists were expected to be friendly and cheerful but not intimate with clients (Aitken, 1948; American Occupational Therapy Association, 1948). Therapists and clients were not to affect each other through the force of their personal attributes. Starting at mid-century, the "therapeutic use of self" (Frank, 1958) became the prevailing philosophical position guiding the therapeutic relationship. Therapists recognized that not only modalities but their own selves could be agents of therapeutic change in their clients. By being role models to their clients and behaving in certain ways, they could help clients change. Although therapists could influence clients, therapists were to remain somewhat professionally detached to ensure that they themselves were not unduly affected by clients.

Starting in the late 1960s with the inception of the human rights, human potential, and consumer movements and continuing into the early 1990s, occupational therapy's view of the therapeutic relationship has been undergoing a major transformation. The profound shift has been toward viewing the relationship as a mutual and collaborative exchange between equals, a perspective exemplified by Yerxa's (1973) work: "The therapist allows himself to feel real emotion as he enters into mutual relation with the client . . . . The authentic occupational therapist is involved in the process of caring and to care means to be affected just as surely as it means to affect" (p. 8).

The current philosophy of the therapeutic relationship has advanced the mutuality perspective to the image of friendship (Peloquin, 1990). This image is revolutionary in that it conveys that the client and therapist together engage in mutually satisfying occupation and interaction (e.g., Clark, 1993). Although the friendship imagery is useful for communicating the depth of respect that a client and therapist can hold for one another, it would be misleading to think that the client–therapist relationship is equivalent to typical social friendships.

Unlike typical friendships, a client and an occupational therapist usually meet and grow to know one another because the therapist is expected to provide a service to the client. This service relationship may arise when it is difficult for the client, because of suffering or impairment, to experience or communicate feelings that contribute to the development of rapport (Kleinman, 1988; Tickle-Degnen & Rosenthal, 1992). Finally, the therapist usually is paid for the services, often not by the client directly, and is accountable to institutional and professional systems that are charged with monitoring therapy and tracking the client's response to therapy.

The view of the relationship being one in which the client and therapist influence one another is consistent with theory and research about how practitioners and clients actually interact with one another in the clinic (Buller & Street, 1992; Mattingly & Fleming, 1994; Tickle-Degnen & Rosenthal, 1992). This work suggests that if either the client or the therapist is not attentive, responsive, or positive—or perceived as such by the other—the interaction will not have high therapeutic rapport.

Experiential and Behavioral Qualities of High Therapeutic Rapport

Health care research findings and clients' autobiographical accounts demonstrate that both the therapist and client contribute to the development of a relationship. The following sections discuss the therapist's and client's rapport qualities.

Therapist's Concentration and Attentiveness

A person who is paying attention to another tends to direct his or her body and eyes toward the other to pick up information from the other person. In therapy, this type of behavior enables the therapist to watch the client and to pick up cues from the client's face and body, sources of much expression of emotion. Therapists also show that they are paying attention to clients by taking the time to sit down and talk with them (Figs. 13-1 and 13-2). Verbal and nonverbal attentiveness has been found to be positively associated with client satisfaction (Hall et al., 1988), test performance (Rosendahl & Ross,

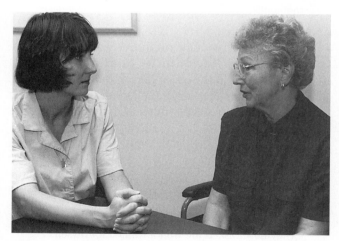

Figure 13-1 Mutual attentiveness by therapist and client forms the basis for effective communication and the development of a successful working relationship.

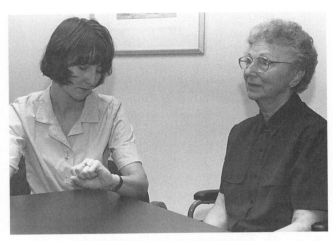

Figure 13-2 The therapist who is distracted by time pressure or other concerns loses the interpersonal connection with the client.

1982), and participation in occupational therapy procedures (Feinberg, 1992).

Paying attention to a client goes beyond conducting a standardized evaluation, and it goes beyond physical attention. It requires listening carefully to what the client has to say about his or her life, the illness, and the experience of intervention (Crepeau, 1991; Kautzmann, 1993; Kleinman, 1988; Peloquin, 1990). Without this kind of attentiveness, the therapist may apply a cookbook intervention that is not individualized to the needs of the client, as happened to McCrum (1998) during rehabilitation following a stroke. During therapy, McCrum felt like a 3-year-old playing with letters of the alphabet:

> "Sitting in my wheelchair with my Day-Glo letter-blocks I could not escape reflecting on the irony of the situation. If only Milan Kundera, Kazuo Ishiguro, or Mario Vargas Llosa, whose texts I had pored over with their authors, could have seen their editor at that moment!"
>
> (p. 139)

Simple tabletop activities in and of themselves are not at fault here. They can be exactly what a client needs. However, in this case, they apparently were not. Therapists usually are well intentioned, but unless their intentions are consistent with what the client perceives to be important, they may be less than beneficial. Reflecting upon her hospital experiences as a child with spina bifida, Saxton (1987) considered the saddest aspect of her experiences to be that so many practitioners were trying hard to help her, yet no one asked and listened to what she herself felt to be important:

> "They never asked me what I wanted for myself . . . . They never asked me if I wanted their help . . . . I just wish all disabled children would say to their helpers: 'Before you do anything else, just listen to me.'"
>
> (p. 55)

Craig (1991) described how her husband's nurse, during each home visit, listened and heard:

> "[S]he began by listening. And anything Ed wanted to tell her was relevant. She let him tell her, in his own way and in his own time, about everything that was happening to his body. And in that way, she came to know his soul."
>
> (p. 241)

Client's Concentration and Attentiveness

Therapists need attention from their clients as well. A client who does not attend to the therapist cannot give or get important information from him or her. Many pathological conditions (e.g., traumatic brain damage and attention deficit disorders) affect the ability to concentrate and therefore interfere with the client's ability to pay attention to others, including the therapist. In addition, people who feel embarrassed (Exline et al., 1965) or anxious (Waxer, 1977) make little eye contact with others. Clients may not be able to engage attentively with a therapist when they are embarrassed or anxious.

Clients may be more involved and attentive when they value their therapy than when they do not. McCrum (1998) did not find value in the form of his therapy, particularly in juxtaposition to his occupation as an editor for brilliant writers. Unfortunately, it appears that the therapist did not engage the client collaboratively in the determination of intervention activities. Despite strong collaborative values and ethics in occupational therapy, research finds that therapists often fall short of fully and collaboratively involving clients and their families in decision making (Brown & Bowen, 1998; Hasselkus, 1991; Northern et al., 1995).

Therapist's Communication and Interpersonal Coordination

It is impossible for even the most attentive therapist to apprehend and feel exactly what the client feels about his or her own illness and life. Likewise, the client cannot fully comprehend the personal experience and role obligations of the therapist. Each is a unique individual with a unique life history and perspective. Despite these differences, the therapist and client can teach each other their personal perspectives through **verbal communication** and **nonverbal communication** (Crepeau, 1991).

The fundamental condition for the therapist to communicate effectively with the client is for the therapist to direct his or her attention to the client. The next step is for the therapist to interpret accurately the client's verbal and nonverbal behavior (Tickle-Degnen & Rosenthal, 1992). This interpretation entails first the observation that another person has behaved and then translation of this observation into an inference about the other's thoughts and emotions (Fig. 13-3). Svidén and Säljö (1993) found that over 18 months the impressions of occupational therapy students about clients became increasingly complex. For example, at a student's first viewing of a client's videotaped behavior, her impression consisted of the following seven words: "It was rather difficult for her psychologically" (p. 495). That

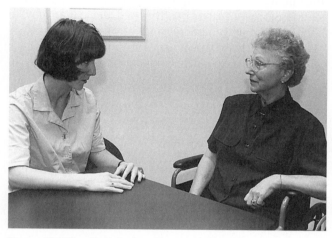

Figure 13-3 The client's backward lean may indicate that she is withdrawing from the therapist or from the information the therapist is giving her. The therapist must determine whether or not the client's behavior is a sign of withdrawal and then whether to adjust her own behavior to maintain rapport. This therapist may decide to become less confrontational, relaxing her posture and making less intense eye contact.

same student's impression 18 months after beginning her training consisted of at least 71 words. It included a description of the client's gaze and vocal behavior and conjectures about the feelings the client may have had, such as hopelessness, confusion, lack of happiness, and embarrassment. By this second viewing, the student had a better articulated and more complex impression of the client and as a result would have been able to engage in a more effective dialogue with the client to confirm or refute elements of the impression.

The research of Marangoni et al. (1995) suggests that the therapist rapidly learns to understand a client's emotions and thoughts, especially if the client gives feedback to the therapist about the accuracy of the therapist's impressions (Research Note). If the client cannot give verbal feedback to the therapist about the accuracy of the therapist's interpretations, the therapist may be able to learn what the client is feeling simply by reflecting on the therapist's own emotions. More than likely, what the therapist feels is similar to what the client feels, because the therapist and client unconsciously and subtly coordinate their bodily and facial movements to one another (Bernieri & Rosenthal, 1991) and literally feel their way into one another's emotions (Hatfield et al., 1994). For example, while working with a client, a therapist may develop a stooped posture and a sad face through a subtle mimicry of the client's behavior. The therapist may begin to have a feeling of dejection in response to the therapist's own bodily and facial pattern of dejection. Typically, individuals are unaware of the

---

 RESEARCH NOTE

Empathic Accuracy in a Clinically Relevant Setting
Marangoni, C., Garcia, S., Ickes, W., & Teng, G. (1995). Journal of Personality and Social Psychology, 68, 854–869.

ABSTRACT

This study addressed three questions regarding empathic accuracy in a clinically relevant setting. First, does the empathic accuracy of a perceiver improve with increased exposure to a target individual? Second, can empathic accuracy be enhanced by providing the perceiver with feedback about the target's actual thoughts and feelings? Third, are there stable individual differences in empathic accuracy that generalize across different targets? The results indicated that although absolute performance levels varied from one target to another, empathic accuracy generally improved with increased exposure to the target. In addition, feedback concerning the target's actual thoughts and feelings accelerated the rate at which the perceivers' empathic accuracy improved. Finally, cross-target consistency in responding revealed stable individual differences in the perceivers' empathic ability.

IMPLICATIONS FOR PRACTICE

► Over time, a therapist is likely to develop increasingly accurate interpretations of a client's thoughts and feelings.

► This accuracy is facilitated if the client gives the therapist feedback about whether or not the therapist's interpretations are accurate. Therefore, the therapist should ask the client if interpretations are correct.

► Some therapists tend to have less difficulty developing accurate interpretations of clients' thoughts and emotions than do other therapists. Therapists should become aware of their own capacity for interpreting others' thoughts and emotions. If they tend to have difficulty with accuracy, they should be careful to clarify consistently their interpretations with the client and compare their interpretations with those of colleagues.

degree to which another person's emotions influence their own and consequently do not reflect on their own emotions to discover what another person's are. Yet if therapists are aware of the possibility of this form of emotional influence, they probably can more accurately detect the unspoken emotions of clients.

After accurate interpretation of a client's message, the next step in effective communication is for the therapist to express his or her emotions and thoughts in a manner that is clear to and beneficial for the client (Tickle-Degnen & Rosenthal, 1992). When a therapist feels positive, hopeful, and engaged in treatment and expresses these feelings in an unambiguous manner, clients tend to have similar reactions (Buller & Street, 1992; DiMatteo et al., 1986; Hall et al., 1995). Nonverbal messages are typically conveyed more rapidly than verbal ones. Watt (1996), a man in severe pain, described his favorite nurse:

> "I believed she would make things better. It was never anything she said. It was something in her face."
>
> (p. 13)

The combination of verbal and nonverbal behavior that the therapist uses to express his or her feelings and attitudes toward the client can profoundly move the client. Brack (Brack & Collins, 1981), a woman with multiple sclerosis, described how her physical therapist conveyed a sense of compassion and hope after a long period of hard work but little progress in therapy. As Brack was waiting for therapy in a line of wheelchairs, she could not suppress her tears of despair and shame at not being able to regain her ability to walk. Her therapist quickly pulled her chair out of the line and wheeled it down to the therapy office, where together they wept:

> "Our eyes met. 'Do you want to quit?' [the therapist] said. 'I know it's tough and you know you may never get any better. But shall we try a little longer?'
>
> Right away I knew I had to. I smiled damply and dried my eyes. What a friend!"
>
> (pp. 71–72)

The therapist in this example did not simply say "Keep trying, I know you can do it." Because she had worked with this client for a long time, she could express her understanding of the client's feelings in a heartfelt and intimate manner, by weeping with the client. Brack continued her description by explaining how she and her therapist kept working at the parallel bars, never giving up. Eventually she was able to walk again. This example demonstrates that effective communication occurs not only through verbal and nonverbal behavior but also through the activities in which the therapist and client engage. The act of engaging in therapy, even when it seems that hope is lost, is a message to the client that hope is *not* lost.

Likewise, messages are conveyed through the tools that occupational therapists offer their clients. When an occupational therapist gives a buttonhook to a client, several messages are offered, among them that the client is capable of using a buttonhook and that dressing independently is a valued goal of the client. In high-rapport interactions, the client is aware of the goals of the interaction and feels control during the interaction. Thus, the performance of activities that are clearly consistent with the client's goals communicates that the therapist understands the client's perspective, and the client may respond with renewed energy and engagement in therapy. Hanlan (1979), a man with amyotrophic lateral sclerosis, wanted to maintain his daily functioning:

> "Of increasing importance to me is the help of occupational therapists . . . . My first O.T., a man with a direct and kind manner, provided me with a buttonhook, so I could button and unbutton my clothing. I had an almost childlike, happy response to discovering this little tool."
>
> (p. 40)

Client's Communication and Interpersonal Coordination

Some clients cannot accurately interpret a therapist's social behavior. Individuals with brain damage, particularly in the right hemisphere, have difficulty perceiving and interpreting social nonverbal cues (Rosenthal & Benowitz, 1986). Among individuals with left hemispheric damage, those with a receptive form of aphasia may be unable to understand the therapist's speech. It is difficult for clients with these types of problems to make sense of the therapist's social overtures and respond appropriately to them. For clients who have interpretation difficulties, the therapist must make frequent multimedia attempts to communicate. For example, the therapist can express information verbally, nonverbally, in written, and in picture form.

Like problems of interpretation, problems of expression can interfere with the development of rapport. Right brain damage and Parkinson's disease have been found to interfere with an individual's ability to express interpretable emotions nonverbally (Brozgold et al., 1998). Clients with expressive aphasia have difficulty communicating their thoughts and needs verbally. For clients with expression difficulties, the therapist must seek information from multiple communication channels, such as through the verbal, facial, and bodily behavior of the client.

Therapist's Enjoyment and Positivity

According to a biological evolutionary perspective, all relationships that require mutual cooperation to achieve beneficial outcomes for individuals begin with signals of intent to do no harm to one another and to cooperate (Preuschoft & van Hooff, 1997). Individuals whose signals express positive feelings inspire cooperative effort, whereas those whose signals express negative feelings inspire disengagement. Consistent with this perspective, a study of occupational therapy students found that those who tended to express negative feelings, as opposed to those who tended to express positive or neutral feelings, had less rapport with their colleagues and were rated as being less clinically skilled by fieldwork supervisors (Tickle-Degnen & Puccinelli, 1999).

Practitioners express their warmth and liking through nonverbal behaviors such as leaning forward and smiling (Figure 13-4). Clients interpret these and other types of friendly verbal and nonverbal behavior as positive and respond with reduced anxiety (Ben-Sira, 1988), increased follow-through with intervention regimens (Feinberg, 1992), and more successful performance (Harris & Rosenthal, 1985). Clients whom their practitioners genuinely like tend to have better therapeutic outcomes than those who are not liked (Gelso et al., 1983).

Peloquin (1993a) has eloquently described how health professionals can act in a manner that distances rather than connects them to their clients and saps their clients' courage. Beisser (1989), a man with polio, found that his dependency on hospital attendants for physical survival had a profound effect on his day-to-day view of himself and the world:

> "Everything that affected them affected me. If I was cared for willingly and without reluctance, I felt good and the world was sunny. If my care was given grudgingly or irritably, in a callous way, powerful feelings of degradation swept over me."
>
> (p. 34)

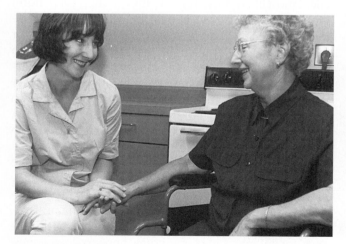

Figure 13-4 The therapist and client show mutual positivity through their facial expressions and physical contact. Social physical contact, like holding a client's hand, is appropriate if it is an expression of professional warmth and the client gains comfort from it. Not all clients like being touched in this manner.

In Beisser's experience (1989), the helpers who enjoyed their work and were nurtured by their relationships with clients were his most effective ones. With them Beisser felt human again, able to reciprocate their warmth and concern. The body of evidence on therapeutic rapport, starting with the seminal work of Rogers (1957), suggests that connecting to clients in a respectful and positive manner contributes to therapeutic effectiveness. The reverse is probably also true: being effective contributes to a feeling of connectedness with clients (Rosa & Hasselkus, 1996).

What may be most important in therapists' expression of positivity toward clients is the genuine feeling and communication of concern and caring (King, 1980). For example, the research findings of Rosenthal et al. (1984) suggest that the tone of voice of a caring therapist is not necessarily uniformly positive and cheerful. Rather, there is an element of anxiety conveyed. It is not easy to achieve a high level of concern and caring in today's health care system, which emphasizes cost containment and adherence to protocol and provides little recognition for caring involvement (Peloquin, 1993b; Sachs & Labovitz, 1994). A supportive system composed not only of the therapist's personal commitment to caring but also of a societal and institutional commitment to caring are needed to sustain a therapeutic level of caring.

Client's Enjoyment and Positivity

Clients who are very anxious or depressed demonstrate relatively little warmth nonverbally. For example, they smile infrequently and make little eye contact. Practitioners, especially those who are inexperienced and unlikely to interpret this behavior as a normal response to illness or a sign of disease, may take personally this lack of warmth by some clients (Tickle-Degnen & Rosenthal, 1992).

Misery from illness may encompass the client's life, reducing the ability to respond warmly to others. As Brack, suffering from multiple sclerosis, noted, " 'Thanks' is a near-forgotten word among us clients as we wallow in our private miseries" (Brack & Collins, 1981, p. 47). From an ethical and professional standpoint, practitioners are expected to rise above petty responses to unpleasant behavior in clients, but unfortunately, they may begin to resent and even hate some of those that they are supposed to help (Gans, 1983).

For example, Beisser (1989) found that his helpers on the polio ward had a powerful form of retribution for clients who were thought to be difficult:

> "You cannot get mad in hospitals. If you do, you may be in trouble . . . . Angry clients come last. So I quickly learned to smile patiently . . . . I had to be careful, for they were more in control of my body than I was."
>
> (p. 19)

Even practitioners who do not engage in this form of retribution may find it hard to work with a client who lacks warmth and happiness. Schindler et al. (1989), for example, found that during a first therapeutic encounter, the more frequently clients gave reports of success and the less frequently they merely described their problems, the more positive the therapists felt.

In occupational therapy, clients may have strong negative reactions to the frustrations of trying to perform what they perceive to be simple tasks, as did Puller (1991), a Vietnam veteran with bilateral upper extremity amputations. He reports, "There were times in OT when I felt like screaming as I tried to learn how to button clothes or to thread a needle" (p. 181). Such frustration is bound to impinge on the client's view of therapy and the therapist, and it should not be ignored. The therapist may have to reevaluate the balance of the emotional costs and physical benefits of particular forms of activity and to confirm that these activities support the client's own goals.

Evidence suggests that practitioners must be careful not to view all expressions of frustration, sadness, or anger as confirmation of pathology (Langer & Abelson, 1974). For example, Widome (1989) described how a nurse responded to an emotional outburst that apparently was Widome's expression of anger at being in the horrible predicament of having cancer. As Widome was walking down a hospital corridor, the nurse asked him how he was feeling:

> "I let loose with a tirade of words . . . . Wouldn't she prefer no life to a thread of existence? . . . The nurse made a notation on my chart that I had made a decision to end my life, that I was considering self-destruction. I was now a marked man—suicidal."
> (pp. 99–100)

Expressions of frustration and anger may be indeed signs of a pathological process that requires diagnosis, or they may be normal responses to the experience of illness and intervention.

Beneficial Effect and High Therapeutic Rapport

Listed next are three of the possible reasons attentive, coordinated, and positive client–therapist interactions may have a beneficial effect on the client's performance and follow-through with intervention:

1. The interaction provides the external scaffolding necessary for skill development, by directing attention to important aspects of a task problem, by communicating the information necessary to solve the problem, and by giving motivational support for pursuing problem solution (Burke, 1986; Tickle-Degnen & Coster, 1995).

2. The interaction reduces disabling anxiety. As the client learns—by communicating with a warm, supportive therapist—to trust the therapist, anxiety is reduced (Ben-Sira, 1988). Anxiety can interfere with therapeutic progress by engulfing the client's attention, leaving limited capacity for focused involvement in therapeutic tasks or by increasing physical tension and interfering with the physical performance of these tasks.

3. The interaction creates a self-fulfilling prophecy of improved performance (Harris & Rosenthal, 1985; Olson et al., 1996). Through verbal and nonverbal communication, a therapist conveys his or her expectations for the progress of a client, with the effect that the client's actual performance conforms to those expectations. Informative, warm, and respectful behavior may affirm to the client that he or she is a capable and valued human being, which mobilizes the client's psychological, intellectual, and physical resources toward fulfillment of the implications of those qualities.

Development of a High Therapeutic Rapport Relationship

All relationships take time to develop. Yet it is fairly well agreed that the critical development of rapport and a **working alliance**, that is, the experience of working together toward mutually agreed-upon goals, is achieved within the first three to five sessions of therapy (Horvath & Luborsky, 1993). First meetings tend to be somewhat superficial and rigidly constrained by role expectations. The therapist most likely performs an evaluation, and the client most likely tries to answer the questions or perform the activities of the evaluation. Individuals seem to be aware implicitly that first encounters are critical for relationship development in that they actively try to control the image they are conveying, while simultaneously and rapidly forming an impression of the other person (DePaulo, 1992). Through close adherence to cultural scripts of friendly, polite behaviors, they offer their identities to one another as valuable and likable (Clark et al., 1996).

In the first meeting, the client may convey private information to the therapist, but the depth of intimacy and mutuality continues to grow over subsequent interactions, although not in a linear fashion (Altman, 1993; VanLear, 1991). A dialectical tension between the desires for intimacy and autonomy appears to manifest itself in a cyclical pattern of intimate and more distant behavior. After the first few therapeutic encounters, there appears to be a period of much fluctuation in the nature of the interpersonal interaction (Lichtenberg, et al., 1998), as if client and therapist are trying out different patterns of relating to one another. It also may be that these fluctuations are a result of shifts between therapeutic work and socializing. There is evidence that the grueling, attentive, task-focused work of therapy requires off-task periods of rest and recovery with opportunities for chit-chat. This chit-chat may serve to affirm the social connection between therapist and client (Hall et al., 1999).

Relationships that endure, whether they be personal or therapeutic, seem to have one primary attribute in common: the ability to control and manage the development of negative emotions (Gottman, 1994; Tracey, 1993). Although individuals in both successful and failing relationships have negative emotions and behavior, in successful relationships, they have interpersonal strategies for rapidly repairing the hurt or negative consequences of these emotions and preventing an escalation of negativity. In failing ones, the individuals are unable to curtail this escalation.

Therapists' and clients' characteristics and conditions in the therapy setting can facilitate or inhibit the development of high rapport. One study (Tickle-Degnen, 1998) found that occupational therapy students who were quiet and empathically concerned attained the highest supervisory ratings in physical rehabilitation settings. Those who were autonomous yet attuned to bodily expressions of emotions attained highest ratings in pediatric settings. Those who were emotionally reactive, especially to facial expressions of emotions, attained highest ratings in psychosocial settings. These results suggest that therapists must adapt their interpersonal styles to different therapeutic contexts. Through self-reflection; feedback from supervisors, colleagues, and clients; and reflective clinical experience, the therapist should be able to learn how to make these adaptations.

Based on the evidence presented here, Box 13-2 gives guidelines for enhancing the development of rapport. It is not the client's responsibility to change to enhance the rapport; it is the therapist's. Therefore, the guidelines are directed at actions the therapist can take.

Typically, therapeutic relationships work toward a planned end to the relationship as goals are achieved or services are no longer needed. As discharge approaches, the therapist should work actively with the client to transform their relationship appropriately, so that the client does not feel abandoned (e.g., Clark, 1993; Klein, 1995). The form this transformation takes depends on the setting. For example, the therapist may help the client to develop other fulfilling relationships in the community or may keep in contact with the client through the phone or occasional clinic visits.

BOX 13-2
PROCEDURES FOR PRACTICE

Therapist Guidelines for Facilitating the Development of High Therapeutic Rapport

Create conditions that maximize therapist's and client's concentration and attention:

- Set aside time to listen to client.
- Reduce distractions in therapy setting.
- Reduce potential for client's embarrassment or anxiety.
- Position own body to see and hear client clearly.
- Position client so that client can see and hear therapist clearly.
- Listen for issues that are most important to client.

Create conditions that maximize therapist and client masterful communication and interpersonal coordination:

- Remain open and sensitive to verbal and nonverbal messages from the client.
- Provide assistance as needed for the client to express emotions and thoughts.
- Check with the client to see whether therapist's interpretation of client's messages is accurate.
- Clearly express emotions and thoughts that are consistent with the needs and goals of the client.
- Check with the client to see whether the client is interpreting therapist's messages accurately.

- Create a challenging and interesting interaction, but one in which the client can interact skillfully.
- Involve the client collaboratively in the development of goals and the planning of intervention.

Create conditions that maximize therapist and client enjoyment and positivity:

- Find a satisfying, fulfilling aspect to every interaction with a client.
- Express genuine concern and caring for the client through verbal and nonverbal behavior.
- Resolve personal problems and fulfill personal social needs outside of the client–therapist interaction.
- Determine whether client's sadness or anger is normal or pathological, and respond appropriately to alleviate suffering.
- Engage client in activities and interaction that are inherently enjoyable for the client.
- During required activities that are not enjoyable, provide periodic opportunities for rest and off-task recovery.
- Manage negativity so that it can be expressed as needed in a constructive manner and does not escalate.

Case Example

Patient Information

Mrs. K., a 75-year-old widow with Parkinson's disease, has entered the adult day treatment program today. She has reluctantly attended at the insistence of her physician and family members, who are concerned with her social isolation and reluctance to take care of basic grooming and self-care needs despite the physical capacity to do so. Upon entering the room, Mrs. K sits in a chair far from the center of activity and stares at the floor. The therapist, who has never met Mrs. K., makes the following observations:

1. Mrs. K. appears, through her choice of seat and position, to desire not to engage with anyone.
2. The client has rigid movements.
3. Mrs. K. has the facial mask associated with Parkinson's disease or the flat affect associated with depression.

Initial Plan

The therapist decides that her first step must be to develop rapport with Mrs. K. to ascertain her needs and whether those needs are likely to be met in the day program. She approaches Mrs. K., introduces herself, and sits close enough to show interest in talking with Mrs. K. but not so close as to appear intrusive. The therapist provides time for Mrs. K. to respond to her and continues her observation of Mrs. K's facial affect, watching for signals of interest or disengagement while expressing respect and caring toward Mrs. K.

Short-Term Goals

1. *Therapist and Mrs. K will attend to one another for a 5- to 15-minute period.*
   The therapist directs her gaze at Mrs. K. and asks questions about a topic that she believes Mrs. K. will enjoy speaking about, such as her children or grandchildren. She finds that she and Mrs. K. are able to sustain a pleasant topic for 5 minutes.
2. *Therapist and Mrs. K will exchange initial orientation information about the program and Mrs. K's interest.*
   While talking with Mrs. K., the therapist begins to learn what Mrs. K. values, some of her interests and opinions. She learns that Mrs. K. sees no reason to groom or get dressed in the morning because she has no planned daily activities outside of the home.

3. *Mrs. K will demonstrate her capacity for showing her emotional response to the therapist.*
   The therapist notes that Mrs. K.'s eye musculature shows little motion and little affective expression, even when Mrs. K. is talking about a favored grandson, although her mouth upturns a bit at the corners. Knowing that this pattern of facial expression during positive emotions is typical of those with Parkinson's disease, the therapist tentatively concludes that Mrs. K. has the capacity to demonstrate positive emotions, yet her expression is ambiguous to the normal social observer.

Revised Goals

1. Mrs. K. will express interest in participating in a 1-hour assessment of her occupational needs.
2. Mrs. K. will communicate information relevant to her occupational needs.
3. Mrs. K. will have a pleasant social interaction with one of the other program participants.

CLINICAL REASONING
in OT Practice

Ethical Dilemma

Mrs. K. continues to refuse involvement in the day program despite the therapist's, the family members', and the physician's insistence for her to be involved. What should the therapist do? What is the therapist's ethical responsibility? How will the therapist's decision affect the therapeutic relationship with Mrs. K.?

When to Refer to Another Therapist

The therapist suspects that one reason that Mrs. K. does not want to be involved in the program is that the therapist has a different ethnicity from that of Mrs. K., and Mrs. K. seems to have a negative attitude toward the therapist's ethnic group. How should the therapist attempt to deal with this possibility? What can be done to promote rapport? At what point and under what conditions should the therapist attempt to refer Mrs. K. to another therapist or program?

Ethics and the Therapeutic Relationship

The Occupational Therapy Code of Ethics (American Occupational Therapy Association, 1994) outlines the key ethical elements of the therapeutic relationship. The code consists of six principles, two of which are covered here because they are the most important to the entire course of the therapeutic relationship:

Principle 1

Occupational therapy personnel shall demonstrate a concern for the well-being of the recipients of their services.

Two elements of this principle are that therapists must (1) provide services in an equitable manner to all individuals and (2) take reasonable precautions to do no harm to the client. A therapist may have fears or negative attitudes about a particular client population, for example, such as individuals with AIDS (Hansen, 1990). Despite these feelings, it is the ethical imperative of therapists to provide services.

Although there is no ethical imperative to feel rapport with clients, the imperative to do no harm suggests that the therapist should make every effort to create optimal intervention conditions for the client. Part of this optimization requires creating a climate of rapport. The therapist should consider changing jobs or clinical specialization if he or she is unable to overcome negative feelings with clients typically seen in a particular setting or specialization area. If these feelings rarely occur and the therapist has made an honest but unsuccessful attempt to support high therapeutic rapport, he or she may consider referring the client to a different therapist. This referral meets the standard of this principle because it demonstrates a concern that the client receive beneficial services.

Another element of this principle is that therapists must maintain relationships that do not exploit the client sexually, physically, emotionally, financially, socially, or in any other manner. Mutuality of feeling, behavior, and goals is critical to the development of a relationship of high therapeutic rapport; however, interdependency or the expectation of reciprocal benefits is not. The therapist who becomes dependent on a client for meeting a personal need is exploitive because of his or her higher power relative to the client's position of vulnerability. Furthermore, although the therapist is ethically responsible for helping the client, the client is not expected to help the therapist in any manner.

Principle 2

Occupational therapy personnel shall respect the rights of the recipients of their services.

One element of the second ethical principle is autonomy. Respect for the client's autonomy requires therapeutic relationships in which clients collaborate to the best of their ability in the determination of goals and priorities during intervention. For clients to be able to collaborate, they must be informed about the nature, risks, and potential outcomes of the intervention and have the opportunity to reject or refuse services or elements of services. This standard is both ethical and consistent with the nature of therapeutic rapport and the effective working alliance (Spencer et al., 1997). Collaborative decisions are self-guiding, carried out not because of external pressures but because of an active feeling of personal control and responsibility (Fig. 13-5).

Other elements of this principle are privacy and confidentiality. During a relationship of high therapeutic rapport, the client may tell the therapist about matters that are private and confidential. The therapist must protect the confidentiality of information by not discussing it in an inappropriate context (for example, in a public elevator conversation) or manner (for example, laughing at the client's capabilities) with a colleague or any other person.

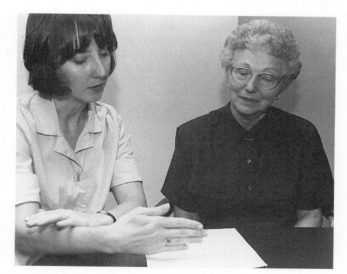

Figure 13-5 In a collaborative relationship, the therapist and client discuss the benefits and risks of participating in various occupational therapy interventions so that the client can make informed decisions about participating in these interventions.

Summary Review Questions

1. What are the elements of high therapeutic rapport?
2. How has the view of the client–therapist relationship changed over time?
3. How are the therapist's experience and behavior related to rapport?
4. How are the client's experience and behavior related to rapport?
5. What are three reasons high rapport may be beneficial for clients?
6. How can the therapist facilitate the development of high therapeutic rapport?
7. What are two ethical responsibilities that a therapist holds in a relationship with a client?

Acknowledgments

The ideas in this chapter evolved during a Mary Switzer Research Fellowship supported by the National Institutes for Disability and Rehabilitation Research. A special thanks to Irene Zombek and Melissa Muns, who searched clients' autobiographies for excerpts. The photographer for this chapter was Robert Littlefield.

References

Aitken, A. N. (1948). Values of occupational therapy in the rehabilitation of the tuberculosis client. *American Journal of Occupational Therapy, 2*, 219–222.

Altman, I. (1993). Dialectics, physical environments, and personal relationships. *Communication Monographs, 60*, 26–34.

American Occupational Therapy Association. (1948). Professional attitudes. *American Journal of Occupational Therapy, 2*, 97–98.

American Occupational Therapy Association. (1994). Occupational therapy code of ethics. *American Journal of Occupational Therapy, 48*, 1037–1043.

Beisser, A. R. (1989). *Flying Without Wings: Personal Reflections on Being Disabled.* New York: Doubleday.

Ben-Sira, Z. (1988). Affective behavior and perceptions of health professionals. In D. S. Gochman (Ed.), *Health Behavior* (pp. 305–317). New York: Plenum.

Bernieri, F. J., & Rosenthal, R. (1991). Interpersonal coordination: Behavior matching and interactional synchrony. In R. Feldman & R. Rime (Eds.), *Fundamentals of Nonverbal Behavior* (pp. 401–432). Cambridge, UK: Cambridge University.

Brack, J., & Collins, R. (1981). *One Thing for Tomorrow: A Woman's Personal Struggle with MS.* Saskatoon: Western Producer Prairie.

Brozgold, A. Z., Borod, J. C., Martin, C. C., Pick, L. H., Alpert, M., & Welkowitz, J. (1998). Social functioning and facial emotional expression in neurological and psychiatric disorders. *Applied Neuropsychology, 5*, 15–23.

Brown, C., & Bowen, R. E. (1998). Including the consumer and environment in occupational therapy treatment planning. *Occupational Therapy Journal of Research, 18*, 44–62.

Burke, J. (1986). Interacting plans in the accomplishment of a practical activity. In D. E. Ellis & W. A. Donahue (Eds.), *Contemporary Issues in Language and Discourse Processes* (pp. 203–222). Hillsdale, NJ: Lawrence Erlbaum.

Buller, D. B., & Street, R. L. Jr. (1992). Physician-client relationships. In R. S. Feldman (Ed.), *Applications of Nonverbal Behavioral Theories and Research* (pp. 119–141). Hillsdale, NJ: Lawrence Erlbaum.

Clark, C. A., Corcoran, M., & Gitlin, L. N. (1995). An exploratory study of how occupational therapists develop therapeutic relationships with family caregivers. *American Journal of Occupational Therapy, 49*, 587–594.

Clark, F. (1993). Eleanor Clarke Slagle Lecture: Occupation embedded in real life: Interweaving occupational science and occupational therapy. *American Journal of Occupational Therapy, 47*, 1067–1078.

Clark, M. S., Pataki, S. P., & Carver, V. H. (1996). Some thoughts and findings on self-presentation of emotions in relationships. In G. J. O. Fletcher & J. Fitness (Eds.), *Knowledge Structures in Close Relationships: A Social Psychological Approach* (pp. 247–274). Malwah, NJ: Lawrence Erlbaum.

Craig, J. (1991). *Between Hello and Goodbye.* Los Angeles: Tarcher.

Crepeau, E. B. (1991). Achieving intersubjective understanding: Examples from an occupational therapy treatment session. *American Journal of Occupational Therapy, 45*, 1016–1025.

Csikszentmihalyi, M. (1990). *Flow: The Psychology of Optimal Experience.* New York: Harper Collins.

DePaulo, B. M. (1992). Nonverbal behavior and self-presentation. *Psychological Bulletin, 111*, 203–243.

DiMatteo, M. R., Prince, L. M., & Hays, R. (1986). Nonverbal communication in the medical context: The physician-client relationship. In P. D. Blanck, R. Buck, & R. Rosenthal (Eds.), *Nonverbal Communication in the Clinical Context* (pp. 74–98). University Park, PA: The Pennsylvania State University.

Exline, R., Gray, D., & Schuette, D. (1965). Visual behavior in a dyad as affected by interview content and sex of respondent. *Journal of Personality and Social Psychology, 1*, 201–209.

Feinberg, J. (1992). Effect of the arthritis health professional on compliance with use of resting hand splints by clients with rheumatoid arthritis. *Arthritis Care and Research, 5*, 17–23.

Frank, J. D. (1958). The therapeutic use of self. *American Journal of Occupational Therapy, 12*, 215–225.

Gans, J. S. (1983). Hate in the rehabilitation setting. *Archives of Physical Medicine & Rehabilitation, 64*, 176–179.

Gelso, C. J., Mills, D. H., & Spiegel, S. B. (1983). Client and therapist factors influencing the outcome of time-limited counseling 1 and 18 months after treatment. In C. J. Gelso & D. H. Johnson (Eds.), *Explorations in Time-Limited Counseling and Psychotherapy* (pp. 87–115). New York: Teachers College.

Gottman, J. M. (1994). *What Predicts Divorce? The Relationship Between Marital Processes and Marital Outcomes* (pp. 409–440). Hillsdale, NJ: Lawrence Erlbaum.

Hall, J. A., Harrigan, J. A., & Rosenthal, R. (1995). Nonverbal behavior in clinician-client interaction. *Applied & Preventive Psychology, 4*, 21–37.

Hall, J. A., Roter, D. L., & Katz, N. R. (1988). Meta-analysis of correlates of provider behavior in medical encounters. *Medical Care, 26*, 657–675.

Hall, J. A., Roter, D. L., & Milburn, M. A. (1999). Illness and satisfaction with medical care. *Current Directions in Psychological Science, 3*, 96–99.

Hanlan, A. J. (1979). *Autobiography of Dying.* New York: Doubleday.

Hansen, R. A. (1990). The ethics of caring for patients with HIV or AIDS. *American Journal of Occupational Therapy, 44*, 239–242.

Harris, M. J., & Rosenthal, R. (1985). Mediation of interpersonal expectancy effects: 31 meta-analyses. *Psychological Bulletin, 97*, 363–386.

Hasselkus, B. R. (1991). Ethical dilemmas in family caregiving for the elderly: Implications for occupational therapy. *American Journal of Occupational Therapy, 45,* 206–212.

Hatfield, E., Cacioppo, J. T., & Rapson, R. L. (1994). *Emotional contagion.* Paris: Cambridge University.

Horvath, A. O., & Luborsky, L. (1993). The role of the therapeutic alliance in psychotherapy. *Journal of Counseling and Clinical Psychology, 61,* 561–573.

Kautzmann, L. N. (1993). Linking client and family stories to caregivers' use of clinical reasoning. *American Journal of Occupational Therapy, 47,* 169–173.

King, L. J. (1980). Creative caring. *American Journal of Occupational Therapy, 34,* 522–528.

Klein, B. S. (1995). Reflections on . . . An ally as well as a partner in practice. *Canadian Journal of Occupational Therapy, 62,* 283–285.

Kleinman, A. (1988). *The Illness Narratives.* New York: Basic Books.

Langer, E. J., & Abelson, R. P. (1974). A client by any other name . . .: Clinician group differences in labeling bias. *Journal of Consulting and Clinical Psychology, 42,* 4–9.

Lichtenberg, J. W., Wettersten, K. B., Mull, H., Moberly, R. L., Merkley, K. B., & Corey, A. T. (1998). Relationship formation and relational control as correlates of psychotherapy quality and outcome. *Journal of Counseling Psychology, 45,* 322–337.

Marangoni, C., Garcia, S., Ickes, W., & Teng, G. (1995). Empathic accuracy in a clinically relevant context. *Journal of Personality and Social Psychology, 68,* 854–869.

Mattingly, C., & Fleming, M. H. (1994). *Clinical Reasoning: Forms of Inquiry in a Therapeutic Practice.* Philadelphia: Davis.

McCrum, R. (1998). *My Year Off.* New York: Norton.

Northern, J. G., Rust, D. M., Nelson, C. E., Watts, J. H. (1995). Involvement of adult rehabilitation patients in setting occupational therapy goals. *American Journal of Occupational Therapy, 49,* 214–220.

Olson, J. A., Roese, N. J., & Zanna, M. P. (1996). Expectancies. In E. T. Higgins & A. W. Kruglanski (Eds.), *Social Psychology: Handbook of Basic Principles* (pp. 211–238). New York: Guilford.

Oxford English Dictionary (compact edition). (1971). Oxford, UK: Oxford University.

Park, R. E., & Burgess, E. W. (1924). *Introduction to the Science of Sociology.* Chicago: University of Chicago.

Peloquin, S. M. (1990). The client-therapist relationship in occupational therapy: Understanding visions and images. *American Journal of Occupational Therapy, 44,* 13–21.

Peloquin, S. M. (1993a). The depersonalization of patients: A profile gleaned from narratives. *American Journal of Occupational Therapy, 47,* 830–837.

Peloquin, S. M. (1993b). The patient-therapist relationship: Beliefs that shape care. *American Journal of Occupational Therapy, 47,* 935–942.

Porszt-Miron, L., Florian, M., & Burton, J. (1988). A pilot study on the effect of rapport on the task performance of an elderly confused population. *Canadian Journal of Occupational Therapy, 55,* 255–258.

Preuschoft, S., & van Hooff, J. (1997). The social function of "smile" and "laughter": Variations across primate species and societies. In U. Segerstrale & P. Molnar (Eds.), *Nonverbal Communication: Where Nature Meets Culture* (pp. 171–190). Mahwah, NJ: Lawrence Erlbaum.

Puller, L. B. (1991). *Fortunate Son.* New York: Grove Weidenfeld.

Rogers, C. (1957). The necessary and sufficient conditions of therapeutic change. *Journal of Consulting Psychology, 21,* 95–105.

Rosa, S. A., & Hasselkus, B. R. (1996). Connecting with patients: The personal experience of professional helping. *Occupational Therapy Journal of Research, 16,* 245–260.

Rosendahl, P. P., & Ross, V. (1982). Does your behavior affect your patient's response? *Journal of Gerontological Nursing, 8,* 572–575.

Rosenthal, R. & Benowitz, L. I. (1986). Sensitivity to nonverbal communication in normal, psychiatric, and brain-damaged samples. In P. D. Blanck, R. Buck, & R. Rosenthal (Eds.), *Nonverbal Communication in the Clinical Context* (pp. 223–257). University Park, PA: Pennsylvania State University Press.

Rosenthal, R., Blanck, P. D., & Vannicelli, M. (1984). Speaking to and about clients: Predicting therapist's tone of voice. *Journal of Consulting and Clinical Psychology, 52,* 679–686.

Sachs, D., & Labovitz, D. R. (1994). The caring occupational therapist: Scope of professional roles and boundaries. *American Journal of Occupational Therapy, 48,* 997–1005.

Saxton, M. (1987). The something that happened before I was born. In M. Saxton & F. Howe (Eds.), *With Wings: An Anthology of Literature by and About Women With Disabilities* (pp. 51–55). New York: Feminist.

Schindler, L., Hohenberger-Sieber, E., & Hahlweg, K. (1989). Observing client-therapist interaction in behaviour therapy: Development and first application of an observational system. *British Journal of Clinical Psychology, 28,* 213–226.

Spencer, J., Davidson, H., & White, V. (1997). Helping clients develop hopes for the future. *American Journal of Occupational Therapy, 51,* 191–198.

Svidén, G., & Säljö, R. (1993). Perceiving clients and their nonverbal reactions. *American Journal of Occupational Therapy, 47,* 491–497.

Tickle-Degnen, L. (1998). Working well with others: The prediction of students' clinical performance. *American Journal of Occupational Therapy, 52,* 133–142.

Tickle-Degnen, L., & Coster, W. (1995). Therapeutic interaction and the management of challenge during the beginning minutes of sensory integration treatment. *Occupational Therapy Journal of Research, 15,* 122–141.

Tickle-Degnen, L, & Puccinelli, N. (1999). The nonverbal expression of negative emotions: Peer and supervisor responses to occupational therapy students' emotional attributes. *Occupational Therapy Journal of Research, 19,* 18–39.

Tickle-Degnen, L., & Rosenthal, R. (1990). The nonverbal correlates of rapport. *Psychological Inquiry, 1,* 285–293.

Tickle-Degnen, L., & Rosenthal, R. (1992). Nonverbal aspects of therapeutic rapport. In R. S. Feldman (Ed.), *Applications of Nonverbal Behavioral Theories and Research* (pp. 143–164). Hillsdale, NJ: Lawrence Erlbaum.

Tracey, T. J. (1993). An interpersonal stage model of the therapeutic process. *Journal of Counseling Psychology, 40,* 396–409.

VanLear, C.A. (1991). Testing a cyclical model of communicative openness in relationship development: Two longitudinal studies. *Communication Monographs, 58,* 337–361.

Waxer, P. H. (1977). Nonverbal cues for anxiety: An examination of emotional leakage. *Journal of Abnormal Psychology, 86,* 306–314.

Watt, B. (1996). *Patient.* New York: Grove.

Widome, A. (1989). *The Doctor/the Client.* Miami: Editech.

Yerxa, E. J. (1973). The 1966 Eleanor Clarke Slagle lecture: Authentic occupational therapy. In American Occupational Therapy Association (Ed.), *The Eleanor Clarke Slagle Lectures: 1955–1972* (pp. 155–173). Dubuque, IA: Kendall/Hunt.

14

Upper Extremity Orthoses

Lisa D. Deshaies

LEARNING OBJECTIVES

After studying this chapter, the reader will be able to do the following:

1. Define and discuss key concepts and terms related to orthoses.
2. Identify major purposes for using orthoses.
3. Explain general precautions relative to the use of orthoses.
4. Identify key factors to consider when selecting the most appropriate orthosis.
5. Given a photograph or illustration, identify the orthosis and a clinical problem for which it may be used.
6. Select an appropriate orthosis for a given diagnosis based on a specific clinical need.

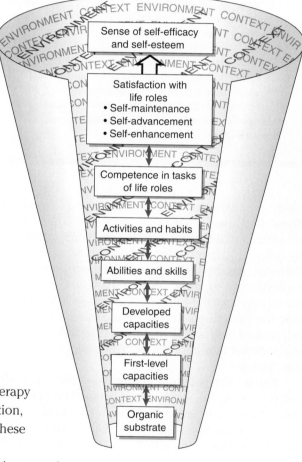

*O*rthoses are often an integral component of occupational therapy for patients with physical dysfunction. Orthotics entails prescription, selection, design, fabrication, testing, and training in the use of these special devices.

Successful use of orthoses is made possible only through an integrated team approach including the patient, his or her significant others, and health care providers. Several rehabilitation professionals bring their expertise to different aspects of the orthotic process. The physician typically prescribes the device. The certified orthotist is an expert in the design and fabrication of permanent orthoses, especially complicated spinal, lower extremity, and upper extremity orthoses used to restore function. The rehabilitation engineer is an expert in technical problem solving involving mechanical and/or electrical solutions to unique needs of patients.

The occupational therapist, as an expert in the adaptive use of the upper extremities in occupational performance tasks, has the major responsibility for the recommendation of appropriate orthoses, the testing and training in the use of orthoses for the upper extremities, and the selection, design, and fabrication of thermoplastic splints. Occupational therapists often collaborate with orthotists and rehabilitation engineers to solve problems encountered by patients in performing their tasks of daily life. The therapist presents the parameters of the problem to these professionals in terms of the patient's abilities and limitations and the functional and psychological goals that the prescribed device should meet or allow. The orthotist or engineer then proposes technical solutions, and together they apply them to the patient and evaluate the outcome.

Finally, the patient and caregivers bring key physical, psychological, social, and functional components to the orthotic process and should be considered the primary members of the team. For the orthosis to be successful, all team members must work in close collaboration.

Kinds of Orthoses

The numerous kinds of upper extremity orthoses vary according to the body parts they include, their mechanical properties, and whether they are custom made or prefabricated.

Classification Systems

An **orthosis** is any medical device applied to or around a body segment to address physical impairment or disability (Lunsford & Wallace, 1997). Orthoses may also be called splints; the American Society of Hand Therapists (ASHT) (1992) validated that the two terms may be used interchangeably. *Brace* and *support* are other commonly used terms for orthoses. One challenge when discussing orthoses is the lack of uniform terminology in the medical literature, which makes it difficult to compare and contrast features and outcomes when a single orthosis may be known by many names.

Before the 1970s there was no standard system for classifying orthoses, and orthoses were identified by proper names or eponyms based on the place of origin or the developer. A classification system was later developed to describe orthoses using acronyms based on the major joints or body parts they include. For example, a thumb carpometacarpal (CMC) support is a hand orthosis (HO); a wrist cock-up splint is a wrist–hand orthosis (WHO); an elbow brace is an elbow orthosis (EO); and a complete support for an arm is a shoulder–elbow–wrist–hand orthosis (SEWHO) (Long & Schutt, 1986; Lunsford & Wallace, 1997). Each classification may contain several types of splints. A wrist cock-up splint and a flexor hinge hand splint are both WHOs, although they serve different purposes.

In an effort to simplify, organize, and describe a standardized professional nomenclature, the ASHT developed the ASHT Splint Classification System in 1992. It classifies splints in terms of their function and the number of joints they secondarily affect. According to this system, a wrist cock-up splint is a wrist extension immobilization, type 0, as no other joints are affected. As this system becomes more widely accepted and used, it will likely serve as a universal language for referral, reimbursement, communication, and research.

This chapter uses the traditional or most commonly used names for the splints it describes.

Basic Types of Orthoses

Mechanical splint properties fall into three categories: static, static progressive, and dynamic. (Colditz, 1995a; Wilton, 1997). The **static splint**, which has no moving parts, is used primarily to provide support, stabilization, protection, or immobilization. **Serial static splinting** can be used to lengthen tissues and regain range of motion by placing tissues in an elongated position for prolonged periods (Bell-Krotoski, 1995; Colditz, 1995a). With this process, splints are remolded as range of motion increases. Because immobilization causes such unwanted effects as atrophy and stiffness, a static splint should never be used longer than physiologically required and should never unnecessarily include joints other than those being treated.

Static progressive splints use nondynamic components, such as Velcro, hinges, screws, or turnbuckles, to create a mobilizing force to regain motion. This type of splinting offers benefits not available with serial static or dynamic splinting, as the same splint can be used without remolding, and adjustments can be made more easily as motion improves.

Dynamic splints use moving parts to permit, control, or restore movement (Colditz, 1995a; Fess & Philips, 1987). They are primarily used to apply an intermittent, gentle force with the goal of lengthening tissues to restore motion. Forces may be generated by springs, spring wires, rubber bands, or elastic cords (Fess & Philips, 1987).

With dynamic splinting to increase range of motion, two concepts are critical. The first is that the force must be gentle and applied over a long time (Brand, 1995; Fess, 1995). Safe force for the hand has been determined to be 100 to 300 g (Brand, 1995; Fess & McCollum, 1998); parameters for proximal joints are not yet clinically defined. Excessive force results in tissue trauma, inflammation, and necrosis.

The second concept is that to be effective and prevent skin problems, the line of pull must be at a 90° angle to the segment being mobilized (Brand, 1995). To ensure this, forces are directed by an outrigger, a structure extending outward from the splint.

Outriggers may be high-profile or low-profile (Fig. 14-1). Each design has distinct advantages and disadvantages. Selection of outrigger design must be based on the specific patient's needs and abilities. High-profile outriggers are inherently more stable and mechanically efficient, require fewer adjustments to maintain a 90° angle of pull, and require less effort for the patient to move against the dynamic force. Low-profile outriggers are less bulky but require more frequent adjustments and greater strength to move against the dynamic force (Fess, 1995).

By allowing motion in the opposite direction, dynamic splints reduce the risk of joint stiffness from immobility, as seen with static splinting. If successful, an increase in passive joint mobility can be expected within 2 weeks (Fess & McCollum, 1998).

In addition to gaining motion, dynamic splints can be used to assist weak or paralyzed muscles. These dynamic splints may be intrinsically powered by another body part or by electrical stimulation of the patient's muscles. Extrinsic power sources, including gas-operated devices and battery-powered motors, have also been used (Long & Schutt, 1986). In practice, these externally powered devices proved to be too complex and difficult to maintain, causing their use to decline (Clark et al., 1997).

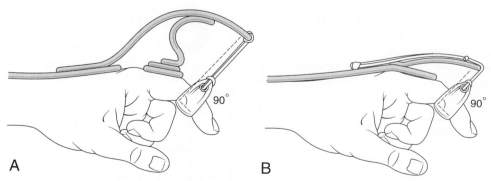

Figure 14-1 Outriggers directing proper 90° line of pull. **A.** High profile. **B.** Low profile. (Adapted with permission from Hunter, J. M., Mackin, E. J., & Callahan, A. D. [Eds.] [1995]. *Rehabilitation of the Hand: Surgery and Therapy* [4th ed.]. St. Louis: Mosby.)

Orthotic Selection

Splinting is one of the most useful modalities available to therapists when used correctly and appropriately (Fess, 1995). Remember, the end result of splinting should always relate to the patient's function. The outcome of successful splinting is that the splint serves its purpose and that the patient accepts and wears it. To meet these ends, the therapist must think critically and often creatively.

The therapist's multifaceted role is to evaluate the need for a splint clinically and functionally; to select the most appropriate splint; to provide or fabricate the splint; to assess the fit of the splint; to teach the patient and caregivers the purpose, care, and use of the splint; and to provide related training as needed. The therapist must take a leadership role to ensure that the treatment team, including the patient and caregivers, work collaboratively in every phase of the orthotic process. The patient and caregivers must be empowered and encouraged to participate actively. The therapist should clearly explain rationales, make clinically sound recommendations, and offer choices to the patient whenever possible. This helps establish each team member's accountability and increases the likelihood that the patient will actually use the splint.

A problem-solving approach to splinting directs the therapist to answer several key questions before splinting proceeds:

▶ What is the primary clinical or functional problem?
▶ What are the indications for and goals of splint use?
▶ How will the orthosis affect the problem and the patient's overall function?
▶ What benefits will the splint provide?
▶ What limitations will the splint impose?

Based on these considerations, the therapist must select or design the most appropriate orthosis. In some cases, the best choice is no orthosis at all.

The growing array of commercial products has led to a greater number of choices. The first is whether the orthosis should be custom fabricated or prefabricated. Materials must also be considered. The therapist must be familiar with properties, benefits, and drawbacks of each. Options abound, with rigid, semirigid, and soft materials available (Breger-Lee, 1995; Canelon, 1995).

When making a splint selection, several key factors must be carefully weighed:

▶ Among the splint-related factors are type, design, purpose, fit, comfort, cosmetic appearance, cost to purchase or fabricate, weight, ease of care, durability, ease of donning and doffing, effect on unsplinted joints, and effect on function.

▶ Patient-related factors include clinical and functional status, attitude, lifestyle, preference, occupational roles, living and working environments, social support, issues related to safety and precautions, ability to understand and follow through, and financial or insurance status.

Several studies have been done on patient's preferences and factors that contribute to splint wear. They show that the following factors may encourage splint wear: flexibility of the splinting regimen and vigorous teaching to enable patients to understand the purpose and wearing schedule (Pagnotta et al., 1998); individualized prescriptions focusing on the patient's comfort and preference (Callinan & Mathiowetz, 1996; Stern et al., 1996); strong family support (Oakes et al., 1970); positive attitudes and behaviors exhibited by health care providers (Feinberg, 1992); and benefits that are immediately obvious to the patient (Groth & Wulf, 1995). Rapport, trust, sensitivity to individual patients' learning styles, trial evaluations, and giving patients the opportunity to voice their concerns and frustrations can also greatly enhance the collaborative process and outcome (Collins, 1999). With the relatively small base of literature on orthotics, therapists must continue to put their clinical judgments and experience to the test and strive for evidence-based practice related to outcomes and factors that influence successful orthotic intervention.

Should problems with splint wear arise (Box 14-1), the therapist should examine both the splint and the wearing schedule. The splint itself may not fit properly or comfortably. The patient's functional demands may outweigh the benefits of splint wearing, or the wearing schedule may be too complex. Actively engaging the patient in the problem-solving process is likely to improve the outcome. Although it is important to strive for the ideal, therapists must remain realistic in the scope of the patient's daily life.

**BOX 14-1
SAFETY BOX**

Orthotic Precautions

The therapist must consider, carefully monitor, and teach the patient and caregiver to report any of these problems related to orthotic use:

▶ Impaired skin integrity (pressure areas, blisters, maceration, dermatological reactions)
▶ Pain
▶ Swelling
▶ Stiffness
▶ Sensory disturbances
▶ Increased stress on unsplinted joints
▶ Functional limitations

Purposes of Orthoses

In this chapter, orthoses are categorized according to several purposes (Box 14-2). Although a specific orthosis is discussed under the category for which it is most commonly used, that purpose may not be its only one. Also, a single orthosis may fulfill several functions simultaneously. The orthoses presented here are by no means an exhaustive list but a representative sampling of commonly used or historically significant orthoses. Inclusion of specific orthoses should not be interpreted as an endorsement of one type over another. Whenever possible, published evidence-based data have been included. As the intent of this chapter is to provide an overview of orthotics, the reader is encouraged to explore the references and resources for more detailed information.

Support a Painful Joint

Pain in a joint or soft tissues can result from a wide variety of causes, including acute trauma, (such as sprains and strains); nerve irritation, (such as carpal tunnel syndrome and ulnar nerve neuritis at the elbow); inflammatory conditions, (such as tendinitis, rheumatoid arthritis); and joint instability (such as degenerative arthritis, ligamentous laxity, shoulder subluxation). When resting a joint is indicated to relieve pain, protect joint integrity, and/or decrease inflammation, supportive orthoses can be used. These orthoses are often worn all day, all night, or both to provide the maximum benefit; or they may be worn only during selected activities. Unless contraindicated, the orthosis should be removed at least once a day for skin hygiene and gentle range-of-motion exercises to prevent loss of joint mobility. The following are common examples of orthoses used for pain relief.

Support a Painful Shoulder or Elbow

Arm slings have been developed to prevent or correct shoulder subluxation or reduce pain in patients who have subluxation caused by brachial plexus injuries,

hemiplegia, and central cord syndrome injuries. Sling designs are numerous, with some commercially available and others fabricated by the therapist.

Certain slings support and immobilize the whole arm. These slings, such as the standard pouch and the double arm cuff sling (Fig. 14-2) restrict motion by keeping the humerus in adduction and internal rotation and the elbow in flexion. Although these slings may take some of the weight off the affected shoulder, downsides are that they place the extremity in a nonfunctional position, reinforce synergy patterns, and fail to provide the patient with the opportunity for motor and sensory feedback (Bobath, 1990; Moodie et al., 1986). Other sling designs support the shoulder but leave the rest of the arm free for function, such as a humeral cuff sling (Fig. 14-3).

Arm troughs, **lapboards**, and half-lapboards are also used to support the painful shoulder when the patient is seated in a wheelchair. These may be more acceptable to patients than slings, and they allow the arm to be ideally positioned with the scapula pulled forward and the hand supported (Bobath, 1990). Lapboards (Fig. 14-4) are generally indicated for patients with poor trunk control or visual field deficits and for those who require greater variability of upper extremity positioning or a work surface. Arm troughs (Fig. 14-5) are used for patients who need a device that does not interfere with wheelchair propulsion or transfer activities (Lange, 1999). The half-lapboard (Fig. 14-6) combines the positive features of both the arm trough and the full lapboard (Walsh, 1987). Full and half-lapboards can be

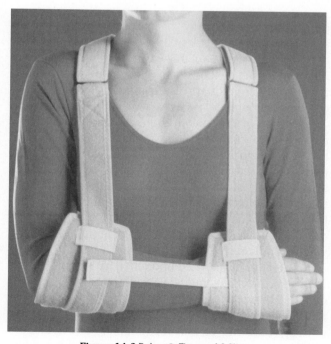

Figure 14-2 Rolyan® Figure-of-8 Sling.

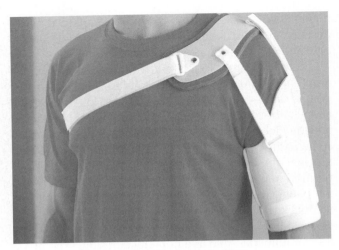

Figure 14-3 Hemi Shoulder Sling.

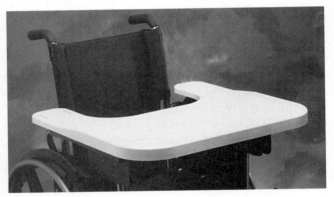

Figure 14-4 Rolyan® Slide-On Adjustable Lap Tray.

sling designs and developed a checklist of 19 desirable and 4 undesirable characteristics to guide the therapist in examining and comparing slings for individual patients. The patient's acceptance of the sling also must be considered. Relative ease of donning and doffing the sling is imperative so the limb is not damaged further from improper wearing. More definitive research on the effectiveness of slings and orthoses in the management of the flaccid or subluxed shoulder is needed, and therapists should carefully consider all options before prescribing slings.

A gunslinger orthosis is another means of supporting a painful shoulder, such as from a brachial plexus injury. This type of orthosis is commercially available or can be custom fabricated for the patient. A commercial gunslinger (Fig. 14-7) can be easily adjusted to position the shoulder and elbow for maximal pain relief. A custom fabricated gunslinger (Fig. 14-8) has the benefit of a

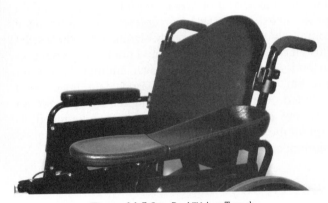

Figure 14-5 Otto Bock™ Arm Trough.

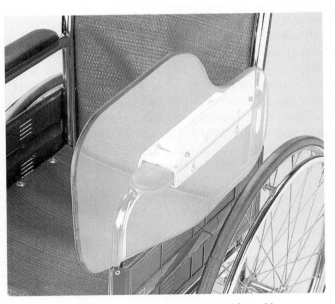

Figure 14-6 Clear Flipaway Armrest in upright position.

purchased commercially or custom fabricated from acrylic or wood. Some designs allow the half-lapboard to be rotated up and out of the way instead of having to be removed from the wheelchair when the patient needs to transfer. Arm troughs are also commercially available or can be custom made.

The use of supports in reducing shoulder subluxation remains controversial. In addition, whether subluxation has a causal relationship to shoulder pain is in question (Zorowitz et al., 1996). There is no consensus as to which type of support is the best in the treatment of shoulder subluxation or whether a support should be used at all. The effects of various sling and support designs have proved variable in multiple studies over the years as summarized by Zorowitz et al. (1995).

Ultimately, it is agreed upon that if a support is to be used, several types should be evaluated on the patient to optimize the reduction of shoulder pain, the function of the affected extremity, and the ease of donning and doffing (Zorowitz et al., 1995). Smith and Okamoto (1981) reviewed more than 22 distinctive hemiplegic

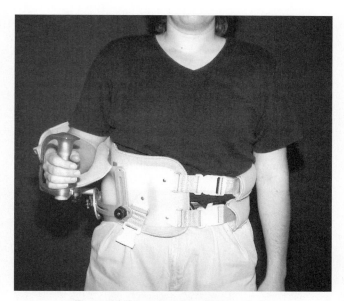

Figure 14-7 Commercial gunslinger orthosis.

much more streamlined design, allowing the patient to wear it under clothing as desired with minor garment adaptations (Lunsford, 1997). Also, this orthosis is much easier to don and doff. It is often the best solution for patients who require long-term or permanent use of a shoulder orthosis.

Commercial neoprene sleeves that provide neutral warmth, gentle compression, and soft dynamic support to the shoulder or elbow are often used to relieve pain from arthritis, tendinitis, sprains, and strains. ***As occupational therapists are expanding their use of supports fabricated from neoprene, it is important to be aware of the potential for dermatological reactions to the material and to teach patients to discontinue use of the support should symptoms develop (Stern et al., 1998).***

The treatment of lateral and medial epicondylitis often entails the use of orthoses to relieve pain and prevent further stress to affected tissues. In both conditions pain reduces grip strength and function. Counterforce braces (Fig. 14-9), of which there are several commercial models, are wide, nonelastic bands designed to reduce stresses on the common forearm extensor or flexor musculature origins (Wilton, 1997). The literature reports wide variation in the success of braces (Wuori et al., 1998). ***Complications can result from the brace being applied too tightly, including nerve compression syndromes. The patient must be carefully taught accordingly.***

A wrist splint placing the wrist in 45° of extension and worn in conjunction with a counterforce brace is often prescribed to rest the forearm musculature (Aiello, 1998). The prescription of orthoses must be based on the

patient's symptoms. It is vital that the cause of the problem and the biomechanics of loading forearm musculature are also addressed in relation to vocational or recreational demands (Wilton, 1997).

Support a Painful Wrist or Hand

Resting hand splints are used to support the wrist, fingers, and thumb. The normal resting position of the hand is determined anatomically by the bony architecture, capsular length, and resting tone of the wrist and hand muscles. This is typically 10 to 20° of wrist extension, 20 to 30° of metacarpophalangeal joint

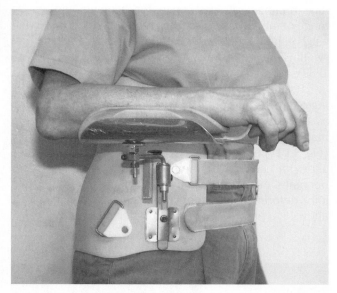

Figure 14-8 Custom-fabricated gunslinger orthosis.

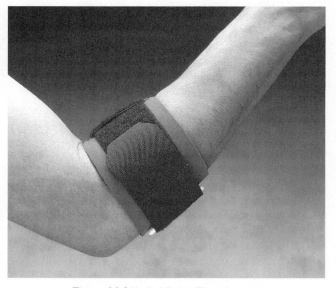

Figure 14-9 VariPad Tennis Elbow Support.

(MCP) flexion, 0 to 20° of proximal interphalangeal joint (PIP) flexion, the distal interphalangeal joints (DIPs) in slight flexion, the thumb CMC in slight extension and abduction, and the thumb MP and IP in slight flexion (Wilton, 1997).

A resting hand splint is commonly prescribed for patients with rheumatoid arthritis. Resting splints can reduce stress on joint capsules, synovial lining, and periarticular structures, thereby decreasing pain (Melvin, 1989) (see Chapter 44). With this population, splinting should be in a position of comfort regardless of whether this is the ideal anatomical position (Fess & Philips, 1987). During an acute exacerbation of the disease, splints are generally worn at night and during most of the day, removed at least once for hygiene and gentle range-of-motion exercises. It is recommended that splint use continue for at least several weeks after the pain and swelling have subsided (Fess & Philips, 1987; Melvin, 1989).

Resting hand splints can be volar or dorsal, depending on needs and preferences. Commercial splints, such as those fabricated from wire–foam (Fig. 14-10) or a malleable metal frame covered by dense foam padding (Fig. 14-11) may be used if the limited adjustments they allow for can provide the patient with a proper fit. This becomes more difficult if the patient has established joint deformities. Custom-fabricated splints (Fig. 14-12) allow for a precise, individualized fit.

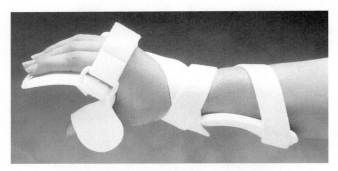

Figure 14-10 LMB Economical Resting Splint.

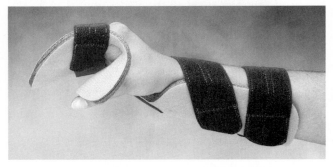

Figure 14-11 Progress™ Functional Resting Splint.

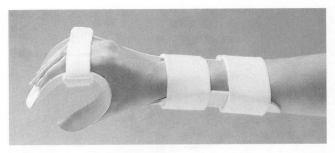

Figure 14-12 Custom thermoplastic resting hand splint.

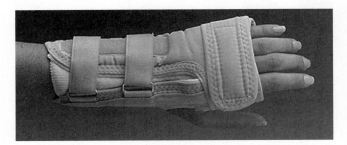

Figure 14-13 Rolyan® D-Ring™ Wrist Brace with MCP Support.

If the thumb or IP joints of the fingers are not painful, a modified resting hand splint (Fig. 14-13) may keep these joints free. This often results in less stiffness related to splint wear, some degree of hand function while the splint is worn, and improved splint wear and comfort.

Although health care professionals generally agree on the benefits of using splints to rest inflamed and painful joints, studies have shown that compliance with wearing resting hand splints as prescribed is less than optimal at approximately 47% (Feinberg, 1992). In a study by Callinan and Mathiowetz (1996), comparing soft versus hard resting hand splints on pain and hand function, results showed that pain was significantly decreased with splint wear and that 57% of patients preferred the soft splint, 33% preferred the hard splint, and 10% preferred no splint. The rate of compliance was greater for the soft splint (82%) than for the hard splint (67%). The authors advocate that therapists provide patients with options relative to comfort and preference to ensure patient satisfaction and improved outcome.

Wrist extension, or cock-up, splints are probably the most commonly prescribed type of orthosis for the upper extremity. Indications for use include sprains, strains, tendinitis, arthritis, carpal tunnel syndrome, wrist fractures following cast removal, and other conditions that cause pain. A wrist splint typically positions the wrist in 10 to 30° of extension, which is thought to be the best position for hand function (Fess & Philips, 1987). A well-fitting splint is one that clears the distal palmar and thenar creases to allow for unrestricted mobility of the fingers and thumb and that conforms to the palm to support the arches of the hand. Wrist splints may be volar (Fig. 14-14), dorsal (Fig. 14-15), or circumferential (Fig. 14-16) and can be custom fabricated or prefabricated. Since these splints are intended to provide wrist support while allowing functional use of the hand, fit and comfort are crucial.

A growing variety of commercial splints are available, with designs and materials offering a range of soft to rigid support. Elasticized wrist orthoses with an adjustable metal stay that slides into a volar pocket (Fig. 14-17) are commonly used because they are cost-effective and readily available. The drawbacks of these splints are they do not fully support the palmar arches,

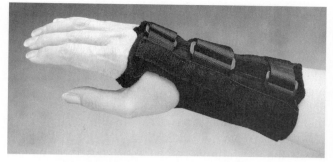

Figure 14-16 Comfort Cool™ D-Ring Wrist Splint.

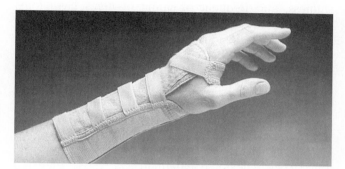

Figure 14-17 Norco™ Wrist Brace.

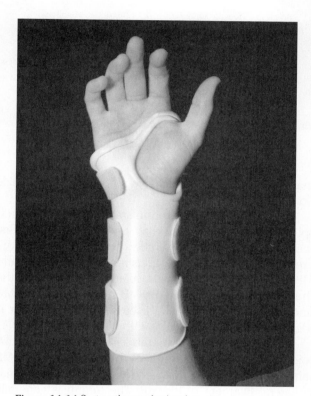

Figure 14-14 Custom thermoplastic volar wrist extension splint.

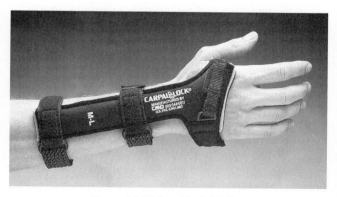

Figure 14-15 Carpal Lock® Splint.

they do not completely clear the palmar and thenar creases, and the metal stay is often prepositioned at a 35 to 45° angle of extension. It is therefore critical to fit and adjust the stay to the desired angle before issuing the splint. Other commercial products are made of wire–foam, neoprene, leather, canvas, and other fabric blends, all of which offer features having distinct advantages and disadvantages.

Several studies have been conducted on the effects on hand function of different styles of wrist extension splints. Carlson and Trombly (1983) reported a decrease in hand function when normal subjects were tested without and then with a static wrist orthosis. Stern (1991) studied hand function speed in normal subjects who wore three styles of custom-fabricated wrist splints and a commercial elastic wrist splint. She found that although all of the splints significantly slowed hand speed, the elastic splint allowed for faster speeds and dexterity than the others. A later study on grip strength and dexterity across five styles of commercial wrist splints concluded that each style impeded power grip and dexterity, but to different extents (Stern, 1996).

Elastic wrist orthoses have been widely used in the treatment of arthritis to stabilize wrists, decrease pain, and improve function. Again, studies have shown conflicting results across different styles of orthoses in grip strength, dexterity, hand function, pain reduction, comfort, security during task performance, and adverse effects of stiffness or muscle atrophy due to orthotic wear (Pagnotta et al., 1998; Stern et al., 1996). In a related study, most of 42 subjects knew their preferred orthosis within a few minutes of wear when given three styles to try (Stern et al., 1997). These studies reinforce the importance of task analysis, having a wide variety of splints to try with each patient, and a careful weighing of the benefits and limitations of splinting.

Another common indication for wrist splinting is carpal tunnel syndrome, a condition caused by median nerve compression, which results in symptoms including pain, sensory disturbances, muscle weakness, swelling, stiffness, and frequent dropping of items. Symptoms often are worse at night or with repetitive activity involving wrist flexion (see Chapter 42). For pain and related symptoms caused by carpal tunnel syndrome, conservative or postoperative treatment often uses wrist splints to prevent the elevation of carpal tunnel pressure by restricting wrist motion (Gelberman et al., 1988).

The ideal position of the wrist to minimize pressure in the carpal tunnel varies according to sources from 10 to 15° of extension (Melvin, 1989) to neutral (Weiss et al., 1995) to slight flexion (Gelberman et al., 1988). There is a consensus that commercial wrist splints, which often place the wrist in excessive extension, may not be of any benefit unless they are modified to a less extended position. Dorsal wrist splints (Fig. 14-15) are often recommended, as they do not create external pressure over the volar wrist.

A long opponens splint (Fig. 14-18), also known as a long thumb spica, can relieve pain from wrist and thumb arthritis or from DeQuervain's tendinitis of the abductor pollicis longus and extensor pollicis brevis. This splint is typically based on the radial aspect of the forearm and extends distally to immobilize the thumb CMC and MP joints. The wrist is generally splinted in slight extension, with the thumb in slight flexion and palmar abduction to enable opposition to the index and middle fingers (Wilton, 1997). If the thumb IP joint or the extensor pollicis longus tendon is involved, the IP joint can be included in the splint as well (Fig. 14-19). Prefabricated splints often provide a softer support, whereas custom-

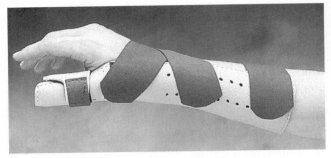

Figure 14-19 Liberty™ Wrist and Thumb Splint.

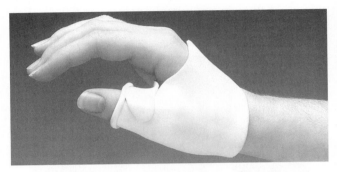

Figure 14-20 Custom thermoplastic short thumb splint.

made thermoplastic splints give more rigid immobilization.

A thumb CMC stabilization splint, or a short thumb spica, is a static splint that encompasses the first metacarpal to provide stability, reduce pain, and increase hand function. It restricts motion of the CMC and MP joints but leaves the wrist relatively mobile and the thumb IP free. A static thumb MP splint allows for CMC and IP motion and can be used when the disorder is localized to the MP joint alone.

Indications for short thumb splints include rheumatoid arthritis or osteoarthritis of the thumb CMC or MP joints or trauma to soft tissues, such as the ulnar collateral ligament of the MP. The thumb is generally positioned to enable opposition to the fingers for function while in the splint, and the splint is most often worn during functional activities that cause or aggravate pain (Melvin, 1995). Commercially prefabricated CMC and MP stabilization splints are often ineffectual because they fit poorly (Melvin, 1995). For a precise fit and rigid support, splints can be custom-fabricated from thermoplastic materials (Fig. 14-20). Newer commercial products made of soft, breathable elastic material have moldable thermoplastic stays to enable a custom fit, combining comfort and ease of fabrication with the required individualized rigid support (Fig. 14-21).

If the thumb or finger IP joints are painful from trauma or arthritis, lateral, dorsal, or volar gutter splints (Fig. 14-22) may be used for pain relief. Silicone-lined

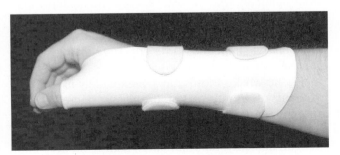

Figure 14-18 Custom thermoplastic long thumb spica splint.

sleeves or pads (Fig. 14-23) can protect painful joint nodules from external trauma.

Pain, volar subluxation, and ulnar deviation of the MCPs are common sequelae of rheumatoid arthritis. MCP ulnar deviation supports may be used to provide stability, realign joints, reduce joint stress, and relieve pain. They may delay the progression of deformity but do not correct or prevent it (Melvin, 1995; Philips, 1989). These supports may be worn alone or incorporated into a resting hand splint.

Prefabricated and custom-designed orthoses with dividers or straps to align the digits include dynamic and static and soft and rigid. Rigid static splints (Fig. 14-24) used to achieve passive correction of deformity can create focal pressure points on the digits. ***It is therefore important not to try to achieve ideal alignment at the risk of creating pressure problems (Melvin, 1989).***

Despite the variety of splint materials and designs, MCP ulnar deviation supports are reported to be not frequently prescribed or used by patients for a variety of reasons (Rennie, 1996). For some patients, immobilization of the MCPs impairs functional use of the hand and may increase stress and pain on the adjacent PIP joints (Melvin, 1995; Philips, 1989). Additionally, bulky or volar-based splints interfere with palmar sensation and impede the ability to grasp objects. However, some patients benefit from the improved digital alignment and pain reduction that supports offer. High patient satisfac-

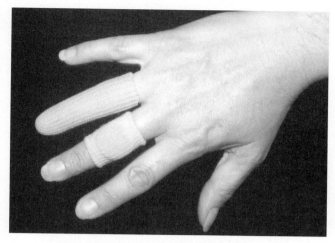

Figure 14-23 Silicone-lined digital sleeve and pad.

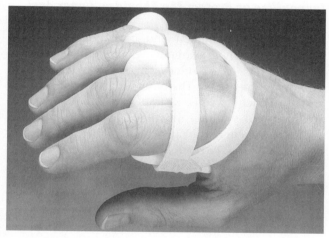

Figure 14-24 LMB Soft-Core™ Wire–Foam™ Ulnar Deviation Splint.

tion rates have been reported for a custom dorsal-based design (Rennie, 1996). Soft ulnar deviation splints are commercially available (Fig. 14-25) or can be custom fabricated (Gilbert-Lenef, 1994). The prime indicator for use and selection of an MCP ulnar deviation support should be the patient's preference (Melvin, 1995).

Immobilize for Healing or to Protect Tissues

Many of the orthoses previously discussed for pain relief can also be used to immobilize for healing or protection following injury or surgery. For example, a gunslinger orthosis used to relieve traction pain associated with a brachial plexus injury can also protect the nerve structures from overstretching during the healing phase. A thumb MP splint that relieves pain from arthritis may also be used while an acutely injured collateral ligament heals. These orthoses are not discussed in detail again; different ones are reviewed.

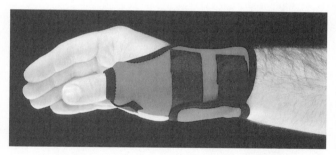

Figure 14-21 Custom-Molded thumb splint.

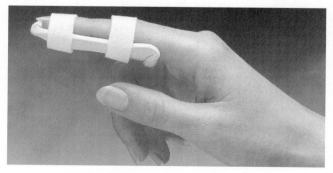

Figure 14-22 Custom thermoplastic volar gutter splint.

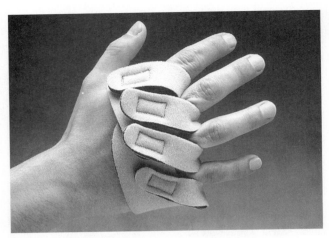

Figure 14-25 Norco™ Soft MP Ulnar Deviation Support.

Immobilize or Protect the Shoulder, Upper Arm, or Elbow

The sling is the simplest and most commonly used device for the upper extremity when there is a need to limit motion of the shoulder yet allow for some motion of the arm on the thorax. The basic arm sling consists of a forearm pouch or cuffs, a strap, and a mechanism for adjusting and securing the strap. Guidelines for sling adjustment are in Box 14-3.

To further limit mobility, shoulder immobilizers (Fig. 14-26) can be used. These devices, which relatively immobilize the shoulder and elbow, are typically used following shoulder surgical reconstructions, arthroplasty, and rotator cuff repair. Immobilizers are more complex than slings, involving strapping that wraps the body to stabilize the arm against the trunk. Several commercial designs are available.

Foam abduction pillows or wedges may be used to maintain the arm at a certain elevation from the body. Abduction braces, sometimes called airplane splints, are commercially available or custom fabricated from thermoplastics. These devices are based on the trunk and can position the shoulder in varying degrees of abduction or rotation, and the elbow in varying degrees of flexion or extension. Commercial braces offer ease of adjustability with the use of wrenches but may need extra padding to prevent skin breakdown. Indications for use include postoperative shoulder repairs, burns, and skin grafts to the axillary region (Long & Shutt, 1986; McFarland et al., 1997).

The treatment of humeral shaft fractures often involves functional fracture bracing (see Chapter 41). A humeral fracture brace (Fig. 14-27) provides external stabilization and alignment of the fracture by compressing surrounding soft tissues while allowing for early mobilization of the shoulder and elbow. These braces may be prefabricated or custom fabricated by the therapist from low-temperature thermoplastics. They are circumferential in design with D-ring straps to allow for a secure closure and size adjustments as edema subsides. They should be lightweight and made of a perforated material for ventilation.

Whether the brace is prefabricated or custom, the therapist should ensure that its distal end does not block elbow flexion motion and that its proximal end does not unnecessarily limit shoulder motion. Excellent results with the use of functional fracture bracing of the humerus has been reported (Wallny et al., 1997).

Casts, splints, and hinged braces can be used to immobilize and protect the elbow following fractures, burns, ligamentous injuries, or surgical procedures. Casts offer rigid immobilization and may be circumferential, posterior, or an anteroposterior bivalve design that

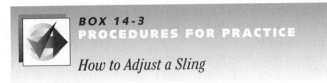

BOX 14-3
PROCEDURES FOR PRACTICE

How to Adjust a Sling

► Place the patient upright.
► Ensure that the elbow is flexed to 90° and is seated properly in the sling, with the hand and wrist also supported as the design allows.
► Adjust the strap or straps so that the arm is comfortably supported.
► Check for comfort.
► Teach patient and caregiver about proper donning and doffing of sling.
► Monitor the axilla and areas where sling straps cross the body for signs of skin breakdown.
► Monitor for signs of edema and joint stiffness.

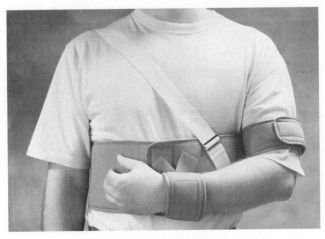

Figure 14-26 Rolyan® Universal Shoulder Immobilizer.

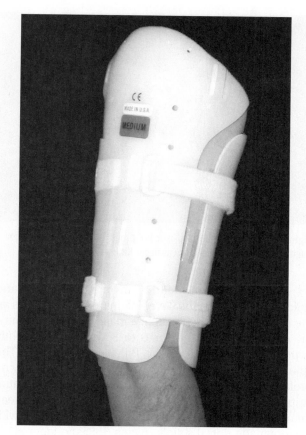

Figure 14-27 Commercial humeral fracture brace.

Unless specifically contraindicated, the antideformity, or safe, position of immobilization is with the wrist in 10 to 30° of extension, the MCPs in 70 to 90° of flexion, the IPs in 0 to 15° of flexion, and the thumb in palmar abduction (Fess & Philips, 1987; Stewart, 1995). This is most often accomplished through a volar custom-fabricated low-temperature thermoplastic splint (Fig. 14-29). If edema is present, the splint should be secured by an elastic wrap or gauze wrap to avoid a tourniquet effect from straps. ***It is crucial never to force joints into the ideal position but to position joints as closely as possible to the ideal and serially revise the splint until the optimal position is realized.***

Antideformity splints are integral to the treatment of acute dorsal hand burns (see Chapter 45). An investigation of the literature found an overall lack of consensus on the design of these splints (Richard et al., 1994). The most commonly recommended position for joints is with the wrist in 15 to 30° of extension, the MCPs in 50 to 70° of flexion, the IPs in full extension, and the thumb in palmar abduction with the IP in slight flexion (Richard & Staley, 1994). Preformed splints are commercially available and may be used if adequate fit can be obtained given the size of the hand and any edema. Custom-fabricated splints, preferably of a perforated material, ensure the best fit. Splints may have to be adjusted daily for optimal fit and maintenance of proper joint positioning. For the grafting and rehabilitation phases of burn

allows the cast to be removed for wound care or range of motion. Hinged braces are frequently used to protect healing ligaments while allowing motion of the elbow. Thermoplastic splints may be anterior or posterior and may be secured by Velcro straps or an elastic wrap. Anterior elbow extension splints (Fig. 14-28) are most commonly used to immobilize and position the elbow following skin grafting.

Immobilize or Protect the Wrist or Hand

The maintenance of normal hand function requires strong tissue repair with free gliding between neighboring structures. Proper positioning of the wrist and hand is critical to prevent complications caused by injury, edema, and tissue healing. Splinting in the early stages of healing can counteract the typical joint contractures of the injured hand that produce the deformities of wrist flexion, MCP extension, IP flexion, and thumb adduction. It is essential to position joints correctly and keep uninvolved joints moving so that they will not stiffen (Stewart, 1995). ***Incorrect application of a splint or improper positioning while in a splint may lead to both joint limitations and tissue damage (Fess, 1995).***

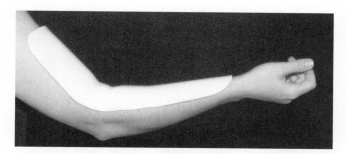

Figure 14-28 Custom thermoplastic anterior elbow extension splint.

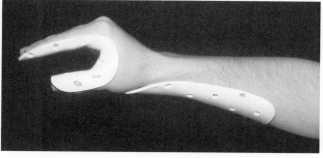

Figure 14-29 Custom thermoplastic "safe position" wrist–hand splint.

treatment, splint design varies with the positions necessary to counteract the contractile forces of the scars.

Wrist splints, as discussed in the previous section, may be used for protection or immobilization of wrists following cast removal or to treat soft tissue injuries. Athletic injuries to the wrist and hand, such as contusions, sprains, strains, fractures, and joint dislocations, often require the use of protective splints to enable the patient to continue participation in sports. As with other splints, selection of material and design should be carefully tailored to the patient's needs. Materials may be thermoplastic, silicone rubber, plaster, fiberglass, cloth tape, or neoprene. Selection should be based on the degree of immobilization required, material durability and breathability, the player's sport position, governing rules of the sport, and the safety of other players (Canelon, 1995).

Treatment of tendon injuries and repairs may involve static positioning to immobilize the tendon for healing or dynamic splinting to protect the tendon while allowing controlled motion to increase tendon repair strength and gliding. Flexor tendon repair protocols vary, but a protective dorsal blocking splint (Fig. 14-30) positioning the wrist and MCPs in flexion and blocking the IP joints in 0° of extension is typically used. Rubber band traction may be added to hold the digits in a flexed position or to enable resistive extension and passive flexion exercises. The splint is usually custom fabricated from low-temperature thermoplastic and is often worn for as long as 6 weeks (Stewart & vanStrien, 1995).

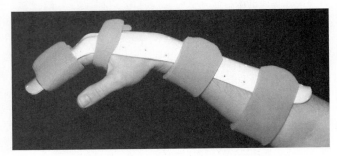

Figure 14-30 Custom thermoplastic dorsal blocking splint.

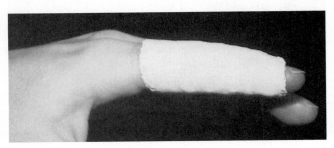

Figure 14-31 Plaster digit cast.

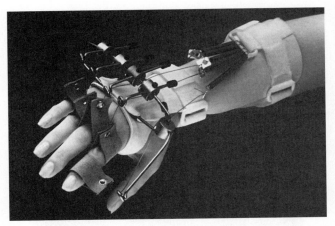

Figure 14-32 Custom thermoplastic low-profile dynamic MCP extension splint using Rolyan® Adjustable Outrigger Kit.

Extensor tendon injuries involve treatment and splinting based on the level of injury. For injuries at the DIP level that may result in a mallet finger deformity, the DIP is immobilized for 6 to 8 weeks in a slightly hyperextended position. The PIP joint is left free. The splints most commonly used are volar based and may be prefabricated or custom fabricated of padded aluminum strips or thermoplastics. Excellent results for the treatment of mallet finger have also been reported with custom-made dorsal splints (Evans, 1995; Foucher et al., 1996). For injuries at the PIP level, treatment includes digital cast (Fig. 14-31) or splint immobilization with the PIP in absolute 0° of extension for 6 to 8 weeks to prevent boutonniere deformity. For more proximal tendon injuries, splinting may involve static positioning, dynamic assists, or both (Evans, 1995).

Splinting is an integral part of postoperative MCP arthroplasty treatment. Early positioning and motion following arthroplasty uses a dynamic MCP extension assist (Fig. 14-32) to support the wrist, control MCP motion, correct the deformity, and assist with extensor power. This controlled stress allows for joint capsule remodeling over time (Kirkpatrick et al., 1996; Melvin, 1989).

Dynamic MCP extension assists may use high-profile or low-profile outrigger designs. They have slings to support the MCPs in neutral extension and deviation and to provide rotatory alignment. The high-profile outrigger has been reported to afford better rotation and to require less force to initiate and maintain motion. The low-profile outrigger is advocated as less obtrusive and equally effective (Melvin, 1995) and as able to provide greater stability to the joints as they move against traction (Wilton, 1997). Outrigger kits are commercially available, or the outrigger may be hand fabricated. The dynamic extension splint may be supplemented by a static positioning splint at night (Fess & Philips, 1987).

To protect digits but allow for stabilization or controlled motion of the MCP, PIP, or DIP joints following injury or surgery, buddy straps (Fig. 14-33) (Jensen & Rayan, 1996), buddy sleeves (Bassini & Patel, 1994), or buddy splints (Lamay, 1994), which connect an injured finger to an adjacent finger, can be used. Common indications for these include stable fractures, PIP joint dislocations, collateral ligament injuries, and staged flexor tendon reconstructions.

Provide Stability or Restrict Unwanted Motion

Orthoses can be helpful in stabilizing joints when their integrity has been compromised by an acute injury or a chronic disease such as arthritis. Stabilization or restriction of motion can often greatly facilitate functional use of a limb.

Stabilize or Restrict Motion of the Shoulder or Elbow

In addition to the purposes previously described, slings, gunslingers, and hinged elbow orthoses can also be used to provide proximal stability that may enable improved distal function.

Stabilize or Restrict Motion of the Wrist or Hand

It is essential to determine the position in which a joint is to be supported relative to hand dominance and task requirements, as specific functional demands vary greatly among individual patients. The wrist is considered by many to be the key to ultimate hand function, and wrist splints are commonly prescribed to provide stability. Dorsal wrist splints allow for the greatest palmar sensation but are least supportive; volar wrist splints are

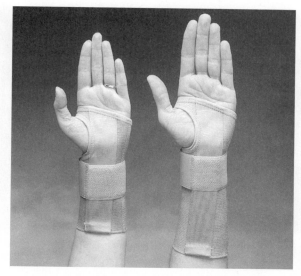

Figure 14-34 Liberty™ Short and Long Elastic Wrist Braces.

most commonly prescribed and provide a moderate amount of stability; and circumferential wrist splints provide the greatest amount of stability (Wilton, 1997).

For optimum mechanical advantage to support the weight of the hand, the forearm portion of the splint should be two-thirds the length of the forearm (Fess & Philips, 1987; Wilton, 1997). Although greater length is believed to add to stability, studies have shown that a longer splint can decrease grip strength, slow finger dexterity, and decrease hand function speeds compared with a shorter wrist splint (Stern, 1996). For smaller or lighter hands and for patients who do not use their hands for high-demand activities, a shorter wrist support (Fig. 14-34) can increase comfort while being less obtrusive than a long splint (Melvin, 1995).

A lumbrical bar is a hand-based orthosis that extends over the dorsal aspect of the proximal phalanges to restrict unwanted hyperextension of the MCPs, which can result from an ulnar or combined median and ulnar nerve injury. By blocking this motion, IP flexion contractures can be prevented and functional hand opening improved as the power of the long finger extensors is transferred to the IPs for extension. Lumbrical bar orthoses using spring wire are commercially available (Fig. 14-35), but these tend to be bulky and limit the ability to grasp objects. Custom-fabricated thermoplastic splints (Fig. 14-36) provide for a more intimate and streamlined fit (Colditz, 1995c; Wilton, 1997).

This same principle of restricting undesired motion is used in a PIP hyperextension block, also known as a swan-neck splint. Swan-neck deformities are common sequelae of rheumatoid arthritis and a possible complication following an extensor tendon injury or repair. These deformities often cause difficulty with hand

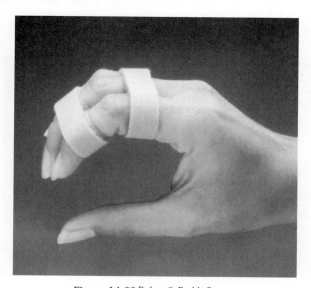

Figure 14-33 Rolyan® Buddy Straps.

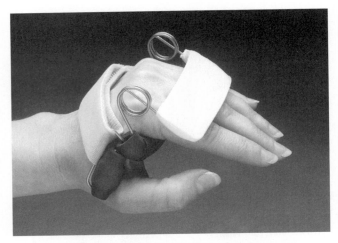

Figure 14-35 LMB MP Flexion Spring.

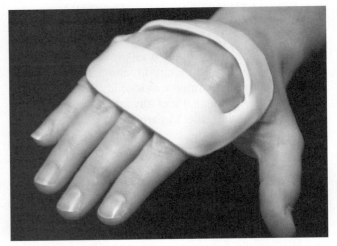

Figure 14-36 Custom thermoplastic lumbrical bar splint.

use their hands in highly demanding tasks. Swan-neck splints can also be used to provide lateral stability to unstable IP joints of the fingers or thumb.

Flexible boutonniere deformities may benefit from boutonniere splinting to block the PIP in a more extended position to allow for greater functional hand opening. These may also be custom made by the therapist or custom ordered from the companies that fabricate swan-neck splints (Fig. 14-39). Since there is direct pressure over the PIP, the dorsal skin must be carefully monitored for signs of breakdown.

Thumb stability is a requirement of almost all prehensile activities, so splinting of unstable thumb joints may have a particular value for function (Fess & Philips, 1987). Instability of the CMC often requires a long thumb splint that crosses the wrist, as shorter splints may not adequately support the CMC. Short thumb spica splints (Fig. 14-20), also known as thumb posts or opponens splints, can provide MP stability and a stable post for pinching. A circumferential design is commonly used; however, problems with marked MP deformity can make donning and doffing of the splint difficult, and direct pressure over the MP may lead to breakdown of fragile skin.

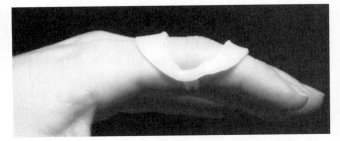

Figure 14-37 Custom thermoplastic PIP hyperextension block.

closure, as PIP tendons and ligaments can catch during motion, and the finger flexors have less of a mechanical advantage to initiate flexion when the PIP is hyperextended. By blocking the PIP in a slightly flexed position, the patient can flex the PIP more quickly and easily.

For short-term use or for trial purposes, custom-fabricated thermoplastic swan-neck splints (Fig. 14-37) may suffice. For long-term use or for use on adjacent digits, commercial swan-neck splints are often recommended, as they are more durable, less bulky, more easily cleaned, and more cosmetically appealing. Custom-ordered ring splints made of silver or gold (Fig. 14-38) are attractive, durable, streamlined, and adjustable for variations in joint swelling, but they are more costly. Prefabricated splints made of polypropylene, also available commercially, offer some of the benefits of silver splints with less cost. Heavy-duty metal splints, such as Murphy ring splints, may benefit patients who

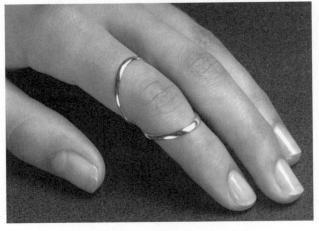

Figure 14-38 Siris™ Silver Swan Neck Splint.

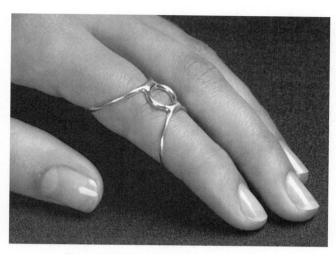

Figure 14-39 Siris™ Silver Boutonniere Splint.

Restore Mobility

Orthoses play an integral role in the restoration of mobility by correcting soft tissue or joint contractures that can occur as a result of poor positioning, trauma, scarring, or increased muscle tone. Devices providing low-load, prolonged stretch have proven to be effective in the contracture management of patients having a neurological or orthopaedic disorder (Hill, 1994; Nuismer et al., 1997). As described earlier in this chapter, different types of splinting may be used: serial static plaster or thermoplastic, dynamic, and static progressive.

A therapist implementing a splinting program to regain motion must understand how splints work to effect positive change. Range of motion is gained not by tissue stretching but by actual tissue elongation from new cell growth (Bell-Krotoski & Figarola, 1995; Fess & Philips, 1987). *The forces used must be gentle and carefully applied, and the tissue must be closely monitored for signs of excessive stress, such as redness and inflammation, which are indicators to mediate or stop treatment.*

Fixed contractures often respond better to **serial casting** than to dynamic splinting. Plaster is an ideal material, as it conforms intimately and is more rigid than thermoplastics. Casts are changed as motion gains are achieved.

Dynamic splinting is more effective when used for early contractures (Bell-Krotoski & Figarola, 1995). It allows for motion in the opposite direction, which helps prevent unwanted stiffness. Splints can also be removed for hygiene and function. Often dynamic splints are worn at night so as not to interfere with use of the limb. However, because of this decrease in wearing time, tissues are not kept under constant tension, and less rapid gains may result. The amount and direction of force must be carefully monitored and adjusted as joint angles change.

Static progressive splinting is often indicated for fixed contractures. It has the advantage of being worn for shorter periods throughout the day, allowing for motion and functional use of the limb.

Restore Mobility of the Shoulder, Elbow, or Forearm

A serial static abduction splint can be used to apply pressure to and elongate burn scars in the axilla. The benefits of wearing this type of splint must be carefully weighed against the complete lack of function that it imposes. For flexion contractures of the elbow, thermoplastic anterior elbow extension splints (Fig. 14-28), serial casts or dropout casts, dynamic elbow extension, or static progressive elbow extension splints can be used.

Serial casting, which typically entails changing the cast weekly, is thought to be most effective with contractures that have been present for less than 6 months (Keenan, 1997). When the contracture is a result of increased tone, such as in the patient with a brain injury, casting is often used in conjunction with nerve blocks or surgical procedures. *Great care must be taken with casting in the presence of severe tone, as pressure areas may develop.*

Dropout casts (Fig. 14-40) use the force of gravity to assist in reducing an elbow flexion contracture. The posterior portion of the cast above the elbow is removed, allowing the forearm to drop into extension. This type of

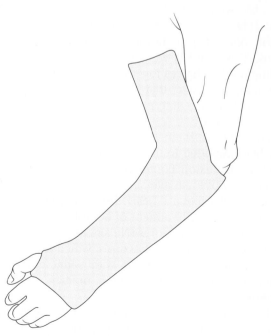

Figure 14-40 Plaster elbow dropout cast.

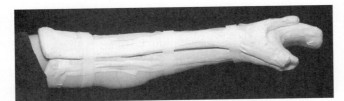

Figure 14-41 Fiberglass anteroposterior elbow splint with wrist and digits included.

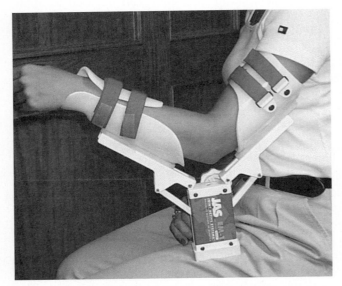

Figure 14-42 JAS Static Progressive Elbow™ Orthosis.

casting is effective only if the patient is upright most of the day.

A bivalved cast, also known as an anteroposterior splint (Fig. 14-41), is often used to maintain range of motion once it is achieved through casting or other means. This splint is well padded, with several straps holding the two halves together. The caregiver must be thoroughly trained so that it is applied properly and in the correct alignment to prevent pressure problems and skin breakdown.

Dynamic or static progressive splints (Fig. 14-42) have been reported to be successful in the treatment of elbow burn flexion contractures when static splinting was not effective. An average of 5 to 10° can be gained per day (Richard et al., 1995). They have also proved to be effective in the treatment of neurological and orthopaedic flexion contractures (Nuismer et al., 1997).

Elbow extension contractures, which are less commonly seen, can be treated with serial casting into flexion, dynamic flexion splinting, or static progressive splinting.

Loss of forearm rotation, often seen following spinal cord injury, peripheral nerve injury, or fracture can be treated with dynamic forearm rotation splinting. Splints

can be custom fabricated (Collelo-Abraham, 1990) or obtained commercially as a preformed product or kit (Fig. 14-43). Altering the direction of force when using these splints can produce supination or pronation. A static progressive supination splint has also been described by Murphy (1990) as achieving favorable results.

Restore Mobility of the Wrist or Hand

Serial short arm casts, with or without the fingers or thumb, can be used in the treatment of flexion or extension contractures related to increased muscle tone. Serial plaster slab splinting (Tribuzi, 1995) can be especially effective in the presence of muscle–tendon unit shortening that can result in the inability to compositely flex or extend the wrist and fingers. Long flexor tightness can develop as a result of the wrist being in a prolonged position of flexion, such as with wrist drop from radial nerve palsy, wrist fracture immobilization, and protective positioning following flexor tendon repair. A plaster slab splint or a volar thermoplastic splint that positions the wrist and fingers in maximum composite extension can help to correct tightness of the long finger flexors.

Serial static thermoplastic wrist splints, dynamic wrist splints (Fig. 14-44), and static progressive wrist splints can be used for limitations in wrist flexion or extension. These may be custom fabricated or pre-

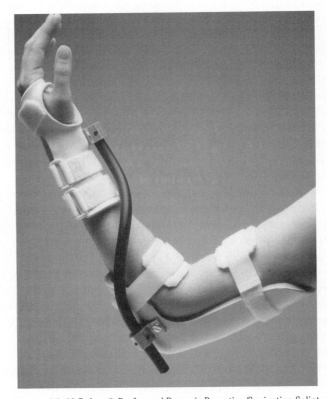

Figure 14-43 Rolyan® Preformed Dynamic Pronation/Supination Splint.

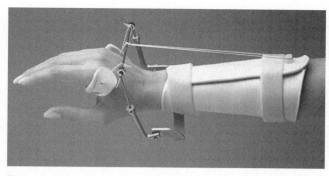

Figure 14-44 Custom thermoplastic dynamic wrist extension splint using Phoenix Wrist Hinge.

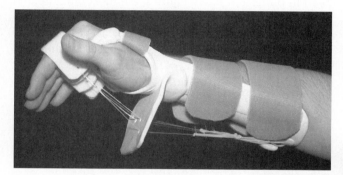

Figure 14-45 Custom thermoplastic dynamic MCP flexion splint.

used to gain composite flexion of all joints, but they have the most effect on the MCPs.

Limited PIP flexion makes grasp difficult, and limited PIP extension interferes with the ability to open the hand in preparation for grasp or to release objects. PIP flexion contractures are a frequent complication of trauma or poor positioning, and extension contractures can be seen following dorsal hand burns or prolonged immobilization for fracture management.

To address these contractures, forearm- or hand-based dynamic thermoplastic splints similar to those designed for MCP flexion and extension can be used by extending the distal part of the splint across the MCP to just proximal to the PIP joint. Immobilizing the MCP applies force to the PIP.

Prefabricated spring wire and spring coil splints are also available to gain flexion or extension range of motion. In a study of prefabricated spring wire (Fig. 14-47) and spring coil (Fig. 14-48) extension splints by Fess (1988), exerted forces were found to vary in the

formed. Dynamic or static progressive component kits can also be purchased commercially. This allows the therapist to custom-mold the splint bases while more easily assembling force units.

Lack of MCP flexion can devastate hand function. Many dynamic splint designs to regain MCP motion are available. Custom-fabricated thermoplastic splints use individual finger loops over the proximal phalanx (Fig. 14-45). Attached to these loops are rubber bands or springs that provide the needed force for sustained tension. An outrigger is used to direct the line of pull at 90°. It is important to clear the distal palmar crease so as not to block full flexion range of motion. These splints may be forearm based or hand based, depending on the mechanical advantage needed, any adhesions, and the patient's wrist strength and stability (Fess & Philips, 1987).

Commercial hand-based dynamic splints use springs, coiled spring wire (Fig. 14-35), or rubber bands to provide flexion force to the MCPs as a unit. These splints are effective only if all MCPs are uniformly stiff. Some force adjustments can be made, but individual finger force amount or angle adjustments are not possible, as they are with custom-made thermoplastic splints having separate finger loops. Finger flexion gloves (Fig. 14-46), which incorporate rubber band traction, can be

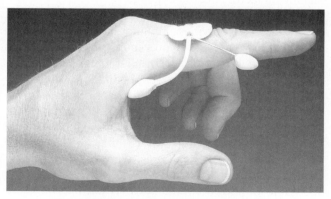

Figure 14-46 Finger Flexion Glove.

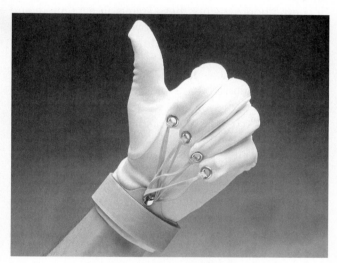

Figure 14-47 LMB Spring Finger Extension Assist.

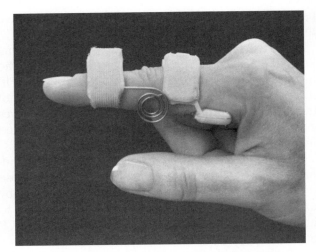

Figure 14-48 Rolyan® Sof-Stretch Coil Extension Splint.

same splint design and to vary also according to the degree of joint contracture. Some forces were alarmingly high, well above recommended limits. Callahan and McEntee (1986) found similar results and expressed concern about whether these splints fit accurately and about forces being distributed over small surface areas as compared with custom-fabricated splints. Designs have since been improved so that tension can be somewhat modified. If used, these splints must be carefully monitored to avoid further joint or tissue damage.

Spring coil extension splints, sometimes called Capener splints, may be custom fabricated and are described in the literature (Callahan & McEntee, 1986; Colditz, 1995b). A study of dynamic splinting in the management of PIP flexion contractures using Capener and low-profile hand-based outrigger splints found the two to be equally effective, suggesting that the patient may prefer the less bulky Capener splint if offered a choice (Prosser, 1996). Additional findings concluded that the longer the flexion contracture was present, the less it resolved and that splint wearing time was a significant factor affecting outcome.

A commercial neoprene dynamic finger extension tube (Fig. 14-49) provides circumferential pressure and a dynamic force into extension via an angled seam on its volar surface. It may also offer other therapeutic values, such as heat, mild joint distraction, and longer tolerable wearing times (Clark, 1997). PIP extension can also be gained though serial plaster casting or splinting.

Thermoplastic gutter (Fig. 14-22) or circumferential splinting and dynamic traction splinting are useful in the treatment of mild contractures, whereas serial plaster digital casting (Fig. 14-31) has been advocated for moderate to severe contractures (Bell-Krotoski, 1995). Plaster casting offers the advantages of intimate confor-

mity, rigidity, breathability, and uniform distribution of pressure. Casting does require the patient's cooperation in keeping the cast dry, and casts have the disadvantage of not being removable for function or motion. For most effective results, casts should be changed every 2 to 7 days (Bell-Krotoski & Figarola, 1995) or sooner if they become loose or wet. The DIP joint may be left free if its motion is not limited. It is at times beneficial to involve the DIP in the cast if increased mechanical advantage is desired for PIP extension. Variations of many of these splints can be used for the treatment of DIP contractures or contractures of the thumb MP or IP.

Adduction contractures of the thumb, commonly seen in burns and nerve injuries, are most often treated with serial static thumb abduction splints, which conform to the first web space (Fig. 14-50). It is important to ensure that abduction forces are directed to the CMC joint by involving as much of the distal aspect of the first metacarpal as possible (Fess & Philips, 1987). Strapping must be designed to apply pressure in the proper direction and to prevent distal migration of the splint. This often requires a strap that crosses the wrist.

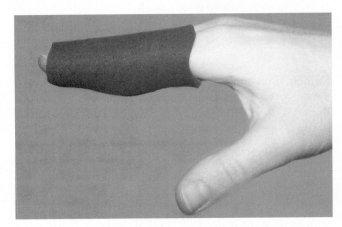

Figure 14-49 Rolyan® Dynamic Digit Extensor Tube™ Splint.

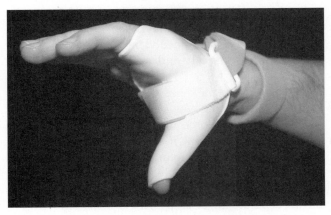

Figure 14-50 Custom thermoplastic thumb abduction splint.

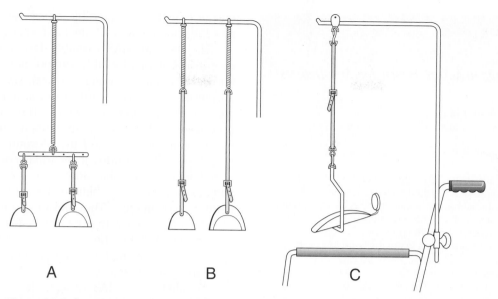

Figure 14-51 Suspension arm devices. **A.** Suspension sling with horizontal bar. **B.** Suspension sling without horizontal bar. **C.** Suspension arm support. (Adapted with permission from Redford, J. B. [Ed.]. [1986]. *Orthotics Etcetera* [3rd ed.]. Baltimore: Williams & Wilkins.)

Substitute for Weak or Absent Muscles

Orthoses are commonly used to assist patients in maximizing the functional use of an affected upper extremity. Orthoses may be used temporarily, as in the case of recovering nerve injuries or neurological diseases such as Guillain-Barré; or they may be prescribed for long-term use, such as in complete spinal cord injury or progressive neuromuscular conditions like postpolio syndrome. They are generally worn only during the day or for specific functional tasks. An orthosis successful in improving the ability to function is often much more accepted and appreciated by the patient than orthoses prescribed for other purposes.

Substitute for Weak or Absent Shoulder or Elbow Muscles

Proximal arm devices can support the shoulder and forearm to encourage motion of weak proximal musculature, allow for distal function, and enable occupational performance as well as prevent loss of motion and provide pain relief.

Suspension arm devices (Fig. 14-51) suspend from above the head, generally on an overhead rod that is mounted to a wheelchair. The arm swings as in a pendulum from straps attached to the overhead rod. The ease of management and low cost have contributed to the long-standing popularity of these devices (Long & Shutt, 1986). The following variations are commercially available and in current use.

The suspension sling has a single strap suspended from the overhead rod. A horizontal balance bar with multiple holes for adjustment of the fulcrum supports separate wrist and elbow cuffs. The suspension sling without horizontal bar has two straps that originate directly from the overhead rod with cuffs to support the elbow and wrist. The suspension arm support has a forearm trough suspended from a single point on the overhead rod. It can also be easily attached to an overhead frame on the patient's bed. Springs of various tensions may be added to the straps that support the limb, allowing a patient with only slight active motion to produce accelerated shoulder movement by bouncing the arm up and down. Suspension devices can be adjusted to allow for certain motions (Box 14-4) but lack the fine adjustment that extremely weak patients may need.

A **mobile arm support** (MAS) (Fig. 14-52) is a mechanical device that supports the weight of the arm and provides assistance to shoulder and elbow motions through a linkage of ball-bearing joints (Long & Shutt, 1986; Lunsford, 1997; Yasuda et al., 1986). The MAS is typically mounted to a patient's wheelchair, but it can also be attached to a tabletop. Their mechanical principles are threefold: (1) use of gravity to assist weak muscles, (2) support of the arm to reduce the load on weak muscles, and (3) reduction of friction by using ball-bearing joints. Criteria for use:

► A defined functional need
► An adequate source of power from neck, trunk, shoulder girdle, or elbow muscles

How to Adjust Suspension Arm Devices

Suspension Arm Sling

▶ For horizontal abduction, rotate the overhead rod laterally.

▶ For horizontal adduction, rotate the overhead rod medially.

▶ For external rotation, move the arm cuffs back on the balance bar to shift weight toward the elbow.

▶ For internal rotation, move the arm cuffs forward on the balance bar to shift weight toward the hand.

▶ For elbow flexion, move the point of suspension backward on the overhead rod to put the hand toward the patient's face.

▶ For elbow extension, move the point of suspension forward on the overhead rod to put the hand away from the patient's face.

▶ For height adjustments, vary the length of the strap or straps that connect to the overhead rod; or raise or lower the bracket on the wheelchair upright.

Suspension Arm Support

▶ For horizontal motion and height adjustments, see list under Suspension Arm Sling.

▶ For elbow flexion, move the rocker arm farther from the trough elbow dial.

▶ For elbow extension, move the rocker arm closer to the trough elbow dial.

▶ Adequate motor control such that the patient can contract and relax functioning muscles

▶ Sufficient passive joint range of motion, with 0 to 90° of shoulder flexion and abduction, 0 to 30° of external rotation, full internal rotation and elbow flexion, and 0 to 80° of pronation preferred

▶ Stable trunk positioning

▶ A motivated patient

▶ A supportive environment that provides the patient with the opportunity and assistance to use the device

Patients who may benefit include those with cervical spinal cord injury, muscular dystrophy, Guillain-Barré syndrome, amyotrophic lateral sclerosis, poliomyelitis, and polymyositis.

Selection of MAS components, assembly of parts, and balance and adjustment of the MAS generally requires postgraduate hands-on training. Balance and adjustment principles are presented in Box 14-5 to give the reader a basic overview and appreciation for what is possible. This does not negate the need for additional training or consultation with experienced therapists to ensure that the best possible adjustments are made to give the patient maximal mechanical advantage.

The standard MAS assembly described in this chapter consists of an adjustable arm positioner bracket (also known as a semireclining bracket), standard proximal and distal arms, a standard rocker arm assembly, and a basic forearm trough (Fig. 14-53). The many commonly used special MAS component parts include the outside rocker arm assembly and the elevating proximal arm (Fig. 14-54). The outside rocker arm (or offset swivel) has a ball-bearing joint that allows for greater freedom in vertical motion, thus facilitating hand-to-mouth or hand-to-table movements. The elevating proximal arm is useful for a patient with poor to fair deltoid strength. As the patient initiates the elevating motion, the rubber band assists allowing the patient to flex and abduct the humerus to a higher level.

An alternative MAS design, the linear MAS (Fig. 14-55), uses linear bearings and straight rods without joints. This streamlines the overall width of the support and lets wheelchairs more easily fit through doorways (Clark et al., 1997).

For a patient who can walk, a gunslinger orthosis can provide both proximal stability and mobility. This type of shoulder–elbow orthosis consists of a metal

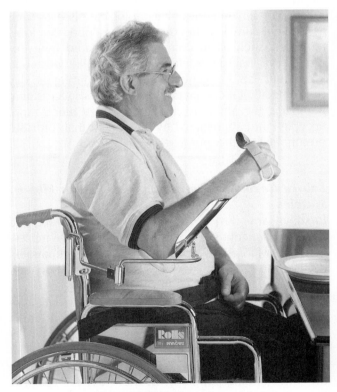

Figure 14-52 Mobile arm support.

BOX 14-5
PROCEDURES FOR PRACTICE

MAS Assembly and Training Principles

How to Assemble and Balance the Standard MAS Assembly

- Assemble tools (Phillips and flathead screwdrivers, Allen wrenches) and MAS parts (bracket, proximal arm, distal arm, rocker arm, trough).
- Inspect ball-bearing components for smooth operation.
- Ensure that the patient is seated properly in the wheelchair, with pelvis well back in chair and trunk in good vertical alignment.
- Fit the trough to the patient's arm by bending the elbow dial toward the radial side of the trough.
- Attach the rocker arm to the trough by placing the screws in the third and fifth holes from the dial.
- Attach the bracket to the wheelchair at approximately the midhumerus level so that it is neutrally rolled[1] and pitched[2].
- Attach the proximal arm to the bracket.
- Attach the distal arm to the proximal arm.
- Attach the trough to the distal arm.
- Balance the arm support to neutral by adjusting the pitch of the bracket and the distal end of the proximal arm so that the bearing tubes are perpendicular to the floor.
- Place the patient's arm in the trough.
- Observe for abnormal shoulder elevation and adjust the height of the bracket as needed to correct it.

[1]Roll is the rotation of the bracket assembly on the wheelchair upright.
[2]Pitch is the tilt of the ball-bearing tube on the bracket assembly.

MAS Hand-to-Mouth Movement Pattern
Instructions to Patient

- Push down on the trough dial while adducting your humerus.
- Externally rotate your shoulder.
- Shift your body weight toward the MAS.
- Straighten up or lean back in your chair.
- Rotate your trunk toward the MAS.
- Turn your head toward the MAS.

Equipment Adjustments to Aid This Motion

- Move the rocker arm farther from the trough elbow dial.
- Pitch the MAS at the bracket assembly toward the wheelchair back.
- Raise the bracket assembly on the wheelchair upright.

MAS Hand-to-Table Movement Pattern
Instructions to Patient

- Lift and internally rotate your shoulder to lower your hand.
- Shift your body weight away from the MAS.
- Roll your shoulder forward.
- Rotate your trunk away from the MAS.
- Tilt or turn your head away from the MAS.

Equipment Adjustments to Aid This Motion

- Move the rocker arm closer to the trough elbow dial.
- Pitch the MAS at the bracket assembly toward the patient's feet.
- Lower the bracket assembly on the wheelchair upright.

MAS Horizontal Abduction and Adduction Movement Patterns
Instructions to Patient

- Shift your body weight in the direction you want to move.
- Rotate your trunk toward the direction you want to move.
- Turn your head briskly in the direction you want to move.

Equipment Adjustments to Aid This Motion

- Roll the bracket assembly on the wheelchair upright toward the patient for adduction.
- Roll the bracket assembly on the wheelchair upright away from the patient for abduction.

MAS Controls Training and Use Training
Controls Training

- Teach the patient the effects of head, trunk, and proximal movements on the movement of the MAS.
- If bilateral MASs are used, begin with one side first.
- Begin with horizontal motions by having the patient practice moving the MAS as far as possible from side to side and front to back.
- Proceed with vertical motions by having the patient practice moving the hand to the table and up to the mouth at various points within the horizontal range.

Use Training

- Teach the patient to use the MAS for specific desired functional activities, such as eating, grooming, writing, keyboarding, page turning, and power wheelchair driving.
- Encourage practice and independent problem-solving skills.

---

forearm trough that is mechanically coupled to a plastic hemigirdle anchored on the patient's pelvis. This device is most useful for patients having good distal function but proximal weakness from brachial plexus injuries, spinal cord injuries, or postpolio syndrome. Prefabricated gunslingers (Fig. 14-7) are commercially available, but for long-term use a custom-designed orthosis (Fig. 14-8) is indicated (Lunsford, 1997).

Depending on the patient's proximal muscle status and specific functional needs, the coupling between the trough and hemigirdle base can be customized to permit a variety of motions, such as glenohumeral internal–

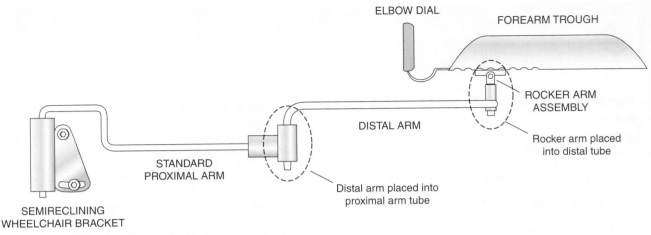

Figure 14-53 Standard components of a MAS.

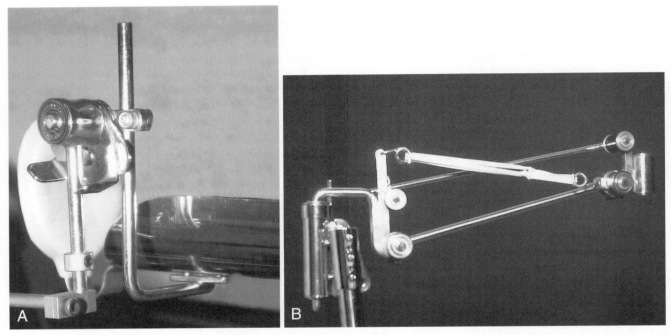

Figure 14-54 Special MAS components: **A.** Outside rocker arm. **B.** Elevating proximal arm.

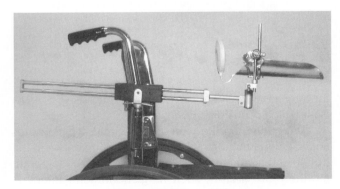

Figure 14-55 Linear MAS.

external rotation and flexion–extension. It can also be made to hold a very weak shoulder in a static position for function, which may be with the hand in midline. If the wrist also has weakness, the trough can be extended to support the hand. Usefulness must be determined for each individual case, considering factors such as acceptance by the patient, ease of donning, cost, and especially functional benefit.

For patients having selective loss of elbow flexion strength, a dynamic elbow orthosis with an elbow flexion assist (Fig. 14-56) may be used. This functional orthosis typically has a spring-loaded elbow mechanism with a ratchet lock. When the patient initiates flexion using residual muscles or compensatory motions, the spring device assists with elbow flexion. A release button allows the elbow to be repositioned into greater flexion or to drop down into extension (Lunsford, 1997).

Substitute for Weak or Absent Wrist or Hand Muscles

The combination of sensory loss and motor imbalance caused by a peripheral nerve injury greatly impairs normal hand function. As Colditz (1995c) points out, it is impossible to build an external device that can substitute for the intricately balanced muscles that a splint attempts to replace. In splinting nerve palsies, the key concept is to understand the patient's condition and neuromuscular status so as to prescribe or design an appropriate splint to increase function. Splints should keep areas of intact sensibility free if possible, should be as simple as possible, and should not immobilize joints unnecessarily. The splinting program must be closely monitored and altered in response to nerve recovery as the patient's muscle status changes (Case Example).

Radial nerve palsy, commonly associated with humeral fractures, can result in the complete loss or partial weakness of wrist, finger, and thumb extensors and weakness of forearm supination and thumb abduction. The loss of wrist extensor strength devastates hand grasp. Not only is the patient unable to position the hand properly, but the inability to stabilize the wrist in extension impairs normal function of the long finger flexors. Loss of extrinsic finger extension is much less of a functional problem, as the unaffected intrinsic muscles can actively extend the IPs. Supporting the wrist in extension is the primary goal of radial nerve splinting,

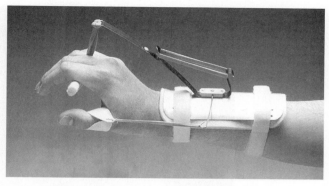

Figure 14-57 Bunnell™ Thomas Suspension Splint.

and the use of a simple static wrist splint may suffice in improving hand function (Fess & Philips, 1987).

Prefabricated radial nerve splints, such as a Thomas suspension splint (Fig. 14-57) or a wire–foam splint, are designed to dynamically extend the wrist, MCPs, and thumb. It is usually preferable not to include the thumb because of the limitation in intrinsic motion it imposes and the danger of stressing the MP collateral ligament through poorly directed forces. Adding individual finger loops to the palmar bar, thus removing bulk in the palm and allowing individual finger motion, can enhance the Thomas suspension splint. The palmar bulk of the wire–foam splint often impedes the ability to grasp large objects. Caution should be used when prescribing a dynamic orthosis, as strong unopposed flexors may easily overcome the dynamic forces trying to hold the wrist and hand in extension, negating functional benefits.

A custom-fabricated radial nerve splint, also known as a Colditz splint, has been designed to allow for partial wrist and full finger motion and a facsimile of a normal tenodesis effect (Fig. 14-58). This splint consists of a low-profile outrigger attached to a dorsal forearm base (Fig. 14-59). Unelastic cords connect the splint base to finger loops. The cord length is adjusted so that when the MCPs actively flex, the wrist is brought into extension. Conversely, when the wrist flexes, the cord tension causes the MCPs to extend. Little training is required for the patient to be able to use the splint functionally, and grasp and release of objects is greatly enhanced. Further advantages of this splint are the maintenance of normal hand arches, the absence of splinting material covering the palm, the low-profile design, and the facilitation of wrist extensor strength as return of nerve function occurs (Colditz, 1995c). Preformed splints and outrigger kits are commercially available.

Splinting in median nerve palsy is geared toward substituting for weak or absent thenar muscles that render the thumb unable to pull away from the palm and oppose to the fingers. This is most often accomplished through a custom-fabricated thermoplastic opponens

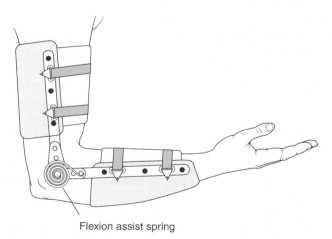

Flexion assist spring

Figure 14-56 Custom dynamic elbow orthosis with flexion assist. (Adapted with permission from Goldberg, B., & Hsu, J. S. [Eds.]. [1997]. *Atlas of Orthoses and Assistive Devices* [3rd ed.]. St. Louis: Mosby.)

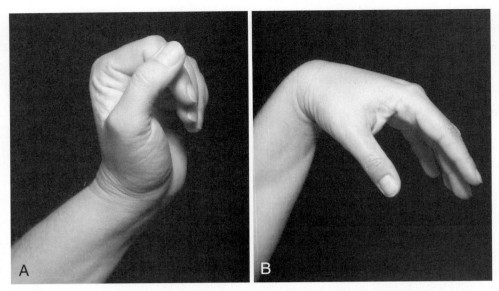

Figure 14-58 Normal tenodesis effect. **A.** When the wrist is extended, the fingers flex. **B.** When the wrist is flexed, the fingers extend.

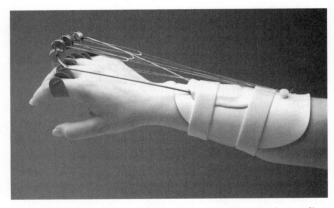

Figure 14-59 Custom thermoplastic radial nerve splint using low-profile Phoenix Extended Outrigger.

splint, which stabilizes the thumb in a position of abduction and opposition to enable pulp-to-pulp pinch (Fig. 14-20). Although such a splint often greatly improves fine motor prehension, this must be individually assessed, as substitution patterns from unaffected thumb muscles may provide sufficient thumb function (Colditz, 1995c; Fess & Philips, 1987). Patients may choose to wear an opposition splint for selected activities only.

In the presence of ulnar nerve palsy, the hand assumes a claw position, or intrinsic-minus position, with ring and small finger hyperextension of the MCPs and flexion of the IPs. This is a result of weakness or loss of lumbrical and interossei muscles, which are responsible for MCP flexion and IP extension. The prime splinting objective is to assist in grasp and release of objects by preventing the claw position. This is accomplished by a lumbrical bar splint, which blocks the MCPs in slight flexion, allowing the force of the unaffected long finger extensors to extend the IPs.

Dynamic splints, such as prefabricated spring wire splints (Fig. 14-35), do not work well, as the spring tension is usually not sufficient to hold the MCPs in flexion when the patient actively opens the hand. Thus, the MCPs hyperextend against the force, which actually strengthens the long extensors and encourages deformity (Colditz, 1995c).

A static custom-molded thermoplastic splint is advocated as the best solution. It should be nonbulky, carefully molded to distribute pressure evenly over the dorsum of the proximal phalanges, and designed so as not to obstruct full flexion of all joints (Colditz, 1995c; Fess & Philips, 1987). The splint may include just the affected ring and small fingers (Fig. 14-60) or may include all fingers to distribute pressure more effectively and comfortably (Fig. 14-36). The latter splint is used in the treatment of combined median and ulnar nerve injuries, which result in the clawing of all four fingers.

For a patient who has only radial nerve function, a custom-fabricated RIC (Rehabilitation Institute of Chicago) tenodesis splint (Fig. 14-61) may be used. This splint can provide minimal hand grasp by harnessing the power of the wrist extensors to bring the thumb, index finger, and long finger into a functional pinch. It has three molded thermoplastic pieces: one to position the thumb, one to position the index and long fingers, and a wrist cuff to serve as the base for connecting a static line from the wrist to the fingers (Colditz, 1995c).

Static orthoses, which allow passive holding of functional implements such as utensils or pens, may also be used in the presence of wrist or hand weakness. Examples include a hand-based universal cuff, an economy wrist support with universal cuff (Fig. 14-62), and a short or long design Wanchik writing splint (Fig. 14-63).

For patients with long-term or permanent loss of muscle function, as is the case in complete spinal cord injury or progressive neuromuscular disease, permanent functional orthoses may be used. These orthoses are fabricated by experienced orthotists from metal and are recommended by occupational therapists for individual patients based on neuromuscular status and specific functional needs. Often these distal orthoses are used in conjunction with proximal ones (such as a MAS) if proximal weakness is also present.

A ratchet wrist-hand orthosis (Fig. 14-64) may be used for patients with weak (below grade 3) wrist extension and finger strength, such as that seen with C5 tetraplegia (see Chapter 43). A thumb post positions the thumb in abduction and in alignment with the index and long fingers, and a finger piece assembly maintains the

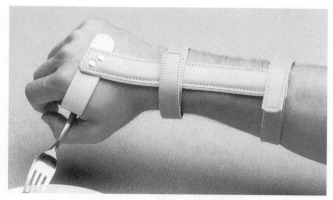

Figure 14-62 Economy Wrist Support with Universal Cuff.

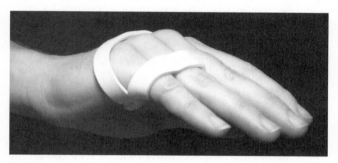

Figure 14-60 Custom thermoplastic lumbrical bar splint for ring and small fingers.

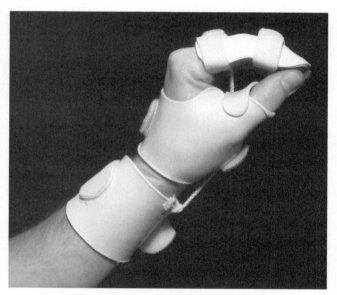

Figure 14-61 Custom thermoplastic RIC tenodesis splint.

index and long fingers in a position for pinch. A ratchet system is used to close the hand in discrete increments. Closing is accomplished by manually pushing the finger piece to flex the fingers against the thumb using the contralateral hand, the chin, or the side of a table or chair. Release is accomplished by a spring that is activated by the press of a release button (Clark et al., 1997; Lunsford, 1997).

For patients with the potential for neurological return at the C6 level, a wrist-action wrist–hand orthosis (Fig. 14-65) can be used as a transition system (Clark et al., 1997). This orthosis allows for free wrist motion, with stops that can be adjusted to limit motion to a prescribed range. When no wrist extensors are present, the wrist is locked into a set position. As recovery occurs and strength increases, progressive range of motion is allowed. Rubber bands are often attached to provide an extensor assist to weak muscles.

A **wrist-driven wrist–hand orthosis** (WDWHO) (Fig. 14-66) may be indicated for patients having 3+ or greater wrist extensor strength, such as a patient with C6 tetraplegia. Using the principle of tenodesis (Fig. 14-58), this type of flexor hinge orthosis transfers wrist extensor power to the fingers for grasping. Active wrist extension operates a mechanical linkage transferring power to flex the index and long fingers against the thumb. A properly adjusted orthosis allows for 1 pound of pinch for every 2 pounds of wrist extensor force. Gravity-assisted wrist flexion opens the hand for release. An activating lever at the wrist controls the size of the opening and the resultant position of prehension to allow for grasp of various size objects and different pinch forces.

Fitting the patient with bilateral WDWHOs may be tempting, but patients do not typically achieve a higher level of function with two orthoses than with one (Clark et al., 1997). Bilateral orthoses are difficult to use, requiring a great deal of balance, coordination, and practice to become successful. If the patient has inadequate proximal strength, it may be difficult to bring the

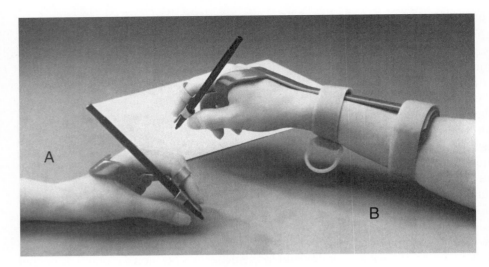

Figure 14-63 Wanchik writing splints.
A. Short design. **B.** Long design.

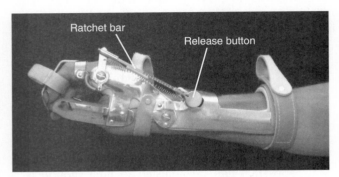

Figure 14-64 Custom metal ratchet wrist–hand orthosis.

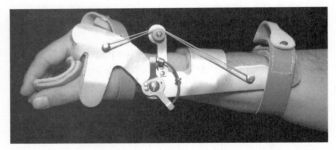

Figure 14-65 Custom metal wrist-action wrist–hand orthosis with rubber band assist.

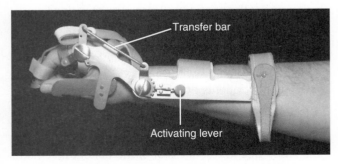

Figure 14-66 Custom metal wrist-driven wrist–hand orthosis.

arms into midline. If sensation has been lost, the patient must rely on visual compensation, which also makes bilateral orthotic use difficult. A patient generally uses one WDWHO, with the contralateral hand serving as a gross assist. Training principles are listed in Box 14-6.

Given the cost and complexity of fabrication and training, follow-up studies have been done to assess whether patients use WDWHOs over the long term after discharge from therapy. Knox et al. (1971) reported a 51% continued use rate; Shepherd and Ruzicka (1991), a 50% rate; and Allen (1971), a 43% rate. Factors that were reported to contribute to continued use are education, commitment, and involving the patient in the orthotic decision-making process (Knox et al., 1971); the ability to don the orthosis easily (Allen, 1971); and adequate training, acceptance, internal motivation, and strong functional or vocational goals (Shepherd & Ruzicka, 1991). In these same studies, reasons for orthotic discontinuation were stated by subjects to be improvement in muscle strength, use of alternative methods or equipment to perform tasks previously done with the WDWHO, poor fit, bulk, and the orthosis taking too long to put on.

Prevent Contractures or Modify Tone

Careful attention to positioning in the presence of wound healing, muscle imbalance, abnormal muscle tone due to stroke or brain injury, or motor disorders such as cerebral palsy is critical in the prevention of loss of range of motion, which can lead to functional or skin hygiene problems. Many of the static splints, casts, and orthoses previously mentioned for immobilization, stabilization, or substitution can be used for this purpose. Examples of these include acute burn immobilization splints to prevent wrist and digital contractures, wrist extension splints to prevent contractures caused by wrist drop, thumb abduction splints to prevent thumb adduction contractures, and lumbrical bar splints to prevent MCP hyperextension and IP flexion contractures.

Ideally, these splints should not limit function, exert excessive stress to soft tissues, or interfere with movement of uninvolved joints. If splints are not required for functional use, often it is possible for patients to wear static positioning splints at night only. In addition to the prevention of contractures, splints may be used to prevent shortening of the muscle–tendon unit. For example, a volar thermoplastic or plaster splint worn at night to position the wrist and fingers in maximum composite extension can help to prevent tightness of the long finger flexors (Tribuzi, 1995).

Lapboards, arm troughs, and suspension arm slings can help to position the upper extremities properly. Bivalved plaster casts or anteroposterior splints (Fig. 14-41) can be used to maintain range of motion, especially in the presence of increased tone. ***Care must be taken to avoid pressure problems by ensuring that casts are properly padded and the skin is closely monitored.***

An inflatable pressure splint (Fig. 14-67), originally designed as an emergency immobilizer for the limbs, has been adopted for use in patients with abnormal tone. When inflated, it provides deep pressure and warmth, and depending on how it is used can either reduce tone in hypertonic extremities or increase tone in hypotonic

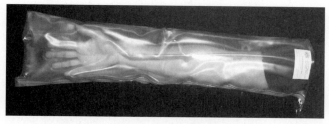

Figure 14-67 Commercial inflatable pressure splint.

extremities. It may be worn as a precursor to movement therapy or during weight-bearing activities to help position the limb. A study of 18 patients with CVA who wore the splint for 30 minutes a day, 5 days per week, for 3 weeks found no significant difference in upper extremity sensation, pain, and motor function between the splinted and control groups, leading the authors to suggest further study as to the long-term effects that inflatable splints may have on tone (Poole et al., 1990).

The use of thermoplastic splinting in the modification of tone in the wrist and hand continues to be controversial in the literature and in practice. A survey of occupational therapists clearly demonstrated the conflicting practices in splinting (Neuhaus et al., 1981). Opponents of splinting argue that splinting may lead to increased muscle tone, joint stiffness, and muscle atrophy and may interfere with treatment aimed at facilitation and functional use. Proponents of splinting contend that splinting can reduce tone (McPherson et al., 1985; Neuhaus et al., 1981).

Literature regarding optimal thermoplastic splint designs and wearing times shows no consensus. Static designs may be volar or dorsal, and comparative studies have been done in attempts to determine quantitatively which design is more effective in tone reduction. A study by McPherson et al. (1982) demonstrated no significant difference between the two basic splint designs and encouraged therapists to reexamine the amount of wearing time prescribed so that tonal reduction occurs without unwarranted secondary stiffness.

A design clinically studied by McPherson (1981) used a dorsal forearm base, volar finger and thumb pans, and finger abductors to position the wrist in 30° of extension, the MCPs in 45° of flexion, the IPs in full extension, the fingers fully abducted, and the thumb in extension and abduction. McPherson reported that splint wearing resulted in a reduction of tone related to the length of time that subjects wore the splint and that the effects of splint wearing were not necessarily permanent.

Common static splint designs include resting pan splints, finger spreaders or abduction splints, and cone splints. Several preformed splints are commercially available (Figs. 14-68 and 14-69), but no clinical studies have been done to establish their fit and effectiveness.

BOX 14-6
PROCEDURES FOR PRACTICE

WDWHO Controls Training and Use Training

Controls Training

► The patient needs to become proficient in basic orthotic skills, such as picking up, placing, and releasing objects of various sizes, textures, densities, and weights.

► Soft medium-sized objects or 1-inch firm, semirough objects are often best to start with; progress to more difficult objects as skill level increases.

► Encourage skills practice from a variety of heights, as the patient may have to learn to abduct and internally rotate the shoulder to approach and handle objects appropriately.

Use Training

► Teach the patient to use the WDWHO to perform specific functional tasks, such as writing, eating, and oral hygiene.

► Have the patient practice activities under various conditions to encourage independent problem solving and spontaneous use of the orthosis.

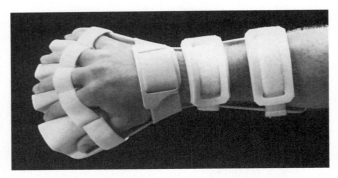

Figure 14-68 Rolyan® Anti-Spasticity Ball Splint with Slot and Loop Strapping.

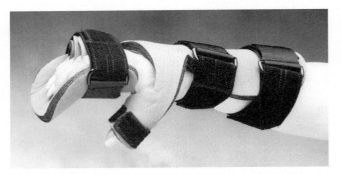

Figure 14-69 Progress™ Dorsal Anti-Spasticity Splint.

Dynamic splint designs have also been developed to reduce tone in the wrist and hand. In a study of 8 subjects, the finding was a greater reduction in hypertonus using a dynamic splint as compared with static splints and passive range of motion (McPherson et al., 1985). Scherling and Johnson (1989) studied the effects of their dynamic splint design on 18 subjects, with all subjects achieving varying degrees of tone reduction with a minimum of 4 hours splint use per day.

Soft splints made of neoprene can be custom fabricated (Casey & Kratz, 1988) or purchased commercially. A hand-based thumb loop can be used to decrease tone and position the thumb out of the palm for function (Fig. 14-70). To position the forearm, a long neoprene strap can be added to the hand splint.

A thermoplastic hand-based inhibitive weight-bearing splint described in the treatment of a child with cerebral palsy and increased flexor tone (Kinghorn & Roberts, 1996) can also be used with adult patients having hypertonicity. This volar splint is custom fabricated to hold the fingers in extension and thumb in radial abduction to enable the hand to be in an optimum position for upper extremity weight-bearing activities (Fig. 14-71).

Splinting may be an effective means of providing a low-cost, noninvasive method for decreasing tone in

some patients but may not be effective in others (Langlois et al., 1991). Continued research on the long-term effectiveness of splinting for tone reduction and the key patient variables that contribute to that effectiveness is needed. Meanwhile, therapists must carefully decide on splint use and monitor outcomes patient by patient.

Specialized Permanent Functional Orthoses

Permanent functional orthoses represent a great investment of time, cost, expertise, and commitment to fabrication, fit, training, and use by the patient–therapist–orthotist team. Proper fit, training, and successful functional use are accomplished only through close collaboration and communication among all who participate in the process. As with all orthoses, this process should begin with careful consideration of functional needs, achievable goals, and education of the patient and significant others in orthotic purpose and selection. Providing the patient with opportunities to interact with

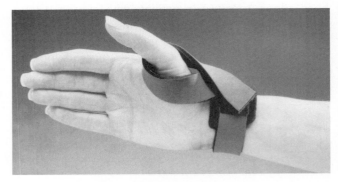

Figure 14-70 Rolyan® Thumb Loop.

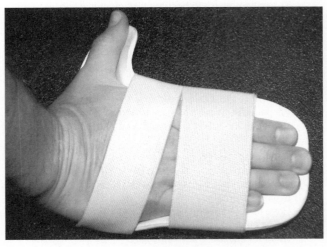

Figure 14-71 Custom thermoplastic hand-based weight-bearing splint.

Case Example

ORTHOTIC INTERVENTION IN A PATIENT WITH PERIPHERAL NERVE INJURY

Patient Information

M. N., a 22-year-old woman 8 weeks post motor vehicle collision, was referred to outpatient occupational therapy for evaluation and splinting of her left arm. She had a brachial plexus traction injury and a humeral fracture, treated with a closed reduction and fracture brace (purpose: to immobilize for healing). Prior to her injury, she was right-hand dominant and employed full time as a secretary.

On initial assessment, these problems were identified as related to her left upper extremity: (1) poor positioning of the entire arm, with Ms. N. using her right arm to hold and support the left arm; (2) absent motor function and impaired sensation throughout; (3) limited passive range of motion of the shoulder in all planes, forearm supination, MCP flexion, and thumb abduction; (4) traction pain in the shoulder; and (5) lack of functional use for any activities.

Recommendations

The occupational therapist recommended orthotic intervention as a key component of Ms. N.'s treatment program. In collaboration with Ms. N. and her mother, who was assisting Ms. N. with transportation to therapy and with other daily tasks, initial orthoses were selected and provided immediately.

Orthotic Intervention: Short-Term Goals

Ms. N. was fitted with a standard pouch sling, which was easy to don and doff and supported the weight of her arm with the goal of pain relief (purposes: to support a painful joint and to protect tissues); and with a custom-fabricated static wrist extension–thumb abduction splint to prevent the loss of wrist extension and to regain MCP flexion and thumb abduction range of motion (purposes: to prevent contractures and to restore mobility).

Orthotic Intervention: Revised Goals

As Ms. N.'s neuromuscular recovery progressed, the following orthoses were used in response to new problems identified:

Week 11: The sling was discontinued, as shoulder and elbow strength had improved to 3 to 3+ and traction pain had resolved. At night Ms. N. wore a custom-fabricated composite wrist and finger extension static splint to prevent long flexor tightness from unopposed finger flexors that had regained 3+ strength (purpose: to prevent contractures).

Week 17: At night Ms. N. wore a custom-fabricated serial static elbow extension splint to regain elbow extension range of motion lost to initial positioning from the sling, an ineffective home range of motion program, and return of unopposed 3+ elbow flexor strength (purpose: to restore mobility).

Week 21: A Colditz radial nerve splint was fabricated to substitute for weak radial nerve muscles and to enhance hand function as long finger flexors and wrist flexors recovered to sufficient strength of 3+. Ms. N. wore this splint during the day to allow functional use of the hand during light tasks (purpose: to substitute for weak or absent muscles).

Week 26: The Colditz radial nerve splint was discontinued, as wrist and long finger extensors had regained 3+ strength. A custom-fabricated thermoplastic lumbrical bar splint for the ring and small fingers was issued to address residual weakness of ulnar nerve intrinsic muscles leading to clawing. Ms. N. wore this splint during the day to assist with hand opening and prevent IP flexion contractures (purposes: to restrict unwanted motion and to prevent contractures).

Week 28: A dynamic forearm rotation splint was fabricated from a commercial kit; Ms. N. wore it at night to regain full supination range of motion initially lost from positioning and an imbalance of forearm rotator muscle strength (purpose: to restore mobility).

Week 36: No further splinting was required, as Ms. N. had full neuromuscular recovery. Ms. N. was able to return to her previous employment with full functional use of her left arm.

This case illustrates how a series of orthoses was used for many purposes through the course of treatment to enable an optimum functional and clinical outcome. It also highlights the need for continual monitoring of the patient's status so that splints may be discontinued as soon as they become unnecessary and new orthoses implemented as different needs arise.

CLINICAL REASONING
in OT Practice

Selecting the Most Appropriate Orthoses for a Patient

Ms. N. is a young, socially active woman who was living independently. What would the therapist anticipate to be Ms. N's primary concerns in orthotic selection? How could the therapist best engage her in the orthotic selection process while determining priorities for her orthotic needs? What are the clinical and functional components that must be closely monitored to determine specific orthotic needs?

experienced users of similar equipment can be quite helpful to the patient, both before the prescription and during training.

A permanent orthosis that is useful to the patient must be valued, accepted, and incorporated into the patient's body image. A prime prerequisite to accep-

tance is that the orthosis allows the patient to do something meaningful that cannot otherwise be done without it (Long & Shutt, 1986; Yasuda et al., 1986). Since the orthosis will be used over the long term, the patient and caregivers must also be told whom to contact should problems arise after the therapy program has ended.

Rancho Los Amigos National Rehabilitation Center   Occupational Therapy Department

MOBILE ARM SUPPORT APPRAISAL

Patient's Name_____   Type of MAS (L)_____

Date Fitted_____   Type of MAS (R)_____

I. PATIENT'S POSITION IN WHEELCHAIR

YES	NO	N/A	Are hips well back in wheelchair?
YES	NO	N/A	Is spine in good vertical alignment?
YES	NO	N/A	Does patient have lateral trunk stability?
YES	NO	N/A	Is wheelchair set-up providing adequate comfort and stability?
YES	NO	N/A	Is patient sitting in maximum upright position possible?
YES	NO	N/A	Does patient have needed hand splints on?
YES	NO	N/A	Does patient meet requirements for passive range of motion?

II. MECHANICAL CHECKOUT

YES	NO	N/A	Are all screws tight?
YES	NO	N/A	Is bracket tightly secured on wheelchair?
YES	NO	N/A	Are all MAS arms and joints freely movable?
YES	NO	N/A	Is proximal arm inserted completely in bracket bearing tube?
YES	NO	N/A	Is distal arm inserted completely in proximal arm bearing tube?
YES	NO	N/A	Is bracket at proper height so shoulder is not forced into elevation?
YES	NO	N/A	Does elbow dial clear lapboard when trough is in "up" position?
YES	NO	N/A	Is patient's hand (in "up" position) as close to mouth as possible?
YES	NO	N/A	Can patient obtain maximum active reach?
YES	NO	N/A	Is patient's arm secured in trough?
YES	NO	N/A	Is trough long enough to give maximum support to forearm?
YES	NO	N/A	Is trough short enough to allow wrist flexion if desired?
YES	NO	N/A	Are trough edges rolled so that they do not contact forearm?
YES	NO	N/A	Is elbow secure and comfortable in elbow dial?
YES	NO	N/A	Is trough balanced correctly?
YES	NO	N/A	During vertical motion, is elbow dial free of distal arm?
YES	NO	N/A	Are vertical stops correctly placed for both up and down motions?
YES	NO	N/A	Are rubber band hooks secured?
YES	NO	N/A	Are rubber bands securely attached?

Figure 14-72 Mobile Arm Support Appraisal Form.   *(continued)*

III. CONTROL CHECKOUT

YES	NO	N/A	Can patient control motion of proximal arm from either extreme?
YES	NO	N/A	Can patient control motion of distal arm from either extreme?
YES	NO	N/A	Can patient control vertical motion from either extreme?
YES	NO	N/A	Have stops been applied to limit motion, if necessary?
YES	NO	N/A	Does patient accomplish maximum horizontal reach in front of body?
YES	NO	N/A	Can patient easily reach mouth?
YES	NO	N/A	Can patient easily reach tabletop?
YES	NO	N/A	Can patient horizontally adduct arm sufficiently to clear doorways?
YES	NO	N/A	Is performance consistent from day to day?

IV. USE CHECKOUT

YES	NO	N/A	Are fine adjustments necessary to enable patient to perform different activities?
YES	NO	N/A	Are there some tasks that patient can perform better without MAS?
YES	NO	N/A	Is patient able to instruct caregivers in how to assemble MAS components?
YES	NO	N/A	Have patient and caregivers been instructed in care of MAS?

Figure 14-72 *(Continued)*

The principles of orthotic training are similar to those of prosthetics. They include testing of fit and mechanics; teaching the patient the names and functions of component parts; care of the orthosis; donning and doffing of the orthosis; controls training; and functional use training. Intensive practice under various conditions to encourage independent problem solving by the patient and skilled spontaneous use is a key element of training. Following is a closer look at two commonly used permanent functional orthoses.

Mobile Arm Supports

As described earlier in this chapter, the MAS (Figs. 14-52 and 14-53) is a mechanical device prescribed to support the weight of an arm and assist weak proximal muscles for function.

Patient and Caregiver Education
If the patient has been actively involved in the decision making, a brief review of the MAS's purpose and capabilities should be sufficient. The patient and caregiver should be oriented to key component names and how they operate. Finally, they should know how to care for and maintain the orthosis.

Assembling and Balancing
Box 14-5 has instructions in how to assemble and balance the standard MAS assembly.

Training and Adjusting
Adaptive equipment or a WHO is commonly used in conjunction with the MAS, and these should be integrated during all phases of MAS training and adjusting. Once the patient is proficient with basic movement patterns, MAS training with all of the activities that the patient is interested in performing should be done. Any of these activities may require various fine component adjustments before final MAS adjustments are completed. Periodic follow-up may be required, especially with a growing child. Box 14-5 has information related to MAS training and adjusting.

Orthotic Checkout
Once final adjustments have been completed, bolts and screws should be checked for a secure fit. A MAS appraisal form (Fig. 14-72) can be used to ensure that all important details are assessed.

Wrist-Driven Wrist–Hand Orthosis

A WDWHO (Fig. 14-65), as previously described, is used to enhance hand function in the presence of distal muscle weakness by using wrist extensor power to enable prehension.

Orthotic Checkout
The therapist must begin with a careful inspection of the orthosis both on and off the patient. Optimal fit is crucial

for maximum function. Ensuring smooth operation of mechanical parts, proper positioning of the digits for pad to pad prehension, and proper location of splint joint axes at the wrist and second MCP is essential. The strength of pinch should be assessed, and the length of the transfer bar should be changed by the orthotist to increase pinch strength as needed.

Straps should facilitate independent application and removal of the orthosis. Loops added to the ends of the straps enable the patient to use the thumb of the other hand to fasten and unfasten them with increased ease.

The patient's ability to don and doff the orthosis is strongly related to independence in activities and to the patient's ultimate acceptance of the device. This is true especially if the patient must remove the orthosis to perform other activities such as propulsion of a wheelchair. Removal of the WDWHO is typically easier than application of it. With training, donning the orthosis can be accomplished in less than a minute (Clark et al., 1997). *Initially, the orthosis should be placed on the patient for no more than 30 minutes. Upon removal, the skin should be carefully checked for any areas of redness. These red areas should be reassessed in half an hour, and if they are still present, the orthosis requires adjustment before the patient can use it.* Once pressure problems have been resolved, wearing time can be gradually increased.

Patient and Caregiver Education

A brief review of the WDWHO's purpose and capabilities should be provided. The patient and caregivers should be instructed in the importance of skin inspection to prevent excessive pressure and skin breakdown. Accordingly, they should also be taught wearing tolerance and the schedule. They should be oriented to key component names and how the components operate prior to orthotic controls training. Finally, they should know how to care for and maintain the orthosis. Education in these areas should be reinforced throughout the orthotic training process.

Controls Training and Functional Use Training

Box 14-6 shows WDWHO controls training and use training.

Summary Review Questions

1. What is the role of the occupational therapist in orthotic rehabilitation?
2. Define orthosis.
3. Name the purposes for which splinting may be used.
4. What are key factors for selecting an orthosis for a particular patient?
5. Discuss factors that may enhance splint wearing and those that may interfere with it.
6. Discuss why a static splint may be chosen and the precautions related to such splints.
7. Describe two dynamic splints and the purposes for which they are used.
8. Select an orthosis to decrease an elbow flexion contracture, discuss the reasons for your choice, and state the principle or principles that it implements.
9. Discuss two types of finger or hand orthoses that assist in restoring function while stabilizing a joint.
10. For which type of patient would you choose a wrist-driven wrist–hand orthosis?
11. Name the basic components of a standard MAS and two diagnostic categories of candidates who may benefit from its use.
12. Describe a treatment session to improve a patient's hand-to-mouth and hand-to-table control of a MAS, and basic adjustments that can be made to the MAS to facilitate these motions.
13. What are the pros and cons of various orthoses designed to modify tone?

Acknowledgments

I thank Y. Lynn Yasuda, MSEd, OTR, FAOTA and Maura Walsh, OTR, CHT for sharing their clinical expertise and advice; Michele Berro, MA, OTR for assisting with obtaining photographs; and Paul Weinreich, Medical Photographer at Rancho Los Amigos National Rehabilitation Center, for his photography and technical support.

I acknowledge the following contributions:

▶ Figures 14-2, 14-4, 14-13, 14-26, 14-32, 14-33, 14-43, 14-44, 14-48, 14-59, 14-63, 14-68, and 14-70 courtesy of the Rehabilitation Division of Smith & Nephew, Inc., Germantown, WI.
▶ Figures 14-3, 14-6, 14-12, and 14-52 courtesy of Sammons Preston, Bolingbrook, IL.
▶ Figures 14-5, 14-7, 14-8, 14-14, 14-18, 14-23, 14-27–14-31, 14-36, 14-37, 14-41, 14-45, 14-49, 14-50, 14-54, 14-55, 14-58, 14-60, 14-61, 14-64–14-67, 14-71, and 14-72 courtesy of Rancho Los Amigos National Rehabilitation Center, Downey, CA.
▶ Figures 14-9–14-11, 14-15–14-17, 14-19, 14-20, 14-22, 14-24, 14-25, 14-34, 14-35, 14-46, 14-47, 14-57, 14-62, and 14-69 courtesy of North Coast Medical, Inc., Morgan Hill, CA.
▶ Figure 14-21 courtesy of AliMed, Inc., Dedham, MA.
▶ Figures 14-38 and 14-39 courtesy of Silver Ring Splint Company, Charlottesville, VA.
▶ Figure 14-42 courtesy of Joint Active Systems, Inc., Effingham, IL.

Resources

Vendors of Splints and Splint Supplies

AliMed, Inc. · 297 High Street, Dedham, MA 02026. 800-225-2610. Fax 800-437-2966.
www.alimed.com

DeRoyal/LMB. · 200 DeBusk Lane, Powell, TN 37849. 800-541-3992. Fax 800-327-0340.
www.deroyal.com

JAECO Orthopedic Specialties, Inc. · P.O. Box 75, Hot Springs, AR 71902-0075. 501-623-5944. Fax 501-623-0159.

Joint Active Systems, Inc. · P.O. Box 1367, Effingham, IL 62401. 800-879-0117. Fax 217-347-3384.

North Coast Medical, Inc. · 18305 Sutter Blvd., Morgan Hill, CA 95037-2845. 800-821-9319. Fax 877-213-9300.
www.ncmedical.com

Otto Bock Medical · 3000 Xenium Lane North, Minneapolis, MN 53441. 800-328-4058. Fax 800-962-2549.
www.ottobockus.com

Sammons Preston · P.O. Box 5071, Bolingbrook, IL 60440-5071. 800-323-5527. Fax 800-547-4333.
www.sammonspreston.com

Silver Ring Splint Company · P.O. Box 2856, Charlottesville, VA 22902-2856. 800-311-7028. Fax 804-971-8828.
www.silverringsplint.com

Smith & Nephew, Inc. · P.O. Box 1005, Germantown, WI 53022-8205. 800-558-8633. Fax 800-545-7758.

3-Point Products, Inc. · 1610 Pincay Court, Annapolis, MD 21401. 888-378-7763. Fax 410-349-2648.

UE Tech · P.O. Box 2145, Edwards, CO 81632. 800-736-1894. Fax 970-926-8870.
www.uetech.com

References

Aiello, B. (1998). Epicondylitis. In G. L. Clark, E. F. S. Wilgis, B. Aiello, D. Eckhaus, & L. Valdata Eddington (Eds.), *Hand Rehabilitation: A Practical Guide* (2nd ed., pp. 175–179). New York: Churchill Livingstone.

Allen, V. (1971). Follow-up study of wrist-driven flexor-hinge-splint use. *American Journal of Occupational Therapy, 25,* 420–422.

American Society of Hand Therapists. (1992). *Splint Classification System.* Chicago: Author.

Bassini, L. B., & Patel, M. R. (1994). Buddy sleeves. *Journal of Hand Therapy, 7,* 257–258.

Bell-Krotoski, J. A. (1995). Plaster cylinder casting for contractures of the interphalangeal joints. In J. M. Hunter, E. J. Mackin, & A. D. Callahan (Eds.), *Rehabilitation of the Hand: Surgery and Therapy* (4th ed., pp. 1609–1616). St. Louis: Mosby.

Bell-Krotoski, J. A., & Figarola, J. H. (1995). Biomechanics of soft tissue growth and remodeling with plaster casting. *Journal of Hand Therapy, 8,* 131–137.

Bobath, B. (1990). *Adult Hemiplegia: Evaluation and Treatment* (3rd ed.). London: William Heinemann Medical.

Breger-Lee, D. (1995). Objective and subjective observations of low-temperature thermoplastic materials. *Journal of Hand Therapy, 8,* 138–143.

Brand, P. W. (1995). The forces of dynamic splinting: Ten questions before applying a dynamic splint to the hand. In J. M. Hunter, E. J. Mackin, & A. D. Callahan (Eds.), *Rehabilitation of the hand: Surgery and Therapy* (4th ed., pp. 1581–1587). St. Louis: Mosby.

Callahan, A. D., & McEntee, P. (1986). Splinting proximal interphalangeal joint flexion contractures: A new design. *American Journal of Occupational Therapy, 40,* 408–413.

Callinan, N. J., & Mathiowetz, V. (1996). Soft versus hard resting splints in rheumatoid arthritis: Pain relief, preference, and compliance. *American Journal of Occupational Therapy, 50,* 347–353.

Canelon, M. F. (1995). Material properties: A factor in the selection and application of splinting materials for athletic wrist and hand injuries. *Journal of Orthopedic Sports Physical Therapy, 22,* 164–172.

Carlson, J. D., & Trombly, C. A. (1983). The effect of wrist immobilization on performance of the Jebsen Hand Function Test. *American Journal of Occupational Therapy, 37,* 167–175.

Casey, C. A., & Kratz, E. J. (1988). Soft splinting with neoprene: The thumb abduction supinator splint. *American Journal of Occupational Therapy, 42,* 395–398.

Clark, D. R., Waters, R. L., & Baumgarten, J. M. (1997). Upper limb orthoses for the spinal cord injured patient. In B. Goldberg & J. D. Hsu (Eds.), *Atlas of Orthoses and Assistive Devices* (3rd ed., pp. 291–303). St. Louis: Mosby.

Clark, E. N. (1997). A preliminary investigation of the neoprene tube finger extension splint. *Journal of Hand Therapy, 10,* 213–221.

Colditz, J. C. (1995a). Therapist's management of the stiff hand. In J. M. Hunter, E. J. Mackin, & A. D. Callahan (Eds.), *Rehabilitation of the Hand: Surgery and Therapy* (4th ed., pp. 1141–1159). St. Louis: Mosby.

Colditz, J. C. (1995b). Spring-wire extension splinting of the proximal interphalangeal joint. In J. M. Hunter, E. J. Mackin, & A. D. Callahan (Eds.), *Rehabilitation of the Hand: Surgery and Therapy* (4th ed., pp. 1617–1629). St. Louis: Mosby.

Colditz, J. C. (1995c). Splinting the hand with a peripheral nerve injury. In J. M. Hunter, E. J. Mackin, & A. D. Callahan (Eds.), *Rehabilitation of the Hand: Surgery and Therapy* (4th ed., pp. 679–692). St. Louis: Mosby.

Collelo-Abraham, K. (1990). Dynamic pronation-supination splint. In Hunter, J. M., Schneider, J. L. H., Mackin, E. J., & Callahan, A. D. (Eds.), *Rehabilitation of the Hand: Surgery and Therapy* (3rd ed., pp. 1134–1139). St. Louis: Mosby.

Collins, L. (1999). Helping patients help themselves: Improving orthotic use. *Occupational Therapy Practice, 4,* 30–34.

Evans, R. B. (1995). An update on extensor tendon management. In J. M. Hunter, E. J. Mackin, & A. D. Callahan (Eds.), *Rehabilitation of the Hand: Surgery and Therapy* (4th ed., pp. 565–606). St. Louis: Mosby.

Feinberg, J. (1992). Effect of the arthritis health professional on compliance with use of resting hand splints by patients with rheumatoid arthritis. *Arthritis Care & Research, 5,* 17–23.

Fess, E. E. (1988). Force magnitude of commercial spring-coil and spring-wire splints designed to extend the proximal interphalangeal joint. *Journal of Hand Therapy, 1,* 86–90.

Fess, E. E. (1995). Splints: Mechanics and convention. *Journal of Hand Therapy, 8,* 124–130.

Fess, E. E., & McCollum, M. (1998). The influence of splinting on healing tissues. *Journal of Hand Therapy, 11,* 157–161.

Fess, E. E., & Philips, C. A. (Eds.). (1987). *Hand Splinting Principles and Methods* (2nd ed.). St. Louis: Mosby.

Foucher, G., Binhamer, P., Cange, S., & Lenoble, E. (1996). Long term results of splintage of mallet finger. *International Orthopaedics, 20,* 129–131.

Gelberman, R. H., Rydevik, B. L., Pess, G. M., Szabo, R. M., & Lundborg, G. (1988). Carpal tunnel syndrome: A scientific basis for clinical care. *Orthopedic Clinics of North America, 19,* 115–124.

Gilbert-Lenef, L. (1994). Soft ulnar deviation splint. *Journal of Hand Therapy, 7,* 29–30.

Groth, G .N., & Wulf, M. B. (1995). Compliance with hand rehabilitation: Health beliefs and strategies. *Journal of Hand Therapy, 8,* 18–22.

Hill, J. (1994). The effects of casting on upper extremity motor disorders after brain injury. *American Journal of Occupational Therapy, 48,* 219–224.

Jensen, C., & Rayan, G. (1996). Buddy strapping of mismatched fingers: The offset buddy strap. *Journal of Hand Surgery, 21,* 317–318.

Keenan, M. A. (1997). Upper extremity orthoses for the brain-injured patient. In B. Goldberg & J. D. Hsu (Eds.), *Atlas of Orthoses and Assistive Devices* (3rd ed., pp. 281–289). St. Louis: Mosby.

Kinghorn, J., & Roberts, G. (1996). The effect of an inhibitive weight-bearing splint on tone and function: A single-case study. *American Journal of Occupational Therapy, 50,* 807–815.

Kirkpatrick, W. H., Kozin, S. H., & Uhl, R. L. (1996). Early motion after arthroplasty. *Hand Clinics, 12,* 73–86.

Knox, C., Engel, W., & Seibens, A. (1971). Results of a survey on the use of a wrist-driven splint for prehension. *American Journal of Occupational Therapy, 15,* 109–111.

Lamay, G. (1994). Buddy splint. *Journal of Hand Therapy, 7,* 30–31.

Lange, M. L. (1999). Positioning the upper extremities. *Occupational Therapy Practice, 4,* 49–50.

Langlois, S., Pederson, L., & Mackinnon, J. (1991). The effects of splinting on the spastic hemiplegic hand: Report of a feasibility study. *Canadian Journal of Occupational Therapy, 58,* 17–25.

Long, C., & Shutt, A. (1986). Upper limb orthotics. In J. B. Redford (ed.), *Orthotics Etcetera* (3rd ed., pp. 198–270). Baltimore: Williams & Wilkins.

Lunsford, T. R. (1997). Upper limb orthoses. In B. Goldberg & J. D. Hsu (Eds.), *Atlas of Orthoses and Assistive Devices* (3rd ed., pp. 195–208). St. Louis: Mosby.

Lunsford, T. R., & Wallace, J. M. (1997). The orthotic prescription. In B. Goldberg & J. D. Hsu (Eds.), *Atlas of Orthoses and Assistive Devices* (3rd ed., pp. 3–14). St. Louis: Mosby.

McFarland, E. G., Curl, L. A., Urquhart, M. C., & Kellam, K. (1997). Shoulder immobilization devices: 3. Abduction braces and pillows. *Orthopaedic Nursing, 16,* 47–54.

McPherson, J. J. (1981). Objective evaluation of a splint designed to reduce hypertonicity. *American Journal of Occupational Therapy, 35,* 189–194.

McPherson, J. J., Becker, A. H., & Franszczak, N. (1985). Dynamic splint to reduce the passive component of hypertonicity. *Archives of Physical Medicine and Rehabilitation, 66,* 249–252.

McPherson, J. J., Kreimeyer, D., Aalderks, M., & Gallagher, T. (1982). A comparison of dorsal and volar resting hand splints in the reduction of hypertonus. *American Journal of Occupational Therapy, 36,* 664–670.

Melvin, J. L. (1989). *Rheumatic Disease in the Adult and Child: Occupational Therapy and Rehabilitation* (3rd ed.). Philadelphia: Davis.

Melvin, J. L. (1995). Orthotic treatment of the hand: What's new? *Bulletin on the Rheumatic Diseases, 44* (4), 5–8.

Moodie, N., Brisbin, J., & Margan, A. (1986). Subluxation of the glenohumeral joint in hemiplegia: Evaluation of supportive devices. *Physiotherapy Canada, 38* (3), 151–157.

Murphy, M. S. (1990). An adjustable splint for forearm supination. *American Journal of Occupational Therapy, 44,* 936–939.

Neuhaus, B. E., Ascher, E. R., Coullon, B. A., Donohoe, M. V., Einbond, A., Glover, J. M., Goldberg, S. R., & Takai, V. L. (1981). A survey of rationales for and against hand splinting in hemiplegia. *American Journal of Occupational Therapy, 35,* 83–90.

Nuismer, B. A., Ekes, A. M., & Holm, M. B. (1997). The use of low-load prolonged stretch devices in rehabilitation programs in the Pacific Northwest. *American Journal of Occupational Therapy, 51,* 538–543.

Oakes, T. W., Ward, J. F., Gray, R. M., Klauber, M. R., & Moody, P. M. (1970). Family expectations and arthritis patients' compliance to a resting hand splint regimen. *Journal of Chronic Diseases, 22,* 757–764.

Pagnotta, A., Baron, M., & Korner-Bitensky, N. (1998). The effect of a static wrist orthosis on hand function in individuals with rheumatoid arthritis. *Journal of Rheumatology, 25,* 879–885.

Philips, C. A. (1989). Management of the patient with rheumatoid arthritis: The role of the hand therapist. *Hand Clinics, 5,* 291–309.

Poole, J. L., Whitney, S. L., Hangeland, N., & Baker, C. (1990). The effectiveness of inflatable pressure splints on motor function in stroke patients. *Occupational Therapy Journal of Research, 10,* 360–366.

Prosser, R. (1996). Splinting in the management of proximal interphalangeal joint flexion contracture. *Journal of Hand Therapy, 9,* 378–386.

Rennie, H. J. (1996). Evaluation of the effectiveness of a metacarpophalangeal ulnar deviation orthosis. *Journal of Hand Therapy, 9,* 371–377.

Richard, R., Shanesy, C. P., & Miller, S. F. (1995). Dynamic versus static splints: A prospective case for sustained stress. *Journal of Burn Care & Rehabilitation, 16,* 284–287.

Richard, R., & Staley, M. (1994). *Burn Care and Rehabilitation: Principles and Practice.* Philadelphia: Davis.

Richard, R., Staley, M., Daugherty, M. B., Miller, S. F., & Warden, G. D. (1994). The wide variety of designs for dorsal hand burn splints. *Journal of Burn Care and Rehabilitation, 15,* 275–280.

Scherling, E., & Johnson, H. (1989). A tone-reducing wrist-hand orthosis. *American Journal of Occupational Therapy, 43,* 609–611.

Shepherd, C. C., & Ruzicka, S. H. (1991). Tenodesis brace use by persons with spinal cord injuries. *American Journal of Occupational Therapy, 45,* 81–83.

Smith, R. O., & Okamoto, G. A. (1981). Checklist for the prescription of slings for the hemiplegic patient. *American Journal of Occupational Therapy, 35,* 91–95.

Stern, E. B. (1991). Wrist extensor orthoses: Dexterity and grip strength across four styles. *American Journal of Occupational Therapy, 45,* 42–49.

Stern, E. B. (1996). Grip strength and finger dexterity across five styles of commercial wrist orthoses. *American Journal of Occupational Therapy, 50,* 32–38.

Stern, E. B., Callinan, N., Hank, M., Lewis, E. J., Schousboe, J. T., & Ytterberg, S. R. (1998). Neoprene splinting: Dermatological issues. *American Journal of Occupational Therapy, 52,* 573–578.

Stern, E. B., Ytterberg, S. R., Krug, H. E., & Mahowald, M. L. (1996). Finger dexterity and hand function: Effect of three commercial wrist extensor orthoses on patients with rheumatoid arthritis. *Arthritis Care & Research, 9,* 197–205.

Stern, E. B., Ytterberg, S. R., Larson, L. M., Portoghese, C. P., Kratz, W. N. R., & Mahowald, M. L. (1997). Commercial wrist extensor orthoses: A descriptive study of use and preference in patients with rheumatoid arthritis. *Arthritis Care & Research, 10,* 27–35.

Stewart, K. M. (1995). Therapist's management of the complex injury. In J. M. Hunter, E. J. Mackin, & A. D. Callahan (Eds.), *Rehabilitation of the Hand: Surgery and Therapy* (4th ed., pp. 1057–1073). St. Louis: Mosby.

Stewart, K. M., & vanStrien, G. (1995). Postoperative management of flexor tendon injuries. In J. M. Hunter, E. J. Mackin, & A. D. Callahan (Eds.), *Rehabilitation of the Hand: Surgery and Therapy* (4th ed., pp. 433–462). St. Louis: Mosby.

Tribuzi, S. M. (1995). Serial plaster splinting. In J. M. Hunter, E. J. Mackin, & A. D. Callahan (Eds.), *Rehabilitation of the Hand: Surgery and Therapy* (4th ed., pp. 1599–1607). St. Louis: Mosby.

Wallny, T., Westermann, K., Sagebiel, C., Reimer, M., & Wagner, U. A. (1997). Functional treatment of humeral shaft fractures: Indications and results. *Journal of Orthopaedic Trauma, 11*, 283–287.

Walsh, M. (1987). Half-lapboard for hemiplegic patients. *American Journal of Occupational Therapy, 41*, 533–535.

Weiss, N. D., Gordon, L., Bloom, T., So, Y., & Rempel, D. M. (1995). Position of the wrist associated with the lowest carpal tunnel pressure: Implications for splint design. *Journal of Bone and Joint Surgery, 77-A*, 1695–1699.

Wilton, J. C. (1997). *Hand Splinting: Principles of Design and Fabrication*. Philadelphia: Saunders.

Wuori, J. L., Overend, T. J., Kramer, J. F., & MacDermid, J. (1998). Strength and pain measures associated with lateral epicondylitis bracing. *Archives of Physical Medicine and Rehabilitation, 79*, 832–837.

Yasuda, Y. L., Bowman, K., & Hsu, J. D. (1986). Mobile arm supports: Criteria for successful use in muscle disease patients. *Archives of Physical Medicine and Rehabilitation, 67*, 253–256.

Zorowitz, R. D., Idank, D., Ikai, T., Hughes, M. B., & Johnston, M. V. (1995). Shoulder subluxation after stroke: A comparison of four supports. *Archives of Physical Medicine and Rehabilitation, 76*, 763–771.

Zorowitz, R. D., Hughes, M. B., Idank, D., Ikai, T., & Johnston, M. V. (1996). Shoulder pain and subluxation after stroke: Correlation or coincidence? *American Journal of Occupational Therapy, 50*, 194–201.

15

Construction of Hand Splints

Nancy Callinan

Nancy Callinan

LEARNING OBJECTIVES

After studying this chapter, the reader will be able to do the following:

1. Describe the anatomical, biomechanical, and mechanical principles applied to splint construction.
2. Identify the properties, benefits, and limitations of various splinting materials.
3. Recognize factors affecting splint wear compliance.
4. Explain design, pattern making, and construction for three splints.
5. Describe the components of a splint checkout.

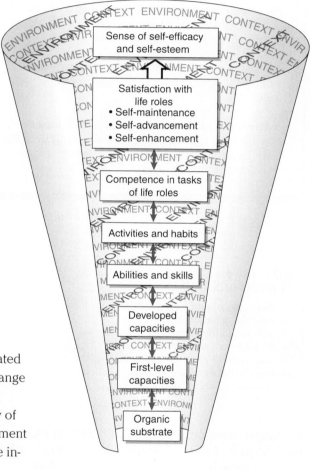

*T*he hand is an incredible tool. Through a carefully orchestrated integration of muscles working together, the hand executes a range of functions from picking a delicate flower to firmly gripping a hammer. If disease or injury disrupts this balance and harmony of muscle power, the hand loses its remarkable skills. This impairment can be treated by splinting to maximize function and return the individual to meaningful occupational performance.

The art and science of occupational therapy are clearly evident in splint construction. In the design and construction of a **splint**, the therapist uses creativity combined with knowledge of the complex anatomy and biomechanics of the hand. An understanding of pertinent mechanical principles is necessary because a poorly designed splint can cause discomfort and further dysfunction of the hand. A thorough understanding of the patient's functional needs and clinical condition is also necessary to ensure that the splint meets the treatment goals. The therapist benefits from appreciation of a variety of splinting materials and their properties in the design and construction of splints.

Splints can have a significant effect on healing tissues and can greatly influence the remodeling of scar tissue. Applying the proper splint at the appropriate stage in healing can significantly influence

GLOSSARY

Dual obliquity—Variance between the length and height of the metacarpals, with the radial side longer and higher than the ulnar side. These relationships must be considered when splinting the hand.

Dynamic splint—A splint that applies a mobile force in one direction while allowing active motion in the opposite direction. The mobile force is applied with rubber bands, elastic thread, or springs.

Fibroblastic phase—Stage of wound healing that follows the inflammatory phase, during which fibroblasts proliferate and initiate collagen production in the healing of tissues.

Haldex gauge—A spring gauge that precisely measures the grams of force for rubber band dynamic traction or torque angle curves.

Inflammatory phase—Phase of wound healing immediately following injury or surgery; characterized by edema and infiltration of leucocytes and macrophages to begin healing of the injured tissues.

Maturation phase—Stage of wound healing that follows the fibroblastic phase; characterized by wound contraction, remodeling, and maturation of the healed tissues.

Serial static splint—A splint with no moving parts designed to be remolded as a contracture improves.

Splint—A device applied to the body to provide protection, positioning, immobilization, restriction, correction, or prevention of deformity for the splinted part; an orthosis.

Static progressive splint—A splint designed to stretch contractures through the application of serially adjusted static force to promote lengthening of contracted tissues.

BOX 15-1
Purposes of Splinting

► Protection of structure at risk of injury
► Positioning for function
► Immobilization for healing
► Restriction of undesired motion
► Correction or prevention of deformity
► Substitution for absent or weak muscles

---

functional outcome. The therapist must thoroughly evaluate the patient and the clinical condition to identify the appropriate splint in the course of rehabilitation.

Splinting is used in conjunction with other treatment strategies to enhance occupational performance. However, the splint may also interfere with functional performance. The therapist must evaluate the effect of the completed splint on the patient during functional activities within the context of the patient's environment to determine whether the splint contributes to the goals of treatment. A splint that impairs performance by causing poor compensatory patterns of movement may necessitate modification of the splint or the wearing schedule. Purposes of splinting are reviewed in Box 15-1.

Anatomical and Biomechanical Considerations in Splinting

The construction of hand splints must take into consideration certain anatomical facts and biomechanical principles.

Anatomical Considerations

Therapists apply a thorough knowledge of anatomy of the hand to their construction of hand splints. The creases of the hand provide landmarks for splint fabrication (Coppard & Lohman, 1996). These creases identify the axis of motion for the corresponding joint. The distal edge of a splint must not extend beyond a crease if motion at that joint is desired (Fig. 15-1). Bony prominences of the hand and wrist (Fig. 15-2) can create pressure points if the splint does not adequately conform to these areas. Potential pressure points are common on the dorsum of the hand and wrist. The arches of the hand (Fig. 15-3): the distal transverse (metacarpal) arch, the proximal transverse (carpal) arch, and the longitudinal arch ensure optimal hand function (Coppard & Lohman, 1996; Tubiana et al., 1996). The splint must conform to these arches to support the functional position of the hand.

The functional position of the hand is 15 to 30° of wrist dorsiflexion, neutral to slight ulnar deviation, 15 to 20° of metacarpophalangeal (MCP) flexion, 10° of flexion at the proximal interphalangeal (PIP) and distal interphalangeal (DIP) joints, palmar abduction of the thumb, and extension of the metacarpophalangeal (MP) and interphalangeal (IP) joints of the thumb (Coppard & Lohman, 1996). This position places the muscles, tendons, and ligaments at a resting length and in position for grasp and prehension (Fig. 15-4). The web space of the thumb allows maximal abduction of the thumb for grasp. Every effort is made to preserve the maximum web space because the size of object that can be grasped depends on the mobility of the thumb web space (Tubiana et al., 1996).

The fingers vary in length and height, with the fingers on the radial side being longer than those on the ulnar side of the hand when the hand is open. The metacarpophalangeal joints on the radial side are higher than those on the ulnar side of the hand when the hand is closed. The therapist must apply this concept of **dual obliquity** to the construction of a splint (Fig. 15-5). That is, the splint must be longer and higher on the radial side of the hand (Fess & Philips, 1987).

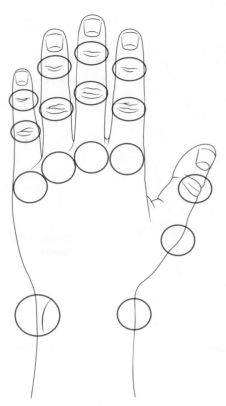

Figure 15-2 Bony prominences can lead to pressure points, especially over the back of the hand. Careful contouring of the splinting material can minimize this problem.

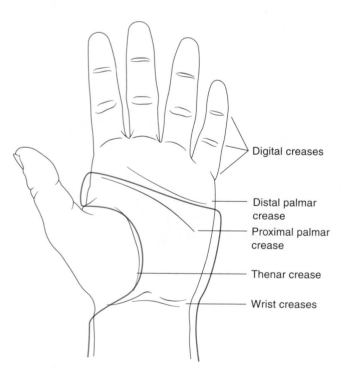

Figure 15-1 Creases of the hand provide landmarks for the distal ends of the splint. For a wrist support splint the distal end of the splint should not block the thenar eminence or distal palmar crease.

Digital creases

Distal palmar crease

Proximal palmar crease

Thenar crease

Wrist creases

The therapist should evaluate sensibility, mobility, motor function, edema, and tone prior to splint design and construction. Sensory deficit in the hand creates a concern: the patient may not be able to feel pressure points or areas of irritation from the splint, which can lead to skin breakdown or injury. In the case of hypersensitivity, the use of a splint can protect the fingertip or hand from unpleasant stimuli. Edema may also indicate the need for close monitoring of splint fit and comfort. As edema diminishes, the splint requires modification or remolding to maintain proper fit. Deficits in mobility may change during the course of splinting, so the splint may have to be modified. Weakness may indicate the need for a dynamic assist splint to prevent muscle imbalance or deformity. As muscle strength improves, the force of the dynamic assist should be adjusted to the patient's needs. Increased or decreased tone may indicate the need for splinting to maintain balance and prevent contracture. As tone changes, the therapist should modify the splint as necessary to meet the goals of treatment. Ongoing assessment helps the therapist identify any need for changes in the splint.

In designing a splint, the therapist must be aware of the natural postures of the hand that affect function. When the hand is held in supination, the wrist is held in

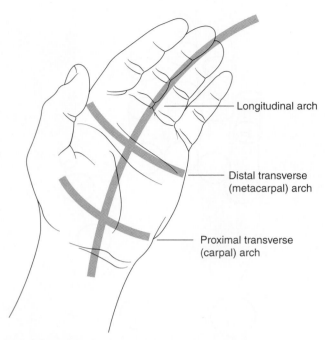

Figure 15-3 Arches of the hand must be supported in splinting.

Longitudinal arch

Distal transverse
(metacarpal) arch

Proximal transverse
(carpal) arch

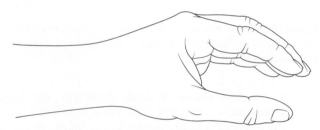

Figure 15-4 Functional position of the hand.

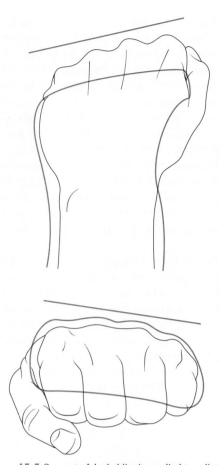

Figure 15-5 Concept of dual obliquity applied to splinting.

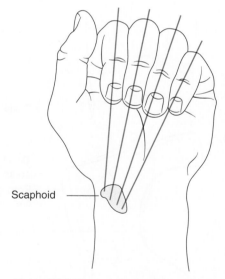

Scaphoid

Figure 15-6 Fingers flex toward the scaphoid.

neutral to slight radial deviation. When the hand is held in pronation, the wrist assumes a more ulnarly deviated posture. These considerations affect fit: if a splint is fitted in supination for a patient who will be using the hand primarily in pronation, the splint may not fit comfortably. Another consideration is that normally during flexion the fingers converge toward the scaphoid bone (Fig. 15-6). Therefore, the application of dynamic assists to finger flexion splints must have the direction of pull toward the radial border of the wrist.

In designing a splint that includes functional positioning of the thumb, the therapist notes the position of the thumb for prehension to the index and middle finger. Typically, the thumb is held in palmar abduction and opposition to these fingers for effective prehension. While forming the splint, the therapist may have the patient hold a pen or other object in the hand to test the ability of the thumb to achieve functional prehension. When designing a splint for the patient with carpal tunnel syndrome, the therapist should be aware of the position of the wrist that produces the lowest pressure in the carpal canal. The ideal position for the wrist is close to neutral, with $2 \pm 9°$ of dorsiflexion and $2 \pm 6°$ of ulnar deviation (Weiss et al., 1995).

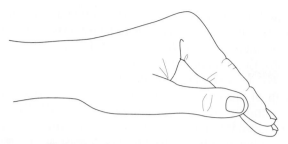

Figure 15-7 Position of safe immobilization.

Biomechanical Considerations

Biomechanical considerations include the effects of healing tissue on the biomechanics of hand use and mechanical principles that affect the design of the splint.

Position of Safe Immobilization

Following injury the hand may stiffen in a nonfunctional position. This position typically includes wrist flexion, MCP extension, and PIP and DIP flexion in a claw position (Bunnell, 1996). The distal transverse arch is flattened. If this position is maintained for long, the hand becomes nonfunctional as a result of shortening of the collateral ligaments. The position of safe immobilization (Fig. 15-7) prevents ligamentous shortening and contracture following injury. This position maintains the length of the collateral ligaments by holding the MCP joints in flexion and the PIP and DIP joints in extension while keeping the wrist in dorsiflexion. Specifically, the wrist is held in 30 to 40° of extension, and the MCP joints are positioned in 70 to 90° of flexion with full extension of PIP and DIP joints (Coppard & Lohman, 1996). This position is also called intrinsic plus, or safe positioning.

Tissue Healing

The therapist should be aware of the phases of wound healing when selecting the splint design for the patient with an injured hand. Splinting applies gentle stress to healing tissues to influence change (Fess & McCollum, 1998). During the **inflammatory phase**, the therapist may use a splint to immobilize and protect the healing tissues. During the **fibroplastic phase** of healing, splints may be used to mobilize healing tissues while protecting them. As the strength of the healing tissues increases and the scar tissue matures in the **maturation phase**, low load force may be applied with splinting. As maturation progresses, the tissues can tolerate an increased amount of stress (Schultz-Johnson, 1996). A splinting program must recognize these changes in healing tissues with appropriate changes in the splint as needed. Exercise programs and functional activity must begin simultaneously with splinting to maximize the benefit.

Influence of Splinting on Scar Remodeling

When mobility is lost to immobilization from casting, injury, or a neurological condition, collagen fibers develop increased intermolecular bonds, which result in dense tissue with relatively little mobility (Bell-Krotoski & Figarola, 1995). This response causes tissues to adapt and shorten, resulting in contracture. Such a limitation in mobility may be treated with splinting. There is some controversy regarding how splinting creates changes in soft tissues (Fess & McCollum, 1998). Is it by stretching existing tissue or the actual production of new tissue? The mechanism of stretching was initially thought to be creep, the elongation of tissues under a prolonged stress over time (Bell-Krotoski & Figarola, 1995; Fess & Philips, 1987). However, if tissues are stretched excessively, they rupture or produce an inflammatory response. Research suggests that ideal tissue remodeling occurs with gentle elongation of tissues. Tissues lengthen and grow if gentle stress is applied. This process is not stretching but rather growth of new tissues to accommodate the stress placed on them (Bell-Krotoski & Figarola, 1995; Brand, 1995). **Dynamic splinting**, **serial static splinting**, and casting are based on this mechanism.

The total end range time (TERT) theory suggests that the amount of increase in passive range of motion of a stiff joint is directly proportional to the amount of time the joint is held at the end of its range (Flowers & LaStayo, 1994). TERT theory states that if a joint is held at the end of its range, the dense connective tissue around the joint grows. This lengthening of tissues increases range of motion. The longer the joint is positioned at its end range, the greater the gain in mobility. Serial static splinting or casting is often used in the application of TERT theory in splinting.

Another theory employs stress relaxation, or static progressive stretch therapy in splinting (Bonutti et al., 1994). This approach elongates tissues through progressive incremental stretch. The static progressive stretch approach applies 30-minute sessions of splint wear with stretch increased every 5 minutes to the patient's tolerance to increase range of motion. **Static progressive splints** apply this theory by applying a low-load force that can be adjusted incrementally. These splints use methods such as MERiT (Maximum End Range Time) components for gradual advancement of the static stress on the splinted part (King, 1993; Schultz-Johnson, 1996).

Torque angle curves provide a consistent method for measuring changes in soft tissues to determine whether splinting is overcoming joint stiffness (Brand, 1995; Breger-Lee et al., 1993). By using a goniometer and a **Haldex gauge** and plotting the data on a graph, a therapist can evaluate the effectiveness of splinting intervention. The Haldex gauge allows the therapist to apply a precise amount of torque for each measurement

(Breger-Lee et al., 1990). The graph displays the joint's response to the force applied with progressive torque on the vertical axis and the range of motion on the horizontal axis. A steep slope of the curve shows the joint is less responsive to splinting than a gradually sloped curve (Flowers & Pheasant, 1988).

Mechanical Principles of Splint Design

The following principles concerning force distribution guide splint design.

Increase the Area of Force Application to Disperse Pressure

Splints apply external forces to the splinted part. Pressure is equal to the amount of force divided by the area of force application (Fess & Philips, 1987; Fess, 1995b). The clinical applications of this principle are: (1) A wide, long splint is more comfortable than a narrow, short one. (2) Contoured pressure over a bone or bony prominence is preferable to uneven or point pressure over the prominence. The therapist must be cautious when padding a splint because it may actually increase a point of pressure if the splint is not well molded to the area.

Increase the Mechanical Advantage to Reduce Pressure and Increase Comfort

The mechanical advantage is the application of parallel force systems with the joint as the axis (A), the distal part

splinted as the resistance (R), the proximal part as the force (F), with the splint acting as a first class lever much like a balanced teeter-totter (Fess & Philips, 1987; Fess, 1995b). Given a constant resistance, the amount of force in the lever system can be decreased by increasing the length of the force arm. In the case of a wrist support splint, the forearm trough is the force arm (FA) and the metacarpal bar serves as the resistance arm (RA) (Fig. 15-8). A longer forearm trough will decrease any pressure caused by the transferred weight of the hand. Mechanical advantage is equal to the FA divided by the RA. In accordance with this principle, the recommended length of the forearm trough is usually two-thirds the length of the forearm (Fig. 15-8). The forearm trough should not be so long as to impede elbow motion, however.

Ensure Three Points of Pressure

The three parallel forces in a first-class lever system, such as a splint, are in equilibrium. The splint acts as a counterforce proximally and distally to the forces of the forearm and hand, respectively. A strap securing the splint at the axis position provides a reciprocal middle force. These parallel reciprocal forces create the three points of pressure (Fess & Philips, 1987, Fess, 1995b). The concept of three points of pressure guides splint design and directs placement of straps for proper force application (Fig. 15-9).

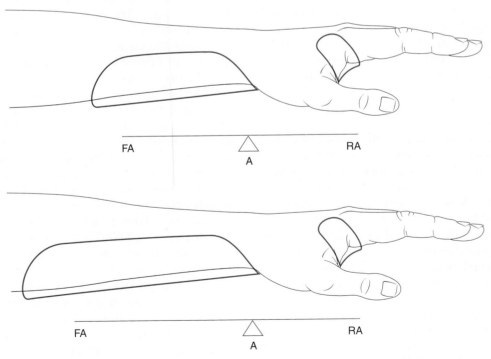

Figure 15-8 Increase the mechanical advantage of the splint by increasing the length of the forearm trough. A, axis; FA, force arm; RA, resistance arm.

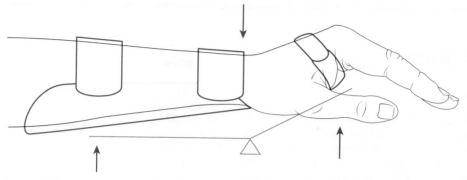

Figure 15-9 Three points of pressure in a wrist support splint.

Add Strength Through Contouring

When a force is applied to a flat piece of material, the material bends. If the same material is molded into a curve, the material can withstand the force more effectively. Contour mechanically increases the material's strength. The splint should follow the contour and extend midway around the part being splinted for maximum comfort and strength (Fess & Philips, 1987). In addition, rounded edges are more comfortable and increase the splint's durability. Curved and contoured edges are preferable to angled or squared edges to conform to the finger lengths, which form a curve, and the other curves throughout the hand, wrist, and forearm.

Perpendicular Traction for Dynamic Splinting

To mobilize a joint through dynamic splinting, the line of pull must be perpendicular to the long axis of the bone being mobilized. Whether using finger loops with an extension outrigger or nail hooks with a flexion pulley, the therapist must maintain a 90° angle of pull to provide the most effective application of force (Fig. 15-10). The perpendicular force application prevents shearing stress and unwanted traction on the joint. As mobility improves, the therapist must make changes in the outrigger to maintain the 90° angle of pull (Fess & Philips, 1987).

Acceptable Pressure for Dynamic Splinting

Forces in dynamic splinting may be applied with rubber bands, elastic thread, or springs (Gyovai & Howell, 1992). The force must not exceed acceptable limits. Low-load forces of 100 to 300g are recommended for dynamic splinting of fingers (Fess, 1995b). Therapists may use lighter forces for the acute stages and heavier forces for treatment of chronic joint contractures (Fess & McCollum, 1998). The therapist must consider the patient's size, condition, and stage of recovery when determining the proper force application. The length and width of the rubber band determine the force of tension. A Haldex gauge (See Resources) can be used in the clinic to determine the exact amount of pressure

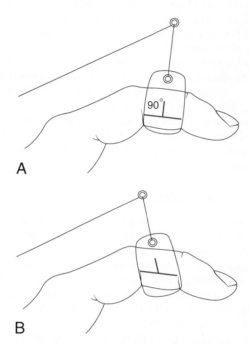

Figure 15-10 Perpendicular angle of pull for dynamic traction: **A.** Correct. **B.** Incorrect.

(force) applied by splinting. Eagerness to achieve results quickly may cause the therapist to use excessive force, which may injure tissue. Effective dynamic splinting of a contracture produces a gain of only 10° per week (Brand, 1995). If dynamic splinting is not enough to remodel tissues or if greater pressure is required, serial casting may be preferable. Serial casts contour intimately to the limb and disperse pressure throughout a larger surface area (Bell-Krotoski & Figarola, 1995).

High- Versus Low-Profile Outriggers

There are advantages and disadvantages to both high- and low-profile outriggers. As improvement occurs, high-profile outriggers generally require fewer adjustments to maintain the 90° angle of pull than the

Case Examples

Mr. J.'s Resting Splint

Mr. J., a 67 year-old right-hand-dominant man, sustained a left cerebral vascular accident with resulting right hemiparesis 3 weeks ago. Prior to the stroke, he was retired but remained active with hobbies, including golf and bridge. When seen by the occupational therapist, he was developing finger flexor hypertonicity that limited his ability to use the limited grasp and release in his right hand. A resting splint was made of Ezeform thermoplastic to hold the fingers and wrist in the maximal extension tolerated. The goal of splinting was to stretch the wrist and finger flexors to allow a more functional position of the hand. Mr. J. wore the splint at night only and performed passive stretch exercises to the finger flexors during the day. He also performed strengthening exercises for the wrist and finger extensors. After 6 months, Mr. J. displayed less flexor tone that limited his active hand use and had developed a more functional pattern of grasp and release. He no longer needed the resting splint. He had regained sufficient grasp and active extension of the fingers to resume his hobbies without modifications.

Mrs. O.'s Thumb (CMC) Splint

Mrs. O. was a 55-year-old right-hand-dominant woman with pain at the base of the right thumb. She had been diagnosed with early osteoarthritis of the trapeziometacarpal joint. Employed as a librarian, she reported pain when grasping books, writing, and turning a key. She also had pain when gardening. A hand-based thumb splint was made of a lightweight perforated thermoplastic (Orfit). Mrs. O. was instructed to wear the splint during activity. She was also instructed in a joint protection program and exercises to perform out of her splint.

She wore the splint at work and applied the joint protection principles at home and in her job. When she was seen for splint strap replacement a year later, Mrs. O. reported that she continued to use the splint for pain at work and in the garden. She also modified her garden tools and used a built-up pen for comfort.

Mr. D.'s Dynamic MCP Extension Assist Splint

Mr. D. was a 29 year-old man who sustained a palmar laceration when cut by sheet metal at work. Six weeks after the superficial wound had healed, he displayed a 45° contracture of the MCP joints, limiting full extension of the fingers. This restricted his ability to lay his hand flat and limited his ability to grasp large objects, jeopardizing resumption of his job in sheet metal fabrication. He had full finger flexion but was limited in grip strength. He was referred to occupational therapy for splinting and exercises. A dorsal wrist cock-up splint of Polyflex II with a dynamic MCP extension assist outrigger supported the fingers in extension while allowing him to use his hand for light functional activities. He was instructed to wear the splint 3 times per day for up to 2 hours as tolerated. As his MCP extension improved, the outrigger was adjusted. Mr. D. also used a static resting splint at night to maintain maximal MCP extension. He was instructed in a home exercise program of stretch and strengthening. Four weeks after he began to wear the dynamic splint, Mr. D.'s MCP extension had improved to within 10° of full extension at the MCP joints. He no longer required use of the dynamic splint, and he returned to his job. He continued to use the static splint at night only for 2 more weeks. At discharge from occupational therapy, he had regained full MCP extension and grip strength. Mr. D. resumed all his previous job duties.

---

low-profile ones (Fess, 1995a,b). Additionally, the high-profile outrigger may require less force to initiate the allowed motion than a low-profile outrigger (Boozer et al., 1994). However, a high-profile outrigger may be cumbersome to the patient returning to work or daily living activities. If a patient has adequate strength of the opposing muscles and can be seen in the clinic for periodic splint adjustment, a low-profile outrigger may be preferable.

Other Considerations in Splinting

Despite the most beautifully designed and constructed hand splint, effectiveness of a splinting program depends on two other factors: compliance and education.

Compliance

Even the most expertly designed and constructed splint will not benefit the patient if the patient does not wear it. Compliance can have a profound influence on the effectiveness of the intervention. Patients' perception of the effectiveness of the splint in achieving the goals of rehabilitation can influence their willingness to wear it (Groth, 1995). Comfort is also an important consideration in ensuring compliance with splint wear. One study showed that patients with rheumatoid arthritis were more compliant with a soft splint than a hard thermoplastic resting splint (Callinan & Mathiowetz, 1996). Comfort means different things to different people. One patient may prefer a lightweight thermoplastic splint, while another is more comfortable with a softly padded splint. The therapist must be attentive to the patient's needs and requests while designing the splint. These considerations should be combined with the therapist's knowledge of the optimal splint design. It is helpful to collaborate with the patient to identify effective options that are acceptable to the patient. Many factors related to design and fabrication can be adjusted to facilitate compliance (Boscheinen-Morrin et al., 1996). Box 15-2 has strategies to increase splint wear compliance.

Education

The therapist must provide adequate instruction to the patient regarding wear and care to ensure proper use of the splint. Patients should be taught the goal and purpose of splinting. It may also be helpful to inform the patients of the consequences of failing to comply with splint wear. Provide written instructions on wear and care. If necessary, provide a diagram of proper application. If the patient has a cognitive deficit, be sure to instruct a caregiver in the proper application of the splint. Include precautions for the patient or caregiver to watch for, including pressure points, edema, and dynamic tension that is too tight. Offer suggestions on adjusting the splint if feasible. Teach the patient how to clean the splint and to keep thermoplastic splints away from heat lest they lose their shape. Make a follow-up visit if you anticipate a change in the patient's status that will necessitate splint modification.

Splint Construction (Box 15-3)

Methods to construct splints from thermoplastic materials are described here. Figures 15-11*A* and 15-12 to 15-20 pertain to a resting splint. Figures 15-11*B* and 15-21 to 15-23 pertain to a hand-based thumb splint. Figures

BOX 15-2
PROCEDURES FOR PRACTICE

Strategies to Increase Splint Wear Compliance

▸ Offer splint options to the patient if possible.
▸ Teach the patient about the benefits of splint wear.
▸ Provide for easy application and removal of the splint.
▸ Make the splint comfortable.
▸ Use a lightweight material if possible.
▸ Immobilize only the joints being treated.
▸ Make the splint cosmetically pleasing to the patient.
▸ If feasible, collaborate with the patient on a wearing schedule.

BOX 15-3
PROCEDURES FOR PRACTICE

Steps of Splint Construction

1. Design splint
2. Select material
3. Make pattern
4. Cut splinting material
5. Heat splinting material
6. Form splint
7. Finish edges
8. Apply straps, padding, and attachments
9. Evaluate the splint for fit and comfort

15-11*C* and 15-24 to 15-29 pertain to a wrist splint serving as a base for a dynamic finger extension outrigger.

Splint Design

Determine the type of splint design by assessing the patient and the clinical condition in reference to the physician's splint order. Consider the goals and purpose of the splint. You can combine this information with an understanding of the patient and any factors that may affect compliance. Also consider relevant cost factors related to custom splint construction. If there is a commercial splint that achieves the same purpose, it may be more cost effective to provide the commercial splint. When time and materials are added up, the custom-made splint is usually more expensive than the commercial splint. However, other factors must be considered in this decision, and cost should not be the only consideration if effectiveness is an issue. Box 15-4 on page 363 has questions to ask when designing the splint.

Material Selection

Selecting the proper material for the splint can be a challenge. It is helpful to become familiar with the properties of various thermoplastics so as to apply the most suitable material for the needs of the patient and the purpose of the splint. You may become biased toward certain materials that are relatively easy to work with, but with experience you will learn to appreciate a variety of materials, each with its own benefits and limitations. Low-temperature thermoplastics have plastic, plastic-like, rubber, or rubberlike bases that give the splinting material its individual characteristics (Breger-Lee, 1995; Breger-Lee & Buford, 1992). Materials with a plastic (polycaprolactone) base, such as Polyform (Smith & Nephew) and NCM Clinic (North Coast Medi-

Text continued on p. 364.

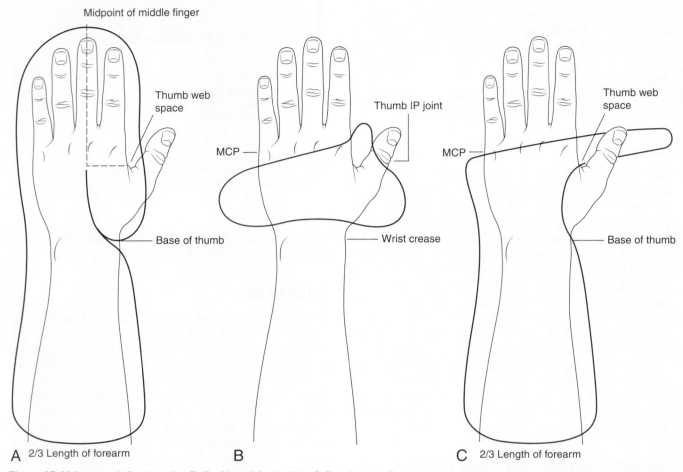

Midpoint of middle finger

Thumb web space

Base of thumb

A   2/3 Length of forearm

MCP

Thumb IP joint

Wrist crease

B

MCP

Thumb web space

Base of thumb

C   2/3 Length of forearm

Figure 15-11 Patterns. **A.** Resting splint. **B.** Hand-based thumb splint. **C.** Dorsal wrist splint.

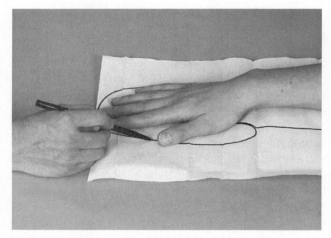

Figure 15-12 Making the pattern for a resting splint on a patient.

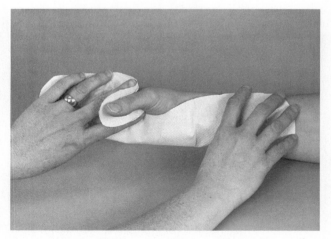

Figure 15-13 Fitting the pattern on the patient.

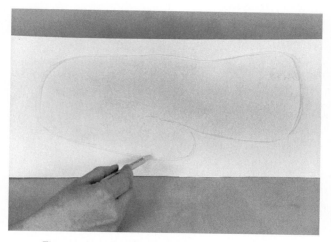

Figure 15-14 Transferring the pattern to thermoplastic.

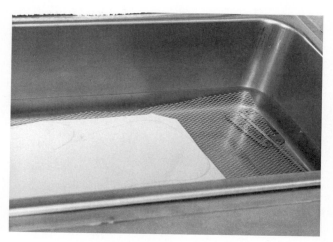

Figure 15-15 Heating the thermoplastic.

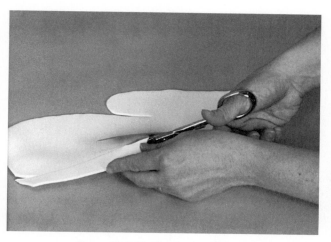

Figure 15-16 Cutting the thermoplastic.

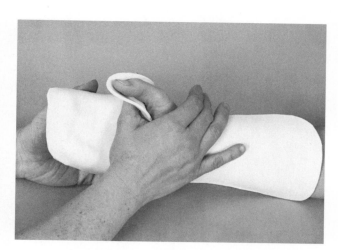

Figure 15-17 Forming the splint on the patient.

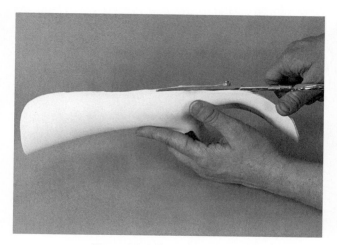

Figure 15-18 Trimming the splint.

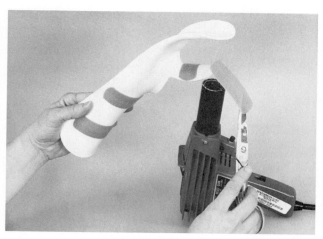

Figure 15-19 Applying straps.

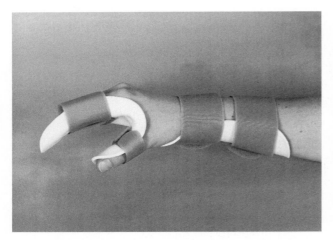

Figure 15-20 Finished resting splint on the patient.

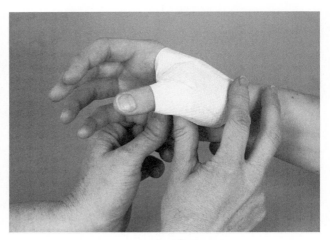

Figure 15-21 Fitting the pattern on the patient for a hand-based thumb splint.

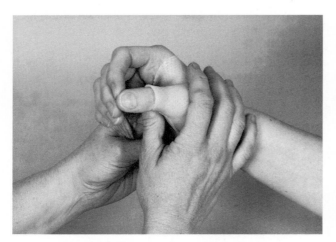

Figure 15-22 Forming the splint on the patient.

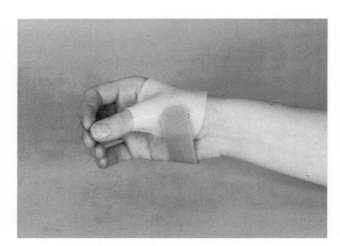

Figure 15-23 Finished splint on the patient.

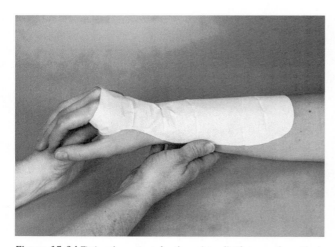

Figure 15-24 Fitting the pattern for the wrist splint base on the patient.

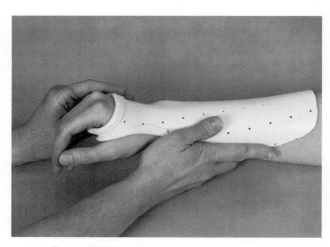

Figure 15-25 Forming the wrist splint on the patient.

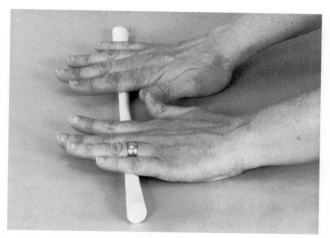

Figure 15-26 Forming the outrigger from splint material scraps.

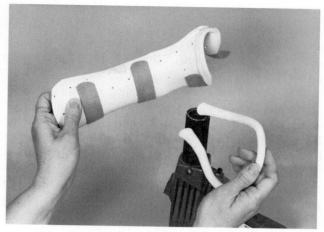

Figure 15-27 Attaching the outrigger to splint base.

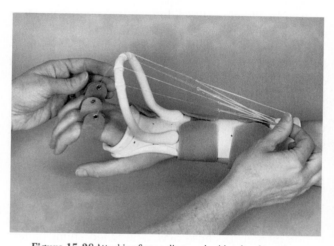

Figure 15-28 Attaching finger slings and rubber band traction.

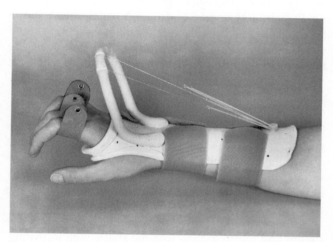

Figure 15-29 Finished dynamic extension outrigger splint on the patient.

BOX 15-4
PROCEDURES FOR PRACTICE

Selecting the Splint Design

- How many joints must be immobilized or mobilized?
- What is the best application? Should the splint be volar or dorsal, ulnar, radial, or circumferential, static or dynamic?
- Should the splint be based on the forearm, hand, finger, or thumb to provide the necessary support for the splinted part?

- Is there a cost-effective commercial splint that achieves the goals?
- Will the patient be able to apply and wear the splint as recommended?
- Which material is best to achieve the purpose of the splint? Does the material affect the design of the splint?

cal) (See Resources for locations of all suppliers) may have fillers that affect their drape and durability. Materials with a rubber (polyisoprene) base, such as Orthoplast (Johnson & Johnson), have less drape and require firmer handling.

An assessment of properties such as rigidity, drape, conformability, surface texture, memory, color, thickness, and perforations help determine the best material for the splint. Table 15-1 outlines some of the properties of various splint materials. The degree of conformability of the splint material determines the handling techniques required (McKee & Morgan, 1998). A material with a high degree of conformability or drape molds easily to the contours of the hand. A material with high conformability is suitable when an intimate contour is desired. However, a material with less drape is preferable in constructing a long arm splint or a splint requiring firm handling techniques. For example, a resting splint for a patient with spasticity may require a high degree of rigidity with low degree of drape. A material with a rubberlike base, such as Ezeform (Smith & Nephew) provides the necessary rigidity without drape, allowing the therapist to use firm handling techniques for fabrication.

The surface texture may also be an important consideration. Some materials have a shiny, smooth surface, while others have texture. Some materials are susceptible to fingerprints. Usually the therapist can control fingerprints by using a smooth, gentle, stroking technique during molding. Some materials have a coating on the surface that resists adhesion. This coating must be removed with a solvent or by scraping the surface before attaching straps or other permanent attachments.

Some materials have memory that allows them to stretch and return to their original shape with reheating. These materials are usually translucent and become transparent when heated to the desired temperature. One example is Aquaplast (Smith & Nephew), which also comes in bright colors.

Many splinting materials are available in a variety of colors. This may be beneficial for ensuring compliance with splint wear in children and teenagers. Allowing patients to select their splint color may improve compliance. Not everybody likes colored splints, however. Many patients prefer a neutral tone. Flesh-tone colors are available in various shades of beige, brown, and black.

Splint materials are also available in a variety of thicknesses. The most commonly used thicknesses are 0.125 and 0.0625 inch. The 0.125-inch material is preferred for rigid forearm-based splints, while the 0.0625-inch material is best suited for hand-based and finger-based splints and circumferential designs. Thinner materials produce lighter-weight splints, which may be better tolerated by some patients. Perforations also affect the weight and rigidity of a splint (McKee & Morgan,

1998). Perforations also provide ventilation, which is especially beneficial in warm weather. Perforations range from microperforation to maxiperforation in some thermoplastics.

Soft, lightweight splint materials are also available. The disadvantages of these splints may be their bulk, lack of rigidity, and relatively short durability (Breger-Lee & Buford, 1991). Soft materials, such as leather, elasticized fabric (Schultz-Johnson, 1992), neoprene (Clark, 1997), silicone rubber (Canelon, 1995; Canelon & Karus, 1995), soft padded fabric with a thermoplastic insert (Callinan & Mathiowetz, 1996), and strapping material (Byron, 1994) may be used for splinting. These materials provide light restriction, which may be desirable for patients who do not tolerate hard thermoplastic splints or for musicians and athletes attempting to reduce harmful motion while continuing to play. The therapist should consider the patient's tolerance to any material being used in splinting. Sensitivity to various materials, such as an allergic contact dermatitis to neoprene (Stern et al., 1998) has been reported in the literature.

High-temperature thermoplastics are also available for rigid splinting. They require use of a band saw for cutting and an oven for heating (Fess & Philips, 1987). These high-temperature thermoplastics have high-impact strength and rigidity but do not contour well, which makes them generally not suitable for hand splinting.

Pattern Making

Once you have decided on the appropriate splint design and material, you will make a pattern. This is an important step because a well-designed splint pattern usually leads to a well-fitting splint. The pattern provides a two-dimensional guide for the three-dimensional splint. The pattern also helps to minimize waste of splint material. Patterns for many commonly prescribed splints are available in splinting textbooks and from splint material manufacturers. Three commonly prescribed splint patterns are demonstrated here (Fig. 15-11). Paper toweling provides an excellent moldable pattern, but any type of paper can be used for the pattern. Place the patient's hand directly on the paper and mark the anatomical landmarks according to the design being used (Fig. 15-12). The pattern must extend beyond the lateral borders of the hand and forearm to allow the splint to form a shallow trough, which will extend halfway around the surface being splinted for adequate support. Extend the forearm trough two-thirds of the length of the forearm. Once the pattern is drawn, cut it out and place it on the patient in the design of the splint (Fig. 15-13 for the resting pan splint, Fig. 15-21 for the thumb splint, and Fig. 15-24 for the dynamic finger

TABLE 15-1
Performance Properties of Selected Low-Temperature Thermoplastics

	Working Temperature	Rigidity Strength	Shrink	Stretch	Drape	Conform Moldable	Bond	Memory	Prints	Comments
Plastic										
NCM Clinic/Precision Splint/RS 3000 (oyster color) (Northcoast/Polymed)	160–170°F	3	1	3	3	3	3	2	3	Easy to work and contour
Polyform/Kay splint (Rolyan/Sammons)	150–160°F	2	1	2+	3	3	3	1	3	Easy to work, mold; do not overheat
Ultraform (Sammons)	160°F	2	2	2	3	2	2	1	2	Nice feel, texture
Aquaplast, Blue Stripe (WFR/Aquaplast)	160–180°F	2	2	3+	3	3	3	2	1	Better cut pattern while translucent
Orthoplast II (Johnson & Johnson)	150–170°F	2	1	3	2	2	3	1	2	Looks, behaves like Multiform
Multiform I & II (Alimed)	150–180°F	3	2	3	3	2	3	1	3–	Inexpensive, easy to work
Plastic and Rubberlike										
NCM Preferred/Custom Splint/JU1000 (Beige) (Northcoast/Polymed)	160–170°F	3	1	2	3	2	2	1	2	Versatile; skin rash w/perspiration
Ultraform 294 (Sammons)	160°F	3	1	1	1	1	2	2	1	Difficult to form
Polyflex II/Kay Splint, Isoprene (Rolyan/Sammons)	160°F	2	1	3	3	3	2	1	2	Good for large, small orthoses; scraps recyclable
Aquaplast (WFR/Aquaplast)	160–180°F	2	3	3	3	3	3	3	2	Need work w/edges, for experienced splint makers
Orfit Soft* (Northcoast)	160–180°F	2	2	3	3	3	3	3	2	Similar to Aquaplast; shrinks less when allowed to cool on patient
Rubberlike										
NCM Spectrum/Ultrasplint/MR 2000 (white) (Northcoast/Polymed)	170°F	2	1	1	1	2	2	1	1+	Reshapes, rolls edges easily
Ezeform/Kay Splint III (Rolyan/Sammons)	170°F	3	1	1	1	2	3	1	1	Good for large orthoses; easy trim edge
Watercolors by Aquaplast (WFR/Aquaplast)	160–180°F	2	2	2	2	3	3	3	2	Great colors, contours nicely
Aquaplast, green stripe (WFR/Aquaplast)	160–180°F	2	2	2	1	2	2	3	1	Less conforming but more rigid for large orthoses
Orfit, Stiff (Northcoast)	135°F	3	2	2	1	2	3	3	1	Increased thickness good for large orthoses
Synergy (Rolyan)	160°F	2	1	1	1	2	1	2	1	Attractive, nice feel; takes effort to contour

(continued)

TABLE 15-1
Performance Properties of Selected Low-Temperature Thermoplastics (Continued)

	Working Temperature	Rigidity Strength	Shrink	Stretch	Drape	Conform Moldable	Bond	Memory	Prints	Comments
RUBBER										
Orthoplast (Johnson & Johnson)	160°F	1	1	1	1	1	3	2	1	Good edges, worse contour
Ultraform Traditions (Sammons)	160°F	2	2						2	Not tested

3, high; 2, moderate (bonds with solvent); 1, little or none. Orfit is not available in the standard 0.125-in. (0.3175-cm) thickness. Orfit soft (0.135-in thick, approximately 0.343 cm) was used to closely approximate the standard thickness as much as possible. Orfit stiff measured 0.164 in. (approximately 0.417 cm).

Note: These ratings are based either on observational and tested data derived at the Gillis W. Long Hansen's Disease Center or from the referenced sources.

(Reprinted with permission from Breger-Lee, D., & Buford, W. E. Jr. [1991]. Update in Splinting Materials and Methods. *Hand Clinics, 7*, 569–585.)

extension outrigger splint). If it fits perfectly, transfer it to the splinting material. If it needs modification, modify it by cutting the pattern down or adding a piece of paper for extra length or width as needed. Check the pattern on the patient to see if it blocks any joints unnecessarily. The splint pattern can be cut back to reduce this restriction if necessary. If the patient is unable to lay the hand flat for pattern drawing because of deformity or spasticity, use the uninvolved hand for pattern making and flip the pattern over for the contralateral side. You can adjust the pattern for edema or any other variation before transferring the pattern.

Transfer the pattern to the splinting material by tracing it onto the plastic (Fig. 15-14). A wax pencil is easy to see and erases easily. An awl can also be used to scratch the pattern onto the plastic. If using a pen or pencil, cut away the marks as you cut out the splint.

Cutting

With a full sheet of splinting material, it is best to cut it to a size that will fit the pattern. Cut the full sheet with a utility knife by scoring it and bending it, then turning the sheet over and scoring it again from the other side. This provides a manageable sheet of thermoplastic. Heat the thermoplastic once the splint pattern is marked (Fig. 15-15). When the material is soft, cut the splint out with sharp straight-edge scissors (Fig. 15-16). By cutting the material after heating, you eliminate the rough edges, which saves time in the finishing step. Hold the material horizontally while cutting to avoid overstretching it. Excessive handling of material can cause fingerprinting. To minimize this problem, lightly hold the material on the edges that will be cut away. Curved scissors may help in cutting out hard-to-reach curved areas.

Precut splinting blanks are available for commonly used patterns. Considering the time to trace and cut the pattern out of a full sheet of splinting material and the potential for wasting material, precut materials may be cost-effective.

Heating Splinting Material

Electric fry pans, splint pans, and hydrocollators can be used to heat the thermoplastic material (Fig. 15-15). It is recommended that the water be at least 1 inch deep if using a fry pan. If using a hydrocollator, be careful not to let the material overstretch or drop to the bottom. Heat pan liners may be helpful with a hydrocollator. The recommended temperature varies between materials (Table 15-1). It is usually best to keep the water at 150 to 160° for most materials. Consult the manufacturer's recommendations for specific materials. Use a thermometer in the water to ensure consistent temperature. The

heating time for most materials is about 1 minute. The therapist should check the material to make sure it is heated uniformly before forming the splint on the patient. The working time for splinting materials also varies. Some of the thinner thermoplastics (0.0625 inch) cool in 1 to 2 minutes. Most of the thicker materials (0.125-inch) have a 3- to 6-minute working time. Since heat guns do not uniformly soften splinting material, they are recommended only for spot heating, minor adjustments, and edge finishing.

Forming the Splint

Once the entire piece of thermoplastic is heated, carefully remove it from the water with a spatula or tongs. The entire piece should feel soft and easily moldable. Lay the material on a towel to dry briefly. If you are rolling the edges to finish them, do so before forming the splint on the patient. Check the temperature of the plastic before placing it on the patient. If the material is too hot, let it cool slightly for the patient's tolerance and comfort. After placing the patient's hand in the desired position, place the splint material on the patient (Figs. 15-17, 15-22, and 15-25). When using a material with draping qualities, it is best to let gravity assist the positioning. If the splint is based on the volar surface, position the hand in supination or a neutral posture. If the splint is dorsal, place the hand in pronation. Because the wrist posture changes slightly in pronation and supination, check the fit of the splint in both these postures before it cools completely. Using smooth and gentle strokes, contour the splint over the arches and bony prominences of the hand. Try not to grip or squeeze the thermoplastic. Materials with a high degree of drape and conformability, such as Polyform, Polyflex II (Smith & Nephew Rolyan), NCM Preferred, and Contour (North Coast Medical), require relatively little handling. Materials with controlled stretch, such as Omega (North Coast Medical), Ezeform, and Synergy (Smith & Nephew Rolyan), require a firmer pressure to create contours and maintain their shape. If making a splint on a spastic extremity or an uncooperative patient, you can use an elastic bandage to assist in holding the splint in place while molding.

When splinting the thumb to allow functional use, it is helpful to have the patient hold a pen lightly or hold the thumb in prehension while the splint is being formed (Fig. 15-22). This ensures functional positioning. At this time it is important to check for any motion that may be unnecessarily restricted. Changes can be made while the splint is forming to reduce any restriction. This is also a good time to check bony prominences for any pressure areas. Light finger pressure can push the material out away from the prominence by rounding out these areas and creating more space for the ulnar styloid or other areas of pressure. You may wish to place a small piece of putty or foam over prominences before splint molding to allow for this enlargement.

While the splint is on the patient, mark the lateral borders if additional material is to be cut away. While the splint is still slightly warm, use your fingernail to mark the trough of the splint so that it extends midway around the forearm. You can also mark distal and proximal edges in this manner and cut away the excess while the material is slightly warm (Fig. 15-18). The warmth facilitates cutting and leaves a nicely finished edge. Flare the proximal edge of the splint away from the skin to prevent a pressure point during wear.

Edge Finishing

Smooth edges are important to prevent pressure points. Cutting the material at the required temperature allows the edges to seal smoothly and not require additional attention. However, with some perforated materials or rough-cut thermoplastics, it may be necessary to smooth the edges. You can achieve a smooth edge by dipping the edge of the splint into the hot water and cutting it to produce a smooth edge or by smoothing it lightly with fingertip pressure after heating it with the heat gun briefly. *The heat gun produces a very hot stream of dry heat. It should never be directed toward the patient's skin*. Remember to set the heat gun on a cool setting before turning it off to avoid damage to the motor. You can eliminate the edge finishing step by cutting the edges so they seal or by rolling edges back after heating the thermoplastic before applying it to the patient. If edges remain slightly rough, you can apply a thin piece of moleskin along the edge to seal it for comfort.

Application of Straps

Straps attach the splint to the patient. Their location must be carefully planned to maintain the best contact with the splint and to provide three-point pressure. Apply adhesive-hook Velcro to the splint and attach the soft-brush Velcro or other foam strapping material to hold the splint securely on the patient. Hook Velcro adheres most effectively if the surface of the splint is prepared for adhesion. Remove the nonstick finish on the thermoplastic by applying a solvent or by scraping the plastic with the sharp edge of the scissors. Then briefly spot-heat the surface of the splint and the sticky side of the Velcro with a heat gun (Fig. 15-19). It is best to place a full piece of sticky-back Velcro on the splint rather than two small pieces on the edges, as repeated pull on the pieces during release of the strap may cause

them to peel off. Strapping materials include colored Velcro, durable foam, and elastic strapping in a variety of widths. Choose the strapping that best secures the splint to the patient comfortably. It is best to round the corners of the strapping material to avoid bending and dog ears (Fig. 15-20).

Padding

To enhance wearing tolerance, you can pad the splint. When padding a splint, allow extra space at the design and molding phase to contour over a bony prominence, avoiding additional pressure in this area. Some padding is applied before forming the splint, some afterward. If the padding is applied to the splinting material before heating, the excess water should be squeezed out before applying the material to the patient. Some thermoplastic material is available with a layer of padding already bonded to it. You can use stockinette liners instead of padding if light protection is desired. Prefabricated cotton or synthetic liners are available commercially. The patient may appreciate use of a light, washable stockinette under the splint to absorb perspiration. Sticky-back moleskin is also available for a thin, soft padding material. Padding should never substitute for a well-fitting splint however. Silicone gel can be used in splints to reduce slippage and to enhance scar remodeling.

Attachments

Outriggers and pulleys can be attached to splints when the splint base is complete. An outrigger provides a base for positioning the 90° angle of pull for dynamic splints or for directing a static progressive force. It can be made by rolling thermoplastic into a tube (Fig. 15-26), by using prefabricated tubes, or by bending wire to the desired position (Coppard & Lohman, 1996). Commercial outriggers are available in high- and low-profile designs. Safety pins and paper clips can also be used for finger outriggers or pulleys (Byron, 1997). When attaching an outrigger or pulley, prepare the surface of the splint first for optimal adhesion by scraping the surface or applying solvent. The outrigger or pulley attachment points should be treated similarly. Using dry heat with a heat gun, heat the surfaces and press them together (Fig. 15-27). They must be held together briefly to ensure adequate bonding. They should not be moved at this time unless repositioning is desired. If the pieces need additional reinforcement, heat another piece of thermoplastic and apply it over the outrigger base attachment. Again, prepare surfaces with dry heat and press them together for effective bonding. Some commercial outriggers can be attached with specially designed thumbscrews.

Dynamic splints may be prone to slide distally because of the traction on the splint. You can control this migration by applying a friction surface on the splint that is in contact with the skin. Microfoam tape (available through Smith & Nephew) has a soft, padded surface that provides light traction to keep the splint in place.

The tension of a dynamic splint is provided by rubber bands, coil springs, or elastic thread. You can attach these to the splint with Velcro tabs, hooks, thumbscrews, or knobs placed proximal to the outrigger on the splint base. Pulleys or line guides can redirect the line of pull as needed for dynamic flexion splinting. Monofilament (fishing line) attached to the rubber band creates a smooth excursion for the rubber band tension as it pulls over the outrigger or under the pulley. The monofilament attaches to a finger sling (Fig. 15-28) or fingernail hook or tab to provide the appropriate tension and 90° angle of pull.

Dynamic splints may incorporate hinges, which provide a movable axis at a joint. Hinges are available commercially or can be made from rivets (Byron, 1994), crimped thermoplastic tubing, or brass fasteners (Dennys et al., 1992).

Evaluating Splint Fit and Comfort

After the splint is finished, have the patient wear it for about 20 minutes and remove it to check for any redness. Redness or blanching of the skin may be an indication that the pressure of the splint is too much (Brand, 1995).

Modify the splint if signs of redness or excessive pressure are present. Then reevaluate fit and comfort (Box 15-5).

Technology is changing rapidly. New materials offer new possibilities for the splinting therapist. By combining skill and creativity with knowledge of new technology and the patient's needs, the therapist can meet the challenges of the future by applying principles of splinting to meet the goals of rehabilitation.

Summary Review Questions

1. Name the steps of splint making in order.
2. Name the creases of the hand and describe their importance in splint construction.
3. What is the difference between the functional position of the hand and the position of safe immobilization in splinting? Give an example of when you would use each.
4. Describe the concept of dual obliquity as applied to splinting.
5. What does *mechanical advantage* mean in splinting? How does it apply to the length of the forearm trough?
6. What are some strategies to enhance compliance with splint wear?
7. Which material would be a good choice for a hand-based thumb splint? Why?
8. What does a splint checkout include?

Acknowledgments

I thank my family, Joe, Sarah, Jacob, and Katie, and my colleagues for their inspiration, support, and encouragement while writing this chapter.

Resources

Alimed Inc. · 297 High Street, Dedham, MA 02026-9135. 800-225-2610. Fax 800-437-2966
www.alimed.com

Johnson & Johnson Orthopaedics, Inc. · New Brunswick, NJ

North Coast Medical, Inc. · 18305 Sutter Blvd., Morgan Hill, CA 95037. 800-821-9319. Fax 877-213-9300
www.ncmedical.com

Polymed Industries, Inc. · Baltimore, MD

Sammons Preston Inc. · 4 Sammons Court, Boling Brook, IL 60440. 800-323-5547. Fax: 800-547-4333
www.sammonspreston.com

Smith & Nephew, Inc. · One Quality Drive, P.O. Box 1005, Germantown, WI 53022. 800-228-3693. Fax 414-253-3066
www.smithnephew.com

BOX 15-5
PROCEDURES FOR PRACTICE

Splint Checkout

Review the splint using these questions as guidelines:

- Does the splint achieve the purpose?
- Does the splint maintain the proper position of the joints? Check angles with a goniometer if necessary.
- Does the splint fit the contours of the hand, the arches, and bony prominences?
- Does the splint restrict or immobilize any joint unnecessarily?
- Is the splint long enough to support the splinted part?
- Are all edges smooth and all possible pressure points relieved?
- Does the splint allow functional use of the hand if allowed?
- Can the patient apply and remove the splint?
- Does the patient understand wear and care instructions?
- Is the splint cosmetically acceptable to the patient?

UE TECH · P.O. Box 2145, Edwards, CO, 81632. 800-736-1894. Fax 970-926-8870

www.uetech.com

WFR/Aquaplast Corp. · Wyckoff, NJ

References

Bell-Krotoski, J. A., & Figarola, J. H. (1995). Biomechanics of soft-tissue growth and remodeling with plaster casting. *Journal of Hand Therapy, 8* (2), 131–137.

Bonutti, P. M., Windau, J. E., Ables, B. A., & Miller, B. G. (1994). Static progressive stretch to reestablish elbow range of motion. *Clinical Orthopedics and Related Research 303*, 128–134.

Boscheinen-Morrin, J., Davey, V., & Conolly, W. B. (1996). *The Hand: Fundamentals of Therapy* (2nd ed., pp. 238–266). Oxford, UK: Butterworth-Heinemann.

Brand, P. (1995). The forces of dynamic splinting: Ten questions before applying a dynamic splint to the hand. In J. Hunter, E. Mackin, & A. Callahan (Eds.), *Rehabilitation of the Hand* (4th ed., pp. 1581–1587). St. Louis: Mosby–Year Book.

Breger-Lee, D. (1995). Objective and subjective observations of low-temperature thermoplastic materials. *Journal of Hand Therapy, 8* (2), 138–143.

Breger-Lee, D., Bell-Krotoski, J., & Brandsma, J. W. (1990). Torque range of motion in the hand clinic. *Journal of Hand Therapy, 3* (1), 7–13.

Breger-Lee, D. E., & Buford, W. E. Jr. (1991). Update in splinting materials and methods. *Hand Clinics, 7*, 569–585.

Breger-Lee, D. E., & Buford, W. L. Jr. (1992). Properties of thermoplastic splinting materials. *Journal of Hand Therapy, 5* (4), 202–211.

Breger-Lee, D. E., Voelker, E. T., Giurintano, D., Novick, A., & Browder, L. (1993). Reliability of torque range of motion: A preliminary study. *Journal of Hand Therapy 6* (1), 29–34.

Boozer, J. A., Sanson, M. S., Soutas-Little, R. W., Coale, E. H., Jr., Pierce, T. D., & Swanson, A. B. (1994). Comparison of the biomechanical motions and forces involved in high-profile versus low-profile dynamic splinting. *Journal of Hand Therapy, 7* (3), 171–182.

Bunnell, S. (1996). Splinting the hand. *Hand Clinics, 12* (1), 173–178.

Byron, P. (1994). Splinting the arthritic hand. *Journal of Hand Therapy, 7* (1), 29–32.

Byron, P. (1997). The Rotterdam splint. *Journal of Hand Therapy, 10* (3), 240–241.

Callinan, N. J., & Mathiowetz, V. (1996). Soft versus hard resting hand splints in rheumatoid arthritis: Pain relief, preference, and compliance. *American Journal of Occupational Therapy, 50*, 347–353.

Canelón, M. F. (1995). Silicone rubber splinting for hand and wrist injuries. *Journal of Hand Therapy, 8* (4), 252–257.

Canelón, M. F., & Karus, A. J. (1995). A room temperature vulcanizing silicone rubber sport splint. *American Journal of Occupational Therapy, 49*, 244–249.

Clark, E. N. (1997). A preliminary investigation of the neoprene tube finger extension splint. *Journal of Hand Therapy, 10* (3), 213–221.

Coppard, B. M., & Lohman, H. (1996). Introduction to splinting: A critical-thinking and problem solving approach. St. Louis: Mosby–Year Book.

Dennys, L. J., Hurst, L. N., & Cox, J. (1992). Management of proximal interphalangeal joint fractures using a new dynamic traction splint and early active motion. *Journal of Hand Therapy, 5* (1), 16–24.

Fess, E. E. (1995a). Principles and methods of splinting for mobilization of joints. In J. Hunter, E. Mackin, & A. Callahan (Eds.), *Rehabilitation of the Hand* (4th ed., pp. 1589–1598). St. Louis: Mosby-Year Book.

Fess, E. E. (1995b). Splints: Mechanics versus convention. *Journal of Hand Therapy, 8* (2), 124–130.

Fess, E. E., & McCollum, M. (1998). The influence of splinting on healing tissues. *Journal of Hand Therapy, 11* (2), 157–161.

Fess, E. E., & Philips, C. A. (1987). *Hand Splinting: Principles and Methods* (2nd ed.). St. Louis: Mosby.

Flowers, K. R., & LaStayo, P. (1994). Effect of total end range time on improving passive range of motion. *Journal of Hand Therapy, 7* (3), 150–157.

Flowers, K. R., & Pheasant, S. D. (1988). The use of torque angle curves in the assessment of digital joint stiffness. *Journal of Hand Therapy, 1* (1), 69–74.

Groth, G. N., & Wulf, M. B. (1995). Compliance with hand rehabilitation: Health beliefs and strategies. *Journal of Hand Therapy, 8* (1), 18–22.

Gyovai, J. E., & Howell, J. W. (1992). Validation of spring forces applied in dynamic outrigger splinting. *Journal of Hand Therapy, 5* (1), 8–15.

King, J. W. (1993). Modification of common treatments in hand rehabilitation. *Journal of Hand Therapy, 6* (3), 214–217.

McKee, P., & Morgan, L. (1998). *Orthotics in rehabilitation*. Philadelphia: Davis.

Schultz-Johnson, K. (1996). Splinting the wrist: Mobilization and protection. *Journal of Hand Therapy , 9* (2), 165–175.

Stern, E. B., Callinan, N., Hank, M., Lewis, E. J., Schousboe, J. T., & Ytterberg, S. R. (1998). Neoprene splinting: Dermatological issues. *American Journal of Occupational Therapy, 52*, 573–578.

Tubiana, R., Thomine, J.-M., & Mackin, E. (1996). *Examination of the Hand and Wrist*. St. Louis: Mosby-Year Book.

Weiss, N. D., Gordon, L., Bloom, T., So, Y., & Rempel, D. M. (1995). Position of the wrist associated with the lowest carpal tunnel pressure: Implications for splint design. *Journal of Bone and Joint Surgery, 77A*, 1695–1699.

16
Wheelchair Selection

Brian J. Dudgeon and Jean C. Deitz

LEARNING OBJECTIVES

After studying this chapter, the reader will be able to do the following:

1. Describe the factors that should be considered in wheelchair selection and explain how they interrelate.
2. Describe the three basic types of wheelchairs and reasons for each to be chosen.
3. Specify measurements typically taken to determine wheelchair and related seating system configurations for a particular individual.
4. Demonstrate knowledge of the components common to many wheelchairs and describe why each merits consideration in wheelchair selection.
5. Discuss the roles and responsibilities of the occupational therapist in wheelchair selection.
6. Suggest how the occupational therapist can facilitate the user's participation in wheelchair selection.

- Sense of self-efficacy and self-esteem
- Satisfaction with life roles
  - Self-maintenance
  - Self-advancement
  - Self-enhancement
- Competence in tasks of life roles
- Activities and habits
- Abilities and skills
- Developed capacities
- First-level capacities
- Organic substrate

"Mobility is a fundamental part of living. Being able to move about, to explore, under one's volitional control is a keystone of independence" (Warren, 1990).

*M*obility is a major part of daily living, facilitating participation in home, work and community settings. Wheelchairs are a focal point for many people with mobility impairments. As such, wheelchair selection and training necessitate consideration of the user's preferences and current and anticipated performance needs, capacities, and environments. The process of evaluating and choosing a wheelchair system as part of functional mobility involves the user, an interdisciplinary team, and equipment suppliers or vendors. Also, family members, primary care providers, and others from the user's work and leisure environments may contribute important information useful in

GLOSSARY

Angle in space—Angle of the seat back in relation to the true vertical when the seat and back are rotated counterclockwise as a unit. Sometimes called orientation, this position may be altered for postural control.

Camber—The amount of angle on the wheels, creating flare-out at the bottom. A 4-6° camber is recommended for push rim convenience and wheelchair width.

Pelvic rotation and obliquity—Asymmetrical position of the pelvis with forward position of one side and/or uneven level of anterior superior iliac spines and ischial tuberosities associated with spinal scoliosis, hip abnormality, or pelvic deformity.

Proximity-sensing systems—Systems that remotely sense the position of a body part (e.g., head) and use that position to control the wheelchair without physical contact between the part of the body used for control and the switch.

Scanning—Control option that presents choices one at a time, grouped or singly, until the desired choice is offered for the user to select by switch activation.

Seat-back angle—The angle of the seat surface relative to the back surface. This angle is typically 90 to 100°. Backrest angles and seat plane angles may be designated separately.

Sip and puff—A system typically involving a dual-action switch, in which one action is controlled by the user sipping on a tube held in the mouth and the second action is controlled by puffing on the same tube. (In wheelchair operation the chair functions can be controlled by patterns of switch closures.)

Third-party payer—Individual or organization (i.e., insurance company) other than the person receiving services that pays for services.

choosing an appropriate wheelchair to meet needs for mobility within and between environments.

Wheelchair selection has a functional orientation that considers multiple factors including the user's (1) needs and goals; (2) home, work, recreational, and other community environments; (3) physical and mental status and anticipated course of impairments; (4) financial and community resources; (5) views about appearance and social acceptability; and (6) interface of the wheelchair system with other assistive technology. Selection issues include current and changing needs of the user and family, training needs for use and maintenance, and anticipated advances in technology. A wide range of wheelchair options are available, but funding and community-based resources for training and servicing of mobility devices often restrict choices.

Some individuals use wheelchairs only occasionally to meet brief transportation needs, while others use them continuously to meet most day-to-day positioning and mobility demands. Especially in the latter case, the events that lead to the need for a wheelchair may be dramatic. For some, acquiring a wheelchair system may create stress or confusion, and this can hinder their contributions to the assessment of needs and selection of a system. Others view the acquisition of a wheelchair as a positive move toward greater independence and freedom, and they make substantial efforts to become informed about choices. In either case, the needs of the user are central to the overall process of selection, prescription, and training, with the wheelchair viewed not just as a means for mobility but as a highly personal

device to be chosen with care and precision (Steins, 1998).

To contribute to the selection, the occupational therapist must have a thorough understanding of the user's personal profile and medical needs, including environment, daily routines, and goals. In addition, the therapist should understand the seating and positioning needs of the individual, wheelchair types, control mechanisms, features, and accessories. Though this information is presented as components, all of these factors interrelate in comprehensive planning for functional mobility through a clinical reasoning process.

Evaluation of the Individual

During evaluation, primary attention is given to user and family goals for use of the wheelchair as part of a comprehensive functional mobility system. Further, the therapist evaluates the skills of the user, the user's ability to develop new skills, and changes expected from the diagnosis (e.g., increased motor impairment). How the user plans to transport the system is also an important consideration. Evaluation of needs should include interview, observation, and examination. Trials with mock seating configurations, control systems and/or self-propulsion methods are often needed to confirm appropriate prescription of these systems. Figure 16-1 outlines evaluation needs; patient-specific information relates to the case example.

The evaluation typically involves both sitting posture and mobility needs. The therapist can best assist in seating and wheelchair selection by understanding the client's personal and medical profiles (Behrman, 1990).

Personal Profile

The client's personal profile includes factors such as age and stature, developmental status, living environment, educational or work planning, recreational pursuits, and other assistive technology needs or uses. Special attention is given to seating and operation of the chair in both private and public environments. Specifically, the therapist should consider factors such as floor surfaces, outdoor terrain, climate, doorways, hall spaces, restroom dimensions, workspace design, transportability, and parking. If a client has used a wheelchair before, it is important for the therapist to determine the user's assessment of pros and cons regarding that wheelchair system. Therapists should recognize that public accessibility is based in part on engineering concepts in which the typical wheelchair user sits at a 19-inch height and propels a manual wheelchair that is 32 inches wide and 48 inches long (Allan & Moffett, 1992). Many people are served well by environmental designs that accommodate this type of user, but others continue to be

---

Sample Wheelchair Evaluation: Needs of the Individual

Client information: Lisa, 17-year-old high-school senior with recent C7 level tetraplegia from traumatic SCI in MVC. Attends evaluation with mother. Inpatient stay in acute rehabilitation unit.

Functional Needs and Goals

Environments of use (home, school, work, community at large): Full-time at home, at school, and in other community locations. Has interest in athletics, high school programs.

Seating needs (time, pressure relief, transfers): Postural support needs for trunk and thighs, cushioning for neurogenic skin. Able to perform push-up pressure relief and independent transfers to/from wheelchair.

Control or propulsion methods (attendant, manual needs, power controls): With postural support and seat belt, self-propels using friction push rims and wheel brakes. May benefit from grade aids for propelling up inclines.

Methods of wheelchair transport (car, van, truck; ground travel, air travel): Family owns full-sized truck and minivan. Lisa has driver's license but has not yet explored or been oriented to adaptive driving.

Physical Examination

Head control: No limitations in mobility when trunk is stabilized.

Sitting balance and spinal deformity: Now Using TLSO.

Pelvic rotation or obliquity: Symmetrical at this time, mobile pelvis, lumbar support through TLSO.

Lower limb mobility: Full PROM, flaccid at rest with periodic spasms into hip adduction, knee extension and ankle plantarflexion. Neurogenic skin below C8 level.

Upper limb mobility: Full PROM, good to normal strength in shoulder, elbow flexion 5/5, extension 4/5, forearm rotation 4/5, wrist extension 4/5, flexion 3/5, finger extension 3/5. Neurogenic skin lateral hand, 4th and 5th fingers.

Wheelchair Sizing Measurements (Fig. 16-2)
Sitting and Balance Needs

Postural support: Now using TLSO for stability, lateral trunk supports for midline positioning. Seat belt and chest harness necessary for support and safety. Explore back cushion contouring when/if TLSO is discontinued.

Cushioning: Solid base of support needed with cushion contour. Tried low-profile Roho and Jay Cushion. Lisa preferred latter for balance, good cushioning effects.

Wheelchair Training Needs

Control or propulsion: Manual propulsion with seating components in place. Enlarged and rubberized friction rim tried and preferred over plain rim or knobs. Wheel camber may assist in hand placement. Needs training for propulsion on level surfaces, maneuvering corners and doorways, all outdoor settings.

Transfers to and from wheelchair and chair, bed, toilet, bathing tub or shower, floor, car: Is beginning transfer training wheelchair to bed using sliding board. Removable armrests and swing-away footrests will enable independence. Will need car transfer training, tub transfer, and floor to wheelchair instruction later.

Wheelchair Maintenance Resources
Lisa expresses interest in learning maintenance routine; father willing to assist as reported by Lisa and her mother. Wheelchair vendor within 15 miles of family home.

Figure 16-1 Evaluation overview. Clinicians address these issues by interview, observation, and physical examination. SCI, spinal cord injury; MVC, motor vehicle collision; TLSO, thoraco-lumbar-sacral-orthosis; PROM, passive range of motion.

constrained by the environment and need individual guidance about making appropriate accommodations. For example, some power wheelchairs have a larger turning radius or excessive weight that limits the user's access to some buildings and/or transportation systems.

Medical Profile

The medical profile includes the user's medical history and physical assessment. The physical assessment should focus on neuromuscular status (e.g., muscle tone, postural control, reflexes, and coordination), musculoskeletal status (e.g., range of motion, deformity, strength, and endurance), sensory status (e.g., anesthetic skin and skin integrity), and physiological status (e.g., temperature regulation, respiration, and cardiopulmonary needs). The therapist should be aware of the client's diagnosis and prognosis, that is, whether the medical condition is temporary, stable, or progressive. Such factors influence choices related to complexity of options and needs for adjustment as well as options for rental, lease, or purchase. For example, if a condition is temporary, a chair may be selected with greater concern for cost factors. In contrast, if a client's condition is chronic and stable, necessitating full-time use of a wheelchair, durability and individualization to meet needs are priorities. If a condition is progressive, a chair that permits a range of adjustments for both seating and wheelchair control may be indicated.

In recent years, wheelchairs have been evaluated using standards promulgated by the American National Standards Institute (ANSI) and RESNA, an interdisciplinary association for the advancement of rehabilitation and assistive technologies, and by direct product comparisons regarding features such as stability, safety, durability, and cost (Cooper et al., 1997). Total cost over the life of the wheelchair is a consideration for users with chronic disability and everyday use. For manual users, some ultralight models appear to have the greatest longevity, or greater years of expected use, in comparison with standard wheelchairs or other lightweight models (Cooper et al., 1999).

Seating and Positioning

Critical to selection of a wheelchair system is the attention given to seating and posture needs of the user. Seating systems have a significant effect on the abilities of the user to perform functional activities and on basic decisions about choice of mobility base types and components. Effective seating has several broad goals that include (1) promoting posture, comfort, physiological maintenance, and tissue protection; (2) accommodating existing deformity; (3) enabling vision readiness

and upper limb function; and (4) enhancing cosmetic appearance and social acceptance. Evaluation and intervention related to positioning often entail participation by team members such as physical therapists to address postural supports, speech therapists to address augmentative communication, and family and others to address daily routines and schedules. Occupational therapists may coordinate these concerns by incorporating the needs and goals of the user and family with medical care concerns in making recommendations and by analysis of functional issues so that recommendations maximize rather than restrict the individual's access to activities in various environments.

Seating Principles: Solid Base of Support

Seating strategies and particular techniques are both age and diagnosis specific (Letts, 1991), although some principles can be applied to meet a variety of needs (Garber & Krouskop, 1997). One such principle is the need to provide the individual with a solid base of support that begins with appropriate pelvic positioning. The sling seat, common to folding and nonsnapping wheelchair cross-brace frames, is the seating element most often criticized, because it tends to create pelvic instability and malalignment of the thighs (Bergen et al., 1990) and is often the primary component of seating modification (Krasilovsky, 1993). A solid seating base is accomplished by stabilizing the pelvis on a firm surface with pressure distributed throughout the buttocks and the full length of each thigh.

Postural Supports

Postural control is influenced by the seat and back surfaces and by orientation adjustments to the **seat-back angle** and the **angle in space** (Fig. 16-2). A sitting position with 90° hip, knee, and ankle positions and with the seat fully upright is sometimes suggested. With a slight anterior tilt to the pelvis, this position distributes weight through the buttocks and thighs, and for some individuals this position inhibits abnormal reflexive responses (Fig. 16-3). Wheelchair frames often have a 95° seat-back angle with a 3 to 5° angle-in-space recline. Hardware that secures the modular seat and the back components to the frame can be used to adjust these angles.

Seat Surfaces and Cushioning

The seat and back surfaces can be planar, precontoured, or custom contoured. Single-plane or flat surfaces are appropriate only for those who need little or no postural support and those who can reposition themselves to

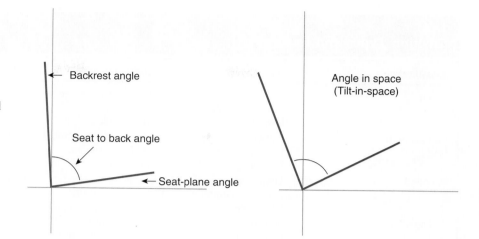

Figure 16-2 Adjustment of seat back angle and angle in space helps to support posture and provide appropriate pressure distribution.

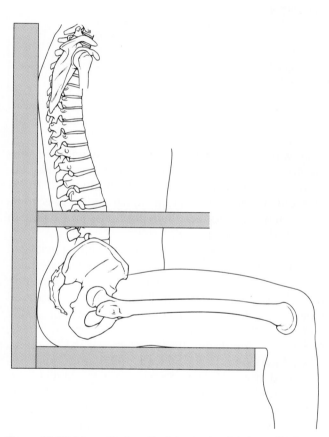

Figure 16-3 Pelvic positioning with slight anterior tilt helps to distribute tissue pressure throughout the buttock and thigh.

maintain balance and comfort. Contoured designs are used to provide added contact for postural support and distribution of pressure. Custom contouring is often necessary for individuals who need accommodation for deformity of the pelvis or spine, those with abnormal muscle tone, and those who have discomfort from lack of support at the lumbar spine. These cushions are fabricated by bead-seat molding, foam-in-place tech-

niques, or other shape-sensing technology (Cooper, 1998).

Cushions are used to reduce peak pressures associated with bony landmarks and to distribute pressure evenly over a large area of skin contact. Shearing forces that compromise circulation can also be reduced by appropriately shaped cushions. Although cushioning relieves skin pressure, factors including postural stability and control, ease of transfers, ability to accommodate deformity, moisture, and maintenance may be as important for some users. Cushioning of the seat and back may call for use of one or more materials such as variable-density foams, honeycomb-shaped plastics, air, gels, custom contouring, and alternating pressure systems. Table 16-1 lists advantages, disadvantages, and examples of each. Selection of surface materials of the cushion also should take into account factors such as heat and moisture, friction, durability, and cosmetic appearance.

Skin should be monitored closely for tolerance when use of any new seat cushion is started. Progressive sitting time schedules along with skin inspection are essential, because no cushion provides sufficient pressure relief during regular use. Properties of materials vary, yet no cushion is considered sufficient in relieving pressure enough to preserve capillary blood flow to compressed tissues while a person is seated. Pressure on sitting surfaces is greatest during manual propulsion (Kernozek & Lewin, 1998), and users should be informed about dynamic factors that may threaten health of skin tissues. Though commercial cushions help to reduce skin pressures (Pellow, 1999), other means of pressure relief are necessary. Assisted or user-performed wheelchair push-ups, side leans, or forward leans may be used for pressure relief needs every 15 to 30 minutes as required. Alternatively, technologies for pressure relief include tilt-in-space mechanisms, use of alternating pressure cushions that continuously cycle high- and low-pressure segments of a cushion (Burns & Betz, 1999),

TABLE 16-1
Cushion Types and Examples

Classification	Advantages	Disadvantages	Example
Foam	Lightweight Easily sized, shaped Low cost	Uneven pressure relief Poor durability Hard to clean	T-Foam by Alimed
Honeycomb	Lightweight Easy cleaning Durability	Uneven pressure relief Difficult to shape New product	Stimulite by Supracor
Air-filled	Lightweight Even pressure relief Little shear	Sitting balance Posture control Puncture and repair	High Profile by Roho
Gel-filled	Self-contouring Posture control Sitting balance	Heavy to move Temperature sensitive Leaking, maintenance	Jay Cushion by Jay Medical
Custom contoured foam	Surface area coverage Reduced shearing Postural control	Expense Longevity with change Reduced weight shift	Contour U, Pindot by Invacare
Alternating pressure systems	Scheduled relief cycle Reduces user effort Contoured	Cost and availability Uneven pressure relief Sitting balance	Dynamic Seating System by Talley Medical

and custom contouring of cushions. The latter show some promise for reducing static seating pressures (Rosenthal et. al., 1996).

Adding Seating System Components

A seatbelt is often recommended because it serves an important role in stabilizing the pelvis as part of a therapeutic positioning or seating system. This anterior support is typically mounted on the wheelchair frame so that it pulls on the pelvis at a 45° angle to the base of the seat back, fitting just under the anterior superior iliac spines. Additional seating supports should be used as needed to improve posture, restrict abnormal movements, and promote head control and voluntary use of the limbs. For example, if sitting balance and abnormal postures are problematic, lateral trunk and thigh supports may be suggested. In addition, use of anterior supports may be necessary across the upper trunk, knee, or ankle for balance and stabilization. Neck and head supports are used to promote good head and neck alignment and are sometimes recommended for safety. Upper extremity positioning also may be a concern, in which case contoured armrests or a wheelchair lap tray can be recommended.

Justification of Seating Systems

Since sitting is a dynamic rather than a static state, seating devices should allow some element of pressure relief and freedom of movement. The principle of *less is more* is recommended when applying specialized seating systems, because as more seating apparatuses are used, freedom of movement tends to diminish. Therefore, only components that maximize individuals' abilities to function, correct their positions, and maintain comfort should be applied.

To justify expenses associated with specialized seating to users and families, the experienced therapist can employ clinical observation and literature reviews to support use of these systems. Improved motor skills (Myhr & von Wendt, 1991; Nwaobi, 1987), comfort and participation (Hulme, Gallacher, Walsh, Niesen, & Waldron, 1987), physiological supports (Nwaobi & Smith, 1986; Stewart, 1991), and functional independence (Hulme, Shaver, Acher, Mullette, & Eggert, 1987; McEwen, 1992; McEwen & Lloyd, 1990; Trefler et al., 1983; Trefler & Taylor, 1991) are widely recognized benefits. However, some therapeutic claims should be viewed cautiously, because specialized seating mostly provides an immediate or prosthetic effect, meaning that it works well only when used. Little evidence can be cited that verifies the beneficial use of seating apparatuses to correct or prevent deformity, speed developmental gains or recovery, or reduce the need for additional therapies (Mac Neela, 1987). Expense justification with the insurance provider must relate to medical necessity. Inappropriate seating and mobility base selection can exacerbate complications and accelerate decline for the user. Functional accessibility and protection of the user from secondary complications that come with immobility or physiolog-

Case Example

WHEELCHAIR SELECTION FOR A STUDENT WITH TETRAPLEGIA

Patient Background

Lisa is a 17-year-old high school senior with C7-level tetraplegia from a traumatic spinal cord injury that she experienced in an automobile crash. She is expected to be a long-term wheelchair user, and has shown in the hospital the ability to propel a manual ultralight wheelchair using friction push rims. Lisa previously was active in soccer and other sports and would like to match her school colors with her wheelchair frame. She was intrigued to learn about competitive wheelchair sports but is inexperienced with independent mobility. Lisa will be using the wheelchair full time at home, at school, and in other community locations.

Recommendations

The care team is preparing a wheelchair prescription and considering these features:

Wheelchair
- ▶ Manual ultralight cross-brace folding frame
- ▶ Purple frame with black upholstery
- ▶ Adjustable axle position with camber control
- ▶ Lift-off desk-length tubular armrests
- ▶ Swing-away fixed-angle footrests with heel loops on flip-up foot plates

- ▶ Vinyl-coated push rims with pneumatic tires and nonpneumatic front casters
- ▶ Grade aids and standard rubber-coated brake levers

Seating
- ▶ Cloth-covered Jay seat cushion with flexible sling back, midscapular height
- ▶ Seat belt and chest strap

CLINICAL REASONING
in OT Practice

Selection of Other Wheelchair Options

Based on Lisa's functional needs, what else should be considered related to wheelchair selection and mobility training? Consider use of other wheelchair accessories, performance in transfers, transportation with the wheelchair, and maintenance of the wheelchair. Under what circumstances might power mobility be considered? What other kinds of activity-specific mobility aids might interest Lisa?

ical risks with seating may be cited for insurance justification.

Wheelchair Types: Mobility Bases

Once the therapist has a comprehensive understanding of the user's personal and medical profile and seating needs, it is important to understand the types and uses of wheelchair systems. Wheelchairs used in everyday activity can be divided into three general categories: (1) attendant-propelled chairs, (2) manual chairs, and (3) power mobility devices (Hobson, 1990). Special-use chairs and attachments to standard mobility bases for participation in recreation and sports also can be considered.

Attendant-Propelled Chairs

Attendant-propelled chairs are designed to be pushed by another individual because of the user's inability to propel or operate manual and power wheelchair systems in a functional or safe manner. This may be necessary for some users on a temporary or circumstantial basis, for example as a means to be mobile on community outings. Attendant assistance also may be a full-time need for individuals who have a diminished cognitive capacity, severe judgment problems, or restricted physical capacity. These chairs may be full size (e.g., those used in skilled nursing facilities) or may be smaller and created for use in limited spaces (e.g., folding stroller types). Attendant-propelled chairs also are used as a substitute for power mobility when the individual's typical mobility system is being repaired or when space constraints preclude power mobility use. When assisting a user in selecting an attendant-propelled chair, it is necessary to consider not only the fit and comfort of the chair for the person who will be seated in the chair but also sizing needs of the person most likely to be pushing it. As with all wheelchairs, attention to transportation of the user and the wheelchair device between environ-

Case Example

WHEELCHAIR SELECTION FOR AN ADULT WITH A PROGRESSIVE DISORDER

Patient Background

Mr. R. is a 48-year-old husband and father with amyotrophic lateral sclerosis (ALS). He is near the end of his ability to walk safely and has quit driving a car. He teaches in a public school and expects to retire at the end of the month. He coaches his children's youth baseball teams. He lacks sufficient strength in his arms to self-propel a wheelchair. To address his needs now for mobility at home, at work, and in the community, a prescription for a wheelchair is being written. Family financial resources are limited.

Recommendations

To address needs within the home, an attendant-propelled wheelchair is needed. A tilt-in-space manual chair that permits full upright to 45° recline is selected along with a foam seat cushion and flexible sling back with a winged headrest. A lap tray is added to enable positioning of the arms and for attachment of communication devices. This chair is requested

through health insurance, and once he is unable to walk safely, it will be used at home and for attending medical appointments.

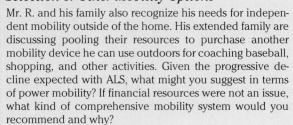

CLINICAL REASONING
in OT Practice

Selection of Other Mobility Options

Mr. R. and his family also recognize his needs for independent mobility outside of the home. His extended family are discussing pooling their resources to purchase another mobility device he can use outdoors for coaching baseball, shopping, and other activities. Given the progressive decline expected with ALS, what might you suggest in terms of power mobility? If financial resources were not an issue, what kind of comprehensive mobility system would you recommend and why?

---

ments needs attention and planning. Besides chairs specifically designed to be attendant propelled, many manual wheelchairs (described later) can be propelled by an attendant.

Manual Chairs

Manual wheelchairs are for those who can propel and brake using the upper limbs (Fig. 16-4). These chairs have a variety of frame types, weights, and transport features. In general, manual wheelchairs have rigid or box frames or folding frames, the latter of which are either free or snapped. Quick-release wheels also may be selected. These characteristics alter the ease of transporting the wheelchair in automobiles. Rigid-frame chairs may provide a smoother ride but can be awkward to load in automobiles. Folding, snap-secured frames with quick-release wheels and detachable front rigging may offer the greatest flexibility for transporting the wheelchair.

The conventional manual wheelchair frame has large rear wheels, used to propel the chair, with smaller caster wheels in the front. Wheelchairs of this design are highly maneuverable and easy to propel, and they allow freedom for tilting, which is necessary when ascending

or descending curbs. Standard designs, sometimes called depot or institutional wheelchairs (Cooper, 1998) weigh at least 50 pounds without specialized seating systems. A distinction can be made between multiuser chairs, often found in health care settings, and single-user or rehabilitation chairs, sometimes designated as lightweight and ultralight chairs. In recent years sturdy lightweight metals and designs have been adapted from sport wheelchairs, resulting in lightweight and ultralight-weight wheelchairs ranging from less than 25 pounds to 40 pounds. Lightweight chairs are often used on a full-time basis. Many new designs allow adjustable wheel positions and seat heights, making it possible to optimize biomechanical efficiency for the user (Masse et al., 1992). Along with reduced weight, these changes can enhance propulsion and ease transport (Brubaker, 1990; Parziale, 1991).

Other types of manual wheelchair designs include the amputee frame for the person with loss of or severely reduced weight of the lower limbs. In this design the rear axle is offset farther behind the seat back than is standard. This concentrates a person's weight farther in front of the rear axle, reducing the risk of the chair tipping backward. Another type of manual wheelchair, although not commonly recommended, is the indoor frame. It has large front wheels, used for propulsion, with smaller casters in back. While this design rolls easily over door sills and rug edges, larger barriers such as curbs are difficult to traverse, and transfers may be awkward because of the forward placement of the large wheels.

Manual propulsion is typically accomplished through hand rims attached to the outside of the large wheels. Optimally, the user is seated so that with shoulders extended to about 120° and elbows fixed, each hand rests at the 12 o'clock position of each hand rim (Brubaker, 1990). Contact with rims generally occurs between the 11 and 2 o'clock positions on each side. Circular steel tube hand rims are common. However, for users who have difficulty with grip, hand rims can be covered with vinyl coating; knobs or other projections can be added to the rims so that grip is not required; and/or gloves or mitts can be worn to improve traction. Gloves and mitts also protect the hands. Hand rims vary in size. Small hand rims, often used on racing chairs, result in a slower and more difficult start but provide for a high top speed that is sustainable with relatively little effort (Ragnarsson, 1990). A common means of maneu-

vering the wheelchair by persons with hemiplegia is to use the more capable side for the hand rim and the leg and foot to steer and provide additional propulsion and braking. This requires removal of the unused footrest and usually requires dropping of the seat or using small-diameter wheels to optimize foot contact with the floor. For the user who plans to propel the wheelchair using only one arm, a chair can be ordered with both hand rims on one side so that each wheel can be controlled independently or together. Learning to maneuver two hand rims on the same side can be perceptually and mechanically difficult. Another option for unilateral control is the single-lever drive. This rare device uses a forward-and-backward motion to propel the chair and rotation of the lever to turn the chair.

Augmentation of manual propulsion and braking systems is available. As an aid to propelling on inclines, hill climbers or grade aid devices restrict the counter-clockwise movement of wheels through a friction stop engaged by a lever on each tire. Speed control and braking to a stop simply depend on slowing wheel rotation by use of the arms or legs. Brakes are used on

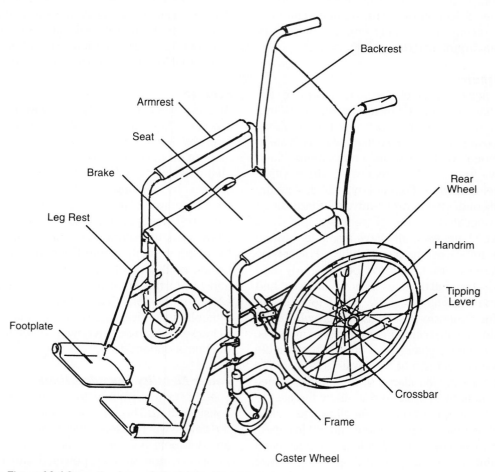

Figure 16-4 Conventional manual wheelchair with component parts.

each large wheel and are engaged through a variable-length single- or dual-action lever, depending on reach and force abilities. Such levers impinge on the tire to resist rolling and require periodic tightening after tire wear. Antirotation locks also can be used on casters. Brakes restrict wheel turning when the chair is parked but are not typically recommended for slowing or stopping. Dynamic braking systems that allow continuous braking on hills or when coming to a stop are available on some wheelchairs in Europe but are not generally available in the United States.

Power Mobility Devices: Motorized Wheelchairs

Power mobility devices are used by individuals (1) who cannot propel a chair using either the hands or the feet, (2) for whom the energy expenditure required to walk or propel a manual chair is contraindicated, (3) who have musculoskeletal complications such as arthritis in upper limb joints, (4) who are prone to repetitive stress injury, and/or (5) who have neuromuscular dysfunction that may cause associated reactions in the lower extremities when the upper extremities are used for manual wheelchair propulsion. There are a number of types of power mobility devices. Selection of power mobility can be a complex task, owing to the many options for wheels, controls, and environmental designs (Field, 1999).

Power Wheelchairs

Conventional power wheelchairs may resemble the manual frame and are powered by motors linked to large rear wheels by belts or gears. Most new power wheelchairs have a power-base design so that the wheels are in effect independent of the seating components. Such bases may have front-, mid-, or rear-wheel drive with a variety of wheel diameters. For each type of design, the wheels may be connected to direct-drive motors through exposed or concealed chains or gear systems. New mid-wheel-drive chairs generally have a smaller turning radius, which improves maneuverability. Power-base wheelchair designs are noted for being sturdy and appropriate for the full-time user both indoors and outdoors. These designs generally allow for ease in changing seating dimensions, such as for a growing child or for an individual with changing seating system needs.

Several power-base chairs have options that enable the user to change seat height or elevate to a standing position independently. Similarly, some manual wheelchairs have manual lever systems that allow the user to rise to a near standing position. These allow the person greater vertical flexibility in movement and environmental accessibility. Consider the individual trying to reach books in a library, working in a shop using power equipment, or confronted with a high counter.

The primary disadvantages of power wheelchairs are that (1) they are large and heavy and may be difficult to maneuver in small spaces and transport from one place to another; and (2) a 5 × 5-foot turning space, as part of standard barrier free-design, may not be sufficient for some power wheelchairs. Typically, van or bus transport of the individual sitting in a power mobility device requires special lifts or ramp devices, and the size of some chairs necessitates a raised roof in these vehicles. Alternatively, the user can transfer into the vehicle and an attendant can load the chair separately by use of a lift or by breakdown of the device into components. Lightweight power wheelchairs are designed to be taken apart for automobile transport. Most of these chairs are built on folding frames and have low-powered motors, making hill climbing and use on uneven surfaces relatively unsuccessful. Assistance with taking apart and reassembling the chair often is required.

Manual Wheelchair With Add-On Unit

Another option for power mobility is the use of an add-on unit on a manual wheelchair to provide power assistance. Such systems can be engaged and disengaged to switch between manual and power mobility. Because a significant amount of weight is added to the chair and units are not easily taken on and off the frame, this option is most commonly suggested to reduce costs or as a trial for a transition to a regular power wheelchair.

Scooter

An increasingly popular type of power wheelchair is the scooter. These are typically three-wheeled, although four-wheeled designs are available, and may have either rear- or front-wheel drive. Most of these designs are characterized by tiller control, wherein users steer the scooter by rotating the front wheel while using a lever-style switch for forward and reverse power. This type of chair is appropriate for the marginal walker and is often used to compensate for a person's inability to travel comfortably within the community. Scooters are usually modular and can be disassembled and loaded in and out of the trunk of a car or the back of a station wagon or van. Steering and control of scooters can be difficult, so individuals with marginal control may be better served by use of a power wheelchair with a variety of control options.

Power Mobility Considerations

Specific factors unique to power wheelchairs require consideration. The therapist should determine whether the device will be used primarily indoors or both indoors and outdoors. A device that is to be used in both settings must have more stability, power, distance capability, and durability than an indoor-only model. In addition, the therapist should consider use and maintenance of the batteries that provide power. Various sizes of deep-cycle lead acid batteries, either wet cell or sealed cell types have different expense, longevity, and needs for maintenance. Other power wheelchair characteristics to consider include noise, braking systems, ride quality, and portability, including ease of assembly and disassembly if appropriate. If the device can be disassembled, the weight and size of each part should be carefully evaluated for transportability.

Selection of appropriate controls for driving is critical. These devices are typically driven using one of two types of options: proportional or microswitch control. Most commonly, a proportional joystick is used in which directions and speeds are linked to angle and magnitude of stick displacement. An alternative is microswitch control activated with a joystick, a multiple-switch array, or a single switch scan. Each switch activation engages a single preset or programmed speed and direction. Microswitch systems require less skilled movement to achieve control, although they are less responsive than proportional control and learning to use them is not simple. Each direction may be controlled by activating a microswitch using a body part (i.e., hand, arm, chin, foot, head, mouth, lips, tongue), and control may be organized through a combination of special techniques such as **sip and puff**, **scanning**, and **proximity-sensing systems** (Fig. 16-5). In special systems, breath may be used for forward and reverse control and proximity sensing switches used to activate

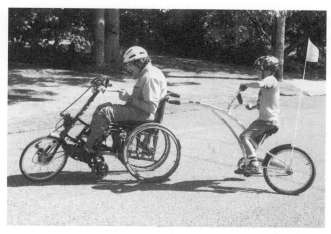

Figure 16-6 Father uses cycling apparatus attached to his everyday-use manual wheelchair for outdoor activity with his children.

turning control. When selecting controls, the therapist should consider adjustment options provided by various systems in relation to the needs to the individual. For example, clients with poor motor control may benefit from programmable electronics so that wheelchair speeds are automatically restricted when turning or so that several levels of control can be programmed for new learning and training in various environments.

Modern power wheelchairs and scooters are electronically braked, meaning that drive wheels do not rotate except under power. Belts or gears are released by levers that allow the chair to roll freely. Parking brakes, like those on manual wheelchairs, may be provided for additional stability and safety.

Activity- or Environment-Specific Wheelchairs

For everyday use, attendant-propelled, manual, or power wheelchairs are selected. However, many users need mobility to overcome unique barriers or for use in recreation and leisure activities that require activity-specific technology (Axelson, 1998). Gurneys allow the individual to lie prone and propel with the upper extremities. Special wheel configurations for power or manual wheelchairs also can be used for ascending or descending stairs. Other special designs for wheelchairs, including those for use at the beach and on other soft and uneven surfaces, are available commercially or may be custom made. For recreation, cycling configurations may be needed. Row cycles are large, low to the ground three-wheeled cycles propelled by a rowing action that activates chain-driven rear wheels. Cycling action also can be added to manual wheelchairs (Fig. 16-6) or be configured as a separate chair for outdoor sport. Sport wheelchairs for racing, basketball, and other competitions are becoming commercially available, but often

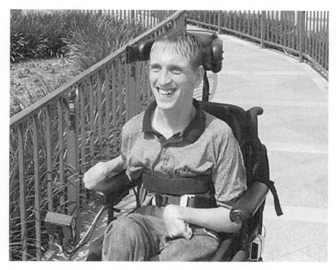

Figure 16-5 College student uses power wheelchair controlled with proximity switches in a head array. Display in front of right armrest provides feedback regarding drive selection, ECU functions, and battery level. A switch on the right side of the head array permits selection of drive and ECU functions. (Courtesy of Adaptive Switch Laboratories, Inc., Spicewood, Texas.)

they require custom manufacturing and expert instruction. For a thorough review of options for using activity-specific or sport and recreation chairs see Cooper (1998).

Wheelchair Sizing and Ergonomic Considerations

Modern wheelchairs are engineered as modular systems, assembled to match the specific physical dimensions of the user. Measurements of the individual form the basis for determining wheelchair frame size, needs for adjustable ranges in component parts, and need for customization to meet special needs.

Sizing

Appropriate size determinations of the wheelchair frame, seat, back, leg rests, and armrests are based on measurements typically taken with the user in an optimally seated position. Alternatively, the therapist can evaluate the individual on a mat in supine or side lying and take careful measurements of distances between key landmarks. These measurements are confirmed for accuracy with the user seated. The user's typical or specialized clothing needs should be considered during measurement. If thoracolumbar bracing or lower limb orthotics and prosthetics are likely to be used in the wheelchair, they should be worn during sizing measurements. Manufacturers of wheelchairs and seating systems have differing standards for measurement and sizing. Typically included are measures of pelvic or hip width; thigh and leg lengths; mid back, mid scapula and

top of shoulder heights; chest and shoulder widths; elbow position; and overall sitting height (Fig. 16-7).

▶ Seat width: The therapist determines the widest point across the hips and thighs and typically adds a total of 5 cm (2 inches) for adequate clearance on the sides. Overall wheelchair width may be dictated by the seat width measure. Because narrower wheelchairs are likely to improve ease of hand rim propulsion and maneuverability, wheelchairs should be as narrow as possible while allowing for comfort, easy repositioning, and transfers.

▶ Seat depth: The therapist, for both the left and right sides, measures the distance from the most posterior part of the buttocks under the thigh to the popliteal fossa of each knee. About 5 cm (2 inches) is subtracted from the measure. This allows as much weight bearing through the thigh as possible without the front edge of the seat pressing into the back of the knee. Right and left leg length discrepancies can be caused by hip dislocation, **pelvic rotation and obliquity**, or other anatomical factors. The shorter side may be used to determine seat depth, or if a greater than 1-inch discrepancy is found, the front seat edge may be offset to accommodate the length of each side.

Selected seat cushion height should be incorporated into further measures of trunk, arm, and leg.

▶ Back height and width: The therapist generally takes three measures from the seat surface upward (1) to the mid back just under the scapula, (2) to the mid scapula or axilla, and (3) to the top of the shoulder. Back height is affected by seat cushions, which

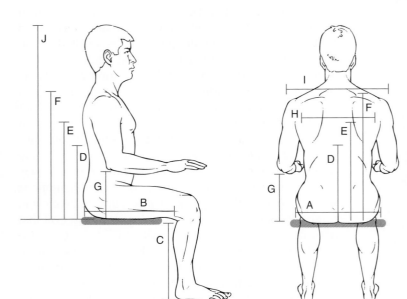

Figure 16-7 Seating measurements. For B to G, all measurements are taken on both right and left sides. A, Hip and thigh width; B, thigh length; C, leg length; D, back height to below scapula; E, back height to mid scapula; F, back height to top of shoulder; G, elbow and forearm height; H, chest width; I, shoulder width; J, sitting height.

TABLE 16-2
Head, Arm, and Leg Supports

Component	Attachment to Frame	Adjustment	Style
Head and neck supports	Fixed or removable	Height, depth, and rotation	Flat, winged, lateral, occipital, or wedged
Armrests	Fixed, swing away and/or removable	Same height or adjustable height	Full length or desk length
Leg rests	Fixed rigid, swing away, and/or detachable	Fixed or telescoping length	Fixed angle or elevating
Calf pad and foot plate	Rigid or flip-up	Variable sizes in pads or straps	Plate, tubular, traction

should be considered in sizing decisions. Height of the chair back is based on the needs for postural stability and freedom of arm movements for propulsion or other functions. For those who exclusively self-propel, a chair back height of 2 to 5 cm (1 to 2 inches) under the tip of the scapula may be preferred. For sporting activities, the optimal back height may be even lower. By contrast, for power wheelchair users, back heights to mid scapula or the top of the shoulder may be necessary to allow use of postural supports for the upper trunk and the head. Chest and shoulder width should be measured in cases of deformity or to determine the space requirements for lateral trunk supports or other trunk positioning devices. Alterations of the standard sling back may be necessary for improving trunk posture by using an adjustable or flexible sling back, contoured backs, or additions of lateral trunk supports.

▶ Seat height and leg rests: Seat height is based on positioning of the individual such that footrests have at least 5 cm (2 inches) clearance from the floor. Use of seat cushions affect this measurement by raising overall seat height. Seat height is determined with the individual's knees and ankles positioned at about 90°. Measurements are taken from under the distal thigh to the heel of the individual's commonly used footwear or shoe. Several centimeters of adjustment are typically available in leg rest lengths to accommodate left- and right-side discrepancies. Unusual leg lengths or hip or knee deformity may necessitate special ordering.

▶ Armrest height: The therapist measures from under each elbow to the cushioned seating surface with the shoulder in neutral, the arms hanging at the sides, and the elbows flexed to 90°. Armrests must provide forearm support with neutral shoulder position but should not obstruct reach to hand rims for propulsion or to brake locks.

Common Components

In addition to overall sizing and seat and back surface, the team and user should consider selection of head and neck rests, armrests, leg rests, and other options. Table 16-2 lists options for head, neck, arm, leg, and foot support. Users should consider armrest stability for performing wheelchair push-ups for pressure release. Detachable or swing-away styles may allow greater ease in sliding board and other sideways transfers and improve access to tables and desks. Guards can be used on armrests to keep clothes from coming in contact with wheels. Attachment of lap trays may require use of full-length armrests or other specialized hardware. The front rigging consists of leg rests and foot plates. Options are selected according to needs for elevation of the calf and foot, ankle position, and stabilization of the leg. Swing-away or detachable front rigging may enable easy transfers and transportability of the wheelchair in and out of vehicles.

Tires can be either pneumatic (air filled), semipneumatic (airless foam inserts), or solid-core rubber and are mounted on spoke or molded wheels. Air-filled tires require regular maintenance but provide a well-cushioned ride and have a shock absorber function that tends to improve comfort and prolong the life of the chair. Semipneumatics provide good cushioning and less maintenance, but tire wear may be more of a problem. Solid-core tires are noted for minimal maintenance and approach the lightweight and low rolling resistance of high-pressure pneumatic tires.

Casters, as either front or rear wheels, vary in diameter, and small ones usually facilitate maneuverability. Pneumatic and semipneumatic caster tires provide some shock absorption for use outdoors and on rough surfaces. Solid-core caster tires are best for use indoors and on smooth surfaces.

Placement of the rear axles can be fixed or adjustable on most manual wheelchairs, especially newer manual lightweight and ultralight styles. Backward placement of the axle tends to increase stability; by contrast, forward placement of the axle decreases stability but increases maneuverability and shortens turning radius. Sometimes rear wheels have a **camber** adjustment. This orients the hand rim for easier propulsion and may slightly widen the wheel base for better stability. Antitipping extensions can be used on a wheelchair to prevent the chair from tipping backward or forward. Typically used on the back, these fixed or adjustable extensions can improve safety during mobility training.

Seatbelts, safety vests, and harnesses vary in design and are used for both safety and positioning. These devices should be considered for individuals who have severe neuromuscular impairments and need control for posture and safety. Restraints may be considered with individuals who have poor judgment, but these should be avoided whenever possible and be regarded separately from seating postural needs. In general, restraint reduction efforts in long-term care facilities are often enhanced by use of appropriate and comfortable seating (Stinnett, 1997).

Frame and upholstery color and material options are numerous. Users can personalize their chair through selections of colors and other styling. Durability, ease of repair, and compatibility of materials with temperature regulation, friction, moisture, and skin protection also require careful planning.

Recline and tilt-in-space options enable postural changes for rest and pressure relief. In attendant-propelled wheelchairs semireclining up to 30° from upright or full reclining up to 90° from upright can be considered. In tilt-in-space systems, the seat and back assembly pivot together. This feature makes the use of postural seating components more stable because the angle between the seat and the back remains unchanged. Power recline systems can be used with conventional or power-base designs. Such systems may involve tilt in space and/or low-shear back recline, both of which provide pressure relief and rest positioning (Hobson, 1992). Tilt-in-space chairs that go back 45 to 60° achieve effective pressure relief under the buttock and thigh and may have other physiological benefits, such as improved respiration (Chan & Heck, 1999). However, these systems may add costs and increase wheelchair size and weight.

Narrowing devices are available for some folding frame manual chairs to reduce chair width temporarily for fitting through doorways. The device mounts on one side of the seat and narrows the chair when a crank is turned.

Other considerations are accessories that optimize use and performance. Lap trays can be used for postural support of the upper limbs and serve a variety of purposes related to functional activity. Other accessories include mounting bags or baskets for storage and carrying, cup or bottle holders for taking fluids, and storage attachments for reacher or walking aids to enhance access and mobility. Some wheelchair users also need other assistive technology, such as communication devices or environmental controls. These devices may be mounted on the wheelchair and operated independently of wheelchair controls or integrated with power wheelchair controllers.

Mobility Training

Mobility training with the wheelchair system is essential, and it may involve other team members, such as the physical therapist. Most users benefit from instruction and practice beyond the training provided by vendors. Once the chair has been provided, a check should be conducted and appropriate training of the user and attendants should commence. This should include review of the user's goals for mobility along with a check of the device for fit and adjustment. Instruction should also be provided regarding (1) use of the chair indoors and outdoors and on a variety of surfaces (e.g., level, incline, and uneven), (2) transfers (e.g., bed, toilet, and car), (3) transport of the wheelchair (e.g., cars, trucks, vans, and buses), and (4) maintenance of the wheelchair (e.g., cleaning the chair, lubricating moving parts, monitoring tire pressure and wear, adjusting brakes, and caring for batteries). Troubleshooting with the wheelchair system ultimately becomes the responsibility of the user and equipment supplier or vendor, but the therapist may advise about problem-solving strategies and organization of maintenance schedules. Throughout training, the therapist emphasizes safety issues, because accidents during day-to-day wheelchair use, though infrequent, do occur, and some appear to be preventable (Calder & Kirby, 1990).

Manual wheelchair users also benefit from instruction about propelling, braking, and transport. Particular attention to hand placement and trunk lean for effective and efficient wheeling can be explored. General consumer use guidelines are available for the user and trainer (Axelson, et al., 1998). Power wheelchair users also need guidance about power functions such as controllers, batteries, and accessory devices. With all wheelchair users, the therapist should provide initial checks; periodic follow-up to address safety issues, fit, and adjustment; and updated information about new options in order to meet the changing needs of the user.

Transportability of the wheelchair system between environments can be especially challenging. As noted, car transfers of the user and loading and unloading of the wheelchair need careful planning. Breakdown of the wheelchair for portability or the addition of special lift accessories to vehicles should be considered during selection. Lifts are often used with vans or buses. In these vehicles, wheelchair tie-downs are necessary as safety mechanisms to keep chairs stabilized when traveling. The necessary style may be determined by wheelchair design. Such devices secure the wheelchair to the base of the vehicle; the individual is independently secured in the wheelchair seat or in another seating device within the vehicle.

Final Determination

In making a final determination regarding seating components, style, size, and control systems, the user and team take a comprehensive and functional view, simultaneously considering the needs, desires, and resources of the user and anticipated advances in technology.

Decision Making and Justification

Costs and related funding issues are critical components of the decision-making process. Expensive technology and options should not be ordered unless justifiable for increased function, health (e.g., skin protection), user satisfaction, or safety. When expensive choices are being considered, it is important to rule out the feasibility of using less costly alternatives. For example, before selecting power mobility, it is important to rule out the feasibility of using a manual chair, because the cost of providing and maintaining a powered system is estimated to be approximately three times that required for a manual system (Warren, 1990). In such cases, appropriate justification must be clearly delineated for users and **third-party payers**. Some users decide to purchase devices or features on their own or seek funding through other sources.

A comprehensive functional mobility system for an individual often includes more than one means of mobility (York, 1989). For example, an individual may benefit from a manual chair for traveling short distances, such as at home, and a power chair for traveling longer distances in the community and at work. Funding sources may pay for only one of these options, but with mobility being unique to different activities, negotiation of options may be explored with health insurance as well as educational and vocational support programs.

The Clinician's Responsibilities

Technology design and products are changing rapidly. Therefore, it is a continual challenge for occupational therapists to remain current. Therapists have a responsibility to keep abreast of new technology, new products, and new product evaluation research. They must be able to provide users with current information on the advantages and disadvantages of various wheelchairs, components, and features. In addition, they must have current knowledge of issues related to availability, serviceability, and performance of various wheelchairs and options (Behrman, 1990). Professional and consumer sources of information about wheelchairs, related options, and manufacturers of mobility systems, controls, and seating systems are useful for product information (see Resources).

Therapists also are encouraged to explore wheelchair standards developed by the Rehabilitation Engineering Society of North America (RESNA) (**www.resna.org**), and the International Standards Organization, ANSI. These voluntary standards for wheelchair developers and manufacturers provide guidelines for product specifications based on uniform measurements and testing. Use of these standards facilitates product comparisons. Besides being aware of wheelchair standards, the therapist also is responsible, in combination with the interdisciplinary team, to develop relationships with appropriate vendors of seating and wheelchair systems.

Wheelchairs, selected through a user-led team, can facilitate participation in multiple environments. Selection of an appropriate wheelchair system results from a clinical reasoning process that considers multiple variables, particularly best fit, function, and the user's preferences. Consumers' satisfaction with seating and mobility systems is critical to program evaluation that addresses outcomes (Weiss-Lambrou et al., 1999). Ragnarsson (1990) stated, "Ultimately, the most important factor in the success of a wheelchair prescription is the user's total level of acceptance and satisfaction with [the] chair as it combines looks, comfort, and function" (p. 8).

Summary Review Questions

1. Who should participate in the wheelchair selection process?
2. What are the three basic types of wheelchairs, and why would each be selected?
3. What factors should be taken into consideration in wheelchair selection?
4. Describe a situation in which the optimal decision for an individual might involve the selection of more than one mobility device.
5. What are the six broad goals of wheelchair seating and positioning?

6. In determining wheelchair and related seating system sizes for a particular individual, what measurements typically are taken?
7. Contrast benefits and limitations of various manual and power mobility frame types.
8. Name and describe two types of controls for power mobility devices. Which would be preferable for a person with cerebral palsy and extremely poor upper extremity control? Why?
9. How can an occupational therapist keep abreast of new product development and research related to these products?
10. How can the occupational therapist facilitate the client's participation in wheelchair selection?
11. Once the wheelchair and seating system have been selected, what is the role of the occupational therapist?

Acknowledgments

We thank and acknowledge the following people for critiquing this manuscript and for contributing their knowledge and expertise: Ann Buzaid, MA, OTR, and Laura Shillam, OTR, Assistive Technology Clinic, University of Washington Hospital and Medical Center, Seattle; and Sharon Greenberg, MOT, OTR, Division of Occupational Therapy, University of Washington.

Resources

Wheelchairs

Accent on Living · P. O. Box 700, Bloomington, IL 61702-0700
www.blvd.com/accent

ABLEDATA · 8401 Colesville Road, Suite 200, Silver Spring, MD 20910
www.abledata.com

Assistive Technology, RESNA · 1700 North Moore St., Suite 1540, Rosslyn, VA 22209
www.resna.org

Exceptional Parent · 555 Kinderkmack Road, Oradell, NJ 07649-1517
www.eparent.com

Mainstream Magazine · P. O. Box 370598, San Diego, CA 92137-0598
www.mainstream-mag.com

New Mobility magazine · 23815 Stuart Ranch Rd., P. O. Box 8987, Malibu, CA 90265
www.newmobility.com

Paraplegia News & Sports 'N Spokes · 2111 East Highland Ave., Suite 180, Phoenix, AZ 85016
www.pva.org

Rehabilitation Engineering Research Center on Wheeled Mobility · University of Pittsburgh, SHRS, 4020 Forbes Tower, Pittsburgh, PA 15260
http://www.wheelchairnet.org

References

Allan, B. L., & Moffett, F. C. (1992). *Accessibility Design for All: An Illustrated Handbook, Washington State Regulations* (5th ed.). Olympia: Washington Council/American Institute of Architects.

Axelson, P. W. (1998). Problem solving through rehabilitation engineering, In D. B. Gray, L. A. Quatrano, & M. L. Lieberman (Eds.). *Designing and Using Assistive Technology: The Human Perspective* (pp. 209–228). Baltimore: Paul H. Brooks.

Axelson, P. W., Chesney, D.Y., Minkel, J., & Perr, A. (1998). *The Manual Wheelchair Training Guide.* Santa Cruz, CA: PAX Press.

Behrman, A. L. (1990). Factors in functional assessment. *Journal of Rehabilitation Research and Development: Clinical Supplement, 2,* 17–30.

Bergen, A. F., Presperin, J., & Tallman, T. (1990). *Positioning for Function: Wheelchairs and Other Assistive Technologies.* Valhalla, NY: Valhalla Rehabilitation.

Brubaker, C. (1990). Ergonometric considerations. *Journal of Rehabilitation Research and Development: Clinical Supplement, 2,* 37–48.

Burns, S. P., & Betz, K. L. (1999). Seating pressures with conventional and dynamic wheelchair cushions in tetraplegia. *Archives of Physical Medicine and Rehabilitation, 80,* 566–571.

Calder, C. J., & Kirby, R. (1990). Fatal wheelchair-related accidents in the United States. *American Journal of Physical Medicine and Rehabilitation, 69* (4), 184–190.

Chan, A., & Heck, C. S. (1999). The effects of tilting the seating system position of a wheelchair on respiration, posture, fatigue, voice volume, and exertion outcomes in individuals with advanced multiple sclerosis. *Journal Rehabilitation Outcome Measures, 3* (2), 1–14.

Cooper, R.A. (1998). *Wheelchair Selection and Configuration.* New York: Demos.

Cooper, R. A, Boninger, M. L., & Rentschler, A. (1999). Evaluation of selected ultralight manual wheelchairs using ANSI/RESNA standards. *Archives of Physical Medicine and Rehabilitation, 80,* 462–467.

Cooper, R. A., Gonzalez, J., Lawrence, G., Renschler, A., Boninger, M. L., & VanSickle, D. P. (1997). Performance of selected lightweight wheelchairs on ANSI/RESNA Tests. *Archives of Physical Medicine and Rehabilitation, 80,* 1138–1144.

Field, D. (1999). Powered mobility: A literature review illustrating the importance of a multifaceted approach. *Assistive Technology, 11,* 20–33.

Garber, S., & Krouskop, T. (1997). Technical advances in wheelchairs and seating systems. *Physical Medicine and Rehabilitation: State of the Art Reviews, 11* (1), 93–106.

Hobson, D. A. (1990). Seating and mobility for the severely disabled. In R. Smith & J. Leslie Jr. (Eds.), *Rehabilitation Engineering* (pp. 193–252). Boca Raton, FL: CRC.

Hobson, D. A. (1992). Comparative effects of posture on pressure and shear at the body–seat interface. *Journal of Rehabilitation Research and Development, 29* (4), 21–31.

Hulme, J. B., Gallacher, K., Walsh, J., Niesen, S., & Waldron, D. (1987). Behavioral and postural changes observed with use of adaptive seating by clients with multiple handicaps. *Physical Therapy, 67,* 1060–1067.

Hulme, J. B., Shaver, J., Acher, S., Mullette, L., & Eggert, C. (1987). Effects of adaptive seating devices on the eating and drinking of children with multiple handicaps. *American Journal of Occupational Therapy, 41* (2), 81–89.

Kernozek, T. W., & Lewin, J. E. (1998). Seat interface pressures of individuals with paraplegia: Influence of dynamic wheelchair locomotion compared with static seated measurements. *Archives of Physical Medicine and Rehabilitation, 79,* 313–316.

Krasilovsky, G. (1993). Seating assessment and management in a nursing home population. *Physical and Occupational Therapy in Geriatrics, 11,* 25–38.

Letts, R. M. (1991). *Principles of Seating the Disabled.* Boca Raton, FL: CRC.

Mac Neela, J. C. (1987). An overview of therapeutic positioning for multiply-handicapped persons, including augmentative communication users. *Occupational and Physical Therapy in Pediatrics, 7* (2), 39–60.

Masse, L. C., Lamontagne, M., & O'Riain, M. D. (1992). Biomechanical analysis of wheelchair propulsion for various seating positions. *Journal of Rehabilitation Research and Development, 29* (3), 12–28.

McEwen, I. R. (1992). Assistive positioning as a control parameter of social-communicative interactions between students with profound multiple disabilities and classroom staff. *Physical Therapy, 72* (9), 634–647.

McEwen, I. R., & Lloyd, L. L. (1990). Positioning students with cerebral palsy to use augmentative and alternative communication. *Language, Speech and Hearing Services in Schools, 21,* 15–21.

Myhr, U., & von Wendt, L. (1991). Improvement of functional sitting position for children with cerebral palsy. *Developmental Medicine and Child Neurology, 33* (3), 246–256.

Nwaobi, O. M. (1987). Seating orientations and upper extremity function in children with cerebral palsy. *Physical Therapy, 67* (8), 1209–1212.

Nwaobi, O. M., & Smith, P. D. (1986). Effect of adaptive seating on pulmonary function of children with cerebral palsy. *Developmental Medicine and Child Neurology, 28* (3), 351–354.

Parziale, J. R. (1991). Standard v. lightweight wheelchair propulsion in spinal cord injured patients. *American Journal of Physical Medicine and Rehabilitation, 70* (2), 76–80.

Pellow, T. R. (1999). A comparison of interface pressure readings to wheelchair cushions and positioning: A pilot study. *Canadian Journal of Occupational Therapy, 66,* 140–149.

Ragnarsson, K. T. (1990). Prescription considerations and a comparison of conventional and lightweight wheelchairs. *Journal of Rehabilitation Research and Development: Clinical Supplement, 2,* 8–16.

Rosenthal, M. J., Felton, R. M., Hileman, D. L., Lee, M., Friedman, M., & Navach, J. H. (1996). A wheelchair cushion design to redistribute sites of sitting pressure. *Archives of Physical Medicine and Rehabilitation, 77,* 278–282.

Steins, S. A. (1998). Personhood, disablement, and mobility technology. In D. B. Gray, L. A. Quatrano, & M. L. Lieberman (Eds.). *Designing and Using Assistive Technology, The Human Perspective* (pp. 29–49). Baltimore: Paul H. Brooks.

Stewart, C. P. (1991). Physiological considerations in seating. *Prosthetics and Orthotics International, 15* (3), 193–198.

Stinnett, K. A. (1997). Geriatric seating and positioning within a wheeled mobility frame of reference in the long-term care setting. *Topics in Geriatric Rehabilitation, 13* (2), 75–84.

Trefler, E., & Taylor, S. J. (1991). Prescription and positioning: Evaluating the physically disabled individual for wheelchair seating. *Prosthetics and Orthotics International, 15* (3), 217–224.

Trefler, E., Nickey, J., & Hobson, D. A. (1983). Technology in the education of multiply-handicapped children. *American Journal of Occupational Therapy, 37* (6), 381–387.

Warren, C. G. (1990). Powered mobility and its implications. *Journal of Rehabilitation Research and Development: Clinical Supplement, 2,* 74–85.

Weiss-Lambrou, R., Tremblay, C., LeBlanc, R., Lacoste, M., & Dansereau, J. (1999). Wheelchair seating aids: How satisfied are consumers. *Assistive Technology, 11,* 43–53.

York, J. (1989). Mobility methods selected for use in home and community environments. *Physical Therapy, 69* (9), 736–747.

Suggested Reading

Batavia, M. (1998). *The Wheelchair Evaluation: A Practical Guide.* Woodburn, MA: Butterworth-Heinemann.

Croteau, C. (1998). *Wheelchair Mobility: A Handbook.* Worcester, MA: Park Press.

Karp, G. (1998) *Choosing a Wheelchair: A Guide to Optimal Independence.* Sebastopol, CA: O'Reilly & Associates.

Mayall, J. K., & Desharnais, G. (1995). *Positioning in a Wheelchair: A Guide for Professional Caregivers of the Disabled Adult,* 2nd ed. Thorofare, NJ: Slack.

Trefler, E., Hobson, D. A., Taylor, S. J., Monahan, L. C., & Shaw, C. G. (1993). *Seating and Mobility for Persons With Physical Disabilities.* Tucson, AZ: Therapy Skill Builders

17

High-Technology Adaptations to Compensate for Disability

Jennifer Angelo and Mary Ellen Buning

LEARNING OBJECTIVES

After studying this chapter, the reader will be able to do the following:

1. Describe the basic components of the AT assessment and team members.
2. Give examples of using AT within occupational functioning.
3. Define key categories of AT.
4. Apply AT to occupational function.
5. Explain the role of AT within occupational therapy practice areas.

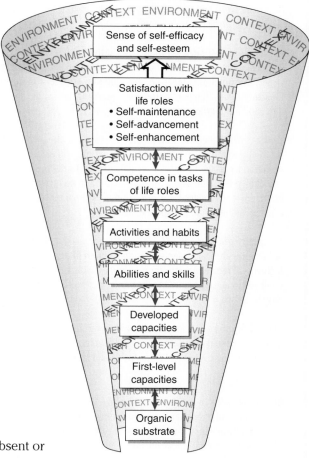

*T*he goal of assistive technology (AT) is to compensate for absent or impaired abilities. Through technology, consumers manage a variety of daily living tasks, participate in life as they choose, and make choices based on their goals and desired roles. Thus, technology supports consumers in occupational performance. As Trombly states in Chapter 1, competent role performance leads to life satisfaction. This is the goal of technology: allowing consumers to engage in occupational performance tasks consisting of meaningful activities that contribute to quality of life. Occupational therapists help consumers overcome functional deficits by understanding their goals and preferences, assessing their abilities, and matching their goals and abilities with appropriate AT solutions. AT devices that match consumers' goals and abilities help them assume or return to meaningful lives.

GLOSSARY

Augmentative and alternative communication (AAC)—A communication system that requires use of something external to the body. Examples include pen and paper, letter or picture communication boards, and communication devices. Devices may be manual or electronic. A communication method, such as letters grouped into words or picture symbols, is used with each system. Consumers often combine vocalizations and gestures to enhance their communication when using an AAC device.

Abbreviation expansion—Software designed to increase typing speed, decrease keystrokes, and decrease errors. Abbreviations are entered into a database. For example, OT is the abbreviation for occupational therapy. The abbreviation is entered instead of the entire word and the software expands the abbreviation into the word or phrase it represents.

Application software—Productivity software that uses the resources of the hardware and operating system to allow the user to perform functional tasks on the computer, such as accounting, illustration, desktop publishing, early learning, personal calendars, and bibliography management.

Array—When the selection method is scanning, the array is the set of options that are presented for selection. The user makes a selection by coordinating switch activation with the presentation of a choice from the array. Some selections in an array open a branch or a secondary array, for example when a punctuation array is opened from an alphabet array.

Computer aided design (CAD)—Software used to design, draft, or lay out technical projects ranging from architecture to manufacturing. Precise measurements can be made. CAD facilitates modifications, and manufacturing and construction costs are easy to obtain.

Dvorak layout—Computer keyboard layout named after its originator. Its design facilitates rapid and efficient keyboarding because it places the most frequently used letters within easy reach.

Electronic aids to daily living (EADL)—Devices that give consumers control of appliances in their environment. This term is favored because it stresses the *task* (i.e., increased independence, safety, communication, and leisure) rather than the *thing* being controlled (i.e., television, telephone, and lights). EADL accurately describes the technology and has helped funding, both here and in Europe.

Environmental control unit (ECU)—Alternative term, still frequently used, for electronic aids to daily living.

E-tran board—Nonvocal communication device in an acrylic window frame with an open space in the center. Communication symbols or letters are placed around the frame in a specific sequence on both sides of the acrylic. The consumer indicates choice by eye gaze. Both communication partners must be trained in its use.

Graphical user interface (GUI)—The software that offers pull-down menus, icons, windows, and dialog boxes to create a visually oriented computer screen. GUIs reduce the cognitive load for computer use and help typical users perform common computer tasks. Adaptations are available to help users with visual impairments.

Infrared (IR)—Light wave outside of (longer than) the spectrum normally detected by the human eye. Sequences of IR code can be interpreted as specific commands by an IR receiver, which executes a command such as volume up or volume down.

Microprocessor—Miniature piece of integrated circuit board that performs a prescribed operation or set of operations. Today not only computers but also automobiles, small household appliances, and consumer products contain microprocessors.

Pixel—Smallest unit of visual display on a computer screen; a dot. These dots combine to form letters, punctuation symbols, or images. A dimension such as 640×480 refers to the number of pixels per given area that a monitor can display. On a color monitor each pixel also carries information about hue and value.

Pneumatic—Switch activation by increasing or decreasing air pressure. Switches that are commonly called sip 'n' puff are pneumatic switches.

QWERTY layout—Common layout for computer keyboards in which the sequential letters in the top left row are QWERTY. This layout originated with mechanical typewriters when it was important to slow typists down so that the strike arms that printed each letter had time to avoid each other.

Radio frequency (RF)—Signaling technology that uses nonpublic bands of RF. It is often used to control appliances and devices in AT or to direct home automation systems.

Scanning—Selection method in which the consumer waits for a choice to be offered rather than actively making a choice. A single switch is used to indicate which of the offered choices is wanted.

(continued)

GLOSSARY (Continued)

Speech synthesizer—Computer peripheral (software, hardware, or a combination) that allows a computer to imitate human speech. Synthesizers are available for many languages.

Transparent access—Quality of a computer adaptation that allows it to be used without special setup, as when an adaptive or mini computer keyboard plugs into the normal computer keyboard port and is immediately available for use.

Tongue-touch keypad (TTK)—Means of direct selection in which the tongue presses one of nine keys imbedded in an interface worn in a dental appliance at the roof of the mouth. Radio frequency signals are sent to an external receiver that can control a computer, drive a wheelchair, or control appliances in the environment. Speech is only mildly affected.

Ultrasound—Sound outside the frequency detected by the human ear. This signaling technology is often used in AT to control appliances or computer-related devices.

Universal design—Design concept used when a built space or a consumer product is accessible or usable by almost all persons. For example, an airport designer considers not only persons using wheelchairs, but those who are elderly, have visual impairments, or do not speak English.

Word prediction—Software that uses rules of recency and frequency to anticipate the word the consumer is beginning to type. It is designed to decrease keystrokes and errors but is not especially effective at increasing typing speed. Word prediction is built into some word processors and is available in some AAC devices.

Context

Social contexts
Familiar peers
Familiar nonpeers
Strangers
Alone

Setting
Home (individual)
Group home
Employment
School
Community

Physical contexts
Light
Sound
Heat

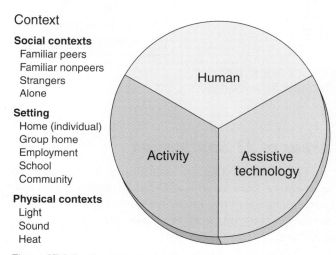

Figure 17-1 The Human Activity Assistive Technology (HAAT) Model. (Modified with permission from Cook, A. M., & Hussey, S. M. [1995]. *Assistive Technologies: Principles and Practice.* Baltimore: Mosby.)

Models

Models serve as analogies and are symbolic representations of difficult-to-visualize elements of a system (Portney & Watkins, 1993). Two models in particular, the Human Activity Assistive Technology Model (Cook & Hussey, 1995) (Fig. 17-1) and the Enabling–Disabling Process (Brandt & Pope, 1997) (Fig. 17-2), represent how AT devices help consumers develop or return to occupational functioning and achieve life satisfaction.

The Human Activity Assistive Technology Model

The Human Activity Assistive Technology (HAAT) Model (Cook & Hussey, 1995), widely used by AT providers, explains the interrelationship between human and nonhuman elements. In this model, *human* refers to an individual attempting to engage in activity. The activity, the fundamental element of the model, is daily living tasks that the individual wishes to accomplish.

The AT portion of the HAAT Model has four sections: the human–technology interface, processor, activity output, and environmental interface. The human–technology interface is the contact between the person and the technology device. The processor, the mechanical or electrical linkage, relays or interprets information from the interface. The activity output includes actions such as opening doors and printing a page of text. The environmental interface adjusts the output of the device in response to input from the environment. The final but essential factor in the HAAT model is the social, cultural, and physical context in which the AT is used. For example, people usually conduct themselves differently at the beach than at a religious ceremony. They may choose to take nonelectronic devices (manual wheelchair and communication board) that cannot be damaged by wind and sand to the beach. They may decide to take a power wheelchair and battery-powered augmentative communication device to a religious ceremony that is indoors and fully accessible. The AT devices must match these different contexts.

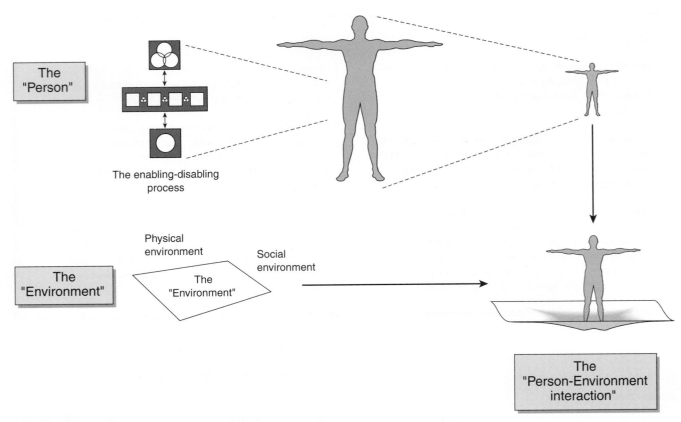

Figure 17-2 The Person–Enviroment Model. (Modified with permission from Brandt, E., & Pope, A. [1997]. Enabling America: Assessing the Role of Rehabilitation Science and Engineering. Washington: National Academy.)

The Person–Environment Interaction Model

The second model, the Person–Environment Interaction Model, depicts an enabling–disabling process (Brandt & Pope, 1997). This model describes a dynamic process that takes place between the individual and the environment. The figure of a human being in the drawing stands on a mat. The mat represents the physical and social environments in which the individual lives. The more severe the impairment, the greater the deflection in the mat. The more the mat deflects, the more the environment must be modified to compensate for the disability created by impairment.

The use of AT devices (i.e., devices used within the environment) and modifications to the environment make the mat more resilient. For example, curb cuts enable consumers using wheelchairs to cross streets and move about freely. Magnifying glasses assist consumers with poor vision to draw insulin into a syringe and monitor their glucose levels independently. A switch connected to a computer with specialized software allows consumers unable to use a computer keyboard to complete work-related tasks.

Areas of AT Application

As occupational therapy contributes in all areas of consumers' lives, so also AT enables performance and participation for consumers in all areas of their lives. AT is used in self-care, work or school, and play or leisure activities.

Self-Maintenance Roles

Many daily activities focus on self care and personal maintenance. Mostly low-tech devices are used in personal grooming activities; however, high tech items, such as electric toothbrushes, WaterPics, and electric shavers, may be used to perform these tasks.

Environmental Controls

It is taken for granted that turning a light on or off or raising the volume when a favorite song is played on the radio increases comfort and enjoyment. Consumers with significant disabilities manage functions such as these through the use of **electronic aids to daily living**

[EADL], also known as **environmental control units [ECU]**. Modifying the on–off switch, the power supply or the control technology, lets the consumer regulate many devices in the environment. Common control technologies are **radio frequency (RF)**, **ultrasound**, and **infrared (IR)** light. Figure 17-3 describes how both simple and complex EADL may be used.

Mobility

Mobility, a basic form of self-maintenance, achieves high ratings from consumers with disabilities as a necessity in everyday life (Verbrugge et al., 1997). It can be used to communicate curiosity, interest in participating, or the wish to be alone. The mobility offered by devices is used when impairment creates limitations in range, comfort, safety, and endurance.

Home Modifications

For consumers with mobility impairments, home modification is usually necessary to allow use of AT devices. It is difficult for a consumer using a wheelchair to cook a meal in a kitchen that has not been modified for wheelchair accessibility. This same consumer will have difficulty using the toilet or managing personal grooming in a standard bathroom with no modifications. **Universal design**, a new inclusive concept in design, incorporates ideas for people-friendly spaces that increase safety and creates spaces usable by all persons.

Computer Access to Support Instrumental Activities of Daily Living

Many instrumental activities of daily living (IADL), such as budgeting, banking, bill paying, correspondence, meal planning, and shopping, can be completed by means of a computer and software, particularly with an Internet connection. Text telephones (TTY) (formerly called telecommunication device for the deaf [TDD]) and hands-free telephones enable calling paratransit organizations, shopping for groceries, and ordering from catalogs over the telephone (see Research Note).

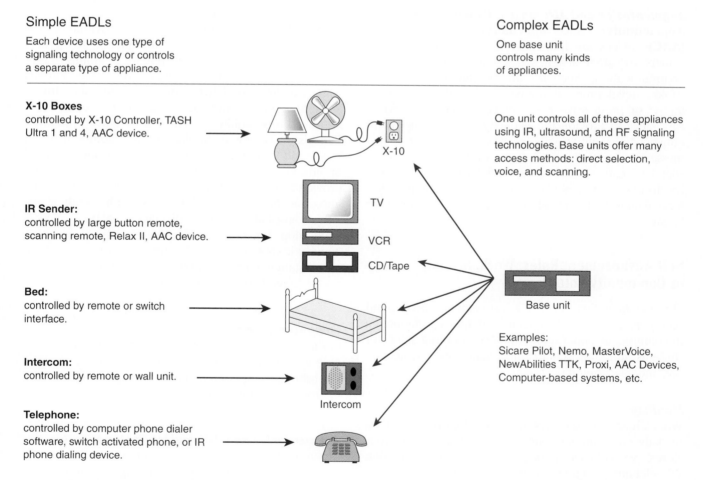

Simple EADLs

Each device uses one type of signaling technology or controls a separate type of appliance.

X-10 Boxes
controlled by X-10 Controller, TASH Ultra 1 and 4, AAC device.

X-10

IR Sender:
controlled by large button remote, scanning remote, Relax II, AAC device.

TV

VCR

CD/Tape

Bed:
controlled by remote or switch interface.

Intercom:
controlled by remote or wall unit.

Intercom

Telephone:
controlled by computer phone dialer software, switch activated phone, or IR phone dialing device.

Complex EADLs

One base unit controls many kinds of appliances.

One unit controls all of these appliances using IR, ultrasound, and RF signaling technologies. Base units offer many access methods: direct selection, voice, and scanning.

Base unit

Examples:
Sicare Pilot, Nemo, MasterVoice, NewAbilities TTK, Proxi, AAC Devices, Computer-based systems, etc.

Figure 17-3 Simple and complex EADL.

RESEARCH NOTE

The Use of Phones by Elders with Disabilities: Problems, Interventions, Costs

Mann, W. C., Hurren, D, Charvat B, & Tomita, M. Assistive Technology, 8, 23–33

ABSTRACT

Recognizing the important role the telephone plays in the life of frail elders, this study sought to gain a better understanding of the problems these elders encounter in using their phones to meet their needs. Starting with a sample of 354 frail elders, it was determined that 35, or just under 10%, were having some difficulty in using of their phones. Of these 35 subjects, 22 were randomly selected for an assessment of their impairments and phone setups in their homes. Interventions were provided to 19 of the 22 subjects, with 2 subjects refusing intervention. At a 6-week follow-up call, all subjects were satisfied with the new phone or phone-related equipment. At a 6-month follow-up, 95% of subjects expressed satisfaction with the intervention.

Average cost of equipment was $70.45; cost of personnel time was significantly higher. Recommendations are made for addressing the phone-related problems of frail elders.

IMPLICATIONS FOR PRACTICE

▶ The telephone is an important piece of technology that facilitates occupational performance.
▶ Telephone-related adaptive equipment must be examined carefully during reviews of technology that assists with independent living and assuming and resuming occupational performance.
▶ Areas where phone-related problems can occur are vision, mobility, fine motor control, cognition, hearing, and safety.

Augmentative and Alternative Communication

Augmentative and alternative communication (AAC) devices are frequently recommended for consumers who are unable to speak or adequately use vocal communication. Speech can be impaired through stroke, developmental apraxia, cerebral palsy, brain injury, or progressive neurological impairment. Some AAC devices provide the capacity to carry on typical conversations, while others assist in relaying a few messages. Generally, AAC devices allow consumers to socialize, call for assistance, direct caregivers, inform health care providers about health issues, initiate plans for activities, and make choices, such as what they want to eat.

Self-Advancement Roles: Work, School, or Community Volunteer

The specific activities of self-advancement roles depend on a person's age and social role. Retirees participating in volunteer activities and employees working at jobs or students attending school find challenges and accomplishments in their daily tasks.

Mobility

Wheelchairs and scooters allow freedom of movement in daily environments—neighborhood streets, schools, stores, workplaces, parks, and recreation facilities. Wheelchairs designed for mobility in rugged environments provide access to areas such as farms, ranches, and the backwoods.

Environmental Access

Assistive technology can play a role in providing access to the environment. Ramps and automatic door openers make entering and leaving public buildings easier whether or not an individual uses a wheelchair. Parents with strollers and delivery persons with hand trucks agree that ramps and automatic door openers have improved the ability to enter and leave buildings. Today's many new technologies make communication easier and faster for everyone. When AT is incorporated or added to these media, the same advantages are provided to persons with sensory, motor, and language impairments. E-mail read by a **speech synthesizer**, TTY, refreshable Braille displays, real-time closed-captioning for conference presentations, teleconferences, videophones for sign language communication, and distance learning all offer opportunities for greater access to work, school, and recreation.

Computer Access

Computers equipped with appropriate adaptations enable writing, accounting, managing databases, desktop publishing, using computer-aided design, searching the Internet, and phoning, faxing, and printing.

Augmentative and Alternative Communication

Communication is essential in school and the workplace. Making choices, demonstrating knowledge, asking questions, forming peer relationships, and getting the job done all occur because of communication. AAC devices can be an effective part of a total communication strategy that includes gestures, speech or vocal sounds, signs, and communication devices.

Self-Enhancement Roles: Recreation and Leisure

Recreational choices reveal who we are as humans. They are chosen according to interest, their challenge characteristics, and their symbolic meaning (Kielhofner, 1997). Recreation and play allows individuals to rehearse new roles, experience themselves in new ways, and escape from the pressures and responsibilities of everyday life. Assistive technology supports people as they engage in self-enhancement roles. While reimbursement streams focus on payment for services that increase independence in work, school, and self-care domains, it is the play and recreation domain that is most clearly associated with motivation and the idealized self. Recreational choices made for their intrinsic and symbolic qualities allow individuals to take on valued images of self as adventurer, connoisseur, or creator (see Chapter 34).

Environmental Controls

Controlling one's environment is an important aspect of recreation and leisure. IR-controlled appliances that are common in home entertainment appliances can be controlled with EADL that learn the IR signals of a particular TV, VCR, or CD player. Switch-adapted toys allow children to learn cause and effect, participate in group activities, develop higher-level motor control, and at times improve cognitive skills. Video games, whether played in stand-alone units connected to a TV or on computers, can be controlled with switches as alternatives for triggers.

Mobility

All types of recreational technologies allow participation and engagement in sports and active recreation. Wheelchairs designed for beaches, tennis courts, or mountain trails allow mobility in specialized environments. Adaptive mobility devices introduced early to children with motor impairments provide independent play and exploration. Water sit-skis and adaptive snow skis like monoskis allow recreational mobility in mainstream recreations. With the increase in accessible facilities in the community, traveling also becomes a possible form of recreation and play.

Computer Access

Computers can be an important source of adaptive leisure. Many Americans enjoy browsing sites on the Internet, playing computer games, and engaging in creative art activities and puzzles on home computers. The Internet can be a means to make travel plans, find accessible accommodations, and rent accessible vans in distant locations.

The AT Assessment Process

The contribution made by a well-chosen and fully used AT device is remarkable. AT's contribution is the result of a skilled, thoughtful, and thorough assessment. A discussion of the elements of this process follows. (Fig. 17-4 is an overview of the AT assessment and intervention sequence.)

Assessments are driven by the consumer's goals and needs (Bain & Leger, 1997; Cook & Hussey, 1995). Goals and needs may also be identified by significant family members or caregivers on behalf of the consumer who has difficulty communicating needs or desires. The AT team attempts to understand and address the consumer's, family members', and caregivers' reasons for and expectations of the assessment. It is important to clear up any misunderstandings about the capabilities of the AT team and the types of AT devices available. Clarifying these issues before beginning the assessment prevents disappointment and creates more realistic expectations.

Consumers, family members, and caregivers come to the assessment with various motivations and needs. For example, young adults may be starting college and need equipment to enhance their ability to complete

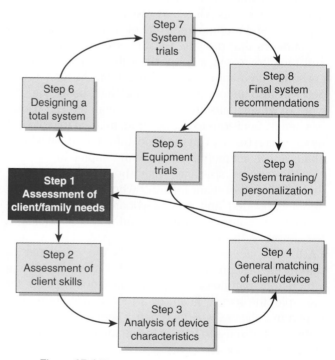

Figure 17-4 Nine steps in the assessment process for AT.

assignments in a timely fashion, obtain information from the Internet, participate in online class discussion, and exchange class notes. Adult consumers may need to update their AT devices to fit the demands of their employment.

In addition to their goals and priorities, the assessment focuses on consumer and family attitudes toward AT. Some people easily adopt technology and incorporate it into tasks and routines. Others resist and even fear it. Some consumers feel that the latest high-technology equipment is not necessary and prefer simpler, more familiar devices. Consumers' religious and cultural background and personal tastes influence the choice of devices. Devices that fit within the personal and cultural context of the consumer and his or her family are more likely to be used than devices that provide the latest in technological sophistication but are outside the realm of the consumer's self-perception. Putting aside personal values, the AT team concentrates on addressing the consumer's goals and preferences.

Team Members

The team consists of a variety of stakeholders and experts. The consumer, family, and caregivers are the team leaders. These individuals will live day in and day out with the equipment; their concerns must be reflected in the AT team's recommendations. Professionals on the team vary according to the consumer's needs.

The seating and positioning expert for the team may be an occupational or physical therapist or a rehabilitation engineer. This AT expert assesses consumers' seating needs and recommends one of several types of seating surfaces that provide a stable, secure, comfortable and pressure-relieving support for the consumer. If the consumer has a mobility impairment, the AT team member will also recommend a wheelchair base. Various types of wheelchairs are available to match the consumer's needs. Decisions to change from manual to powered mobility can be made at this time. Information on wheelchairs and assessment is provided in Chapter 16.

The access specialist may be an occupational therapist or other team member who is knowledgeable about expanded and mini keyboards, joysticks, computer head controls, switches, and software packages that improve the use of computers, AAC devices, and EADL. The access specialist assists the consumer in finding the best possible access methods by determining which body part he or she has the most control over, for example, the hands, head, or a foot. Furthermore, this expert investigates whether control is improved through enhancers (discussed later in the chapter) such as typing sticks or head sticks.

A teacher or special educator may be on the team if the consumer is a student. The teacher or special educator describes schoolwork tasks that the student has difficulty performing. This information helps the AT team understand the issues and recommend solutions to support educational tasks.

A vocational rehabilitation counselor may be on the team for a consumer who is actively looking for employment. The vocational rehabilitation counselor describes specific tasks to be performed on the job and helps with funding.

A speech pathologist with expertise in AAC directs the team when the focus of the assessment is communication. This professional evaluates the consumer for both verbal and written communication needs and potential. Depending on the consumer's age, cognition, and linguistic competence, the speech pathologist determines the types of symbol sets that will be most useful for communication. The speech pathologist relies on the access assessment results to determine how the consumer will use sophisticated or simple augmentative communication devices. The recommended interventions depend on the consumer's goals, environments, and cognitive ability and may include several communication methods in addition to an AAC device.

A rehabilitation engineer may be on the team if the consumer has complex needs and off-the-shelf solutions are not likely to be effective. He or she may also serve consumers with severe impairments needing to integrate several pieces of technology. For example, some consumers have reliable control only over a finger or eyebrow. Using this finger or eyebrow and an input method (i.e., switch) these consumers drive wheelchairs, control AAC devices, and operate word processors on computers.

A social worker is sometimes part of the team. The social worker may seek out appropriate funding sources or help consumers and significant others come to terms with the disability through counseling.

Rehabilitation technology suppliers (RTS) (previously known as vendors) play an important role on the AT team. AT teams do not necessarily have access to all of the devices they would like to have on hand for assessments. When the team wants to evaluate devices they do not have, they call the RTS who carries the device. The RTS can demonstrate devices and may be able to lend devices for assessment. Many AT teams have positive, close working relationships with a variety of suppliers. These working relationships facilitate smoothly functioning evaluation centers and help consumers later with follow-up and product adjustments.

The AT Assessment

Prior to the assessment, the AT team needs to understand the consumer's goals, the family members' and caregivers' goals, and the consumer's strengths and weaknesses. This information is captured either through an intake questionnaire or a videotape or telephone interview. The answers to the questionnaire and videotape give the team a realistic picture of the consumer's motor control and possibly the environments where the consumer will use the devices. Having this information prior to the assessment gives the team time to prepare devices and/or borrow equipment. Areas commonly addressed in assessments follow.

Seating

To achieve the best results for the entire assessment, optimal seating is mandatory. Results for the rest of the assessment will not indicate the consumer's true ability if he or she uses a seating system that does not provide adequate support (see Chapter 16).

Sometimes it is not possible to address seating issues before the rest of the assessment. When this happens, a seating simulator can be used. A seating simulator has an adjustable back, sides, armrests, lateral supports, pommels, and foot supports. The risk in using a seating simulator instead of the consumer's personal seating system is that it may be difficult to duplicate the control the consumer had in the seating simulator. Therefore, whenever possible the *best* solution is to assess consumers in their own appropriately fitting seating system and wheelchair.

Another important factor to determine early in the assessment is where and in what positions the consumer spends most of the time. Asking these questions at the beginning of the assessment avoids recommending access methods that the consumer can use with nearly full accuracy in the wheelchair only to find out that at home the consumer spends most of the time on the floor, in a beanbag chair, or in a lounge chair. Once seating issues have been resolved, motor control for access is typically addressed.

Motor Control

Ideally, access methods, such as touch typing, are effortless. Effortlessness comes after practicing and refining the skill. For the typist, it seems the fingers know the words as they rapidly move across the keys. Attention is on the thoughts the typist wishes to enter into the word processor rather than individual keystrokes. To reach effortlessness, it is important to narrow access methods to those that the consumer is able or potentially able to activate consistently and reliably.

The therapist first identifies potential anatomical sites for access by evaluating range of motion and fine motor coordination. Often consumers and their family members and caregivers know the body parts over which the consumer has most control and can provide this information. Usually the hands and fingers are assessed first, as they are the preferred method for interacting with objects (Cook & Hussey, 1995). If the consumer is unsuccessful at accurately using his or her hands or fingers, head movements may be assessed next. Consumers who have limited control over their upper extremities sometimes have control over head movements. If the consumer is only partly successful at using his or her head to indicate a selection, the consumer may have more control over eye movements. The assessment may continue with evaluating the potential for volitional control of the feet, knees, or other sites that can interface with access devices. The best two or three sites should be considered at this point in the assessment.

Evaluating range of motion helps to determine the range a consumer has for accessing a keyboard, switch, and other input devices. Assessment boards are easily constructed and useful when assessing range of motion and coordination (Box 17-1). To evaluate range of motion the therapist uses an assessment board. Using one body part, the therapist asks the consumer to point to the squares on the board's perimeter with a finger,

BOX 17-1
PROCEDURES FOR PRACTICE

Preparing Range of Motion and Fine Coordination Assessment Boards

Materials needed:

▶ Two pieces of poster board measuring approximately 11 by 17 inches each
▶ Permanent marker
▶ Ruler
▶ Clear plastic-coated contact paper

Directions:

1. Using the permanent marker and ruler, mark off one of the poster boards into a 2-inch grid.
2. Mark the other poster board into a 1-inch grid.
3. Number the squares on each poster board sequentially.
4. Place clear contact paper over each poster board.

The poster boards are now ready to be used during the assessment. The plastic covering protects the boards against moisture. Also, stickers can be placed and removed repeatedly from the poster boards without damaging them.

Some consumers are motivated to touch specific squares with colorful, eye-catching stickers or small food items, such as Cheerios. Consumers whose cognition is intact can point to requested numbers printed in each square. Duplicating a small version of the grid on an assessment form allows the therapist to shade in the squares on the grid with the locations or numbers that the consumer easily reached. This assessment tool is further described in *Assistive Technology for Rehabilitation Therapists* (Angelo, 1997).

hand, head (using a head pointer), or toe depending on which anatomical site is being evaluated. Using the grid printed on the assessment form, the therapist indicates the areas the consumer should reach. Assessing range helps the therapist get an idea of the types of access devices the consumer can use successfully. For example, if the consumer easily reaches the perimeter of the poster board grid, a normal computer keyboard may be useful. Conversely, if the consumer can reach only squares in the middle of the grid and close to the midline, the access method needs to use this area.

To assess coordination, the therapist asks the consumer to point to specific squares on the perimeter and in the middle of one of the poster boards. Accuracy in pointing to specific squares gives the therapist an idea of the consumer's coordination. If the board with 1-inch squares was used first and accuracy is sufficient using one or more of the anatomical sites, the therapist proceeds with the assessment. If the accuracy is only fair with all anatomical sites, the test is repeated using the 2-inch grid. If the results do not clearly indicate the consumer's pointing ability with at least one anatomical site, the therapist may ask the consumer to try a head pointer or hand-held device to assist with accuracy. Figure 17-5 shows a consumer using a head pointer to operate an augmentative communication device.

Once pointing trials with three or four anatomical sites are completed with some consistency, compare the results. Comparisons help determine which anatomical site the consumer uses most consistently and accurately. The therapist asks the consumer to point to the same six squares in the same order using each anatomical site being tested. Keeping all the variables identical except for the anatomical site, the therapist determines which anatomical site offers the consumer the best

In direct selection, all items in the selection set are available at any time. Examples of direct selections are computer keyboards, telephone keypads, and calculator keypads. The advantage of direct selection is that it is intuitive. If an individual presses a K on the keyboard, he or she can expect to get a K on the visual display. Also, it is usually faster than using indirect selection. The disadvantage is that direct selection requires coordination and some range of motion, depending on the size of each item in the selection set.

At times trying to press just the right key is too difficult for some consumers with limited motor control. For example, the A key on a computer keyboard may be too far away, or the consumer may repeatedly press the Q or Z key when trying for the A key.

With indirect selection (also known as scanning), only one item of the set is available at any given time. Examples are the numbers used to set the time on a digital clock and moving through the numbers on a radio dial to select a specific station. The advantage is that the consumer needs only consistent and reliable control over one movement, such as an eyebrow, the forehead, one finger, or a toe. The disadvantage is that it is much slower to use than direct selection. Visual tracking skills and the ability to sequence are needed, as is a high level of attention. Also, it is considered to be cognitively more difficult than direct selection.

control. The consumer is asked whether he or she agrees with which site provided the most control. If the consumer feels more comfortable using another body part, the therapist and consumer should discuss this and come to agreement on which site should be the primary access site.

Direct Versus Indirect Selection Methods

Once the anatomical site has been determined, the types of access devices can be reviewed. This evaluation helps assess whether the consumer can use direct selection or indirect selection (Box 17-2). If a consumer effortlessly uses an anatomical site to point, direct selection is probably most appropriate. However, if the consumer cannot accurately and consistently point with any of the anatomical sites, the therapist should assess the consumer's ability to press a single switch for indirect selection.

The goal for the indirect selection assessment is to identify anatomical sites with which the consumer can activate a switch consistently without unintentionally pressing it. To assess indirect selection, a variety of single switches are placed near the anatomical sites used in the

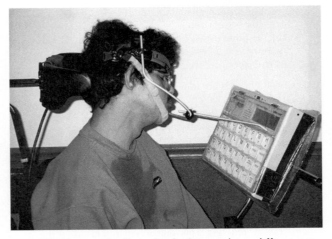

Figure 17-5 An example of how a head pointer can be used. Here a man uses it as an input method with a communication device.

coordination assessment. Table 17-1 describes several commonly used switches along with typical activation methods. As with direct selection, the hands or fingers may be assessed first, followed by the head and other body sites.

Switch Assessment

Switch mounting is critical for success when using single-switch access. Poorly mounted switches create frustration and lead to disuse. Switches are mounted so they remain in place. This provides for consistent and reliable switch pressing throughout use. The switch mount must be easily secured in the proper position. Mounts with obvious connections to wheelchairs or desks are far more likely to be used correctly than those that have complicated attachments. Furthermore, switch mounting must be easily removed so that it does not interfere with other activities, such as transfers and eating.

The type of switch depends on the anatomical site chosen to control it. A variety of switches are shown in Figure 17-6. For example, consumers having control over one finger may best use a small, sensitive switch. In contrast, a foot switch mounted near a wheelchair footrest has to be rugged, as it must withstand use from shoes and impact when the wheelchair is in motion. Some consumers have control over an anatomical site

that is bony, such as the back of the hand. In this case, a switch with a covering that cushions and protects the skin from abrasion is appropriate.

Regardless of the type of switch recommended, it should provide feedback so the consumer knows whether the movement was successful. Usually this feedback is auditory, but it may be visual. Switches

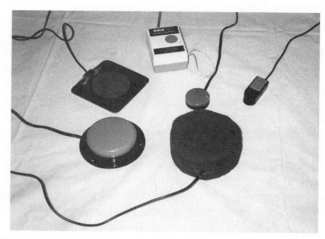

Figure 17-6 A variety of commonly used switches. Starting at the bottom and moving clockwise: Soft switch, Jelly Bean, Plate, String, Snap, and Microlite.

TABLE 17-1
Common Switches and Activation Method

Category and Specific Switches	Company	Primary Activation Site
No Physical Contact		
IST switch (infrared)	Words+	Eye
Eyegaze	LC Technologies	Eye
Eyecan	H. K. Eyecan, Ltd.	Eye
Adjustable proximity switch	Adaptive Switch Laboratory	
Adjustable photoelectric switch	Adaptive Switch Laboratory	
Untouchable Buddy	TASH	Arm, hand, head, foot
Physical Contact, No Pressure		
Pneumatic (also known as sip & puff)	Prentke Romich	Mouth
P-switch	Prentke Romich	Any volition and consistent muscle contraction
Pressure		
Single rocking lever	Prentke Romich	Arm, hand, head, foot
Tongue switch	Prentke Romich	Tongue
Wobble	Prentke Romich	Arm, hand, head
Jelly bean switch	Ablenet	Arm, hand, head, foot
Specs switch	Ablenet	Arm, hand, head, foot
Big red	Ablenet	Arm, hand, head, foot
Wobble	Zygo	Arm, hand, head, foot
Bass	Don Johnston	Arm, hand, head, foot

activated through head movements should produce quieter auditory feedback than switches activated with anatomical sites farther away from the ears. A noisy switch mounted near the ear that is used for several hours can be annoying and tiring.

Six occupational therapists with expertise in AT participated in a focus group to develop a list of the 10 most important considerations for switch access (Angelo, 2000). In the control category, the therapists indicated that the most important considerations were reliability of response, ability to perform timed responses, ability to activate and deactivate the switch within a given time frame, and endurance (the ability to sustain a force and to apply that force repeatedly over time). In the ease of movement category, therapists said that tasks should be performed volitionally, easily, and efficiently and that past performances with positive outcomes should be considered. The therapists also indicated that context was important. Assessments should be conducted in the environment where the consumer routinely performs the task. Finally, switch safety should be considered. Switches should have rounded corners, and all wires should be secured so that they do not become entangled with fingers, pointing devices, or other equipment (Box 17-3).

BOX 17-3
PROCEDURES FOR PRACTICE

Switch Assessment

1. Identify the anatomical sites for switch activation over which the consumer has most control. No timing is involved in this step.
2. Evaluate the consumer's ability to wait a specific length of time (1 to 5 seconds) before activating the switch. Being able to activate the switch within the appropriate time is critical for using indirect selection effectively. Inability to wait the appropriate length of time (i.e., activating the switch prematurely) leads to selection errors.
3. Evaluate the consumer's ability to maintain contact with the switch. Some switches must be held down for a specific length of time before the switch activates. This activity also shows the consumer's ability for inverse scanning.
4. Evaluate the consumer's ability to release the switch on command. Releasing the switch at the appropriate time indicates whether the consumer can make accurate selections during scanning. Errors in selection occur when the switch is released too soon or too late.
5. Once one or more anatomical sites have been identified for accurate switch pressing, the AT team determines which type of switch is most appropriate and how best to mount the switch.

This concept is further described in Cook & Hussey (1995).

Cognition

Cognition is usually evaluated informally during AT assessments (Cook & Hussey, 1995). The consumer's attention span, reading level, short- and long-term memory, and ability to follow instructions and sequence tasks should all be noted. Determining these abilities helps the AT team determine which devices are appropriate to the consumer's cognitive ability (see Chapter 8).

Visual Acuity and Visual Perception

The primary reason for AT assessment may be blindness or visual impairment and this will guide many aspects of the assessment. Otherwise, it is important to assess visual acuity and perception of all consumers. During an AT assessment, eye range of motion, conjugate eye movements, visual field cuts, tracking, **scanning**, and figure–ground discrimination are assessed. Assessments such as the *Motor Free Visual Perception Test* (Colarusso et al., 1996) and the *Test of Visual Perception Skills* (Gardiner, 1993), which directly test visual perception, may help determine the consumer's abilities (see Chapter 7).

The team needs to know about the consumer's visual acuity. They assess it by asking the consumer to identify symbols, letters, or icons of different sizes. This information helps to determine the appropriate size of symbols for communication boards and displays on other AT devices. In addition to size, the team determines the contrast. Some consumers need high contrast between the symbol and background. Consumers with visual impairments sometimes prefer light colored letters or symbols on a dark background. Finally, the distance from the eye to the screen should be evaluated to determine optimal viewing.

If the AT team suspects an acuity problem, without exception a referral should be made to a qualified optometrist or ophthalmologist. If problems remain after the vision examination, a referral to an optometrist specializing in visual perceptual dysfunction may be necessary.

Once acuity issues have been resolved, eye range of motion (visual field) should be assessed. This means assessing how far to the right, left, up, and down the consumer can move his or her eyes. For consumers using indirect selection methods, the ability to track (follow a target with the eyes) and scan (find a specific target in a field of targets) must be determined.

Assessing conjugate eye movement provides useful information. A simple way is to ask the consumer to follow an object as it is brought toward his or her nose. If the eyes do not converge, the AT team should determine which eye is dominant and give that eye preference during the assessment and when equipment is set up for use.

Next, determine whether there is visual field loss. A field cut can occur in the center, blocking out central vision, in multiple spots, or within any quadrant of the visual field. This information is helpful for determining the location of the visual display. Tracking is assessed in conjunction with field loss. Delays in eye movement, a midline jerk, or regions where the consumer loses the object being followed can indicate a visual field loss. Once the performance of the visual system and the ability to track are known, scanning can be assessed. If tracking is impaired, activities that encourage the development of tracking skills, such as simple cause-and-effect software under the control of a single switch, can be used to encourage development of tracking. Auditory scanning or providing an audible cue prior to item selection is another possibility.

Scanning in general means the ability to search visually for objects. In AT assessments it means that the consumer can find the correct word, icon, or object in a series of objects or an array. More information on scanning is provided in Box 17-4.

Figure–ground discrimination should also be assessed to determine how well the consumer can distinguish objects in the foreground from those in the background. The AT team needs this information to ensure that objects used in a visual display are easily recognized and that the background is not competing with the objects in the foreground. Sometimes objects (icons, words, or symbols) have to be placed farther apart or the background simplified to reduce visual stimulation.

Finalizing the Match Between User and Technology

By this time in the assessment, the AT team has a clear idea of the consumer's motor, cognitive, visual, and visual perception abilities. The AT team should have two or more combinations of AT devices, input devices, mounts, and control enhancers that they think closely match the consumer's abilities. Trials of two to three devices with the control interface and control enhancers allow the consumer to become familiar with the equipment and determine how comfortable he or she feels when using it.

Once devices, control interfaces, and control enhancers options have been narrowed to two or three choices, a more extensive trial of each is conducted. As previously mentioned (Angelo, 2000), this trial, if not the entire assessment, should be in the environment where the consumer will use the equipment. Using the system in the actual or intended environment—home, workplace, or school—uncovers problems that may not emerge during center-based trials. Noise, desks that are too small for equipment, tables that are too low and

---

BOX 17-4
Basic Scanning Modes

Automatic
The consumer presses the switch to initiate scanning. The cursor highlights items in the selection set one at a time. The consumer presses the switch as the desired item is highlighted.

Inverse
The consumer presses the switch to initiate scanning. However, the consumer must maintain switch closure for the cursor to move across the selection set. When the desired item is highlighted, the consumer releases the switch, indicating the choice.

Step
The consumer presses the switch to move to the next item in the selection set. The cursor moves to the adjacent item each time the switch is pressed. A selection is made when the cursor dwells on an item and the consumer refrains from pressing the switch.

---

bump knees when the consumer tries to get a wheelchair underneath, and lights that are too dim or that glare on the display can be addressed and solutions identified. This trial should occur *before* submitting recommendations and a final equipment list. A trial in the environment where the equipment will be used ensures the best recommendations possible and increases the likelihood that the devices will actually be used and not abandoned.

The AT Intervention Process

The specifics of AT recommendations are guided by the consumer's needs, goals, capacities, abilities, and desired roles. Broad categories of AT solutions include control enhancers, computers, AAC devices, and EADL.

Control Enhancers

AT devices alone usually do not provide enough support for consumers to engage in occupational roles. Consumers also need the support of low-technology aids, that is, control enhancers. The term *control enhancer*, first used by Cook and Hussey (1995), refers to aids that enhance or extend a consumer's physical control. Examples of control enhancers are head pointers, hand-held pointing devices (pencils, pointers with built-up handles, typing sticks, Wanchik writers), mouth sticks, wrist rests, and arm supports. Control enhancers also include placement of interface devices (keyboards and switches) and visual displays. Adjusting the height, angle, and distance of the interface devices and visual display can assist consumers to reach their potential in using AT devices. For example, control is enhanced by adjusting keyboard placement, angle, and height for consistent and accurate control over key pressing and the screen height and distance to provide optimal viewing. Control enhancers support using devices efficiently and without fatigue. Comparing several control enhancers helps determine the best fit between the consumer and the AT devices.

Adaptive Computer Access

A discussion on computer adaptation methods to meet the needs of consumers with disabilities should start with a review of the basic parts and functions of a computer. Box 17-5 has a brief overview of the inside workings of a

computer. The discussion of methods for improving computer access is based on its two major human interfaces: input and output.

Input

Input, the first component, is the means by which instructions are given to the computer. These instructions usually come from standard input devices, such as keyboards and mice. However, several other devices are available for consumers who have difficulty with or cannot use these standard input devices. All operating systems now include accessibility options. These control panel options allow easy adaptation to the conventional

---

BOX 17-5
Parts of a Computer

Application Software
The software that coordinates with the operating system and the hardware to create the tools that allow people to be productive with computers. Application software ranges from drawing and early-learning software for children to advanced statistical and mathematical programs for scientists. Nearly everyone is familiar with application software such as word processors, spreadsheets, and databases.

Central Processing Unit (CPU)
The part of a computer that is often called hardware; it includes circuit boards, microprocessors, timing clocks, disk drives, and a cooling fan. The electronics within the CPU follow programmed instructions to respond in specific sequences to commands received from a combination of software and user commands. The speed of the computer, measured in megahertz, and the computing power of the microprocessor dictate how efficiently a computer can sequence instructions and perform calculations.

Computer Peripherals
Additions to the CPU that customize the computer's capacities to meet the computing requirements of the end user. This includes modifications to input and output of the computer. Flat monitors, telephone and cable modems, page scanners, plotters for creating technical drawings, trackballs and joysticks, digital cameras, color printers, voice recognition microphones, and video cameras that capture moving images for transmission across Internet connections are just a few examples of computer peripherals.

Cursor
The element of the computer interface that indicates where an action will occur. For example, the blinking cursor in a word processing document shows where a letter will be added or a word inserted. The computer mouse or the arrow keys move the cursor on the screen.

Interface
Technology that adds new capabilities to a computer. The most common is adding more random access memory (RAM) to a computer. Adding RAM creates more functional workspace for storing data. This allows the consumer to work with larger, more powerful applications or with several applications at the same time. Adding more powerful circuit boards allows a

computer to take on additional capacities. For example, a network card allows a computer to be connected to a network like those found in workplaces and universities. Other cards add advanced multimedia or calculation capacity to standard computers. As computers become more powerful and more commonly used in networks, many peripherals, now considered options, will become standard.

Operating System
The underlying software that allows the computer to process applications software. Operating systems are designed to work with specific microprocessors. Today computers commonly use a graphical user interface (GUI, pronounced gooey) to interact between the user and the operating system. GUIs use the analogy of desktops, pages, file folders, and wastebaskets to help users perform basic file management tasks. Icons, which represent documents and tasks, can be selected, moved, or copied by clicking and dragging them with a mouse. The two main operating systems, or platforms, in use today are Windows and Macintosh. Other operating systems are primarily used within large systems and are usually managed by computer information systems professionals.

Memory and Storage
Memory that is built into the circuit boards and is used for routine computer tasks. The amount of active memory or random-access memory (RAM) available varies with the task. When writing a paper or building a Web page, RAM remembers the words and pictures in consideration until the user saves them. Information stored in RAM can be lost if the power goes off or if the computer is shut down before work is saved. Computers commonly save the user's work in hard drives, floppy disks, and storage areas on networks so it can be retrieved or revised at another time.

Random Access Memory (RAM)
The main memory, where the computer keeps a record of the task in process. Once transferred or saved to a storage device (e.g., hard, floppy, or zip drive), the task is recorded. The contents of RAM can be lost if power is interrupted or the computer freezes up.

Software
Instructions written in a computer language that communicates with and drives processes within hardware.

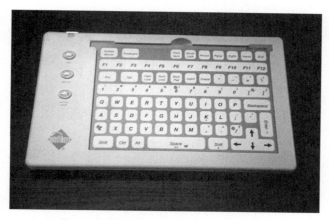

Figure 17-7 Intellikeys keyboard (Intelli Tools).

keyboard that aid one-handed typing or compensate for minor tremors or poor coordination.

Alternative Keyboards

Consumers who have difficulty using a standard keyboard even with adaptations should consider alternative keyboards. Most alternative keyboards provide **transparent** computer access; that is, the computer thinks the input is coming from a standard computer keyboard.

Several commercial products are included in this category. Some are flexible and can be used in a variety of ways. Others have narrow applications. One flexible keyboard, Intellikeys (Figure 17-7), works with Windows or Macintosh computers. It comes with a set of standard overlays that are instantly detected by the keyboard through bar code sensors. Overlays range in layout designs from those meeting the needs of early learners to advanced computer users. Sensitivity and acceptance rates are easily adjusted, and key guards can facilitate key pressing accuracy. The keyboard also allows mouse control to be assumed by arrow keys if the consumer cannot manage a mouse. Because the keyboard is made up of multiple switches that are pressure sensitive rather than mechanical, custom overlays with hot spots, or keys that vary in size, can also be created. Software that comes with the keyboard allows developing overlays for consumers with minimal range of motion or cognitive skills. The keyboard is 11×17 inches. Fairly good range of motion is needed to reach all of the keys.

For consumers with limited range of motion, smaller keyboards are a solution. The Datalux (Figure 17-8) has a small, compact keyboard layout. Another keyboard that uses technology similar to the Intellikeys but is smaller is the TASH Mini, sized as 5×6 inches. Fingers or a head stick don't have to move far to reach all keys. Like Intellikeys, it uses keys that are pressure sensitive rather than mechanical. The TASH Mini arranges keys in a layout that either places the most-used keys in the center

of the keyboard or in normal **QWERTY** layout. Keys can also control mouse movements.

Another small keyboard is the Magic Wand. The consumer holds a metal stylus and touches the appropriate key on the keyboard with this stylus. No force is required. A chordic keyboard like the BAT personal keyboard is operated by pressing keys with either the right or left hand but not both. Multiple finger combinations, like chords on a piano, are used to enter all of the alphanumeric characters. Macros (small programs that run inside an application) can execute special commands and keyboard shortcuts; however, usually a pointing device, such as a mouse or trackball, is also necessary.

Trackballs

Though mice are the most common computer pointing device, trackballs offer some important advantages to consumers needing adaptation. Because the ball remains stationary in a base, the hand can rest in one place, increasing proximal stability for the fingers. The trackball is generally more forgiving of poorly coordinated movements than the mouse. Some consumers with poor coordination who cannot control a mouse can control a trackball. Furthermore, some consumers can control a trackball through foot or toe movements. Trackballs usually come with software that allows adjusting the ratios between ball movement and mouse speed. Clicks and double clicks can be linked to buttons on the right or left side of the trackball base. Another technology for mouse pointing is the track pad. A fingertip moves and taps a 1.5–inch-square pad to direct the cursor.

Mouse Emulation

When hands cannot control a mouse, the head can be used. The cursor is controlled through head movements, and mouse clicks are produced with a switch, often a

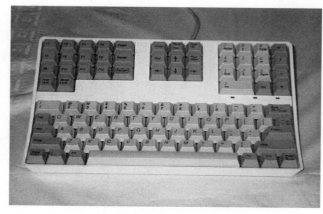

Figure 17-8 Datalux keyboard.

pneumatic switch, also known as a sip–puff switch. HeadMaster Plus is a small, highly accurate mouse emulator that functions through a lightweight sensor mounted on glasses or a headset. It is connected to a battery-powered pager-sized control box that works for 8 to 10 hours before recharge is necessary. This allows consumers with power wheelchairs to attach the control box to the wheelchair and have drive-up independence with a computer. Using IR technology with right and left button clicks provided by an external switch or the built-in sip–puff switch, the HeadMaster Plus allows **pixel**-to-pixel accuracy and smooth cursor movement. Other head-controlled devices are the HeadMouse and the Jouse. The HeadMouse uses an infrared optical sensor mounted on top of the monitor to track a tiny, disposable reflective dot that is placed on the consumer's forehead, eyeglasses, or hat. An external switch or auto click software is used for mouse clicks. Jouse, a joystick mouse operated by mouth, provides for quick and precise cursor action. The Jouse is mounted on the desktop near the computer. The consumer pulls up to the computer, positions his or her head comfortably and is ready to begin computer tasks. A built-in sip–puff switch activates mouse buttons. Typing can be achieved with Morse code or an on-screen keyboard. All of these head-controlled devices allow use of **graphical user interface (GUI)**-based programs like **computer assisted drawing (CAD)**, desktop publishing, and graphic design. Text entry is accomplished through software that creates an on-screen keyboard.

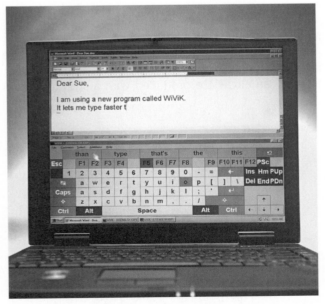

Figure 17-9 WiVik 2, a movable, resizable on-screen keyboard that lets the user transparently enter text into Windows using any pointing device. Distributed by Prentke Romich.

On-Screen Keyboards

On-screen keyboards, sometimes called virtual keyboards, are created through software and are displayed on the computer monitor (Figure 17-9). They are mostly used with head-controlled mice or joysticks and occasionally with trackballs. Keys are activated by clicking on them or by hovering over them with the cursor, dwelling for a user-defined amount of time. Since rate is comparable only to that of a one-finger typist, on-screen keyboards are usually packaged with **word prediction** or **abbreviation expansion** software. Word prediction software uses rules of recency and frequency to project the word the typist is beginning to spell; optimally configured, it saves keystrokes. Word prediction works well in this application. The consumer's eyes are already focused on the computer monitor. Abbreviation expansion lets the consumer easily establish shortcuts to frequently used phrases or personal information, such as BTW for by the way.

Touch Screens

Like the trackball, touch screens are used for mouse emulation. Selecting or interacting with this software entails touching an item displayed on the computer screen. Touch screens are used when the cognitive demands for computer tasks must be kept low, such as when working with young children or adults with cognitive impairments. Touch screens are commonly used in public kiosks.

Voice Recognition

Voice recognition technology has made rapid advances since its development. Originally seen as a tool for performing data entry in manufacturing environments where the hands were busy, its application for consumers with disabilities was quickly recognized. Consumers with significant motor impairments who had speech, even with mild dysarthria, were able to train voice models and write independently using a computer. Though early versions required that each word be spoken separately, today systems use continuous speech recognition. Sophisticated software and high-performance microphones compare sound input with probable words. Voice recognition demands good literacy skills. Consumers compare what is written on the screen to what was spoken. At present it is not ideal for hands-free control of computer or mouse functions, and it requires a quiet place. Voice recognition has been adopted widely by people without disabilities. Therefore, the cost has decreased dramatically.

Optical Character Recognition

Optical character recognition (OCR) was developed originally to save secretaries the work of retyping documents. It has also helped consumers with visual impairments or learning disabilities gain greater access to printed materials. OCR uses a flatbed page scanner to capture an image. The OCR software analyzes the page and recognizes it as alphanumeric characters or an image. Documents recognized as text can be spoken, converted to large print, sent to a Braille printer, or sent through translation software. It is available in stand-alone adaptive solutions like the Arkenstone Open Book or by attaching the required components to a personal computer. Special education programs use this technology to convert paper worksheets and tests to digital documents. Students complete the assignments using adaptive computer access. Naturally, the accuracy of the recognition process is critical for success. Accuracy rates of 99% are achieved with high-quality printed materials.

Eye Gaze

Some consumers with severe motor impairments, such as those with high-level spinal cord injury or brainstem stroke, can use eye gaze strategies. There are several approaches to this technology. VisionKey uses a small interface attached to eyeglass frames to read the position of the eye in relation to a 49-position keyboard within the viewer's field of vision. By directing one eye, the consumer types or selects characters or commands from the keyboard. The selection is highlighted to confirm the consumer's choice. The selected characters are viewed on a computer screen by the other eye. The advantage of this solution is that it moves with the consumer's head to maintain an eye-to-sensor alignment. Another approach to eye gaze uses a sensor mounted on a computer monitor. Quick Glance and LC Technology both use this approach. The camera lens focuses on one eye to interpret the eye's movement in relation to the head. Software processes the movement to determine where the consumer is looking and moves the cursor to that point. Mouse clicks are performed with either a slow eye blink or a hardware switch. On-screen keyboards are used for word processing, EADL, and speech synthesizers. The consumer's head must be kept stationary so the eye remains in the sensor's field of view. Recalibration is needed if the head moves outside this range. LC Technology's system uses a second monitor to display **application software**, with the first monitor being used for computer input. Eye gaze technology was very expensive in the past, but newer products have brought competition and reduced prices.

Morse Code

When consumers have few motor control sites, an option that may be proposed is Morse code. Though Morse code brings up images of pretelephone days, it is a useful means for sending data to a computer and other devices.

The consumer must have control and endurance at one motor site, such as a finger or eyebrow, and the cognitive ability to learn and remember the codes. One or two switches can be used. Consumers with the motoric ability to initiate both long and short signals use one switch. Consumers who are limited in motoric ability use two switches, one for dit and one for dah. Once the code is sent, the computer converts it to alphanumeric characters, keyboard shortcuts, or operating system macros. Using Morse code, consumers compose text, use spreadsheets, and browse the Internet. Other strategies may be more useful for mouse control, but mouse directions and clicks can also be sent. Unaided consumer rates of 20 words per minute are common. Morse code can be paired with word prediction. However, this slows down the rate of sending codes, as the consumer must stop and look at a word prediction list.

Tongue-Touch Keypad

Another strategy used when there are few motor control sites is the **tongue-touch keypad (TTK)**. When the tongue has good motor control, it is used to touch one of nine keys imbedded in an orthodontic appliance on the roof of the mouth. A battery-powered ultrasound transmitter in the TTK sends the signal to the controller of a power wheelchair, an EADL, or a computer. Software that accompanies the TTK interprets the signal to allow total control of the operating system and **application software**. Each switch embedded in the TTK corresponds to a cell in a 3×3 matrix. When one of the nine cells is selected, the computer accepts the input and enlarges that cell in the matrix to offer nine additional choices.

Scanning

Scanning is the input method of last resort, which is not to diminish its importance. Because it involves waiting, inefficiencies are inherent in the process. Software that presents the type of scanning array appropriate to the computing task must be installed on the computer and configured for the user. Scanning arrays can be developed to control computer applications, EADL, and augmentative communication devices.

Output

Once a computer receives input, the central processing unit (CPU) and its software perform the requested task. CPUs deliver the same output regardless of how the input is communicated to the processor.

Output is the product that a computer delivers on the screen, printed page, or as sound. Output may be a final product, dialog boxes, or alert sounds played as a computer reports about processing data. Because of the formats in which output is presented, consumers with

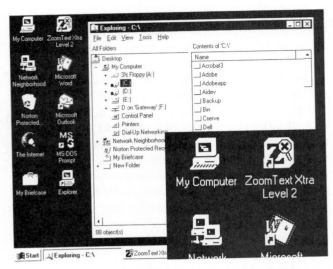

Figure 17-10 Enlargement of computer monitor using Zoomtext.

sensory impairments do not have equal access to them. This leads to the other category of adaptations to computers—adaptations to output.

Screen

Most computer output is interpreted visually, so most adaptations to output are used by consumers with visual impairments. The range of visual impairments is actually quite broad, stretching from field deficits and color blindness to low vision and total absence of light perception. Thus, there is a broad range of adaptations. Some are as simple as reducing the amount of light coming from the screen. A simple solution is reversing the screen contrast so that the letters are a light color on a dark background. This adaptation is possible by using features in the operating system to modify the default settings.

Large Print. Increasing the size of objects on the screen is an option accomplished by one of several methods. One approach is to use a larger monitor but keep the resolution low. If the resolution of a 17-inch monitor capable of displaying 1280×1024 pixels is set to 640×480, everything displayed on the screen is magnified by two.

Screen enlargement software provides a more powerful solution. Many software packages magnify the screen 2 to 16 times. An example of a screen enlargement program, Zoomtext, is shown in Figure 17-10. The software provides the option of viewing a section of text on the screen at a chosen level of magnification. The software can also return the screen to regular-size text so the entire screen can be viewed. Software that offers options such as panning through sentences or highlighting words as they are read by a text-to-speech synthesizer allows the auditory system to compensate for visual deficit. Most screen enlargement software also allows

consumers to set up default colors, which is helpful if particular colors or color contrasts enhance the consumer's remaining vision.

Text to Speech. In the absence of usable vision, the next level of adaptation is software that substitutes entirely for vision not only within application software but also within the operating system. Consumers with visual impairments were first successful with computers with the disk operating system (DOS). They memorize text commands and function independently. As mentioned earlier, most computers today depend on GUIs with highly visual interfaces, icons, and pull-down menus. Though the rise of the GUI was forecast to be the end of computing for the blind, this has not occurred (Buning & Hanzlik, 1993; Schrier, 1993; Vanderheiden, 1989). Applications generically called screen readers allow the consumer with no vision to send the mouse to locations on the screen while listening to a synthesizer read menu choices, text in dialog boxes, and paragraphs in word-processed documents. In most cases, the mouse and reading functions are controlled by the number pad on the keyboard or by a separate keypad. Consumers can set up preferences for pronunciation of special words and the rate of speech.

Refreshable Braille. The percentage of consumers who can read Braille continues to drop; it now includes fewer than 10% of consumers with blindness (American Printing House for the Blind, 1994). This concerns many in the blind community, who know that reading Braille is highly correlated with literacy and high academic achievement. Refreshable Braille is an innovative adaptation that overcomes several problems associated with Braille documents, such as the bulk of thick paper and inability to search them quickly or correct errors (Cook & Hussey, 1995). The refreshable Braille display is produced by pins that protrude and recess to create tactile dots. The dots change according to the character the software tells them to represent. Computer Braille uses eight dots rather than the usual six, conveying additional information in each cell (e.g., underlining).

The refreshable Braille display extends from the lower edge of the computer keyboard. Braille-reading consumers using a computer check their work by moving their fingers from the QWERTY keyboard to the refreshable Braille display. A 40-character Braille display represents half of a line of 80-character text displayed on the computer monitor. The consumer controls which line of Braille is displayed and moves through and edits text by sending the text cursor to the correct Braille cell.

Because the Braille display modifies the computer output, it presents the output for any computer-based task. This means the Braille display can also present the text in a Web page, the figures in a column, the text in a table, or the notation in a math formula. Additional information is communicated, and consumers using Braille displays have access to more information than they do when using text-to-speech computer output modifications.

Paper

People commonly take away the products of a computer work session in print form. What adaptations are possible if text printed on paper cannot be read?

Large Print. Consumers with low vision may convert documents to large print. Certain fonts, such as serif fonts (each character has a little flourish at the ends) are easier for the eye to recognize than sans serif text. Sans serif text is unornamented and is read more accurately by OCR systems with fewer recognition errors. In most word processing applications it is easy to select all of the text in a document and change the font and size before printing the document.

Braille Print. Similarly, instead of sending a word processor document to a conventional printer, a document can be sent to a Braille embosser, which punches Braille characters into heavy paper. Braille printers vary in quality from those designed for personal use to those that print hundreds of pages a day. Combining technology with OCR systems to create Braille versions of documents eliminates a tedious job for Braille transcriptionists and has made it easier to produce documents in Braille.

Auditory Signals

Hearing impairment also creates a need for modifying computer setups. Operating systems commonly offer the option of having the menu bar flash as a substitute for alert sounds. Computers, being highly visual tools, do not require other adaptations. However, as multimedia, particularly sound, becomes a larger part of the World Wide Web experience, it is more important to include the option for a text description of a sound feature, particularly when it is important in conveying the full message of a Web page.

Augmentative and Alternative Communication

AAC provides temporary or permanent assistance with written or verbal communication (American Speech Language and Hearing Association [ASHA], 1989). The several communication methods can be divided into two groups, unaided and aided. Unaided communication systems include sign languages, gestures, facial expressions, and looking up for yes and down for no.

Aided communication systems use physical objects to transmit or receive messages (ASHA, 1991). Though both types are needed for effective communication, aided communication systems will be our focus, with discussion organized around key characteristics of these devices.

Nonelectronic Communication Systems

Aided communication systems can be categorized in several ways, nonelectronic or electronic, nonvocal or vocal output, and dedicated or nondedicated devices. Nonelectronic devices include devices that function without batteries or electricity. Examples of nonelectronic aids are pencil and paper and alphabet, symbol, or picture boards and books. These aids vary in size from fitting into a shirt pocket to covering the top of a wheelchair lap tray. They can be used nearly anywhere, since maintenance is minimal and no electricity is required. However, these devices do not have storage capability, and unique messages cannot be prepared ahead of time. When messages can be prepared ahead of time and stored, as in electronic devices, they can be delivered at the convenience of the consumer and the communication partner. Electronic devices also have the advantage of being able to get the attention of others through a vocalization or a sound. Their disadvantages are increased weight (anywhere from approximately 0.5 pound to 10 pounds) and the need for regular battery charging.

Synthesized or Digitized

Electronic AAC devices provide voice output. Aids with voice output use either digitized or synthesized speech. Digitized speech devices work like tape recorders. Human voice recordings of specific messages are stored on microchips within the device. Usually speakers of the same gender and roughly the same age are used to make the recordings, so that devices of consumers sound the way they might sound if they could use their own voices. Devices using digitized speech can provide anywhere from a few seconds to a few minutes of voice output. A disadvantage of digitized speech is that it requires a lot of memory for storage. For this reason, it is used to deliver short messages when messages will change frequently or when storage of a few messages is needed.

Synthesized speech requires less electronic memory. Microprocessor-based programs in the device follow rules of pronunciation for the spoken language and convert text to vocal output (synthesized speech) following those rules. Exceptions, such as proper names, can be programmed to the pronunciation rules. High-quality speech synthesizers at low cost are available, giving consumers choices in vocal personality and gender. Synthesized speech is available in several languages.

Though most devices come with stored words and phrases, they are easy to customize. Customization is accomplished by using the keyboard to enter new words and phrases and following the sequence for storing new vocabulary. Synthesized speech offers independence and flexibility. Consumers can add words and sequence them in any combination.

Static or Dynamic

Visual displays for electronic communication devices are either static or dynamic. Static displays do not change appearance as the consumer uses them. To give the consumer more communication options on static displays, strategies such as levels (layers) for words or visually rich icons with multiple meanings are used. Particular words, such as those for mealtime, may be grouped on a specific level. With the level strategy, some areas on the displays are reserved for navigating between levels. The multiple-meaning icon strategy keeps all communication options on one level. Icons are pictures that represent a concept. A careful scheme for associating words or phrases with pictures allows a consumer to produce both standard and novel utterances. With static displays, commands and icons remain in the same place. This allows the consumer to develop automatic sequences for messaging.

While consumers engage in conversations, dynamic displays change in response to anticipated communication needs. Imagine that it is lunchtime and a friend asks the consumer, "Where do you want to go for lunch?" The consumer turns to the device, which provides a menu of topics, such as greetings, mealtime, school, and vacation. The consumer selects the food icon. The screen changes to present a different set of choices: foods and restaurants. The consumer selects restaurants. Once again the screen changes and presents a new set of selections, including Dave's Bar-B-Q, Dairy Delite, McDonald's, the China Palace, and Pizza Hut. The consumer selects the restaurant where he would like to have lunch and the stored associated sentence or words are produced.

Dynamic displays offer some advantages, since only a smaller set of options that are closer to the theme of a conversation are presented. This is an excellent strategy for presenting words used infrequently in conversation. However, core vocabulary, the words and phrases that are part of *all* speech regardless of the topic, may be left behind on previous pages. Some devices are designed so that this separation is minimized. The cognitive load of retrieving pages can be high. Therefore, groupings of topics or vocabulary should be logical. Figure 17-11 shows the DynaMyte, an augmentative communication device with dynamic display capabilities.

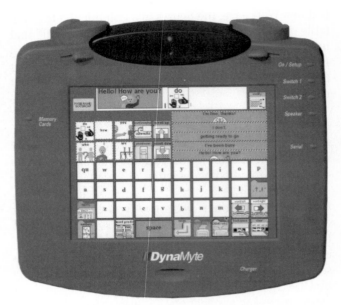

Figure 17-11 Dynamyte communication device.

Dedicated or Nondedicated

AAC devices can be dedicated or nondedicated. Dedicated devices function solely as communication devices. These devices may or may not produce audible messages, connect to a computer, or print messages. Nondedicated devices serve as communication aids while providing additional functions. Some nondedicated devices are software loaded onto a computer. The advantage is that the consumer has a fully functioning computer that can be used for word processing and other tasks as well as an AAC device. Separation between dedicated and nondedicated devices was common in the past, but as microprocessors increase in power and decrease in size, most of the more powerful AAC devices offer computerlike functions. Many control EADL devices too.

Vocal or Nonvocal

Devices also vary by whether they have nonvocal or vocal output. As with nonelectronic devices, when using nonvocal output aids, the consumer must get the attention of the communication partner before beginning the message. The communication partner must be looking at the communication aid before communication can begin. For some nonvocal output devices, communication cannot take place unless the partner understands the system. Vocal aids mean that the device speaks the message. These devices are vocal output communication aids (VOCA). VOCAs include digitized and synthesized speech. Examples of nonvocal output devices include alphabet boards, picture boards, drawings, photographs, symbols and **E-tran boards**.

Orthography or Representation

When consumers use the alphabet and spell messages to the partner, the alphabet can be arranged in one of several ways, depending on the need. Typical layout arrangements are alphabetical, QWERTY, and frequency. Alphabetical order is used when the team anticipates that the consumer will continue to use cognitively simple devices and probably not move on to devices with more options. The QWERTY arrangement, the typical alphanumeric keyboard, is appropriate for consumers using or expecting to use a computer.

The third strategy is arranging the letters by frequency of use, maximizing control and efficiency. Consumers who point to the letters or scan use this strategy. With pointing, the most frequently used letters are placed where the consumer can most accurately and consistently point. Letters used less frequently are placed in the periphery. Placing the most frequently used letters where the consumer has the best accuracy facilitates use of the device and the flow of communication. Scanning **arrays** should be designed so that the commonly used letters or words are offered as the first or second choice.

Symbol systems are used with both vocal and nonvocal output systems. Symbols may be drawings, icons, or figures specifically developed for communication systems and designed to represent concepts. There is little similarity among representational systems, and each approach has its followers and preferred methods for introduction and use. Examples of published symbol sets are Picture Communication Symbols, PicSyms, MinSpeak, and Blissymbolics. Information on these and other symbol sets can be found in *Augmentative and Alternative Communication* (Beukelman & Mirenda, 1992).

Electronic Aids to Daily Living

EADL provide alternative independent control of the electrical devices in an environment, most often at home. The name has recently changed from environmental control unit (ECU) to EADL as a more accurate description of the function of this technology and to improve reimbursement from funding sources by relating its use to functional outcomes (M. Lange, 1999, personal communication). The term *environmental control unit* stresses what is being controlled (i.e. television, telephone) rather than stressing the task (i.e. increased independence, safety, communication, leisure). EADL give access to devices such as lights, telephone, audiovisual or home entertainment appliances, beds, intercoms, thermostats, door locks, and window curtains.

This type of technology is increasingly commonly used by consumers without disabilities. In new home construction this technology is called home automation and is marketed as a means to save money by remotely regulating sprinklers, lights, and thermostats.

EADL can be activated either through direct access, like pressing a button on a garage door opener, or through indirect methods (scanning). Because most direct-access methods were developed for the mass market, this type is usually inexpensive and found in electronics stores. If motor impairments prevent the use of direct selection, a specialized AT product must be used. The same criteria used for determining an access method for computer or AAC device apply to choosing an access method for EADL.

Categories of EADL Control Technology

EADL let the consumer control electrical items without having to move to the appliance or interact with its typical controls. Anyone who has used a TV remote understands that convenience and ease are also a motivation for controlling an appliance remotely. Occupational therapists might recommend an EADL device to consumers needing help managing fatigue, pain, and mobility or manipulating knobs, dials, and buttons.

Some appliances only need simple on–off control signals, while others need more complex control signals. For example, turning a light on or off requires a simple on–off signal, but setting the channel on a television set or opening curtains halfway requires more complex control signals. EADL control signals can be transmitted by several methods: through the building's electrical wiring; IR, ultrasound, and RF transmitters and receivers; or a combination of these modes. Certain technologies lend themselves to specific kinds of appliance control.

Use of the building's electrical wiring for control of electrical appliances is convenient for appliances such as lights or fans, which require only simple on–off control signals. Such appliances are plugged into a small coded switch module that is plugged into the wall outlet. A control box, also plugged into an electrical outlet somewhere in the consumer's house, sends a signal with the module code and the on–off signal over the wiring system. The receiver module detects the signals and switches electrical power to the plugged-in appliance. The quantity of codes and variety of modules available make it possible to turn electrical systems off and on throughout a home or apartment. The variety of control boxes ranges from simple hardwired push-button switches to sophisticated computer-controlled interfaces. These devices are known collectively as X-10 modules and controllers.

IR light transmitters are also used to generate control signals. Sometimes IR transmitters are used with X-10 controllers and sometimes without. IR light control signals are invisible to the human eye. The control signal is interpreted by an IR receiver and translated into the correct function. Most television remote control works on this principle, and since it sends a light beam, it must be pointed directly at the television and have a clear line of sight. Various patterns of IR light are coded to direct the appliance to perform specific functions. IR tends to be used in applications that require multiple adjustments, such as television sets, VCRs, and CD players.

Ultrasound controllers work in a similar manner, but control signals are transmitted via sound waves rather than light waves. The ultrasound controllers transmit at an inaudible frequency. Since sound waves disburse readily in home environments, ultrasound controllers do not need a line of sight and can travel farther (up to 200 feet), though they are blocked by walls and other obstacles. Ultrasound is used in some simple EADL devices that send on–off signals to IR receiver modules.

RF control signal transmitters are another option. RF signals are less affected by obstacles such as walls but are sometimes susceptible to interference from other radio frequencies. Devices using RF usually offer the consumer a choice of bands to bypass interference on heavily used channels. That is, the consumer can change the frequency band or channel so as not to turn on devices in the neighbor's house. RF transmitters and receivers are often used to open garage doors and unlatch front doors. They are also frequently the controller of choice to use with an X-10 control system.

Simple EADL

Simple EADL give simple control over electrical devices. They can contribute to learning cause and effect, increasing personal control, and developing responsibility. Simple EADL can be set up to work in momentary mode—work only as long as the switch is activated—or latched mode—stay on until the switch is pressed again to turn off the device. Many appliances can be con-

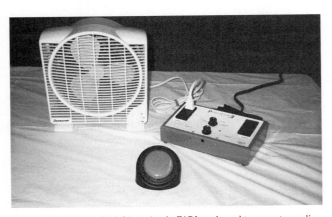

Figure 17-12 Power Link 3 is a simple EADL tool used to operate appliances. Here it is used with a fan.

nected and operated by this method. One simple EADL is the appliance interface, which can be easily incorporated into early-learning fun in the kitchen. Using a single switch, consumers can participate in cooking by turning on small appliances, such as blenders and popcorn poppers. Figure 17-12 shows the Power Link 3 being used with an infrared switch to operate a fan. Therapists can build on this skill and set up other simple switch-controlled EADL interfaces that send ultrasound signals to bedroom lights or fans to provide control over personal space. Phones that scan phone numbers or picture phones, which combine speed dial with large buttons that hold a photo, give modified phone access with simple interfaces. More complex devices like the Relax II unit learn IR codes and provide control over one home entertainment system.

Complex EADL

Consumers who have significant impairments or who desire control over more appliances within their environment need complex EADL devices with sophisticated functions. These exist as dedicated EADL devices, as components of a computer-based system, and as a system within AAC devices.

Dedicated devices (e.g., Nemo, Quartet, Proxi, Sicare Pilot) perform complex adjustments to multiple systems within a consumer's environment. Some use voice commands; others use scanning input to take commands from the consumer. They respond and transmit control signals to systems in the environment using a combination of transmission technologies based on what is best for the task being controlled. These systems can activate intercoms, unlock doors, and dial the phone. Consumers should be aware of their vulnerability in power outages and either install uninterruptible power supplies or have a 911 auto-dial backup system.

Systems with similar capacity can be found in computer-based EADL. Computer software such as Words+ transmits a signal to a control box, which sends IR to a phone, appliance, entertainment center, or X-10 module. Computer-based systems are ideal for work settings where consumers are already interacting with their computers. This same feature may be limiting if the consumer must go to the computer to interact with an appliance.

Many top-end AAC devices include EADL functions. A subset of icons like the ones the consumer uses in the AAC device can activate IR signals either directly to an IR-controlled appliance or to an intermediary device that forwards signals on to X-10 modules or telephone dialers. AAC devices can be customized so functions can be added as the consumer gains skill and confidence.

CLINICAL REASONING
in OT Practice

AT Related to Self-Maintenance Roles

Claire, a 65-year-old widow, is experiencing increased disruption in her daily living routines as her macular degeneration gets worse. She depends on her daughter, Jean, to stop by her apartment daily to assist her with visual tasks. Claire is upset because Jean's husband has taken a new job in another state and they will be moving soon. Jean has heard that there are low vision aids that might help restore her mother's self-sufficiency and has encouraged her mother to seek occupational therapy assistance. Claire's goals include restoring her independence with food preparation instructions, bill paying, and reading correspondence, the TV guide, and the Senior Activity schedule.

► What kind of AT solution might allow Claire to regain some of her self-sufficiency and ease her daughter's mind about moving away?
► What pieces of equipment would assist Claire in her environment?
► What would help ensure a good "fit" between Claire and the equipment?

Sensory Accommodations

Many microprocessor-based aids help people with sensory impairments manage their daily living environments.

Closed-Circuit Television

Consumers with low vision and limited interest in computer-based adaptations may accept closed-circuit television (CCTV) systems. A television camera is mounted and focused on a surface where the consumer places the printed material he or she wants to read, such as a recipe, invoice, magazine article, or greeting card. The camera sends the image of the document to a TV monitor mounted at the consumer's eye level. Screen magnification and contrast can be set to the consumer's needs. This technology has become lighter and more portable. Some systems use the consumer's own television set. Consumers using CCTVs daily find that they enable independence in many daily living tasks.

Braille Note Takers and Writers

For consumers with visual impairment, portable microprocessor-based note takers combine many productivity tools. This small keyboard comes with either a 6-key Braille keyboard or a full QWERTY keyboard. Some models offer speech feedback through an earphone; others offer review through a single Braille cell that refreshes under the consumer's finger. Consumers record notes from meetings and later upload them to a computer or print them directly to a paper or Braille printer. These devices also contain calendars, appointments, addresses, and phone numbers. Some offer stopwatch and timer functions.

Closed Captioning

Real-time closed captioning is an excellent accommodation for consumers with hearing impairments. This system combines a court reporter's stenography skills for capturing spoken language with a computer for processing the text. This technology projects or displays the speaker's words as readable text. It is often used for keynote speakers at large conferences or in office meetings where participants are gathered around a table.

Environmental Access and Universal Design

AT devices enable participation and control only when environments are accessible to consumers and their devices. Independent power mobility offers no advantage in places without ramps and rooms where doorways are too narrow to accommodate the wheelchair. Consumers using AAC devices cannot communicate if people will not listen to them.

Since people who use AT devices are not always permitted to show that their devices enable them to compensate for their physical or sensory impairments, the Americans with Disability Act (ADA) supplies the force of federal law to facilitate their opportunities (see Chapters 10 and 36).

Funding

Obviously, this equipment costs money. At times, inexpensive solutions can be found to enhance the consumer's occupational performance, but often the equipment is costly. AT enables consumers to participate in roles that might otherwise be denied to them. Therefore, the consumer's abilities, needs, and specific occupational goals should drive the assessment, *not* the availability of funding. The compelling need for an AT device or services should *drive* the search for funding.

AT Should Drive the Funding Process

The consumer's goals may require AT devices that are totally beyond his or her financial resources. When funding drives the assessment, expensive solutions are not reviewed and the consumer is offered only solutions that are more within his or her means. If the best solution

Case Example

MR. S. REGAINS CONTROL THROUGH ASSISTIVE TECHNOLOGY

Patient Information

Mr. S., an active and extroverted 29 year old, sustained traumatic brain injury 4 months ago in a collision with an automobile while he was riding his bicycle home from work. Despite wearing a helmet, he sustained damage to the right motor cortex, which affects motor control on the left side of his body, his dominant side. At the time of his referral to the Center for Brain Injuries (CBI) AT program, fractures, bruises and abrasions were healed and his walking was steadily improving. He was able to rise to stand from a passenger car seat, transfer to a heavy-duty rolling walker, and walk 20 to 25 feet before resting. Handwriting and short-term memory were still impaired, but fortunately, spoken language, spatial awareness, and social skills were intact.

The registered nurse assigned to Mr. S.'s care had considerable advocacy and case management skills experience. She realized that assistive devices could make a significant improvement in Mr. S.'s independence. Therefore, prior to discharge from the hospital, she requested a home accessibility assessment. The occupational therapist made a home visit and recommended modifying doorways and entrances in the house, adding grab bars to the bathroom, rearranging bedroom furniture, and reorganizing the clothes closet to facilitate dressing. As a result of these changes, Mr. S. regained a significant level of independence in self-care.

Prior to the injury, Mr. S. was in his fifth year of working for a firm that provided environmental planning and resource use consultation to construction companies and small manufacturers in a three-county region. His responsibilities included meeting clients, determining their goals and needs, and working with the field staff to perform specific tests and measurements. He summarized findings, wrote reports, tracked time and charges, and participated in ongoing planning meetings as needed by the contractor. His company supervisor is eager for Mr. S. to return to work; however, it is not yet clear whether he will be able to perform all of his previous duties.

Mr. S. was referred to CBI for assessment of AT that may facilitate his return to work. Although the hospital rehabilitation team included an occupational therapist, physical therapist, and speech language pathologist, none of these professionals had experience with AT. With this knowledge Mr. S.'s wife approached the Department of Vocational Rehabilitation (DVR) and was pleased to discover AT expertise was available at the CBI program. (The car driver's auto insurance continued to cover Mr. S.'s outpatient rehabilitation services.) Additionally, DVR was eager to accept Mr. S. as a new client because of his strong desire to return to work. Eligibility and application forms were completed, and Mr. S. had an introductory interview at CBI.

Assessment

Mr. L., the occupational therapist at CBI, made Mr. S. feel comfortable right away, and Mr. S. began talking about his job. Mr. L. realized that using a computer to write reports and letters and run data analyses were essential to Mr. S.'s job. It was clear too that mobility would be an issue if Mr. S. was going to meet clients in a variety of locations. He also realized that a visit to Mr. S.'s job site and an interview with Mr. S.'s supervisor would be necessary to give him a complete understanding of Mr. S.'s job functions. The rest of the appointment was spent assessing Mr. S.'s hand skills (speed, accuracy, range of motion, bilateral coordination) and visual perception skills.

Recommendations

As the session concluded, Mr. L. engaged Mr. S. in a conversation to set goals and discuss alternatives. They agreed that evaluating adaptations to maximize Mr. S.'s ability to use the computer would be the top priority. A schedule was established. Mr. S. would come to CBI three times weekly over the next 4 weeks.

Short-Term Goals

1. Mr. S. will participate in a 2-week trial of a scooter. Mr. L. realized that power mobility might be important if Mr. S. was going to meet the demands of his job. Although hesitant, Mr. S. agreed to a trial during his final 2 weeks at CBI.
2. As a means to keep his employer and DVR counselor involved in the AT process, Mr. S. will use his evolving computer skills to prepare a weekly summary of accomplishments at the program.
3. Mr. S. will participate in evaluation and selection of adaptations that optimize computer access.

Since using a computer was a key component of Mr. S.'s job, relearning to use one became the primary goal. Mr. S.'s physical limitations made it difficult for him to use a standard keyboard with both hands. Impaired sensation, weakness, and lack of independent finger movement on Mr. S.'s left hand made touch-typing nearly impossible. Watching his hands, working to achieve independent finger movement and continually refocusing between the screen and the paper he was typing from was fatiguing and distracting. Mr. L. thought of two methods to resolve this issue. The first was for Mr. S. to continue working on bimanual typing skills in the hope that sensation and motor control would return. Mr. L. knew this would be a long-term goal. As part of this approach he would also choose one of several adaptations that accommodates a one-handed typist, such as software that converts a standard keyboard into a one-handed model or a special one-handed keyboard that substitutes chording patterns for all keystrokes.

The other approach was to use voice recognition for general text entry and allow Mr. S. to edit errors with keystrokes made with his nondominant right hand. He could control the cursor using a trackball with the same hand. Any concerns about the appropriateness of voice recognition could be addressed with a visit to the office and/or asking Mr. S. about whether his office was in a cubicle or an enclosed room. Background noise, frequent interactions with coworkers, and distractions would limit the usefulness of voice recognition as an adaptive strategy.

Intervention

When Mr. S. came in for his first AT work session at CBI, Mr. L. discussed these issues with him. Mr. S. immediately expressed interest in the voice recognition solution. He told Mr. L. that voice recognition was already being used as an efficiency tool by some of his colleagues, and he was eager to explore a solution that could be used almost immediately to help him be productive. Since others in his office used the software, he knew he could get technical support for problems. The engineering and simulation software that he uses at work relies heavily on mouse movements. Therefore, Mr. S. was willing to review several right hand–controlled trackballs as a solution. Mr. L. introduced the issue of adequate seating and computer ergonomics. Mr. S. realized that a proper chair and armrests would allow him to work at maximal efficiency.

Mr. L. helped Mr. S. get started on creating voice files and learning voice command basics. He had difficulty learning the commands for correcting voice recognition errors. He realized that he would have to be patient not only with his altered learning style but also with retraining his non-dominant right hand. At the end of the first session Mr. S. felt frustrated and overwhelmed, but after a few more sessions, he saw improvement. He realized he was acquiring new skills and one step built upon the previous steps. At the end of the first week he wrote the required summary about what he had learned. Mr. L. asked Mr. S. whether he would also consider writing an article about his recovery for the CBI newsletter, which would be published in 2 weeks. Mr. S. was doing so well by the end of the fifth session that he wrote the story of his recovery. Mr. L. suggested that he find and review an article on the environmental impact of a proposed new road in town. Mr. S. agreed, knowing that he was beginning to make progress toward his long-term goal, returning to work.

When Mr. S. realized that the combination of voice recognition and the trackball almost completely compensated for his poorly controlled left hand, he began to think of the advantages of adapting his home computer. Mr. and Mrs. S. used the computer to send e-mail messages to distant family members and surf the Web to keep up with biking gear and vacation opportunities. Mr. L. told him that he would be able to use voice recognition for e-mail by implementing a cut-and-paste technique and that URLs could be typed with his right hand and then bookmarked.

Mr. L. arranged for a 2-week rental of a four-wheel scooter, which the DVR counselor thought was a reasonable expense. Four-wheel scooters are more stable than three-wheel scooters and have reduced likelihood of tipping on unpaved and uneven surfaces. One disadvantage of the four-wheel scooter is that it requires a larger turning radius. This would test Mr. S.'s ability to plan and execute turns. The plan was for Mr. S. to use the scooter inside CBI during the third week and during the fourth and final week take it out in the community on his two excursion days. A certified occupational therapy assistant (COTA) on the CBI staff traveled with Mr. S. as he practiced using the scooter for visiting a nearby public library, meeting Mrs. S. for lunch, and using public transportation. The COTA offered instructions and taught him some community travel skills.

Mr. S. realized almost immediately that the scooter could make a big difference to him. His 3 months of restricted mobility had been difficult, and he wanted more than anything to return to his active lifestyle. Sure, he would have to get used to the new image he would project as friends and acquaintances saw him driving the scooter rather than riding his bicycle. But for now, he was willing to make that adjustment. A scooter allowed him to conserve his energy yet still gave him the opportunity to transfer easily, stand to reach high items, and take steps within safe and accommodating environments like his office or the kitchen. After his first community outing he reported to Mr. L. that he wanted him to write a letter of justification to the DVR counselor requesting funding for a scooter. He knew it would create the margin he needed to be successful in his return to work.

Mr. L. introduced the issue of transporting the scooter. Though it could be disassembled for placement in the trunk, Mr. S. could not do this independently, and it was too heavy for Mrs. S. When Mr. L. realized that Mr. and Mrs. S. already owned a minivan (purchased to support their interest in biking) he recommended the installation of a hydraulic lift that could grasp the scooter fully assembled and lift it into the rear of the van. This would allow Mr. S. to use his rolling walker or the side of the van for support as he walked forward to his seat in the van. For now Mrs. S. was willing to drive Mr. S. to work each morning. They had determined that on days that Mr. S. needed to get to an appointment with a client, their retired neighbor would drive the van. The scooter could get Mr. S. to locations near the office, as most sidewalks in town had curb cuts. A driving evaluation and Mr. S.'s need for driving adaptations could be assessed in the future.

During the fourth week Mr. L. and Mr. S. made a visit to Mr. S.'s workplace to finish device recommendations and equipment layout. Mr. L. measured Mr. S.'s cubicle and desk. He also noted the orientation of the desk in the cube and the noise level. With this information, Mr. L. recommended a flexible desk-mounted gooseneck microphone to be used with the voice recognition system. Even when he was speaking softly, the unidirectional microphone would pick up Mr. S.'s voice rather than environmental noise, and it could be easily moved out of the way with one hand for conversations or phone calls. Mr. L. also recommended an ergonomically designed chair and a forearm rest for Mr. S.'s right arm for support and to reduce fatigue as he used the trackball. The chair had a five-wheel base for stability and a long back providing head support when Mr. S. needed to rest his head while using the voice recognition software. The chair's seat height was adjustable, so Mr. S. could place his feet flat on the floor. Also the seat depth was adjustable, providing a 1-inch extension that accommodated Mr. S.'s long thighs. The armrests were adjustable to provide proper forearm support.

Mr. L. could also see the need for a copy stand next to the computer monitor. The copy stand allowed Mr. S. to review his notes while writing reports with the voice recognition system. Having the paper at eye level next to the monitor would reduce eye strain and neck fatigue and allow him to work for longer periods. Mr. L. suggested that a reference book Mr. S. used frequently be placed above on a shelf on the right side of the desk so it was always available.

The phone seemed best placed near Mr. S.'s right side next to the trackball so when phone calls came in he could answer them immediately. Mr. L. recommended that a new telephone with speed dial and an optional headset should be purchased to allow optimal telephone use. Mr. L. knew it was difficult to hold the receiver and dial the phone or jot down notes using only one hand.

Mr. L. knew that Mr. S. would be able to handle the computer-related aspects of his job. This left issues related to architectural access and using a scooter. Mr. L. looked over the facility and realized that modifications would be needed at the building's entrance and in the employees' bathroom. He made some suggestions and gave Mr. S.'s supervisor the number of the American's with Disabilities (ADA) Technical Assistance Center. The boss was relieved to know that an Internal Revenue Service (IRS) allowance for small businesses provided a tax credit to cover the expenses related to facility changes to accommodate a worker with a disability. He was eager to get Mr. S. back to work and agreed to get the project started and come up with a short-term solution while the work was being done.

Finally, prior to discharge from CBI, Mr. S. began to think about resuming bike riding (triggered when he saw an article in the lobby at CBI about adaptive hand cycles). He realized that this kind of bike would bypass his problem with balance and allow him to return to biking with friends. Actually he had seen a man riding one these bikes just last year on Ride the Rockies and had admired his grit. He would just need to get back to work and start putting some money aside for this new goal.

Discharge Plans and Recommendations

Mr. L. and Mr. S. had accomplished a great deal during their 4 weeks together. Mr. L.'s experience made him realize that Mr. S. would face unforeseen challenges as time went on. He and Mr. L. worked out a schedule for ongoing support. Mr. L. set up an appointment for a 2-week postdischarge visit to Mr. S.'s work site. At that time they would evaluate Mr. S.'s progress and if needed would use one or two visits to resolve any work-related or adaptive equipment issues. In his discharge recommendations to DVR, he recommended keeping Mr. S.'s case open for 3 and 6-month consultations to assess the quality and stability of Mr. S.'s progress, his success with adaptive strategies and equipment at work, and his continued adjustment to employment.

CLINICAL REASONING
in OT Practice

Roles of Various Stakeholders in AT Assessment and Treatment

Many people, including Mr. and Mrs. S., the registered nurse at the hospital, occupational therapist making the home visit, DVR counselor, employer, therapist, and COTA at CBI were involved in availing Mr. S. of AT necessary for his resumption of self-identified important roles. How did each person influence the availability of AT following Mr. S.'s discharge? What sorts of communication mechanisms facilitated this process? Consider the various levels of AT expertise represented in this team and contribution of each individual relative to his or her knowledge.

---

facilitates the consumer's occupation but is expensive, the assessment team needs to document that the solution will best meet the consumer's goals and present a strong case to the funding agency.

Legislation and Funding for AT

On November 13, 1998, President Clinton signed into law the Assistive Technology Act (ATA) of 1998 (PL 105-334), which affirms technology devices as valuable tools for individuals with disabilities. This act extends the original Tech Act funding (PL 103-218, the Technology-Related

Assistance Act of 1988, as amended), which places AT education and advocacy resources in all 50 states and 6 territories. These projects are directed (1) to increase public awareness of the benefits of AT devices and services, (2) to promote interagency coordination to improve AT funding, (3) to provide technical assistance and training, and (4) to provide outreach support to community-based organizations that assist individuals in finding funding and using AT. Congress recognizes the natural links between people and the role they play in society. These relationships make good starting points for finding the appropriate funding for a consumer.

Workers

Vocational rehabilitation agencies, federally funded in each state, are responsible for helping consumers get the training, education, services and AT they need to become employable. Vocational rehabilitation is a major funder for AT for working-age persons.

The ADA makes it unlawful to exclude persons with disabilities from public services, transportation, telecommunications, and employment. To help pay for reasonable accommodation for an employee or prospective employee with a disability, a business can apply for a Credit for Small Businesses, which allows tax credit. Expenditures to make a workplace accessible include computer adaptations and remodeling bathrooms (Mendelson, 1996).

Social Security helps consumers with disabilities who are returning to work or who want to begin work. Certain work-related expenses resulting from the impairment may be deducted when counting worker earnings against the Supplemental Security Income maximum allowable earned income. Consumers receiving Social Security can set aside some of that money to achieve employment without losing benefits.

The Internal Revenue Service allows workers to take a tax write-off for health care and miscellaneous work expenses. AT is deductible under the definition of medical care, which includes amounts paid "for the diagnosis, care, treatment or prevention of disease or for the purpose of affecting any structure or function of the body." Other tax provisions enable employed consumers with disabilities to deduct work-related expenses, like AT, from their gross income. A tax credit can also be taken when the expenses incurred by a taxpayer for the care of a dependent who has one or more disabilities frees the taxpayer to work (Mendelson, 1996).

Of course workers with health insurance can use their health insurance to fund some kinds of AT. Most health insurance plans use the criterion of medical necessity to decide whether to fund the AT device or service. This means that they are more likely to cover a wheelchair or prosthesis than a computer adaptation. Policies must be carefully reviewed individually, as insurance plans vary as to what is and is not covered.

Older Adults and Unemployed Adults

Medicare is the primary funder for older adults and those on permanent disability. Medicare is not a strong payment source for most AT. Items that Medicare pays for must fall into certain predesignated categories and must have an approved Medicare number. Most of the durable medical equipment paid for by Medicare cannot be categorized as high-tech or AT devices. Wheelchairs are a significant expenditure by Medicare, but any kind of wheelchair other than a basic model must be clearly justified in a statement of medical necessity. Because Medicare is the primary payer, other health insurance pays the 20% remaining only if Medicare pays. In early 2001, Medicare expanded coverage to include funding for AAC devices and services. If an older adult can pay for the AT device with private funds, Medicare outpatient services may reimburse occupational therapists for AT-related services to increase independence in IADL.

Unemployed adults with disabilities are generally eligible for Medicaid. Because Medicaid is administered at the state level and each state interprets the regulations independently, coverage varies from state to state.

Injury- and Illness-Related Causes

Health insurance can become a source of reimbursement for AT devices and services when the need for AT devices is the result of an injury or illness. Health insurance at present is primarily offered by managed care organizations and health maintenance organizations. Many large health organizations hire case managers to coordinate rehabilitation resources in complex cases. It is clear that consumers who have strokes, head or spinal cord injuries, or progressive neurological disease benefit from AT devices and services. However, teaching a case

---

CLINICAL REASONING
in OT Practice

AT Related to Self-Advancement Roles

Eighteen months ago, George experienced a spinal cord injury at the C5-6 level secondary to a motor vehicle collision. Currently, George's biggest frustration is the limited recovery of motor skills in his arms. He can shrug his shoulders, flex and extend his elbows, and pronate and supinate his forearms. However, he has limited grasp and release. After extensive rehabilitation and a significant episode of reactive depression, George seems receptive to some ideas that will help him manage his limitations. Prior to the injury, he worked as a graphic designer. Currently, he is receiving full disability as a result of the injury. The firm he worked for completely transitioned to computer-aided design (CAD) last year. His employer has expressed willingness to make a PC and software available to George at home. The employer's hope is that George might, with adaptations, training, and vocational exploration, be able to return to his former position at work. The computer mouse and digitizing pad were George's primary graphics tools. Keyboarding was used occasionally for correspondence and the textual elements of designs.

▸ What AT solutions could help George reengage in computer-aided design?
▸ How would control enhancers be useful to George?
▸ How much training will be needed to ensure that George will be successful?
▸ Where should the training take place?

manager about the potential of AT to increase independence and enable a return to occupation remains an important function of occupational therapy practice.

When trauma or negligence is the source of an injury that necessitates the use of AT, a financial settlement or a trust fund can be the source of reimbursement for AT devices and services. In this case, the occupational therapist may direct a letter of justification to a judge or trustee.

Consumer Loans

Obtaining a loan is a typical way to purchase products. State Tech Act projects have information on low-interest loan programs. Banks and credit unions are required to offer consumers with disabilities loans that take their special financial circumstances into consideration.

Charity

When all other sources fail, there are still bake sales, raffles, car washes and appeals to service clubs and civic organizations as a means of funding AT devices.

Justification Letters

With the knowledge gained from the consumer-centered assessment, the consumer's trial use of a device, interviews with significant others, and a possible home visit, the occupational therapist is in a strong position to lay a clear case of need for AT devices. This document is called a letter of justification or in some cases a letter of medical necessity. A physician's prescription is needed for all requests in medical model services and generally accompanies the therapist's letter of justification. With education- or work-related funding sources another form of "prescription" may be needed.

The occupational therapist uses knowledge of the relationship between clinical assessment data and the predicted or potential outcomes for the consumer. Using clear writing, case data, and sometimes photographs or videotape footage of the consumer successfully using the device, the therapist presents how the cost of AT devices will be offset by an increase in function, engagement in education, employability, and/or greater independence. It is important to tailor the letter to the funding source. For example, in requests for funds from Medicaid, AT devices and services must be justified as *medically* necessary. In contrast, when applying for services under the Individuals with Disabilities Education Act (IDEA), the letter must demonstrate that the devices are *educationally* necessary.

A letter of rejection doesn't necessarily mean no. Many private and public sources of funding use a system of appeals to weed out groundless requests. First, get the notice of refusal in writing; then prepare for the appeal. The mandate for funding AT is clear, but agencies and organizations still attempt to avoid financial responsibility by raising objections. A clear, logical letter of justification has won many appeals for AT devices and services.

Roles of Occupational Therapists With AT Intervention

Even when occupational therapists have developed a bag of tricks for using AT with average consumers, some consumers will still have needs that call for referring them to an AT center. Referral to experts requires putting the interest of the consumer first. Consumers with complex problems may need the integration of multiple solutions to allow them to arrive at their functional goal. Use referring to an expert (probably in a large metropolitan area or a large facility) as an opportunity to learn more about AT yourself. Your consumer will need someone's assistance integrating a complex solution into everyday tasks and routines. You will have a chance to learn and advance your AT practice knowledge as well.

Specific roles for the professionals within the AT assessment team have already been discussed. Some other possible roles for occupational therapists are now presented.

AT Specialist

Occupational therapists with AT service delivery experience usually strive for the assistive technology provider (ATP) credential. This certification, offered through the Rehabilitation Engineering and Assistive Technology Society of North America (RESNA),validates an individual's knowledge and qualifications in AT. RESNA is an interdisciplinary association of people with a common interest in technology and disability whose purpose is to improve the potential of people with disabilities to achieve their goals through the use of technology. The RESNA ATP credential sets a standard for entry level of expertise for AT practice. Professionals with ATP credentials are expected to adhere to a code of ethics, to practice in a consumer-centered manner, and to continue to gain competence in their area of AT service provision.

Consultant

Some occupational therapists have developed consulting practices in which they advise organizations on program development, change issues, quality improvement, and planning (Jaffe & Epstein, 1992). Many organizations need assistance to implement AT service delivery within their educational, rehabilitation, governmental, or private sector organizations. Occupational therapists with consulting skills and knowledge of AT solutions can offer an important service that can lead to greater opportunities for future AT consumers.

Product Development Team and Product Testing

With their broad clinical knowledge of consumers' needs and challenges and their comfort with functional tasks and environments, occupational therapists make strong contributions to engineering and research teams. Engineers and others with technical expertise appreciate working with occupational therapy clinicians because a prototype product ready for testing or manufacture is more likely to achieve its intended purpose of improving function.

Continuing Education

One thing is certain: AT is *always* changing. Any professional practicing in this area must make a commitment to continuing education. RESNA and other organizations continuously offer education (see Resources). University courses, as well as sessions at annual conferences, weekend workshops and on-line courses allow occupational therapy practitioners to pick up the knowledge and skills needed to incorporate AT into a range of practice settings. Listserves like those offered by AOTA, RESNA and university programs allow novice practitioners to use the expertise and help of experienced AT practitioners to solve practical problems. Hiring staff development expertise is another way for a group of practicing therapists to begin to incorporate more AT into a specific practice settings.

Summary Review Questions

1. What are the various roles the occupational therapist can play on an AT team?
2. Describe the main points of the HAAT and Enabling-Disabling Process models.
3. Define high and low technology.
4. List the steps in an AT assessment.
5. List several input and output devices, other than a keyboard and standard mouse, and describe who might use them.
6. Explain the main methods that EADL use to transmit signals from the input device to the control box.
7. Where could consumers look for funding for AT devices?

Resources

Suppliers

Ablenet · 1081 Tenth Ave. SE, Minneapolis, MN 55414. 800-322-0956. 612-379-0956. Fax 612-379-9143
E-mail: CustomerService@ablenetinc.com
www.ablenetinc.com

Adaptive Switch Laboratories, Inc. · 125 Spur 191, Suite C, Spicewood, TX 78669. 800-626-8698. 830-798-0005. Fax: 830-798-6221
E-mail: info@asl-inc.com
www.asl-inc.com

Arkenstone · Virtual Assistive Technology Center, NASA Ames Moffett Complex, Building 23, P.O. Box 215, Moffett Field, CA 94035-0215. 800-444-4443. Fax 650-603-8887. TDD: 800-833-2753
E-mail: info@arkenstone.org
www.arkenstone.org

Datalux Corporation · 155 Aviation Dr., Winchester, VA 22602. 540-662-1500. 800-328-2589. Fax 540-662-1682
www.datalux.com

Don Johnston Incorporated · 26799 West Commerce Drive, Volo, IL 60073. 800-999-4660. 847-740-0749. Fax 847-740-7326
E-mail: info@donjohnston.com
www.donjohnston.com/

Dragon Systems, Inc. · 320 Nevada Street, Newton, MA 02460. 800-437-2466. 617-965-5200. Fax 617-965-2374
E-mail: info@dragonsys.com
www.dragonsys.com/

DynaVox Systems Inc. · 2100 Wharton Street, Pittsburgh, PA 15203. 888-697-7332. Fax 412-381-6860
E-mail: sales@dynavoxsys.com
www.sentient-sys.com/

Eye Control Technologies · PO Box 2317, Corvallis, OR 97339. 888-865-5535. 541-753-6645. Fax 541-753-6689
E-mail: sales@eyecontrol.com
www.eyecontrol.com/home/entry.html

Freedom of Speech, Inc. · 2344 Nicollet Ave. S. #400, Minneapolis, MN 55404. 612-544-3333. Fax 612-872-7374
E-mail: fos@freedomofspeech.com
www.freedomofspeech.com

H.K. Eyecan, Ltd. · 36 Burland St., Ottawa, Ontario, Canada K2B 6J8. 613-860-0333. 800-356-3362. Fax 613-596-4300
E-mail: Eyecan@cyberus.ca
www.cyberus.ca/~eyecan/

Humanware · 6245 King Road, Loomis, CA 95650. 800-722-3393
E-mail: webmaster@humanware.com
www.humanware.com/

Intelli Tools · 55 Leveroni Ct. Ste 9, Navato, CA 94949. 415-382-5959. 800-899-6687. Fax 415-382-5950
E-mail: info@intellitools.com
www.intellitools.com

LC Technologies, Inc. · 9455 Silver King Court, Fairfax, Virginia 22031-4713. 703-385-7133. 800-393-4293. Fax 703-385-7137
E-mail: requests@eyegaze.com
www.lctinc.com/

Madenta Inc. · 3022 Calgary Trail South, Edmonton, Alberta, Canada T6J 6V4. 780-450-8926. Fax 780-988-6182
E-mail: sales@madentec.com
www.madenta.com/

Prentke Romich Company · 1022 Heyl Road, Wooster, OH 44691. 800-262-1984. 330-262-1984. Fax 330-263-4829

PRC Regional Consultants · 800-848-8008
E-mail: info@prentrom.com
E-mail: customer-feedback@prentrom.com
www.prentrom.com/index.html

Synapse Adaptive · 1 Stop Speech Recognition & Adaptive Technology, 3095 Kerner Blvd., Suite S, San Rafael, CA 94901. 888-285-9988. Fax 415-455-9801
E-mail: info@synapseadaptive.com
www.synapseadaptive.com

RJ Cooper & Assoc. · 24843 Del Prado #283, Dana Point, CA 92629. 949-661-6904. Fax 949-240-9785
E-mail: info@rjcooper.com
www.rjcooper.com/

TASH Inc. · Unit 191 Station Street, Ajax, Ontario, Canada L1S 3H2. 905-686-4129. 800-463-5685. Fax 905-686-6895
E-mail: tashcan@aol.com
www.tashinc.com

Words+ Inc. · 1220 West Avenue J, Lancaster, CA 93534-2902. 661-723-6523. 800-869-8521. Fax 661-723-2114
E-mail: info@words-plus.com
www.words-plus.com/mn

Zygo Industries, Inc. · P.O. Box 1008, Portland, OR 97207. 503-684-6006. 800-234-6006. Fax 503-684-6011
E-mail: zygo@zygo-usa.com
www.zygo-usa.com

Research and Development Centers

Center for Applied Special Technology · 39 Cross Street, Suite 201, Peabody, MA 01960. 978-531-8555. 978-538-3110. TTY 978-531-0192
E-mail: cast@cast.org
www.cast.org/

Trace Research & Development Center · University of Wisconsin-Madison, 5901 Research Park Boulevard, Madison, WI 53719-1252. 608-262-6966. Fax 608-262-8848
E-mail: web@trace.wisc.edu
www.trace.wisc.edu/

Disability Information Resources

American Foundation for the Blind · 11 Penn Plaza, Suite 300, New York, NY 10001. 212-502-7600
www.afb.org/

Equal Access to Software and Information · Access to Information for Persons with Disabilities, c/o TLT Group, P.O. Box 18928, Rochester, NY 14618. 716-244-9065
E-mail: EASI@TLTGROUP.ORG
www.rit.edu/~easi/

Family Village · Waisman Center, University of Wisconsin-Madison, 1500 Highland Ave., Madison, WI 53705-2280
E-mail: familyvillage@waisman.wisc.edu
www.familyvillage.wisc.edu/

Job Accommodation on the Web · West Virginia University, P. O. Box 6080, Morgantown, WV 26506-6080. Voice, TTY 800-526-7234
www.janweb.icdi.wvu.edu/

LD Online · c/o WETA, 2775 South Quincy St., Arlington, VA 22206
E-mail: ldonline@weta.com
http://www.ldonline.org/

Poor Richard's Publishing (LD Resources) · LD Resources, 202 Lake Rd., New Preston, CT 06777. 860-868-3214
E-mail: richard@ldresources.com
www.ldresources.com

W3C Disabilities Developments Page · Organization: World Wide Web Consortium
E-mail: jbrewer@w3.org
www.w3.org/pub/WWW/Disabilities/

WebABLE!
www.webable.com

World Institute on Disability Home Page
www.wid.org/

Organizations

American Foundation for the Blind · 11 Penn Plaza, Suite 300, New York, NY 10001. 800-232-5463. 212-502-7661. TDD 212-502-7662. Fax 212-502-7777
E-mail: afbinfo@afb.net
www.afb.org/

American Occupational Therapy Association · Technology Special Interest Section
www.aota.org/members/area3/index.asp.

Blindness Resource Center · The New York Institute for Special Education, 999 Pelham Parkway, Bronx, New York 10469. 718-519-7000 Ext. 315. Fax 718-231-9314
E-mail: ilumin@earthlink.net
www.nyise.org/blind.htm

Center for Accessible Technology · 2547 8th St. 12A, Berkeley, CA 94710. 510-841-3224
E-mail: info@cforat.org
www.cforat.org

Closing the Gap · P.O. Box 68, 526 Main St., Henderson, MN 56044. 507-248-3294. Fax 507-248-3810
E-mail: info@closingthegap.com
www.closingthegap.com

Council for Exceptional Children · 1920 Association Drive, Reston, VA 20191-1589. 888-CEC-SPED (800-232-7733). TTY (text only) 703-264-9446. Fax 703-264-9494
E-mail: service@cec.sped.org
www.cec.sped.org/

Disabled People's International · 101-7 Evergreen Place, Winnipeg, Manitoba, Canada R3L 2T3. 204-287-8010. Fax 204-453-1367. TTY: 204-284-2598
E-mail: dpi@dpi.org
www.escape.ca/~dpi/

Do-It Program · University of Washington, Box 354842, Seattle, WA 98195-4842
E-mail: doit@u.washington.edu
www.washington.edu/doit
Voice, TTY 206-685-DOIT (3648)
Voice, TTY, from Washington state only, outside Seattle 888-972-DOIT (3648). Fax 206-221-4171. Voice/TTY, Spokane office 509-328-9331

National Center for the Dissemination of Disability Resources · 211 E. Seventh St., Room 400, Austin, TX 78701-3281. 800-266-1832. 512-476-6861. Fax 512-476-2286
www.ncddr.org/

RESNA (The Rehabilitation Engineering & Assistive Technology Society of North America)
www.resna.org

References

American Printing House for the Blind (1994). *Distribution of Federal Quota Based on the January 4, 1993 Registration of Eligible Students*. Louisville, KY: Author.

American Speech Language and Hearing Association (1989). Competencies for speech-language pathologies providing services in augmentative communication. *American Speech-Language-Hearing Association, 31*, 107–110.

American Speech Language and Hearing Association (1991). Report: Augmentative and alternative communication. *American Speech-Language-Hearing Association, 33 (Supplement 5)*, 9–12.

Angelo, J. (1997). *Assistive Technology for Rehabilitation Therapists*. Philadelphia: Davis.

Angelo, J. (in press). Factors affecting single switch efficiency in assistive technology. *Journal of Rehabilitation Research & Development, 37*, 591–598.

Bain, B. K., & Leger, D. (1997). *Assistive Technology: An interdisciplinary approach*. New York: Churchill Livingstone.

Beukelman, D. R., & Mirenda, P. (1992). *Augmentative and Alternative Communication*. Baltimore: Paul H. Brookes.

Brandt, E., & Pope, A. (1997). *Enabling America: Assessing the Role of Rehabilitation Science and Engineering*. Washington: National Academy.

Buning, M., & Hanzlik, J. (1993). Adaptive computer use for a person with visual impairment. *American Journal of Occupational Therapy, 47*, 998–1008.

Colarusso, R., Hammill, D., & Mercier, L. (1996). *Motor-Free Visual Perception Test—Revised*. Novato, CA: Academic Therapy.

Cook, A. M., & Hussey, S. M. (1995). *Assistive Technologies: Principles and Practice*. Baltimore: Mosby.

Gardiner, M. (1993). *Test of Visual-Motor Skills*. Burlingame, CA: Psychological and Educational.

Jaffe, E., & Epstein, C. (1992). *Occupational Therapy Consultation: Theories, Principles and Practice*. St. Louis: Mosby–Year Book.

Kielhofner, G. (1997). *Conceptual Foundations of Occupational Therapy*. Philadelphia: Davis.

Mendelson, S. B. (1996). *Tax Options and Strategies for People with Disabilities*. New York: Demos Vermande.

Portney, L., & Watkins, M. (1993). *Foundations of Clinical Research: Applications to Practice*. Norwalk, CT: Appleton & Lange.

Schrier, E. (1993). The future of access technology for blind and visually impaired people. *Journal of Visual Impairment and Blindness, 84*, 520–523.

Vanderheiden, G. (1989). Nonvisual alternative display techniques for output from graphics-based computers. *Journal of Visual Impairment and Blindness, 83*, 383–390.

Verbrugge, L., Rennert, C., & Madans, J. (1997). The great efficacy of personal and equipment assistance in reducing disability. *American Journal of Public Health, 97*, 384–392.

18
Physical Agent Modalities

Alfred G. Bracciano and Don Earley

LEARNING OBJECTIVES

After studying this chapter the student will be able to do the following:

1. Describe the three phases of wound healing and types of pain.
2. Identify the professional issues related to physical agents.
3. Define and discuss superficial and deep heat agents.
4. List the precautions in the use of physical agents.
5. Describe the clinical application of electrotherapeutic modalities.

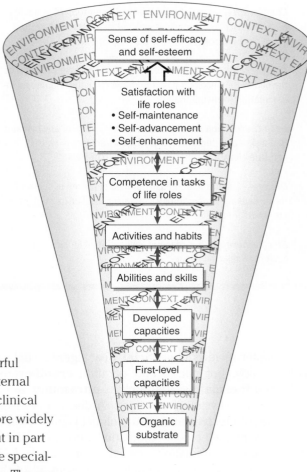

*T*he profession of occupational therapy has a long and colorful history, adapting and changing in response to internal and external issues and challenges. The use of physical agents as a part of clinical practice, though still somewhat controversial, has become more widely accepted within the profession. This transition has come about in part because of changes in health care delivery, expanded practice specialization, and service delivery in hand therapy and orthopaedics. The use of physical agents as a part of clinical practice has been motivated by the need to facilitate outcomes and healing in our patients as quickly and cost-effectively as possible. As increasing numbers of occupational therapists use physical agents to facilitate occupational function in their patients, the need for training and education to understand how and why these agents work is crucial.

This chapter provides a broad overview of the physical agents commonly used by occupational therapists. Physical agents are most often used as part of the treatment to address pain, edema, muscle weakness or guarding, and loss of function or sensation. This chapter discusses pain theories and wound healing. This information, often overlooked by therapists, is vital to determine which type of agent would be most efficacious and at which point in treatment and healing it should be applied.

GLOSSARY

Acute pain—Rapid onset of pain relative to a biological function associated with tissue trauma.

Chronic pain—Recurring or persistent pain, often poorly localized; may be associated with anguish, apprehension, depression, or hopelessness.

Conduction—Exchange of energy, for example heat or cold when two surfaces are in contact with each other.

Convection—Conveyance of heat by the movement of heated particles, such as air or water molecules, across the body part being treated, creating temperature variations.

Cryotherapy—Application of a superficial cold agent to part of the body. Often used for pain relief and reducing edema and inflammation following trauma.

Deep thermal agent—Therapeutic application of any modality to the skin and underlying soft tissue structures to cause a temperature elevation in tissue up to a depth of 5 cm.

Dosage—Amount and intensity of heat delivered to selected tissue causing temperature variations; classified as mild, moderate, or vigorous.

Electrotherapy—Therapeutic application of an electrical current to selected tissue.

Impedance—Amount of resistance to ultrasound waves.

Inflammation—Cellular and vascular response in affected tissue that follows injury or abnormal stimulation; the initial phase of the healing process. The body's attempt to rid itself of bacteria, foreign matter, and dead tissue and to decrease blood loss.

Physical agent modality—Treatment technique that uses heat, light, sound, cold, electricity, or mechanical devices.

Proliferation—Formation of new collagen tissue and epithelium in the intermediate stage of wound healing.

Referred pain—Pain occurring in an area different from the source of injury or disease.

Remodeling—Third phase of wound healing; dynamic process with maturation of new collagen tissue within the wound.

Superficial heat agents (SHAs)—Therapeutic application to the skin of any modality that raises the temperature of skin and superficial subcutaneous tissue to a depth of 1 cm.

Ultrasound—Deep heat modality; application of sound waves to soft tissue, causing thermal and nonthermal effects; sound having a frequency greater than 20,000 Hz.

The chapter reviews **superficial heat agents**, such as hydrotherapy, hot packs, and paraffin; **cryotherapy**; and **deep thermal agents**, such as **ultrasound**, along with their biophysiological effects. A discussion of the principles of **electrotherapy** and clinical application of neuromuscular electrical stimulation and transcutaneous electrical stimulation are also presented. It is beyond the scope of this chapter to present all of the information needed to use physical agents safely and effectively. The intent of this chapter is to provide a basic description of physical agents and their potential for incorporation into clinical practice to facilitate occupational function. The reader is encouraged to continue learning through review of other texts and materials and through further academic preparation and education.

Physical agent modalities are interventions or technologies that produce a response in soft tissue through the use of light, water, temperature, sound, or electricity. Physical agents may include paraffin baths, cold packs, hot packs, fluidotherapy, contrast baths, ultrasound, whirlpool, neuromuscular electrical stimulation (NMES), and transcutaneous electrical nerve stimulation (TENS) (American Occupational Therapy Association, 1997). The American Occupational Therapy Association (AOTA) (1992) supports the use of physical agents as an adjunctive method of treatment that can be used preparatory to or in conjunction with purposeful activity or occupation. Physical agents are used to remediate capacities which allows reacquisition of abilities that may enhance participation in activities of daily living and role performance. Use of physical agents without application to functional outcome or occupational performance is not considered occupational therapy treatment. Though other health professions may also use physical agents as part of their treatment protocols, the occupational therapy profession's distinct approach focuses on occupational performance issues at the level of the person and environment.

Competency and Regulatory Issues

The AOTA (1997) contends that the selection, application, and adjustment of physical agents is not entry-level practice; it requires continued training and education as the therapist's career progresses. Occupational therapists who use physical agents must have documented knowledge of the theoretical background and the technical skill necessary for their safe and proper application. Skill and training in these interventions can be accomplished through fieldwork experience, on-the-job training, postprofessional or graduate education, in-service training, or continuing education. The AOTA (1993) states that course work in the following areas is necessary before using physical agents: anatomy and physiology; principles of chemistry and physics related to the properties of light, water, temperature, sound and electricity; the physiological, neurophysiological, and electrophysiological changes that occur with the use of physical agents; and the response of normal and abnormal tissue to the agents. Occupational therapists who use physical agents have an ethical and legal obligation to obtain appropriate training in the use of these interventions. It is important that education and training in physical agents provide the therapist with more depth and breadth of knowledge than the mere technical skill of application.

Therapists must be critical consumers of continuing education course work, which may be provided by a manufacturer or sales representative during in-service training. (See Resources for a list of manufacturers and vendors.) Many therapists use physical agents and technologies without the foundations necessary to safely incorporate them into clinical practice and clinical reasoning. Without a thorough grounding in the fundamentals of physical agents, occupational therapists become mere technicians, applying physical agents incorrectly, at the wrong time in the treatment process, or without regard to facilitating occupational function.

Occupational therapists who use physical agents as part of their clinical practice also need to know local, state, and institutional rules and guidelines, which may restrict or limit the use of physical agents. Some states, including Florida, Georgia, and Minnesota, have specific training and competency standards that are regulated by licensing boards. All occupational therapists who will be using these agents should contact their state regulatory board and be able to defend their training and expertise to their colleagues and clients.

Wound Healing and Pain

Physical agents have been defined as treatment techniques that use heat, light, sound, cold, electricity, or mechanical devices. They include electrical therapeutic modalities that induce heat or electrical current beneath the skin. In addition to course work related to the properties of light, water, temperature, sound, and electricity, occupational therapists using physical agents should have a thorough understanding of the wound healing process, classification of pain, and biophysiology of these agents so as to apply them in a timely, appropriate, and safe manner.

Normal Wound Healing

An understanding of wound healing and an appreciation for the sequence of events that follows an injury are necessary to determine the appropriate intervention to facilitate healing. Tissue and wound healing is a complex process affected by both physical and psychological components. In the healthy individual, the body's attempt to heal itself in response to an injury is well ordered and sequenced. The stages of healing and repair may overlap, but they consist of three primary phases: inflammatory, proliferative, and **remodeling**.

Phase I: Inflammatory
The inflammatory phase is the initial response to an injury; it is both vascular and cellular. The inflammatory response is the body's attempt to rid itself of bacteria, foreign matter, and dead tissue and to decrease blood loss. The inflammatory response may be associated with changes in skin color (red, blue, purple), temperature (heat), turgor (swelling), sensation (pain), and loss of function. Acute **inflammation** usually lasts for 24 to 48 hours and is completed within 7 days, though a subacute phase may last for 2 weeks.

Phase II: Proliferative
The proliferative phase of recovery is also known as the fibroplastic, granulation, or epithelialization phase. At this point the injured area is filled with new connective tissue and the wound is covered with new epithelium (**proliferation**). The primary components of this stage of healing are granulation, epithelialization, and wound contraction. This phase overlaps the inflammatory phase, continuing until the wound is healed. Wound contraction, which is caused by the forming of red granulation tissue, shrinks the affected area. It begins approximately 5 days after the injury. It is complete approximately 2 to 3 weeks post injury. Fibroblasts are responsible for fibroplasia and collagen synthesis. Cross-linkages of the collagen tissue provides the wound with its tensile strength and durability (Scheurmann, 1982). The proliferative phase is complete when epithelialization has covered the wound, a collagen layer has formed, and initial remodeling is achieved.

Phase III: Remodeling

Remodeling is also known as the maturation phase. This stage begins about 2 weeks after injury and may continue for a year or more. Remodeling is characterized by a balance of collagen synthesis and collagen lysis, formation and breakdown. During this time the scar becomes more elastic, smoother, and stronger. If collagen synthesis exceeds collagen lysis, hypertrophic scarring or keloids may occur. As remodeling continues, the collagen fibers assume the characteristics of the tissue they are replacing.

Wound Assessment

Internal and external factors, such as presence of foreign objects, infection, nutrition, and medications may slow or affect the healing process; they are most significant in elderly people (Mulder et al., 1995). When treating open wounds, therapists should obtain baseline information on the wound's appearance prior to treatment. Documentation should include the anatomical location and area of wound, the size and shape of the wound, the color of any dead or necrotic tissue; a description of the exudate (purulent, with pus or a milky look; serous [clean, yellowish]; serosanguinous [pinkish]; any granulation tissue or epithelialization; and a description of the surrounding intact skin (erythema, heat, pain, edema).

Physical agents applied at the appropriate sequence and phase during wound healing can accelerate healing and resolution of the injury. Appropriate selection of the type and depth of penetration of the thermal agent may significantly affect the healing process at a cellular level.

Pain Perception

Many of the clients seen by occupational therapists report pain as one of their primary complaints, which may limit their ability to participate in occupational tasks. By using physical agent technologies to treat pain in our clients, we may be able to integrate them more fully into their primary roles and activities, improving outcomes and quality of life. Understanding the pain experience informs clinical reasoning and influences our selection of physical agents.

Nociceptors (sensory receptors specific to pain), which have variable thresholds, identify potential or actual tissue damage and respond to mechanical distortion, variations in the chemical components, and thermal changes in the tissue fluid. There are several ascending tracts that transmit pain signals to the brain.

Pain occurs when there is a noxious event, such as injury or inflammation, to an area of the body causing an excitation of the nociceptors in somatic or visceral tissue (Hakim, 1995). Pain is characterized as being acute or chronic and can be referred, that is, felt in an area of the body other than the site of injury.

▶ **Acute pain** has a biological function; it lasts from seconds to days, acting as a warning that injury has occurred or that something is wrong. Acute pain is closely associated with tissue damage and nociception occurring with a rapid onset. Physical agents are indicated as a part of the treatment approach in patients with acute pain.

▶ **Chronic pain** recurs or persists for a long time. It may be associated with anguish, apprehension, depression, or hopelessness. Chronic pain is often poorly localized, without an underlying cause being fully identifiable. Chronic pain pervades the individual's life. Physical agents are usually ineffective in consistently relieving pain for patients with chronic pain. Chronic pain affects an individual's occupational functioning, affecting society, the economy, employment, and health care systems.

▶ **Referred pain** occurs at an area different from the source of the injury or disease, that is, not where the nociceptors were stimulated. These irritable points, sometimes known as trigger points, can be located through palpation.

Physical agents such as heat, sound, compression, cold, or electricity may all reduce the effects of pain and can influence healing in soft tissue injuries. Selection of the correct intervention or physical agent is based on a thorough evaluation of the patient and on the diagnosis, treatment goals, clinical experience of the therapist, and the goals of the patient.

Incorporating Physical Agents Into a Typical Occupational Therapy Treatment

Physical agents are used as a precursor to functional activity to facilitate occupational performance. The therapist determines which physical agents will help achieve the patient's goals. For example, a patient with rheumatoid arthritis may have pain and limited movement. Paraffin to both hands and wrists may alleviate the patient's pain and stiffness prior to training with adaptive equipment for self-care activities.

Before administration of any modality, the therapist questions the patient as to any untoward negative response to physical agents applied in previous treatment and reviews whether the patient has any contraindications for the selected agent. Prior to administration of the physical agent, the therapist informs the patient as to the procedure, expected outcome, and subjective sensation that the patient may feel during the treatment. Skin integrity is always evaluated prior to administration of physical agents and immediately preceding the intervention. Documentation should be clear and concise, stating the modality used, parameters or settings, sequence in the course of treatment, and patient's response (Box 18-1). Therapists also assess the effectiveness of the modality on a session-by-session basis. If the modality fails to provide the desired outcome or if the patient has discomfort or negative results, the modality should be discontinued.

Superficial Heat Agents

A superficial heat agent (SHA) is any modality applied to the skin that raises skin and superficial subcutaneous tissue temperature. The objectives of heat are to decrease pain and stiffness, improve range of motion and tendon excursion, improve viscosity of synovia, and promote healing and relaxation. Conditions that may benefit from heat include muscle spasm, subcutaneous adhesion, sympathetic nervous system disorders, contractures, neuromas, chronic arthritis, trauma, wounds, and subacute and chronic inflammation. Superficial heat has a therapeutic effect at depths of up to 1 cm (Kaul, 1994). If a depth greater than 1 cm is desired, ultrasound should be considered.

Treatment Planning

In planning treatment that involves heat, one typically considers general and specific **dosage** guidelines, primary effects, and modality selection.

Dosage Guidelines

General dosage guidelines provide a starting point for selection of agent and for application parameters. Specific dosage guidelines guide application based on specific characteristics of the patient. For example, the dose temperature must be considered when selecting a

SHA, as it influences the physiological responses. Also, the physiological responses depend on the extent of the temperature elevation within the tissue. Elevation of tissue temperature in turn depends on the rate and duration (continuous or intermittent) at which the heat is applied, the area of tissue exposed to the heat, and the mechanism of transferring heat to the body— **conduction** (the exchange of energy when two surfaces are in contact) or **convection** (the conveyance of heat through movement of heated particles, such as air or water) (Hoban, 1993). Consideration of these guidelines during occupational therapy facilitates application of safe and effective dosages of heat (Earley, 1999).

Consideration of the phases of soft tissue healing and the acuteness or chronicity of the impairment also influences the dosage of heat, which ranges from mild to vigorous. A mild dose implies a minimal elevation in tissue temperature, with the primary benefits related to the somatosensation of warmth. Many conservative home remedies provide this mild dosage. A moderate dose causes an increase in tissue temperature of approximately 6°F and a moderate increase in blood flow. A vigorous dose implies a marked increase in blood flow with substantial tissue temperature elevation, up to 14°F. Box 18-2 lists precautions and contraindications of SHAs. One should be especially vigilant with moderate and vigorous doses of heat and monitor skin color and respiratory status.

Primary Effects of Superficial Heat Agents

The four primary effects of superficial heat agents are analgesic, vascular, metabolic, and connective tissue responses. Each has different dosage guidelines.

► The analgesic effect influences pain symptoms. Heat acts selectively on free nerve endings, tissues, and peripheral nerve fibers, which directly or indirectly reduces pain and elevates pain tolerance (Michlovitz, 1990). A mild to vigorous dose is required to obtain an analgesic effect.

► Vascular effects aid in pain relief and in decreasing muscle spasm. At 6°F of tissue temperature elevation, substances such as histamines are released in the bloodstream, resulting in vasodilation. This increased blood flow reduces ischemia, muscle spindle activity, and tonic muscle contractions, decreasing pain. Moderate dosage is needed to obtain these effects.

► Metabolic effects influence tissue repair and aid pain relief. Increases in blood flow and oxygen within the tissues bring a greater number of antibodies, leukocytes, nutrients, and enzymes to injured tissues. Pain is reduced by the removal of byproducts of the inflammatory process. Nutrition is enhanced at the cellular level, and repair occurs. A

BOX 18-2
SAFETY BOX

Superficial Heat Agents

Precautions	Contraindications
▶ Edema	▶ Impaired sensation due to skin graft or scar
▶ Diminished sensation	▶ Tumors, cancer
▶ Compromised circulation	▶ Advanced cardiac disease (body inadequately dissipates heat)
▶ Use of anticoagulant medications	▶ Acute inflammation, acute edema
	▶ Deep-vein thrombophlebitis
	▶ Pregnancy (systemic effects of circulating blood on fetus are unclear)
	▶ Bleeding tendencies
	▶ Infection
	▶ Primary repair of tendon or ligament
	▶ Semicoma or impaired cognitive status
	▶ Rheumatoid arthritis: vigorous dosages of heat can exacerbate joint inflammation

(Schmidt, 1979).

mild to vigorous dosage of heat is needed to facilitate the metabolic effects, depending on the acuity of the wound or soft tissue condition.

▶ Improvement in the properties of collagen and extensibility of tissues occurs when heat is combined with passive or active mobilization and/or engagement in occupation. This connective tissue response occurs during an 8- to 10-minute window after the application of heat (Norkin & Levangie, 1992). Reduced joint stiffness and increased range of motion also occur. A moderate to vigorous dose is needed to achieve these benefits.

Selection of Superficial Heat Agents

The choice of modality depends on the treatment objective, the location and surface area of the involved structure, and the desired dosage and tissue temperature. Other considerations include whether moist or dry heat is desired, the positioning of the extremity in a nondependent or intermittently dependent position, and whether active or passive participation by the patient is desired (Earley, 1999). The acuity or chronicity of the

patient's condition is also an important factor. Injuries in the acute phase (24–48 hours) should be treated with cryotherapy, not heat. Wounds in the remodeling stage of recovery, on the otherhand, would be treated with higher dosages of heat to facilitate the remodeling process by helping the collagen fibers to align themselves in a symmetrical fashion.

Clinical Use of Specific Superficial Heat Agents

As previously mentioned, superficial heat is primarily transmitted through conduction and convection. Hydrotherapy and fluidotherapy are examples of convection agents while hot packs and paraffin are categorized as conduction agents.

Whirlpool Baths and Hydrotherapy

The whirlpool bath is effective with open wounds, status post fractures, inflammatory conditions, peripheral vascular disease, and peripheral nerve injuries. Whirlpool is considered an active SHA; its primary advantage is that the therapist can see and have immediate access to the body part being treated, and the client can actively participate in exercises. Water temperature can be set to the desired temperature, 100 to 104°F, and the degree of agitation of the water can be controlled to act as a soft tissue massage and/or resistance for exercise. If wounds or excessive skin dryness are present, cleansing and debridement can aid healing. Proper disinfecting must be used.

Fluidotherapy

Fluidotherapy uses fine particles of ground corn husks suspended in a hot air stream to heat the extremity (Borrell et al., 1980). Temperature is controlled by a thermostat, with most conditions requiring a temperature between 105 and 118°F. Temperature settings depend on the dosage of heat needed and the extremity being treated. The force of the air and particles circulating within the machine can be graded via the blower speed, facilitating mobilization and desensitization.

The advantage of fluidotherapy is the ease of implementation and the therapist's access to the client's extremity while in the unit, allowing for passive or active assistive range of motion or manual therapy.

Hot Packs

Hot packs, or hydrocollator packs, are forms of moist heat that come in a variety of sizes. They heat large areas of the body and adequately cover contoured areas of the body, such as the shoulder. The temperature of the hot pack is typically 104 to 113°F. Hot packs are generally easy to use and require minimal maintenance. **It is important to ensure that a dry padding is used between the hot pack and the skin to avoid burns,** even though it cools as the treatment progresses. Hot packs help to reduce pain and muscle spasms and to improve connective tissue extensibility. Although a hot pack is considered a passive treatment, a positional sustained stretch of the tissue being treated can be accomplished during the treatment.

Paraffin

Paraffin is used to provide a high degree of localized heat to smaller joints. It is primarily used to decrease stiffness, improve range of motion, and relieve pain. Healed amputations, arthritis, strains, and sprains are a few conditions that benefit from paraffin. Paraffin allows for an even distribution of heat to the treatment surface, reducing the viscosity of the synovia and hence decreasing stiffness and pain associated with arthritis.

The wrap or glove technique is the most popular method of application. The therapist should always check the temperature of the paraffin before use to ensure a safe temperature and avoid burns. The client immerses the extremity in the bath and withdraws it to allow the paraffin to harden. This gloving process is repeated approximately 10 times, depending on the client's tolerance to heat. The extremity is then wrapped in a plastic bag followed by a towel to retain the heat and is left on for 20 minutes (Fig. 18-1). At the end of treatment, the paraffin is removed and discarded.

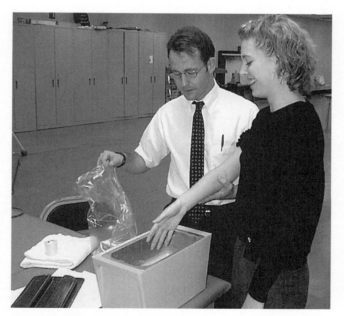

Figure 18-1 Application of paraffin to increase pain-free AROM of the digit interphalangeal joints. The extremity will be wrapped in a plastic bag and then a towel.

Passive stretching of joints can be accomplished with an elastic wrap secured prior to the dipping. This form of treatment can be used in conjunction with paraffin to maximize the benefits of mobilizing and remodeling connective tissue.

Cryotherapy

Cryotherapy is the application of a superficial cold agent to relieve pain and to reduce in edema and inflammation following trauma. It is the application of any substance to the body that results in withdrawal of heat from the body, lowering the temperature of the tissue. Tissue temperature change and biophysical effects of cooling are related to the time of exposure, the method used to cool the tissue, and the conductivity of the tissue. **Be careful when considering the length of exposure to the cold agent, as changes in skin temperature occur quickly, and tissue may be damaged before the desired biophysical effects are achieved.**

Purpose and Effects

The clinical use of cold is based on physiological changes resulting from tissue temperature reduction. Cold is used in the management of acute trauma because it affects arteriolar vasoconstriction, reducing bleeding; decreases metabolism and vasoactive agents such as histamine, thereby reducing inflammation and swelling; and elevates the pain threshold. In most acute traumas, cold is used with compression and elevation.

There are four methods for administering cold treatment: cold packs, ice cubes, cold baths, and controlled cold-compression units. Application of cold provides an anesthetic or numbing effect, and the patient may initially report a cold, aching, or burning sensation. As with any thermal agent, monitoring of the skin is essential to avoid damage to the tissue, and caution is advised for patients with decreased sensation or mentation.

Indications and Precautions

Cryotherapy is easy to apply and is indicated for a number of treatment conditions. The most common use for cryotherapy is in the treatment of acute injury and inflammation (Fig. 18-2). Other conditions and indications for the use of cold include edema, pain post exercise (combined with compression, exercise, and massage), arthritic exacerbation, acute bursitis or tendinitis, spasticity, and acute or chronic pain secondary to muscle spasm.

The physiological effects of cold can last for several hours. Rewarming of the tissue takes approximately 20 minutes. Care should always be used when applying

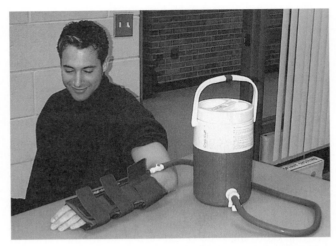

Figure 18-2 Application of cryotherapy for distal extremity edema and inflammation.

cold, and skin condition should be monitored to avoid frostbite and tissue damage. Box 18-3 lists contraindications to cryotherapy.

Therapeutic Ultrasound

Therapeutic ultrasound is deep heat via acoustic energy that is inaudible to the human ear. The ultrasound beam itself does not transmit heat. Heat accumulates in the tissue because of the conversion of energy absorbed from the sound wave in continuous-mode or high-intensity ultrasound. Therapeutic ultrasound has two primary effects on tissue: thermal and nonthermal, or acoustic. Both can be used to facilitate healing and ultimately improve occupational function (Bracciano, 1999).

In the thermal mode, ultrasound is a deep-heating agent capable of elevating tissue temperatures to a depth of 5 cm or more. A frequency of 1 MHz provides deeper penetration than 3 MHz. Nonthermal ultrasound does not elevate tissue temperature but provides secondary cellular effects, such as increased cellular permeability and diffusion. Ultrasound is acoustic energy that is used in medicine for diagnosis and tissue destruction and in rehabilitation to help restore and heal soft tissues.

Physical Principles

Standard ultrasound units consist of a power supply, oscillator circuit, transformer, coaxial cable transducer, and ultrasound applicator. The generator uses alternating current as a power source, converting electrical energy into ultrasonic energy. Inside the applicator a

crystal, consisting of natural quartz or synthetic material, contracts or expands in response to alternating current (Fig. 18-3). The vibration of the crystal generates the sound waves, which are transmitted to a small volume of tissue, causing the tissue molecules to vibrate. Ultrasound travels poorly through air, so a lubricant is used to maintain contact between the transducer and the tissue, ensuring that the energy is dispersed into the tissue (Fig. 18-4).

Ultrasound can be transmitted, absorbed, reflected, and refracted depending on the type of tissue and the angle of the wave. The rate at which the sound wave travels depends on the density of the molecules of the tissue. There is an inverse relationship between absorption and penetration. If the molecules are close together or compressed, the rate is less, as less energy is absorbed because the molecules resist compression. When the sound waves are generated rapidly and dispersed into the tissue, the molecules in the waves' path are pushed

BOX 18-3
SAFETY BOX

Cryotherapy

Avoid cryotherapy with patients who exhibit the following:

► Peripheral vascular disease or any circulatory compromised area
► Cold sensitivity, Raynaud's phenomenon
► Multiple myeloma, leukemia, systemic lupus (cryoglobinemia is a disorder of abnormal protein formation that can lead to ischemia in these individuals)
► Cold urticaria/intolerance; can occur with rheumatic diseases, following crush injuries and amputations

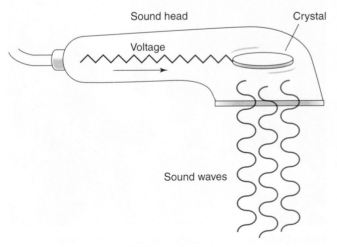

Figure 18-3 Production of ultrasound.

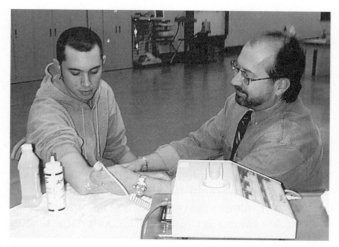

Figure 18-4 Application of nonthermal ultrasound for acute elbow lateral epicondylitis.

back and forth by the alternating phases of successive waves until the wave runs out of energy. This type of wave, moving in one direction, compressing and decompressing the molecules in its way, is termed a longitudinal wave. If the movement of the soundwaves is at right angles to the propagation of the wave, a shear wave is created in solid substances. Clinically, shear waves occur when the wave encounters bone, causing the wave to be deflect along the periosteum. This may cause heating of the outer covering of the bone but is negligible in terms of tissue temperature elevation (Bracciano, 1999).

Each tissue in the body transmits and absorbs ultrasound according to its unique properties. These properties are known as absorption coefficients, with body fluids such as blood and water having the lowest **impedance** (or resistance to ultrasound waves) and lowest acoustic absorption coefficient. Bone possesses the highest impedance and absorption coefficient, making it a good absorber of ultrasound energy (Kimura et al., 1988).

Energy Distribution

The spread of ultrasound waves into tissue is affected by the frequency and size of the crystal. The intensity of the beam of energy varies within the sound wave; this phenomenon is the beam nonuniformity ratio (Allen & Batye, 1978; Kimura et al., 1988). These higher areas of intensity are in part responsible for hot spots, which can be prevented by moving the sound head during treatment.

The intensity of the beam of energy is a significant factor in determining tissue response. In general, the higher the intensity, the greater the tissue temperature elevation. Intensity is documented as watts per square centimeter. The duty cycle determines the overall

amount of acoustic energy a patient receives and plays a role in determining tissue response (Fig. 18-5). The duty cycle is a percentage or ratio of time that the ultrasound energy is actually being introduced into the body. A 50% duty cycle provides twice as much acoustic energy as a 25% duty cycle, as the on-time is twice as long. Consider a hose with a squeeze nozzle, analogous to the ultrasound transducer. If the handle is squeezed and held, water is released in a stream from the hose—constant energy. If the handle is squeezed and released rapidly, the water is turned on and off, or pulsed. The same concept holds for ultrasound. When the sound wave is on 100%, the sound wave and energy are constant. When the sound energy is turned on and off rapidly, the sound wave is pulsed and is described in terms of a ratio of the cycle. Whether to use continuous or pulsed ultrasound depends on the pathology, stage of wound healing, and amount of area being treated (Fyfe & Parnell, 1982).

Energy is absorbed from the ultrasound beam in proportion to the density of the tissue, with protein-dense structures, such as scar, joint capsules, ligaments, tendons, and bones, most apt to absorb the ultrasound energy. Because ultrasound can target specific areas of the body, therapists can heat dense or deep-lying tissues (Binder, 1985).

Effects on Tissue: Thermal Versus Nonthermal Ultrasound

A number of physiological effects occur with thermal ultrasound. They include increased metabolic rates of tissue, increased blood flow and tissue permeability, increased viscoelasticity of connective tissue, elevation of pain thresholds, and increased enzymatic activity, which may stimulate the immune system. Thermal ultrasound may increase joint range of motion, facilitate

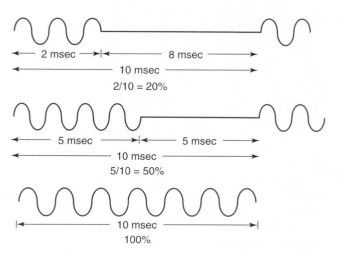

Figure 18-5 Duty cycles determine the on time of the ultrasound

tissue healing, decrease muscle spasm and pain, and decrease chronic inflammatory process (Dyson & Suckling, 1978; Enwemeka, 1989). The heating effects of ultrasound can be decreased by pulsing the sound waves or by decreasing the intensity. When these methods are used, cellular or mechanical changes occur.

Nonthermal ultrasound causes increased cellular permeability and diffusion and a variety of second-order effects that facilitate tissue repair (Dyson & Pond, 1970).

The effects of nonthermal ultrasound on tissue healing occur with short treatment duration along with lower intensities, 0.1 and 0.2 W/cm², pulsed at 20% duty cycle. A frequency of 1 MHz provides deeper penetration, up to 5 cm, than 3 MHz, which penetrates approximately 1 cm. Treatment sessions should be repeated every 24 to 48 hours to facilitate tissue repair.

Nonthermal effects of pulsed ultrasound occur at the cell membrane due to stable cavitation, acoustic streaming, and micromassage (Apfel, 1989). Acoustic streaming occurs with the unidirectional movement of the body fluids that cause currents which exert force and structural changes in the cell membrane along with increased permeability. Second-order effects of nonthermal ultrasound are due to the destabilization of the cellular membrane. Secondary effects of pulsed ultrasound may include an increase in phagocytic activity; increase in the number and motility of fibroblasts, resulting in enhanced protein synthesis; increased granular tissue; and improved angiogenesis, facilitating wound contraction. Low-intensity pulsed ultrasound may also accelerate fracture healing in tibial and Colles fractures (Lehmann & Guy, 1971).

Clinical Use of Ultrasound

A thorough evaluation of the patient is necessary to identify problems and to set treatment goals prior to using ultrasound. It is essential to determine the location, stage of healing, depth, and anatomical location of the injury and the area and type of tissue to be treated. Superficial conditions, for example epicondylitis, are best treated using a frequency of 3 MHz. If a thermal effect is not needed, such as in a subacute condition or superficial pathology, low intensities can be used with a pulsed sound wave. Acute conditions should be treated for shorter periods than chronic conditions, and smaller areas of tissue require less time than larger areas (Bracciano, 1999).

Ultrasound may also be used before functional activity for prophylactic pain-relieving effects. Thermal ultrasound (100% duty cycle, high intensities) can be used to heat tissue and increase its length. Combining thermal ultrasound with positional stretch, splinting, functional activities, or manual therapy may be effective in stretching the heated tissue through a pain-free range of motion following application of ultrasound.

Acute conditions are best treated with lower-intensity dosages, 0.1 to 0.5 W/cm²; the patient is unlikely to feel any warmth at this low level. Subacute conditions can be treated using a low-intensity dosage, 0.5 to 1 W/cm²; chronic conditions and those requiring a thermal effect require a setting between 1 and 2 W/cm². Patients may report some degree of warmth during the treatment but should not report any pain, discomfort, or burning. If these symptoms occur, the intensity should be reduced, the sound head should be moved more quickly, or ultrasound gel should be added if an inadequate amount is causing an uncomfortable tingling sensation or vibration.

Phonophoresis

Phonophoresis is the use of ultrasound to facilitate the delivery of topically applied drugs or medication to selected tissue. Though it is frequently used, there are questions as to the effectiveness of phonophoresis because of variability in outcomes associated with inconsistent treatment parameters, such as intensity of sound waves and transmission characteristics of the conducting gel. Intensities of 1.5 W/cm² are effective for both the thermal and nonthermal effects of ultrasound as part of phonophoresis. A low intensity, 0.5 W/cm², may be more effective for treating acute injuries (Bracciano, 2000). Many hydrocortisone creams commonly used in the clinic (1% or 10% hydrocortisone in a thick white cream base) do not transmit ultrasound and this method of delivery is ineffective (Henley, 1991; Masse, 1996). Dexamethasone sodium phosphate mixed with a sonic gel transmits ultrasound effectively and can be formulated by a pharmacist. Following phonophoresis, a dressing can be used to seal the area and prevent moisture from escaping.

Precautions for Use of Ultrasound

Clients should be monitored during ultrasound, and any pain or discomfort may indicate that the intensity is too high or there is an inadequate amount of gel. Ultrasound should never be applied over the eye, the heart, the pregnant uterus, or the testes. Sonification to malignant tissue should also be avoided. Caution must be used when applying ultrasound over areas of decreased circulation and avoided over areas of thrombophlebitis. High intensities and application over the growth plates in children should also be avoided (Sicard-Rosenbaum et al., 1995). When using ultrasound as a thermal agent, one must follow general contraindications and

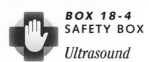

BOX 18-4
SAFETY BOX

Ultrasound

Precautions	Contraindications
▶ Unhealed fracture sites	▶ Suspected deep-vein thrombophlebitis
▶ Primary repair of a tendon or ligament	▶ Bleeding and edema; areas with tendency to hemorrhage
▶ Marked demineralization/osteoporosis	▶ Where sensation is reduced or if a person cannot report heat sensations accurately
▶ Plastic and metal implants	▶ In the very old and very young, because of compromised body temperature regulation
	▶ Skin or lymphatic cancers; tumors or malignancies
	▶ Over a cardiac pacemaker or surrounding adjacent tissue
	▶ Pregnancy
	▶ Infected areas
	▶ Epiphyses of growing bone
	▶ In conjunction with radium or radioactive isotopes treatment for cancer within 6 months
	▶ Over the heart
	▶ Over eyes
	▶ Over testes
	▶ Over carotid sinus and cervical ganglion
	▶ Over the spinal column or where there is inadequate protection over spinal cord, such as after laminectomy

precautions for any thermal modality. Box 18-4 lists precautions and contraindications for ultrasound.

Electrotherapy

Electrotherapy has been used since the time of the early Romans. The growth of electrical stimulation in recent years is due to the research of Melzak and Wall (1965) and their gate theory of pain and to advances in technology. Electrotherapy is the application of electrical stimuli to accomplish any of a variety of therapeutic purposes and goals. Frequently used applications include neuromuscular electrical stimulation (NMES),

transcutaneous electric nerve stimulation (TENS), electrical stimulation for tissue repair (ESTR), functional electrical stimulation (FES), electrical muscle stimulation (EMS), and iontophoresis. (Clinical application of commonly used modalities will be discussed later.)

▶ NMES uses pulsating alternating current to activate muscles through stimulation of intact peripheral nerves to cause a motor response. Stimulation of the nerve is used to decrease muscle spasm, for muscle strengthening, and for its effect on muscle pumping, which can reduce edema. NMES stimulation of innervated muscle can also be used for muscle reeducation and to prevent atrophy.

▶ FES is neuromuscular electrical stimulation to activate targeted muscle groups for orthotic substitution or to facilitate performance of functional activities (Fig. 18-6). FES is often used with individuals who have shoulder subluxation or foot drop after a stroke.

▶ TENS describes the wide variety of stimulators used for pain control. TENS uses surface electrodes with the goal of sensory analgesia rather than a motor response.

▶ EMS is electrical stimulation of denervated muscle to facilitate viability and to prevent atrophy, degeneration, and fibrosis of the fibers. EMS may facilitate nerve regeneration and muscle reinnervation while decreasing muscle atrophy.

▶ Iontophoresis is the use of low-voltage direct current to ionize topically applied medication into the tissue. Iontophoresis is often used in the treatment of

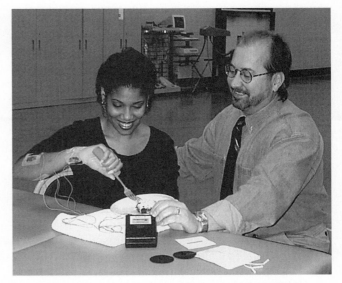

Figure 18-6 FES for the extrinsic flexor and extensor muscle groups to facilitate grasp for self-feeding.

Case Example

USE OF SHAs TO FACILITATE RESUMPTION OF SELF-ADVANCEMENT ROLES

Patient Information

Mr. J. is a 33-year-old father of three young children. He incurred an injury to his dominant right hand while working in the maintenance department of a local hospital. He sustained musculoskeletal, vascular, and nervous tissue injuries in addition to amputation of his third and fourth distal phalanges when his hand became entangled in a power takeoff. A week after surgery, Mr. J. was referred to occupational therapy for wound management, range of motion as tolerated, and splinting.

Phase 1 of Treatment

Following evaluation and assessment and after suture removal, initial treatment consisted of whirlpool at a tepid temperature, 90°F, with mild agitation. Whirlpool gently cleaned and debrided the hand and wounds and facilitated healing. Three and a half weeks post surgery, during the subacute phase of healing, the wounds closed and greater range of motion was warranted. Whirlpool continued to be the modality of choice, as edema was minimal and the patient could actively elevate his extremity and flex and extend the digits during the treatment.

The initial short-term goals in this phase consisted of (1) continued wound healing and edema reduction; (2) improved active range of motion.

Phase 2 of Treatment

During the subacute stage, skin integrity continued to improve, edema was reduced, and all aspects of the musculoskeletal injuries were healed. Fluidotherapy was now the SHA of choice, providing moderate to vigorous doses of heat while allowing Mr. J. to move his hand and fingers during treatment. This was a motivating factor for Mr. J., for he was beginning to use his hand and was anxious to return to his preinjury roles

and employment. Mr. J. benefited from the desensitization effects of the modality, which normalized hyperesthesia. As Mr. J. participated in functional job-simulated occupations, he recognized the positive thermal effects of heat to the persistent stiffness in his hand. Paraffin was used prior to participation in job-simulated activities. The thermal effects of the paraffin were complemented by a sustained passive composite flexion stretch obtained with an adhesive elastic wrap prior to the paraffin dip. Revised short-term goals in this stage consisted of (1) optimize active range of motion and pain desensitization so that he can independently perform simulated job tasks; (2) demonstrate right-hand function adequate for return to work.

SHAs allowed Mr. J. to maximize his participation and performance in treatment, and he returned to his position in the maintenance department without restrictions within 8 weeks of beginning outpatient occupational therapy.

CLINICAL REASONING
in OT Practice

Impact of Wound Healing in Physical Agent Selection

Mr. J.'s traumatic injury included soft tissue damage and traumatic amputation of the third and fourth distal phalanges. The phases of the healing process are overlapping and dynamic. Edema becomes a concern in these types of injuries.

How were the effects of edema compensated for during the application of thermal agents? Why were superficial heat agents used during treatment? How could deep thermal agents, such as ultrasound, have been incorporated into the treatment process, and why?

---

inflammatory conditions or for scar formation and management.

► ESTR, also known as high-voltage galvanic stimulation (HVGS) or HVPC, has been used for wound healing but is complicated and controversial. Medicare initially discontinued reimbursement for HVGS but reinstated it after much discussion and argument with the American Physical Therapy Association (APTA). Because of its complexity for entry-level clinicians, it is not reviewed in this chapter.

Principles of Electricity

To use electrotherapy in occupational therapy practice, clinicians need working knowledge of the principles of current, duration, rise and decay time, frequency, duty cycle, and current modulation and ramp time.

Current

Electric current is the movement of ions or electrons, which are charged particles, from one point to another in order to equalize the charge. Current, measured in amperes, occurs when there is an imbalance in the number of electrons in two distinct locations. Voltage, measured in volts, is the potential or electromotive force that drives the current. Current flows from an area of high electron concentration (cathode, or negative pole) to an area of less concentration (anode, or positive pole). Opposition or resistance to current flow is measured in ohms. Ohm's law states that voltage is proportional to both current (I) and resistance (R), such that $V = I \times R$. For clinical application, three specific forms, direct current (DC), alternating current (AC), and pulsatile current, are used (Fig. 18-7).

Direct Current

DC is unidirectional, with the electrons moving continuously in one direction and the electrodes maintaining their polarity. DC flow, characterized by the square wave, can cause chemical reactions in the body and facilitate the ionization of medication through the skin.

Alternating Current

AC is characterized by periodic changes in the direction of the current flow. The current is uninterrupted and bidirectional, without any true positive or negative pole. Household electricity uses AC. Hertz is the number of times the current reverses direction in 1 second (cycles per second).

Pulsatile Current

Pulsed current is the term used when the electron flow is periodically interrupted. These interrupted currents can flow in one direction (monophasic) or two directions (biphasic). In pulsed current, the current is interrupted for very short periods of milliseconds or microseconds. Most stimulators can be classified under one of three wave forms: monophasic, biphasic, or polyphasic.

▶ Monophasic wave forms have a single phase to each pulse, with the current flow unidirectional and either negative or positive. A monophasic pulse has a pulse duration averaging 40 to 60 msec.
▶ Biphasic currents have two opposing phases in a single pulse, with the lead phase of the pulse above the baseline and the final phase below. Biphasic pulses may be symmetrical or asymmetrical, with a phase duration between 25 and 250 seconds.
▶ Polyphasic waveforms consist of a burst of three or more phases, a series of pulses delivered as a single charge. This current is also known as interferential or Russian current. There have been many claims as to the uniqueness of this type of current, though there

are no confirmed physiological advantages to this type of waveform.

Duration

For monophasic current, phase and pulse duration are synonymous, referring to the length of time between the beginning and end of one phase of the pulse. For biphasic currents, the pulse duration is equal to the total of the two phase durations, including the intrapulse

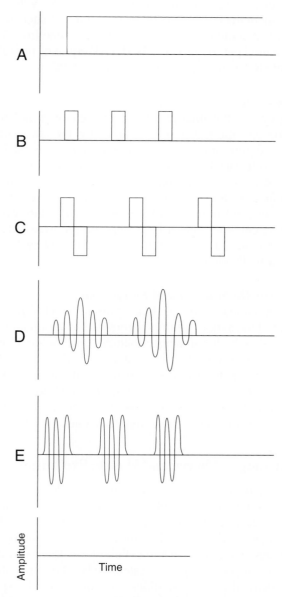

Figure 18-7 Commonly used electrotherapeutic current wave forms. **A.** Direct current. **B.** Monophasic pulsed. **C.** Biphasic pulsed. **D.** Interferential beats. **E.** Russian bursts.

interval. As phase duration increases, comfort levels decrease. Shorter pulse and duration result in better conductivity of the current with less impedance (Currier, 1993).

Rise Time and Decay Time

Rise time is the amount of time needed for the amplitude to go from 0 volts to peak. The rate of rise is related to the ability of the amplitude to excite nervous tissue.

Frequency

The number of pulses or wave forms repeated at regular intervals is the pulse or stimulus frequency. The pulse frequency consists of the number of pulses or cycles per second delivered to the body. The rate of successive electrical stimuli is adjustable and may range from 1 to 120 stimuli per second (1 to 120 Hz). Frequency may also be labeled as the pulse rate (Robinson, 1995).

Duty Cycle

Duty cycle is the amount of time between the stimulation period and the rest period. That is, it is the ratio of the time the current is on to the time the current is off. The duty cycle may be expressed as a percentage or a ratio. For example, a treatment protocol in which electrical stimuli are delivered for 10 seconds followed by a 50-second off period is expressed as a 1:5 duty cycle. Duty cycle is important in determining muscle fatigue. As the patient's condition improves, the duty cycle can be gradually increased.

Current Modulation and Ramp Time

Changes to the current or to the pulse characteristics are referred to as modulation. Current can be modulated by modifying the frequency, amplitude, or duration. Ramping is a change of the pulse intensity or duration of the pulse. Ramp time is the time required for successive current stimuli to reach the desired amplitude. Rampdown, the gradual decrease of the intensity, describes the movement of the peak amplitude back to zero.

Physiology of Nerve and Muscle Excitation

In addition to a working knowledge of electrical principles, clinicians using electrotherapy must understand the physiology of nerve and muscle excitation. The application of electrical current causes physiological changes at both a local and cellular level; these changes can occur segmentally or systemically. The application of electrical current modifies the body's physiological response and physiochemical effects.

Human tissue is either excitable or nonexcitable. Excitable tissues, such as nerves and muscles, can initiate and propagate an action potential if the stimulation parameters are sufficient. Stimuli must be sufficiently intense and long-lasting to cause the ions to shift across the resting membrane and depolarize the cell. Depolarization of the neural or muscle cell occurs quickly, and the sudden alteration in the cell membrane's electrical potential is known as an action potential. Action potentials are an all-or-none occurrence and, once started, are carried along the cell membrane. Following depolarization, if a membrane becomes hyperpolarized, it may be unable to discharge an action potential, and accommodation occurs.

Propagation

Tissues with high water content, such as muscle and nerve, transmit electricity better than those with lower water content, such as bone, fascia, and adipose tissue. The diameter of the fiber and degree of myelination are also factors affecting the rate of propogation of action potentials. Conduction is faster in myelinated fibers and in large-diameter fibers, which offer less resistance to the conduction of current. More intense stimuli, achieved by increasing the stimulus duration and amplitude, is needed to depolarize smaller-diameter nerves and denervated muscle membrane (Mehreteab & Weisberg, 1994). Large-diameter nerves are associated with nonnoxious cutaneous sensory modalities and motor nerves linked to large motor units. The small-diameter cutaneous sensory nerves are associated with pain pathways. As the amplitude and pulse duration increase, so do the number of nerve fibers recruited. The strength–duration curve in Figure 18.8 describes the relationship between the amplitude and duration of the stimulus needed to depolarize the membranes of various types of nerves to achieve a response (Mehreteab & Weisberg).

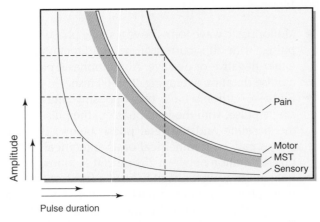

Figure 18-8 Strength–duration curve of an electrical stimulus. MST, maximum sensory threshold.

When the cell membrane or tissue receives an unchanging stimulus over time, the cell membrane begins to adapt to the stimulus and requires higher levels of stimulation to trigger an action potential; this is termed accommodation. Following stimulation and generation of an action potential in a nerve cell membrane, the membrane needs a short period to recover its excitability. This recovery time is known as the absolute refractory period.

Electrically Stimulated Movement

The diameter of the nerve, depth of the nerve, and duration of the pulse affect a nerve's response to electrical stimulation. Sensory nerves are stimulated first, followed by motor nerves, then pain fibers (Fig. 18-8), finally leading to excitation of the muscle fibers. Though pain fibers are superficial in relation to motor nerves, they also have a smaller diameter and a greater resistance to electrical current flow. Motor nerves reach threshold, and if there is sufficient intensity, contraction of all muscle fibers attached to that nerve (motor unit) occur before pain is felt. Stimulation of the skin surface causes an activation of sensory receptors before motor or pain nerves (Baker et al., 1988). Smaller motor units are recruited at varying and slowly increasing frequencies followed by larger motor units. If the stimulus frequency is sufficient, the muscle twitch contraction becomes fused in synchronous rapid succession, and the contraction becomes tetanic.

In a voluntary contraction, smaller motor units are recruited first, followed by the larger motor units as contraction strength increases. This gradual, asynchronous sequence allows for fine motor control, with the larger fibers being recruited as increased strength or speed is needed. This type of recruitment allows smooth, controlled movement. In electrically stimulated movement patterns, however, the reverse occurs, with larger motor units being recruited first in a synchronous pattern. This causes electrically stimulated muscle to fatigue more rapidly and limits the finely controlled quality of functional movement.

Treatment Planning Specific to Electrotherapy

Before incorporating electrotherapy into treatment, clinicians make decisions about the type of electrical stimulator to use and placement and size of electrodes.

Parameters of Electrical Stimulation Devices

The many stimulators available are offered with a variety of poorly supported claims by both manufacturers and clinicians. Research has been equivocal, and the clinician must critically evaluate the claims against the research-based outcomes of electrotherapeutic interventions.

Stimulators can be classified as having high or low voltage. Low-voltage units function at 1 to 100 volts. High-voltage units have an output of up to 500 volts. Wave forms are classified as being unidirectional or bidirectional (monophasic or biphasic) and further divided into continuous DC or pulsed, which is interrupted DC or AC.

The depth of current penetration is related to the peak amplitude. With biological tissue, the higher the voltage applied, the larger the current that will be passed through the tissue.

Electrodes

Electrodes are the contact point providing the current flow from the stimulation device to the body. The electrode acts as an interface with the skin surface, the point where the electron–ion conversion occurs. Electrodes should offer little resistance to the current flow. A variety of electrodes are commercially available. Common electrode material includes carbon–rubber electrodes, which are silicon rubber impregnated with small carbon particles; metal- or foil-backed electrodes; sponges over metal plates; karaya gum electrodes; and self-adherent polymer electrodes. The self-adhering electrodes may be reusable and do not require strapping or taping, making them convenient to use.

Metal- or foil-backed electrodes are used with sponges or conductive polymers to provide even conductivity throughout the electrode surface. This type of electrode may be preferred in high current density applications, such as with medium-frequency neuromuscular stimulation. Adequate contact with the skin is crucial, and complete coverage of the electrode with gel, if used, is necessary.

Electrodes should be examined before each use and changed when necessary. Electrodes degrade with use and become unable to conduct the current efficiently. Therapists should look for cracking and worn spots in the rubber–carbon electrodes or excessive dryness in self-adhering electrodes and replace them as needed. With frequent use, carbon–rubber electrodes may develop nonconductive areas because of the absorption of dirt, skin oil, or electrode gel and depletion of the carbon rubber. This may cause "hot spots," areas of high current density, that may be uncomfortable for the patient and cause skin burns. A biting or stinging sensation during electrical stimulation may be caused by uneven conductivity, and the electrodes should be replaced.

Regardless of the type of electrode used, proper skin care and hygiene is necessary to prevent skin irritation or breakdown. This factor becomes critically important for clients who are using the stimulators on a home program or when there is prolonged placement and use of the electrodes.

Electrode Size

Current density is inversely related to the electrode size. As the electrode size decreases or the contact area of the electrode decreases, the current density increases which is an explanation for "hot spots" mentioned above. As the current density increases, there is a greater perception of the stimulation beneath the electrode along with a greater physiological response due to the charge transfer. **Excessive current density under an electrode can lead to discomfort or skin burns.**

Because of the inverse relationship between electrode size and current density, smaller electrodes require less current to stimulate tissue, and large electrodes generally produce a stronger contraction with decreased pain or discomfort. Electrode size is determined by the size of the targeted tissue.

Electrode Placement

As the current density is greater in superficial layers of the skin, the distance between the electrodes also influences the depth of the current flow. When the electrodes are close together, the current passes superficially, and when the electrodes are farther apart, the current penetrates deeper.

Location and orientation of electrodes must also be considered when stimulating muscles. Small electrodes can be used to obtain an isolated contraction from smaller muscles, such as those of the hand. Larger electrodes disperse the current into the tissue and are less specific in stimulating isolated muscles. Care should be taken when applying and selecting location of the electrodes, as those closely spaced may increase discomfort.

There are two primary methods of electrode placement for electrical stimulation, monopolar and bipolar. Simply put, the terms identify whether one lead and electrode is placed over the targeted tissue or if both leads and electrodes are placed over the area. The monopolar technique uses one stimulating electrode, which is placed over the targeted area. The other lead and electrode are placed over an area that is not affected by stimulation; this is the dispersive, or nontreatment, electrode. In the monopolar technique, only one pole or side of the circuit (active electrode) of the electrical stimulator is used to stimulate the target area. The dispersive electrode completes the electrical circuit and can be placed away from the target area. The dispersive electrode is often larger, minimizing the current density

and perception of sensory stimulation. Monopolar techniques are most often associated with trigger- and acupuncture-point stimulation.

Bipolar techniques consist of both electrodes placed over the target area to cause stimulation of the tissue. Because both electrodes or sides of the circuit are in contact with the targeted area, the current flow is more local, and the stimulation is perceived under both electrodes of the circuit. Most often, the electrodes are the same size, and this technique can be used to stimulate large muscles or muscle groups. Bipolar techniques are often used to activate muscles atrophied because of disuse or to obtain stronger contraction (neuromuscular facilitation) to increase limited movement.

Clinical Use of Electrotherapy

The unique applications and indications for each type of electrotherapy are discussed in turn.

Electrical Stimulation

Electricity has been advocated in the treatment of a variety of body systems and for a plethora of conditions, including joint swelling and inflammation, joint dysfunction, tissue healing, muscle reeducation, circulatory disorders, postural disorders, pelvic floor disorders, fracture healing, and pain management. There are a number of claims for electrical stimulation along with a variety of protocols and applications, some objective but many unsubstantiated, and the clinician should take a systematic and objective approach to its use.

Functional Electrical Stimulation

FES, the use of NMES as a replacement for orthotics, has been an effective adjunct in facilitating occupational function, most notably positional stability and mobility. Stimulation of innervated paretic or paralyzed muscles can decrease dependence on slings, splints, or orthotics through the development of increased strength and endurance of the paretic musculature. FES has been effectively used with hemiparetic clients who display shoulder subluxation during the flaccid phase of recovery and also to facilitate grasp-and-release activities (Eckerson & Axelgaard, 1984; Phillips, 1989)

In the hemiplegic client, gravity stresses the shoulder capsule, stretching the ligamentous capsule. When muscle tone and voluntary control develop at the shoulder, normal glenohumeral alignment may not recur during resting muscle tone because of ligamentous laxity. Slings may be helpful to establish glenohumeral alignment, but stimulation of the posterior deltoid and supraspinatus muscles may be more effective in improving normal shoulder integrity (Baker & Parker, 1986; Griffin & Reddin, 1981).

Use of FES for maintaining shoulder integrity by preventing subluxation and reeducating muscles, can be an effective adjunct to splinting and facilitate occupational function. Clearly outlining and teaching the client and caregivers in a home program is vital to ensure continuity and carryover.

Neuromuscular Electrical Stimulation

NMES has a variety of clinical uses as an adjunct to occupational therapy treatment. NMES is defined as the "use of electrical stimulation for activation of muscle through stimulation of the intact peripheral nerve" (American Physical Therapy Association, 1990, p. 29). Whereas NMES is often erroneously referred to as "functional" electrical stimulation, FES actually refers to the use of NMES as a substitute for an orthosis to assist with a functional activity, such as standing or holding an object. NMES can be used for strengthening and endurance, range of motion, facilitation of muscle function, management of muscle spasms and spasticity, edema reduction, and orthotic substitution. Clinical use of NMES requires a partially intact or intact peripheral nerve, and its use with primary muscle disease or muscular dystrophy is questionable.

Maintain Muscle Mass

NMES can be a successful adjunct to conventional treatment in individuals with limited traumatic or orthopaedic injuries. There is a relationship between training intensity and strength gains, and improving muscle strength is based in part on the overload principle. The overload principle refers to the fact that for strength gains to occur, the body must be subjected to greater levels of stress than it is accustomed to. To accomplish this, the therapist must increase the load, frequency, or duration of the exercise or activity. Clients who are deconditioned or have areas of weakness may benefit from NMES to improve endurance of the targeted muscle. Isometric strengthening using NMES produces better results than conventional isometric exercises alone but is most effective when paired with functional goals and movements (Baker, 1993).

Maintain or Gain Range of Motion

Neurologically impaired patients often develop spasticity as a consequence of their injury. Range of motion techniques and positioning are often part of the overall training and education program for family members and caregivers. Unfortunately, clients with moderate to severe spasticity often have difficulty following through on these techniques and can develop limitations affecting their occupational function. Hemiplegic patients with chronic moderate spasticity in the wrist or finger flexors may be appropriate candidates for this intervention. For these individuals, the stimulus should ramp up and be sufficiently intense to allow for a slow stretch without increasing spasticity due to a quick stretch or jerk (Baker, 1993). Ramp-up times should be extended to 6 to 8 seconds or longer, and proper positioning or blocking of other muscles should be considered. Serial casting or splinting of the extremity can be an effective adjunct to NMES. The use of NMES is effective as part of a home program, since it reduces the spasticity and allows the caregiver to carry out passive range of motion several times daily.

For the orthopaedic client, range of motion may be limited by contractures secondary to immobilization or pain. NMES may be used to improve joint range of motion if the limitation is due to intrinsic soft tissue shortening as opposed to a bony block or biomechanical limitation. The technique should maintain a low-intensity stretch for a few seconds. Serial casting and splinting of the extremity may add to the effectiveness of this treatment.

Management of Spasticity

The effectiveness of NMES for the treatment of spasticity depends in part on the underlying disease causing the spasticity. The response of NMES with a spastic spinal cord injury may be different from that with a brain injury or multiple sclerosis. The variability of abnormal tone may only result in a temporary interruption of the motor neuron excitability with short term treatment effects. Stimulation of a spastic muscle in the neurologically impaired client using a high frequency causes a response similar to fatiguing the muscle (Vodovnik et al., 1984).

NMES also affects spasticity by stimulating the muscle antagonist to the spastic muscle which inhibits the spastic muscle, allowing range of motion exercise. Heat or ice and serial casting or splinting paired with functional movements and activities may enhance the therapeutic response.

Orthopaedic patients may have pain–spasm cycles caused by local spasm of a particular muscle or group. Decreasing the pain–spasm cycle through the application of NMES to the area improves and enhances range of motion and occupational performance.

Facilitate Voluntary Control

NMES has been used frequently for muscle reeducation and facilitation, particularly with neurological injuries and orthopaedic injuries post surgery. Facilitation and retraining can be effective for patients suffering from disuse atrophy, muscle weakness, and pain. In neurologically involved patients, the sensory feedback loop becomes distorted or impaired.

The goal of NMES for facilitation and reeducation is to incorporate the stimulation with voluntary contraction, functional movement and activity, and sensory feedback (Bracciano, 2000). The intent of NMES for facilitation and reeducation is to flood the central nervous system with sensory and kinesthetic information linked to an anticipated motor response. A variety of functional activities incorporating the desired motor response should be used to ensure adequate carryover of the response. For example, a stroke patient who is working on grasp and release should be provided with a variety of objects consisting of various shapes, sizes, and weights to hold and release. Placement of the objects should require movements to various heights and locations.

Transcutaneous Electrical Nerve Stimulation

Pain is one of the most common complaints that cause patients to seek medical care. Adequate pain management facilitates occupational function (Fig. 18-9). TENS can be used to manage pain in musculoskeletal disorders. The two primary theories on which the modulation of pain with TENS is based are the gate control theory (Melzack & Wall, 1965) and the endorphin theory (Bonica, 1990).

Treatment applications using electrical stimulation for pain control employ pulsed or alternating current with a variety of stimulation patterns. The type of stimulation is based on the neurological response to the stimulation. The four primary types of stimulation frequently employed include subsensory level, sensory level, motor level, and noxious level. Stimulation sites for electrode placement are based on the problem areas and goals for the patient. Optimal electrode placements should correlate with the structures and sources of pain and include motor points, trigger points, and acupuncture points. TENS units are often used at home, and the therapist should explain the purpose of the equipment and instruct the patient in its operations and precautions, with written and pictorial instructions. Through application of TENS for sensory analgesia, the patient may better perform functional activities and movements that foster independence and function.

Iontophoresis

Iontophoresis is a method of topically delivering a medication or ionized drug to an area of tissue by using direct electrical current. Iontophoresis is noninvasive, essentially painless, and an effective way to administer

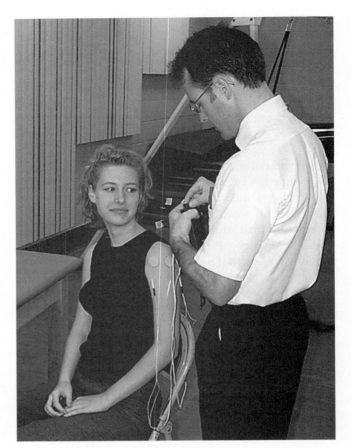

Figure 18-9 Application of TENS to the shoulder for acute pain.

medications to local targeted tissues. Occupational therapists frequently use iontophoresis in the treatment of inflammatory conditions such as epicondylitis, carpal tunnel syndrome, glenohumeral bursitis, ulnar nerve inflammation, and wrist tendinitis and tenosynovitis. Therapists using iontophoresis should thoroughly understand the pathophysiology of the condition, the wound healing process, and medications being used. Caution must be used whenever using iontophoresis, as medications may cause an allergic or anaphylactic reaction. Patients should **always** be asked whether they have any known allergies, sensitivities, or reactions to foods or medications. Documented orders should always be obtained from the patient's physician prior to using iontophoresis (Bracciano, 2000).

Physical agents should never be the single method or treatment approach in occupational therapy treatment. When used judiciously after taking into account the diagnosis, healing process, and phase of recovery, physical agents can make a valuable contribution to occupational therapy, facilitating outcomes and occupational performance.

Case Example

USE OF NMES TO FACILITATE RESUMPTION OF SELF-ADVANCEMENT ROLES

Patient Information

Mr. R. is a 43-year-old man who had a left middle cerebral artery thrombosis 4 weeks before his initial outpatient assessment. Mr. R. is married, with four children aged 4 to 13, employed as an editor of a local newspaper, and actively involved as a Boy Scout troop leader and with his church as a lector. Mr. R. returned for outpatient occupational therapy when he "began to move the fingers" of his right hand. Assessment findings were that Mr. R. displayed active flexion and extension of his fingers and a weak gross grasp. He could actively extend his wrist to neutral but was unable to stabilize the wrist functionally, which limited his ability to produce a functional grasp or to maintain higher-level prehension patterns. Mr. R. is independent in activities of daily living using one-handed techniques but has begun to use his right hand as a gross assist and to stabilize objects. Mr. R. is eager to return to his job at the newspaper, although this will require fine motor dexterity to use the computer keyboard and to manipulate papers. The primary therapist who completed the evaluation believes that with the developing return and given the patient's youth, an aggressive treatment protocol including NMES would benefit the patient. She had never used NMES and decided to refer the patient to a colleague in the occupational therapy department who has had extensive academic training and continuing education in physical agent modalities and their application.

Recommendations

The occupational therapist recommended three treatment sessions per week for 3 weeks. Based on the evaluation and input from Mr. R. and his wife during the assessment, the following treatment goals were established: (1) improve strength and active range of motion in the right hand and upper extremity; (2) improve prehension patterns and object manipulation; (3) return to employment with work site modifications as needed. The treatment plan included neuromuscular facilitation techniques and activities to facilitate and strengthen movement patterns and functional independence as well as NMES.

Short-Term Goals

NMES was incorporated in the treatment plan to facilitate voluntary movement in the right wrist extensors. Short-term goals for Mr. R. included (1) ability to hold a 6 inch object, such as a brush, with stimulation on; (2) active grasp and release of a fork during a hand-to-mouth pattern with stimulation on; (3) manipulation of objects of varying weights and sizes with stimulation on, progressing to intermittent stimulation as needed.

NMES electrodes were placed on the forearm to provide balanced wrist extension without ulnar or radial deviation. Electrode placement and stimulation parameters initially included finger flexion to provide a stronger grasp and were decreased as voluntary control and strength developed. Treatment time using NMES was initially 20 minutes per session, but duration was increased to 30 minutes after a week, when progress was noted. A variety of motor patterns and activities were used to provide the patient with visual, kinesthetic, and cutaneous feedback and to coordinate the stimulation with volitional prehension. Activities were graded to include different patterns of upper extremity positioning during stimulation of the wrist extensors and by using a variety of weights, lengths, and types of objects.

Treatment Outcome

Using NMES as an adjunct to occupational activities, Mr. R. progressed quickly, developing improved distal control of the hand and fingers. NMES activities were incorporated into his home exercise program after 2 weeks of clinical use. Mr. R.'s wrist control, strength and finger dexterity improved to the point that occupational tasks in the clinic included retraining, without NMES, on the computer keyboard preparatory to his return to employment. Writing was also an integral part of his treatment. As his strength, endurance, and coordination improved, Mr. R. returned to work part-time after 4 weeks and had gradually returned to full employment at 8 weeks.

CLINICAL REASONING
in OT Practice

Referral for Physical Agents

Mr. R. was referred for additional therapy when he began to develop voluntary control of his affected hand. Because of his age and occupational roles and responsibilities, Mr. R. was eager to return to his premorbid occupational status and function as quickly as possible.

Why was NMES paired with functional movements and activities? What qualifications should occupational therapists have to use physical agents as part of the treatment process? If the therapist was unfamiliar with the therapeutic intervention, NMES, how might the therapist obtain appropriate training and education in the modality? Whom would the therapist contact to determine state regulations regarding use of NMES in occupational therapy practice?

Summary Review Questions

1. Identify and discuss the three phases of wound healing. Why is the phase of wound healing a significant factor in selection of a specific physical agent modality as an adjunct to treatment?
2. Discuss the types of pain and their effect on occupational function.
3. Define and discuss superficial and deep heat agents. Identify indications and contraindications for application of deep heat agents and their effect on occupational function.
4. List the most frequently used applications of electrotherapy.
5. Discuss AOTA's position on physical agents and how physical agent modalities can be incorporated into a comprehensive treatment program.
6. Define and discuss therapeutic ultrasound and its thermal and nonthermal effects.
7. List precautions and contraindications for superficial heat agents and cryotherapy.

Resources

AliMed · 297 High St., Dedham, MA 02026-1935. 800-225-2610

American Occupational Therapy Association · 4720 Montgomery Lane, Bethesda, MD, 20824. 800-729-2682

American Physical Therapy Association · 1111 North Fairfax Street, Alexandria, VA 22314-1488

The Chattanooga Group, Inc. · 4717 Adams Rd., P.O. Box 489, Hixson, TN 37343-4001. 800-592-7329

Comfort Technologies, Inc. · P.O. Box 7, Pittstown, NJ 08867. 800-321-STIM (7846)

Dynatronic · 7030 Park Centre Dr., Salt Lake City, UT 84121-6618. 800-874-6251

Empi, Inc. · 1275 Grey Fox Rd., St. Paul, MN 55112. 800-328-2536

Henley Healthcare · 120 Industrial Boulevard, Sugarland, TX 77478. 281-276-7000

Metler Electronics · 1333 S. Claudina St., Anaheim, CA 92805-6235. 800-854-9305

Neoforma
www.neoforma.com

North Coast Medical · 187 Stauffer Boulevard, San Jose, CA 95125-1042. 800-821-9319

Smith and Nephew, Inc. · One Quality Drive, P. O. Box 1005, Germantown, WI 53022-8205. 800-558-8633

Sammons Preston · P. O. Box 5071, Bolingbrook, IL 60440-5071. 800-323-5547

References

Allen, K., & Battye, C. (1978). Performance of ultrasound therapy equipment in Pinellas county. *Physical Therapy, 54*, 174–179.

American Occupational Therapy Association (1997). Physical Agent Modalities: Position Paper. *American Journal of Occupational Therapy, 51*, pages 1090–1091.

American Occupational Therapy Association. Commission on Education Physical Agent Modalities Task Force (1993). Educational Preparation for use of physical agent modalities in occupational therapy (report). Rockville, MD: Author.

American Physical Therapy Association Section on Clinical Electrophysiology (1990). *Electrotherapeutic Terminology in Physical Therapy*. Alexandria, VA: Author.

Apfel, R. (1989). Acoustic cavitation: a possible consequence of biomedical uses of ultrasound. *British Journal of Cancer, 45* (Suppl. V), 140–146.

Baker, L. L. (1993). *Neuromuscular Electrical Stimulation: A Practical Clinical Guide* (3rd ed). Downey CA: Rancho Los Amigos Research and Education Institute.

Baker, L. L., Bowman, B. R., & McNeal, D. R. (1988). Effects of wave form on comfort during neuromuscular electrical stimulation. *Clinical Orthopedics, 223*, 75–85.

Baker, L. L., & Parker, K. (1986). Neuromuscular electrical stimulation of the muscles surrounding the shoulder. *Physical Therapy, 66*, 1930-1937.

Bonica, J. J. (1990). *The Management of Pain*, Volumes 1 and 2 (2nd ed.). Malvern, PA: Lea & Febiger.

Borrell, R. M., Parker, R., Henley, E. J, Masley, D., & Repinecz, M. (1980). Comparison of in vivo temperatures produced by hydrotherapy, paraffin wax treatment, and fluidotherapy. *Physical Therapy, 60*, 1273–1276.

Bracciano, A. (2000). *Physical Agent Modalities: Theory and Application for the Occupational Therapist*. Thorofare, NJ: Slack.

Bracciano, A. (1999). Therapeutic ultrasound: Sound information for the occupational therapist. *OT Practice, 4* (1), 20–25.

Currier, D. (1993). Effects of electrical and electromagnetic stimulation after anterior cruciate ligament reconstruction. *Journal of Orthopedic and Sports Physical Therapy, 17*(4), 177–184.

Dyson, M., & Pond, J. (1970). The effect of pulsed ultrasound on tissue regeneration. *Physiotherapy, 64*, 105–108.

Dyson, M. & Suckling, J. (1978). Stimulation of tissue repair by ultrasound: A survey of mechanisms involved. *Physiotherapy, 64*, 105–108.

Earley, D. (1999). Superficial heat agents: A hot topic. *OT Practice, 4* (1), 26–30.

Eckerson, L. F., & Axelgaard, J. (1984). Lateral electrical surface stimulation as an alternative to bracing in the treatment of idiopathic scoliosis. *Physical Therapy, 64*, 483.

Enwemeka, C. (1989). The effects of therapeutic ultrasound on tendon healing. *American Journal of Physical Medicine and Rehabilitation, 68*, 283–287.

Fyfe, M., & Parnell, S. (1982). The importance of measurement of effective transducer radiating area in the testing and calibration of therapeutic ultrasonic instruments. *Health Physics, 43*, 377–381.

Griffin, J., & Reddin, G. (1981). Shoulder pain in patients with hemiplegia: A literature review. *Physical Therapy, 61*, 1041–1045.

Hakim, M. H. (1995). Pain and its measurement. *Hamdard, 38*, 86–90.

Henley, E. (1991). Transcutaneous drug delivery: Iontophoresis, phonophoresis. *Critical Reviews in Physical Medicine and Rehabilitation, 3*, 139–151.

Hoban, C. (1993, October 1). Therapeutic heat. Michigan Occupational Therapy Association Annual Conference. East Lansing, MI.

Kaul, M. P. (1994). Superficial heat and cold. *The Physician and Sports Medicine, 22*, 65–74.

Kimura, I., Gulick, D., Shelly, J., & Ziskin, M. (1988). Effects of two ultrasound devices and angles of application on the temperature of tissue phantom. *Journal of Orthopedic and Sports Physical Therapy, 27,* 27–31.

Lehmann, J., & Guy, A. (1971). Ultrasound therapy. In J. Reid & M. Sikov (Eds.), *Interaction of Ultrasound and Biological Tissues* (pp. 141–152). DHEW Publication FDA 73-8008. Washington: Government Printing Office.

Masse, J. (1996). Phonophoresis. *Sports Medicine, 10,* 4–6.

Mehreteab, T., & Weisberg, J. (Eds.). (1994). *Physical Agents: A Comprehensive Text for Physical Therapists.* Norwalk, CT: Appleton & Lange.

Melzack, R., & Wall, P. D. (1965). Pain mechanisms: A new theory. *Science, 150,* 971–979.

Michlovitz, S. L. (1990). *Biophysical Principles of Heating and Superficial Heat Agents: Thermal Agents in Rehabilitation* (2nd ed.). Philadelphia: F. A. Davis Co.

Mulder, G., Brazinsky, B. A., & Seeley, J. (1995). Factors complicating wound repair. In: J. M. McCulloch & L. C. Kloth (Eds.), *Wound Healing Alternatives in Management.* (2nd. ed., pp. 45–59). Philadelphia: F. A. Davis.

Norkin, C., & Levangie, P. (1992). *Joint Structure and Function: A Comprehensive Analysis.* (2nd ed.). Philadelphia: F. A. Davis.

Phillips, C. A. (1989). Functional electrical stimulation and lower extremity bracing for ambulation exercise of the spinal cord injured individual: A medically prescribed system. *Physical Therapy, 69,* 842–849.

Robinson, A. (1995). *Clinical Electrophysiology* (2nd ed). Norwalk, CT: Appleton & Lange.

Schmidt, K.L. (1979). Heat, cold and inflammation. *Rheumatology, 38,* 391–404.

Schuermann, D. (1982). The nature of wound healing. *Association of Operating Room Nurses Journal, 35,* 1067–1077.

Sicard-Rosenbaum, L., Lord, D., & Danoff, J. (1995). Effects of continuous therapeutic ultrasound on growth and metastasis of subcutaneous murine tumors. *Physical Therapy, 75,* 3–13.

Vodovnik, L., Bowman, B. R., & Hufford, P. (1984). Effects of electrical stimulation on spinal spasticity. *Scandinavian Journal of Rehabilitation Medicine, 16,* 29–34.

19

Planning, Guiding, and Documenting Therapy

Mary Vining Radomski

LEARNING OBJECTIVES

After studying this chapter, readers will begin to do the following:

1. Describe essential elements in effective documentation.
2. Articulate and analyze their own thinking as they provide occupational therapy services.
3. Differentiate between anticipated therapy outcomes and long- and short-term goals.
4. Appreciate the importance of collaboration with the client in treatment planning.
5. Consider a variety of treatment approaches in planning therapy.
6. Make a commitment to maintaining their own professional competence.

*T*he caliber of the clinician's thinking about each step in the occupational therapy process will set the stage for either inspired intervention or treatment that is rote, uninteresting, and ineffective. One might argue that the ongoing behind-the-scenes thinking about assessment and treatment (known as clinical reasoning) is at least as important as what happens between the client and therapist in a typical 30-minute session.

Clinical documentation chronicles clinical reasoning about occupational therapy diagnosis (Rogers & Holm, 1991), therapy plans, actions, and results. For many clinicians (often including this author), documentation is the price paid for otherwise interesting work. Documentation, however, can be the vehicle through which clinicians think out loud: a map for planning treatment and a compass for monitoring results and shifting course.

This chapter is structured on these two parallel dimensions of occupational therapy practice (Fig. 19-1): internal clinical reasoning (screening, assessing, planning, intervening, monitoring, discontinuing treatment) and external communication (documenting assessment and treatment). The

GLOSSARY

Accreditation—A determination by an accrediting body than an eligible health care organization complies with established standards (JCAHO, 1999).

Comorbidities—Medical problems typically unrelated to the treatment diagnosis that affect the anticipated outcome and/or the treatment approach.

Continuum of care—A system of services of varying intensity that address the ongoing or intermittent needs of persons with disabilities; ranging from acute medical intervention to rehabilitation to subacute rehabilitation to home health services to outpatient treatment to community wellness opportunities (CARF, 1999).

Evidence-based practice—Methods and mind-set that integrate research study evidence into the clinical reasoning process (Tickle-Degnen, 1999).

Goal—Narrowly defined end result of therapy to be achieved in a specified time (Bryant, 1995). Goals are usually designated as long- or short-term.

Joint Commission on Accreditation of Healthcare Organizations (JCAHO)—Founded in 1951, an independent, not-for-profit organization dedicated to improving quality of care in various health settings (JCAHO, 1999).

Length of stay—Total number of days between the date the patient is admitted to the hospital and the date he or she is discharged.

Outcome—Anticipated end result of therapy, given the client's characteristics, expected length of stay or therapy duration, and resources (funding, social support).

Rehabilitation Accreditation Commission (CARF)—Founded in 1966, a national organization whose mission is to promote the quality, value, and outcome of rehabilitation services through a consultative accreditation process that centers on enhancing the lives of persons served (CARF, 1999).

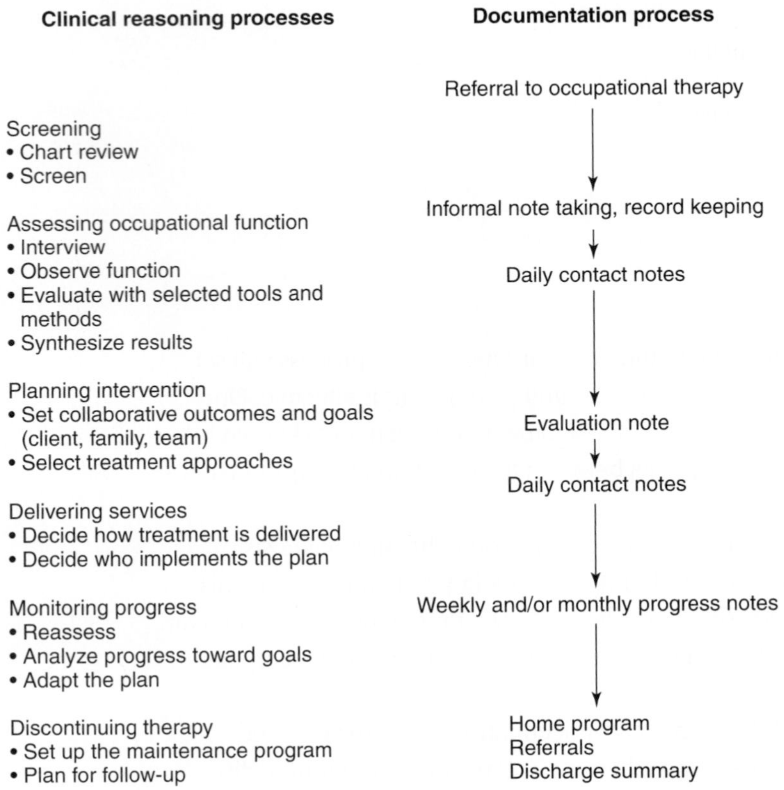

Clinical reasoning processes

Screening
• Chart review
• Screen

Assessing occupational function
• Interview
• Observe function
• Evaluate with selected tools and methods
• Synthesize results

Planning intervention
• Set collaborative outcomes and goals (client, family, team)
• Select treatment approaches

Delivering services
• Decide how treatment is delivered
• Decide who implements the plan

Monitoring progress
• Reassess
• Analyze progress toward goals
• Adapt the plan

Discontinuing therapy
• Set up the maintenance program
• Plan for follow-up

Documentation process

Referral to occupational therapy

↓

Informal note taking, record keeping

↓

Daily contact notes

↓

Evaluation note

↓

Daily contact notes

↓

Weekly and/or monthly progress notes

↓

Home program
Referrals
Discharge summary

Figure 19-1 Occupational therapy documentation reflects the therapist's clinical reasoning throughout the course of providing services.

chapter concludes with a discussion of the ways therapists use these processes to improve their clinical competence.

Clinical Reasoning

According to Schell (1998), clinical reasoning is "the process used by practitioners to plan, direct, perform, and reflect on client care" (p. 90). This process is ongoing and developmental. It begins as the therapist first reads a patient's referral; extends through assessment, treatment, and discharge; and continues as the clinician reflects on the process and results of intervention with this individual in planning services for another.

As therapists make decisions and plans for assessment and treatment, they simultaneously employ at least four lines of clinical reasoning (Schell, 1998):

▶ Scientific reasoning—Logical thinking about the nature of the patient's problems and optimal course of action in treatment.
▶ Narrative reasoning—Thinking in story form to place the patient's functioning in the context of his or her background and broader experience.
▶ Pragmatic reasoning—Practical thinking about logistics and practical aspects and circumstances of delivering services to this patient.
▶ Ethical reasoning—Idealistic thinking about what should be done on behalf of this individual.

Clinical reasoning is a dynamic process, influenced by the clinician's experience, personal situation, and background (Rogers & Holm, 1991; Schell, 1998). For example, a middle-aged therapist with elderly parents and an equally experienced therapist with young children may arrive at different assessment conclusions and develop different treatment plans for an 80-year-old patient recovering from a pelvic fracture because of their different life experiences. Similarly, the characteristics of settings in which occupational therapists work shape clinical reasoning (Rogers & Holm, 1991). Physical, financial, and personnel resources influence assessment tools and methods, and multidisciplinary teams establish informal rules about the boundaries of each discipline's contribution (Rogers & Holm, 1991). **Evidence-based practice** minimizes the personal and environmental biases in the clinical reasoning process.

Evidence-Based Practice

Evidence-based practice is "the conscientious, explicit, and judicious use of current best evidence in making decisions about the care of individual patients. [It integrates] individual clinical expertise with the best available external clinical evidence from systematic research" (Sackett et al., 1997, p. 2).

Evidence-based practice includes both method and mind-set. The method is made up of seven steps: (1) Write an answerable clinical question. (2) Gather best evidence to answer the question, including clinical assessment findings, systematic reviews from the literature, and primary studies. (3) Evaluate the validity and clinical usefulness of the gathered evidence. (4) Synthesize the findings. (5) Communicate with various stakeholders, including client and family, about evidence as it relates to assessment or treatment. (6) Apply findings to practice. (7) Monitor, evaluate, and document the results (Sackett et al., 1997; Tickle-Degnen, 2000a). Whyte (1998) suggests that apart from the methodology, evidence-based practice should not occur as occasional mammoth reviews but as habits of thinking and doing that pervade the way the clinician practices.

While evidence-based practice is increasingly emphasized in the literature, because of characteristics of rehabilitation research and attitudes of clinicians, it may not yet have infiltrated day-to-day practice. Whyte (1998) described challenges to evidence-based practice in rehabilitation based on the fact that many treatments do not lend themselves to controlled clinical trials. Subjects in well-designed studies tend to be unrealistically homogeneous and do not have the confounding problems or severity of impairments typical of many rehabilitation patients (Whyte, 1998). He advised clinicians to use studies based on single-subject experimental designs to guide decision making when more rigorous research is not available.

Dubouloz et al. (1999) studied occupational therapists' perceptions of evidence-based practice. The eight therapists who participated in this qualitative study put more emphasis on knowledge gained from clinical experience and consultation with others than on research literature. Participants did not seem to link research to clinical practice. They "based their practice decisions on clients' input and previous experience as these sources were seen as crucial to competent practice, whereas knowledge from research was seen as primarily important in confirming the effectiveness of practice to non-clients" (Dubouloz et al., 1999, p. 537).

Tickle-Degnen (1999) cautioned against practice based solely on evidence from clients and peers: "A particular weakness of unsystematic gathering of evidence is that human beings tend to gather evidence during their daily lives in such a manner as to confirm their own assumptions and beliefs" (p. 539).

Clinical Documentation

Occupational therapists contribute information to medical records in a number of formats: source-oriented medical records, organized in sections according to the department providing care; integrated medical records in chronological order; and problem-oriented medical records organized according to four components, database, complete list of problems, plans for each problem, and progress notes (Robertson, 1997). SOAP notes are typically used to report progress in problem-oriented medical records (Robertson, 1997). (SOAP is an acronym for the four parts of a progress note: subjective, objective, assessment, plan.) Obviously, occupational therapists contribute documentation that complies with the structure of the medical records established for their specific work settings.

Clinical documentation in occupational therapy provides a chronological record of the client's status and condition related to occupational functioning and details the course of therapeutic intervention (American Occupational Therapy Association [AOTA], 1995). It reflects the clinician's reasoning and serves as the basis for judging the appropriateness, effectiveness, and necessity of intervention (AOTA, 1995).

In the course of their daily work, occupational therapists produce a number of reports, including daily contact notes, evaluation summaries, weekly or monthly progress notes, and discharge summaries (Table 19-1). Documentation formats include computerized records, checklists, forms, and narrative notes. Regardless of format, to communicate in these documents, therapists must be clear about their target audience (McGuire, 1997; Robertson, 1997). That is, who will read this note and what do they need or want to know about the occupational therapy work with this patient? Clinicians aim to provide succinct descriptions of functional status, anticipated outcome, and progress to date, so that a single document meets a number of stakeholders' information needs. The reading audience may include members of the treatment team, who want to know how best to collaborate; the third-party payer, who wants to decide whether to pay for services; the accrediting agency, such as **Joint Commission on Accreditation for Healthcare Organizations (JCAHO)** or **Commission on Accreditation of Rehabilitation Facilities (CARF)**, which want to determine whether quality services are provided at your institution; the legal system, which wants evidence in malpractice litigation; and the client and significant others, who want to understand the care (Robertson, 1997).

McGuire (1997) outlined six principles that reflect excellent standards for occupational therapy documen-

tation. She suggested that clinical documentation addressing these principles meets the information requirements of a variety of stakeholders, including Medicare, the largest third-party payer in the United States. After stating each principle, I briefly summarize McGuire's recommendations for clinical documentation (Fig. 19-2).

1. Focus on function. Clinicians describe the client's previous or premorbid level of function in key areas, review his or her current status, and/or provide estimates of potential improvements or outcomes as a result of therapy.
2. Focus on underlying causes. Clinicians "combine medical knowledge with observation and task analysis to identify specific impairments that restrict or limit occupational function" (McGuire, 1997, p. 439).
3. Focus on progress. Clinicians describe clients' progress toward goals according to objective measures, details of careful observation, and/or standardized levels of independence (Box 19-1).
4. Focus on safety. Many stakeholders look to the occupational therapist to provide information about the client's safety and competence in self management, self-advancement, and self-enhancement roles.
5. State expectations for progress or explain slow progress or lack of progress. Occupational therapists must "document a continued expectation that the patient's condition will continue to improve significantly in a reasonable and generally predictable amount of time" (McGuire, 1997, p. 441). Therapists need to document setbacks that delay progress, such as medication changes, medical complications, and social disruptions.
6. Summarize needed skilled services. Occupational therapists avoid detailing the specific therapeutic interventions used during a given treatment session or period but emphasize the provision of skilled services. Skilled services include evaluations; direct intervention, such as training in techniques or strategies; task modification; selection or construction of equipment or orthotics; and instructions to the patient or caregiver about maintenance programs.

Providing Occupational Therapy Services

Clinical reasoning and documentation pervade each aspect of providing occupational therapy services: screening, assessing, planning, intervening, monitoring, and discontinuing treatment.

TABLE 19-1
Overview: Types of Occupational Therapy Documentation

	Purpose	Typical Formats	Content	When to Document
Contact, treatment, or visit note	Brief account of individual session	Short narrative note, checklist, or flow sheet	Amount of time spent evaluating or treating the client Brief characterization of intervention (e.g., ADL instruction, strengthening, compensatory strategy training) Description of client's response relative to short-term goals	After each evaluation or treatment session
Evaluation report	Detail assessment findings; interpret results; estimate outcomes of intervention, goals, time frame, treatment plan	Observations and findings recorded on a form Handwritten or typed report	Background information Referral source, services requested, date of referral Dates of evaluation sessions and time invested Summary of medical history, secondary problems, comorbidities Precautions and contraindications Premorbid or prior level of occupational function Client's report of problems and priorities Assessment results Summary and analysis of assessment findings Projected outcomes of therapy, goals, and time frame Statement of client's participation in goal setting General description of treatment plan, including approach and recommended frequency of sessions	After completing assessment, synthesizing results, and collaborating with client about goals
Progress report	Summary of progress toward goals, interventions, updated goals and treatment plan	Form or checklist with section for handwritten comments Flow sheet as used with clinical pathways Handwritten or typed report	Dates of service and dates of progress period Number of treatment sessions during progress period Overview of activities, techniques, modalities Summary of instructions to client or family Description of adaptive equipment issued or recommended Client's response to intervention specific to goals Recommendations regarding continuation of therapy Revised goals and time frame for achievement Revised treatment plan (approach, recommended frequency of sessions) Client's participation in goal setting for therapy	Weekly or monthly, depending on setting
Discharge report	Review of occupational therapy assessment, intervention, and outcome.	Form or checklist with section for handwritten comments Flow sheet as used with critical pathways Handwritten or typed report	Dates of referral, service initiation and discontinuation Total number of evaluation and treatment sessions Summary of client's progress towards each therapy goal Overview of interventions employed specific to each goal Description of maintenance program and discharge instructions Recommendations for follow-up, maintenance programs, referrals to other services or agencies	After the last session in an episode of care

Sources: Allen, C. A. (1997). Clinical reasoning for documentation. In J. D. Acquaviva (Ed.), *Effective Documentation for Occupational Therapy* (2nd ed., pp. 53–62). Bethesda, MD: American Occupational Therapy Association; AOTA (1995). Elements of clinical documentation (revised). *American Journal of Occupational Therapy*, 49, 1032–1035; Wilson, D. (1997). Clinical reasoning for documentation. In J. D. Acquaviva (Ed.), *Effective Documentation for Occupational Therapy* (2nd ed., pp. 1–3). Bethesda, MD: American Occupational Therapy Association.

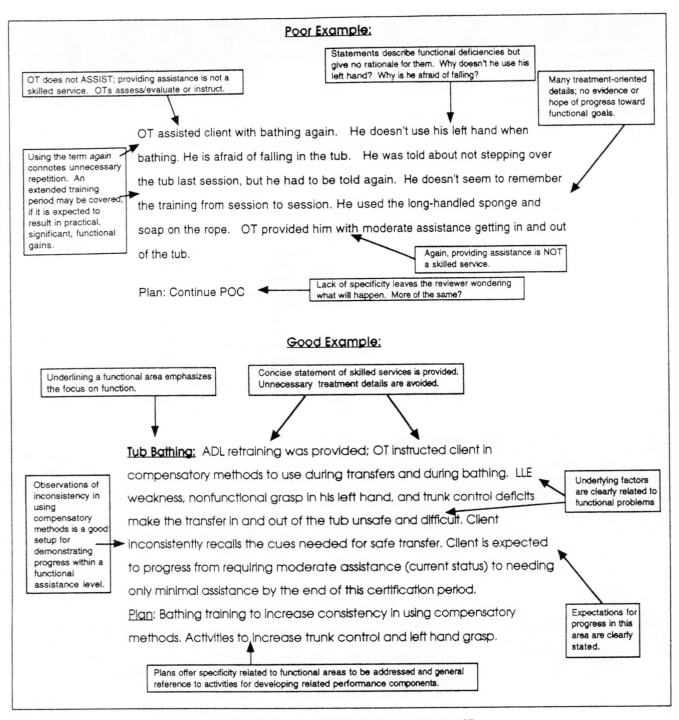

Figure 19-2 Features of effective progress notes. ADL, activities of daily living; LLE, left lower extremity; OT, occupational therapist; POC, plan of care. From "Documenting Progress in Home Care" by M. J. McGuire, 1997, *American Journal of Occupational Therapy, 51*, p. 444. Copyright 1997 by the American Occupational Therapy Association. Reprinted with permission.

BOX 19-1
Medicare Definitions of Level of Assistance

Total Assistance
Patient needs 100% assistance by one or more persons to perform all physical activities and/or requires cognitive stimulation to elicit a functional response to an external stimulation (e.g., swallow when food is in mouth).

Maximal Assistance
Patient needs 75% assistance by one person to perform physically any part of a functional activity and/or needs cognitive stimulation to perform gross motor actions in response to direction.

Moderate Assistance
Patient needs 50% assistance from one person to perform physical activities or constant cognitive assistance to sustain or complete simple repetitive activities safely.

Minimum Assistance
Patient needs 25% assistance by one person for physical activities and/or periodic cognitive assistance to perform functional activities safely.

Standby Assistance
Patient needs supervision of one person to perform new activity adapted by the therapist for safe and effective performance.

Independent Status
Patient requires no physical or cognitive assistance to perform functional activities.

Trombly, C. A. (1995). Planning, guiding, and documenting therapy. In C. A. Trombly (Ed.). *Occupational Therapy for Physical Dysfunction* (4th ed. pp. 29–40). Baltimore: Williams and Wilkins.

Screening

People are referred for occupational therapy if they have impairments, activity limitations, or participation restrictions; are at risk in these areas; or need help promoting health (Moyers, 1999). A physician's order or referral is prerequisite to beginning services covered by third-party payers.

Screening is defined as reviewing information relevant to a prospective patient to determine the need for further evaluation and intervention (Moyers, 1999). Therapists gather this information through chart review and a brief interview.

Chart Review and Brief Interview
Occupational therapists review relevant documents in the patient's medical record before beginning assessment or treatment. Other team members' assessments (e.g., the physician's history and physical, social service or psychology intake notes, nursing assessments) help the therapist create a preliminary clinical image related to disease, severity of illness or disorder, **comorbidities**, age, sex, and personal and social background (Rogers & Holm, 1991). After the chart review, the occupational

therapist typically meets the patient and/or significant other to introduce himself or herself, informs them of the referral, and briefly describes the nature of occupational therapy and the anticipated services. The purpose of this conversation is to ensure the appropriateness of the referral and obtain preliminary agreement to participate. The conversation may take place during the first few minutes of the initial assessment session, as with outpatients or patients receiving home care, or be a brief encounter in the patient's hospital room, with the assessment scheduled to take place later.

Documentation Requirements: Referral to Occupational Therapy Services
A physician's order should include the following information: the patient's diagnosis (underlying disorder, disease, or injury that contributes to occupational dysfunction); the treatment diagnosis (the likely impairment contributing to occupational dysfunction); the actual or estimated date of recent change in the level of function; a request for evaluation or treatment; the date, and the physician's signature (Allen et al., 1997).

If the screening suggests that the referral to occupational therapy is inappropriate or the client or family defers participation, the clinician records that orders were received and a screen was performed and explains why further assessment and treatment appear unwarranted.

Assessing Occupational Function: The Four Elements

Various aspects of occupational therapy assessment have been detailed elsewhere in this text (see Chapters 3 to 10). The discussion that follows sets the four elements of assessment—interview, observation of function, evaluation, and synthesis of results—in the broader schema of providing occupational therapy services, and it emphasizes the clinical reasoning dimensions rather than specific tools or methods.

Interview
Using a structured interview, the clinician identifies the client's needs and goals in the context of his or her life (Fisher, 1998). Fisher extolled the value of this aspect of the assessment process:

> "This step is critical, and it must occur, even under the pressures of cost containment, reduced duration of care, staff cuts, and increased accountability. In fact, there is some evidence that taking more time, initially, to establish client-centered performance will result in overall outcomes being enhanced and overall costs reduced."
>
> (Fisher, 1998, pp. 515–516)

Observe Function

The occupational therapist observes the client performing one of the activities described as important and problematic to generate hypotheses regarding underlying impairments or inefficiencies that interfere with function. For example, while observing a client with stroke get dressed, the clinician looks for cues that point to underlying causes of performance problems (hypothesizing, for example, that difficulty locating socks, shirt, and shoes is due to left neglect).

Evaluate With Selected Tools and Methods

Based on observations of functional performance and resultant hypotheses regarding underlying causes, therapists use selected evaluation tools and methods to verify and quantify the existence of impairments or inefficiencies. In fact, clinicians evaluate only performance components, impairments, or inefficiencies suspected of impeding occupational function rather than casting a wide net to identify all possible deficits, as in the past.

Synthesize Results

Occupational therapists study assessment findings to draw conclusions about the client's competence and quality of occupational function. The client's strengths and weaknesses, likely underlying causes or explanations for performance problems, and potential barriers and enablers to improved functioning become the basis of the hypothesis for treatment (Opacich, 1991). The hypothesis for treatment reflects the therapist's understanding of the client's problems. While it may change as treatment gets under way, the hypothesis for treatment guides the selection of the treatment approach (Opacich, 1991).

Documentation Requirements: Record Keeping and Notes

Occupational therapists typically jot notes regarding client performance during the assessment. Sometimes these forms or protocols ultimately go directly into the medical record. Worksheets are also used for data collection (with the typed or handwritten summary produced for the medical record upon completion of the assessment). Some occupational therapy assessments and treatment plans are completed after just one evaluation session, in which case the therapist generates the documentation described in the next section. When the assessment spans multiple sessions, daily contact notes are recorded in the medical record.

Planning Intervention

After formulating a hypothesis for treatment, the occupational therapist plans intervention. Clinical reasoning is involved in estimating outcomes, setting goals, and selecting treatment approaches and methods.

Estimate Outcomes and Set Collaborative Goals

An **outcome** of therapy is an anticipated end result, given a specific set of parameters (Bryant, 1995). Outcomes are chosen in part according to expected **length of stay** or anticipated number of outpatient or home-based sessions and the type of funding available. The contemporary rehabilitation environment often requires clinicians to identify key expected outcomes for and with persons served, measure these outcomes, and determine how outcomes can be achieved in a resource-wise or cost-effective manner (Cope & Sundance, 1995). Interdisciplinary rehabilitation teams often establish client-specific outcomes for a given episode of care, with each discipline setting goals that contribute to these core outcomes.

Moyers (1999) described four multidimensional outcomes of occupational therapy intervention: (1) function (performance component function); (2) occupational performance (independence in activities of daily living [ADL], work, play); (3) health and well-being (symptom status improvement, prevention of disability); and (4) quality of life (purposeful participation in community life, emotional well-being, balance of activity and rest, life satisfaction). Global outcomes of occupational therapy intervention can also be identified according to resumption of self-maintenance, self-advancement, and self-enhancement roles.

In projecting outcomes of treatment, occupational therapists are urged to look beyond functional independence or relearning of physical skills as the superordinate aims of occupational therapy (Radomski, 1995) and help clients attain wholeness, autonomy, meaning, and purpose in their daily lives (Crabtree, 2000).

Predicting outcomes of therapy forces clinicians to answer two key questions in treatment planning: (1) In what broad ways will this client's life, health, and functioning improve as a result of therapy at this point in the recovery or adaptation process? (2) How long will it take to realize these benefits? The answers require an appreciation for the **continuum of care** and a realization that not every dysfunction, impairment, or inefficiency can or should be addressed within a given episode of care. For example, resumption of self-maintenance roles may be an appropriate occupational therapy outcome for a stroke patient with good family support who is expected to receive inpatient rehabilitation for 2 to 3 weeks. On the other hand, resumption of self-advancement roles would probably not be an appropriate outcome of inpatient rehabilitation. Occupational therapy services to promote work readiness can likely be provided more cost-effectively when the individual is an

TABLE 19-2
Example of Establishing Short-Term Goals

Long-Term Goal: Independence in Lower Extremity Dressing	
Short-Term Goals Based on Performance	Short-Term Goals Based on Task Analysis
Trunk flexion and BUE forward reach adequate for LE dressing Cognitive-perceptual skills adequate for positioning clothing during LE dressing Endurance adequate for safety and independence during LE dressing Compensatory methods and appropriate use of adaptive equipment for safe, independent LE dressing	Client will properly place trousers over feet for donning. Client will spontaneously dress LLE before RLE. Client will pull up trousers from a supported standing position. Client will demonstrate proper use of sock donner and long-handled shoe horn and complete LE dressing in 5 minutes without becoming SOB.

BUE, both upper extremities; LE, lower extremity; LLE, left lower extremity; RLE, right lower extremity; SOB, short of breath.
From "Documenting Progress in Home Care" by M. J. McGuire, 1997, *American Journal of Occupational Therapy, 51,* p. 483. Copyright 1997 by the American Occupational Therapy Association. Reprinted with permission.

BOX 19-2
PROCEDURES FOR PRACTICE

Linking Long- and Short-Term Goals to Anticipated Rehabilitation Outcomes

Mr. B. is a 20-year-old man with C8 tetraplegia beginning multidisciplinary inpatient rehabilitation. The following examples of outcome and long- and short-term goals are not meant to be exhaustive lists of intervention plans but rather to illustrate the linkage between global outcome projections and therapy plans.

► Projected outcome of rehabilitation stay: In 8 weeks, Mr. B. will resume self-maintenance roles, requiring no more than occasional physical assistance from family members to manage in the home environment.

► Examples of long term occupational therapy goals (to be achieved in 8 weeks):
1. Mr. B. will perform upper body dressing independently and require no more than moderate assistance for lower body dressing.
2. Mr. B. will use adaptive equipment to feed himself independently.

► Examples of short term occupational therapy goals (to be achieved in 2 weeks):
1. Mr. B. will don a pullover shirt with no more than general verbal cues.
2. Mr. B. will participate in the evaluation of various types of adaptive equipment for self-feeding and use selected aids to feed himself independently after setup by therapist.

within a month of a stroke. Treatment planning based on anticipated outcomes of therapy not only reflects good stewardship, it is required by accreditation bodies, such as CARF (2000).

Long- and Short-Term Goals

Once the occupational therapist and client conceptualize global outcomes of therapy, they work backward to establish a sequence of long- and short-term goals to get there (Cope & Sundance, 1995). A **goal** is a measurable, narrowly defined end result of therapy to be achieved in a specified time (Bryant, 1995). Long-term goals reflect what will be achieved by the time the client is discharged from treatment or discharged to the next level of care on the continuum (Moorhead & Kannenberg, 1997). In occupational therapy, long-term goals always relate to expectations of the client's functional skills and/or resumption of roles. Short-term goals are the small steps that cumulatively result in long-term goal achievement. Short-term goals are based either on expected improvements in performance components that ultimately contribute to improved function or on the client's improved ability to perform portions of the functional task (McGuire, 1997). Table 19-2 compares these two types of short-term goals.

A client's occupational therapy goals are always linked to a predicted outcome. Box 19-2 illustrates how long- and short-term goals support realization of outcomes. Box 19-3 describes how to use goal attainment scaling to measure progress.

Collaborating With Clients to Set Goals

Collaborative goal setting is not only an accreditation requirement of CARF (2000) and JCAHO (1999), it may enhance the process if not the results of therapy. Spencer et al. (1997) suggested that collaborative goal setting

outpatient. Furthermore, resumption of work roles typically occurs after the patient achieves medical stability, approaches maximal restoration of function, and begins the adjustment process, none of which is likely to occur

BOX 19-3
Goal Attainment Scaling

Goal attainment scaling is a method of evaluating the effectiveness of therapy that produces a quantitative index of the client's progress over time and means by which one client's progress can be compared with that of other clients in the same program (Ottenbacher & Cusick, 1990). Goal attainment scaling was developed for use in mental health (Kiresuk & Sherman, 1968) and has been used to measure change as a result of cognitive rehabilitation (Rockwood et al., 1997) and brain injury rehabilitation (Joyce et al., 1994; Trombly et al., 1998).

For each goal, a 5-point behavioral scale is constructed as shown below. Ottenbacher and Cusick (1990) provided an excellent summary regarding how quantitative outcome data can be calculated and interpreted.

Client's problem area: She relies on other people to make transportation arrangements for her.

Predicted Attainment	Score	Goals
Most favorable outcome	+2	Patient accurately makes her own transportation arrangements without supervision or assistance.
Greater than expected outcome	+1	Patient accurately makes her own transportation arrangement with occasional cueing.
Expected outcome	0	Patient accurately makes her own transportation arrangement with ongoing supervision.
Current status	−1	Patient is provided with information about transportation arrangements made for her
Least favorable outcome	−2	Patient cannot successfully use transportation information provided for her.

enables the client to develop hope for the future. Ponte-Allan and Giles (1999) examined the relationship between types of goals set by stroke inpatients and the results of therapy. They compared patients whose goals were functional, independence-oriented statements to those whose goals were general, less functional statements or who made no goal statements at all. While there were no differences in age, sex, side of lesion, or levels of disability at admission, patients who had functional goals had higher discharge scores on the *Functional Independence Measure* for grooming, upper and lower extremity dressing, and toilet and tub transfers.

Clients' expectations of therapy depend on their previous experience in similar situations, background, experiences of friends and relatives (Wade, 1999), state of health and mind, and long-held priorities and values. Occupational therapists should not assume they know clients' goals, values, or priorities for treatment. Kane et al. (1997) found that professionals in long-term care and recipients of services placed different importance on various aspects of disability. Consumers viewed dependency in instrumental activities of daily living (IADL) as more of a loss than the professionals did, whereas professionals were more concerned about consumers' inability to perform basic self-care activities.

Collaborating with clients in goal setting is a critical counterbalance to therapist-biased expectations and priorities in treatment planning (Box 19-4). Therapists need to teach clients how to participate in goal setting

(Nelson & Payton, 1997), probing for concerns, goals, and ideas. Patients may expect medical professionals to tell them what to do rather than ask for their input. Asking such an individual, "What are your occupational therapy goals?" is likely to be met with a perplexed look and a vague response. As one client put it, "Asking one question about goals on an initial evaluation is probably not adequate" (Nelson & Payton, 1997, p. 582).

Select Treatment Approaches and Methods

In Chapter 1, Trombly describes two broad therapy approaches that aim to improve clients' effectiveness and satisfaction with occupational roles: remedial therapy and adaptive therapy. Before proceeding with intervention, occupational therapists consider the client's strengths and weaknesses based on assessment findings to select a treatment approach that will achieve expected outcomes and meet collaborative goals for therapy. In so doing, clinicians consider the extent to which a given treatment approach places demands on the client's metaprocessing abilities (self-awareness, self-monitoring, motivation), therapy time needed to improve occupational function, and potential for generalization of results.

Remedial Therapy

Remedial therapy aims to restore an impaired capacity or ability with the expectation that this improvement will bring about general change in the client's activities, tasks, and roles. For example, a therapist may base the treatment plan for a patient with an incomplete C8 spinal cord injury on the premise that if upper extremity strength is optimally restored, the patient will not only become independent in grooming but also be more efficient with meal preparation and work tasks. Remedial approaches typically address performance components (AOTA, 1994a). In general, remedial therapy places low demands on metaprocessing, but as it aims to fix underlying impairments, it may be somewhat slow to affect occupational function. For some clients, especially the recently injured, it is difficult to determine whether improvements can be attributed to remedial therapy or naturally occurring physiological recovery.

Adaptive Therapy

Adaptive therapy is employed when (1) a remedial approach does not result in full restoration of a client's premorbid capacities and abilities or (2) the client wants to optimize his or her level of independence while continuing to work toward restoration of fundamental capacities and abilities. For example, an inpatient with hemiplegia receives remedial therapy to improve upper extremity strength and function after a stroke but also learns one-handed dressing tech-

niques (adaptive therapy) to facilitate independent discharge to home. Adaptive therapy entails three possible therapy actions: changing the context, reestablishing habits and routines, and acquiring new skills and strategies.

Changing the Context. Context changes focus on changing factors that are external to the client to improve occupational function (changing the demands of the task or environment, changing the tools used, changing the social supports or expectations). For example, using a Rangetimer, which automatically turns off the stove at a predetermined time, may allow a person with memory impairment to cook without an undue safety risk. Installing grab bars in a client's bathroom may dramatically increase the client's ability to carry out self-maintenance tasks. Negotiating changed work responsibilities with an employer may enable a newly injured worker to keep his or her job. Changing the context generally places low metaprocessing demands on the client and can result in rapid improvements in occupational function, especially changes to physical aspects of context. The effects of intervention, however, are often task specific and do not necessarily generalize to other activities, tasks, and roles.

BOX 19-4
PROCEDURES FOR PRACTICE

Suggestions for Collaborating With Clients to Set Meaningful Occupational Therapy Goals

▶ Incorporate life history information into the assessment process so that you can get a glimpse of what the client has found meaningful and important during his or her life (Spencer et al., 1997). Awareness of the client's personal context enables the clinician to discuss, frame, or propose possible therapy outcomes and goals in ways that the client will understand.

▶ Appreciate that clients' ability to identify and advance their goals for therapy is influenced by where they are in recovery and adaptation. Individuals who are acutely ill or whose hospitalization has insulated them from the real-world effects of new disabilities often cannot anticipate the challenges that await them in the community. Outpatients and home-based clients are typically better able to articulate needs and hopes for therapy because of their experiences with performance gaps.

▶ Consider the broad continuum of care (inpatient to home health to outpatient to work reentry) as you aim to match the right goals with the right time frame by asking, "What does the person both value and need from occupational therapy at this point in his or her recovery?"

▶ Appreciate that most clients are unfamiliar with occupational therapy and what we have to offer them and therefore cannot independently generate goals for

therapy. The therapist sometimes facilitates collaborative goal setting by proposing a menu of possible goals to address in therapy and modifying that list with the client.

▶ Acknowledge the influence of cognitive function on a person's capacity to set goals. For a person to establish a meaningful goal, he or she must first accurately appraise his or her status and compare it to past or premorbid performance. The individual must be able to imagine what is both possible and likely (given present condition and status) and how much time and effort are required to attain what is envisioned. Solicit input from family if the client cannot independently determine or communicate his or her goals for therapy.

▶ If you cannot arrive at consensus of broad therapy outcomes, try to agree on short-term goals. For example, a client who is 3 months post brain injury wants only to work toward resuming work as an air traffic controller, a broad outcome the clinician views as unrealistic. Instead of haggling over what the future may or may not hold for this individual (which dampens energy, hope, and motivation), the client and therapist agree that to return to work, the client must independently get ready each morning; therapy work begins there.

Reestablishing Habits and Routines. With enough repetition and consistency, people perform many daily occupations efficiently and accurately with little or no conscious attention (that is, automatically). For example, most people have a consistent procedure for morning hygiene and dressing that rarely changes from one day to the next. These routines or habits let people expeditiously carry out frequently performed activities with minimal attentional load. After a disabling injury or illness, many clients need assistance either to reestablish existing routines or to create new ones that better match changed capacities and abilities. (Chapter 29 is a detailed discussion of how habits and routines are reestablished or created.)

Clients need to be motivated or at least compliant enough to carry out a consistent series of steps necessary to reestablish habits and routines but do not necessarily need deep awareness of deficits or understanding of the rationale of this approach. Because there is virtually no expectation of generalization (e.g., reestablishing a morning self-care routine will have no effect on efficiency with which one does the laundry), clients should work on reestablishing habits and routines in the environment in which those routines will be used.

Acquiring New Skills and Strategies. Occupational therapists teach clients new skills and strategies that allow them to compensate for permanent or temporary impairments. For example, a person with lower extremity weakness or paralysis acquires new skills for moving from the wheelchair to bed. An individual with multiple sclerosis learns energy conservation strategies that allow her to optimize her productivity; a client with brain injury learns techniques that help him get to appointments on time despite ongoing memory impairment. (Chapter 12 discusses how people learn new skills and strategies.)

Learning new skills and strategies generally takes longer to affect occupational function than, for example, changing elements of the physical context. However, acquiring the skills to transfer in and out of a wheelchair may have benefits that generalize to a variety of activities and tasks, thus enabling performance of a number of occupational roles. To benefit from this approach, clients must appreciate the importance of the new skills and strategies, be motivated to participate in training, and be capable of recognizing opportunities in which the new skills and strategies can be employed.

Determining the Optimal Treatment Approaches

Evidence-based practice methods can be used to determine optimal treatment approaches for a specific client. After articulating an answerable clinical question and gathering available evidence, clinicians evaluate the evidence to make decisions about the best approach. They judge its quality based on classes of the evidence, such as randomized controlled studies, case–control research, case series, and expert opinion (Whyte, 1998). Furthermore, they evaluate the validity of a study's results by asking the following questions: (1) Were patients randomly assigned to experimental and control conditions, and was the randomization concealed? (2) Were all patients who started the study accounted for at its conclusion? (3) Were patient's outcomes analyzed in the groups to which they were randomized? (4) Were the patients and clinicians blind to the experimental and control conditions? (5) Did all treatment groups receive comparable treatment except for the treatment under study? (6) Is my patient similar to those enrolled in the study? (Sackett et al., 1997; Whyte, 1998)

The rehabilitation literature does not always conclusively point to a singular treatment approach for a given set of problems. In such cases, Radomski and Davis (1999) suggest that clinicians weight the amount of treatment time and effort devoted to various treatment approaches, based on the best available evidence and the client's capacities, abilities, goals, and resources. They proposed the concept of a treatment fraction—the deliberate distribution of treatment efforts across appropriate treatment approaches to achieve goals. For example, with a woman acutely recovering from Guillain-Barré syndrome, the treatment fraction might look something like this: 40% of therapy efforts directed at remedial therapy (intervention focusing on improving strength and endurance); 35% for acquiring skills and strategies, such as learning modified self-care methods and energy conservation strategies; 25% for changing the context (helping the patient make her home more accessible). When she returns to therapy as an outpatient, the treatment fraction changes: 20% of the therapy time is devoted to remedial therapy; 20% to changing the context (helping the patient's family shift roles and responsibilities around the patient's changing abilities); 25% to acquisition of skills and strategies; and 35% to reestablishing habits and routines. The distribution is dramatically different for a client with Alzheimer's disease; the therapist may choose to devote 80% of therapy time to changing the context (adapting the home environment and coaching significant others regarding how to respond when their loved one is confused) and 20% to establishing behavioral routines. There are no hard and fast rules for the correct weighting of therapy time and efforts. However, the treatment fraction illustrates the importance of deciding how to spend therapy resources in pursuit of the client's goals rather than exclusively subscribing to one approach or mindlessly shifting focus session by session.

Required Documentation: Evaluation Note

An occupational therapy evaluation note is added to the medical record when assessment and treatment planning are complete. Table 19-1 shows the purpose of this document and what must be included.

Delivering Services

Once therapists collaboratively determine therapy outcomes, goals, and approaches, treatment begins. Clinicians continue to make decisions regarding how the treatment is delivered (one-to-one or group treatment) and by whom. The exception is when a clinical pathway dictates a predetermined therapy course that dovetails with intervention of other team members (Box 19-5).

How Treatment Is Delivered: Individual or Group Sessions

Occupational therapy occurs during one-to-one sessions with the client or in dyads or small groups. While clinicians must be sensitive to costs associated with providing services, they base scheduling decisions on each client's unique needs and goals rather than solely the clinician's convenience or profit.

Individual Treatment

Clinicians typically schedule individual sessions for assessment and reassessment. Individual sessions are also appropriate when client's privacy must be protected, such as during ADL training or when the client seems particularly vulnerable or in need of emotional support. Patients who are easily distracted, such as those in early phases of recovery from brain injury, are also best treated individually.

Group Treatment

Groups typically consist of clients engaged in parallel activities, such as performing individualized exercise regimens at the same time and place, or in collaborative activity, such as preparing a meal together. Clients tend to be grouped according to similar goals, treatment, or education needs or similar diagnoses, conditions, or limitations. Beyond its value from an economic standpoint, group treatment offers many benefits to clients. Group therapy can facilitate the exchange of social support and encouragement among clients as they derive hope for their own futures from observing others master similar challenges.

Who Delivers Treatment

Economic trends in health care require that the most appropriate person perform therapy tasks to optimize efficiency (Russell & Kanny, 1998). Occupational therapists make decisions about who will carry out the treatment plan (occupational therapist, occupational therapy assistant, and/or occupational therapy aide). Occupational therapists orchestrate the treatment plan and are ultimately responsible for service delivery (AOTA, 1999a). They typically spend their time conducting evaluations, identifying problems, planning solutions, and supervising implementation (Dunn & Cada, 1998; Glantz & Richman, 1997). Occupational therapy assistants spend most of their time delivering direct service and documenting results (Dunn & Cada; Glantz & Richman).

Required Documentation: Daily Contact Notes

Each time the client is seen for assessment and treatment, the clinician documents the contact (Table 19-1).

Monitoring Progress

Clinicians constantly monitor clients' response to intervention and their progress toward goals. At regular intervals, typically weekly for inpatients and at least monthly for outpatients, clinicians formally reassess status relative to goals, analyze barriers and enablers to progress, evaluate effectiveness of the treatment approach, and make decisions about continuing, modifying, or discontinuing treatment. If short-term goals are met but long-term goals are not, the short-term goals are upgraded (Moyers, 1999). If short-term goals are not met or performance has leveled off, the therapist examines and possibly modifies the treatment approach, reflects on the caliber of his or

---

BOX 19-5
Critical Pathways

Critical Pathway (Care Map)
Optimal schedule of key interventions from various disciplines for a specific diagnosis or procedure in order to achieve desired patient outcomes in a defined period of time (Dykes, 1997). A critical pathway is a multidisciplinary plan in that it outlines all the tests, procedures, treatments, and teaching that the patient is expected to need during hospitalization (Dykes). The treatment team documents the patient's status as compared to the plan directly on the critical pathway, with deviations recorded as a variance. A basic assumption underlying the critical pathway is the 80–20 rule; that 80% of patients follow a predictable path all of the time and 20% do not (Dykes). Critical pathways provide consistency of care for most but not all patients. They are not meant to be followed blindly and can always be modified to meet the needs of individual patients (Dykes). Figure 19-3 is a portion of a critical pathway used after total knee replacement surgery.

PLACE BAR CODE HERE

PATIENT NAME:

ORTHO PAIN MANAGEMENT/ANALGESICS ROUTINE PROTOCOL:
(If patient is on Ortho Pain Protocol)

1. Assess and document pain q̄ 2h while awake. If pain is mild for 24 hours, assess q̄ 4h.
3. For unsatisfactory pain control **increase** each **scheduled** dose of morphine or hydromorphone by half (50%) of the total PRN milligrams given since the last **scheduled** dose.
4. For excessive side effects or mild pain (e.g., pain ≤ 3/10 for 12 hours), decrease **scheduled** dose by half (50%).
5. Discontinue scheduled morphine or hydromorphone when pain has been mild for 12 hours and patient tolerating other analgesics.
7. Oral "step down" analgesic(s). To begin when IV or PCA opioid is being tapered.
8. When pain is mild and patient using ≤ 3 tablets PRN during the previous 24 hours, discontinue scheduled opioid doses and give 1 to 2 tablets every 3 to 4h PRN.

LOS GUIDELINES: *(does NOT include DOS)*
If patient DC plan is to go home with or without home care, plan on a **4 day LOS.**
If patient DC plan is to go to an extended care facility, plan on transfer after a **4 day LOS.**
Referral/DC instruction forms initiated **DAY BEFORE DISCHARGE.**

I&O / IV PROTOCOL:
Continue I&O for 48 hr. p̄ IV d/c'd.
Convert to SL when tolerates PO adequately.
Discontinue SL if:
- Antibiotics completed
- No transfusion necessary
- Pt. tolerating diet

ACTIVITY PROTOCOL

KEY:	DOS	POD #1	POD #2	POD #3	Remainder of Stay
✓ completed intervention, move to next intervention (IN PEN) △ change Ⓐ assist Ⓘ independent c̄ with s̄ without q̄ every AEB as evidenced by B/4 before BR bedrest/bathroom d/c discontinue DC discharge LOS length of stay OOB out of bed pt. patient PT physical therapy RT related to SBA stand by assist SR siderail SS social service W/A when awake	**ACTIVITY PLAN:** Dangle or up to commode x1 with assist of 2 HOB up as tol Turn as tol **NO PILLOW UNDER KNEE** CPM/immobilizer as ordered **Pt:** BID **HYGIENE:** Pt. able to assist with upper body hygiene, full assist with lower body, back cares Remove TEDs for cares BID	**ACTIVITY PLAN:** Transfer with assist of 1-2 for meals and therapy as ordered Use walker/transfer belt Elevate/support operated leg while sitting **NO PILLOW UNDER KNEE** If CPM ordered: use as directed If immobilizer ordered: increase 5-10 degrees/day, use 1-2 hour 2-3 x/d Quad sets and SLRs QID **Pt:** BID **HYGIENE:** Pt. able to assist with upper body hygiene, full assist with lower body, back cares Remove TEDs for cares BID	**ACTIVITY PLAN:** Transfer with walker and assist of 1-2 for meals and therapy Ambulate in room x2 Use walker/transfer belt Up in chair/commode Elevate/support operated leg while sitting Sit for short intervals with feet on floor QID **NO PILLOW UNDER KNEE** If immobilizer ordered: use as directed, wear at HS only, if pt. can SLR If CPM ordered: Increase 5-10 degrees/day, Use QID for 1 hour intervals Quad sets and SLR's QID Accomplish bed mobility without use of SR/trapeze **Pt:** BID **OT:** Referral prn **HYGIENE:** Pt. indep with upper body, assist with lower body Remove TEDs for cares BID	**ACTIVITY PLAN:** Transfer with walker/crutches and standby or assist of 1 Ambulate to BR No use of commode in room Up in chair for all activities, keep feet on floor Ambulate outside of room **NO PILLOW UNDER KNEE** If immobilizer ordered: wear at HS only, if pt. can SLR If CPM ordered: Increase 5-10 degrees/day, Use QID for 1 hour intervals Quad sets and SLRs QID Independent bed mobility **Pt:** BID **OT:** ADL eval prn **HYGIENE:** Assist with lower extremities prn Remove TEDs for cares BID	**ACTIVITY PLAN:** Progress towards independence in bed mobility, transfers, ambulation, with walker/crutches **NO PILLOW UNDER KNEE** If CPM ordered: increase CPM 5-10 degrees/day to 90 degrees Use 3-4 times/day for minimum 1 hour intervals Progress to independent exercise program **PT:** Based on pt. need **OT:** Based on pt. need **HYGIENE:** Progress towards independence and shower before D/C

Figure 19-3 The activity protocol from a critical pathway used after total knee replacement surgery. (Reprinted with permission from Abbott-Northwestern Hospital, Minneapolis, MN.)

her skills with the treatment methods, looks for transient explanatory factors, consults with experts, and/or considers discontinuing therapy.

Required Documentation: Weekly and/or Monthly Progress Notes

Progress notes document the formal examination of the client's progress toward treatment goals (Allen, 1997). Table 19-1 details information in progress reports. For outpatients with Medicare, therapists also must complete monthly recertification forms also detailing the patient's progress toward goals, which must be signed by the patient's physician every 30 days.

Discontinuing Therapy

Therapy is discontinued when goals have been met, the client's performance has leveled off or deteriorated in such a way that he or she is not benefiting from services, or the client chooses to stop. Ideally, the client and family participate in discharge planning, which entails setting up a maintenance program, referring to other services, and/or planning for follow-up.

- ▶ Set up the maintenance program. Clients and families receive instructions that allow them to extend the benefits of treatment after discharge. Therapists typically provide written and oral information regarding continued exercise, recommended equipment, and strategies or techniques that optimize function.
- ▶ Refer to other services. Many clients who discontinue occupational therapy at one site continue treatment at another level of care. For example, often persons receiving inpatient rehabilitation receive additional occupational therapy in long-term care facilities, through home health agencies, or as outpatients. To continue treatment seamlessly, therapists pass information along to the next tier of intervention. Therapists may also identify areas of need that are outside their scope of practice or competence and refer clients to appropriate disciplines or specialists.
- ▶ Plan for follow-up. Implicit in treatment plans geared to addressing the right issues at the right time in a client's recovery and adaptation is the expectation that the therapist will not treat all possible problems during a given episode of care. A scheduled occupational therapy follow-up session is a mechanism by which the clinician can screen for the need for more services. A follow-up session is necessary when the client improves, regresses, or anticipates changed needs or goals or when the social or environmental

context changes (Moyers, 1999). Some clients are ambivalent about discontinuing occupational therapy: recognizing lack of progress but fearing abandonment and stalled recovery or deterioration. Planned follow-up assures clients that occupational therapy services will be available to them if needed in the future.

Required Documentation: Home Program, Referrals, Discharge Summary

Not only are written home programs and referrals provided to the client and referral source, these reports are added to the medical record. The discharge summary provides an overview of services provided, outcomes, and recommendations (Table 19-1). Allen (1997) suggested that creating this document can be a reflective process for the clinician, who considers goals met or not and factors contributing to or interfering with progress.

Using Practice Experience to Improve Competence

You, as an occupational therapy professional, are ultimately responsible for assessing, improving, maintaining, and documenting your own competence to practice (AOTA, 1999b; Youngstrom, 1998). Competence has many dimensions, including knowledge, critical reasoning, interpersonal abilities, performance skills, and ethical reasoning (AOTA, 1999b). Like occupational therapy services, continuing competence entails assessment, goal-directed action, and documentation.

Self-Assessment: Reflecting on Practice

The cornerstone of continuing competence is reflection on yourself and your practice. Therapists deliberately and regularly take stock of their status and determine their growth edges. Clinicians interested in growth ask for feedback from peers and formally review their own performance. Schell (1992) recommended that clinicians annually outline their strengths, areas needing improvement, accomplishments of the past year, and goals for the coming year (Box 19-6).

Goal-Directed Action

Having assessed your professional strengths and weaknesses, you have many ways to improve your competence, including the following:

- ▶ Participate in your professional national and state occupational therapy associations. During volunteer service you will encounter other occupational therapists who are committed to their profession and their own growth.

► Establish a mentoring relationship. Mentors benefit from the relationship as they expand into new areas of practice, and protégés benefit from coaching and intellectual stimulation (Smith, 1992).

► Keep a journal to document information and questions; to reflect on ideas, concerns, and beliefs; and ultimately to identify learning needs (Tryssenaar, 1995).

► Start a journal club at work in which clinicians regularly read and discuss articles relevant to occupational therapy practice.

► Videotape your work. Slater and Cohn (1991) described an occupational therapy department that formed two-member teams to interview, observe, and videotape each other. Before videotaping a treatment session, the clinician was interviewed and asked to tell his or her story of the patient and what he or she expected to accomplish during the session. After videotaping treatment, the clinician was again interviewed, describing what actually occurred. The interviews and videotaped session were used as part of larger group discussions about clinical reasoning.

► Volunteer for medical record reviews and audits. By reviewing the documentation of others and submitting your documentation to the same scrutiny, you will learn how you can make your documentation clearer and more useful.

Documentation

Crist et al. (1998) recommended that occupational therapists use "transitional portfolios" (p. 729) to plan and document their professional competence. More than a résumé or a curriculum vitae, the transitional

Case Example

DETERMINING ONE'S CLINICAL COMPETENCE

Background

Ms. C. is an occupational therapist working in a small physical disabilities setting at a suburban hospital in the Midwest. She has 5 years of experience, having been working in long-term care for 1 year and for 4 years in her present position. She serves both inpatients and outpatients, primarily with orthopaedic or neurological problems.

The Referral

Mrs. K. is a 50-year-old woman with a diagnosis of left postmastectomy lymphedema with multiple infections and fibrosis. Mrs. K. underwent mastectomy for left breast cancer 15 months ago and had 20 of her lymph nodes removed on the left side. She had chemotherapy and irradiation and is now considered cancer free. She recently saw her oncologist with complaints of left upper extremity swelling and aching heaviness in the arm and across the chest and back. She reported difficulty with fit of clothing on the left, which causes her increasing embarrassment at work. Her sleep is also disturbed because of left arm discomfort. She is referred to outpatient occupational therapy for evaluation and treatment of lymphedema, including manual lymph drainage, compressive bandaging, fitting of custom compressive garments, and instruction in home exercises and skin care.

Self-Reflection on Clinical Competence

While Ms. C. had previous experience treating cancer patients, instructing in self-care, home management, and work simplification strategies, she had no specific training in the area of lymphedema management. Because this new area of practice interested her, she searched the internet for information. She readily found information on lymphedema and its treatment (**www.cancer.org**) and guidelines for contacting a lymphedema treatment center, information about training programs, and names of clinicians with specialized training (**www.lymphnet.org**). She searched the National Library of Medicine (**www.nlm.nih.gov**) for abstracts of research regarding treatment of lymphedema.

Having some preliminary information, Ms. C. used AOTA Standards of Continuing Competence, summarized in Box 19-6, to assess her competence to treat Mrs. K. She concluded that she did not have the knowledge, critical reasoning, or performance skills necessary to assess and treat Mrs. K. She used information from her Internet search to refer Mrs. K. to another facility with specially trained therapists and decided to pursue training herself to make these services available to patients at her hospital.

BOX 19-6
PROCEDURES FOR PRACTICE

Analyzing Your Competence

Clinicians use the answers to the following questions based on AOTA Standards of Competence (1999b) and Code of Ethics (1994b) to guide their response to an unfamiliar diagnoses, conditions, or problems. These documents help clinicians determine whether they are competent to provide independent assessment and treatment or supervised assessment and treatment or should refer the client to someone with more expertise.

▸ Knowledge
  1. Do I have adequate and up-to-date theoretical knowledge about this diagnosis, condition, or problem?
  2. Do I know about any legislative, legal, or regulatory issues specific to this client's diagnosis, condition, or problem?
  3. Do I know of any contraindications or precautions associated with treating this diagnosis, condition, or problem?
▸ Critical reasoning
  1. Will I be able to recognize the appropriate response to treatment?
  2. Will I be able to recognize potentially harmful primary or secondary effects of treatment?
  3. Will I be able to decide how to respond to untoward responses to treatment?

▸ Interpersonal abilities
  1. Am I competent to discuss the pros and cons of various methods to assess and treat this diagnosis, condition, or problem with the client?
  2. Am I competent to collaborate with other professionals specific to this diagnosis, condition, or problem?
▸ Performance skills
  1. Is specialized training or certification required or recommended for treating this diagnosis, condition, or problem?
  2. Am I skilled at using modalities, devices, or technology required to treat this diagnosis, condition, or problem?
  3. Is the client at risk for harm associated with inappropriate treatment of this diagnosis, condition, or problem?
▸ Ethical reasoning
  1. Is my motivation to assess or treat this client influenced by personal gain or profit?
  2. Is there any conflict of interest related to my decision to treat or assess this client?

portfolio houses artifacts of completed and exemplary work (certificates of attendance, awards, articles), in-process projects and plans for professional development, and a reflective journal with ideas, goals, feelings about one's reading, research, and work experiences. By systematically collecting and organizing information and artifacts specific to accomplishments, progress, and goals, occupational therapists take responsibility for their present and future professional competence.

Summary Review Questions

1. Describe specific aspects of occupational therapy documentation that you think are critical information for various target audiences.
2. Summarize ways a clinician's bias may affect clinical reasoning during each phase of providing occupational therapy services.
3. Draft two long-term and two short-term occupational therapy goals for a hypothetical client with multiple sclerosis whose anticipated outcome of therapy is to return to clerical work.

4. Write a brief statement (fewer than 25 words) that you could use to describe occupational therapy to a new client as a prelude to collaborative goal setting.
5. Compare and contrast the treatment fractions of two clients receiving occupational therapy services: a woman with amyotrophic lateral sclerosis and a woman with acute traumatic brain injury.
6. Ask an occupational therapy colleague for feedback about your competence in areas of knowledge, critical reasoning, interpersonal abilities, performance skills, and ethical reasoning. Summarize your strengths and identify areas for growth.

References

Allen, C. (1997). Clinical reasoning for documentation. In J. D. Acquaviva (Ed.), *Effective Documentation for Occupational Therapy* (2nd ed., pp. 53–62). Bethesda, MD: American Occupational Therapy Association.

Allen, C., Foto, M., Moon, T., Wilson, D., & Thomas, V. J. (1997). Understanding the medical review process. In J. D. Acquaviva (Ed.), *Effective Documentation for Occupational Therapy* (2nd ed., pp. 63–73). Bethesda, MD: American Occupational Therapy Association.

American Occupational Therapy Association (1994a). Uniform terminology for occupational therapy (3rd ed). *American Journal of Occupational Therapy*, 48, 1047–1059.

American Occupational Therapy Association (1994b). Occupational therapy code of ethics. *American Journal of Occupational Therapy*, 48, 1037–1038.

American Occupational Therapy Association (1995). Elements of clinical documentation (revision). *American Journal of Occupational Therapy*, 49, 1032–1035.

American Occupational Therapy Association (1999a). Guide for supervision of occupational therapy personnel in the delivery of occupational therapy services. *American Journal of Occupational Therapy*, 53, 592–594.

American Occupational Therapy Association (1999b). Standards of Continuing Competence. *American Journal of Occupational Therapy*, 53, 599–600.

Bryant, E. T. (1995). Acute rehabilitation in an outcome-oriented model. In P. K. Landrum, N. D. Schmidt, & A. McLean (Eds.), *Outcome-Oriented Rehabilitation* (pp. 69–93). Gaithersburg, MD: Aspen.

CARF (1999). *1999 Medical Rehabilitation Standards Manual*. Tucson, AZ: Author.

CARF (2000). *2000 Medical Rehabilitation Standards Manual*. Tucson, AZ: Author.

Cope, D. N., & Sundance, P. (1995). Conceptualizing clinical outcomes. In P. K. Landrum, N. D. Schmidt, & A. McLean (Eds.), *Outcome-Oriented Rehabilitation* (pp. 43–56). Gaithersburg, MD: Aspen.

Crabtree, J. (2000). What is a worthy goal of occupational therapy? *Occupational Therapy in Health Care*, 12, 111–126.

Crist, P., Wilcox, B. L., & McCarron, K. (1998). Transitional portfolios: Orchestrating our professional competence. *American Journal of Occupational Therapy*, 52, 729–736.

Dubouloz, C., Egan, M., Vallerand, J., von Zweck, C. (1999). Occupational therapists' perceptions of evidence-based practice. *American Journal of Occupational Therapy*, 53, 445–458.

Dunn, W., Cada, E. (1998). The national occupational therapy practice analysis: Findings and implications for competence. *American Journal of Occupational Therapy*, 52, 721–728.

Dykes, P. C. (1997). Designing and implementing critical pathways: An overview. In P. C. Dykes & K. Wheeler (Eds.), *Planning, Implementing, and Evaluating Critical Pathways* (pp. 8–25). New York: Springer.

Fisher, A. G. (1998). Uniting practice and theory in an occupational framework. *American Journal of Occupational Therapy*, 52, 509–521.

Glantz, C. H., & Richman, N. (1997). OTR-COTA collaboration in home health: Roles and supervisory issues. *American Journal of Occupational Therapy*, 51, 446–452.

Joint Commission on Accreditation of Healthcare Organizations (1999). *Comprehensive Accreditation Manual for Hospitals*. Oakbrook Terrace, IL: Author.

Joyce, B. M., Rockwood, K. J., & Mate-Kole, C. C. (1994). Use of goal attainment scaling in brain injury in a rehabilitation hospital. *American Journal of Physical Medicine and Rehabilitation*, 73, 10–14.

Kane, R. L., Rockwood, R., Finch, M., & Philip, I. (1997). Consumer and professional ratings of the importance of functional status components. *Health Care Financing Review*, 19, 11–22.

Kiresuk, T. J., & Sherman, R. E. (1968). Goal attainment scaling: A general method for evaluating comprehensive community mental health programs. *Community Mental Health Journal*, 4, 443–453.

McGuire, M. J. (1997). Documenting progress in home care. *American Journal of Occupational Therapy*, 51, 436–445.

Moorhead, P., & Kannenberg, K. (1997). Writing functional goals. In J. D. Acquaviva (Ed.), *Effective Documentation for Occupational Therapy* (2nd ed., pp. 75–82). Bethesda, MD: American Occupational Therapy Association.

Moyers, P. A. (1999). The guide to occupational therapy practice. *American Journal of Occupational Therapy*, 53, 247–322.

Nelson, C. E., & Payton, O. D. (1997). The planning process in occupational therapy: Perceptions of adult rehabilitation patients. *American Journal of Occupational Therapy*, 51, 576–583.

Opacich, K. J. (1991). Assessment and informed decision-making. In C. Christiansen & C. Baum (Eds.), *Occupational Therapy: Overcoming Human Performance Deficits* (pp. 356–372). Thorofare, NJ: Slack.

Ottenbacher, K. J., & Cusick, A. (1990). Goal attainment scaling as a method of clinical service evaluation. *American Journal of Occupational Therapy*, 44, 519–525.

Ponte-Allan, M., & Giles, G. M. (1999). Goal setting and functional outcomes in rehabilitation. *American Journal of Occupational Therapy*, 53, 646–649.

Radomski, M. V. (1995). There is more to life than putting on your pants. *American Journal of Occupational Therapy*, 49, 487–490.

Radomski, M. V., & Davis, E. S. (1999). *Cognitive Compensatory Strategies: From Treatment to Function*. Workshop presented for the Minnesota Occupational Therapy Association, Minneapolis.

Robertson, S. C. (1997). Why we document. In J. D. Acquaviva (Ed.), *Effective Documentation for Occupational Therapy* (2nd ed., pp. 29–38). Bethesda, MD: American Occupational Therapy Association.

Rockwood, K., Joyce, B., & Stolee, P. (1997). Use of goal attainment scaling in measuring clinically important change in cognitive rehabilitation patients. *Journal of Clinical Epidemiology*, 50, 581–588.

Rogers, J. C., & Holm, M. B. (1991). Occupational therapy diagnostic reasoning: A component of clinical reasoning. *American Journal of Occupational Therapy*, 45, 1045–1053.

Russell, K. V., & Kanny, E. M. (1998). Use of aides in occupational therapy practice. *American Journal of Occupational Therapy*, 52, 118–124.

Sackett, D. L., Richardson, W. S., Rosenberg, W., & Haynes, R. B. (1997). *Evidence-Based Medicine*. New York: Churchill Livingstone.

Schell, B. B. (1992). Setting realistic career goals. *Occupational Therapy Practice*, 3, 11–20.

Schell, B. B. (1998). Clinical reasoning: The basis of practice. In M. E. Neistadt & E. B. Crepeau (Eds.), *Willard & Spackman's Occupational Therapy* (pp. 90–100). Philadelphia: Lippincott.

Slater, D. Y., & Cohn, E. S. (1991). Staff development through analysis of practice. *American Journal of Occupational Therapy*, 45, 1038–1044.

Smith, B. C. (1992). Mentoring: The key to professional growth. *Occupational Therapy Practice*, 3, 21–28.

Spencer, J., Davidson, H., & White, V. (1997). Helping clients develop hopes for the future. *American Journal of Occupational Therapy*, 51, 191–198.

Tickle-Degnen, L. (1999). Organizing, evaluating, and using evidence in occupational therapy practice. *American Journal of Occupational Therapy*, 53, 537–539.

Tickle-Degnen, L. (2000). Communicating with clients, family members, and colleagues about research evidence. *American Journal of Occupational Therapy*, 54, 341–343.

Trombly, C. A. (1995). Planning, guiding, and documenting therapy. In C. A. Trombly (Ed.), *Occupational Therapy for Physical Dysfunction* (pp. 29–40). Baltimore: Williams & Wilkins.

Trombly, C. A., Radomski, M. V., & Davis, E. S. (1998). Achievement of self-identified goals by adults with traumatic brain injury: Phase I. *American Journal of Occupational Therapy*, 52, 810–818.

Tryssenaar, J. (1995). Interactive journals: An educational strategy to promote reflection. *American Journal of Occupational Therapy, 49,* 695–702.

Wade, D. T. (1999). Goal planning in stroke rehabilitation: How? *Topics in Stroke Rehabilitation, 6,* 16–36.

Whyte, J. (1998). *Evidence-Based Rehabilitation: Why Not Cloud the Issue With Facts!* Paper presented at the meeting of the American Congress of Rehabilitation Medicine, Seattle, WA.

Wilson, D. (1997). If I had known then what I know now . . . . In J. D. Acquaviva (Ed.), *Effective Documentation for Occupational Therapy* (2nd ed., pp. 1–3). Bethesda, MD: American Occupational Therapy Association.

Youngstrom, M. J. (1998). Evolving competence in the practitioner role. *American Journal of Occupational Therapy, 52,* 716–720.

20

Optimizing Abilities and Capacities: Range of Motion, Strength, and Endurance

Jeanne Jackson, Julie McLaughlin Gray, and Ruth Zemke

LEARNING OBJECTIVES

After studying this chapter, the reader will be able to do the following:

1. State the biomechanical and physiological mechanisms that underlie therapeutic exercise and occupation.
2. Apply the methods of movement, positioning, and compression to prevent limitation of range of motion.
3. Apply the principles of the biomechanical approach to increase range of motion, strength, and endurance as needed for occupational performance.
4. Apply these principles to the selection of occupations as a means for treating range of motion, strength, and/or endurance problems.
5. Design treatment goals and therapy for clients who have problems with range of motion, strength, and/or endurance to enhance occupational performance.

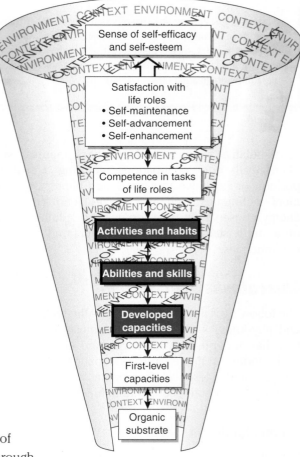

*A*ccording to the Model of Occupational Functioning, a goal of occupational therapy is to foster competency and self-esteem through participation in life occupations (Trombly, 1995). Biomechanical and physiological principles that relate to movement can provide guidelines for treatment when participation in occupation is threatened because of limitations in the capacities of range of motion (ROM), strength, or endurance. For example, occupational therapists use these principles to assist in remediating impairments from acute injuries or compensating for chronic disability to enable occupation. Occupational therapists also use these principles in preventing illnesses and conditions such

---

GLOSSARY

Ankylosis—Pathological stiffening of a joint due to fibrotic changes in the bones and/or tissues surrounding the joints.

Concentric contraction—Muscle contraction that moves a limb segment in the direction of the muscle pull.

Contracture—Static shortening of muscle and connective tissue that limits ROM at a joint.

Cross-bridge—ATP segment that moves and reconnects actin and myosin fibrils during muscle contraction.

Eccentric contraction—Muscle contraction that applies a breaking force to a movement produced by an opposing force (e.g., gravity) or resistance because the direction of the muscle pull is opposite the actual movement.

Fibromyalgia syndrome—Disorder that causes tenderness and stiffness in the muscles. Associated symptoms include sleep problems, malaise, memory and cognitive problems, depression, anxiety, headaches, skin rashes, urinary tract problems, and temperature dysregulation (Melvin, 1996).

Heterotopic ossification—Formation of new bone material in an abnormal site, such as adjacent muscle (Salter, 1999).

Kinematics—Study of the form of motion, describing movement paths in terms of the amount and direction of displacement in meters, velocity or speed in meters per second, and acceleration or rate of change of speed in meters per second squared of body segments. Joint angle changes in a given direction are also kinematic characteristics.

Kinetics—Study of forces, including static forces that balance or stabilize, and dynamic forces that mobilize.

Parameter—Variable that can be manipulated.

Torque—Product of force x perpendicular distance between the force and the axis of rotation.

---

as cumulative stress trauma and back injuries, which often result from occupations requiring a sustained position or repetitive motions (see Chapter 36). Treatment techniques such as joint protection principles, energy conservation, positioning, and splinting all rely on an understanding of biomechanical and physiological principles.

Musculoskeletal System

The following is a simple overview of the biomechanical and physiological elements of the musculoskeletal system that underlie ROM, strength, and endurance. This basic understanding enables occupational therapists to analyze and prescribe therapeutic occupations and exercise to promote occupational function.

Biomechanical Aspects

The biomechanical aspects of human movement are described in terms of **kinematics** and **kinetics**. Kinematics describes the trajectory, or path, of motion in temporal and spatial terms. Kinematic analysis addresses the amount and direction of movement, speed, and acceleration of body segments and joint angles (Luttgens & Hamilton, 1997; Soderberg, 1997). Researchers have used these quantitative kinematic descriptors to de-

scribe the movement of infants (Fetters & Todd, 1987), motor-impaired children (Downing et al., 1991), adults with cerebral palsy (McPherson et al., 1991) and adults who have had cerebrovascular accidents (Trombly, 1992). Therapists use this information for structuring occupation and designing exercise programs.

Kinetics addresses the underlying forces that cause motion or maintain stability (Luttgens & Hamilton, 1997; Norkin & Levangie, 1992). These forces may be internal to the body, such as muscle contraction or the elasticity of structural and connective tissue, which enable us to engage in our daily occupations. Forces of movement or stability may also be external to an individual, such as wind that moves (force) a sailboat, the friction of grass (force) slowing down a golf ball, the friction of the carpet (force) against a moving wheelchair, or the weight of a spoon (force), which may limit self-feeding in an individual with muscle weakness. Gravity is perhaps the greatest external force, most unnoticeable and constant, that affects all human movement. It is the gravitational pull on the body, body segments, and other objects that gives them weight. The gravitational attraction of an object to the earth resists upward movements of that object (Greene & Roberts, 1999). Therapists must be aware of these various forces when developing treatment plans using therapeutic occupations and/or exercise programs.

The following is an example of forces, stability, and motion in occupation. While dining, a person grasps a glass filled with a beverage and lifts it to take a sip. This task requires both stability and motion. Initially, muscles in the trunk and shoulder girdle (internal forces) cocontract to provide proximal stability, allowing for controlled distal mobility. To raise the glass, muscle contractions of the elbow flexors, for example the biceps, act as an internal force that overcomes external forces, which include the weight (thus taking into account gravity) of the bony levers (forearm and hand) and the glass. The biceps contraction causes rotary motion, or flexion, of the elbow joint. Rotary motion occurs when each point on the bone segment (ulna and radius) moves through an arc at the same time at a constant distance from the axis (elbow joint) (Norkin & Levangie, 1992). The arc formed by that rotary movement is called the ROM of that joint. To cause rotation, the biceps must have enough strength to overcome the external forces.

To analyze the movement in this scenario, one must also consider **torque**. Torque is the effectiveness of a force in causing rotary movement (Greene & Roberts, 1999; Norkin & Levangie, 1992). In rotary movements, torque depends on (1) the amount of force applied and (2) the distance of the force from the axis of movement. Thus, in mathematical terms the torque of a force is equal to the amount of force applied times the perpendicular distance between the line of force and the axis of rotation [T = F(ld)] (Luttgens & Hamilton, 1997; Smith et al., 1996). In relation to the example of taking a sip, the torque of the biceps (effort force) is equal to the force the muscle can produce times the perpendicular distance from its insertion on the radius to the axis of motion or elbow joint (Fig. 20-1A). The torque of resistance force (the glass and forearm) is equal to the resistance force (weight of glass and forearm) times the perpendicular distance between the glass and the axis of movement or elbow joint (Fig. 20-1B). In this case,

biceps torque is greater than the torque of the forearm and glass, so flexion can occur.

The concept of torque shows that the placement of an object either closer to or farther from the axis of rotation changes its efficiency to cause rotary movement, even though the object's weight remains constant. Therapists use this concept in a number of situations. For example, a short reacher as opposed to a long one requires less force of the patient's upper extremity muscles to pick up an object. With a long reacher the object provides more resistance torque because the distance between the object and the person's joint (axis of movement) is greater than with the short reacher. Likewise, when assisting a patient to perform a stand-and-pivot transfer from the wheelchair to bed, a therapist stands close to the patient as they both pivot and the therapist lowers the patient to a sitting position. The patient provides less resistance torque (the weight of the patient times the perpendicular distance between the patient and the therapist's back) when he or she is close to the therapist. This in turn requires less effort force by the therapist's back muscles for raising, maintaining the position during the pivot, and lowering the patient to the bedside. This body mechanic principle for protecting stress on one's back (i.e., holding objects close to one's center of gravity when lifting or transporting) can be explained by this principle of torque. (See Chapter 32 for more information on body mechanics.)

In biomechanical terms, rotary movement is analyzed as one of three types of lever systems. A lever system consists of a rigid bar (such as a bone), an axis of rotation (such as a joint), and two forces, effort and resistance. Effort is the force that causes movement, and resistance is the force that tends to keep the object from moving.

A first-class lever is a system in which the effort and resistance forces lie on either side of the axis of rotation (Norkin & Levangie, 1992). A common example of a

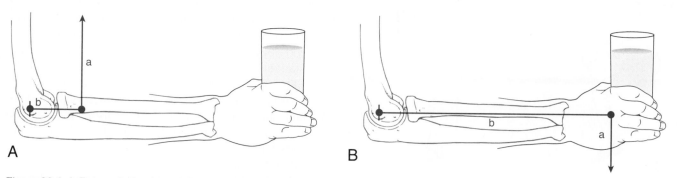

Figure 20-1. A. Torque of effort force. *a*, Line of pull of effort force (elbow flexors). *b*, Perpendicular distance between the insertion of the elbow flexors and the axis of rotation. **B.** Torque of resistance force. *a*, Line of pull of resistance force (weight of glass and forearm). *b*, Perpendicular distance between the resistance force and the axis of rotation.

first-class lever is the seesaw (Fig. 20-2*A*). As one can envision, a seesaw would remain in balance, with no movement, if two children of the same weight sat the same distance from the axis. This balance, or equilibrium, is maintained because the torque (weight of child 1 times the perpendicular distance from child 1 to the axis of rotation) on one side of the seesaw equals the torque (weight of child 2 times the perpendicular distance from child 2 to the axis of rotation) on the opposite side of the seesaw. In essence they balance, and there is no movement. If one of the children is heavier, he or she must move closer to the axis to maintain that balance (Fig. 20-2*B*).

In second- and third-class levers the effort and resistance force lie on the same side of the axis (Norkin

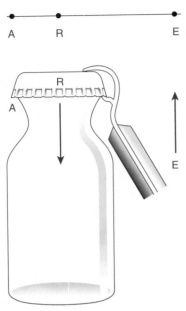

Figure 20-3 Top. Schematic drawing of a second-class lever. **Bottom.** Second-class lever depicted by using a bottle opener to remove the cap from a bottle. *A*, axis; *R*, resistance force (tightly secured cap); *E*, effort force (force from bottle opener to open cap).

& Levangie, 1992). A second-class lever system, such as a bottle opener or a wheelbarrow used to carry compost in a garden, is a system in which the resistance force lies closer to the axis of rotation than does the effort force (Fig. 20-3). With a bottle opener, the resistance force is the force of the cap that is tightly connected to the bottle. The effort force is a person's hand lifting the end of the opener to release the cap. This lever system allows a relatively small amount of force to overcome strong resistance. Second-class lever systems explain the tools used frequently in occupations when mechanical advantage is required, such as an extended handle on a faucet.

In third-class lever systems the effort force lies closer to the axis than does the resistance force (Norkin & Levangie, 1992) (Fig. 20-4 Top). The example of bringing a glass to one's mouth represents a third-class lever. The elbow joint is the axis; the biceps is the effort force; and the combined weight of the forearm and glass is the resistance force (Fig. 20-4 Bottom). In contrast to the stability of first-class levers and the mechanical advantage of second-class levers, third-class levers produce greater speed and ROM. For this reason, most of the muscles in the human body work in third-class lever systems when they contract concentrically to produce speed and ROM needed to engage in occupation.

The mechanical aspects of the musculoskeletal system promote both stability and mobility to provide the basis for action in occupation. The potential work capacity of the various muscles of the body also depends

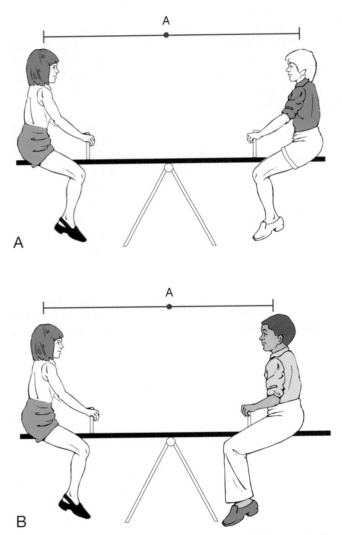

Figure 20-2 A. First-class lever system. Balanced equilibrium depicted by children on a seesaw. Both children weigh 60 pounds and they are equidistant from the axis. **B.** First-class lever system. The heavier child must be closer to the axis of the seesaw to maintain the equilibrium.

on the force they can generate and the distance over which they can shorten. In other words, the resulting work depends not only on biomechanical factors but also on physiological factors.

Physiological Aspects

The contractile portion of skeletal muscle is within the myofibrils of the muscle, where adenosine 5+ triphosphate (ATP) creates **cross-bridges** between the actin and myosin filaments. According to the sliding filament theory, muscle contraction occurs when the ATP cross-bridges are broken, actin is pulled over the myosin, and new cross-bridges are developed (Fig. 20-5) (Norkin & Levangie, 1992; Smith et al., 1996). As this sequence continues, tension is generated and the muscle shortens (**concentric contraction**). In a lengthening contraction (**eccentric contraction**) the opposite process occurs (Box 20-1).

A muscle's strength and endurance depend on multiple factors. Muscle strengthening results in both hypertrophy and more effective neural patterns and neural motor connections (Brody, 1999a; Segal, 1990). Muscle size is increased when an activity stresses the muscle's ability to produce tension and force. As the load or duration increases, some motor units fatigue, requiring recruitment of others. The demand for recruitment of motor units ultimately leads to the growth of the muscle fiber through myofibrillar changes, namely an increased number of sarcomeres or myosin and actin filaments. The more actin and myosin filaments avail-

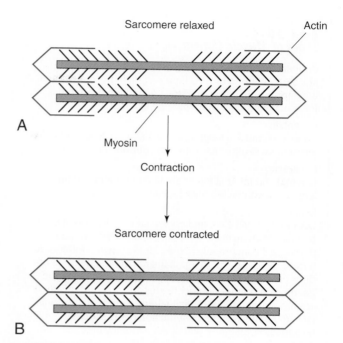

Figure 20-5 Schematic of actin and myosin cross-bridges during muscle relaxation and contraction. **A.** Relaxed muscle. **B.** Contracted muscle. (Adapted with permission from Hall, C. M., & Brody, L. T. (1999). Functional approach to therapeutic exercise for physiological impairments. In C. Hall & L. Brody (Eds.), *Therapeutic Exercise Moving Toward Function* (pp. 45–46.). Philadelphia: Lippincott Williams & Wilkins.)

able, the more cross-bridges can develop, creating more tension or strength in the muscle. For example, pianists increase finger strength by practicing musical pieces that stress (through vigor or duration) their hand musculature. As a piano player continues, or more challenging chords are used, actin and myosin filaments are generated to increase strength as needed. In contrast, when muscles are not used, myosin and actin filaments are lost, resulting in weakness.

Neural change, namely increased synchrony of motor unit activation, also contributes to muscle strength (Segal 1990; Shankar, 1999). Individual motor units, which make up muscles, fire according to the all-or-none principle of neural propagation. When all of the required motor units of the hand and finger muscles needed to press a key on the piano fire in synchrony, more tension is generated than when those same motor units fire asynchronously. Remember that in addition to muscle size and synchrony of motor unit firing, psychological factors such as motivation to perform an occupation affect effort exerted which contributes to muscle strength.

Muscle endurance is the ability of a muscle to sustain or perform repeated contractions over time (Brody, 1999a; Smith et al., 1996). Muscle endurance

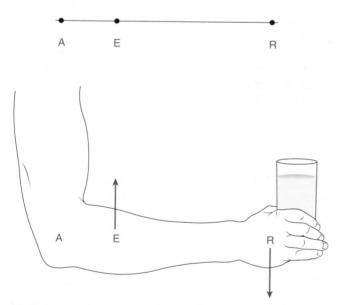

Figure 20-4 Top. Schematic drawing of a third-class lever. **Bottom.** Third-class lever, depicted by lifting a filled glass. *A*, axis; *E*, effort force (elbow flexors); *R*, resistance force (weight of glass and forearm).

BOX 20-1
Types of Muscle Contractions

Concentric
Muscle shortens to move a limb section in the direction of the muscle pull. In a concentric contraction the internal force of the muscle overcomes the external resistance.

Eccentric
Contracted muscle lengthens to act as a brake against an external force to allow for a smooth controlled movement.

Isometric
External and internal forces are in equilibrium and the length of a contracted muscle remains the same.

Example
Lowering a filled 10-pound cookie jar from the top of the refrigerator uses an eccentric contraction of the shoulder flexors and concurrently of the scapula upward rotators. Returning the cookie jar to top of the refrigerator before mom finds out you have eaten the cookies requires concentric contractions of the shoulder flexors and concurrently the scapula upward rotators. Maintaining a grasp on the cookie jar exemplifies isometric contraction of the shoulder horizontal adductors and the distal upper extremity muscles.

---

relies on a number of factors, such as the ability of the central and peripheral nervous system to relay messages from the limbic, premotor, and association cortices to the muscles and the ability of the lungs, capillaries, and muscles to transport and uptake oxygen, which is needed for metabolic and enzymatic processes (Brody, 1999b; Smith et al., 1996). At times muscle endurance is intricately related to the cardiovascular system. In fact, occupations that require cardiovascular endurance, such as tennis, also require muscular endurance. However, some occupations, such as those requiring maintained postural control, require muscle endurance without cardiovascular endurance. (For a more detailed understanding of the cardiac and pulmonary systems, see Chapter 47).

In general, improvement in muscle endurance requires availability of more oxygen. When heart rate increases, so does the amount of oxygen the person can take in, in a given amount of time, and dispense to the muscles (VO_2) (Brannon et al., 1993). The muscles require oxygen to break down ATP into the chemical energy needed for actin and myosin to form cross-bridges and thus create a muscle contraction (Smith et al., 1996). Local muscle fatigue is often related to impaired capillary systems interfering with the transportation of blood (oxygen) to the muscles, insufficient storage of glycogen, and/or a disruption of the metabolic process that breaks ATP into chemical energy (Brody, 1999b).

Biomechanical Approach to Treatment

Based on these biomechanical and physiological principles, occupational therapists can design treatment programs to address ROM, strength, and endurance problems affecting occupation. Ultimately the remediation or prevention of these limitations is aimed at ensuring the individual's occupational functioning.

Goal: To Maintain or Prevent Limitations of Range of Motion

ROM assessments provide guidelines for the typical ranges available at various joints in the human body. However an individual's actual ROM at any joint is determined by the physical constitution of the body and the person's typical occupations. For example, a waiter who carries platters of food with one hand throughout the work shift probably has greater wrist extension ROM than most others. Functional ROM is the range necessary to perform daily occupations. Occupational therapists are concerned with preventing ROM limitations that interfere with daily occupations.

Principle: Immobilization Reduces Range of Motion

Many ROM limitations can and should be prevented. When a joint remains immobilized, changes in the muscle (loss of muscle fiber and change in the number and length of sarcomeres), and connective tissue (disorganized synthesis of new collagen, ligament weakness, and elastic stiffness) and disruption of the workings of the synovial fluid, synovial membrane, and articular cartilage create limitations in ROM (Brody, 1999a; Soderberg, 1997). Tendons and ligaments change biochemically and lose tensile strength in the absence of motion and stress. With immobilization, muscle filaments lose their ability to slide, which is necessary for contraction. Edema and developing viscosity of fluid can increase the circumference of a joint and limit ROM (Brody, 1999a; Soderberg, 1997). Prolonged swelling leads to fibrotic changes and adhesions in the edematous tissue that result in contractures (Hertling & Kessler, 1996). Changes begin as early as 24 hours of immobilization. As a result of these underlying changes, a joint maintains only the range through which it is moved on a regular basis.

Patients who cannot move their own joints and for whom motion is not contraindicated need passive ROM exercises and proper positioning to maintain their available ROM. For example, when a patient is in a coma or unable to move because of paralysis, ROM should be maintained to enable a return to occupations when recovery occurs. Also when an agonist muscle is significantly weaker than its antagonist, the uneven tension between the two muscles may create a **contracture**. Furthermore, maintaining ROM can prevent discomfort, skin breakdown, hygiene problems, and difficulty in caring for the person. Occupational therapists are ultimately concerned with limitations in ROM that affect a client's ability to perform occupations.

Methods

The methods occupational therapists use to prevent those limitations in ROM include compression, positioning, and movement through full ROM.

Compression

Compression is used to prevent ROM limitations secondary to edema. Edema can be controlled by compression with elastic strip or tubular bandages. The occupational therapist must take care to apply these correctly so they do not constrict circulation in the more distal part of the extremity. *Skin color is observed regularly to confirm that circulation is preserved.* Coban (3M, St. Paul, MN), a self-adhesive elastic bandage, is wrapped around the part spirally in a distal to proximal direction and the edges are overlapped by at least 25% of the width of the material so that the fluid can flow evenly back toward the body and not be trapped in pockets of unwrapped tissues (Enos et al., 1984). Tubigrip (Mark One Health Care Products, Philadelphia, PA) is a tubular elastic support bandage that provides graduated constant pressure support when the correct size is applied. Compression is most effective in eliminating edema when combined with positioning and passive or active movement of the limb.

Positioning

When a person's limb is too weak to resist gravity, positioning in a resting or functional position is essential to avoid development of deformities, minimize edema, and maintain ROM gained in treatment. Positions of function are encouraged, and all nonfunctional positions are avoided throughout the day and night. For example, therapists using the neurodevelopmental treatment (NDT) approach may position a person in bed on the hemiplegic side, a functional position because it frees the nonhemiplegic side for various functions, such as arranging the blankets and answering the phone (Davies, 1985). This position promotes sensory input and awareness, and elongation and relaxation of the muscles on the hemiplegic side. Positioning can be accom-

plished by the use of orthoses, pillows, rolled towels, and positioning boards, among other things. For example, elevating a patient's edematous hand by use of a pillow assists the fluid to drain back to the body.

In spite of prevention, sometimes contractures and consequent **ankylosis** are unavoidable because of the disease process. In these instances positioning, splinting, and bracing are used to ensure that ankylosis occurs in as nearly a functional position as possible. A functional fixed position is one that allows the person to manage self-care and other functional tasks. For example, the functional position of the hand and wrist is slight (10–30°) extension of the wrist, opposition and abduction of the thumb, and semiflexion of the finger joints. If a patient's hand contracts in that position, the person can still use it to hold objects. If, however, the hand contracts in a fully flexed position, it not only is nonfunctional but also presents a hygiene problem. Likewise, a hand that fuses in an extension contracture has no holding capacity. When positioning a patient, the occupational therapist must be vigilant in anticipating eventual outcomes of prolonged immobilization that may compromise occupational performance.

Movement Through Full Range of Motion

The methods used for movement through full ROM, referred to as ranging, are (1) teaching the patient to move the joints that are injured, immobilized, or edematous and (2) passively moving the joints if the patient cannot. For specific instructions see Resources (*Home Rehabilitation Exercise: Shoulder, Elbow, Forearm, Wrist and Hand*). The ranging technique for active ROM (AROM) and passive ROM (PROM) are similar. Twice daily each involved joint is slowly and gently moved three times from one limit of motion to the other. In AROM, the patient actively performs the desired motion. In PROM, the therapist gently moves the patient's limb through the desired motion, paying particular attention to planes of motion and joint biomechanics. For example, the therapist pays special attention to the scapulohumeral rhythm when ranging the shoulder girdle. By moving the scapula with one hand and the humerus with the other, the therapist ensures that they are moving in synchrony (Figure 20-6). Attention to this alignment during movement of the scapula and humerus eliminates injury to the glenohumeral joint, bursae, capsule, and ligaments. As previously mentioned, the joint maintains only the range through which it is moved, and therefore, the therapist or patient must move a limb through the full available range or it will not be maintained. *Exception: A person who has tetraplegia and will rely on tenodesis action for grasp (see Chapter 43) must be ranged in the following*

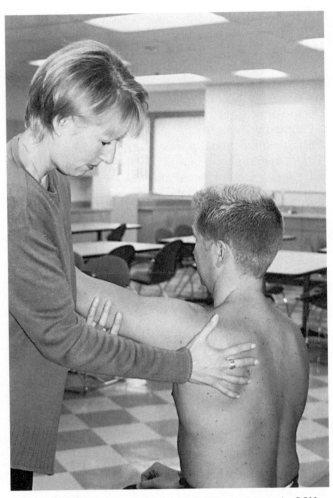

Figure 20-6 Facilitation of glenohumeral rhythm during passive ROM.

manner to allow finger flexor tendons to develop necessary tightness for grasping. When flexing the fingers, the wrist must be fully extended, and when extending the fingers, the wrist must be fully flexed.

PROM can also be performed by external devices, such as battery-operated continuous passive motion (CPM) machines. CPM machines are commercial orthoses used to maintain ROM and prevent postoperative swelling by continually moving the joint from one limit of motion to the other (Salter, 1999; Slater, 1993). See Bunker et al. (1989), Gelberman et al. (1991), LaStayo (1995), and LaStayo et al. (1998) for additional information on the use of CPM with the upper extremities.

AROM is preferred to PROM for reduction of edema because the contraction of the muscle helps pump the fluid out of the extremity. However, if AROM is not possible, PROM can aid in reducing edema. Positioning of the edematous extremity above the heart during distal PROM is recommended to aid in venous return.

Occupational therapists often structure activities to provide AROM to prevent limitations in ROM. For example, the patient may use his or her hemiplegic upper extremity in weight bearing for balance and postural stability while shaving to maintain the ROM in wrist and finger extension. Another example is the *ROM Dance Program* (see Resources). The *ROM Dance Program*, devised by Harlowe and Yu, is a 7-minute movement program modeled after t'ai chi chuan that incorporates joint motion in all ranges while the dancer listens to a poem that is meant to evoke pleasurable images. Although the ROM dance was developed for people with rheumatoid arthritis, it has been used with other populations, including the well elderly (Mandel et al., 1999).

Goal: To Increase Range of Motion

If limitations in ROM impair a patient's ability to function independently in occupations or are likely to lead to deformity, treatment to increase ROM is indicated. Whereas some significant limitations of ROM can be ameliorated or corrected by occupation and exercise, some cannot. Problems that can be changed include contractures of soft tissue, such as skin, muscles, tendons, and ligaments. Problems that cannot be changed through these means include bony ankylosis or arthrodesis, long-standing contractures in which there are extensive fibrotic changes in soft tissue, and severe joint destruction.

Occupational therapists may treat ROM limitations, using the principle of stretch, to help a patient develop the capacities needed to perform occupations. If ROM limitations cannot be reduced, occupational therapy becomes compensatory, focusing on providing techniques and/or equipment to enable participation in life occupations.

Principle: Stretch

Stretch is a process by which tissue is lengthened by an external force, usually to eliminate tightness that has the potential to cause a contracture. Stretch produces change only if done to the point of maximal stretch, defined as a few degrees beyond the point of discomfort, and held there for a few seconds. The force, speed, direction, and extent of stretch must be controlled (Shankar, 1999). The force must be enough to put tension on the tissue but not enough to rupture it. Different tissues tolerate stretch differently; tight muscles can be stretched more vigorously than tight joints (Kottke, 1990). The speed should be slow to allow the tissue to adjust gradually. The direction of stretch is exactly opposite to the tightness. The stretch is applied to the point of maximal stretch.

Gentle stretching that achieves small increments of

gain over time is more effective than vigorous stretching aimed at large, rapid gains. As a protective mechanism, connective tissue resists quick, vigorous stretching, which is therefore ineffective or injurious (Kottke, 1990). The method of moving gently to the point of maximal stretch and holding that position allows connective tissue, which has plasticity, to adapt to new requirements and adjust its length gradually over time. ***Residual pain after stretching indicates that the stretch was too forceful and caused tearing of soft tissues or blood vessels*** (Kottke, 1990). It is clinically recognized that maintained stretching is most effective; however, gains are also noted using briefly held stretch, usually 15 to 30 seconds (Brody, 1999a; Kisner & Colby, 1990). A study of healthy subjects found that 15 seconds of passive stretch was as effective as 2 minutes (Hallum & Medeiros, 1987).

Methods

There are two types of stretching, active and passive. In active stretching the muscle contraction is the source of the force, and in passive stretching an external force is applied.

Active Stretching

An occupational therapist's expertise lies in using occupations for treatment, in this case as a means of reaching the goal of increasing ROM. The use of occupation for stretching is empirically based on the idea that a person involved in an interesting and purposeful activity will gain greater range, because he or she is relaxed, is not anticipating pain, is motivated to complete the task, and therefore is likely to move as the activity demands.

The therapist and patient choose a life occupation that has significance to the patient. Because occupations can be performed using a number of muscle patterns, the therapist must determine how the patient completed the activity prior to injury. If the activity, as naturally performed by the patient, requires stretching the soft tissues that are shortened, it can be used as a form of active stretching. Occupations used as a means to increase ROM must provide a gentle active stretch by use of slow, repetitive isotonic contractions of the muscle opposite the contracture, or by use of a prolonged passive stretched position of the contracted tissue. In both types of stretch the requirement is that the range be increased slightly beyond the limitations. If the contracture existed before the limb was immobilized, active stretch is not likely to be effective; that is, if the patient was free to move and did not during daily activities, it is unlikely that gains will be made using activity to correct the contracture. Because people move in individually characteristic ways and because they frequently compensate by using available range in

adjacent joints, the therapist must carefully monitor the patient's motions. The therapist cannot assume that the activity itself will evoke the desired response in all persons. Reasonable adaptations of the occupation may sometimes be used to elicit the desired motions. Examples of adaptations are adjusting the size of a handle to stretch finger flexors or extensors and increasing the incline of a drafting table to achieve greater shoulder ROM while drawing.

Outcome studies have demonstrated gains in ROM through participation in active exercise programs and occupations. For example, subjects who participated in the ROM dance made significant gains in ROM compared with control subjects who did a traditional home program (Van Deusen & Harlowe, 1987). Another example is the use of *Simon*, an electric game that produces sound and light patterns, to increase range of shoulder motion of posttraumatic brain-injured patients (Sietsema et al., 1993). When compared with arm reach exercises, the use of the game elicited significantly greater ROM for 20 adult subjects than did arm reach exercises.

Exercises that increase the range of shortened tissue are the proprioceptive neuromuscular facilitation (PNF) techniques called contract–relax (CR) and agonist contraction (AC) (Brody 1999a; Voss et al., 1985). CR involves a maximal isometric contraction of the tight muscle, usually performed at the point of limitation. The muscle is contracted maximally for approximately 2 to 5 seconds against resistance provided by the therapist and then relaxed. During the relaxation phase, the therapist moves the part in the direction opposite to the contraction and holds it (Brody 1999a). For example, if there is a contracture of elbow flexors, the elbow is extended to its limit. The patient is instructed to contract the flexors isometrically and maximally, then relax, at which moment the therapist smoothly extends the elbow into greater range. The CR is repeated until as many increments of gain as possible are achieved. The AC sequence entails a maximal stretch of the tight muscle followed by an isotonic contraction of the muscle opposite the tight muscle. Using AC in the above example of elbow flexion contracture, the therapist moves the patient's limb into extension and the patient contracts the triceps to stretch the biceps further. Some therapists use a combination of CR and AC, or CRAC (Brody, 1999a). Again, in the case of elbow flexion contracture, the biceps is contracted against maximal resistance provided by the therapist. The biceps is then relaxed and the patient contracts the triceps.

Therapists have typically used a variety of stretching techniques, including those described here. Based on a review of studies spanning 20 years, Brody (1999a) concluded that no one technique has been demonstrated to have greater benefit over the others.

Passive Stretching

Passive stretching is often done by a physical therapist; however, occupational therapists may have to perform passive stretching prior to engagement in occupation. Techniques for passive stretching may include manual stretch and the use of orthotic devices, such as splints or casts, to provide controlled passive stretching (see Chapter 14). The procedures for manual stretching by the therapist are outlined in Box 20-2. Box 20-3 lists precautions.

Some patients can perform passive stretching of soft tissue contractures themselves. Activities such as the ROM dance, which includes some passive stretching, can be integrated into their daily occupations. Occupational therapists can modify the ROM dance to provide the necessary active and passive stretches to meet the patient's needs. Therapists must remember that with any method to increase rather than maintain ROM, the patient's limb must move to the point of maximal stretch.

Goal: To Increase Strength

If limitations in a patient's strength prevent engagement in occupations or may lead to a deformity, treatment aimed at increasing strength is warranted. Weakness can be deforming if the muscles on one side of a joint are significantly weaker than their antagonists or if the weakness prohibits the person from moving the limb and/or maintaining a functional position.

BOX 20-2
PROCEDURES FOR PRACTICE

Manual Stretching Methods

- ▶ Provide a relaxing environment for the patient.
- ▶ Describe manual stretching, noting that it involves tolerable pain.
- ▶ Use motions identical to motions used in ROM evaluation (see Chapter 4).
- ▶ Stabilize the bone proximal and distal to the joint that is to be moved to avoid any compensatory movement.
- ▶ Move the bone smoothly, slowly, and gently to the point of maximal stretch (mild discomfort indicated verbally or facially by the patient).
- ▶ Make sure the movement is in the line of pull of the muscle.
- ▶ Encourage the patient to assist in moving the limb if possible.
- ▶ Hold the limb at the point of maximal stretch 15 to 30 seconds (Brody, 1999a).
- ▶ Relief of discomfort should immediately follow the release of stretch.

BOX 20-3
SAFETY BOX

Safety Precautions Related to Passive Stretching

- ▶ Inflammation weakens the structure of collagen tissues; therefore, those tissues must be stretched cautiously with slow, gentle, motion (Kottke, 1990).
- ▶ Sensory loss prevents the patient from monitoring pain; thus, the therapist must pay particular attention to the tension of the tissues being stretched.
- ▶ Overstretching must be avoided because it causes internal bleeding and subsequent scar formation that may eventually ossify. Overstretching can lead to heterotopic ossification.

Principle: *Increase Stress To Muscle*

Muscle strength increases when the muscle is stressed to the extent that additional motor units are recruited and the muscle hypertrophies (Shankar, 1999; Smith et al., 1996). For muscles to hypertrophy and strengthen they must be stressed to the point of fatigue. Occupation or exercise parameters that may be manipulated to increase stress to a muscle include type of contraction, intensity or load, duration of contraction, rate or velocity of contraction, and the frequency of exercise.

Methods
Occupations and Exercise

Occupations, exercise, or both can be used to increase strength. Therapists may find that various occupations provide sufficient opportunities for muscle strengthening and are more effective at maintaining the patient's interest and motivation than exercise alone. At other times therapists may develop an exercise program specifically targeted to strengthen certain muscles needed for occupation. This exercise may also be combined with occupation in a number of ways. Exercise may be used as a warmup to occupation, or occupation may be introduced to enhance carryover of the strength gained by exercise. Research demonstrates that strengthening programs that encompass similar characteristics to the desired occupation or outcome in terms of contraction, speed, and position yield the best transference of strengthening results (Morrissey et al., 1995). Carefully prescribed therapeutic occupations can strengthen muscles in situations closely approximating their intended uses.

For some individuals, an exercise program may be a valued occupation in and of itself. In these cases, exercise can be used as a therapeutic occupation designed to address the individual nature of the performance, the meaning of exercise for that person, and the context in which that person typically exercises. In this instance, the occupational therapist may use the therapeutic occupation of exercise to remediate any performance component. For example, weightlifting can be used with a patient who has a brain injury not only to increase strength but also to enhance attention, memory, and organizational skills (see Chapters 29 and 39).

Grading Muscle Strength Parameters

When prescribing a strengthening program, therapists can manipulate the exercise or occupational **param-**eters. DeLorme (1945) and DeLorme and Watkins (1948) developed exercise programs based on principles of resistance and repetition to increase muscle strength. DeLorme's classic method, progressive resistive exercise, continues to be used today in its original or modified form. Progressive resistive exercise is a program in which a person lifts 50%, then 75%, and finally 100% of his or her repetition maximum (RM). RM is the maximum weight a person can lift with coordination through full ROM 10 times. Each exercise set (50%, 75%, and 100%) is done 10 times. Box 20-4 has guidelines

BOX 20-4
PROCEDURES FOR PRACTICE

Guidelines for a Strengthening Program

Type of Exercise	Definition	Muscle Grades	Procedures
Isometric	Exercise in which a weak muscle is isometrically contracted to its maximal force 10 times with rest periods between each contraction.	Trace (0) The force of contraction is not sufficient to move the part	Provide a stimulating environment Explain procedures Instruct the patient to contract the weak muscle ("hold"). External resistance applied by the therapist may help the patient isolate the contraction to the weak muscle or muscle group. Patient holds contraction at maximum effort as long as possible. Repeat 10 times with a rest between each contraction. Increase duration of maximal contraction as patient improves. ***Maximal isometric contraction is contraindicated for patients with cardiac disease.***
Isotonic Assistive (Active assistive ROM)	Exercise in which a weak muscle is concentrically or eccentrically contracted through as much ROM as patient can; therapist and/or external device provides assistance to complete motion.	Poor minus (2–) Fair minus (3–) The muscle can move only through partial available range in either a gravity-eliminated or against-gravity plane.	Provide a stimulating environment. Explain procedures. For a 2– muscle, position limb to move in a gravity-eliminated plane. For a 3– muscle, position the limb to move against gravity. Patient moves weak muscle through as much range as possible. Therapist provides external force to complete motion. Although this seems similar to PROM, it differs because patient actively attempts to contract weak muscle.
Isotonic active (active ROM)	Patient contracts muscle to move part through full ROM	Poor (2) Fair (3) Muscle can move through full available range in either gravity-eliminated or against-gravity plane.	Provide a stimulating environment. Explain procedures. For a 2 muscle, position the limb to move in a gravity-eliminated plane. For a 3 muscle, position the limb to move against gravity. Patient moves weak muscle through full available ROM. Patient repeats motion for 3 sets of 10 repetitions with rest break between sets.

(continued)

BOX 20-4
PROCEDURES FOR PRACTICE

Guidelines for a Strengthening Program (Continued)

Type of Exercise	Definition	Muscle Grades	Procedures
Isotonic active resistive (active resistive ROM)	Patient contracts muscle to move part through full available ROM against resistance.	Poor plus (2+) Fair (3) Fair plus (3+) Good (4) Good plus (4+)	Provide a stimulating environment. Explain procedures. For a 2+ or 3 muscle, position limb to move in gravity-eliminated plane. For a 3+ or above muscle, position limb to move against gravity. Therapist determines appropriate amount of resistance, which is the most a patient can lift through 10 repetitions with smooth controlled movement. Patient moves weak muscle through full available ROM against resistance[a]. Patient does 3 sets of 10 repetitions with varying resistance and rest break between sets.

Resistance can be provided by weights either held in patient's hand or strapped around moving part. Resistance can also be provided by tools and materials of activity.

Case Example

MS. M.'S EXPERIENCE OF FIBROMYALGIA

Patient Information

Ms. M. is a 40-year-old woman who was the executive administrator of a large computer company. She lives at home with her partner and her high-school-aged son from a previous marriage. Her partner is a lawyer in a small law firm that requires at least 10- to 12-hour days. Ms. M. is a high-powered, motivated woman who not only enjoyed but was energized by the various people with whom she interacted at her job and the diverse assignments she supervised. When Ms. M. returned home from work, she often used household occupations as a means of changing from her high-energy level to a more relaxed state. Ms. M. by no means felt she was responsible for keeping the house in order. She shared this equally with her partner and also her son. Ms. M.'s partner worked on Sundays, providing Ms. M. unscheduled time alone except for weekly worship. Ms. M. was adamant that at least one day of the weekend be spent engaging in social occupations with her partner. Relationships are essential in her life.

Ms. M. began to complain of pain, tenderness, and stiffness in her muscles, a skin rash on her arms, difficulty sleeping, extreme fatigue, and increased anxiety followed by depression in January 2000. She was diagnosed with **fibromyalgia syndrome** (Melvin, 1996) in February and took a disability leave of absence from work. She was referred to outpatient occupational therapy because she had difficulty performing her daily occupations. Following an occupational therapy evaluation that included this history, these problems were identified: (1) poor sense of life coherence due to loss of occupations; (2) lack of daily routine because of the loss of her ability to engage in her usual occupations; (3) depression and anxiety due to an unpredictable future and lack of daily routine; (4) inability to complete ADL and IADL because of fatigue and pain.

Recommendations

The occupational therapist recommended two treatment sessions each week for 8 weeks. Ms. M. and the therapist established the following long-term treatment goals: (1) Ms. M. will establish a new routine of daily occupations. This will provide her a sense of continuity in life and decrease her anxiety and depression. (2) Ms. M. will carry out her hygiene, self-care, dressing, and showering independently

(continued)

without discomfort. (3) Ms. M. will perform selected household activities independently without discomfort. (4) Ms. M. will design and carry out an individualized fitness program to reduce the disease symptoms that interfere with her occupations.

Short-Term Goals

► Ms. M. will carry out a morning stretching program 5 days per week. The occupational therapist worked with Ms. M. in adapting the ROM dance to maintain upper extremity range, stretch her limbs, and enhance her mood. Ms. M. performed this stretching program each morning. She used her creativity to design her own dances to target specific tender muscles.

► Ms. M. will cook independently, incorporating energy conservation and pacing techniques. Ms. M. identified baking as a top priority that required high energy. To decrease the stress of baking, the therapist taught her energy conservation techniques to use while baking. Together the therapist, Ms. M., and her partner modified the kitchen (i.e., put heavy pots and pans on the counters, purchased a high stool for sitting while cooking) to allow for less energy expenditure and muscle stress (bending and lifting) while maintaining the aesthetic appearance of the kitchen.

► Ms. M. will identify three possible daily occupational routines for low-, moderate-, and high-energy days. The therapist assisted Ms. M. in understanding how her daily occupations contribute to her health and self-esteem. Ms. M. completed a 1-week diary of her occupations in which she reported not only the activities but their significance, the emotions they evoked, and the physical and cognitive stress or enhancement they provided. Her therapist

helped her set priorities for self-care and home management for days when she had varying levels of energy. Occupations were ranked in terms of energy they required, pain they caused, stretch and muscle conditioning they provide, her experience of the occupation as a chore or a stress releaser, and the importance of getting the occupation done. The therapist also helped Ms. M. learn to buffer high-energy occupations with restful occupations, such as reading the newspaper or watching the news on television. Ms. M. used her knowledge about occupation to develop and practice a variety of daily routines that met her alternating patterns of energy depletion, pain, and muscle hypersensitivity.

Revised Goals

► Ms. M. will do aerobic exercises three times a week for general muscle endurance.

► Ms. M. will identify weekend occupations for herself and her partner that are consistent with her energy level, pain, and mood.

CLINICAL REASONING
in OT Practice

Effects of Endurance and Strength on Performing Occupations

The therapist developed an exercise program to assist Ms. M. in building the strength and endurance needed to carry out her daily occupations. How would the strengthening program differ from the program to build endurance? How could Ms. M. use occupation to build strength? How could Ms. M. use occupation to increase her endurance?

---

for setting up a therapeutic exercise or occupation program. Although these guidelines are for exercise programs, the principles can be used in designing a routine of occupations to be used for strengthening.

The type of contraction—concentric, eccentric, or isometric—is established by the demands of the task and assistance provided by the therapist (Box 20-1). Isometric contraction of a muscle at resting length can produce the most forceful contraction. *However, when the patient has hypertension or cardiovascular problems, isometric contraction should be avoided, because isometric contraction of either large or small muscles increases blood pressure and heart rate (Brannon et al., 1993; Luttgens & Hamilton, 1997)* (see Chapter 47). Also, more weight can be lowered by a given muscle during an eccentric contraction than can be lifted concentrically or held at any one point. A corollary is that less effort is exerted

when lowering a given weight that when lifting it. Regardless, the type of contraction should mirror what is required by the patient's occupations, because transfer of effects of training is unlikely between isometric and isotonic training programs (Hall & Brody, 1999; Morrissey et al., 1995). Occupational therapists commonly use occupation to build strength.

In the context of strengthening, the intensity of occupation or exercise refers to the amount of resistance offered and therefore includes gravity. The intensity or resistance should be increased over time for strengthening. For example, Ms. M., who has poor musculature but needs upper extremity strengthening to accomplish her daily tasks, can begin by washing her face side-lying in bed (reduced effect of gravity) until she can complete the task upright. Ms. M.'s occupational therapist can set up the task to be accomplished in bed and assist Ms. M. to bring her hand to her face so that she washes with her

Case Example

MR. G.'S RECOVERY FROM BACK INJURY

Patient Information

Mr. G., a 46-year-old man with a landscaping career, sustained a back injury when he tripped over his 2-year-old son's play lawnmower, lost his balance, and fell on the grass. Initially he had pain in his lower back and a sharp tingling sensation down his leg. Medical examination revealed that he had severely sprained his back muscles in the fall and had exacerbated pain because of previous bone spurs on the lumbar spine and a degenerating disc at L5-S1. Mr. G. was prescribed a brief period of bed rest and given medication for pain and muscle relaxation. Following this medical intervention, Mr. G. was referred to outpatient occupational therapy for exercises and instruction in how to perform his daily occupations so that his back pain would be relieved or minimized and further back injury would be prevented.

Mr. G.'s therapist conducted an interview and observed to ascertain which occupations were particularly significant in Mr. G.'s life, which occupations created pain, and how he performed them. Mr. G. described two main roles in his life, work (landscaping) and child care. Mr. G. explained that he and his partner both work outside the home in paid employment and share the child care and household responsibilities. Mrs. G. works part time at a travel agency. Although she has a flexible schedule, she usually goes to the office at least two evenings per week, so that Mr. G. is required to take care of their three children, Eliza, aged 4, and Tom and Pat, aged 2. Mr. G. is performing his self-care occupations with moderate assistance from his wife and with severe discomfort. He required maximal assistance for all home and child care occupations. He had not performed any other leisure or work occupations at the time of the evaluation.

Mr. G. is the sole owner of his landscaping business and has five experienced gardeners working for him. The occupations of his job: (1) He managed the finances, which requires sitting at a computer for approximately 5 hours, two to three times per month. (2) He designed landscapes, which required sitting at a drawing table for 3 to 4 hours at a time. (3) He consulted with the client and nursery personnel to design the landscape and buy the plants. These tasks required driving, creativity, communicating, and at times bending and lifting heavy pots. (4) He supervised the gardeners, which often entailed working with them to plant or lay down cement, stones, birdbaths, and other heavy garden fixtures.

Mr. G.'s evening schedule consists of cooking dinner, changing diapers, bathing the children, dressing them for bed, playing with them, and emotionally supporting them. The children love to play rough-and-tumble with their daddy. Multiple piggy-back and horsey rides are an expected part of play time. Furthermore, each parent has developed a special bedtime activity. Mrs. G. reads a book and Mr. G. pulls them on a cardboard train around the house and deposits each child in his or her bed.

Recommendations

The occupational therapist recommended two treatment sessions per week for five weeks. In collaboration with his wife and the therapist, Mr. G. set the following long-term goals: (1) Change or delete certain daily occupations to prevent further injury. (2) Learn proper body mechanics during daily occupations to relieve strain on his back. (3) Perform self-care, home, child care and landscaping occupations independently without pain.

Short-Term Goals

► Mr. G. will explore his options for avoiding some of the physically stressful occupations at his landscaping business and will enact a reasonable plan. The therapist and Mr. G. discussed various scenarios about his business. The most feasible option was to increase the responsibilities of two of the gardeners and give them a pay raise so that he would no longer purchase or carry heavy plants or help with planting. By eliminating these tasks and using proper body mechanics for the other tasks, Mr. G. could maintain his landscaping business.

► Mr. G. will pick up his children, incorporating good body mechanics 75% of the time. Initially, Mr. G. stopped his child care and household responsibilities. The therapist taught Mr. G. the principles of body mechanics, such as holding objects close to the body when lifting, keeping the back straight and using the leg muscles to lift, and avoiding simultaneous bending and twisting when moving items from one place to another. Mr. G. practiced and was successful with these techniques with various items around the house. He applied these principles to lifting his children, paying close attention to facing his child, being close to his child, and lifting with his legs. Although this technique worked, Mr. G. also taught his children to climb up on his lap, where he could position them well and use his leg muscles to stand up.

Revised Goals

▶ Mr. G. will analyze his body movements and change them to reflect good body mechanics during cooking, diapering, and playing with the children.

▶ Mr. G. will perform his computer work and landscape designing independently, incorporating proper body mechanics, pacing, energy conservation, and joint protection.

CLINICAL REASONING
in OT Practice

Prevention of Back Injuries While Lifting

While alone at work, Mr. G. had to lift a large, heavy box of office supplies from the floor to his desk. How might a therapist instruct Mr. G. to position the box to lessen the force on his back when lifting the box? Using the concept of torque, how might the therapist justify the positioning of the box?

---

muscles in a gravity-eliminated plane. Ms. M. may next attempt to wash her face sitting upright in a chair in the bathroom, moving the extremity against the resistance of gravity. The therapist can further increase the intensity by adding various weighted tools, such as a light puff, a washcloth, and a washcloth and bar of soap. The therapist can continue to increase the intensity through more resistive occupations, such as dressing, making a bed, washing a car, gardening, or playing basketball to increase strength gradually.

In this situation, resistance is graded by adding a load to the extremity (i.e., tools such as a washcloth, different textured clothing, or the resistance of dirt on a car) or by changing the plane of movement (i.e., gravity eliminated to against gravity). The duration of occupation can also be graded by increasing the need for muscle contraction through time spent in activity. A patient who is very weak may not even be able to finish washing his or her face in bed. The therapist can manipulate the rest breaks during the activity or complete a portion of the activity to increase the duration of the patient's participation. In this example, the treatment goal may be for the patient to take an entire bath or complete other occupations that take longer.

The occupational therapist must gradually increase the rate or velocity of contraction, described as the number of repetitions per period of time, according to the patient's abilities and comfort. As research suggests (Morrissey et al., 1995), the velocity of muscle contraction in training should eventually match the velocity of muscle contraction that is required in the patient's occupational routine. Finally, the frequency of exercise periods can also be graded for added strength benefit.

Goal: To Increase Endurance

Exercise programs designed to increase muscle endurance rather than muscle strength require somewhat different design. The following describes the underlying principles and guidelines for those modifications.

Principle: Less Than Maximal Resistance Over Time

In ordinary daily occupations that are lightly resistive, motor units are activated asynchronously. After a motor unit ceases activity, the muscle fibers recover to some degree while fellow units take their turn. Fatigue occurs more slowly with light resistive movements than with maximal contraction, in which many more units must contract simultaneously without the opportunity to recover. Doing repetitive concentric or eccentric contractions against less than maximal resistance increases endurance through less glycogen depletion and improved oxidative capacity of muscle fibers. Exercise to increase muscle endurance therefore uses moderately fatiguing activity for increasingly long periods with intervals of rest to allow metabolic recovery (DeLateur & Lehmann, 1990).

Method
Grading Occupations to Increase Endurance

One of the most dramatic examples of adaptability of the muscular system is the extent to which muscle endurance can be improved by engaging in mild activity with increased amounts of repetition. To increase endurance, therapists guide patients to engage in longer periods of occupation at 50% of their maximal capacity. Occupation or exercise used to build endurance is graded by

RESEARCH NOTE

Benefits of Leisure-Time Physical Activity on the Cardiovascular Risk Profile at Older Age

Mensink, G. B., Ziese, T., & Kok, F. J. (1999). *International Journal of Epidemiology, 28,* 659–666

ABSTRACT

Background: Intensity, frequency, and duration of physical activity may contribute in various ways to the maintenance of cardiovascular health. Their relative importance may change at different stages in life, and this should be taken into account for activity recommendations.

Methods: The relationship of frequency and duration of leisure time physical activities with cardiovascular risk factors was studied in 4942 male and 5885 female participants aged 50 to 69, of German Cardiovascular Prevention Study (1984–1991).

Results: After adjustment for several possible confounders, women with modest levels (2–12 times per month, 0.5–2 hours per week) of moderate to vigorous activity (at least 5 kcal/kg/hour) had significantly lower systolic blood pressure (−1.8%), resting heart rate (−3.1%) and body mass index (−3.2%) than sedentary women. Beneficial differences increased with frequency and duration of activity. Light activities (3–4.5 kcal/kg/hour), conducted at least 5 times a week, were significantly associated with favorable lower diastolic blood pressure (−1.4%), resting heart rate (−2.3%) among women, and body mass index (women −2.9%, men −2.2%) among both genders. Recommended activity levels (at least 5 times, at least 3.5 hours weekly) were associated with a lower prevalence of multiple risk factors.

Conclusion: For sedentary elderly, even less physical activity than currently recommended is likely to improve the cardiovascular risk profile.

IMPLICATIONS FOR PRACTICE

▶ A unique expertise of occupational therapy is the design and prescription of purposeful and meaningful activity—occupation—to enhance and promote health. Along these lines, occupational therapists frequently use therapeutic occupation to improve an individual's ROM, strength, and endurance. This study supports the notion that a variety of daily activities, even those performed at low intensities, have the potential for such health-promoting benefits as an improved cardiovascular risk profile.

▶ More specifically, the study demonstrates the observable and measurable effects of an occupation on the cardiovascular system. Occupational therapists can use this research to develop interventions and effectiveness studies that systematically monitor and analyze the multiple benefits of occupation-based treatment.

▶ Occupational therapists should be aware of the variety of activities available for strengthening, endurance building, fitness, and overall health promotion. They should complete a thorough occupational history to learn which activities in the patient's background may provide interest and exercise benefits. Through careful activity analysis and monitoring, occupational therapists can frequently use meaningful and purposeful activity to enhance strength and endurance, achieving the additional cognitive, psychosocial, and spiritual gains these activities may be designed to provide.

For additional references demonstrating the effects of occupation on various systems contributing to health, see Glass et al. (1999), Hassmen & Koivula (1997), Lan et al. (1998), Naylor et al. (2000), and Shephard (1997).

---

increasing the exercise period, which is done either by raising the number of repetitions of a concentric or eccentric contraction or by lengthening the time an isometric contraction is held. The occupational therapist can also increase the frequency of engaging in occupation or exercise if patients are not ready to increase duration times.

Occupational therapists provide the patients with interest-sustaining occupations that can be graded along the dimension of time or repetition. For example, patients who are interested in board games such as backgammon or chess may increase the number of games they play or the length of time they play. Occupational therapists can also work with patients to schedule their everyday routines so that they gradually increase the amount of time they engage in occupations throughout the day and/or gradually increase the duration of engagement in one particular occupation. Remember, to increase muscle endurance the therapist must increase the number of repetitions of a specific motion, not just an activity. Programming for cardiovascular endurance specifically with patients who have cardiopulmonary problems is discussed in Chapter 47.

Summary Review Questions

1. What are the physiological aspects of muscle contraction?
2. Give an example of a third-class lever system in the body. What is the force arm (effort force)? What is the resistance arm (resistance force)?

3. Explain lifting a handled shopping bag in terms of torque.

4. Analyze the forces, stability, and motions required to put a can of soup on the shelf at nose height.

5. How should passive stretching treatment be modified if the patient acknowledges residual pain after treatment?

6. What parameters can be manipulated to alter stress on the muscle to increase strength?

7. What are the necessary characteristics of exercise or occupation required to increase muscle endurance?

8. Plan a therapeutic occupation program to strengthen a patient who has generalized poor (2) upper extremity musculature. Revise the program to accommodate changes in the patient's musculature from poor (2) to fair (3).

9. Differentiate between a therapeutic occupation program designed to strengthen muscles and one designed to increase muscle endurance.

10. Following replacement of the PIP joint of the ring finger, the patient's finger and hand are edematous. What treatment choices does the occupational therapist have?

Resources

Harlowe, D., & Yu, P. (1993). *ROM relaxation: Body awareness & breathing*. Distributed by The ROM Institute, 3601 Memorial Dr., Madison, WI 53704.

Harlowe, D., & Yu, P. (1993). *The ROM dance: Seated version*. Distributed by The ROM Institute, 3601 Memorial Dr., Madison, WI 53704.

Lee, K., & Marcus, S. (1990). *Home Rehabilitation Exercises: Shoulder, Elbow, Forearm, Wrist, and Hand* (English). American Occupational Therapy Association. www.aota.org.

References

Brannon, F. J., Geyer, M. J., & Foley, M. W. (1993). *Cardiac Rehabilitation: Basic Theory and Application* (2nd ed.). Philadelphia: Davis.

Brody, L. (1999a). Mobility impairment. In C. M. Hall & L. T. Brody (Eds.), *Therapeutic Exercise: Moving Toward Function* (pp. 87–111). Philadelphia: Lippincott Williams & Wilkins.

Brody, L. T. (1999b). Endurance impairment. In C. M. Hall & L. T. Brody (Eds.), *Therapeutic Exercise: Moving Toward Function* (pp. 70–86). Philadelphia: Lippincott Williams & Wilkins.

Bunker, T. D., Potter, B., & Barton, N. J. (1989). Continuous passive motion following flexor tendon repair. *Journal of Hand Surgery, 14-B*, 406–411.

Davies, P. M. (1985). *Steps to Follow: A Guide to the Treatment of Adult Hemiplegia*. Berlin: Springer-Verlag.

DeLateur, B. J., & Lehmann, J. F. (1990). Therapeutic exercise to develop strength and endurance. In F. J. Kottke & J. F. Lehmann (Eds.), *Krusen's Handbook of Physical Medicine and Rehabilitation* (pp. 480–519). Philadelphia: Saunders.

DeLorme, T. (1945). Restoration of muscle power by heavy resistance exercises. *Journal of Bone and Joint Surgery, 27*, 645–667.

DeLorme, T., & Watkins, A. L. (1948). Technics of progressive resistance exercise. *Archives of Physical Medicine and Rehabilitation, 29*, 263–273.

Downing, A., Martin, B., & Stern, L. (1991). Methods for measuring the characteristics of movements of motor-impaired children. *Assistive Technology, 2*, 131–141.

Enos, L., Lane, R., & MacDougal, B. A. (1984). Brief or new: The use of self-adherent wrap in hand rehabilitation. *American Journal of Occupational Therapy, 38*, 265–266.

Fetters, L., & Todd, J. (1987). Quantitative assessments of infant reaching movements. *Journal of Motor Behavior, 19*, 147–166.

Gelberman, R. H., Nunley, J. A., Osterman, A. L., Breen, T. F., Dimick, M. P., & Woo, S. L.-Y. (1991). Influences of the protected passive mobilization interval on flexor tendon healing: A prospective randomized clinical study. *Clinical Orthopaedics, 264*, 189–196.

Glass, T. A., deLeon, C. M., Marottoli, R. A., & Berkman, L. F. (1999). Population based study of social and productive activities as predictors of survival among elderly Americans. *British Medical Journal, 31*, 478–483.

Greene, D. P., & Roberts, S. (1999). *Kinesiology: Movement in the Context of Activity*. St. Louis: Mosby.

Hall, C. M., & Brody, L. T. (1999). Impairment in muscle performance. In C. M. Hall & L. T. Brody (Eds.), *Therapeutic Exercise: Moving Toward Function* (pp. 43–69). Philadelphia: Lippincott Williams & Wilkins.

Hallum, A., & Medeiros, J. M. (1987). Effect of duration of passive stretch on hip abduction range of motion. *Journal of Orthopedic and Sports Physical Therapy, 18*, 408–415.

Hassmen, P., & Koivula, N. (1997). Mood, physical working capacity and cognitive performance in the elderly as related to physical activity. *Aging (Milano), 9*(1–2), 136–142.

Hertling, D., & Kessler, R. (1996). The wrist and hand complex. In D. Hertling & R. M. Kessler (Eds.), *Management of Common Musculoskeletal Disorders: Physical Therapy Principles and Methods* (3 ed., pp. 243–284). Philadelphia: Lippincott.

Kisner, C., & Colby, L. A. (1990). *Therapeutic Exercise: Foundations and Techniques* (2nd ed.). Philadelphia: Davis.

Kottke, F. J. (1990). Therapeutic exercise to maintain mobility. In F. J. Kottke & J. F. Lehmann (Eds.), *Krusen's Handbook of Physical Medicine and Rehabilitation* (4th ed., pp. 436–451). Philadelphia: Saunders.

Lan, C., Lai, J. S., Chen, S. Y., & Wong, M. K. (1998). 12-month Tai Chi training in the elderly: Its effect on health fitness. *Medicine and Science in Sports and Exercise, 30*, 345–351.

LaStayo, P. C. (1995). Continuous passive motion for the upper extremity. In J. M. Hunter, E. J. Makin, & A. D. Callahan (Eds.), *Rehabilitation of the Hand: Surgery and therapy* (4th ed., pp. 1545–1560). St. Louis: Mosby.

LaStayo, P. C., Wright, T., Jaffe, R., & Hartzel, J. (1998). Continuous passive motion after repair of the rotator cuff: A prospective outcome study. *Journal of Bone and Joint Surgery, 80-A*, 1002–1011.

Luttgens, K., & Hamilton, N. (1997). *Kinesiology: Scientific Basics of Human Motion* (9th ed.). Madison: Brown & Benchmark.

Mandel, D., Jackson, J., Zemke, R., Nelson, L., & Clark, F. (1999). *Lifestyle Redesign: Implementing the well elderly program*. Bethesda: American Occupational Therapy Association.

McPherson, J., Schild, R., Spaulding, S., Barsamian, P., Transon, C., & White, S. C. (1991). Analysis of upper extremity movement in four sitting positions: A comparison of persons with and without cerebral palsy. *American Journal of Occupational Therapy, 45*, 123–129.

Melvin, J. L. (1996). *Fibromyalgia Syndrome: Getting Healthy*. Bethesda, MD: American Occupational Therapy Association.

Morrissey, M. C., Harman, E. A., & Johnson, M. J. (1995). Resistance training modes: Specificity and effectiveness. *Medicine and Science in Sports and Exercise, 27*, 648–660.

Naylor, E., Penev, P. D., Orbetya, L., Janssen, I., Ortiz, R., Colecchia, E. F., Keng, M., Finkel, S., & Zee, P. C. (2000). Daily social and physical activity increases slow-wave sleep and daytime neuropsychological performance in the elderly. *Sleep, 23*(1), 87–95.

Norkin, C., & Levangie, P. K. (1992). *Joint Structure and Function: A Comprehensive Analysis* (2nd ed.). Philadelphia: Davis.

Salter, R. B. (1999). *Textbook of Disorders and Injuries of the Musculoskeletal System* (3rd ed.). Baltimore: Williams & Wilkins.

Segal, R. S., & Wolf, S. L. (1990). Morphological and functional consequences for therapeutic exercise. In J. P. Basmajian & S. L. Wolf (Eds.), *Therapeutic Exercise* (5th ed, pp. 1–48). Baltimore: Williams & Wilkins.

Shankar, K. (1999). *Exercise Prescription*. Philadelphia: Hanley & Belfus.

Shephard, R. J. (1997). What is the optimal type of physical activity to enhance health? *British Journal of Sports Medicine, 31*, 277–284.

Sietsema, J. M., Nelson, D. L., Mulder, R. M., Mervau-Scheidel, D., & White, B. E. (1993). The use of a game to promote arm reach in persons with traumatic brain injury. *American Journal of Occupational Therapy, 47*, 19–24.

Slater, R. B. (1993). *Continuous Passive Motion (CPM): A Biological Concept for the Healing and Regeneration of Articular Cartilage, Ligaments, and Tendons: From Its Origination to Research to Clinical Application*. Baltimore: Williams & Wilkins.

Smith, L. K., Weiss, E. L., & Lehmkuhl, L. D. (1996). *Brunnstrom's Clinical Kinesiology* (5th ed.). Philadelphia: Davis.

Soderberg, G. L. (1997). *Kinesiology: Application to Pathological Motion* (2nd ed.). Baltimore: Williams & Wilkins.

Trombly, C. (1992). Deficits of reaching in subjects with left hemiparesis: A pilot study. *American Journal of Occupational Therapy, 46*, 887–897.

Trombly, C. A. (1995). Theoretical foundation for practice. In C. A. Trombly (Ed.), *Occupational Therapy for Physical Dysfunction* (4th ed. pp. 15–27). Baltimore: Williams & Wilkins.

Van Deusen, J., & Harlowe, D. (1987). The efficacy of the ROM Dance Program for adults with rheumatoid arthritis. *American Journal of Occupational Therapy, 41*, 90–95.

Voss, D. E., Ionta, M. K., & Myers, B. J. (1985). *Proprioceptive Neuromuscular Facilitation: Patterns and Techniques* (3rd ed.). Philadelphia: Harper & Row.

21

Optimizing Motor Behavior Using the Occupational Therapy Task-Oriented Approach

Julie Bass-Haugen, Virgil Mathiowetz, and Nancy Flinn

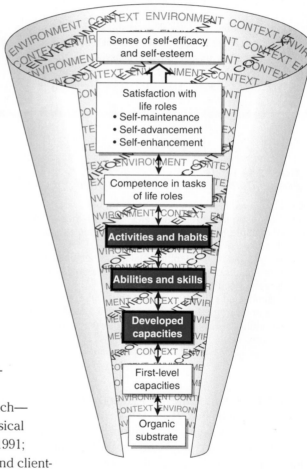

LEARNING OBJECTIVES

After studying this chapter, the reader will be able to do the following:

1. Name the treatment principles of the Occupational Therapy (OT) Task-Oriented Approach.
2. Discuss personal and environmental factors that may be major influences on occupational performance.
3. Define the terms unique to the OT Task-Oriented Approach.
4. Explain the roles of the client and the therapist in the OT Task-Oriented Approach.

*T*he OT Task-Oriented Approach emerges from a systems model of motor behavior and is influenced by recent developmental and **motor learning** (skill acquisition) theories. Two primary bodies of knowledge serve as the basis for the approach— task-oriented approaches that have been discussed in the physical therapy and exercise science literature (e.g., Davis & Burton, 1991; Horak, 1991) and OT models that that are occupation-based and client-centered (Christiansen & Baum, 1997; Law et al., 1997; Trombly, 1995). In particular, the model of occupational functioning (Trombly, 1995) contributes to an emphasis on roles and tasks in the OT task-oriented approach. The model of occupational functioning clearly influences the occupational therapy systems model of motor behavior depicted in Figure 5-3.

Before reading further, review the model, theories, assumptions, and basic evaluation ideas related to this approach in Chapter 5 and principles of learning in Chapter 12. This chapter examines

GLOSSARY

Attractor—Preferred but not obligatory pattern of motor behavior that emerges from the interaction of a unique person with a particular task and environment.

Blocked practice—Practice that consists of drills and requires many repetitions of the same task in the same way (Schmidt, 1991).

Closed task—A task with stable environmental conditions and consistency from one trial to the next.

Collective variable—Fewest number of variables or dimensions that describe a unit of behavior quantitatively.

Continuous task—Repetitive task without a clear beginning or end.

Control parameter—Variable that shifts behavior from one preferred pattern to another and does not control the change but acts as agent for reorganization of behavior (Heriza, 1991)

Degrees of freedom—Elements that are free to vary.

Discrete task—Task involving movements with a recognizable beginning and end.

Motor learning—Acquisition of general strategies for solving movement problems in a variety of contexts.

Open task—Task in which some features of the environment are in motion or unstable and there is variation from one trial to the next.

Part learning—Practice of separate steps of a task.

Phase shift—Transition, often nonlinear, from one preferred qualitative coordinated pattern to another (Heriza, 1991).

Random practice—Practice of tasks that vary randomly within the session (Schmidt, 1991).

Serial tasks—Tasks with connected discrete movements.

Whole learning—Practice of a task in its entirety.

BOX 21-1
Assumptions for the OT Task-Oriented Approach

- ► Functional tasks help organize motor behavior.
- ► Occupational performance emerges from the interaction of multiple systems that constitute the unique characteristics of the person and environment.
- ► After CNS damage or other changes in personal or environmental systems, clients' behavioral changes reflect attempts to achieve functional goals.
- ► Practice and active experimentation with varied strategies and in varied contexts are needed to find the optimal solution for a motor problem and develop skill in performance.

---

specific treatment strategies related to the assumptions of this approach (Box 21-1).

Many ideas (e.g., occupational performance, person, environment) presented as part of the OT Task-Oriented Approach are as old as occupational therapy itself. However, recent motor behavior literature provides a stronger theoretical basis for using purposeful and meaningful tasks as the primary treatment modality. The development of this approach is still evolving. The motor behavior, physical therapy, and adapted physical education literature is examined for identification of principles and key concepts related to task-oriented

approaches. Similarly, the OT literature on client-centered, occupation-based models is used to frame the task-oriented approach in an OT context. There is limited but growing empirical support for the assumptions and treatment principles of this approach. Further development of the OT Task-Oriented Approach and empirical research will provide direction for future practice.

Because this approach suggests that the client have active involvement in treatment, it may have limited applications in acute settings and for clients with significant cognitive impairments. However, some aspects of the OT Task-Oriented Approach (e.g., use of real objects and natural environments, focus on meaningful tasks and functional goals) are appropriate even in these situations.

Treatment Principles and Practices

The treatment principles and general treatment goals are listed in Box 21-2 and are described next. Box 21-3 summarizes general indicators used to determine when to discontinue treatment.

Client-Centered Focus

A client-centered focus is an integral aspect of the OT Task-Oriented Approach.

Adopt a Client-Centered Focus in Treatment

Many therapists refer to the art and science of OT. The art of the OT Task-Oiented Approach is the identification of interventions for the unique needs of each client, taking into account unique personal and environmental sys-

tems and roles that have importance and meaning for the individual. Thus, treatment planning cannot be prescriptive. No cookbook strategies are correct for every person in every environment. This may seem overwhelming to the student who is trying to process much

---

BOX 21-2
PROCEDURES FOR PRACTICE

Treatment Principles of a Task-Oriented Approach

Client-Centered Focus

- ▶ Adopt a client-centered focus in treatment.
- ▶ Elicit active participation of the client during treatment.

Occupation-Based Focus

- ▶ Use functional tasks as the focus in treatment.
- ▶ Select tasks that are meaningful and important in the client's roles.
- ▶ Analyze the characteristics of the tasks selected for treatment.
- ▶ Describe the movements used for task performance.
- ▶ Determine whether the movement patterns are stable or in transition.
- ▶ Analyze the movement patterns and functional outcomes of task performance.

Person and Environment

- ▶ Identify the personal and environmental factors that serve as major influences on occupational performance.
- ▶ Anticipate that the personal and environmental variables influencing occupational performance will change.
- ▶ Address critical personal and environmental systems to cause change in occupational performance.
- ▶ Treat neural and nonneural factors of the sensorimotor

system that interfere with optimal occupational performance.
- ▶ Adapt the task or broader environment to promote optimal occupational performance.
- ▶ Use natural objects and natural environments.

Practice and Feedback

- ▶ Structure practice of the task to promote motor learning.
- ▶ Design the practice session to fit the type of task and learning strategies.
- ▶ Provide feedback that facilitates motor learning and encourages experimentation with solutions to occupational performance problems.
- ▶ Optimize occupational performance given the constraints on the person and environment.

General Treatment Goals

- ▶ Discover the optimal movement patterns for task performance.
- ▶ Achieve flexibility, efficiency, and effectiveness in task performance.
- ▶ Develop problem-solving skills by clients so they can identify their own solutions to occupational performance problems in home and community environments.

BOX 21-3
PROCEDURES FOR PRACTICE

Discontinuing Treatment

The therapist looks for one or more of these indicators to assist in determining when it is appropriate to discontinue treatment:

- ▶ The client is satisfied with performance of occupations and related roles.
- ▶ The client spontaneously uses efficient and effective movements that are stable but flexible in functional tasks.
- ▶ The client has developed independent and effective skills for solving occupational performance problems in the home and community.

- ▶ The client uses movement patterns and demonstrates functional outcomes of task performance that are optimal given the constraints on the person and environment.
- ▶ The client easily reverts to long-standing obligatory or irregular movement patterns after an intervention is withdrawn.
- ▶ The client does not demonstrate more optimal movements patterns or improved task performance after critical personal or environmental systems have been systematically modified.

new information. However, these challenges in practice can be the very things that make OT so exciting and rewarding.

In the OT Task-Oriented Approach, assessment and the planning of treatment should look different for each client. This may sound obvious to the student who has had limited experience in clinical settings. However, it has been shown that in practice assessment, documentation and treatment activities often do not reflect the priorities and meaningful occupations identified by clients (Neistadt, 1995a, 1995b).

Elicit Active Participation of the Client During Treatment

Clients should have an active role in treatment. They should guide selection of tasks for treatment and contribute to finding solutions for occupational performance problems. Clients who are actively engaged in their treatment show achievement in self-identified goals (Trombly et al., 1998), increased functional independence at discharge, and discharges to less restrictive environments (Gibson & Schkade, 1997).

There are several ways to facilitate active participation in treatment. Provide user-friendly instructions on how to practice tasks outside of the therapy session and structure clients' environments to facilitate this practice (Ada et al., 1990). Create therapeutic environments that are conducive to active learning by attending to both organizational and physical structures of the setting. An environmental analysis can assist in determining whether the broader environment promotes passivity or active involvement in treatment. Characteristics of an active learning environment are summarized in Box 21-4.

Teach clients the principles of task analysis (Higgins, 1991) and how to evaluate their own performance in terms of the outcomes of their efforts and the efficiency and effectiveness of their movement patterns. Involve clients in graphing their results and recording progress toward functional goals (Ada et al., 1990). A goal of therapy is to help clients understand the movement patterns and the performance contexts that contribute to optimal performance for given tasks (Burton & Davis, 1992). The therapist promotes understanding of personal capabilities and limitations and encourages exploration of modifiable environmental resources (Higgins, 1991). These strategies assist clients in developing skills needed for solving motor problems in their home and community.

Give skilled clients permission to solve their own motor problems and to use movement patterns that are the most functional for them, regardless of how these strategies are perceived by others (Burton & Davis, 1992; Latash & Anson, 1996). When clients become skilled in task analysis and solving motor problems, the therapist

---

BOX 21-4
Characteristics of an Active Learning Environment

▶ Create an environment that encompasses the common challenges of everyday life.
▶ Develop learning contracts that describe shared rehabilitation goals.
▶ Develop a cohesive team that is committed to active learning.
▶ Require clients to communicate their need for help in specific tasks to staff.
▶ Give clients control over when and where they are to be transported.
▶ Give able clients responsibility for routine housekeeping.
▶ Arrange chairs in small circles in reception and common areas.
▶ Provide opportunities for practice outside of therapy.
▶ Provide written instructions, audiotapes, videotapes, and diagrams for practice.
▶ Organize the environment to match the level of performance.
▶ Illustrate progress to clients.

Ada, L., Canning, C., & Westwood, P. (1990). The patient as active learner. In L. Ada & C. Canning (Eds.), *Key issues in Neurological Physiotherapy* (pp 99–124). Boston: Butterworth Heinemann.

---

can celebrate their participation in various tasks and autonomy in learning (Higgins, 1991). This is true even when clients' solutions are not traditional or identical to the strategies therapists would recommend. For example, Mattson, a wheelchair racer with a C6-7 spinal cord lesion, found he could propel faster using a backhand stroke that maximized use of his remaining muscle groups (Burton & Davis, 1992). This technique was unconventional, but Mattson's performance dramatically improved, and soon afterward many other wheelchair racers were using the same technique. Thus people may use unique movement patterns because they require the least amount of energy and are an efficient means of achieving a functional goal (Kamm et al., 1990).

Occupation-Based Focus

The intervention plan for the OT Task-Oriented Approach is occupation-based.

Use Functional Tasks as the Focus in Treatment

The goal of treatment for motor behavior problems is to enable clients to do the things they want to do now and in the future. Thus, at each point from the initial evaluation to recording progress to discharge to follow-up the determination of the effectiveness of interventions is performance on functional tasks. The interventions themselves also emphasize the practice of real functional tasks.

There is renewed interest in functional tasks and goals in clinical and basic research. Neurological recovery from central nervous system (CNS) dysfunction requires task-related training (Dobkin, 1998), and functional disability is one of the most important predictors of discharge outcomes (Brodie, Holm, & Tomlin, 1994). Thus, recently developed evaluations in OT emphasize measures of functional task performance. Treatment protocols for motor behavior problems emphasize using functional tasks (Burton & Davis, 1992; Carr & Shepherd, 1998) as both the means and ends in the treatment process (Gray, 1998; Trombly, 1995).

Many studies have examined the effect of functional goals on motor behavior. Thelen and Fisher (1983) studied kicking behavior in 3-month-old infants. They found that kicking increased when a mobile was tied to the leg by way of a control line. Adults with hemiplegia have demonstrated more repetitions of movement patterns when an occupation-based activity was used rather than rote exercise (Hsieh et al., 1996). Research is also beginning to support the idea that occupation-based interventions are more effective than other interventions in addressing impaired performance components such as coordination (Flinn, 1999; Neistadt, 1994; Trombly & Wu, 1998). Finally, functional tasks are preferred by many clients over other types of treatment activities (Zimmerer-Branum & Nelson, 1995).

The results of these studies support the idea that therapists' interventions for motor behavior problems should revolve around meaningful occupations and functional goals. The functional goals of interest in OT are broad. Basic activities of daily living (ADL) and instrumental activities of daily living (IADL) tasks are important. However, the tasks should also address functional tasks in other self-maintenance, self-advancement, and self-enhancement roles. See the Research Note.

Select Tasks That Are Meaningful and Important to the Client's Roles

The importance of many functional tasks is unique to the individual. What is important to one person may not be important to another. So how do therapists determine the key tasks for a given individual? They should consider a client's occupational roles and the meaning of these roles to the person (see Chapter 3). Life satisfaction is not determined by successful completion of a random set of functional tasks (e.g., changing a diaper and taking out the garbage). Satisfaction or reward comes from the feeling that roles are fulfilled (e.g., parent and homemaker). Roles are defined by the client in terms of the tasks and related activities that are interesting or important (Fisher & Short-DeGraff, 1993; Pollock, 1993; Trombly, 1993, 1995). For example, two clients may view the role of parent differently. One may identify washing a child's clothing as a key functional

---

RESEARCH NOTE

Treatment-Induced Cortical Reorganization After Stroke in Humans
Liepert, J., Bauder, H., Miltner, W. H. R., Taub, E., & Weiller, C. (2000). Stroke, 31, 1210–1216

ABSTRACT

The purpose of this study was to evaluate reorganization of the motor cortex in individuals with stroke who had received constraint-induced movement therapy. Thirteen subjects with stroke in the chronic stage participated in a 12-day period of constraint-induced movement therapy. They used the affected arm exclusively in a variety of tasks during the therapy period. Focal transcranial magnetic stimulation was used to map the cortical motor output area of a hand muscle on both sides before and after treatment. Results showed that before treatment, the affected hand muscle had a significantly smaller cortical representation area than the contralateral side. After treatment, the cortical representation of the affected hand muscle was significantly enlarged. There was also a corresponding improvement in motor performance of the affected limb. In follow-up studies to 6 months after treatment, motor performance remained improved and the cortical area sizes in the two hemispheres became almost identical and close to the normal condition. This study supports a therapy-induced improvement in movement and long-term alteration in brain function after stroke.

IMPLICATIONS FOR PRACTICE

▶ Individuals use whatever movements are possible and needed to achieve functional goals. In constraint-induced movement therapy, individuals use the affected arm for task performance when the unaffected arm is not available.

▶ The motor cortex demonstrates neuronal plasticity after stroke even in the chronic stage.

▶ Constraint-induced movement therapy programs that incorporate a variety of tasks may influence cortical reorganization after stroke and improve movements and performance.

task, whereas another may view playing touch football as more important. These two functional tasks vary greatly in their environments and in the motor behaviors required to achieve the functional goals.

The consideration of roles also helps the occupational therapist tap into the personal motivations of clients for performing particular tasks. When a client is motivated to change motor behaviors, it usually reflects an internal desire to perform, acquire, or accomplish something (Crutchfield & Barnes, 1993). This motivation may occur because the degree of skill in performance is not personally satisfactory (Higgins, 1991) or because of other personal and environmental influences (Lewthwaite, 1990). In summary, select tasks that are within the realm of capabilities, are goal oriented, have meaning for the clients, and motivate them.

Finally, the therapist must consider that role change is a likely outcome of CNS dysfunction, including a loss of some previous roles and acquisition of new roles (Hallett et al., 1994). Thus, temporal information on past, current, and future roles can guide the treatment planning process and help identify related occupations. Chapters 3 and 5 provide guidelines for considering occupational roles and occupational functioning along a continuum of time (Law et al., 1990).

Analyze the Characteristics of the Tasks Selected for Treatment

After a specific task has been selected for treatment, a task analysis is necessary because clients' capabilities vary and different tasks require different skills. Task analysis entails an examination of the task requirements and the personal capabilities to determine whether there is a match that permits task performance. If there is no match, the occupational therapist plans interventions that address the problems of the client or the characteristics of the environment or both. The outcome of a task analysis helps the therapist design appropriate motor learning experiences and select practice and feedback strategies that fit the nature of the task. Several classification schemes may be useful in task analysis (Davis & Burton, 1991; Gentile, 1987; Schmidt, 1988).

In Schmidt's (1988) classification, tasks and the required movements for tasks are described as **discrete**, **serial**, or **continuous**. Skilled performance in a continuous task is generally retained even when there are periods when practice is impossible (Crutchfield & Barnes, 1993). For example, most people learn to ride a bike when they are quite young. As an adult, they may go through long periods when there is no opportunity to practice this skill. However, once you learn to ride a bike, you easily remember it later after only brief practice. On the other end of the continuum are tasks requiring discrete movements. Many skilled movements used in sports with balls (e.g., hitting, slam dunking, and

pitching) are discrete: they have a definite beginning and end. Frequent practice of the movements is required to maintain skill at a high level. Neither discrete nor continuous tasks are easily broken into steps, as serial tasks are.

Gentile (1987) proposed a taxonomy of tasks based on characteristics of the environment and a person's actions during task performance. The environment is described in terms of its characteristics and variability in these characteristics from one performance to the next. The environment, which includes objects, supporting surfaces, and other people, may be stationary or in motion during a given task. In addition, there may be variation or consistency in these environmental characteristics from trial to trial. When the environment is stationary during performance and does not change from one trial to the next, the task is a **closed task**. Signing your name on a check at a desk is a closed task, because the environment is generally stable and unchanging. In an **open task**, some features of the environment are in motion and vary from one performance to the next. These tasks are complex and place many demands on the person, because the performance context is unstable and changes for different trials. Driving a car is an open task (Poole, 1991) because the driver must process the motions of other cars, pedestrians, and the broader performance context (e.g., snow or rain). Furthermore, these features of the environment vary dramatically from one trip to another.

The function of a person's actions is the second dimension in Gentile's (1987) taxonomy. This dimension consists of the person's actions during task performance and includes body orientation and object manipulation. In a given task, body orientation might require stabilization or transport. For example, during a word processing task, the trunk and lower extremities primarily provide stability. In a tennis match, however, the trunk and lower extremities move or transport toward the ball. Actions are also analyzed in terms of whether the upper extremities provide stability or manipulate objects. For example, the upper extremities help maintain balance and are part of the postural support system when a person walks on a wet kitchen floor. In this situation there is no object manipulation. In washing the floor, however, arms and hands are used for object manipulation (e.g., mop or sponge). The complete taxonomy proposed by Gentile combines the environmental context and the function of the action dimensions and results in 16 categories of tasks.

Describe the Movements Used for Task Performance

A description of the preferred movement patterns that emerge for a given task in a given context helps guide treatment. Preferred movement patterns, or **attractors**,

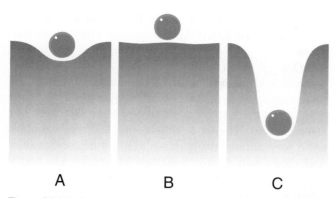

Figure 21-1 Various attractor states. **A.** Shallow well, stable and flexible attractor state. **B.** No well, no attractor state. **C.** Deep well, stable and inflexible attractor state.

are ordinarily stable and the optimal way to achieve a functional goal because they are efficient and effective (Kamm et al., 1990). A preferred movement pattern can be illustrated by how a marble moves on different surfaces (Fig. 21-1). The wells in the figure depict the stability of the patterns (Thelen, 1989). The marble on a surface with a shallow well (Fig. 21-1A) illustrates optimal movement patterns used for everyday tasks. The movements tend to be stable, just as a marble would tend to fall into the same well. However, this well is shallow enough that the marble can move out of it, signifying how a person can modify movements or use a new movement pattern if there is a change in the person or environment.

For example, how would you describe movements used to write your name? One characteristic is that there is a fair amount of consistency in the way a person moves as he or she writes. These preferred movements are usually the best movements for a given situation (e.g., writing on paper with a pencil at a desk). There may be some variations in the ways people move in this situation, but the movements do not vary widely. However, there is also some flexibility in movements, so that if a needs arises (e.g., one has a blister on a finger or wants to use a stick to write in the sand) a person can temporarily or permanently change the movements used to complete the task. Many clients with CNS damage show good motor recovery and resumption of movement patterns similar to this example. They resume stable but flexible performance of tasks in their daily lives (Fig. 21-1A).

Clients in the acute stage of recovery often use movement patterns that show little stability (Fig. 21-1B). Their performance is similar to the movement patterns represented by a marble on a flat or bumpy surface—very irregular and unpredictable. It may appear that there is no preferred movement pattern. Every time they do a task, they do it in a different way. As a result, task performance is not efficient or effective. This is similar to

the movement patterns seen the first few times a new sport is tried.

Other clients seem obligated to perform a task in only one way (Fig. 21-1C). In this situation, the well is so deep that a large perturbation or disturbance would be needed to dislodge the marble or to change the preferred movement pattern. Performance is likely to revert to this pattern soon after treatment. This movement pattern may be effective for task performance in one context, but the person may be unable to achieve functional goals in varied contexts because there is no flexibility in movement patterns. For example, a client may use a flexor pattern for all tasks that require reaching. This pattern may be effective when the arm is only an assist in some bilateral reaching tasks; however, most reaching tasks require complex and varied motor skills. For these tasks, the client may be unable to adapt movements and so unable to achieve the functional goals. These obligatory patterns are often observed in persons years post CNS damage.

Determine Whether the Movement Patterns Are Stable or in Transition

The next step is to determine whether the movement patterns are stable or in transition. This information is important because it helps the therapist identify the optimal times to provide treatment and the strategies necessary to produce a change in the preferred movement patterns (Kamm et al., 1990; Scholz, 1990). The beginning of a transition period may coincide with aging, CNS damage, a new environment, or many other factors. Data on movement patterns are gathered by analyzing task performance and by constructing an individual developmental profile of previous changes in motor behavior (Thelen, 1989). The therapist observes performance of the same task several times in the same context and then in different contexts. Intervention is not needed if the preferred movement pattern is relatively efficient and effective for a given task and is stable but flexible so that it can be modified for different contexts. On the other hand, if there is no preferred movement pattern or if the pattern is fixed, the therapist may consider treatment to facilitate change in movement patterns and occupational performance.

If the movement patterns are in transition, there is increased variability in the movements used to complete a task and increased susceptibility to change or perturbation by the influence of some personal or environmental systems. In addition, movement patterns take longer to return to a stable state if perturbed (Heriza, 1991). These findings mark a potential transition period or **phase shift** and may be characterized as a marble on a smooth or bumpy surface (Fig. 21-1B). When the movement patterns are unstable or in transition, therapists are generally more likely to facilitate a change to different patterns—ones, it is hoped, that are more efficient and effective in achieving the task goal. Remediation of motor behavior problems should begin before the movement patterns fall into obligatory, stereotyped patterns (Kamm et al., 1990).

If the movement patterns are stable in a particular performance context, it may be more difficult to produce a change in the way the task is performed in that context. In this scenario, change in movement patterns is less likely, and the person is apt to return easily to the preferred pattern, even if it is possible to produce a temporary change. This stability may be characterized as preferred but flexible (Fig. 21-1*A*) or obligatory (Fig. 21-1*C*). For example, neuromotor synergy patterns may represent the stable, obligatory movement patterns of a damaged system. If the movement patterns have been obligatory or irregular for a long time, interventions may not effect a change to other movement patterns. In this case, perhaps only a trial period of therapy is warranted.

Analyze the Movement Patterns and Functional Outcomes of Task Performance

An analysis of movement patterns will help estimate stability and flexibility, understand changes, and prevent fixation of movement patterns (Kamm et al., 1990; Scholz, 1990). Scholz used an example to illustrate two strategies for evaluating the stability of movement patterns. Consider the gait of a child with cerebral palsy. The preferred pattern for this child may be a bunny hop, and a goal of therapy may be to move toward a reciprocal pattern of walking. One quantitative measure of movement patterns may be the relative phase of the hip motions as measured by videography. That is, are the hip motions in the same phase (both in flexion) or in opposite phases (one in flexion and the other in extension)? The therapist analyzes the fluctuations in the relative phase when the child is using the preferred pattern, the bunny hop. Next, this pattern is perturbed by slowing the locomotion or by imposing a physical restraint on one lower extremity. The therapist learns the child's movement patterns for this task by analyzing how much slowing or restraint is needed to change to a reciprocal pattern and how long it takes to return to a bunny hop after the critical factors are removed.

The first strategy is to look at fluctuations in one or more quantitative measures of movement patterns during task performance. The second strategy is to determine what happens when the therapist tries to disturb or perturb the movement patterns by changing some critical personal or environmental factors. Therapists ask themselves how much change is necessary to disturb the pattern and how long it takes for the movement pattern to return to the previous state. The quantitative measures of movement patterns are **collective variables**, and the critical factors influencing behavior are **control parameters**.

One of the challenges in the OT Task-Oriented Approach is identification of collective variables, the measures of movement that can describe in simple terms all of the systems that cooperate to produce movements (Heriza, 1991; Thelen & Ulrich, 1991). These variables are a way of objectively measuring the motor behavior and changes in motor behavior. Therapists are beginning to discover ways to measure the outcomes of functional performance. However, sometimes OT interventions are not intended to result in a substantial change in the outcome. For example, a client may have achieved moderate independence in bathing but still not have optimal performance. The goal in OT may be to help change the movement patterns used for getting out of the tub so that performance is more safe and efficient. Thus, measures are needed to document progress in motor performance as well as levels of independence.

Recent motor behavior research may help to identify these potential measures of occupational performance. Slow reaction times, slow movement times, increased variability in performance, movement trajectories with discontinuities, and rate or speed limitations have been noted in disorders of movement (Campbell, 1991; Corcos, 1991). One measure that is easy to use in treatment is time (time to begin the task, time to complete the task, and time until movement patterns regress to previous pattern after being perturbed). As videography and movement analysis become more accessible in clinical settings, occupational therapists may measure the relative timing of one motion with respect to another (relative phase), the curvature or straightness of movements (trajectories), the distance and direction of movement (displacement), and the speed or constancy of speed (velocity, accelerations, and decelerations) (Corcos, 1991; Fetters, 1991; Heriza, 1991; Scholz, 1990). Finally, movement pattern categories or comprehensive descriptors of movement may help to describe sequences of movements and natural variation in movement patterns for certain tasks. For example, VanSant (1991) described unique movement pattern categories of the upper extremities, lower extremities, and axial region used by different age groups for a variety of righting tasks.

Person and Environment

The interventions used in the OT Task-Oriented Approach address personal and environmental systems to enable optimal occupational functioning.

Identify the Personal and Environmental Factors That Serve as Major Influences on Occupational Performance

The therapist begins treatment planning by examining tasks that were difficult for the person to perform and describing the preferred movement patterns for these tasks. The therapist then identifies the personal and environmental systems that support optimal functional performance and those that contribute to ineffective performance (Letts et al., 1994). The interactions of these systems are also important (Shepherd, 1992) (see Chapter 5). Part of the OT process, then, is making systematic changes in personal characteristics (e.g., attention and positioning) and environmental context (e.g., size of object and stability of base of support) and observing the effect on occupational performance. This process can help identify one or several critical factors (control parameters) that can cause a shift in motor behavior.

A qualitative analysis (observation and description) also may be used to describe the interactions of person and environment on task performance. For example, VanSant (1991) identified the personal systems used for activities requiring righting (e.g., rising from a bed and getting up from a chair or the floor). She found that the preferred movement patterns for these activities are influenced by body dimensions (e.g., ratio of leg length to body length; size of body relative to bed or chair; height; weight; body build and topography), age, gender, and activity level. Thelen (1989) studied treadmill stepping in infants and found that neurological and morphological maturation and the postures of the leg were the critical factors influencing the movements used. Velocity has been identified as a control parameter in the locomotion patterns used by people and animals (Scholz, 1990). If a horse is forced to increase its speed, changes in movements associated with a walk, trot, and gallop can be observed (Crutchfield & Barnes, 1993). Such studies are critical in helping occupational therapists identify the critical systems inherent in performing particular tasks.

It may seem impossible to identify only a couple of systems from the multiple systems and subsystems that influence motor performance. However, occupational therapists already do this, using quantitative and qualitative analysis. Consider the task of placing items on a shelf above shoulder level. Now imagine, or better yet actually try, placing various items on the shelf. Consider the different movement patterns used to lift an empty paint can and a full paint can to the high shelf. What is the critical factor that explains the change in movement patterns when lifting an empty can versus a full can? It is the weight of the can relative to arm strength. What is the critical factor that explains the change in movement patterns when lifting a tennis ball versus a beach ball in the same task (assuming weight is held constant)? In this situation, it is the size of the object relative to hand size. Both of the critical factors in these examples are performer-scaled variables (Davis & Burton, 1991), or parameters that link a characteristic of the person (e.g., strength or hand size) to a characteristic of the object that is used in the task (e.g., weight or size).

Thelen (1989) stated that it is also important to consider unobvious and distantly related factors as possible critical factors. She described studies showing that the onset of crawling, a motor skill, is an influential factor in cognitive, affective, and social changes in children. The ability to move to another environment is a critical factor that can cause a dramatic change in the problem-solving, communication, and play behaviors of children.

One last clinical example is used to propose other systems that might serve as critical factors. In one long-term care setting, health care professionals were wondering why older men who had had cerebrovascular accidents were not achieving independence in dressing. One therapist hypothesized that it was loss of automatic reactions and postural control. Other therapists proposed that motor planning problems or general loss of strength and endurance explained the performance deficit. Again, all of these systems did indeed influence motor behavior. However, a family member revealed that the critical factor for the motor behaviors related to dressing was the culture of the residents. That is, most residents in this setting were members of a culture that did not place value on independence in self-care for older adults, especially men who had disease-related impairments. In fact, it was an expectation that women in the extended family would come to the residence every day to complete ADL.

There are several purposes in relating these examples. One is to challenge therapists to use creativity and common sense in treatment. For given individuals with given tasks, the critical factors may be neural or nonneural sensorimotor components (e.g., soft tissue contracture, muscle weakness, and abnormal muscle tone). However, occupational therapists sometimes neglect important factors like a different culture and look only at performance components that seem directly related to the motor behaviors. No system automatically deserves more attention than any other system unless research indicates otherwise.

Anticipate That the Personal and Environmental Variables Influencing Occupational Performance Will Change

The critical variables influencing motor behavior change over time. CNS damage affects each system differently relative to occupational performance. This idea is illustrated in Figures 21-2 and 21-3, which depict hypothetical

Case Example

MR. B.: APPLICATION OF THE OT TASK-ORIENTED APPROACH

Client Information

Mr. B., 55 years old, had a left cerebral vascular accident with resultant right hemiparesis 6 months ago. He is on disability status from his job as an administrator at a junior college. His medical and social history is further described in Chapter 5. His goal in outpatient rehabilitation is to participate in a trial of the student counseling aspect of his administrative job to determine whether he has potential to return to work.

OT will work on tasks related to his role as mediator in student issues. The following tasks were identified as important for success in this role: contact student to gather information and set up meeting; review documentation; meet the student in a conference room; discuss issue with student; document discussion; return to office; write, copy, and send report on the outcome to student and others as needed.

It was agreed that documenting the discussion during the meeting was a critical component of the role and had to be addressed. During a simulation of a meeting, a number of problems related to performance of this task were evident: slow movement in bringing his chair close to the table; slow movement in bringing his arm to rest on top of the table; slow movement and limited endurance in grasping a regular pen; decreased speed and accuracy and increased variation in cursive writing.

Critical factors impairing performance were the weight of the conference room furniture, decreased strength (power) in shoulder flexion, and decreased strength (power) and endurance in palmar pinch. Critical factors suggesting improved future performance were adequate budget for needed supplies and furniture, Americans With Disabilities Act support for return to work, desire to appear capable to handle task, good cognitive skills, and supportive secretary.

Recommendations

The occupational therapist recommended three 1-hour treatment sessions at the college. The first session was to take place immediately. The second session would take place after supplies and furniture arrived, and the third session would take place about a week after the second session. (Separate recommendations were developed for other tasks related to his role as mediator.)

Short-Term Goals

The occupational therapist and Mr. B. established these short-term goals: At the end of two sessions, Mr. B. will independently (1) adjust furniture in the conference room to prepare for task performance; (2) use a tape recorder to record the discussion; (3) record notes during a 5-minute discussion with sufficient completeness and accuracy for development of a report.

During the first session, a conference room chair with adjustable height, wide armrests, and swivel seat was ordered. A tape recorder with voice activation, adjustable speed, and an internal microphone was requisitioned. Felt-tip pens with a textured grip were acquired. Several adapted pens and pen holders were lent to Mr. B. for a trial period. A practice session of writing using various pens and grasps was conducted. Mr. B. also helped design a home program of additional tasks that would strengthen targeted muscle groups in the right hand. The tasks included reaching for the spices needed for each meal, organizing cupboards, buttering bread, and writing down recipes.

During the second session, Mr. B. practiced a variety of ways to position himself for efficient writing. He learned to adjust the chair and use the swivel feature to position the chair close to the table before sitting. When moving from standing to sitting, Mr. B. could use his right arm as an assist by placing it on the table as he lowered himself. Mr. B. was instructed in and practiced operation of the tape recorder. Use of the left hand was better for manipulation of the small buttons on the recorder when efficiency in performance was needed. The occupational therapist observed Mr. B.'s right-handed writing using different devices and timed (1) bringing right arm from lap to table, (2) picking up pen, and (3) completing specified writing task. Summary feedback was provided after each performance. The home program was adjusted to promote practice of positioning self and operating the recorder and to increase the task demands related to targeted muscle groups. Finally, the occupational therapist worked with Mr. B. and the secretary to develop a template and some codes for recording discussions and reducing the writing requirements during the discussion.

During the third session, Mr. B. demonstrated all components of the task. He practiced variations in task performance. Mr. B. was instructed in strategies for analyzing his own performance. Increased speed in bringing the right arm from the lap to the table was noted. Movement time for picking up the pen was still slow. It was agreed that the left hand would pick up the pen and hold it vertical to allow an easier and quicker grasp by the right hand. The right palmar pinch had increased in strength and endurance sufficiently to enable completion of a 10-minute writing task with the felt-tip pen. The home program was adjusted to promote practice of use of codes in simulated discussions and to continue work on tasks related to targeted muscle groups.

Revised Goal

Within 4 weeks, Mr. B. will independently record notes during a 15-minute discussion with sufficient completeness and accuracy for development of a final report.

CLINICAL REASONING
in OT Practice:

Mr. B.

▸ What information could you use to determine whether Mr. B.'s optimal performance of the writing task is with his left or right hand?

▸ What other personal or environmental factors might influence Mr. B.'s performance in a discussion with a real student (see assessment of Mr. B. in Chapter 5)?

▸ What might be some future changes in the personal or environmental factors influencing performance, given what you know about Mr. B.?

▸ How would you determine when performance is optimal and when to discontinue treatment for this particular goal?

---

changes in systems and subsystems over time for a unique person. The *y* axes represent the system's degree of positive or negative influence on occupational performance, and the *x* axes represent these changes over time from onset of CNS damage to the rehabilitation stage to discharge or home. Some systems are highly affected immediately after CNS damage, while other systems become more important later. For example, the physical environment in Figure 21-2 may become a more important variable when the person returns home. The home may or may not support performance of previous occupational roles and tasks. In rehabilitation settings, the physical environment is designed for persons with physical disabilities and thus may not be as important because the setting is so unlike the natural environment. Systems that influence occupational performance at one time may not be the critical systems at other times. Figure 21-3 shows the effects of neural and nonneural components of muscle tone at different points in time. Based on our clinical experience, neural factors (e.g., spasticity) are important immediately after the onset of CNS damage but have less of an effect on performance later. The influence of nonneural factors (e.g., soft tissue contracture), however, is almost the reverse.

A client's occupational performance at any one time reflects the interaction of all of these systems. The critical variables at a given time may vary greatly, depending on the characteristics of the person and environment. What is effective for one client may not be effective for the next client with similar CNS dysfunction. In addition, systems that enhance performance at one time may interfere with it later (Kamm et al., 1990). What is effective early in treatment may not be effective later. Therapists must identify the major influences on motor behavior at a specific time for a specific person and anticipate changes in the critical variables.

Address Critical Personal and Environmental Systems to Change Occupational Performance

After a critical personal or environmental factor is identified, the therapist alters this personal or environmental characteristic until a shift in motor behavior is observable. Relatively small changes in a critical personal or environmental system may produce large changes in the movement patterns used for a task (Thelen, 1989). For example, putting an infant in water (Thelen, 1989) or an adult on a treadmill with partial body weight support (Hesse et al., 1995) dramatically affects walking. Forcing use of an affected arm by constraining the other arm (Morris, 1997; Wolf et al., 1989) or application of a splint to provide wrist support (Kamm et al., 1990) may change the upper extremity movement patterns and thus change occupational performance. The goals of OT are to help individuals identify and use critical factors that support optimal performance and to determine the optimal value for producing the best performance outcome (Burton & Davis, 1992).

Treat Neural and Nonneural Factors of the Sensorimotor System That Interfere With Optimal Occupational Performance

Studies show that many subsystems of the sensorimotor system, not just neural subsystems, may have a role in motor behavior after CNS damage. For example, increases in muscle strength are related to improved functional performance in clients with hemiparesis (Andrews et al., 1981; Bohannon, 1986). Sabari (1991) described an inability to dissociate the scapula from the thorax or the pelvis from the lumbar spine, weakness of specific muscles, inability to counteract gravitational forces, abnormalities in muscle tone, and incorrect timing of components within a movement as possible sensorimotor factors constraining movement in a hemiplegic

Case Example

MRS. M.: APPLICATION OF THE OT TASK-ORIENTED APPROACH

Client Information

Mrs. M. is 34 years old and married with two children, 6 and 9 years old. She was diagnosed with relapsing or remitting multiple sclerosis 3 years ago, although she had various intermittent symptoms for at least 10 years before the diagnosis. She has had two exacerbations in the past 3 years lasting 3 to 4 weeks. Primary symptoms were severe fatigue, blurred vision, constant tingling and numbness in both hands, muscle weakness in both arms, and leg weakness so severe she couldn't walk. Both times she recovered to her previous level of function. When in remission, Mrs. M. reports tingling in her left, nondominant hand and left arm weakness; occasionally her left leg gives out, resulting in a momentary inability to bear weight. Her main concern is the daily fatigue that comes on suddenly, like hitting the wall, which also makes the other symptoms worse. She fatigues in the afternoon, although she works until 4:00, picks up her children from after-school programs, and makes dinner. In the evening, her left arm is frequently so weak she cannot use it, and she is too fatigued to move off the couch. If she attends an evening event, it takes an entire day of rest to regain the energy and strength in her left arm.

Her husband works in retail, with hours on weekends and many evenings. He is usually home in the morning to prepare and clean up after breakfast and get the children off to school. He does all of the grocery shopping and other miscellaneous errands. Mrs. M. does the evening meal preparation, laundry, and housekeeping. Evening meal preparation is valued as a meaningful task in her role as a mother but is challenging because of her fatigue at the end of the day. Laundry is difficult because the machines are in the basement and she makes frequent trips up and down the stairs. She has difficulty carrying the large basket full of clothes because of the weakness in her arm. Sometimes she drags the basket up the stairs with her right arm. Vacuuming is easier because she has a small carpeted living room and can vacuum using her right arm. She gets her housework done on Saturday morning and sleeps most of the afternoon because of fatigue.

She works as an office receptionist, recently reducing her work schedule from full time to 3 days per week. The job requires phone work, word processing, and occasional filing. She sits most of the time. Her employer knows she has multiple sclerosis but did not make work accommodations, since she has not requested any.

Mrs. M. used to enjoy bicycling, gardening, and needlework but has not participated in any of these activities in 2 years. Needlework is hard because of her weak grip, and if she does anything more than her usual work activities, she says, "I pay for it the next day."

Mrs. M. wants to continue working because they need the money. She also believes it is important to have regular dinners with her children to provide stability, since her husband is often absent in the evenings.

Recommendations

The occupational therapist recommended two 1-hour treatment sessions at home to address Mrs. M.'s goals related to working and meal preparation. The first session took place immediately. The second session took place after Mrs. M. completed a trial of modifications to her routine and environment.

Short-Term Goals

The occupational therapist and Mrs. M. established these short-term goals: Within two weeks, Mrs. M. will (1) satisfactorily complete 3 work days a week without reporting excessive fatigue and (2) prepare a meal 3 evenings a week without reporting excessive fatigue.

During the first session, the therapist asked Mrs. M. to outline the activities of her day and week and indicate when fatigue was most severe. They discussed principles of energy conservation and identified specific strategies that she would try during the next 2 weeks. Examples include taking frequent rests before feeling tired, planning the day, and developing a daily and weekly schedule to improve efficiency. In consultation with the occupational therapist, Mrs. M. decided to ask her employer to allow her to take a 10-minute break every hour and a half rather than her usual lunch break. She also asked permission to bring an incline chair to work so she could rest comfortably during her breaks. Before making dinner, Mrs. M. would take a 10-minute rest as soon as she came home and delegate table preparation to the children while she cooked. In addition, the children would prepare one simple course for the meal (e.g., salad) and clear the table and load the dishwasher.

During the second session, Mrs. M. reported on her work and meal preparation using the modified routine. She reported decreased fatigue for these two occupations. Additional strategies were suggested for further modifying the routine and environment.

Revised Short Term Goal

Within 1 month, Mrs. M. will engage in one self-enhancement task a week without affecting her ability to do necessary tasks and without excessive fatigue.

CLINICAL REASONING
in OT Practice

Mrs. M.

▶ What information did the therapist likely use to determine that fatigue was a critical variable for Mrs. M.?

▶ What are some additional personal or environmental factors to address in the future?

▶ How would you measure progress toward the revised short-term goal?

▶ What other goals would you like to explore in collaboration with Mrs. M.?

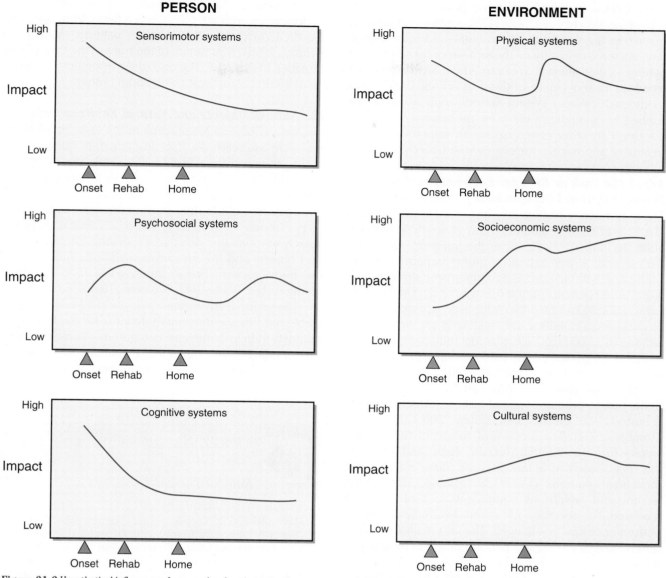

Figure 21-2 Hypothetical influences of personal and environmental systems on occupational performance for a unique person at different times (at onset, during rehabilitation, and at home).

arm. Significant sensorimotor deficits in the unaffected upper extremity of individuals who have had cerebrovascular accidents have also been documented (Desrosiers et al., 1996).

These sensorimotor factors offer alternative explanations for the movement patterns used by clients. For example, a client with hemiparesis may use a flexor pattern for reaching or lifting because of muscle weakness. A person without CNS damage uses this pattern, too. Imagine lifting a very heavy object, say a television. Describe the positions of the arms. The arms are pulled in close to the body (a flexor pattern), because arm strength relative to the weight of the object requires use of a biomechanically efficient pattern (a short resistance

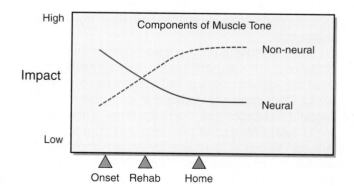

Figure 21-3 Hypothetical influences of neural and nonneural components of muscle tone on occupational performance at different points in time (at onset, during rehabilitation, and at home).

arm). Clients may use this same pattern when lifting something as light as a feather. Their limited arm strength relative to the weight of the feather—and more important, the force of gravity on the arm—require an efficient pattern as they attempt to control the many **degrees of freedom** in movement of the arm (Flinn, 1995). Thus biomechanical and system factors, such as those described by Spaulding (1989) for prehension and those discussed in other chapters, are an important part of treatment approaches for clients with CNS dysfunction.

Adapt the Task or Broader Environment to Promote Optimal Occupational Performance

The performance context is as important as the personal characteristics in treatment (Dunn et al., 1994; Fisher & Short-DeGraff, 1993). Consider the following examples. People with lower extremity motor impairments can scuba dive without special equipment and do so as well as any other person (Burton & Davis, 1992). On the other hand, walking can be difficult for even a person without physical impairments if the walking is attempted at an altitude of 15,000 feet. What factors influence motor behavior in these two examples? In both cases, the ability or inability to perform a task is context dependent.

There are various ways to alter the physical context of the task to promote optimal task performance (Davis & Burton, 1991; Gentile, 1987; Gillen, 2000; Sabari, 1991; Trombly, 1994). The slope and height of the support surface may be adjusted. The size, shape, and texture of the object used in a task may be varied to alter the movement patterns (Fuller & Trombly, 1996). Size, length, and weight of equipment or tools may be modified. The accuracy and speed requirements for task performance can be changed. The information required or provided as part of task performance can be adjusted in terms of timing, precision, and abstractness of the response. These adaptations are similar to the compensatory strategies described in other OT approaches. In the OT Task-Oriented Approach, the therapist explores modifications of the physical performance context to promote optimal functional performance, not simply to compensate.

Systems other than the physical context must also be considered. Heriza (1991) and Thelen (1989) emphasized the importance of social influences on motor behavior. They reviewed studies that show that infants' locomotion changes and develops faster when there is social reinforcement of the behaviors. The social and cultural context of performance is also emphasized in several recent approaches (Dunn, 1993; Spencer et al., 1993). Therapists themselves are part of the broader environment in occupational performance (Newell, 1998). They coach clients to help them discover and adopt optimal patterns of task performance (Scholz, 1996). They structure the learning activities and provide feed-

back to help clients achieve reliable, stable, and efficient performance without prohibiting clients from identifying their own optimal movement patterns (Masters & Polman, 1996). A summary of the roles of the therapist is provided in Box 21-5. The role of environmental systems on motor behavior must be explored further.

Use Natural Objects and Natural Environments

Use natural objects for practice of the task. Simulations and rote exercise do not produce the same movement patterns as tasks using real objects. Studies of persons with stroke showed more efficient, direct, smooth, and planned movements in reaching tasks enriched with natural objects than in the condition without objects (Trombly & Wu, 1998; Wu et al., 1998). Other research supports the idea that the greater the number of real objects and the greater the symbolic information, the more performance is improved (Lin et al., 1998; Mathiowetz & Wade, 1995; Wu et al., 1998).

Use natural environments to help clients develop stable but flexible movement patterns for the tasks and contexts in their home and community (Burgess, 1989). The rehabilitation unit should simulate the real-life setting as much as possible if interventions cannot be

BOX 21-5
PROCEDURES FOR PRACTICE

Roles of Therapist

Many roles for the therapist are proposed in the literature (Burton & Davis, 1992; Gentile, 1992; Heriza, 1991; Higgins, 1991; Kamm et al., 1990). All are important in helping the client to become autonomous in solving motor problems.

- Collaborate with the client in selecting a variety of tasks for practice.
- Modify the task initially so the learner can succeed.
- Teach task analysis, structure learning opportunities, provide feedback, and facilitate understanding of unique personal and environmental systems that promote optimal performance.
- Provide ungeneralizable solutions that the client can memorize if the client cannot learn using this approach.
- Coach the client during learning by directing the focus to the functional outcome, suggesting movements to try, recording progress, and assisting with decision making when new challenges arise.
- Alter the personal and environmental factors and identify optimal times to change movement.
- Provide manual guidance if necessary, but allow some elements to vary so that the client can experiment with movement patterns.
- Fade assistance provided through handling as soon as possible.

provided in the actual situation (Mulder, 1991; Poole, 1991). Therapeutic modules (Stahl, 1993) simulate community-based environments. Many rehabilitation units have apartments with ordinary home furniture. Other resources of the institution can also simulate community settings (e.g., gift shop, cafeteria, and chapel).

Practice and Feedback

The design of practice sessions and characteristics of feedback are important in interventions based on the OT Task-Oriented Approach.

Structure Practice of the Task to Promote Motor Learning

Until recently, motor learning, or the outcome of practice, was primarily measured in terms of observable changes in performance during or immediately after practice. Our goal for the outcome of practice, however, is that clients can perform better once they leave treatment. Research in motor learning (Schmidt, 1991) shows that measurement outcomes of the performance during practice are not the same as later performance. If the goal is to improve motor performance over the long term, the effectiveness of the practice must be evaluated in terms of later performance.

Some practice sessions include drills that require clients to perform many repetitions of the same task in the same way (Schmidt, 1991). This is called **blocked practice**. For example, for dressing, the client is presented a series of steps that must be practiced again and again in the same manner. Recent studies have examined the type of practice that is most beneficial for changing the capability for later performance. These studies (Hanlon, 1996; Schmidt, 1991) suggest that practice of tasks should vary randomly (**random practice**); that is, therapists should ask clients to try a variety of dressing tasks within one session. One thing to remember when adopting a random practice approach is that performance during the practice session may actually look worse than performance after blocked practice. This is acceptable because the goal is to enhance motor learning or the capability for later performance rather than change observable behaviors during a practice session.

Variation of the context within a task is also an important component of practice (Jarus, 1994; Keshner, 1991; Lee et al., 1991; Mulder, 1991; Sabari, 1991; VanSant, 1991). Manipulation of task dimensions such as support surfaces, objects, equipment, task demands, and required information are examples of strategies to vary the context (Davis & Burton, 1991). Varied contexts promote development of preferred movement patterns for specific contexts and flexibility in movement patterns

for different contexts (Heriza, 1991; Thelen, 1989). The client who practices only in a narrow context learns only a limited number of solutions. However, the client who practices the task in many contexts learns many solutions and can vary performance (Higgins, 1991). Bernstein (1967) summarized this principle by stating that people need repetition without repetition.

Design the Practice Session to Fit the Type of Task and Learning Strategies

Research shows that different types of tasks require different types of practice sessions to facilitate learning (Winstein, 1991). Practice may require the client to practice the task in its entirety (**whole learning**), in separate steps (**part learning**), or in some combination of whole and part learning. Winstein (1991) studied weight shifting with part learning to improve locomotion, a continuous task, in persons with hemiparesis. She found that persons in the treatment group using part learning did improve in the symmetry of standing posture but showed no significant improvement over a control group in actual locomotion. Whole learning rather than part learning is generally recommended for both continuous and discrete tasks (Crutchfield & Barnes, 1993). Separate practice (i.e., part learning) of the discrete components of a serial task is beneficial. Kerr (1982) stated that the complexity of the task should also be taken into consideration. When the task is relatively simple, whole learning is recommended. Part learning is suggested for more complex tasks.

The stages of learning have been described as discovery (cognitive), mastery (associative), and generalization (autonomous) (Fitts & Posner, 1967; Higgins, 1991). Many clients are in the discovery stage as they develop an understanding of the task, identify the performance problems, and find a general solution for their new capabilities. This stage is characterized by slow performance, clumsiness, and self-imposed rigidity or freezing of body parts to control all degrees of freedom that are normally free to vary in high levels of skill. In this stage, clients attempt to exert control over some parts of the body to learn the influence of changes in their personal systems and relationships to the environment (Higgins, 1991). Later stages of learning help the client refine the solutions identified in the discovery stage and generalize these solutions to other tasks. The behaviors in these later stages are more consistent, more accurate, faster, and better coordinated (see Chapter 12).

Therapists must also consider the type of learning that the practice session will elicit (Gentile, 1998). Explicit (declarative) learning requires conscious learning of the rules for task performance and is more generalizable because it is not very context dependent. Implicit (procedural) learning requires learning how to do the task on an unconscious level. This type of learning is facilitated by structuring the environment and practice of the task. Chapter 12 provides additional detail on these aspects of learning.

Provide Feedback That Facilitates Motor Learning and Encourages Experimentation With Solutions to Occupational Performance Problems

If the goal is to have clients rely on intrinsic feedback for task performance in the future, careful planning of the extrinsic feedback during treatment is important. Using intuition and earlier perspectives on feedback, therapists often assume that frequent, immediate, and consistent feedback is best. Lee et al. (1991), Schmidt (1991), and Winstein (1991) reviewed results of studies on appropriate feedback strategies related to the knowledge of results or the outcome of performance. Studies of people without motor problems suggested that feedback should be less frequent, scheduled randomly or intermittently, faded over time, and given as summary information or when performance is outside a given error range. These feedback strategies resulted in better retention of motor skills over time than frequent, immediate, and consistent feedback. Preliminary studies of individuals post stroke (Merians et al., 1995) indicate that reduced frequency of feedback improved performance consistency but not accuracy. Further research on feedback with subjects having motor problems is needed. Therapists should carefully analyze the effect of their feedback on individual clients' performance.

Optimize Occupational Performance Given the Constraints on the Person and Environment

> "Optimization in the process of therapeutic intervention should be directed at a functional outcome rather than a peripheral motor pattern [with the primary goal of OT] to promote learning in a functionally significant context so that adaptive solutions are developed and optimized by the CNS with respect to a certain activity."
>
> (Latash & Anson, 1996, p. 98)

After CNS damage, clients may have to learn strategies for task performance given personal limitations. When clients understand the idea of the task, their personal limitations and capabilities, environmental resources, and a basic solution to the problem, they may begin to practice the task. The inefficient and ineffective movements sometimes seen at this time are consistent with the limited understanding and control one has during the early stages of learning and at the lower levels of skill (Higgins, 1991). Perhaps the client simply needs further practice and time to develop skill. However, therapists must identify ineffective movement patterns that are hindering optimal task performance or contrib-

uting to future problems in personal and environmental systems. Mulder (1991) added one more caution regarding the analysis of preferred patterns: The achievement of functional outcomes is probably more important to the client and family than the therapist's goal of "normal" movement patterns. Again, a client-centered approach focused on meaningful occupations and roles is important.

Limitations and Future Directions

A consideration of limitations and future directions is important in the discussion of any occupational therapy approach.

Limitations

There are some limitations to the OT Task-Oriented Approach. It is not yet fully developed or refined, and efficacy studies must be done. It is also difficult to simulate natural environments or some work and leisure tasks in many clinical settings. However, as therapy clinics are remodeled and new clinics are designed, there is potential to create more natural environments in the hospital. This limitation suggests that therapy interventions should ideally occur in clients' home, school, leisure, and work settings whenever possible. The increased pressure to shorten hospital stays and the increased development of community-based treatment programs should support this trend. Another limitation of this approach relates to communication problems when using concepts that originate outside of OT and the testability of an approach based on abstract, complex ideas (Horak, 1991).

Future Directions

All treatment approaches evolve over time. Clinical practice and research will test the assumptions and treatment principles of this approach. Some assumptions and principles will be supported and developed further. Others will not be supported and may be dropped or modified. The OT Task-Oriented Approach provides occupational therapists with new ideas about the remediation of motor behavior problems. Basic and clinical research is needed. Development of evaluation tools and measures of change is critical. Identification of critical factors influencing occupational performance and measures of motor behavior will lead to more effective treatment strategies. Further testing of this approach with persons having CNS dysfunction and other motor behavior problems is needed to provide additional support for its use in practice. The authors challenge the reader to join us in this process.

Summary Review Questions

1. What are the treatment principles of the OT Task-Oriented Approach?
2. What does *attractor* mean? Describe the characteristics of the different movement patterns illustrated by Figure 21-1 in terms of attractor states. Give examples of these patterns that might be observed in clients who are attempting to achieve functional goals.
3. What are optimal and less than optimal times for producing a change in motor behavior?
4. What are some strategies for making the treatment process more client centered and unique to the characteristics of the person and environment?
5. What is the role of the client in the OT Task-Oriented Approach? The therapist?
6. How is change in motor behavior measured?
7. What are some possible measures of performance, and how are they important in determining whether optimal performance is achieved?
8. What are critical variables (i.e., control parameters) or systems of the person and environment, and how should they be used in treatment to facilitate optimal performance?
9. What are the characteristics of skilled and optimal performance, and how can therapists facilitate development of these characteristics in their clients?
10. Describe feedback that facilitates development of skill in performance and an optimal solution to a motor problem.
11. Why are natural objects and environments important to use in finding the optimal solution for a motor problem and develop skill in performance?

References

Ada, L., Canning, C., & Westwood, P. (1990). The patient as active learner. In L. Ada & C. Canning (Eds.), *Key issues in Neurological Physiotherapy* (pp 99–124). Boston: Butterworth Heinemann.

Andrews, K., Brocklehurst, G. C., Richards, B., & Laycock, P. J. (1981). The rate of recovery from stroke and its measurement. *International Rehabilitation Medicine, 31,* 155–161.

Bernstein, N. (1967). *The Coordination and Regulation of Movements.* Oxford, UK: Pergamon.

Bohannon, R. W. (1986). Strength of lower limbs related to gait velocity and cadence in stroke patients. *Physiotherapy Canada, 38,* 204–206.

Brodie, J., Holm, M., & Tomlin, G. (1994). Cerebrovascular accident: Relationship of demographic, diagnostic, and occupational therapy antecedents to rehabilitation outcomes. *American Journal of Occupational Therapy, 48,* 906–913.

Burgess, M. K. (1989). The issue is: Motor control and the role of occupational therapy: Past, present, and future. *American Journal of Occupational Therapy, 43,* 345–348.

Burton, A. W., & Davis, W. E. (1992). Optimizing the involvement and performance of children with physical impairments in movement activities. *Pediatric Exercise Science, 4,* 236–248.

Campbell, S. K. (1991). Framework for the measurement of neurologic impairment and disability. In M. J. Lister (Ed.), *Contemporary Management of Motor Control Problems: Proceedings of the II STEP Conference* (pp. 143–154). Alexandria, VA: Foundation for Physical Therapy.

Carr, J. H., & Shepherd, R. B. (1998). *Neurological Rehabilitation: Optimizing Motor Performance.* Oxford: Butterworth-Heinemann.

Christiansen, C., & Baum, C. (1997). *Occupational Therapy: Enabling Function and Well-Being.* Thorofare, NJ: Slack.

Corcos, D. (1991). Strategies underlying the control of disordered movement. *Physical Therapy, 71,* 25–38.

Crutchfield, C. A., & Barnes, M. R. (1993). *Motor Control and Motor Learning in Rehabilitation.* Atlanta: Stokesville.

Davis, W. E., & Burton, A. W. (1991). Ecological task analysis: Translating movement behavior theory into practice. *Adapted Physical Activity Quarterly, 8,* 154–177.

Desrosiers, J., Bourbonnais, D., Bravo, G., Roy, P.-M., & Guay, M. (1996). Performance of the "unaffected" upper extremity of elderly stroke patients. *Stroke, 27,* 1564–1570.

Dobkin, B. (1998). Activity-dependent learning contributes to motor recovery. *Annals of Neurology, 44,* 158–160.

Dunn, W. (1993). The issue is: Measurement of function: Actions for the future. *American Journal of Occupational Therapy, 47,* 357–360.

Dunn, W., Brown, C., & McGuigan, A. (1994). The ecology of human performance: A framework for considering the effect of context. *American Journal of Occupational Therapy, 48,* 595–607.

Fetters, L. (1991). Measurement and treatment in cerebral palsy: An argument for a new approach. *Physical Therapy, 71,* 244–247.

Fisher, A., & Short-DeGraff, M. (1993). Nationally speaking: Improving functional assessment in occupational therapy: Recommendations and philosophy for change. *American Journal of Occupational Therapy, 47,* 199–201.

Fitts, P. M., & Posner, M. I. (1967). *Human Performance.* Belmont, CA: Brooks/Cole.

Flinn, N. (1995). A task-oriented approach to the treatment of a client with hemiplegia. *American Journal of Occupational Therapy, 49,* 560–569.

Flinn, N. (1999). Clinical interpretation of effect of rehabilitation tasks on organization of movement after stroke. *American Journal of Occupational Therapy, 53,* 345–347.

Fuller, Y., & Trombly, C. (1996). Effects of object characteristics on female grasp patterns. *American Journal of Occupational Therapy, 51,* 481–487.

Gentile, A. M. (1987). Skill acquisition: Action, movement, and neuromotor processes. In J. H. Carr, R. B. Shepherd, J. Gordon, A. M. Gentile, & J. M. Held (Eds.), *Movement Science: Foundations for Physical Therapy in Rehabilitation* (pp. 93–154). Rockville, MD: Aspen.

Gentile, A.M. (1992). The nature of skill acquisition: Therapeutic implications for children with movement disorders. In H. Forssberg & H. Hirschfeld (Eds.), *Movement disorders in children* (pp. 31–40). Basel: S. Karger.

Gentile, A. M. (1998). Implicit and explicit processes during acquisition of functional skills. *Scandinavian Journal of Occupational Therapy, 5,* 7–16.

Gibson, J. W., & Schkade, J. (1997). Occupational adaptation intervention with patients with cerebrovascular accident: A clinical study. *American Journal of Occupational Therapy, 51,* 523–529.

Gillen, G. (2000). Improving activities of daily living in an adult with ataxia. *American Journal of Occupational Therapy, 54,* 89–96.

Gray, J. M. (1998). Putting occupation into practice: Occupation as ends, occupation as means. *American Journal of Occupational Therapy, 52*, 354–364.

Hallett, J. D., Zasler, N., Maurer, P., & Cash, S. (1994). Role change after traumatic brain injury. *American Journal of Occupational Therapy, 48*, 241–246.

Hanlon, R. E. (1996). Motor learning following unilateral stroke. *Archives of Physical Medicine and Rehabilitation, 77*, 811–815.

Heriza, C. (1991). Motor development: Traditional and contemporary theories. In M. J. Lister (Ed.), *Contemporary Management of Motor Control Problems: Proceedings of the II STEP Conference* (pp. 99–126). Alexandria, VA: Foundation for Physical Therapy.

Hesse, S., Bertelt, C., Jahnke, M. T., Schaffrin, A., Baake, P. L., Malezic, M., & Mauritz, K. (1995). Treadmill training with partial body weight support compared with physiotherapy in nonambulatory hemiparetic patients. *Stroke, 26*, 976–981.

Higgins, S. (1991). Motor skill acquisition. *Physical Therapy, 71*, 123–139.

Horak, F. B. (1991). Assumptions underlying motor control for neurologic rehabilitation. In M. J. Lister (Ed.), *Contemporary Management of Motor Control Problems: Proceedings of the II STEP Conference* (pp. 11–27). Alexandria, VA: Foundation for Physical Therapy.

Hsieh, C., Nelson, D., Smith, D., & Peterson, C. (1996). A comparison of performance in added-purpose occupations and rote exercise for dynamic standing balance in persons with hemiplegia. *American Journal of Occupational Therapy, 50*, 10–16.

Jarus, T. (1994). Motor learning and occupational therapy: The organization of practice. *American Journal of Occupational Therapy, 48*, 810–816.

Kamm, K., Thelen, E., & Jensen, J. L. (1990). A dynamical systems approach to motor development. *Physical Therapy, 70*, 763–775.

Kerr, R. (1982). *Psychomotor learning*. New York: CBS.

Keshner, E. (1991). How theoretical framework biases evaluation and treatment. In M. J. Lister (Ed.), *Contemporary Management of Motor Control Problems: Proceedings of the II STEP Conference* (pp. 37–47). Alexandria, VA: Foundation for Physical Therapy.

Latash, M. L., & Anson, J. G. (1996). What are "normal movements" in atypical populations? *Behavioral and Brain Sciences, 19*, 55–106.

Law, M., Baptiste, S., McColl, M., Opzoomer, A., Polatajko, H., & Pollock, N. (1990). The Canadian Occupational Performance Measure: An outcome measurement protocol for occupational therapy. *Canadian Journal of Occupational Therapy, 57*, 82–87.

Law, M., Cooper, B. A., Strong, S., Stewart, D., Rigby, P., & Letts, L. (1997). The person-environment-occupation model: A transactive approach to occupational performance. *Canadian Journal of Occupational Therapy, 63*, 9–23.

Lee, T., Swanson, L., & Hall, A. (1991). What is repeated in a repetition? Effects of practice conditions on motor skill acquisition. *Physical Therapy, 71*, 150–156.

Letts, L., Law, M., Rigby, P., Cooper, B., Stewart, D., & Strong, S. (1994). Person-environment assessments in occupational therapy. *American Journal of Occupational Therapy, 48*, 608–618.

Lewthwaite, R. (1990). Motivational considerations in physical activity involvement. *Physical Therapy, 70*, 808–819.

Lin, K.-C. Wu, C.-Y., & Trombly, C. (1998). Effects of task goal on movement kinematics and line bisection performance in adults without disabilities. *American Journal of Occupational Therapy, 52*, 179–187.

Masters, R. S. W., & Polman, R. C. J. (1996). What are normal movements in any population? *Behavioral and Brain Sciences, 19*, 81–82.

Mathiowetz, V. G., & Wade, M. (1995). Task constraints and functional motor performance of individuals with and without multiple sclerosis. *Ecological Psychology, 7*, 99–123.

Merians, A., Winstein, C., Sullivan, K., & Pohl, P. (1995). Effects of feedback for motor skill learning in older healthy subjects and individuals post-stroke. *Neurology Report, 19*, 23–25.

Morris, D. M. (1997). Constraint-induced movement therapy for motor recovery after stroke. *Neurorehabilitation, 9*, 29–43.

Mulder, T. (1991). A process-oriented model of human motor behavior: Toward a theory-based rehabilitation approach. *Physical Therapy, 71*, 157–164.

Neistadt, M. (1994). The effects of different treatment activities on functional fine motor coordination in adults with brain injury. *American Journal of Occupational Therapy, 48*, 877–882.

Neistadt, M. (1995a). Methods of assessing clients' priorities: A survey of adult physical dysfunction settings. *American Journal of Occupational Therapy, 49*, 428–436.

Neistadt, M. (1995b). Treatment activity preferences of occupational therapists in adult physical dysfunction settings. *American Journal of Occupational Therapy, 49*, 437–443.

Newell, K. M. (1998). Therapeutic intervention as a constraint in learning and relearning movement skills. *Scandinavian Journal of Occupational Therapy, 5*, 51–57.

Pollock, N. (1993). Client-centered assessment. *American Journal of Occupational Therapy, 47*, 298–302.

Poole, J. L. (1991). Motor control. In C. B. Royeen (Ed.), *AOTA Self-Study Series: Neuroscience Foundations of Human Performance* (Monograph 11, pp. 1–31). Rockville, MD: American Occupational Therapy Association.

Sabari, J. S. (1991). Motor learning concepts applied to activity-based intervention with adults with hemiplegia. *American Journal of Occupational Therapy, 45*, 523–530.

Schmidt, R. A. (1988). *Motor Control and Learning: A Behavioral Emphasis* (2nd ed.). Champaign, IL: Human Kinetics.

Schmidt, R. A. (1991). Motor learning principles for physical therapy. In M. J. Lister (Ed.), *Contemporary Management of Motor Control Problems: Proceedings of the II STEP Conference* (pp. 49–63). Alexandria, VA: Foundation for Physical Therapy.

Scholz, J. (1990). Dynamic pattern theory: Some implications for therapeutics. *Physical Therapy, 70*, 827–843.

Scholz, J. (1996). How functional are atypical motor patterns? *Behavioral and Brain Sciences, 19*, 85–86.

Shepherd, R. B. (1992). Adaptive motor behaviour in response to perturbations of balance. *Physiotherapy Theory and Practice, 8*, 137–143.

Spaulding, S. (1989). The biomechanics of prehension. *American Journal of Occupational Therapy, 43*, 302–306.

Spencer, J., Krefting, L., & Mattingly, C. (1993). Incorporation of ethnographic methods in occupational therapy assessment. *American Journal of Occupational Therapy, 47*, 303–310.

Stahl, C. (1993). Rehab in the rain or in a rowboat: New environments bring the outdoors indoors. *Advance for Occupational Therapists, 9*, 14–15.

Thelen, E. (1989). Self-organization in developmental processes: Can systems approaches work? In M. R. Gunnar & E. Thelen (Eds.), *Systems and Development* (pp. 77–117). Hillsdale, NJ: Lawrence Erlbaum.

Thelen, E., & Fisher, D. M. (1983). The organization of spontaneous to instrumental behavior: Kinematic analysis of movement changes during very early learning. *Child Development, 54*, 120–140.

Thelen, E., & Ulrich, B. D. (1991). Hidden skills. *Monographs of the Society for Research in Child Development, 56* (Serial 223). Chicago: University of Chicago.

Trombly, C. (1993). The issue is: Anticipating the future: Assessment of occupational function. *American Journal of Occupational Therapy, 47,* 253–257.

Trombly, C. A. (1994). Purposeful activity. In C. Trombly (Ed.), *Occupational Therapy for Physical Dysfunction* (4th ed., pp. 237–254). Baltimore: Williams & Wilkins.

Trombly, C. A. (1995). Occupation: Purposefulness and Meaningfulness as Therapeutic Mechanisms. *American Journal of Occupational Therapy, 49,* 960–972.

Trombly, C., Radomski, M. V., & Davis, E. S. (1998). Achievement of self-identified goals by adults with traumatic brain injury: Phase I. *American Journal of Occupational Therapy, 52,* 810–818.

Trombly, C., & Wu, C.-Y. (1998). Effect of rehabilitation tasks on organization of movement after stroke. *American Journal of Occupational Therapy, 53,* 333–344.

VanSant, A. (1991). Life-span motor development. In M. J. Lister (Ed.), *Contemporary Management of Motor Control Problems: Proceedings of the II STEP Conference* (pp. 77–83). Alexandria, VA: Foundation for Physical Therapy.

Winstein, C. J. (1991). Knowledge of results and motor learning: Implications for physical therapy. *Physical Therapy, 71,* 140–149.

Wolf, S. L., Lecraw, D. W., Barton, L. A., & Jann, B. B. (1989). Forced use of hemiplegic upper extremities to reverse the effect of learned nonuse among chronic stroke and head-injured patients. *Experimental Neurology, 104,* 125–132.

Wu, C.-Y., Trombly, C., Lin, K.-C., & Tickle-Degnen, L. (1998). Effects of object affordances on reaching performance in person with and without cerebrovascular accident. *American Journal of Occupational Therapy, 52,* 447–456.

Zimmerer-Branum, S., & Nelson, D. (1995). Occupational embedded exercise: A choice between occupational forms by elderly nursing home residents. *American Journal of Occupational Therapy, 49,* 397–402.

22

Optimizing Motor Control Using the Carr and Shepherd Approach

Joyce Shapero Sabari

LEARNING OBJECTIVES

After studying this chapter, the reader will be able to do the following:

1. Identify key concepts and principles from movement science that have influenced Carr and Shepherd's approach to optimizing motor performance.
2. Describe the key factors that contribute to optimal movement and explain how therapeutic interventions can influence each of these key factors.
3. Interpret scores from the *Motor Assessment Scale* and practice using this tool to assess motor performance.
4. Analyze movement during functional task performance to determine occupational therapy treatment goals.
5. Develop individualized treatment plans to assist patients in reaching their optimal motor function in the areas of standing up and sitting down, balance, walking, and reach and manipulation.

*M*otor impairments are significant obstacles to the desired achievement of occupational and role performance of many individuals who have sustained disease or damage to the central nervous system (CNS). Occupational therapists provide intervention to assist these people in (1) optimizing their motor function and (2) integrating their improved motor skills into enhanced performance of functional activities that provide independence and meaning to their daily lives.

Carr and Shepherd, Australian physical therapists, are among a growing group of physical therapists (Duncan & Lai, 1997; Lister, 1991), occupational therapists (Mathiowetz & Bass Haugen, 1994; Trombly & Wu, 1999), and movement scientists (Gentile, 1998; Shumway-Cook & Woollacott, 1995) who apply principles of motor control and learning to practical rehabilitation interventions for people

---

GLOSSARY

Adaptive features—Physiological, mechanical, and functional changes that develop as a person's neuromuscular system attempts to function within the constraints of negative features associated with CNS dysfunction.

Attractor state—Preferred pattern of organization within a system.

Control parameter—Variable that when changed will influence changes in a system's pattern of organization.

Degrees of freedom—Number of elements that are free to vary within a system, hence must be controlled.

Kinematics—Description of movement in terms of direction, speed, and position of body segments.

Kinetics—Description of movement in terms of forces required.

Manual guidance—Hands-on physical cueing by a therapist to provide kinesthetic information about a movement strategy.

Negative features—Losses in motor function directly attributable to CNS pathology.

Positive features—Exaggerations of normal phenomena after CNS pathology due to release of primitive centers from inhibitory hierarchical control.

Practice—Opportunity to develop skill through engagement in tasks that require problem solving and implementation of effective motor strategies.

Postural adjustments—Automatic, anticipatory, and ongoing muscle activation that enables individuals to maintain balance against gravity, optimal alignment between body parts, and optimal orientation of the head, trunk, and limbs in relation to the environment.

---

with motor difficulties due to CNS dysfunction. Carr and Shepherd's ideas are entirely compatible with the OT Task-Oriented Approach presented in Chapter 21. A major difference is that Carr and Shepherd's approach is designed exclusively to improve motor control. Thus, Carr and Shepherd provide specific guidelines for assessing and treating this category of performance component deficits but do not discuss guidelines for enhancing individuals' participation in occupations or social roles.

Carr and Shepherd's specific strategies for helping individuals reach optimal potential in motor control provide a foundation for a critical component of occupational therapy intervention. These strategies are particularly applicable to clients who are coping with residual motor impairments after stroke or traumatic brain injury. The strategies may also be useful in interventions with clients who face challenges presented by a progressive neurological condition such as multiple sclerosis or Parkinson's disease.

Clients who demonstrate potential to improve motor control deserve the opportunity to learn to perform motor tasks with efficiency, fluidity, and versatility. Carr and Shepherd's approach provides occupational therapists with practical guidelines for the following:

▶ Assessment of motor function during task performance
▶ Analysis of motor performance to determine key limiting factors that are amenable to change through therapeutic intervention

▶ Prevention or reduction of these key limiting factors through direct intervention and client education
▶ Design of activities to be used as therapeutic challenges that stimulate development of effective movement strategies
▶ Adaptation of the physical environment to promote maximum function by each individual
▶ Assistance for individuals in developing strategies for approaching and mastering the motor challenges of new activities they may wish to perform in the future.

Theoretical Framework

The framework on which Carr and Shepherd's approach is based includes the dynamical systems theory of motor control, the plasticity of the CNS, and the maladaptive biomechanical changes that occur after CNS injury. Principles of motor learning guide the therapist in structuring the therapeutic environment to maximize patients' recovery of motor function.

Dynamical Systems Theory and CNS Plasticity

A principle of dynamical systems theory, described in Chapters 5 and 21, is that organisms demonstrate an inherent capacity to self-organize throughout life (Perry, 1998). Plasticity (Kolb, 1995) is a system's capacity to reorganize after disruption and to adapt to functional demands. Although damaged neural tissue does not structurally regenerate, plasticity in the mammalian CNS has been well documented (Lee & van Donkelaar, 1995). Neuroscience research (Aizawa et al., 1991; Rossini et al., 1998) has shown that functional improvements after brain lesions are associated with changes in metabolic activity or patterns of neural connections in brain regions that were previously inactive during performance of the function under study. A critical factor common to all situations in which CNS plasticity has been observed is the presentation of environmental opportunities for animal or human research participants to attempt to perform functional tasks previously mediated by the impaired system (Butefish et al., 1995; Johansson, 1996). Environmental challenges serve as the impetus for dynamic reorganization of an injured CNS.

Carr and Shepherd's approach assumes that therapeutic challenges have the potential to influence how a person's neuromuscular system will reorganize itself after injury to the CNS. Furthermore, they recognize that voluntary movements are initiated by functional task goals (Jeannerod, 1990; Willingham, 1998) and are influenced by the spatial and force characteristics of goal objects (Mathiowetz & Wade, 1995; Trombly & Wu, 1999). Therefore, functional task demands are used instead of exercise to provide graded motor challenges.

Dynamical Systems Theory: Attractor States and Control Parameters

Chapters 5 and 21 introduce the term **attractor state**, which refers to a preferred pattern. According to dynamical systems theory (Kamm et al., 1990), people develop preferred movement patterns for various categories of motor performance. Attractor states for activities ranging from handwriting to a golf swing cast a unique and identifiable imprint on each individual's style of performance.

The flexibility of an attractor state is characterized, in a schematic presentation, by the depth of its well (see Fig. 21-1). Movement patterns with shallow wells are extremely unstable. They are inconsistent; they vary each time the task is performed. Movement patterns with deep wells are extremely stable. Deep well patterns make it difficult for the person to achieve versatility in task performance. Neither shallow nor deep attractor wells allow for optimal motor function. When one's neuromuscular system is functioning efficiently, the preferred patterns are characterized by attractor wells that are deep enough to allow for consistent performance but shallow enough to allow sufficient flexibility to deal with varying task and environmental demands.

Control parameters are variables that, when changed, influence changes in motor behavior (Perry, 1998). External control parameters, such as task requirements or features in the environment, frequently elicit variations in performance. In the case of efficient

handwriting, the type of pen and the writing surface influence a person's motor strategies for executing the task. Internal control parameters, such as body alignment, muscle length, and muscle strength, also influence motor behavior. Postural asymmetry or mobility limitations impose constraints that limit a person's choices regarding motor performance. Although Carr and Shepherd do not typically use the terms *attractor states* and *control parameters*, Fig. 22-1 illustrates how these concepts are critical to understanding and implementing their approach. Early in the intervention, internal control parameters for each individual are identified as obstacles to efficient movement. Interventions for preventing or reducing these obstacles to efficient movement are discussed later in this chapter.

Impairments of Interest to Rehabilitation Professionals

Typically, neuroscientists, physicians, and therapists have categorized the motor characteristics of CNS dysfunction as **positive features** or **negative features**. Positive features are exaggerations of normal phenomena due to release of spinal or brainstem reflexes from hierarchical inhibitory control. Positive features of stroke and brain injury include spasticity and hyperreflexia. Since the 1960s, the medical and therapy professions have considered positive features to be the major obstacle to improved clinical function. However, there is no clinical or experimental evidence to support this view (Carr et al., 1995). Furthermore, research findings are increasingly supporting the view that negative features of brain dysfunction are more important than positive features in causing motor disability. Negative features, which include weakness, fatigability, slowness, and impaired dexterity are due to impairments in recruitment

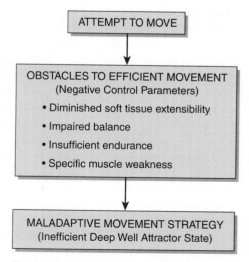

Figure 22-1 Development of maladaptive strategies.

and firing rate modulation of motor neurons (Ada et al., 1996).

Carr and Shepherd have introduced a third category of features associated with upper motor neuron dysfunction. **Adaptive features** are physiological, mechanical, and functional changes in muscle and other soft tissues that develop in response to immobility, disuse, and attempts to move within the constraints of weakness. For occupational therapists, who typically use the term *adaptive* to connote behaviors that are effective in coping with environmental demands, Carr and Shepherd's term may seem misleading. *Secondary impairment*, which indicates areas of dysfunction that are not directly caused by the neurological pathology (Sabari, 1998), is synonymous with Carr and Shepherd's term *adaptive features*. When muscles are immobilized in their shortened position, physiological changes include the loss of sarcomeres and remodeling of connective tissue (Carr et al., 1995; O'Dwyer et al., 1996). Subsequently, muscles undergo mechanical changes of shortening and stiffening. As illustrated in Fig. 22-1, abnormal movement patterns are not necessarily manifestations of spasticity or reflex disinhibition. Rather, they can be explained as functional adaptations to movement demands in the presence of negative symptoms.

Carr and Shepherd advocate early therapeutic intervention after stroke or brain injury to prevent or minimize the adaptive features of central nervous dysfunction. In particular, active and passive mobility is introduced early to prevent and reduce muscle stiffness and shortening.

The Therapeutic Environment

The therapeutic environment is established to facilitate relearning of effective strategies for performing functional movement.

Therapist as Coach

The patient–therapist relationship in Carr and Shepherd's approach is one of active, collaborative mentoring with regard to motor performance. Therapists must have extensive knowledge about the kinetic and kinematic features of movement, both as performed by individuals with intact neuromuscular systems and as frequently observed in people demonstrating specific motor dysfunction, such as hemiparesis or ataxia. Therapists apply this knowledge when assessing performance, setting goals, structuring **practice** sessions, and providing feedback and instruction. The therapist's critical goals as coach are (1) to encourage performance of the most important mechanical features within a given category of motor tasks and (2) to discourage behavioral adaptations that have limited effectiveness.

Treatment is viewed as a teaching–learning process. Learning proceeds most smoothly when the patient has a clear idea of the motor goal and which strategies are appropriate or inappropriate for reaching that goal. Carr and Shepherd recommend that therapists routinely ask patients to describe or demonstrate, with another body segment if necessary, the specific movements required to achieve a task. This provides therapists with a clear understanding of what patients think they are being asked to do. Instructions can then be modified to ensure that each patient and therapist are actually working toward the same goal.

Carr and Shepherd recommend four strategies for providing information to patients. Therapists choose the most appropriate combinations of these strategies to suit the needs of individual patients.

1. Oral instruction is a useful teaching strategy, but only when words are kept to a minimum. The therapist identifies the most important aspect of the movement on which the patient will concentrate during task performance. Oral instructions presented in terms of an object goal are easier to follow than abstract directions to move. For example, "Touch the checker" is more likely to elicit active forward reach than "Reach forward." Of course, oral instructions are replaced or reinforced by nonverbal communication if the patient demonstrates difficulty understanding spoken language.

2. Visual demonstration is generally provided through the therapist's own performance of the task, with a focus on one or two components most important to the patient's development of control. Carr and Shepherd report success with photographs of a patient's maladaptive alignment during task performance and with stick figure drawings that indicate the essential task components (Carr & Shepherd, 1987). These strategies seem particularly effective in teaching tasks that are inherently sequential, such as rising from supine to sitting, standing up, and sitting down.

3. **Manual guidance** helps to clarify the model of action by passively guiding the patient through the path of movement or by physically constraining inappropriate components. During attempts at task-related forward reach, the therapist may provide passive movement to the scapula, with simultaneous cues over the acromion for the patient to limit elevation of the entire shoulder girdle. When a patient attempts to sit down, the therapist's manual guidance behind the shoulders reinforces the concept that the individual must move the upper body forward to achieve the necessary hip and knee flexion for smooth, controlled descent.

4. Accurate, timely feedback about quality of performance helps the individual learn which strategies to repeat and which to avoid. The therapist reserves positive comments for actual improvements in performance. If effort is rewarded in the same way as success, the person receives confusing feedback about the correctness or incorrectness of the motor strategy in question.

Practice

Theories about motor skill acquisition emphasize the active problem-solving aspects of learning (Schmidt, 1992). Correspondingly, Carr and Shepherd's approach views the individual as an active participant whose major goal in rehabilitation is to relearn effective strategies for performing functional movement.

Instead of learning specific movements, participants in Carr and Shepherd's program learn general strategies for solving motor problems. Rather than performing exercises without functional goals, patients practice tasks that require mild variations in movement patterns during successive repetitions. Furthermore, limb movements and **postural adjustments** are always learned simultaneously and in the context of task performance. Whole task performance is emphasized, rather than practicing component parts of tasks.

Carr and Shepherd believe that practice is a critical component to motor skill development. Because patients learn what they practice, it is important that they not revert to compensatory movement strategies during daily activities outside of therapy. Carr and Shepherd emphasize that significant motor improvements are achieved only if patients practice movement according to the therapist's guidelines throughout each day. Therefore, the therapist structures a practice program for each patient to reinforce activities performed during therapy

sessions. Friends and relatives learn effective ways to assist the patient in this program. The therapist provides clear written directions, photographs, drawings, and/or performance checklists to ensure that the additional practice is consistent with the motor strategies promoted during therapy.

Treatment is task specific and based directly on movement analysis of the patient's performance of that task. The therapist continues to reevaluate and analyze the patient's performance throughout each treatment session to make ongoing decisions about intervention. If performance does not improve, the therapist checks the original analysis of the patient's problems and considers whether the training approach should be modified.

Finally, practice includes opportunities for task analysis and motor problem solving through the introduction of novel activities that require application of a particular motor strategy the person has learned in a different context.

Intervention

The next section presents the general framework for intervention using the Carr and Shepherd approach and more specific information for treatment of four key areas of functional movement: standing up and sitting down, balance, walking, and reaching for and manipulating objects.

General Framework

An understanding of factors that contribute to optimal motor performance (Fig. 22-2) is key to applying Carr and Shepherd's framework to occupational therapy intervention. Implicit in their model is a recognition that

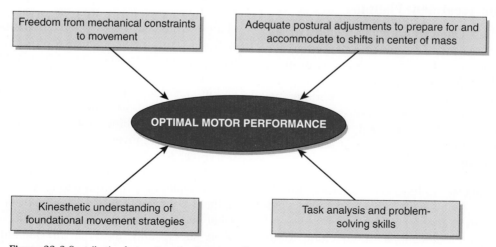

Figure 22-2 Contributing factors to optimal motor performance.

positive and negative features of motor impairment may not be amenable to change through rehabilitation. Therapeutic challenges can certainly assist patients in learning to use their available muscle function, but no known interventions can facilitate muscle firing in the absence of required physiological substrates. Fortunately, therapists can play a critical role in preventing and reducing the adaptive features associated with CNS motor dysfunction. In addition, in our role as coaches, we can assist patients in developing cognitive skills that will enable them to optimize their available levels of motor control.

Carr and Shepherd (1998) present a framework for assessing and improving four general categories of motor performance: standing up and sitting down, walking, reach and manipulation, and balance. For each of these areas, they provide these guidelines for therapists:

▶ Anticipate, prevent, and reduce mechanical constraints that are likely to interfere with performance.
▶ Understand the **kinematics** and **kinetics** that research has shown to accompany typical performance by individuals with intact musculoskeletal function.
▶ Understand how research has shown the kinematics and kinetics of performance to differ in individuals with CNS dysfunction.
▶ Understand how postural adjustments are integrated into efficient task performance.
▶ Structure activities to provide graded challenges to anticipatory and ongoing postural adjustments.
▶ Structure activities that help patients develop a kinesthetic understanding of fundamental movement strategies.
▶ Structure activities that will help patients develop motor task analysis and problem-solving skills.

Evaluation and Treatment Planning

As with the OT Task-Oriented Approach, clinical evaluation is a detailed analysis of the patient's performance of selected tasks in each of the four categories of motor performance. Therapists observe patients as they perform functional activities and compare performance with critical kinematic features that are associated with these tasks (Box 22-1). This observation enables therapists to develop individualized treatment plans, which include the following:

▶ Stretching exercises to lengthen shortened muscles and enhance mobility at body segments where limitations were noted
▶ Environmental modifications or coaching to improve postural alignment

BOX 22-1
PROCEDURES FOR PRACTICE

Assessment

During task observation, the therapist assesses performance for the following:

▶ Evidence of mobility impairments at specific joints
▶ Missing or limited components (e.g., lack of anterior pelvic tilt, hip flexion, ankle dorsiflexion when rising to stand)
▶ Incorrect timing of components within a movement pattern (e.g., inappropriate interplay among extrinsic and intrinsic finger muscles during attempts at grasp)
▶ Evidence of weakness or paralysis of specific muscles (e.g., weakness in quadriceps on attempts to stand up)
▶ Compensatory motor behavior (e.g., elevation of the entire shoulder girdle on attempts to reach forward)

▶ Exercises and activities designed to strengthen muscles that are innervated but weak
▶ Verbal and kinesthetic instruction about key foundational strategies to improve performance
▶ Practice of key fundamental strategies in a variety of other tasks
▶ Practice of the observed task in varying conditions, incorporating newly acquired mobility, muscle strength, and foundational strategies

Patients are active participants in the analysis of their performance. This allows therapists to see how well each person can detect movement problems. In addition, this self-analysis encourages individuals to develop insight about their own movement, develop problem-solving skills, and understand the goals of the treatment program.

Although Carr and Shepherd recommend using a qualitative assessment style as a guide to treatment planning, they have developed a quantitative scale that is useful for documenting progress and conducting research. The *Motor Assessment Scale (MAS)* (Carr et al., 1985, revised: J. Carr & R. Shepherd, personal communication, 1994) consists of eight movements: supine to side-lying, supine to sitting on the edge of the bed, balanced sitting, sitting to standing, walking, upper arm function, hand movements, and advanced hand activities (Box 22-2). As indicated in Box 22-2 and discussed in Chapter 5, each motor activity is scored on a 7-point ordinal scale ranging from 0 to 6. A score of 6 indicates optimal behavior. The *MAS* has enjoyed support in the rehabilitation literature (Gresham et al., 1995) and has been successfully used as an outcome measure in published efficacy studies of clinical intervention (Ada &

BOX 22-2
PROCEDURES FOR PRACTICE

Abridged Criteria for Scoring MAS

The score assigned on each item is the highest criterion met on the best performance of three. A 0 score is assigned if the patient is unable to meet the criteria for a score of 1.

Supine to Side-Lying to Intact Side

1. Pulls self into side-lying with intact arm, moving affected leg with intact leg.
2. Moves leg across actively and lower half of body follows. Arm is left behind.
3. Lifts arm across body with other arm. Moves leg actively; body follows in a block.
4. Actively moves arm across body; rest of body follows in a block.
5. Rolls to side, moving arm and leg; overbalances. Shoulder protracts and arm flexes.
6. Rolls to side in 3 seconds. Must not use hands.

Supine to Sitting on Edge of Bed

1. After being assisted to side-lying, lifts head sideways; cannot sit up.
2. Side-lying to sitting on edge of bed with therapist assisting movement.
3. Side-lying to sitting on edge of bed with standby help assisting legs over side of bed.
4. Side-lying to sitting on edge of bed with no standby help.
5. Supine to sitting on edge of bed with no standby help.
6. Supine to sitting on edge of bed within 10 seconds with no standby help.

Balanced Sitting

1. Sits only with support after therapist assists.
2. Sits unsupported for 10 seconds.
3. Sits unsupported with weight well forward and evenly distributed.
4. Sits unsupported with hands resting on thighs; turns head and trunk to look behind.
5. Reaches forward to touch floor 4 inches in front of feet and returns to starting position.
6. Sitting on stool, reaches sideways to touch floor and returns to starting position.

Sitting to Standing

1. Gets to standing with help (any method).
2. Gets to standing with standby help.
3. Gets to standing with weight evenly distributed and with no help from hands.
4. Gets to standing; stands for 5 seconds, weight evenly distributed, hips and knees extended.
5. Stands up and sits down with no help; even weight distribution; full hip and knee extension.
6. Stands up and sits down with no help 3 times in 10 seconds; even weight distribution.

Walking

1. Stands on affected leg with hip extended; steps forward with other leg (standby help).

2. Walks with standby help from one person.
3. Walks 10 feet alone. Uses any walking aid but no standby help.
4. Walks 16 feet with no aid in 15 seconds.
5. Walks 33 feet, picks up small sandbag from floor, turns around, walks back in 25 seconds.
6. Walks up and down four steps with or without an aid three times in 35 seconds. May not hold rail.

Upper Arm Function

1. Supine, protracts shoulder girdle. Tester places arm in 90° flexion and supports elbow.
2. Supine, holds shoulder in 90° flexion for 2 seconds. (Maintains 45° external rotation and 20° elbow extension.)
3. From position in level 2, flexes and extends elbow to move palm to forehead and back.
4. Sitting, holds arm in 90° shoulder flexion with elbow extended, thumb pointing up, for 2 seconds. No excess shoulder elevation.
5. Achieves position in level 4; holds for 10 seconds; lowers arm. No pronation allowed.
6. Standing, arm abducted 90°, with palm flat against wall. Maintains hand position while turning body toward wall.

Hand Movements

1. Sitting, lifts cylindrical object off table by extending wrist. No elbow flexion allowed.
2. Sitting, forearm in midposition. Lifts hand off table by radially deviating wrist. No elbow flexion or forearm pronation allowed.
3. Sitting, elbow into side, pronates and supinates forearm through three-quarters of range.
4. Sitting, reaches forward to pick up 5-inch ball with both hands and puts ball down. Ball placement requires elbow extension. Palms stay in contact with ball.
5. Sitting, picks up plastic foam cup from table and puts it on table across other side of body.
6. Sitting, continuous opposition of thumb and each finger more than 14 times in 10 seconds.

Advanced Hand Activities

1. Reaches forward arm's length; picks up pen top; releases it on table close to body.
2. Picks up a jellybean from teacup with eight jellybeans and places it in another cup. Cups are at arm's length.
3. Draws horizontal lines to stop at a vertical line 10 times in 20 seconds.
4. Makes rapid consecutive dots with a pen on a sheet of paper. (Picks up and holds pen without assistance; at least 2 dots per second for 5 seconds; dots, not dashes).
5. Takes a dessert spoon of liquid to the mouth, without spilling. (Head cannot lower towards spoon).
6. Holds a comb and combs hair at back of head. (Shoulder is externally rotated, abducted at least 90°; head is erect.)

Used with permission from J. Carr & R. Shepherd, personal communication, 1994.

Westwood, 1992; Dean & Mackey, 1992; Nugent & Schurr, 1994). Positive aspects of the tool include its ease of administration, high reliability (Poole & Whitney, 1988), high concurrent validity compared to selected items on the *Fugl-Meyer Assessment* (Poole & Whitney, 1988), and its emphasis on functional task performance. In addition, occupational therapists have found that use of the *MAS*, with its structured format of task observation, is helpful in focusing and sharpening their observational skills (Kieran et al., 1999). Preliminary analysis of the upper limb items, using Rasch analysis, provides support for the scoring criteria hierarchy on the upper arm item but indicates that some elements of the scoring criteria hierarchies for the *MAS*'s two hand items may demonstrate problems in content validity (Kieran et al., 1999).

Standing Up and Sitting Down

Carr and Shepherd argue that the stand pivot transfer is typically overemphasized in neurorehabilitation. For patients who demonstrate potential to walk, learning how to stand up and sit down has greater functional implications and is more natural to learn than traditional transfer techniques.

Treatment to enhance a patient's ability to stand up and sit down improves that person's sitting posture, sitting and standing balance, functional reach, and gait. Each of these aspects of motor performance demands ability to appreciate how one's own body alignment and dynamic movement affect one's center of mass. In addition, each of these categories of functional activity demands a balance of mobility and stability in the pelvis, trunk, and limbs.

Essential Features of Performance

There are two phases to the normal kinematics of standing up. During the preextension phase (Shepherd & Gentile, 1994), or forward phase (Ada et al., 1993), the hips flex to move the center of mass forward. In the extension phase, or upward phase, the hips and knees extend to move the center of mass upward to final standing alignment. Each phase is characterized by kinematic and kinetic requirements. Force requirements are most important during the extension phase. These are met via contractions in the extensors of the ankle, knee, and hip. The kinetic requirements of standing up are similar to those of the stance phase during gait. To ensure that the limb does not collapse, a decrease in force at one joint can be compensated for by an increase at the other joints.

Several kinematic features during the preextension phase influence the amount of force needed during the extension phase. Forward foot placement has been found to interfere with both phases of standing up (Shepherd & Koh, 1996). Therefore, Carr and Shepherd recommend that people with CNS movement dysfunction prepare for standing by placing their feet behind an imaginary perpendicular line drawn down from the knees (Carr & Shepherd, 1998). Trunk position during preextension, determined by flexion at the hips, significantly affects the kinematics and kinetics of the extension phase. In subjects with normal movement, failure to flex forward at the hips lengthens the extension phase, increases muscle force requirements during the extension phase, and changes the order of movement during the extension phase from knee–hip–ankle to hip–knee–ankle (Shepherd & Gentile, 1994). Therefore, forward flexion at the hips is emphasized in treatment as a key element to standing up and sitting down.

Arm movement also affects the mechanics of rising to stand. Active arm flexion naturally accompanies the onset of leg extension and contributes to maximizing available extensor force in the lower limb (Carr & Gentile, 1994). Forward motion of the arms and upper body assists in establishing momentum prior to the extension phase. This momentum decreases the amount of lower limb force required to lift the body up against gravity to the erect standing posture. To capitalize on this momentum, Carr and Shepherd recommend that patients learn to complete the task of standing up with no pause between the preextension and extension phases. Therefore, unless there are safety considerations, they advise that patients practice the task in its entirety.

Finally, Carr and Shepherd believe that it is important to give patients opportunities to strengthen their leg muscles through activity performance. They caution against using the common strategy of teaching patients to push down with their arms to assist themselves in standing up. This may be useful in the short run as a compensatory technique to reduce force requirements at the hip, knee, and ankle. However, this strategy denies patients the opportunity to improve their muscle strength.

Assessment and Treatment

Box 22-3 provides the essential factors of Carr and Shepherd's program for developing the ability to stand up. Passive muscle lengthening may be necessary if patients demonstrate mobility limitations in ankle dorsiflexion, knee flexion or extension, hip flexion or extension, or sagittal-plane pelvic motion. Whole-task practice is important to assist patients in developing necessary sequencing and timing during functional performance.

Sitting down from standing has several similarities to standing up but is a different activity that must be practiced as well. Because there is no momentum to reduce force requirements, additional muscle strength (particularly in knee extensors) is needed just before the body mass is lowered onto the seat. Carr and Shepherd

BOX 22-3
PROCEDURES FOR PRACTICE

Sit to Stand

Strategic Movement Components
- Initial foot placement (knee and ankle <90°)
- Forward motion of upper body (requires sufficient ankle dorsiflexion and hip flexion; trunk remains erect)
- Sequential extension at the knee, hip, and ankle
- Relatively equal contributions by both lower limbs

Environmental Modifications
- Raise seat to decrease lower limb force requirements.
- Grade seat to lower heights as strength in leg extensors improves.
- Use chair without arms; chair arms tend to encourage habitual use of hands.
- Select chair that allows for placing the feet back (knee and ankle flexed to less than 90°).

recommend that when learning to stand, patients be instructed to stop the movement and reverse their direction for a few degrees. This will help them develop control over changing from concentric to eccentric muscle activity.

Balance

Balance is the ability to maintain an upright posture against the dynamically changing effects of gravity on our body segments. Postural control mechanisms enable us to maintain balance by ensuring that our body's center of mass remains within the base of support (Ghez, 1991). During daily activities, a person's center of mass can be displaced in three ways: (1) by an external force applied to the body, as occurs during contact sports; (2) by external movement of the support surface, as occurs when we sit or stand in a moving vehicle; and (3) during performance of activities requiring self-initiated movement of the head, limbs, or trunk (Carr & Shepherd, 1998).

Typically, for persons with motor impairments due to CNS dysfunction, balance challenges arising from self-initiated movement are more important to daily function than are balance challenges arising from external perturbations. Although traditional neurobehavioral approaches have focused on improving postural reactions to external perturbations, there is no evidence that these improvements have any positive effect on balance during self-initiated postural challenges.

Postural adjustments are both task and context specific. Studies have shown that muscle activation patterns for balance control vary according to (1) the position of the person, (2) the task being performed, (3)

the context in which the activity occurs, and (4) the person's perception of which body part is in contact with the more stable base of support (Nashner, 1982; Nashner & McCollum, 1985). Therefore, Carr and Shepherd advocate that postural adjustments be learned only in the context of task performance. Furthermore, balance training in one position or during performance of one task is not likely to generalize to improved postural control in other contexts (Shepherd, 1992).

Essential Features of Performance

Effective balance requires adequate function in sensory and motor systems (Box 22-4). Sensory processing of visual, vestibular, tactile, and proprioceptive information allows a person to maintain continuous and dynamic awareness about the body's center of mass and alignment between body segments. Muscle contractions of appropriate amplitude and timing allow for predictive and ongoing force production to match the changing influence of gravity during motor performance. Sufficient joint mobility and muscle length allow the necessary movements to be generated through their full ranges of motion.

Individuals with impairments in these areas are likely to develop adaptive strategies that may seem effective in the short run but that have long-term maladaptive influence on balance and other motor function (Box 22-4). When people feel unable to maintain their balance in posturally threatening situations, one such strategy is to constrain movement at selected body parts and thus decrease the number of motor elements or **degrees of freedom** the CNS must control. Individuals with postural adjustment deficits as a result of CNS dysfunction may feel insecure about their ability to maintain balance, even in routine sitting or standing positions. The strategy of fixating one's pelvis on the lumbar spine or the scapula on the thorax has short-term benefits for enhancing the person's sense of postural

BOX 22-4
Impairments Underlying Balance Dysfunction

Negative Features Affecting Balance Dysfunction
- Impairments in muscular force and timing
- Impairments in sensory processing (visual, tactile, proprioceptive, vestibular)

Adaptive Features Affecting Balance Dysfunction
- Avoiding all shifts in center of mass
- Shifting weight away from a paretic limb
- Using hands for support
- Stiffening the body
- Soft tissue shortening

security. A negative consequence is that these patterns lead to soft tissue shortening and difficulty disassociating the scapula and pelvis from adjacent proximal structures. This lack of sufficient mobility at the limb girdles subsequently limits the normal kinematics of upper and lower extremity movement. Figure 22-3 illustrates how immobility and muscle shortening interact in a self-perpetuating cycle.

The strategies of shifting weight away from a paretic leg, unnecessarily widening the base of support, or using one's hands excessively for support present further obstacles to using and improving available muscle strength and sensory processing skills. In addition, they contribute to additional problems in gait and in using the upper limbs to their maximum potential. Carr and Shepherd's approach seeks to prevent the development of these maladaptive strategies through the early introduction of techniques to enhance balance and postural security.

Assessment and Treatment
Balance is assessed through observational analysis as the person performs self-initiated movements in sitting and standing. These include the following:

► Looking in a variety of directions (e.g., up at the ceiling, behind oneself)
► Reaching forward, sideways, and down to the floor to pick up objects
► Walking in various conditions

Balance training overlaps with each of Carr and Shepherd's three other areas of functional performance. Patients are presented with activities that offer graded challenges to their ability to shift their center of mass over the base of support. Prior to activity engagement, the therapist ensures that joint mobility and postural alignment are maximized. Box 22-5 lists the critical activity elements that therapists manipulate in structuring activity-based balance training. These general guidelines provide occupational therapists with limitless possibilities for creative activity synthesis based on each patient's interests, goals, and level of function. The outcomes study (Dean & Shepherd, 1997) highlighted in

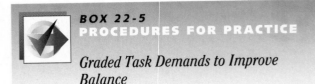

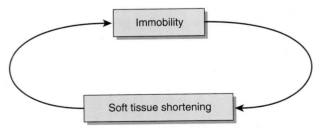

Figure 22-3 Cycle of immobility and soft tissue shortening.

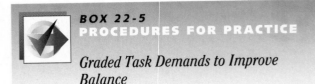

BOX 22-5
PROCEDURES FOR PRACTICE

Graded Task Demands to Improve Balance

Position of the Person
► Size and shape of base of support (foot placement, seating or standing surface)
► Initial alignment of body segments

Object Placement
► Position determines direction of weight shift; moving laterally more difficult than moving forward
► Distance

Object Characteristics
► Weight
► Size; greater challenge to balance when both hands must be used

Temporal Demands
► Stationary object—increasing demands on speed of performance
► Moving object—increasing the speed at which the object moves

this chapter's Research Note provides support for the clinical efficacy of these interventions.

Walking
Walking, a critical component of daily task engagement, is a reasonable expectation for many individuals with CNS dysfunction. Occupational therapists work with patients who wish to improve their performance in kitchen and bathroom activities and in leisure or work pursuits. In each of these contexts, the occupational therapist must help patients reach their optimal walking potential.

Essential Features of Performance
Successful walking requires production of a basic locomotor rhythm, support and propulsion of the body in the desired direction, dynamic balance control of the moving body, and the ability to adapt movement to changing environmental demands and goals (Carr & Shepherd, 1998).

Research on individuals with no musculoskeletal impairments has revealed remarkable consistency among people in the kinematic aspects of gait. Patterns of muscle use, however, vary widely. Besides differing between subjects, the kinetics of gait may vary within a single subject, depending on walking speed and fatigue. Furthermore, a natural redundancy in the motor system for walking readily allows for compensation by stronger muscles when specific muscles are weak.

Walking forward in a uniform direction is achieved through repetitive performance of sequential gait cycles. Each cycle begins when the heel of one foot makes contact with the ground. As that leg supports the body weight, it rocks forward until its only ground contact is at the toes. Simultaneously, the other leg swings forward until its heel makes contact with the ground. Double support is the brief period when both feet are on the ground. Immediately after double support, the first leg swings forward while the second leg supports the body weight. One gait cycle is completed when the heel of the first foot touches the ground once again.

For purposes of description, the gait cycle for each leg is divided into a stance phase and a swing phase. Box 22-6 shows the subdivision of these phases of the gait cycle. Basic knowledge about the motor requirements during each phase of the gait cycle guides therapists in their interventions for patients with CNS dysfunction.

The essential components of motor activity during the stance phase include extensor muscle activity at the hip, knee, and ankle; smooth alternation of eccentric and concentric muscular activity in knee and ankle muscles; muscle activity in the gluteus medius at mid-stance to prevent excessive downward tilt of the pelvis on the side of the swinging leg; and ongoing postural

---

BOX 22-6
The Gait Cycle

Stance Phase
▸ Weight–load acceptance: from heel contact to foot flat on ground
▸ Midstance: from foot flat on ground to heel off of ground
▸ Pushoff: weight moving forward onto toes and foot preparing to leave ground

Swing Phase
▸ Liftoff (early swing): leg swings forward with foot clearing the ground.
▸ Reach (late swing): leg decelerates and prepares for heel contact.

RESEARCH NOTE

Task-Related Training Improves Performance of Seated Reaching Tasks After Stroke: A Randomized Controlled Trial

Dean, C. M., & Shepherd, R. B. (1997). Stroke, 28, 722–728

ABSTRACT

After a stroke, the ability to balance in sitting is critical to independence. Although impairments in sitting balance are common, little is known about the effectiveness of rehabilitation strategies designed to improve it. The purpose of this randomized placebo-controlled study was to evaluate the effect of a 2-week task-related training program aimed at increasing reaching distance and the contribution of the affected lower leg to support and balance.

Twenty subjects at least 1 year after stroke were randomized to an experimental or control group. The experimental group participated in a standard training program involving practice of reaching beyond arm's length. The control group received sham training: completion of cognitive-manipulative tasks within arm's length. Reach while sitting was measured before and after training using electromyography, videotaping, and two force plates. Variables tested were movement time, distance reached, vertical ground reaction forces through the feet, and muscle activity. Subjects were also tested on sit-to-stand, walking, and cognitive tasks. Nineteen subjects completed the study.

After training, experimental subjects could reach significantly faster and farther, significantly increase load through the affected foot, and increase activation of the affected leg muscles compared with the control group ($p < .01$). The experimental group also improved in sit-to-stand. The control group did not improve in reaching or sit-to-stand. Neither group improved in walking. This study provides strong evidence of the efficacy of task-related motor training to improve the ability to balance during seated reaching activities after stroke.

IMPLICATIONS FOR PRACTICE

▸ After a stroke, sitting balance can be improved through opportunities to practice reaching to grasp objects with the unaffected hand under variable conditions.
▸ Providing patients with task-related challenges to use self-initiated balance adjustments is an effective method for improving sitting balance and performance in rising to stand.
▸ When self-initiated balance adjustments are not challenged, patients do not improve sitting balance or sit-to-stand.
▸ Individuals recovering from stroke need opportunities to sit without external supports and to challenge self-initiated balance adjustments by reaching to grasp objects, with variations in object location and weight, seat height, movement speed, and extent of thigh support on the seat.

Case Example

MR. M.: LEFT CEREBROVASCULAR ACCIDENT

Patient Information

Mr. M. was a 70-year-old man who sustained an infarct to his left middle cerebral artery 4 weeks before his referral for home-based occupational therapy. After hospitalization and inpatient rehabilitation, he returned home to his apartment in a building with an elevator. After occupational therapy assessment in his home, these problems were identified:

1. Mild difficulties with bed mobility and sitting balance because of limitations in thoracolumbar dissociation and pelvic mobility.
2. Need for contact guard and occasional minimal assist in rising to stand from sitting because of limitations cited above.
3. Insecure balance in standing.
4. Inability to use his dominant right arm for any task. Testing revealed intact proprioceptive and tactile sensation and ability to perform all active movements of the shoulder, elbow, forearm and wrist with therapist support and positioning. However, all individual movements required great effort, and he could not combine movements at multiple arm segments to meet the demands of functional tasks. Although he could perform finger flexion and extension, he was unable to achieve functional grasp and could not oppose his thumb to his other fingers.
5. Inability to independently perform self-care activities requiring advanced skills in sitting or standing balance, standing up or sitting down, or use of both arms. He relied on assistance from a home health attendant to perform toileting activities in sitting or standing, get onto and off a tub seat, dress himself, cut meat, shave himself to his own high expectations, and prepare any food.

Initial *MAS* scores are indicated in Figure 22-4.

Recommendations

The occupational therapist recommended two treatment sessions each week for 6 weeks and in collaboration with Mr. M. established the following long-term treatment goals: (1) Mr. M. will safely and independently stand up and sit down from a variety of seating surfaces and will perform functional tasks while standing. (2) Mr. M. will use his right arm and hand during task performance. (3) Mr. M. will safely and independently perform all activities in which he engaged prior to the stroke and will have sufficient motor and task analysis skills to attempt performing new activities.

Short-Term Goals

The following goals were set for the first 3 weeks of occupational therapy treatment:

1. **Mr. M. will achieve full, fluid, active motion at the right scapula, the thoracic and lumbar spine, and the pelvis.** Treatment focused on teaching Mr. M. exercises in lying supine and sitting that provided soft tissue stretch to improve mobility in: scapular protraction and upward rotation, thoracolumbar dissociation, and pelvic mobility. The OT taught Mr. M. to appreciate which planes of motion should be available in his scapulae, trunk, and pelvis and encouraged Mr. M. to design activities that would elicit movements at each body segment in all available planes of motion. Mr. M. also learned to determine optimal alignment of body segments for various body postures and functional tasks. Achievement of this goal enabled Mr. M. to attain full independence in bed mobility and facilitated his performance in tasks requiring sitting balance, standing balance, sit-to-stand, and right upper arm control.

2. **Mr. M. will maintain sitting balance during activities requiring self-initiated movements of his head, limbs, and trunk and will independently stand up and sit down from a variety of seating surfaces.** Mr. M. improved his balance by using his improved mobility at the trunk and pelvis and practicing unilateral and bilateral reach and grasp in sitting and standing. He improved his ability to stand up and sit down from a variety of seating surfaces in his home after the OT identified the major control parameters influencing his initial performance (Figs. 22-5 and 22-6) and helped him improve his performance strategy (Figs. 22-7 and 22-8).

3. **Mr. M. will use his right arm and hand as an assist to his left during a variety of functional tasks. He will achieve this by improving his control over increasing numbers of degrees of freedom at the right shoulder, elbow, forearm, and hand.** Mr. M. began by practicing holding his shoulder at 90° flexion while supine, with decreasing external support from the therapist. As soon as he demonstrated ability to hold his shoulder in this position, the therapist added one new movement demand at a time, while Mr. M. maintained his shoulder in this position. Examples of new movement demands included scapular motions, elbow motion, wrist motion, lateral pinch to grasp a tissue, and rotational movements at the GH (glenohumeral) joint. Mr. M. practiced

varying movement combinations as homework, and he progressed to controlling these combined motions while sitting, a position with greater gravitational demands. Mr. M. accomplished his earliest hand activities while resting his right hand in his lap and reaching down and forward or down and to the side. He practiced a variety of bimanual tasks, such as ripping paper, operating a vacuum cleaner (Fig. 22-9 *A*), buckling a belt, and holding his face in position while shaving. Unilateral tasks included grasping tissues (Fig. 22-9 *B*), operating a television remote control, applying lotion to his left forearm, and using cylindrical grasp to pick up a variety of items in his home. On reevaluation, he could achieve lateral pinch and pad-to-pad pinch. He developed active control of thumb flexion and began to demonstrate thumb opposition.

Revised Goals (See Fig. 22-4 for MAS scores after 3 weeks of treatment)

1. Mr. M. will be able to perform activities requiring right thumb opposition and individual finger movements. He will be able to perform all hand activities, regardless of what shoulder position is required for a given task.

2. Mr. M. will be able to perform activities requiring the integration of standing balance, bilateral use of his upper limbs, and unilateral use of his right arm and hand while holding a cane in his left hand.

CLINICAL REASONING
in OT Practice

Assessing Sit to Stand

Analyze Mr. M.'s performance in Figures 22-5 and 22-6 to determine which factors contributed to his difficulty in rising to stand. What interventions would you use to assist him in improving his ability to rise to standing to the level of function illustrated in Figures 22-7 and 22-8?

---

adjustments to balance the body mass over a dynamically changing base of support.

For those with hemiparesis, clinical problems in the stance phase interfere most with functional walking, because stance phase activity allows for effective swing by the nonparetic leg and prepares the paretic leg to swing with maximal efficiency (Carr & Shepherd, 1998). Thus, Carr and Shepherd recommend that treatment after stroke or head injury focus on improving patients' ability to master the stance phase of the gait cycle.

Since the goals of the swing phase are (1) to clear the foot from contacting the ground as the leg swings forward and (2) to prepare the leg to assume a stance position as it reaches the end of its swing forward in space, the essential components of motor activity during the swing phase are fluid pelvic mobility, including lateral pelvic tilt as weight is shifted from the current leg onto the other leg and pelvic rotation to allow the swinging leg to advance forward; sufficient hip, knee, and ankle (dorsi) flexion to shorten the leg for foot clearance as the leg swings forward; and knee extension and ankle dorsiflexion just prior to heel contact to ensure that the heel, rather than the flat foot or the toes, will strike the ground to initiate the stance phase.

Assessment and Treatment

Walking is evaluated through observation and comparison of each patient's performance against a list of essential components, or critical kinematic features, of walking. Observation from both the sagittal and coronal

Motor Assessment Scale

Patient's Name: *Mr. M.*

	Pre-treatment Score	Re-evaluation Score
1. Supine to side lying	4	6
2. Supine to sitting over side of bed	5	6
3. Balanced sitting	4	6
4. Sitting to standing	3	5
5. Walking	3	5
6. Upper arm function	1	6
7. Hand movements	3	5
8. Advanced hand activities	0	3

Figure 22-4 Mr. M.'s *MAS* Scores (See Case Example).

planes is essential for appropriate analysis. Although Carr and Shepherd encourage therapists to be attentive to the kinematic aspects of gait, they recognize that subtle changes in kinematic behaviors do not constitute legitimate outcomes. Thus, they recommend that therapists assess the following objective variables before and after treatment: stride length, step length, stride width, time spent in double support, walking velocity, and use of arms for support and balance (i.e., the patient's need

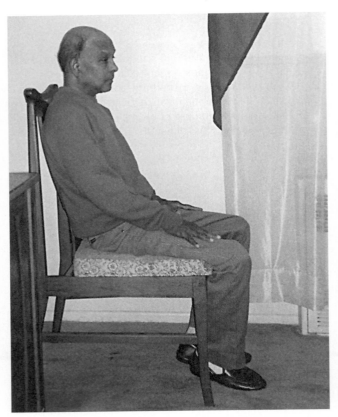

Figure 22-5 Early preextension phase of standing up: Mr. M.'s initial evaluation.

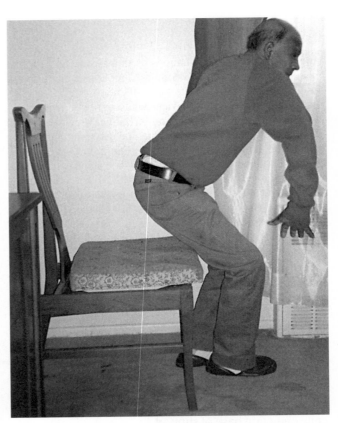

Figure 22-6 Extension phase of standing up: Mr. M.'s initial evaluation.

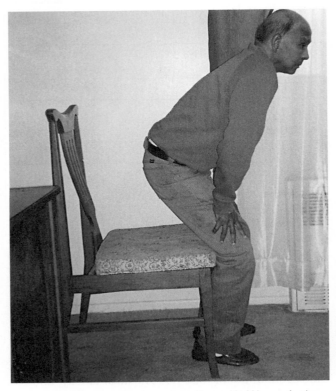

Figure 22-7 Preextension phase of standing up: Mr. M.'s reevaluation.

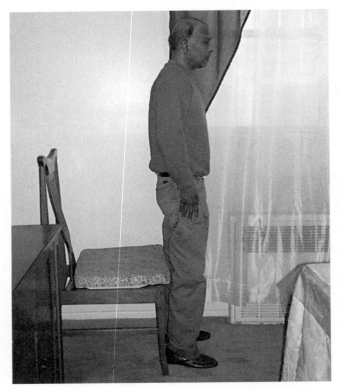

Figure 22-8 Extension phase of standing up: Mr. M.'s reevaluation.

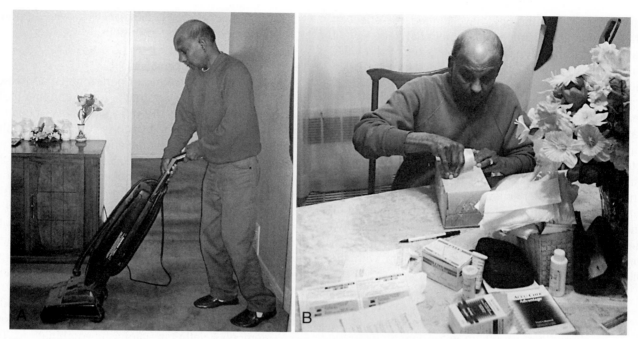

Figure 22-9 Functional task practice during occupational therapy sessions: **A.** Standing. **B.** Seated.

for walking aids). Scores on the walking item of the *MAS* have been used to provide research support for the efficacy of Carr and Shepherd's approach to improving walking after stroke (Dean & Mackey, 1992).

Treatment goals are to prevent soft tissue shortening; improve muscle strength and control for support, propulsion, balance, and toe clearance; and improve rhythm and coordination during functional walking. Treatment methods include active exercises to lengthen shortened muscles, training to improve force generation and speed of muscle contraction, and actual practice walking and stair climbing. Occupational therapists expand on Carr and Shepherd's goals to include graded, functional walking practice during performance of upright activities.

Reach and Manipulation

The arm and hand function as a single unit in reach and manipulation, with the hand beginning to open for grasp at the start of a reaching action (Jeannerod, 1990). In many activities, the upper body or even the entire body is an integral component of this single coordinated unit. Clearly, reach and grasp are not exclusively upper limb activities. All reaching actions from sitting or standing are preceded and accompanied by postural adjustments. When objects are beyond arm's reach, shifts in total body alignment contribute to functional performance.

Essential Features of Performance

Forward reach in sitting entails (1) anterior movement of the pelvis, (2) flexion of the trunk at the hips, and (3) active use of the legs to aid in balancing by creating an active base of support. Reaching sideways while sitting is more challenging than reaching forward, since the base of support is smaller. Reaching while standing requires (1) establishment of an appropriate base of support with one's feet and (2) shifting body weight and center of mass toward the direction of the goal object.

Therapeutic interventions for individuals with CNS dysfunction must inherently combine evaluation and treatment of balance with assessment and training of reach and manipulation. Carr and Shepherd caution against waiting until patients achieve a certain level of balance before introducing therapeutic tasks to improve reach and manipulation. Similarly, they caution against waiting until patients demonstrate a specified level of shoulder function before assessing for and providing treatment to improve hand skills.

A New Perspective on Conceptualizing Therapeutic Intervention

Traditionally, upper limb function after serious stroke or traumatic brain injury has been associated with poor outcomes (Nakayama et al., 1994). Carr and Shepherd suggest that several factors, in addition to the direct extent of neural pathology, have limited the effect of rehabilitation interventions on functional recovery of reach and grasp. They agree with Taub and Wolf (1997) that during the flaccid period immediately after brain injury, patients learn to rely exclusively on the unaffected arm for performing one-handed activities. This "learned nonuse" (Taub et al., 1993), combined with inappropriate therapeutic intervention for the upper limb, results in insufficient opportunity to practice activity with the paretic arm. In addition, the effects of immobility on soft tissue extensibility limit active motor function even further. Finally, Carr and Shepherd debunk some common beliefs that prevail among rehabilitation professionals. They recommend that therapists shed unsubstantiated beliefs about recovery of motor control after brain injury and replace them with the following assumptions:

1. Recovery does not necessarily proceed in a proximal to distal sequence. Rather, therapists and patients should consistently monitor emerging muscle strength in all segments of the upper limb.
2. There is no reason to wait until patients demonstrate shoulder stability and control before presenting therapeutic challenges to hand function. Rather, the presentation of activities requiring limited grasp may provide valuable therapeutic challenges that can help organize emerging shoulder function.
3. Therapeutic challenges to active limb use need not be postponed until spasticity is inhibited. In fact, evidence indicates that the hypertonus, or resistance to passive movement, that many clinicians associate with spasticity is in most patients typically due to muscle shortening and increased stiffness (Carr et al, 1995). Therefore, Carr and Shepherd do not advocate the use of any procedures aside from those that preserve or enhance soft tissue extensibility for reducing spasticity as a means to enhancing active, functional use of the upper limb.
4. There are no universal patterns of muscle linkages associated with recovery of motor function after brain injury. Rather, research has shown that abnormal patterns of motor performance are related to each patient's distribution of muscle weakness combined with the mechanical demands of each task (Trombly, 1992, 1993). For example, the pattern of shoulder elevation combined with retraction of the shoulder girdle, which is often seen when individuals attempt to flex or abduct a hemiparetic shoulder, is not directly linked to the neural pathology. Rather, it is an adaptive use of available muscle strength against gravitational force. Thus, interventions to improve motor patterns are based on individualized analyses of each patient's abilities, and activities are

presented as graded challenges to provide opportunities for developing motor skills.

The Degrees of Freedom Problem

Of the four categories of motor performance addressed by Carr and Shepherd's approach, reach and manipulation are characterized by the greatest number of degrees of freedom. This provides us with exceptional flexibility in tailoring reach and manipulation to the contextual demands of different tasks and environments. At the same time, this freedom of choice increases the complexity of motor demands during upper limb activities (Latash & Latash, 1994). Many people with stroke or head injury demonstrate a capacity to perform singular motions of a paretic upper limb when assisted by a therapist. However, their inability to control multiple degrees of freedom results in an inability to use the arm for functional reach or grasp (Sabari, 1991).

One effective strategy observed in people who move with ease is to reduce the degrees of freedom by linking some elements together in synergistic combinations. The kinesiology of normal movement is characterized by several synergistic combinations in the upper limb and trunk (Levangie & Norkin, 2001). Some examples are:

▶ Combined action of rotator cuff muscles to assist the deltoid during glenohumeral (GH) flexion and abduction
▶ Upward rotation of the scapula that accompanies GH flexion and abduction (scapulohumeral rhythm)
▶ Shifts in body weight and pelvic orientation that accompany reaching motions of the upper limb
▶ Synergistic combinations between GH and forearm rotators for efficient positioning of the hand in space
▶ Synergistic contraction of the wrist extensors during grasp patterns requiring forceful finger flexion

After stroke or head injury, many persons lose their ability to implement these synergistic linkages automatically. The critical goals of intervention to improve reach and manipulation skills:

▶ Minimize movement obstacles presented by weakness and immobility.
▶ Teach foundational movement combinations that underlie efficient reach and grasp.
▶ Provide graded opportunities to practice controlling an increasing number of degrees of freedom during exercise and activity performance.

Assessment and Treatment

Like other evaluations in Carr and Shepherd's approach, clinical assessment of reach and manipulation is achieved through detailed observation of each patient's attempts to perform selected functional tasks. Therapists use their knowledge about the kinetics and kinematics of upper limb function to develop hypotheses as to which deficits may be serving as control parameters to limiting the versatility or efficiency of motor strategies. Most motor dysfunction can be attributed to specific muscle weakness, muscle stiffness and length changes, and/or adaptive strategies developed to compensate for these impairments. Shoulder pain may also be a significant control parameter to efficient reach. (Box 22-7 lists ways to prevent secondary impairments at the shoulder.) Therapists test their hypotheses through direct assessment of muscle strength and length and through patients' responses to interventions designed to modify adaptive strategies.

Training is individualized and based on the hypotheses developed during observation of functional task performance. Early control of weak muscles is facilitated by finding an optimal length for muscle contraction and by positioning the limb so that gravity assists rather than resists the muscle. An example also used in the neurodevelopmental treatment (NDT) approach is to elicit early contraction of the deltoid with the person lying supine with the shoulder flexed to 90°. In this position gravity provides a stabilizing force on the shoulder. Therefore, activation of fewer motor units is required for the individual to hold the arm and move it slightly from this position. Shortened muscles are lengthened by slow, passive stretch by the therapist, family members, or patients themselves. Therapists make patients aware of inefficient adaptive strategies and provide them with opportunities to perform a variety of reach and grasp activities using alternative movement strategies. Box 22-8 summarizes the motor components essential to reach and manipulation. Therapists consider these components when synthesizing and grading therapeutic tasks.

BOX 22-8
Essential Components to Functional Arm Use

Reaching

Forward
Flexion at shoulder

Sideways
Abduction at shoulder

Backward
Extension at shoulder

▶ Appropriate scapular motion (upward rotation and abduction for forward and sideways reach; downward rotation and adduction for backward reach)
▶ Elbow extension and varying amount of shoulder external rotation
▶ Opening of hand aperture between thumb and fingers
▶ Extension of wrist
▶ Pronation and supination appropriate to object orientation

Grasping
Preparation to grasp:

▶ Extension of wrist and fingers
▶ Abduction and opposition at thumb carpometacarpal joint
▶ Finger abduction for large objects

Grasp: Closure of thumb and fingers around object

Holding

▶ Flexion and extension of wrist while holding object
▶ Lifting, placing, and rotating objects of various sizes, shapes, and weights

Manipulating

▶ Flexion and extension of fingers
▶ Flexion and opposition at carpometacarpal joints of thumb and fifth finger
▶ Independent finger flexion and extension (e.g., keyboard depression)

Adapted with permission from Carr, J. H., & Shepherd, R. (1998). *Neurological Rehabilitation: Optimizing Motor Performance.* Oxford: Butterworth-Heinemann.

BOX 22-7
SAFETY BOX

Preventing Secondary Impairments at the Shoulder

▶ Prevent muscle shortening of adductor and internal rotator muscles; provide stretch through positioning or passive motion.
▶ Minimize downward gravitational force on soft tissue around glenohumeral joint.
▶ Avoid passive humeral flexion or abduction without appropriate concomitant scapular motion.
▶ Avoid any passive movement of the arm by individuals unfamiliar with scapulohumeral interactions.

Carr and Shepherd recognize that many patients with hemiparesis may rely excessively on one-handed performance of daily tasks, even when they demonstrate potential to use their affected arm and hand. They support the use of constraint-induced movement therapy (Taub & Wolf, 1997) when appropriate. In addition, they recognize that bimanual tasks provide a natural framework for encouraging active use of available hand function.

Actual training in grasp and manipulation is achieved through varied task-related practice of both unilateral and bilateral activities. Sensory training is provided naturalistically through opportunities to manipulate objects with various shapes, sizes, and textures in the context of task performance. They suggest a variety of interventions to augment training, including specialized feedback, functional electrical stimulation, mental practice, and the use of orthoses. Intensity of practice can be increased through the use of relatives as training coaches, constraint-induced movement therapy (Taub & Wolf, 1997), and access to computer-driven games. Dean and Mackey's (1992) study provides research support for the efficacy of Carr and Shepherd's approach in improving upper limb and hand function.

Occupational therapists are particularly qualified to synthesize activities designed to provide graded challenges to reach and manipulation. In addition, occupational therapists excel at designing individualized orthotic and environmental adaptations to facilitate task performance while providing opportunities to develop functional skill to each person's maximal potential.

Carr and Shepherd's approach to optimizing motor control is well suited for use and adaptation in occupational therapy. Occupational therapists who apply these ideas use their skills in analyzing the kinematic and kinetic requirements of specific activity performance to develop individualized goals and treatment. In addition, occupational therapists using this approach structure tasks and environments to assist patients in developing efficient motor strategies and motor problem–solving skills. Finally, occupational therapists provide meaningful practice that enables individuals to use their available motor function to its fullest potential in daily activity performance.

Summary Review Questions

1. What are the relationships between control parameters, negative features and adaptive features of CNS dysfunction, and attractor states?
2. How are the principles of activity analysis and synthesis applied when implementing Carr and Shepherd's approach?
3. Which kinematic features of the preextension phase of standing up influence the ease with which a person will perform the extension phase?
4. Why do Carr and Shepherd lay greater emphasis on assessing and intervening to improve postural adjustments than postural reactions?
5. What are the essential components of the stance phase and swing phase of the gait cycle? How can occupational therapists structure interventions to assist patients in walking to their optimal potential?
6. How can occupational therapists structure interventions to assist patients in controlling increasing numbers of degrees of freedom when performing reach and manipulation tasks?

7. What specific mechanical constraints are likely to affect a person's ability to stand up and sit down? To maintain balance during activity performance? To walk during activity performance? To perform activities requiring reach, grasp, and manipulation?
8. What foundational movement strategies are likely to assist a person's ability to stand up and sit down? To maintain balance during activity performance? To walk during activity performance? To perform activities requiring reach, grasp, and manipulation?
9. Provide specific examples of postural adjustments that are likely to assist a person's ability to stand up and sit down, to maintain balance during activity performance, to walk during activity performance, and to perform activities requiring reach, grasp, and manipulation.
10. How can occupational therapists assist patients in developing their task analysis and problem-solving skills in the context of functional movement?

References

Ada, L., O'Dwyer, N., Green, J., Yeo, W., & Neilson, P. (1996). The nature of the loss of strength and dexterity in the upper limb following stroke. *Human Movement Science, 15*, 671–687.

Ada, L., O'Dwyer, N., & Neilson, P. D. (1993). Improvement in kinematic characteristics and coordination following stroke quantified by linear systems analysis. *Human Movement Science, 12*, 137–153.

Ada, L., & Westwood, P. (1992). A kinematic analysis of recovery of the ability to stand up following stroke. *Australian Physiotherapy, 38*, 135–142.

Aizawa, H., Inase, M., Mushiake, H., Shima, K., & Tanji, J. (1991). Reorganization of activity in the supplementary motor area associated with motor learning and functional recovery. *Experimental Brain Research, 84*, 668–671.

Butefish, C., Hummelsheim, H., Denzler, P., & Mauritz, K. H. (1995). Repetitive training of isolated movements improves the outcome of motor rehabilitation of the centrally paretic hand. *Journal of the Neurological Sciences, 130*, 59–68.

Carr, J. H., & Gentile, A. M. (1994). The effect of arm movement on the biomechanics of standing up. *Human Movement Science, 13*, 175–193.

Carr, J. H., & Shepherd, R. B. (1987). *A Motor Relearning Program for Stroke* (2nd ed.). Rockville, MD: Aspen.

Carr, J. H., & Shepherd, R. (1998). *Neurological Rehabilitation: Optimizing Motor Performance.* Oxford: Butterworth-Heinemann.

Carr, J. H., Shepherd, R. B., & Ada, L. (1995). Spasticity: Research findings and implications for intervention. *Physiotherapy, 81*, 421–429.

Carr, J. H., Shepherd, R. B., Nordholm, L., & Lynne, D. (1985). Investigation of a new motor assessment scale for stroke patients. *Physical Therapy, 65*, 175–180.

Dean, C. M., & Mackey, F. (1992). Motor assessment scale scores as a measure of rehabilitation outcome following stroke. *Australian Physiotherapy, 38*, 31–35.

Dean, C. M., & Shepherd, R. B. (1997). Task-related training improves performance of seated reaching tasks after stroke: A randomized controlled trial. *Stroke, 28,* 722–728.

Duncan, P. W., & Lai, S. M. (1997). Stroke recovery. *Topics in Stroke Rehabilitation, 4,* 51–58.

Gentile, A. M. (1998). Implicit and explicit processes during acquisition of functional skills. *Scandinavian Journal of Occupational Therapy, 5*(1), 7–16.

Ghez, C. (1991). Posture. In E. R. Kandel, J. H. Schwartz, & T. M. Jessell (Eds.), *Principles of Neural Science* (3rd ed., pp. 596–608). Norwalk, CT: Appleton & Lange.

Gresham, G. E., Duncan, P. W., Stason, W. B., Adams, H. P., Adelman, A. M., Alexander, D. N., Bishop, D. S., Diller, L., Donaldson, N. E., Granger, C. V., Holland, A. L., Kelly-Hayes, M., McDowell, F. H., Myers, L., Phipps, M. A., Roth, E. J., Siebens, H. C., Tarvin, G. A., & Trombly, C. A. (1995). *Post-Stroke Rehabilitation.* (AHCPR Publication 95-0662). Rockville, MD: U.S. Department of Health and Human Services.

Jeannerod, M.(1990). *The Neural and Behavioral Organization of Goal-Directed Movements.* Oxford, UK: Clarendon.

Johansson, B. B. (1996). Environmental influence on outcome after experimental brain infarction. *Acta Neurochirurgica [Suppl], 66,* 63–67.

Kamm, K., Thelen, E., & Jensen, J. L. (1990). A dynamical systems approach to motor development. *Physical Therapy, 70,* 763–775.

Kieran, O. P., Lim, A. L., & Sabari, J. S. (1999). Using the *MAS* to measure functional recovery of the hemiplegic arm. Academic Annual Assembly Abstracts. *Archives of Physical Medicine and Rehabilitation, 80,* 1138.

Kolb, B. (1995). *Brain, Plasticity and Behavior.* Mahwah, NJ: Lawrence Erlbaum.

Latash, L. P., & Latash, M. L. (1994). A new book by N. A. Bernstein: "On dexterity and its development." *Journal of Motor Behavior, 26,* 56–62.

Lee, R. G., & van Donkelaar, P. (1995). Mechanisms underlying functional recovery following stroke. *Canadian Journal of Neurological Sciences, 22,* 257–263.

Levangie, P. K., & Norkin, C. C. (2001). *Joint structure and function: a comprehensive analysis* (3rd ed.). Philadelphia: F. A. Davis.

Lister, M. J. (1991). *Contemporary Management of Motor Control Problems: Proceedings of the II Step Conference.* Alexandria, VA: Foundation for Physical Therapy.

Mathiowetz, V., & Bass Haugen, J. (1994). Motor behavior research: Implications for therapeutic approaches to central nervous system dysfunction. *American Journal of Occupational Therapy, 48,* 733–745.

Mathiowetz, V., & Wade, M. G. (1995). Task constraints and functional motor performance of individuals with and without multiple sclerosis. *Ecological Psychology, 7,* 99–123.

Nakayama, H., Jorgensen, H. S., Raaschou, H. O., & Olsen, T. S. (1994). Recovery of upper extremity function in stroke patients: The Copenhagen Stroke Study. *Archives of Physical Medicine and Rehabilitation, 75,* 852–857.

Nashner, L. M. (1982). Adaptation of human movement to altered environments. *Trends in Neurosciences, 5,* 358–361.

Nashner, L. M., & McCollum, G. (1985). The organization of human postural movements: A formal basis and experimental synthesis. *The Behavioral and Brain Sciences, 8,* 135–172.

Nugent, J. A., & Schurr, K. A. (1994). A dose-response relationship between amount of weight-bearing exercise and walking outcome following cerebrovascular accident. *Archives of Physical Medicine and Rehabilitation, 75,* 399–402.

O'Dwyer, N. J., Ada, L., & Neilson, P. D. (1996). Spasticity and muscle contracture following stroke. *Brain, 119,* 1737–1749.

Perry, S. B. (1998). Clinical implications of a dynamic systems theory. *(American Physical Therapy Association) Neurology Report, 22,* 4–10.

Poole, J. L., & Whitney, S. L. (1988). Motor assessment scale for stroke patients: Concurrent validity and interrater reliability. *Archives of Physical Medicine and Rehabilitation, 69,* 195–197.

Rossini, P. M., Caltagirone, C., Castriota-Scanderbeg, A., Cicinelli, P., Demartin, M., Pizzella, V., Traversa, R., & Romani, G. L. (1998). Hand motor cortical area reorganization in stroke: A study with FMRI, MEG and TCS maps. *Neuroreport, 9,* 2141–2146.

Sabari, J. S. (1991). Motor learning concepts applied to activity-based intervention with adults with hemiplegia. *American Journal of Occupational Therapy, 45,* 523–530.

Sabari, J. (1998). Application of learning and environmental strategies to activity based treatment. In G. Gillen & A. Burkhardt (Eds.), *Stroke Rehabilitation: A Function-Based Approach* (pp. 31–46). St. Louis: Mosby.

Schmidt, R. A. (1992). *Motor Performance and Learning: Principles for Practitioners.* Champaign, IL: Human Kinetics.

Shepherd, R. B. (1992). Adaptive motor behaviour in response to perturbations of balance. *Physiotherapy Theory and Practice, 8,* 137–143.

Shepherd, R. B., & Gentile, A. M. (1994). Sit to stand: Functional relationship between upper body and lower limb segments. *Human Movement Science, 13,* 817–840.

Shepherd, R. B., & Koh, H. P. (1996). Some biomechanical consequences of varying foot placement in sit-to-stand in young women. *Scandinavian Journal of Rehabilitation Medicine, 28,* 79–88.

Shumway-Cook, A., & Woollacott, M. (1995). *Motor Control: Theory and Practical Applications.* Baltimore: Williams & Wilkins.

Taub, E., Miller, N. E., Novack, T. A., Cook, E. W., Fleming, W. C., Nepomuceno, C. S., Connell, J. S., & Crago, J. E. (1993). Technique to improve chronic motor deficit after stroke. *Archives of Physical Medicine and Rehabilitation, 74,* 347–354.

Taub, E., & Wolf, S. L. (1997). Constraint induced movement techniques to facilitate upper extremity use in stroke patients. *Topics in Stroke Rehabilitation, 3,* 38–61.

Trombly, C.A. (1992). Deficits of reaching in subjects with left hemiparesis: A pilot study. *American Journal of Occupational Therapy, 46,* 887–897.

Trombly, C. A. (1993). Observations of improvement of reaching in five subjects with left hemiparesis. *Journal of Neurology, Neurosurgery, & Psychiatry, 56* (1), 40–45.

Trombly, C. A., & Wu, C. Y. (1999). Effect of rehabilitation tasks on organization of movement after stroke. *American Journal of Occupational Therapy, 53,* 333–344.

Willingham, D. B. (1998). A neuropsychological theory of motor skill learning. *Psychological Review, 105,* 558–584.

23

Optimizing Motor Behavior Using the Bobath Approach

Kathryn Levit

LEARNING OBJECTIVES

After studying this chapter, the reader will be able to do the following:

1. Identify the major problems that result from stroke.
2. Describe the major principles underlying the neurodevelopmental treatment (NDT)–Bobath approach to stroke rehabilitation.
3. Discuss the role of muscle tone and postural control in the production of normal movement and describe how problems in these areas contribute to impaired occupational functioning post stroke.
4. Integrate NDT/Bobath concepts and techniques with the occupational functioning model.
5. Develop an OT treatment plan for a patient with acute stroke using NDT/Bobath principles and techniques.

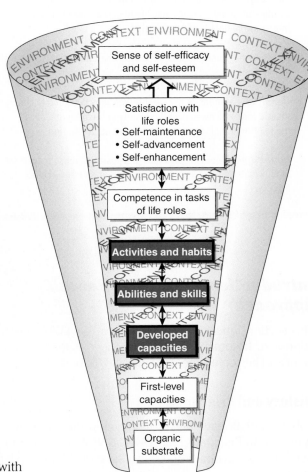

K. Bobath and B. Bobath developed a treatment approach designed to increase normal movement patterns in children with cerebral palsy and adults with acquired hemiplegia. Their treatment is known as the Bobath approach or NDT. NDT/Bobath treatment focuses on restoring normal movements and eliminating abnormal movements. The occupational functioning model usually describes this type of treatment as preparatory because it is directed toward establishing sensorimotor performance components that are prerequisites for function. This chapter introduces the NDT/Bobath approach to the treatment of adults with hemiplegia. A complete description of the treatment approach and its techniques can be found in Bobath (1990). Davies (1985) and Eggers (1984) provide information on using the approach to improve occupational functioning.

GLOSSARY

Abnormal coordination—Patterns of muscle activation, timing and sequencing that deviate from normal, resulting in inefficient, stereotyped movement patterns.

Abnormal tone—Muscle tone that is higher or lower than normal.

Associated reactions—Involuntary and nonfunctional changes in limb position and muscle tone associated with difficult or stressful activities.

Facilitation—Manual techniques and other processes including tactile and verbal feedback used to help the patient achieve a more normal quality of movement.

Flaccidity—Muscle tone that is lower than normal. Also known as hypotonicity.

Handling—Manual, hands-on interventions designed to change muscle tone and normalize the quality of the patient's movements. Handling is used for inhibition and facilitation.

Inhibition—Manual techniques and positions used to decrease or eliminate the effects of spasticity and/or abnormal reflex activity.

Key points of control—Hand placements on the patient's trunk and extremities used to allow the therapist to influence the quality of the patient's posture and movement. Often divided into proximal and distal key points.

Loss of postural control—Inability to use automatic patterns of muscle activation that maintain the center of gravity within a stable base of support both at rest and during movement.

Placing response—Part of the normal system of postural adjustments to changes in position, characterized by maintaining a position when support is removed.

Reflex-inhibiting pattern (RIP)—Position that counteracts the pull of spastic muscles. Used to inhibit abnormal tone and to facilitate more normal patterns of muscle activation.

Spasticity—Muscle tone that is higher than normal and resists passive stretching; also known as hypertonicity.

Introduction to the NDT/Bobath Approach

This section introduces the reader to the NDT/Bobath approach. It contains a brief overview of the development and key components of the NDT/Bobath approach.

History and Principles

Bobath and Bobath began to develop their treatment approach in England in the 1940s. B. Bobath, trained in Germany as a gymnast and remedial movement specialist, went to England to avoid persecution and found work as a physical therapist. When treating adults with hemiplegia, she noted the abnormal stiffness in their affected extremities, their asymmetrical body postures, and the nonfunctional stereotyped patterns of movement in their involved side. B. Bobath tried to help her patients regain functional use of their hemiplegic side. She assumed that the abnormal patterns of muscle tone and motor control were the major impairments interfering with normal motor control of the trunk, arm, and leg. Through trial and error, B. Bobath developed techniques for decreasing abnormal reflex activity and muscle tone

and for increasing control of normal patterns of movement on the hemiplegic side of the body. These techniques were based on her knowledge of normal kinesiology, not the developmental sequence.

B. Bobath discovered that she could help her patients with hemiplegia move more freely and function with less compensation by decreasing the abnormal tone in their affected side. She also found that when spasticity decreased, her patients could acquire improved control of posture and movement on their affected side and could use these new patterns for function. Based on these clinical findings, Bobath developed a new model for treating adults with hemiplegia. Her approach involved the use of manual techniques to eliminate abnormal tone and movement and retrain normal patterns of coordination in the affected trunk, arm, and leg. Because her goal was to restore movement and function on the affected side, she specifically rejected both traditional compensatory approaches that neglected the potential for function in the hemiplegic side and other neurophysiological approaches that encouraged abnormal movement and reflex activity.

As B. Bobath developed the treatment techniques, neurologist K. Bobath reviewed research in neurology and neurophysiology to develop a scientific basis for his wife's treatment. B. Bobath's claims that her treatment could change spasticity and restore normal movement responses were controversial, and K. Bobath used research findings to support her discoveries. Because the clinical techniques developed first, K. Bobath presented his scientific rationale in hypothetical terms, describing it as an explanation for, not the basis of, intervention.

Bobath and Bobath called their treatment approach a living concept because they expected it to change and develop over time. They made many changes to the treatment process to make it more active and functional. They also made an effort to update their theory by adding new scientific explanations for certain aspects of their treatment. While controversial when first introduced, many of the assumptions of Bobath and Bobath are now an accepted part of stroke rehabilitation, and the approach is widely used throughout the world (Rast, 1999). However, because the writings of K. Bobath rely on models of nervous system function and movement control that are now out of date, the NDT/Bobath approach has been the target of criticism (Gordon, 1987). Since the deaths of the Bobaths in 1990, the Neurodevelopmental Treatment Association in the United States and similar groups in other countries have been working to update the theoretical basis for NDT/Bobath treatment (Box 23-1).

Definitions of Terms and Constructs

Bobath and Bobath developed their approach to address the motor problems associated with **hemiplegia**, or loss

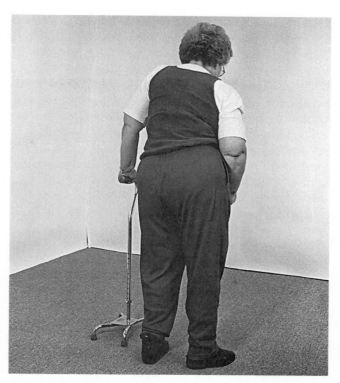

Figure 23-1 Patient showing poor postural control while walking with a cane.

of muscular control on one side of the body. According to them, hemiplegia is associated with two categories of motor problems: the loss of normal movement responses and the development of abnormal tone and movement. They hypothesized that these two sets of problems cause the abnormal patterns of coordination and functional limitations common to patients with hemiplegia. They also believed that treatment that addressed these problems would improve movement control on the hemiplegic side, hence occupational performance. These assumptions are discussed separately in the sections that follow.

Movement Control Problems After Stroke

Bobath and Bobath described the loss of normal movement responses as the first type of motor impairment associated with hemiplegia. Patients with hemiplegia may demonstrate **loss of postural control**, or inability to activate muscles automatically to maintain the body in balance at rest and during movement, and **loss of selective movement control** of the muscles controlling movement of the hemiplegic arm and leg. Loss of postural control is associated with difficulty shifting weight, maintaining control against gravity, and activating equilibrium responses when balance is challenged. These problems lead patients to rely on adaptive equipment to substitute for poor balance (Fig. 23-1). Loss of

---

BOX 23-1
NDT Philosophy

The NDT Instructors Group approved the following statement of NDT Philosophy in May, 1998 (Bierman, 1998).

The Neurodevelopmental Treatment (NDT)/Bobath approach is a "living concept." It is a problem-solving approach that involves the treatment and management of movement dysfunction in individuals with CNS pathophysiology. The person is addressed as a whole, and intervention is individualized to meet his/her specific goals. NDT is an interactive process among the individual, care givers, and members of the interdisciplinary team.

The overall goal of treatment and management is the enhancement of the individual's capacity to function. To achieve this goal, the practitioner addresses quality of movement utilizing principles of movement science. Treatment involves active participation of the individual, and direct handling to optimize function with gradual withdrawal of direct input by the therapist. The NDT approach contributes to a person's independence and quality of life.

selective movement control prevents patients from using the hemiplegic arm, resulting in reliance on one-handed techniques for task performance. Bobath and Bobath suggested that patients who adopt these asymmetrical compensations learn to neglect the potential for recovery on the hemiplegic side. These compensations also contribute to the development of abnormal, asymmetrical patterns of posture and movement.

Bobath and Bobath identified **abnormal tone** as the second motor problem interfering with movement control and function in hemiplegia. Abnormal tone refers to alterations in muscle tension. After a stroke, muscle tone on the hemiplegic side may be higher or lower than normal. Patients demonstrate **flaccidity**, or hypotonia, when muscle tone is lower than normal. Flaccidity is generally present immediately after the stroke. **Spasticity**, or hypertonia, develops gradually in selected muscles of the affected trunk, arm, and leg and is characterized by excessive muscle stiffness and slow effortful movements. Spasticity is often accompanied by **associated reactions**, which are involuntary, nonfunctional changes in limb position associated with the performance of difficult or stressful activities. For example, the hemiplegic arm may assume a flexed position when the patient walks (Fig. 23-2). According to Bobath and Bobath, spasticity interferes with sequencing of muscle activity on the hemiplegic side, contributing to abnormal patterns of coordination.

Bobath and Bobath believed that these two categories of motor impairment result in the stereotyped nonfunctional movement patterns and functional limitations associated with hemiplegia. In their writings, the Bobaths also emphasized that sensory disturbances may contribute to abnormal coordination and decreased motor control. They hypothesized that patients with hemiplegia have forgotten how to move in normal patterns of coordination. They suggested that this sensory disturbance may result in loss of normal movement responses, even when muscles are sufficiently strong to support movement. The loss of the sensory memory for movement may also contribute to abnormal patterns of coordination, because patients may initiate and sequence muscle activity inappropriately. Thus, while their treatment approach was designed to address problems with tone and movement, the Bobaths recognized that sensation was necessary for motor coordination and motor learning.

Neurodevelopmental Treatment of Patients With Stroke

NDT/Bobath treatment uses a specific set of manual techniques to address the problems of tone and movement control and to provide sensory messages about how movement is organized and executed. These techniques have the goals of preventing or eliminating abnormal patterns of coordination, retraining normal movement responses, and increasing functional use of the hemiplegic side (Box 23-2). B. Bobath used her hands on the patient's body to produce therapeutic changes in tone and movement. She called this treatment **handling** to reflect the manual hands-on quality of her treatment. Initially, handling was relatively static, requiring the use of reflexes and positioning to produce changes in muscle tone. As the approach evolved, handling became a more dynamic process in which the handling activates movement patterns in the patient that both decrease abnormal tone and coordination and reeducate normal movements.

The NDT therapist uses handling to provide specific tactile, proprioceptive, and kinesthetic messages that help organize the quality of the patient's movement and influence the status of relevant impairments, such as

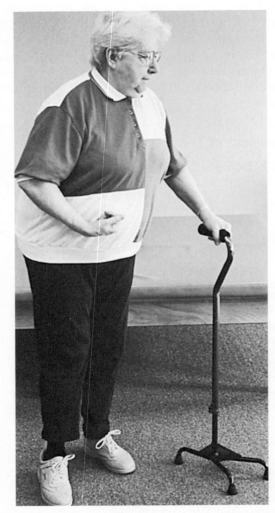

Figure 23-2 Patient showing associated reaction in the hemiparetic arm while walking.

used to activate automatic postural responses and trunk control, and to train weight-bearing and non–weight-bearing movements in the arm and leg. Occupational therapists may also use facilitation techniques to intro-

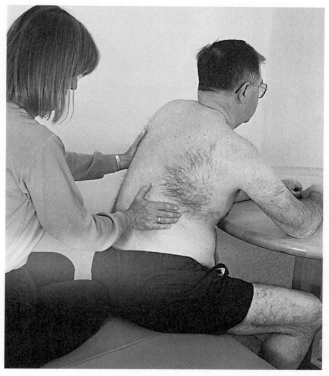

Figure 23-3 Therapist's hands showing key points of control on the trunk.

spasticity and flaccidity. While Bobath and Bobath did not specifically identify impairments such as subluxation and contracture as contributing to abnormal coordination, these impairments may present mechanical blocks to normal movement and are also addressed through handling. B. Bobath found that certain hand placements, which she called **key points of control**, are most effective for controlling the patient's movement. During treatment, the therapist selects key points that give maximal control over the patient's problems and the movement pattern the therapist wishes to influence. Proximal key points are used to influence posture and movement of the trunk, shoulder girdle, and hip, and distal key points are used to control the position of the distal extremities (Fig. 23-3).

Handling is used for two types of techniques: **inhibition** and **facilitation** (Box 23-3). Inhibition techniques are used to address problems of abnormal tone and abnormal coordination. The NDT/Bobath therapist uses inhibition to decrease spasticity and block or eliminate abnormal patterns of movement. Inhibition techniques often use **reflex-inhibiting patterns (RIPs)**, a term for patterns that counteract the pull of tight or spastic muscles. The NDT/ Bobath therapist uses RIPs to establish a normal tonal state prior to teaching normal movement. B. Bobath believed that therapists should not attempt to retrain normal movement responses until spasticity was minimized, because spasticity prevents normal patterns of reciprocal muscle activation.

When muscle tone is normalized through inhibition, the NDT therapist uses facilitation techniques to train normal movement patterns. Facilitation techniques are

duce and practice new strategies for performing functional activities in occupation-as-means or occupation-as-end. During facilitation, the therapist establishes light contact with appropriate key points of control and moves the patient in normal patterns that are important for function. The patient actively participates in this movement-based treatment, even though the therapist initially controls the quality and characteristics of the movement. The therapist uses this handling to teach the patient the sensation of normal movement and to allow the patient to practice movements that cannot be performed independently. As the patient learns to perform the desired movements, the therapist gradually gives the patient more control until the patient moves without input from the therapist.

In cases of flaccid hemiplegia, facilitation techniques may be combined with stronger stimulation techniques to increase muscle tone and muscle contractions. These techniques provide strong proprioceptive input to the muscle via tapping or quick stretch. Stimulation techniques must be used carefully to avoid producing an abnormal response. Once muscle contraction is established, the therapist returns to facilitation with the goal of using the muscle contraction in a normal movement.

Relationship to Occupational Functioning

Bobath and Bobath assumed that improvements in the status of sensorimotor performance components would result in improved occupational performance. They noted that when patients learn new movements, they often spontaneously use these movements functionally without further treatment. For example, when NDT techniques are used in the acute phase, patients may spontaneously use their improved trunk control to adjust the foot pedals on the wheelchair or put on a shirt without need for practice or instruction. However, since remediation of lower-level functional prerequisites may not automatically result in improved occupational performance (Trombly, 1995), the NDT/Bobath approach also uses aspects of occupation-as-means and occupation-as-end.

In occupation-as-end, the patient is directly engaged in learning an activity or task. After a stroke, occupational therapists use occupation-as-end to teach self-care skills such as dressing and bathing or mobility activities such as rolling, transfers, and wheelchair propulsion. NDT therapists have developed compensatory occupation-as-end techniques for activities such as dressing, grooming, and bed mobility. These methods are designed to maintain symmetry and bilaterality and to encourage patients to shift their weight actively and incorporate their involved extremities into task perfor-

mance. The NDT/Bobath approach rejects the use of one-sided compensations, emphasizing instead that patients should perform these tasks in ways that use the hemiplegic side and prevent spasticity. Examples of the use of NDT/Bobath techniques in occupation-as-end are discussed later in the chapter.

In occupation-as-means, the therapist uses activities therapeutically to influence impairments and provide opportunities for motor learning and practice. The NDT therapist frequently uses actual tasks or parts of tasks in occupation-as-means treatment to increase postural control. For example, with the patient sitting, the therapist may use activities that require weight shifts over the body's base of support to increase control of the postural muscles of the trunk and the lower extremity (Fig. 23-4). Similarly, the therapist may structure cooking or grooming tasks to practice use of the hemiplegic arm to support weight while standing or to train the use of the hemiplegic arm in bilateral grasp.

Activities for occupation-as-means should be used to strengthen normal movement control of the muscles of the hemiplegic side. They should incorporate movement patterns that the patient can perform independently but that are not automatic enough to be used easily in daily life. Activities that are too difficult for the patient to perform normally or that result in undesirable patterns of movement should be avoided. However, the NDT therapist may use facilitation to help the patient practice an activity that cannot be performed independently. For example, the therapist may help maintain weight bearing on the hemiplegic arm while the patient practices reaching with the uninvolved arm or may assist the hemiplegic hand to grasp while the patient practices lifting a cup to the mouth. Some examples of NDT occupation-as-means activities are included in the treat-

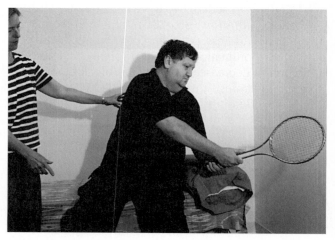

Figure 23-4 Patient swinging a tennis racquet to increase control of trunk.

BOX 23-4
PROCEDURES FOR PRACTICE

NDT/Bobath Evaluation and Treatment Planning

1. Identify abilities and functional capabilities. Include movements of both the arm and leg, postural patterns of the trunk, and functional independence in life skills. How does the patient accomplish these functions?
2. Identify functional limitations, including functions that the patient cannot perform that are necessary for improved independence and quality of life.
3. Determine what problems interfere with movement control and functional performance, such as these:
   ▶ Abnormal tone
   ▶ Abnormal coordination
   ▶ Loss of postural control
   ▶ Loss of selective movement control
   ▶ Sensation
4. Establish functional goals and treatment goals:
   ▶ Identify the functions that the patient will be able to learn to perform within an established time frame. Indicate whether performance will involve compensation or use of the involved side with normal coordination.
   ▶ Identify the impairments that you will need to address to meet the functional goal.
   ▶ Based on the patient's response to handling, determine where to begin treatment. What techniques of inhibition and facilitation will be used?

Adapted with permission from Bobath, B. (1990). *Adult Hemiplegia: Evaluation and Treatment* (3rd ed.). London: Heinemann; and from Ryerson, S., & Levit, K. (1997). The shoulder in hemiplegia. In R. Donatelli (Ed.), *Physical therapy of the shoulder* (3rd ed., pp 205–228). New York: Churchill Livingstone.

tact with the patient, the therapist observes the patient's behavior to gather information about typical posture, preferred movement patterns, and spontaneous use of the hemiplegic side. The therapist also observes how the patient performs activities of daily living (ADL), transfers, and bed mobility. The therapist notes whether the patient spontaneously uses the affected side or relies on compensations that reflect asymmetry and neglect. The therapist also watches to see whether the patient demonstrates abnormal tone and coordination on the hemiplegic side. These problems will be addressed in treatment.

Although these initial observations yield important information, the most important aspect of the NDT assessment is the evaluation of motor patterns and the patient's response to being moved. These tests are described briefly next. A more detailed description of the tests can be found in Bobath (1990).

The NDT therapist uses handling to identify the normal patterns of movement that are present on the hemiplegic side and the abnormal patterns that are contributing to the patient's movement problems and functional limitations. The therapist also uses handling to determine the patient's response to sensory input. To assess movement control, the therapist moves the patient into postures and movement sequences that are important for occupational performance. For example, the therapist tests postural control by facilitating trunk movements, equilibrium reactions and protective responses (Fig. 23-5) with the patient sitting and standing.

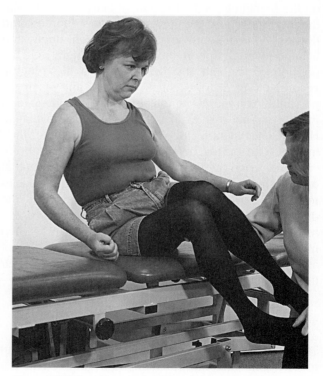

Figure 23-5 Therapist using handling to test equilibrium reactions.

ment section of this chapter. Eggers (1984) provided a complete description for using occupation-as-means within an NDT framework.

Evaluation and Treatment Planning

The NDT/Bobath approach uses assessment to gather information about the patient's movement control and functional status, the problems interfering with use of the hemiplegic side, and the patient's response to handling (Box 23-4). This information is used to set treatment goals and plan treatment activities. This section reviews the important components of this system of evaluation and treatment planning.

Assessment in the NDT/Bobath Approach

The NDT therapist gathers assessment information through a variety of procedures. During the initial con-

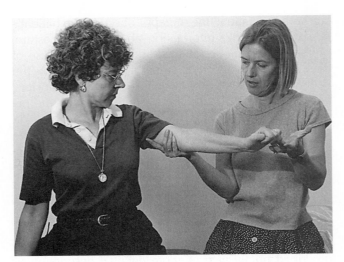

Figure 23-6 Therapist using placing to assess control of the hemiparetic arm.

The therapist also uses handling to test selective control of arm and leg movements by moving proximal and distal limb segments in varying combinations of joint movement. The therapist uses information about the patient's balance and spontaneous movements gained in the observational stage of assessment to select the movement patterns to be assessed via handling.

Handling provides the therapist with specific sensory information about the quality and strength of the patient's movements. When movement control is present on the hemiplegic side, the patient actively assists with the movement, and the movement seems effortless and flowing. If the therapist stops the movement briefly and lightens manual support, the patient will briefly hold the position. B. Bobath referred to this as the **placing response** (Fig. 23-6). Facilitation is easy and placing is possible when muscle tone is in the normal range and muscle strength is available to support movement. However, facilitation and placing are not possible when muscle tone on the hemiplegic side is abnormal. For example, when the therapist facilitates movements that oppose the pull of spastic muscles, the spastic muscles resist the movements, and movements that go in the direction of spastic activity are performed with excessive assistance. Similar problems with facilitation arise when muscle tone is hypotonic. Patients with flaccidity do not assist movements or show the placing response. Their limbs feel heavy and floppy during facilitation.

Treatment Goals for the Stages of Recovery

The NDT/Bobath therapist uses the information about muscle tone and movement control gathered in the evaluation to establish treatment goals. NDT therapists establish several types of goals. The therapist sets functional goals to be achieved through practice of occupation-as-means or occupation-as-end. In addition, the NDT therapist establishes goals that relate to motor problems, such as spasticity, that will be inhibited and movements on the hemiplegic side to be facilitated. The exact goals depend on the patient's problems, level of functional independence, movement control, and reasons for seeking treatment.

In acute-care or inpatient rehabilitation settings, most patients have impairments such as weakness and loss of muscle control and are dependent in most self-care activities. At this stage of recovery, NDT goals focus on increasing independence in life tasks, preventing the development of abnormal tone and abnormal movements, and increasing motor control on the hemiplegic side. To accomplish functional goals, the NDT/Bobath therapist introduces and practices adapted techniques for ADL, bed mobility, transfers, and wheelchair management. These NDT occupation-as-end techniques are designed to increase occupational performance while preventing learned neglect, postural asymmetry, and associated reactions. For example, the therapist may train the patient to sit up in bed from lying on the hemiplegic side to introduce weight bearing on the hemiplegic arm and leg (Fig. 23-7). The therapist also uses positioning, range of motion exercises, and inhibitory treatment techniques, such as supine scapula mobilization and weight bearing on the hemiplegic arm, to maintain muscle length and prevent spasticity. The therapist uses facilitation to increase muscle control in

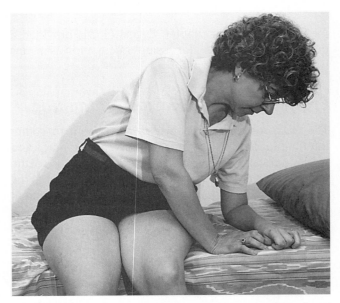

Figure 23-7 Patient practicing sitting up using the hemiparetic arm for support.

postural adjustments and selective movements of the arm.

As patients recover from strokes, their problems change, and so do the treatment goals. Although some patients remain flaccid on their hemiplegic side or recover motor control without developing abnormal tone, many develop spasticity in some muscles. Spasticity first appears as an associated reaction in conjunction with patients' efforts to become more independent in self-care activities and with early attempts at walking. Abnormal posturing of the arm and leg is more common, and the spastic muscles develop increased resistance to passive stretch. Patients with spasticity are usually able to use compensatory patterns for gross motor patterns like rolling and sitting up and for some ADL. Their trunk control has improved enough to allow sitting and standing without loss of balance and walking with a brace and cane. However, their trunk posture is often asymmetrical, with less weight taken on the hemiplegic leg. The patient with spasticity may also have regained sufficient muscle control in the hemiplegic arm to move it, but abnormal coordination and excessive stiffness prevent skilled functional use (Fig. 23-8).

NDT treatment goals for the patient with spasticity include inhibiting abnormal tone and movement, increasing normal movement responses, and improving occupational performance by incorporating the hemiplegic side into task performance. The therapist uses inhibition techniques to address specific problems with abnormal tone, abnormal coordination, and associated reactions. Treatment should also include use of facilitation to increase postural control in sitting and standing and to develop selective movement control in the hemiplegic arm and hand. Because patients at this stage of recovery are functionally independent in many tasks, functional goals may include training of new tasks, decreasing compensations in tasks that are performed independently, and increasing functional use of the hemiplegic arm and hand. For example, to increase functional independence for a patient who shaves with his uninvolved hand while sitting, the therapist may either teach him to perform this task while standing or train him to use the hemiplegic hand to apply shaving cream.

Many patients with hemiplegia do not progress beyond the problems associated with spasticity and fail to develop normal movement control in their hemiplegic side. However, some patients never develop spasticity in the involved side, and others recover movement control. These higher-level patients walk well without postural asymmetry because they have better trunk control and are able to support weight on their hemiplegic leg. They also show improvements in motor control of the hemiplegic arm and may be able to use the arm for weight

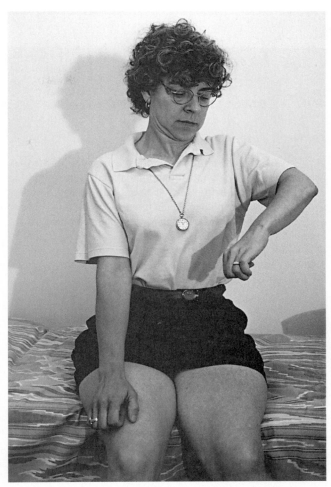

Figure 23-8 Patient moving arm that demonstrates abnormal pattern of coordination.

support and to hold objects that are placed in the hand. In spite of the good motor recovery, problems opening the hand to initiate grasp and release and maintaining good elbow extension during reaching may persist. These patients may also complain of problems with the accuracy and speed of movement that make it difficult to use the arm for function. NDT goals for higher-level patients focus on improving coordination of the hemiplegic arm and hand, especially in the patterns necessary for reach, grasp, and manipulation, and decreasing compensation. The therapist may use facilitation, occupation-as-means, and occupation-as-end to achieve these goals.

Treatment Techniques: Integrating NDT/Bobath into OT Practice

The NDT/Bobath approach is most effective when used by all members of the rehabilitation team, so that nurses; physical, occupational, and speech therapists; and fam-

Case Example

MR. R: BOBATH/NDT APPROACH TO TREATMENT OF STROKE

Patient Information

Mr. R., a 64-year-old retired economist 2 months post stroke, was referred to outpatient occupational therapy after treatment in a rehabilitation center and at home. Mr. R. had a severe stroke that resulted in flaccidity in the muscles of the left trunk, arm, and leg and loss of balance in sitting and standing. At the time of the evaluation, the patient and his wife were living with a daughter and her family because of the demands associated with his care. The occupational therapy assessment identified the following problems:

- Dependence in ADLs and IADLs due to loss of postural control
- Severe pain in left shoulder and edema of the left hand
- Failure to attend to the left side of the body or to position the left arm for safety or comfort
- Nonfunctional left arm and hand due to flaccidity

Recommendations

The occupational therapist recommended 2 therapy sessions per week for 8 weeks. Mr. R.'s insurance company authorized 16 30-minute sessions. In consultation with Mr. R. and his daughter, the occupational therapist established the following treatment goals, which were motivated by the patient's desire to return to his own home:

- Increase independence in dressing and bathing with compensations that increase the use of the left side
- Eliminate shoulder pain and hand edema
- Increase automatic attention to the left arm during functional activities
- Train wheelchair management and transfers
- Increase functional use of the left arm in forearm weight bearing in sitting

Short-Term Goals

- **Mr. R. will be able to sit unsupported on a firm chair and initiate trunk weight shifts in anteroposterior, lateral, and rotational planes without loss of balance.** The therapist determined that Mr. R. lacked sufficient control of trunk movements in sitting to dress safely. During treatment, she worked to increase control of trunk movements in the patterns necessary for upper and lower body dressing and grooming. She also used weight bearing at a table to increase trunk control so that Mr. R. would learn to support weight on his affected left arm and activate muscles in his trunk and shoulder girdle. The therapist taught Mr. R. and his daughter how to practice

these trunk movements at home. She also changed the way the daughter helped Mr. R. transfer to increase weight bearing on the left leg and appropriate activity in trunk extensor muscles. As trunk control improved, Mr. R. could use his uninvolved right arm to put on his shirt while sitting without loss of balance. He also could independently manage his wheelchair locks and foot pedals. Visual neglect of the left side decreased, as he was able to turn his head to the left without loss of balance.

- **Mr. R. will wear the prescribed shoulder support and hand splint while he is out of bed and perform edema massage and shoulder exercises three times a day.** The therapist removed the elevated arm trough from the patient's wheelchair because it increased shoulder pain. She showed the patient's daughter how to use a pillow to position the arm in the wheelchair. Mr. R. was fitted with a commercial shoulder brace for use during walking. This brace supported the subluxation but did not position the elbow in flexion. The therapist also fabricated a wrist splint that supported the wrist in neutral but did not contain a finger platform. The patient and daughter were instructed to stop all exercises that caused pain. They were taught how to massage the hand to decrease edema. In addition, the therapist taught Mr. R. how to move his arm in small ranges, supporting the left hand in the right using the modified clasped hand grasp, and how to position the arm in bed. The treatment was successful. Hand edema began to decrease immediately, and the hand was no longer painful to the touch after three treatments. The therapist also could passively move the arm below 60° of shoulder elevation without pain in supine when supporting the shoulder joint. The therapist changed the massage and passive exercise program to reflect these improvements. She also introduced transfers and rolling using the clasped-hand technique to incorporate the left arm into the activity.

- **Mr. R. will actively assist with dressing.** Mr. R.'s daughter was used to dressing her father while he lay in bed. The therapist recommended that they start dressing with Mr. R. seated in a straight chair with arms. One treatment session was devoted to teaching Mr. R.'s daughter how to assist dressing while encouraging her father to be active and assist the task. The daughter initially supported the left arm and assisted trunk weight shifts. As her father grew more confident, she provided less physical assistance but continued to give verbal cues. The therapist introduced occupation-as-end dressing when Mr. R. had sufficient trunk control to perform necessary weight shifts without loss of balance and when pain no longer limited passive movements of the left arm.

Revised Goals

▶ Mr. R. will perform upper body and lower body dressing activities independently while sitting in a straight chair.

▶ Mr. R. will attend to the position of his left arm at all times and will position the arm appropriately without verbal reminders.

▶ Mr. R. will support weight on the left forearm in sitting at a table and use this pattern functionally in activities such as eating, reading and writing.

▶ Mr. R. will transfer independently from the wheel chair using the clasped-hands technique.

CLINICAL REASONING
in OT Practice

Effects of Physical Impairments on ADL Performance

At the time of his evaluation, Mr. R. could not dress himself. His daughter was dressing and undressing him. The occupational therapist wanted to start training him to dress immediately, as independent self-care was a major long-term goal. Her plan was to develop a dressing plan for Mr. R. and his daughter to use at home. This plan would begin with support and assistance from the daughter, with the daughter gradually withdrawing this assistance as Mr. R. developed better control of the movement components necessary for independence.

What impairments contributed to Mr. R.'s loss of functional performance? What support and assistance are most important during the first dressing sessions? How do you teach Mr. R.'s daughter to assist upper body dressing during the early phase of treatment? How can she assist lower extremity dressing?

Selection of Shoulder Support for Subluxed Shoulder

The occupational therapist prescribed the use of a shoulder support for Mr. R.'s left arm. She expected the support to decrease shoulder pain by stabilizing the joint position while Mr. R. was sitting and walking. The therapist wanted to use a support that conforms to NDT principles. Would the therapist choose a traditional bucket sling for Mr. R.? Why might this sling be undesirable? What features should the therapist look for in selecting an appropriate sling?

---

ily members all use a similar approach to management. However, occupational therapists can have a significant effect on tone and movement by integrating NDT principles and techniques into OT practice, even when other professionals use a differing treatment approach.

The next section describes ways to integrate NDT concepts and techniques into rehabilitation of the hemiplegic arm and into ADL. The Neurodevelopmental Treatment Association offers postgraduate training courses for physical and occupational therapists interested in learning more about this approach to treatment (see Resource).

Treatment of the Hemiplegic Arm

The NDT/ Bobath approach to treatment of the hemiplegic arm is designed to address impairments such as abnormal tone, pain, subluxation, and the loss of movement control. Specific impairments are treated using inhibition techniques such as reflex-inhibiting patterns, scapula mobilization, trunk rotation, and weight bearing. NDT therapists also use facilitation to reeducate selective arm movements, to teach the patient to use the arm for weight bearing, and to increase skilled use of the hand. While inhibition of abnormal responses is generally done before facilitation of normal movements, the line between inhibition and facilitation is often indistinct, as techniques such as weight bearing can be used for both inhibition and facilitation. The amount of treatment time devoted to inhibition versus facilitation varies according to severity of problems and treatment goals, but both techniques are generally used in every treatment session.

Inhibition in Arm Treatment

Inhibition is an important part of the NDT approach to movement reeducation because normal movements cannot be facilitated in the presence of abnormal tone and reflex activity. NDT therapists use inhibition with patients who have spasticity to decrease the amount of tension in the muscle, restore normal resting lengths to muscles that are habitually shortened and stop excessive or unwanted muscle contraction. Bobath and Bobath described inhibition of spasticity as the process of **normalizing tone**, because after treatment the spastic arm feels flexible and light rather than stiff and heavy, and it can follow guided movement more normally.

Reflex inhibiting patterns (RIPs) are one the main techniques for inhibiting spasticity in the hemiplegic arm. Since flexor spasticity in the arm is concentrated in

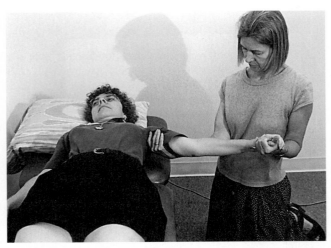

Figure 23-9 Therapist using a RIP to inhibit flexor spasticity.

BOX 23-5
PROCEDURES FOR PRACTICE

Inhibition of Spasticity in the Hemiplegic Arm using RIP

1. Position patient in sitting.
2. Place hands on the hemiplegic arm using proximal and distal key points of control. Patient's arm will be in a flexed, adducted position.
3. Correct adduction of the humerus first, leaving the elbow in flexion.
4. Maintain the humerus in neutral rotation by the side of the body and use pressure on top of the forearm to extend the elbow gradually. If the forearm is supinated, pronate it first.
5. When the tension in the biceps has decreased, slide your hand from top of the forearm to the wrist and hand. Extend the wrist to neutral first, leaving the fingers flexed.
6. When tension in the wrist flexors has decreased, open the fingers, keeping the wrist in a neutral position.
7. Maintain the arm in an extended position and proceed to weight bearing or guided movement.

shoulder elevators and internal rotators and elbow, wrist, and finger flexors, it is inhibited with a RIP that includes shoulder girdle depression and shoulder external rotation, elbow and wrist extension, and an open hand (Fig. 23-9). When muscles in the hemiplegic arm are spastic, they resist lengthening, and the therapist must move slowly and systematically to bring the arm into the full RIP (Box 23-5). Once spasticity in the arm has decreased, the therapist begins to retrain selective movements using facilitation. The next section discusses this process. Bobath (1990) also described the use of trunk rotation

and shoulder mobilization in supine, and the use of weight bearing to inhibit flexor spasticity in the hemiplegic arm.

In acute rehabilitation, most patients exhibit low tone and weakness rather than spasticity. In this setting, NDT therapists use inhibition techniques instead of traditional techniques, such as range of motion and stretching, to maintain muscle length and normal joint mechanics in the shoulder girdle and arm and to prevent spasticity and abnormal coordination. The therapist places the hemiplegic arm in an extended position that maintains passive length in the flexor muscles of the arm and holds this position while facilitating normal movement responses. If the hemiplegic arm has little or no spasticity, it does not resist moving into the RIP. Because the muscles of the arm provide no resistance, the therapist must be careful not to overstretch the wrist and hand while using this technique (Box 23-6).

The therapist and nurse should help the patient position the flaccid arm in patterns that maintain muscle length in elbow extension and shoulder girdle abduction and external rotation. For example, when the patient lies supine in bed, the hemiplegic arm should be positioned with the elbow in extension, the shoulder and forearm in neutral rotation, and the hand and wrist supported so that they do not fall into flexion (Fig. 23-10). This position is preferable to allowing the patient to rest the arm on the chest, where it lies in flexion. While the patient is in the wheelchair, lap boards or pillows should support the hemiplegic arm. These wheelchair aids support the weight of the hemiplegic arm and help prevent both shoulder subluxation and spasticity. Positioning techniques are used less frequently as the patient recovers motor control in the hemiplegic arm.

BOX 23-6
SAFETY BOX

Avoiding Overstretch of the Flaccid Arm

The therapist must be careful to avoid overstretching the flaccid muscles of the hand and wrist during inhibition, facilitation, and upper extremity weight bearing.

▶ Avoid positioning the wrist in maximal extension or flattening the palm of the hand.
▶ Do not pull the hemiplegic thumb into hyperextension or hyperextend the metacarpal joints of the fingers, as this may result in hypermobility of these small joints.
▶ Use a distal grip that maintains the wrist joint in neutral or slight extension and supports the transverse arches of the palm. The therapist may let the patient's fingers flex when the palm and wrist are supported.

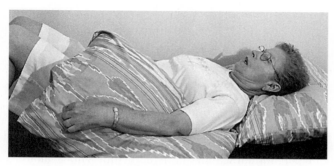

Figure 23-10 Hemiplegic arm correctly positioned for sleeping.

Facilitation

Facilitation techniques are designed to restore normal movement responses and to prevent learning abnormal patterns of coordination. Facilitation includes teaching the patient to support weight on the hemiplegic arm, teaching the patient to perform selective movements of the hemiplegic arm in patterns important for function, and providing opportunities to practice functional use of the arm in occupation-as-means. Facilitation in occupation-as-end is discussed in the next section.

Weight-Bearing Movements

Weight bearing is one of the most important aspects of NDT treatment of the hemiplegic upper extremity because it can be used to maintain muscle length, normalize tone, and increase activity in the muscles of the trunk and arm (Ryerson & Levit, 1997b). In the NDT/Bobath approach, weight bearing is a dynamic process. Rather than statically propping on a rigid arm, the patient is taught to activate muscles in the trunk by moving body weight over the stable arm. This movement of the trunk automatically produces changes in the position of the hemiplegic arm relative to the trunk, actively lengthening and shortening muscles, and results in changing patterns of muscle activation in the arm. Since use of the arm for weight support does not require fine motor control, even patients with severe weakness and loss of motor control can learn to use their hemiplegic arms in weight bearing. Thus, weight bearing is used to facilitate muscle activity in the hemiplegic arm and to increase functional use of that arm.

The NDT therapist generally begins to train weight bearing by teaching the patient to accept weight on the hemiplegic arm with forearms on a table (Ryerson & Levit, 1997a). This pattern is important for activities that are commonly performed at a table, such as eating, reading, and writing (Fig. 23-11). Extended arm (elbow) weight bearing is more difficult for the patient because it requires control of the elbow and wrist joints as well as control of the trunk and shoulder girdle. NDT therapists often train extended arm weight bearing with the hemiplegic arm by the side of the body when the patient is sitting. This position is used functionally for supporting the trunk and to assist with standing up. As the patient improves balance control in standing, the therapist may also train extended arm weight bearing in that position, so that the patient learns to use the hemiplegic arm for support while working in the kitchen or bathroom.

Selective Arm Movements

Facilitation of arm movements is another important part of arm treatment (Box 23-7). The NDT therapist uses this aspect of facilitation to give the patient the sensation of normal movement, teach normal patterns of initiation and sequencing, and reeducate and strengthen normal movements to be used for function (Ryerson & Levit, 1997a). Facilitation is really a system of guided move-

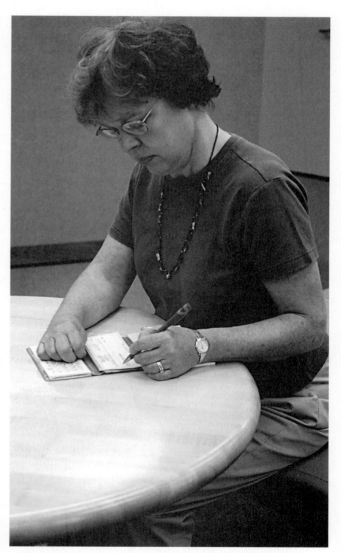

Figure 23-11 Patient using hemiparetic arm to support weight and provide stability while writing.

BOX 23-7
PROCEDURES FOR PRACTICE

The Process of Facilitation

1. Restore alignment of the segments to be moved using key points of control.
2. Assist the desired movement using light hands.
3. Proceed slowly and feel for the patient's response.
4. Repeat movements until patient can actively assist.
5. Lighten messages of your hands so that the patient moves with less assistance. Give verbal feedback during this phase.
6. Gradually withdraw control. The patient's movement control may decline but should not produce an abnormal response.
7. Provide practice opportunities through use of activities (occupation-as-means) or home exercises.

ment. In the acute stage, the therapist uses proximal and distal key points to establish normal alignment in the arm and maintains this control while moving the patient's arm in normal patterns that are important for functional use of the arm. The patient is encouraged to assist with the movement when possible. As the patient begins to assist, the therapist first lightens, then removes a portion of the control, giving the patient the opportunity to take partial control of the movement. The therapist uses the information from handling to decide where and when to let go, so that the quality of the patient's movement pattern stays relatively consistent when the therapist withdraws control. Handling provides the patient with sensory messages that teach the timing and sequencing of arm movements. The active assistive quality of facilitation also helps to decrease the excessive effort that many hemiplegic patients use to initiate movements of their involved side.

Arm Treatment With the Patient Supine. The NDT therapist often begins to facilitate normal patterns of arm movement with the patient supine. Supine is the easiest position for patients with low tone and weakness to control their arms because the bed or mat provides postural stability. Treatment of the supine patient is also easier for the therapist, as the stable position of the patient's trunk makes it easier to maintain normal scapulohumeral rhythm while lifting the hemiplegic arm into flexion and abduction.

To facilitate arm movements in supine, the therapist begins by making sure that the hemiplegic shoulder joint is correctly aligned by repositioning the humeral head in the fossa if the joint is subluxated. Then, using proximal and distal key points on the arm, the therapist extends

the hemiplegic elbow and brings the patient's shoulder into flexion (Fig. 23-12). The therapist should make sure that the scapula rotates easily before bringing the arm above 60° of forward flexion. If the therapist thinks spasticity or muscle tightness is blocking scapula movement, scapula mobilization can restore normal joint mechanics before bringing the arm into elevation. Patients feel pain in the hemiplegic shoulder during facilitation when the humerus is not seated in the fossa or when normal scapulohumeral rhythm is not available. Therefore, the therapist must correct shoulder joint alignment and maintain normal joint mechanics while facilitating arm movements in any position to avoid traumatizing the shoulder joint (Box 23-8).

When the hemiplegic arm can be raised above 90° of flexion without pain, the therapist begins to use guided movement as facilitation to increase muscle activity. As the therapist feels the patient begin to assist or follow her movements, she asks the patient to try to

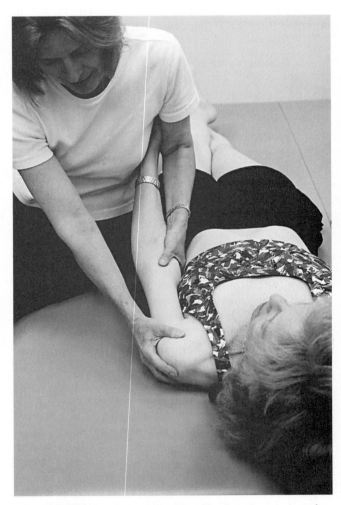

Figure 23-12 Therapist corrects position of hemiparetic arm prior to facilitating arm movements.

The therapist must reposition the subluxed shoulder joint before active or passive movements of the arm are attempted. Correcting the subluxation entails moving the scapula into neutral or slight upward rotation and lifting the humerus so that it rests in the glenoid fossa. The therapist should maintain the shoulder joint in this corrected position during treatment of the arm. To restore normal joint mechanics,

► The therapist places one hand under the axilla to support the inferior portion of the shoulder joint and the other hand on the patient's scapula. The therapist uses this hand placement to correct the position of the upper trunk and to rotate the scapula upward.
► Holding the corrected shoulder position with one hand, the therapist moves the other hand to the distal humerus and lifts the humerus up into the glenoid fossa.
► If the humerus is internally rotated, the therapist moves the humerus into neutral rotation.
► The therapist checks that the scapula is mobile on the thorax before moving the arm above 60° of forward flexion or abduction. If the scapula cannot rotate freely, scapular mobility should be restored before moving the humerus into elevation.
► The therapist maintains correct scapulohumeral rhythm during arm treatment.

hold the arm in position. B. Bobath called this technique **place and hold** because it is based on the normal placing response. Place and hold can be practiced with the shoulder and elbow in varying positions so that the patient develops control of proximal and distal arm movements (Fig. 23-13). As the patient develops the ability to place the arm in supine and to move in small ranges without letting the arm fall, handling is lightened or removed to allow opportunities for independent practice.

Arm Movements With the Patient Sitting. As soon as the patient begins to assist with facilitated movements in supine, the therapist should begin to practice guided movements of the arm with the patient is sitting. Subluxation of the glenohumeral joint is more common in sitting than supine because the muscles of the hemiplegic arm are too weak to hold the scapula in the correct position on the trunk and because the loss of trunk control also affects scapula alignment (Ryerson & Levit, 1997a, 1997b). The therapist must reduce the subluxation before beginning facilitation and maintain this corrected position during arm treatment. (Figs.

23-14 to 23-16). Initially, the therapist uses this control over the shoulder girdle during guided movements of the arm to strengthen normal patterns of coordination and prevent pain. As strength and control increase, the therapist gradually withdraws this control.

The NDT therapist uses facilitation to reeducate or strengthen movements that are difficult for the patient to perform without assistance. The movements of shoulder flexion or shoulder abduction with elbow extension are usually the most difficult because they go against the pattern of muscle return. The therapist facilitates these extended arm movements to establish this difficult pattern of coordination and to prevent the patient from learning to use flexor spasticity to move the arm. However, to use the arm for function, the patient must initiate arm movements with different combinations of shoulder and elbow movements. To do this, the therapist uses facilitation of elbow flexion and extension so that the patient gains control of elbow movements outside the pattern of mass flexion.

Using Occupation-As-Means in Arm Treatment

The NDT therapist uses occupation-as-means activities to practice and strengthen movement control in the hemiplegic arm and to combine movements of the arm with trunk weight shifts. The therapist uses handling to introduce these activities but should withdraw this control as quickly as possible, letting the patient practice without assistance. Occupation-as-means activities can be set up with the hemiplegic arm in weight bearing. For example, the patient may play checkers on the treatment mat while weight bearing on the hemiplegic arm or rinse dishes in the sink with the unaffected hand while maintaining the hemiplegic arm on the counter

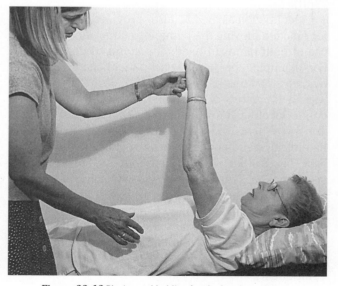

Figure 23-13 Placing and holding for the hemiparetic arm.

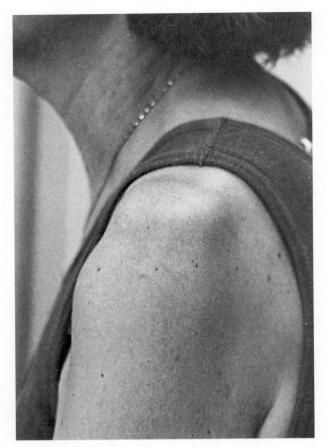

Figure 23-14 Close-up of shoulder showing glenohumeral subluxation.

Occupation-As-End Treatment

Occupational therapists incorporate NDT/Bobath principles and techniques into occupation-as-end training of ADL and other tasks by using specific compensations that support the goals of handling. These NDT/Bobath compensations are designed to incorporate the involved arm into task performance and increase or maintain trunk symmetry by encouraging active trunk movements. NDT therapists also use these compensations to prevent spasticity and abnormal coordination in the hemiplegic arm. The NDT therapist selects the occupations to be trained according to the patient's level of functioning and the goals for independence. Therapists who deliver services in hospitals or at home probably focus on retraining basic ADL, such as bathing, dressing, and toileting, and tasks such as rolling in bed and transfers. However, as patients regain their independence in these occupations, therapists may incorporate NDT principles into occupation-as-end training of vocational tasks, such as using a computer mouse, or leisure activities, such as golf or swimming.

Gross motor activities such as rolling in bed, sitting up, and standing up are important functional tasks that

(Fig. 23-17). These activities help the patient learn to use the hemiplegic arm to provide support and balance. The patient may also practice using weight bearing on the arm to inhibit associated reactions during dressing (Fig. 23-18).

Occupation-as-means also provides opportunities for practice moving the hemiplegic arm or coordinating use of both hands in bilateral patterns of coordination. For example, the hemiplegic patient may strengthen reaching patterns of the hemiplegic arm by practicing wiping the table or washing a window. To practice control of elbow movements, the therapist may facilitate arm movements while the patient holds an object in the hemiplegic hand and practices bringing it to the body or face (Fig. 23-19). Bilateral coordination is reinforced by tasks such as carrying a tray or pushing a vacuum cleaner. The therapist selects tasks for occupation-as-means according to the movement components embedded in them. The practice of these meaningful activities is expected to generalize to increased functional use of the hemiplegic arm in other tasks that use similar components.

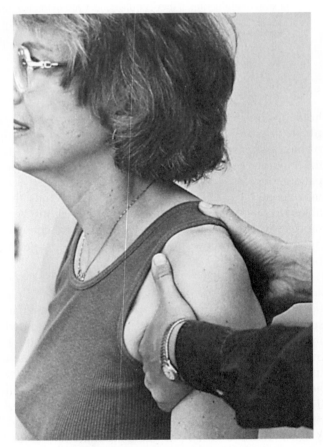

Figure 23-15 Therapist correcting subluxation.

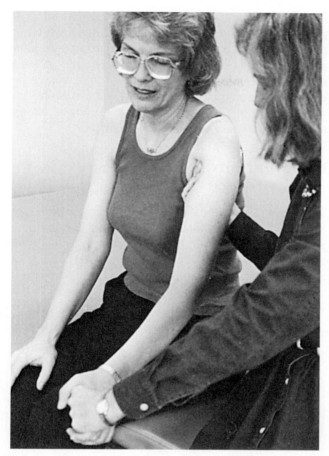

Figure 23-16 Therapist controlling subluxation while facilitating arm movement.

are introduced in acute treatment. When the patient cannot move the hemiplegic arm, the NDT therapist trains specific compensations designed to prevent neglect of the arm during these activities and prevent abnormal coordination or one-sided compensations. For example, the NDT therapist teaches the patient to interlace the fingers of both hands, keeping palms together and thumbs facing up, when it is necessary to move the arm. This clasped-hand grip helps patients to maintain the hemiplegic forearm in midposition and the wrist in extension and to move the arm forward with elbow extension, avoiding the pattern of flexor spasticity. Patients who have difficulty interlacing the fingers may grasp the ulnar side of the hemiplegic wrist and place the uninvolved thumb in the palm of the hemiplegic hand.

The therapist teaches patients to use the clasped-hand grip for self-ranging activities in sitting and supine, rolling, and standing up. For example, the therapist teaches rolling to the uninvolved side by having the patient clasp the hands, reach both hands toward the ceiling with extended elbows, then initiate rolling by turning the head and reaching both arms across the body (Fig. 23-20, *A* and *B*). This technique ensures that the hemiplegic arm does not get left behind the body and that the patient will not turn in bed by pulling on the bed rails. Similarly, having the patient clasp hands before coming to standing prevents an associated reaction in the hemiplegic arm, maintains symmetry in the trunk, and prevents the patient from pushing up with the unaffected arm.

The NDT therapist also uses compensatory techniques to incorporate the hemiplegic arm into activities such as dressing and grooming. Flexor posturing of the arm during task performance is a major problem for some patients. Typically the arm postures when the patient is struggling or using excessive effort. After the task is complete, the arm may remain in this flexed position. The NDT therapist introduces compensations during life tasks to maintain symmetry in the trunk and maintain the hemiplegic arm in extension. For example, to prevent posturing of the hemiplegic arm while the patient puts on a shirt, the patient may be taught to flex

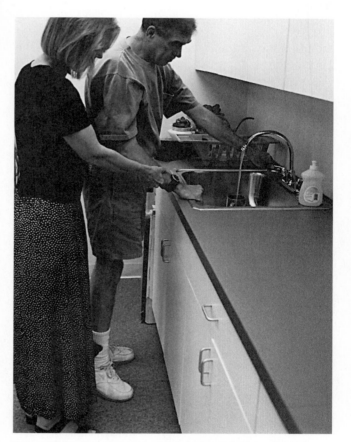

Figure 23-17 Therapist helps maintain the hemiparetic arm in weight bearing while the patient rinses the dishes at the sink.

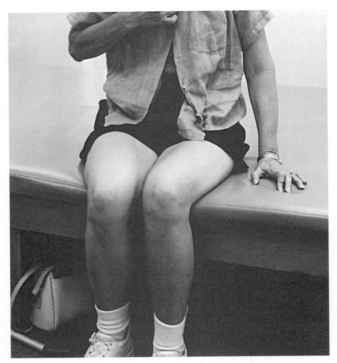

Figure 23-18 Patient uses hemiparetic arm in weight bearing while dressing.

the trunk forward and reach the hemiplegic arm to the floor before putting it into the shirt sleeve (Fig. 23-21) (Davis, 1990). This technique passively maintains extension in the arm. As control of the arm improves, the patient may learn to place the hemiplegic arm in a position of extended weight bearing on the bed during tasks such as buttoning the shirt, when the arm is most likely to posture.

Although functional training is designed to promote independent task performance, the NDT therapist initially uses handling in combination with verbal instructions and demonstrations to teach the patient what is expected. The NDT therapist uses handling to structure the task, so that the patient has only to control the movement of one body segment during task practice. Handling is a particularly important part of occupation-as-end training in the acute phase, since patients at this stage of recovery have problems controlling both trunk and arm position (Van Dyck, 1999).

For patients with poor sitting balance, the NDT therapist may assist the movement of the trunk during task practice. For example, the therapist may use his or her hands on the patient's trunk to provide stability and maintain weight on the hemiplegic hip while the patient leans forward to don shoes (Fig. 23-22). Or the therapist may assist the upper extremity in task performance while the patient performs the necessary trunk movements

independently. For example, the therapist may facilitate the correct shoulder and elbow movements while the patient holds the deodorant stick in the hemiplegic hand and applies it to the uninvolved side. As the patient's movement control increases and task performance becomes more automatic, the therapist withdraws physical assistance. At this point, verbal feedback may be offered to help improve the patient's performance.

Contributions to Psychosocial Adjustment

The emphasis that the NDT/Bobath approach places on functional recovery in the hemiplegic side has potential psychosocial as well as physical benefits to patients who have had strokes. In contrast to traditional rehabilitation approaches, whose emphasis on compensatory use of the uninvolved side suggests that the hemiplegic side will not recover, the NDT/Bobath approach, with its

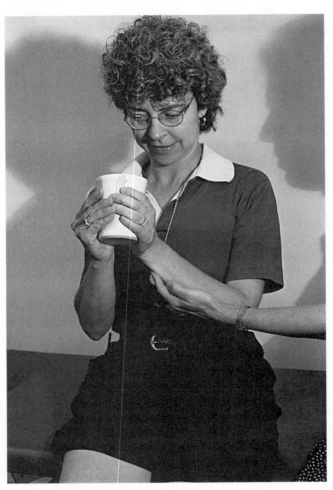

Figure 23-19 Therapist facilitates elbow flexion while the patient grasps cup with both hand and brings it to the mouth.

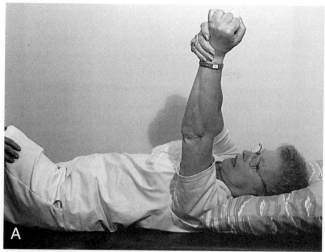

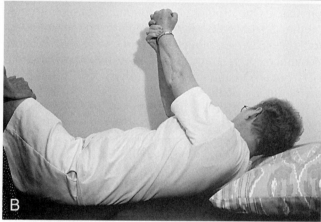

Figure 23-20 A. Patient lifts hemiplegic arm. **B.** Patient turns the arms and upper trunk to roll to the uninvolved side.

emphasis on treating the hemiplegic side, offers stroke patients a very different message. From the early days of rehabilitation, NDT therapists help stroke patients relearn functional tasks in ways that make use of the existing motor patterns in the trunk, arm, and leg. They also use treatment to increase control of movement in the affected side. These treatment activities give the hemiplegic patient realistic hopes of functional recovery, may contribute to a more positive attitude toward the disability, and engender positive outcome expectancies.

Efficacy and Outcomes Research

A literature search of the NDT/Bobath approach to stroke rehabilitation identified a small body of research comparing the effectiveness of this approach with that of other therapeutic interventions. Salter et al. (1991)

compared the functional status of patients receiving NDT treatment with that of patients receiving traditional treatment during inpatient rehabilitation. Eighty patients with a diagnosis of cerebrovascular accident received either traditional rehabilitation or NDT from nurses and therapists. There were no significant differences in length of stay or functional status at discharge. While the NDT group had significantly higher functional scores on toileting, they also had higher scores on this measure at admission, suggesting that this difference is not a valid treatment effect.

Wagenaar et al. (1990) used an alternating treatment design to compare the efficacy of NDT with that of Brunnstrom's movement therapy approach in promoting functional recovery post stroke. The authors expected large differences in efficacy between the two approaches because of their contrasting approaches to treatment but found no major differences in functional

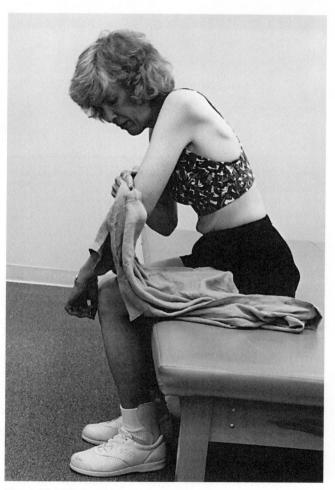

Figure 23-21 Patient using compensation to put the hemiparetic arm in the sleeve.

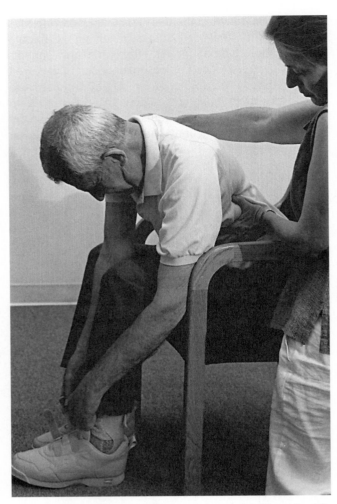

Figure 23-22 Therapist using handling techniques to provide trunk stability while the patient fastens his shoes.

recovery associated with type of treatment. One patient made greater progress in walking speed during the Brunnstrom phases, but this result did not generalize to other patients or to other measures of functional performance. The authors reported that motor recovery, not treatment, was most highly correlated with upper extremity function and walking status. Similar results were reported by Basmajian et al. (1987) in a study comparing the results of an NDT-based intervention with a program of cognitive and behavioral training.

Sunderlund et al. (1992) compared the results of traditional British therapy that they identified as Bobath with the results generated by an enhanced therapy regime consisting of more frequent treatments, home exercises, and behavioral methods designed to increase motor learning. The subjects were 132 stroke patients randomly assigned to the Bobath or enhanced treatment

groups. Measurements at 6 months post stroke showed small but significant differences between the groups. Patients receiving enhanced treatment had greater improvements in strength and range and speed of movement than those receiving only Bobath treatment. This treatment effect was most pronounced in the patients with initial mild levels of impairments. Despite the differences in upper extremity control, the two groups did not differ significantly in ADL performance at 6 months, suggesting that the improvements in arm movement associated with the enhanced program did not translate directly into functional changes.

These studies provide some evidence that NDT/Bobath treatment produces changes in motor control and function. However, they fail to demonstrate the superiority of NDT/Bobath over other treatment approaches. One problem contributing to this failure may be the lack of availability of standardized measurement tools sensitive to the changes in movement control, postural responses, and muscle tone that may result from NDT/Bobath treatment. A second problem is related to methodology of the studies themselves. For example, both Salter et al. (1991) and Waganaar et al. (1990) used patients with acute strokes and did not attempt to match the two groups on type or severity of stroke, suggesting that problems with study design and the confounding effects of spontaneous recovery may influence their findings.

Hafsteinsdottir (1996) reviewed eight studies conducted between 1983 and 1990 that compared effectiveness between NDT and one or more other treatment approaches. Although all but one study found no difference between approaches, Hafsteinsdottir concluded that all of the studies had major limitations that affected the validity of their results. Given the small number of existing studies, the relatively small sample sizes, and the problems with measurement and study design, the conclusion that NDT/Bobath is no more effective than other treatment approaches is questionable. More research using larger and more varied patient populations, better study design, and expanded measurement tools will be necessary before the question of effectiveness can be completely answered.

Barriers to Effectiveness

The effectiveness of NDT/Bobath techniques in producing functional improvements may be limited by the NDT therapist's need to provide excessive assistance and control during handling. NDT handling has been criticized by motor learning theorists as too passive and lacking in opportunities for independent practice (Gordon, 1987). This criticism may be valid. While B. Bobath described handling as involving active participation by the patient, she also stressed that the therapist should control the quality of movement and prevent abnormal movements. Her emphasis on movement quality has resulted in a perception among NDT therapists that patients should not be encouraged to move independently until they are able to use normal patterns of muscle activation. This restriction may limit the patient's functional recovery, as Sunderlund and colleagues demonstrated that patients who received instruction in home exercises in addition to Bobath treatment showed greater improvements in functional control of their hemiplegic arms than patients who received only Bobath treatment. NDT therapists and clinical instructors are aware of this problem and are changing the practice of handling to provide more opportunities for independent practice.

Summary Review Questions

1. What do Bobath and Bobath say are the major problems after stroke?
2. Define the following terms: facilitation, inhibition, and handling. How are these procedures used to treat adult hemiplegia?
3. How do Bobath and Bobath define postural control? What problems are associated with loss of postural control?
4. Explain why abnormal tone is a major problem requiring occupational therapy treatment.
5. List several ways to control spasticity.
6. What is the overall goal of NDT/Bobath treatment for stroke patients? How does this goal relate to the practice of occupational therapy?
7. Describe several ways occupational therapists may incorporate NDT/Bobath concepts into ADL training.
8. How do the goals of treatment differ for patients with low-tone and patients with spasticity?
9. Why is weight bearing on the arm important for function? List several ways to use upper extremity weight bearing in treatment.
10. Describe a treatment program to increase movement and function in the hemiplegic arm if the patient has flexor spasticity.

Resource

NeuroDevelopmental Treatment Association
A resource for NDT continuing education courses and literature about NDT/Bobath approach for adults and children. · 1550 S. Coast Highway, Suite 201, Laguna Beach, CA 92651
e-mail: ndta@alderdrozinc.com
www.ndta.org

References

Basmajian, J., Gowland, C., Brandstater, M., Swanson, L., & Trotter, J. (1987). Stroke treatment: Comparison of integrated behavioral physical therapy vs traditional physical therapy programs. *Archives of Physical Medicine and Rehabilitation, 63,* 267–272.

Bierman, J. (1998). NDT theoretical overview. *NDTA Network, 10,* 3.

Bobath, B. (1990). *Adult Hemiplegia: Evaluation and Treatment* (3rd ed.). London: Heinemann.

Davies, P. (1985). *Steps to Follow.* New York: Springer-Verlag.

Davis, J. (1990). The Bobath approach to the treatment of adult hemiplegia. In L. Williams Pedretti & B. Zoltan (Eds.), *Occupational Therapy Practice Skills for Physical Dysfunction* (pp. 351–362). St. Louis: Mosby.

Eggers, O. (1984). *Occupational Therapy in the Treatment of Adult Hemiplegia.* Rockville, MD: Aspen.

Gordon, J. (1987). Assumptions underlying physical therapy intervention: Theoretical and historical perspectives. In J. Carr, R. Shepherd, J. Gordon, A. Gentile, & J. Held (Eds.), *Movement Science: Foundations for Physical Therapy in Rehabilitation* (pp. 1–30). Rockville, MD: Aspen.

Hafsteinsdottir, T. (1996). Neurodevelopmental treatment: Application to nursing and effects on the hemiplegic stroke patient. *Journal of Neuroscience Nursing, 28,* 36–47.

Rast, M. (1999). NDT in continuum: Micro to macro levels in therapy. *Developmental Disabilities Special Interest Section Quarterly, 2,* 1–3.

Ryerson, S., & Levit, K. (1997a). *Functional Movement Re-education.* New York: Churchill Livingstone.

Ryerson, S., & Levit, K. (1997b). The shoulder in hemiplegia. In R. Donatelli (Ed.), *Physical Therapy of the Shoulder* (3rd ed., pp. 205–228). New York: Churchill Livingstone.

Salter, J., Camp, V., Pierce, L., & Mion, I. (1991). Rehabilitation nursing approaches to cerebrovascular accident: A comparison of two approaches. *Rehabilitation Nursing, 16,* 62–66.

Sunderland, A., Tinson, D., Bradley, E., Fletcher, D., Langton Hewer, R., & Wade, D. (1992). Enhanced physical therapy improves recovery of arm function after stroke. *Journal of Neurology, Neurosurgery & Psychiatry, 55,* 530–535.

Trombly, C. (1995). Occupation: Purposefulness and meaningfulness as therapeutic mechanisms. 1995 Eleanor Clark Slagle Lecture. *American Journal of Occupational Therapy 49,* 960–972.

Van Dyck, W. (1999). Integrating treatment of the hemiplegic shoulder with self-care. *OT Practice, 4,* 32–37.

Wagenaar, R., Meijer, O., van Wieringen, P., Kuik, D., Hazenberg, G., Lindeboom, J., Wichers, F., & Rijswijk, H. (1990). The functional recovery of stroke: A comparison between neurodevelopmental treatment and the Brunnstrom method. *Scandinavian Journal of Rehabilitation Medicine, 22,* 1–8.

24

Optimizing Motor Behavior Using the Brunnstrom Movement Therapy Approach

Catherine A. Trombly

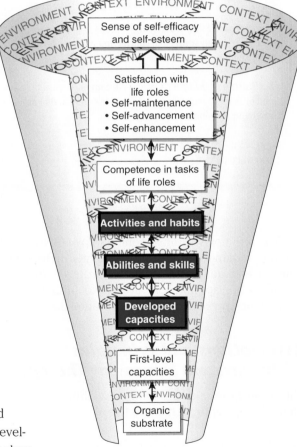

LEARNING OBJECTIVES

After studying this chapter, the reader will be able to do the following:

1. State the assumptions that underlie Brunnstrom's movement therapy.
2. List the six stages of recovery for the upper extremity and for the hand.
3. State the treatment principles of this approach.
4. Describe the treatment procedures to facilitate movement control in the trunk and upper extremity of hemiparetic patients using this approach.
5. Suggest functional activities suitable to encourage practice of movement behavior at various stages of recovery.

*B*runnstrom, a physical therapist, was particularly concerned with impaired motor control following stroke. Her method of developing this treatment approach gives therapists insight into the behaviors of a master clinician. In developing movement therapy, Brunnstrom experimented with trial-and-error application of procedures that she derived from motor control literature and from observations of patients. She paid careful attention to the patient's motor and verbal reactions to each procedure, interpreted those reactions in light of her knowledge of motor control and development, and adjusted the procedure accordingly. Successful procedures were replicated patient to patient.

GLOSSARY

Associated reaction—Involuntary movements or patterned, reflexive increases in muscle tone and limb position on the hemiplegic side that occur in stressful situations. They are commonly seen when movement is resisted, when the patient exerts effort, or when the patient fears loss of balance.

Assumption—Supposition that something is true; foundation of a theory.

Extensor synergy—For the upper extremity: scapular protraction, shoulder horizontal adduction and internal rotation, elbow extension, and forearm pronation. For the lower extremity: hip extension, adduction, and internal rotation; knee extension, plantar flexion and inversion of the ankle; and plantar flexion of the toes.

Facilitate—To make easier.

Facilitation—State of readying neurons to depolarize and propagate an impulse or to make contraction of a muscle or a reflex response more likely.

Facilitation techniques—Manual treatment techniques and hand placements used to increase muscle tone and to produce movement responses.

Flaccidity—State of lacking tone; limb feels limp and falls into place when not supported.

Flexor synergy—For the upper extremity: scapular elevation and retraction, shoulder abduction and external rotation, elbow flexion, and forearm supination. For the lower extremity: hip flexion, abduction, and external rotation; knee flexion; ankle dorsiflexion and inversion; and dorsiflexion of the toes.

Inhibit—To make more difficult.

Inhibition—State of hyperpolarization of neural cell membrane decreasing likelihood of propagating an impulse or to make contraction of a muscle or a reflex response less likely.

Inhibition technique—Manual treatment techniques and movement patterns used to decrease spasticity and stop abnormal movement patterns.

Practice—Repetition with the intent to improve.

Spasticity—State of excess tone and hyperactive response to stretch. If moderately to severely spastic, the limb feels tight and is difficult to move into position.

Synergy—Patterned movements of the entire affected limb in response to a stimulus or to voluntary effort.

The principles of movement therapy and the evaluation and treatment procedures presented here are summarized and adapted from Brunnstrom (1970), which describes her approach in detail. No further development of the approach has occurred since then.

Assumptions and Principles of Brunnstrom Movement Therapy

The **assumptions** that underlie the Brunnstrom Movement Therapy approach are as follows:

- In normal motor development, spinal cord and brainstem reflexes become modified and their components rearranged into purposeful movement through the influence of higher centers.
- Because reflexes and whole-limb movement patterns are normal stages of development and because stroke appears to result in "development in reverse," reflexes and primitive movement patterns should be used to **facilitate** the recovery of voluntary movement post stroke. Brunnstrom (1956) believed that no reasonable training method should be left untried. She stated, "It may well be that a subcortical motion synergy which can be elicited on a reflex basis may serve as a wedge by means of which a limited amount of willed movement may be learned" (p. 225).
- Proprioceptive and exteroceptive stimuli can be used to evoke desired motion or tonal changes.
- Recovery of voluntary movement post stroke proceeds in sequence from mass stereotyped flexor or extensor movement patterns to movements that combine features of the two patterns and finally to discrete movements of each joint at will. The stereotyped movement patterns are called limb synergies. **Synergy** in this sense refers to patterned movements of the entire limb in response to a stimulus or to voluntary effort.
- Newly produced correct motions must be practiced to be learned.
- **Practice** within the context of daily activities enhances the learning process.

The principles of this approach derive from these premises. They are listed in Box 24-1.

Evaluation

Evaluation using the Brunnstrom movement therapy approach is appropriate for persons who have had a stroke and who have occupational dysfunction secondary to sensorimotor impairments. If the occupational therapist determines that the patient cannot carry out activities and tasks that are important to the roles that the patient wants, needs, or is expected to do, the therapist observes the patient's attempts, and if it is indicated, assesses the patient's sensorimotor status (Box 24-2).

Sensation

The sensory evaluation precedes the motor evaluation. The patient's ability to recognize movements of the affected arm and to localize touch in the hand without looking are especially noted, because they are associated with better eventual recovery of voluntary movement of the arm and hand, respectively. See Chapter 6 for evaluation procedures. Results of the sensory evaluation guide choice of **facilitation** modalities that the therapist may use to improve movement or alert the

therapist to encourage the patient to substitute visual feedback for lost movement or position senses.

Tonic Reflexes

Tonic reflexes are assessed to determine whether they can be used in early treatment to initiate movement when none exists. The primitive tonic brainstem reflexes that may be present include the symmetrical and asymmetrical tonic neck reflexes, tonic labyrinthine reflexes, and tonic lumbar reflexes. The evaluation of these reflexes is described in Box 24-3. The complete reflex response may not be manifest; however, a change in tone does occur if the patient's movement is under reflex control. A change in tone is gauged by comparing the amount of resistance to passive stretch in the test condition to that in a neutral condition.

Associated Reactions

Associated reactions are involuntary movements or patterned, reflexive increases of tone in muscles that would be expected to contract to cause the movement. Associated reactions are triggered by effortful voluntary movement (Boissy et al., 1997). They are seen in the involved extremities of stroke patients when other parts of the

---

BOX 24-1
PROCEDURES FOR PRACTICE

Principles of Brunnstrom's Movement Therapy

► Treatment must progress developmentally, from evocation of reflex responses to willed control of voluntary movement to automatic functional motor behavior.

► When no motion exists, facilitate it using reflexes, **associated reactions**, proprioceptive facilitation, and/or exteroceptive facilitation to develop muscle tension in preparation for voluntary movement.

   ► Elicit reflex responses and associated reactions in combination with the patient's voluntary effort to move, which produces semivoluntary movement; this allows the patient to feel the sensory feedback associated with movement and the satisfaction of having moved to some degree voluntarily.

   ► Proprioceptive and exteroceptive stimuli also assist in eliciting movement. Resistance, a proprioceptive stimulus, promotes a spread of impulses to other muscles to produce a patterned response (associated reaction), whereas tactile stimulation (exteroceptive) and muscle or tendon tapping (proprioceptive) facilitate only the muscles related to the stimulated area.

► When voluntary effort produces a response, ask the patient to hold (isometric) the contraction. If successful, ask for an eccentric (controlled lengthening) contraction and finally a concentric (shortening) contraction.

► Even when only partial movement is possible, stress reversal of movement from flexion to extension in each treatment session.

► Reduce or drop out facilitation as quickly as the patient shows evidence of volitional control. Drop out facilitation procedures in order of their stimulus–response binding. Reflexes, in which the response is stereotypically bound to a certain stimulus, are the most primitive and are dropped out of treatment first. Responses to exteroceptive stimulation are least stereotyped, and therefore, tactile stimulation is eliminated last. No primitive reflexes, including associated reactions, are used beyond stage III.

► Place emphasis on willed movement to overcome the linkages between parts of the synergies. Willed movement means that the patient is trying to accomplish it. Patients may be more successful if you ask them to do familiar movements involving a goal object (Trombly & Wu, 1999; Wu et al., 2000).

► Have the patient repeat correct movement, once elicited, to learn it. Practice should include functional activities to increase the willed aspect and to relate the sensations to goal-directed movement.

body are resisted during movement or when the patient makes an effort to move. Associated reactions are evaluated to determine which can be used to facilitate movement when no voluntary movement exists.

Basic Limb Synergies

Limb synergies are instances of associated reactions. They may occur reflexively or as early stages of voluntary control when **spasticity** is present. When the patient initiates a movement of one joint, all muscles that are linked in synergy with that movement automatically contract, causing a stereotyped movement pattern.

In the upper extremity, the **flexor synergy** is composed of scapular retraction and/or elevation, shoulder abduction and external rotation, elbow flexion, and forearm supination (Fig. 24-1 and Fig. 23-8). Position of the wrist and fingers is variable. Elbow flexion is the strongest component of the flexor synergy and the first motion to appear or to be facilitated. Shoulder abduction and external rotation are weak components. Shoul-

der hyperextension may be seen when abduction and external rotation are weak, although it is not considered part of the flexor synergy. Flexor synergy can be evoked when no movement exists by applying resistance to shoulder elevation or elbow flexion of the uninvolved upper extremity.

The **extensor synergy** of the upper extremity is composed of scapular protraction, shoulder horizontal adduction and internal rotation, elbow extension, forearm pronation, and variable wrist and finger motion, although wrist extension and finger flexion may be seen (Fig. 24-2). The pectoralis major is the strongest component of the extension synergy; consequently, shoulder horizontal adduction and internal rotation are the first motions to appear or to be facilitated. Pronation is the next strongest component. Elbow extension is a weak component. Extensor synergy can be evoked when no movement exists by applying resistance to horizontal adduction of the uninvolved upper extremity, which is equivalent to **Raimiste's phenomenon**.

Upper extremity flexor synergy usually develops before extensor synergy. When both synergies are developing and spasticity is marked, the strongest components of the flexion and extension synergies sometimes combine to produce the typical upper extremity posture in hemiplegia: the arm is adducted and internally rotated, with the elbow flexed, forearm pronated, and the wrist and fingers flexed.

The lower extremity flexor synergy is composed of hip flexion, abduction, and external rotation; knee flexion; dorsiflexion and inversion of the ankle; and dorsiflexion of the toes. In this synergy, hip flexion is the strongest component; hip abduction and external rotation are weak components. The lower extremity extensor

---

BOX 24-2
PROCEDURES FOR PRACTICE

Evaluation in the Brunnstrom Movement Therapy Approach

Determine the following:

1. Proprioceptive and exteroceptive sensory status
2. Effect of tonic reflexes on the patient's movement
3. Effect of associated reactions on the patient's movement
4. Level of recovery of voluntary motor control

BOX 24-3
PROCEDURES FOR PRACTICE

Evaluation of Brainstem Reflexes

Reflex or Reaction	Stimulus	Response
ATNR	Turn head 90° to one side; repeat to the other side.	Increase in extensor tone of limbs on the face side and flexor tone on the skull side.
STNR	1. Flexion of the head 2. Extension of the head	1. Flexion of arms and extension of legs. 2. Extension of arms and flexion of legs.
TLR	1. Prone position 2. Supine position	1. Increased flexor tone in arms and legs. 2. Increased extensor tone in arms and legs.
Tonic lumbar	Rotate upper trunk in relation to the pelvis	Increased flexor tone in the upper extremity and increased extensor tone in the lower extremity on the side toward which the trunk is turned. Opposite picture on the side opposite to the direction of rotation.

ATNR, asymmetrical tonic neck; STNR, Symmetrical tonic neck; TLR, tonic labyrinthine.

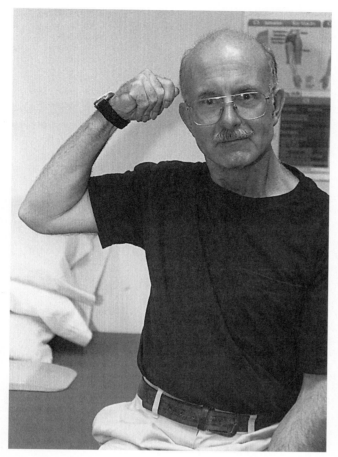

Figure 24-1 Flexor synergy. This patient lacks the supination component of the flexor synergy.

synergies, Brunnstrom identified other associated reactions that she used in the early stages of treatment:

► Resistance to flexion of the uninvolved leg causes extension of the involved extremity, and resistance to extension of the uninvolved leg causes flexion of the involved extremity. Recently this has been verified electromyographically (Fujiwara et al., 1999).

► Resisted grasp by the uninvolved hand causes a grasp reaction in the involved hand. This is an example of mirror synkinesis.

► Attempt to flex the involved leg or resistance to leg flexion causes a flexor response in the involved arm. This reaction is called homolateral synkinesis.

► Actively or passively raising the affected arm above the horizontal causes the fingers to extend and abduct. This is Souque's phenomenon.

► Resistance to abduction or adduction of the unaffected lower limb results in a similar response in the opposite affected leg. This is Raimiste's phenomenon.

synergy is composed of hip extension, adduction, and internal rotation; knee extension; plantar flexion and inversion of the ankle; and plantar flexion of the toes. Hip adduction, knee extension, and plantar flexion of the ankle with inversion are all strong components. Weak components of this synergy are hip extension, hip internal rotation, and plantar flexion of the toes. Ankle inversion occurs in both lower extremity synergies.

The lower extremity extensor synergy is dominant when the person is standing, because of the strength of this synergy combined with the influences of the positive supporting reaction and stretch forces against the sole of the foot that elicit plantar flexion.

Other Associated Reactions Identified by Brunnstrom

The brainstem reflexes listed in Box 24-3 are associated reactions that Brunnstrom and other therapists used to evoke some movement when no movement existed but spasticity was present in hemiparetic limbs. In addition to these brainstem reflexes and to the basic limb

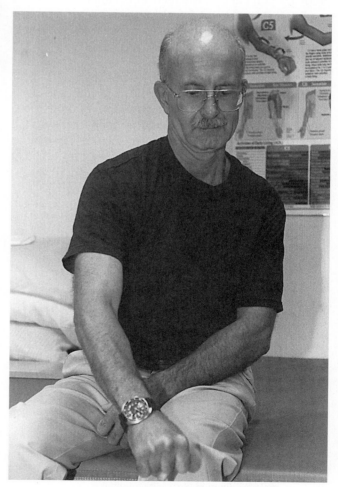

Figure 24-2 Extensor synergy.

Level of Recovery of Voluntary Movement

The level of motor recovery is evaluated using a tool that sequences motor performance after stroke from reflex to full voluntary control. In preparation for evaluation, the patient is made physically and psychologically comfortable. Each motion is demonstrated to the patient, who does it with the unaffected extremity before attempting to do it with the affected one. That allows the therapist to be certain that the person understands the request. Instructions should be given in functional terms. For example, to test the flexor synergy of the upper extremity, say "Touch your ear," and for the extensor synergy, "Reach out to touch your [opposite] knee" (Brunnstrom, 1966). No facilitation is used during the evaluation.

The Brunnstrom Stages

Box 24-4 lists the six stages of recovery of the proximal upper extremity and the hand that Brunnstrom (1970) identified. Although on average stroke patients proceed through these stages, recovery of a particular patient may stop at any stage. To date there are no reliable ways to predict which patients will recover voluntary movement.

Brunnstrom stages I to VI are useful to designate summarily the status of voluntary control. The patient is reported to be in the stage at which he or she can accomplish all motions specified for that stage (Box 24-4). Because progress is gradual, sometimes the patient is in transition between stages. If the patient has completed one stage but is just beginning to be able to do the motions of the next stage, many therapists report the level as II going on III, III going on IV, and so on. The upper and lower extremities and the hand may all be in different stages of recovery at a given time.

The stages were quantified in Brunnstrom's original evaluation, the *Hemiplegia Classification and Progress Record* (Brunnstrom, 1966). That instrument was valid in that it reflected both observations made by Twitchell (1951) of the recovery process of 118 patients with acute and chronic strokes and Brunnstrom's (1970) own observations of 100 patients. No data exist concerning the reliability of this assessment, but it can be assumed to be low because the rating scales were not operationally defined.

The Fugl-Meyer Assessment of Motor Function

The *Fugl-Meyer Motor Function Assessment* (*FMA*) (Fugl-Meyer et al., 1975) is a widely used adaptation of Brunnstrom's *Hemiplegia Classification and Progress Record*. Fugl-Meyer et al. defined 50 details of movement across Brunnstrom's six levels of recovery.

The patient's ability to do the requested movement is scored according to the degree of completion. The *FMA* uses an ordinal-level scoring system in which each detail is rated 0, cannot be performed; 1, can be partly performed; or 2, can be performed faultlessly. For example, when asked for a flexor synergy response, if the patient can bring the hand only as far as the mouth rather than to the ear, the score is 1. When the patient's response is incomplete, as in this example, it is necessary to observe the patient's repeated attempts to determine the specific weak areas of the synergy or movement pattern.

Total score ranges from 0, flaccidity, to 100, normal motor function, for the upper and lower extremities. The subtests may be used independently; Table 24-1 shows the upper extremity subtest. The total score for the upper extremity is 66. The score can also be recorded as

---

BOX 24-4
Stages of Recovery of the Upper Extremity

Arm
I. Flaccidity: no voluntary movement or stretch reflexes
II. Synergies can be elicited reflexively; flexion develops before extension; spasticity developing.
III. Beginning voluntary movement, but only in synergy; increased spasticity, which may become marked
IV. Some movements deviating from synergy:
  a. Hand behind back
  b. Arm to forward horizontal position
  c. Pronation and supination with the elbow flexed to 90°. Spasticity decreasing.
V. Independence from basic synergies:
  a. Arm to side horizontal position
  b. Arm forward and overhead
  c. Pronation and supination with elbow fully extended. Spasticity waning.
VI. Isolated joint movements freely performed with near normal coordination. Spasticity minimal.

Hand
I. Flaccidity.
II. Little or no active finger flexion.

III. Mass grasp or hook grasp. No voluntary finger extension or release.
IV. Semivoluntary finger extension in a small range of motion. Lateral prehension with release by thumb movement.

V. Palmar prehension
  Cylindrical and spherical grasp (awkward).
  Voluntary mass finger extension (variable range of motion).

VI. All types of prehension (improved skill).
  Voluntary finger extension (full range of motion).
  Individual finger movements.

TABLE 24-1

Fugl-Meyer Assessment of Motor Function: Upper Extremity Subtest

3/15/96

Patient Name _Mrs. G_   **Date** _1/27/96_

Shoulder/Elbow/Forearm

Stage	Instruction	Response	Scoring Criteria	
I & II. Reflex activity	Tap the biceps and finger flexor tendons	_2_ Stretch reflex at elbow and/or fingers	0 = no reflex can be elicited 2 = reflex can be elicited	2
	Tap the triceps tendon	_2_ Stretch reflex		2
III. Voluntary movement within synergy	Flexor synergy "Turn your affected hand palm up and touch your ear"	Flexor synergy _2_ Shoulder retraction _2_ Shoulder elevation _2_ Shoulder abduction to 90° _1_ Shoulder external rotation _2_ Elbow flexion _1_ Forearm supination	(for each of 9 details) 0 = cannot perform 1 = can perform partly 2 = can perform faultlessly	2 2 2 2 2 2
	Extensor synergy "Turn your hand palm down and reach to touch your unaffected knee"	Extensor Synergy _1_ Shoulder adduction & internal rotation _0_ Elbow extension _1_ Forearm pronation		2 2 2
IV: Voluntary movement mixing flexor and extensor synergies	"Show me how you would put a belt around you [or tie an apron]"	_0_ Affected hand moves to lumbar spine area	0 = cannot perform 1 = hand must actively pass anterior-superior iliac spine 2 = faultless	1
	"Reach forward to take [object held in front of patient]"	_0_ Reaches into 90° of shoulder flexion	0 = elbow flexes or shoulder abducts immediately 1 = if these occur later in motion 2 = faultless	0
	"Put your arm to your side & bend your elbow. Turn your palm up & down."	_0_ Pronates and supinates forearm with elbow at 90° and shoulder at 0°	0 = if cannot position arm or cannot pronate or supinate 1 = shoulder and elbow joints correctly positioned and beginning pronation & supination seen 2 = faultless	0
V: Voluntary movement outside of synergies	"Turn your palm down and reach over here to touch [object held out to side]"	_NT_ Abducts shoulder to 90° with elbow extended to 0° & forearm pronated	0 = initial elbow flexion or loss of pronation 1 = partial motion or elbow flexes and forearm supinates later in motion 2 = faultless	NT
	"Reach as high as you can toward the ceiling"	_NT_ Flexes shoulder from 90 to 180° with elbow in 0°	0 = elbow flexes or shoulder abducts immediately 1 = if these occur later in motion 2 = faultless	NT
	"Reach your arm directly forward and turn your palm up & down"	_NT_ Flexes shoulder to 30-90°; extends elbow to 0°; and supinates and pronates	0 = if cannot position arm or cannot rotate 1 = correct position and beginning rotation 2 = faultless	NT
VI: Normal Reflex Activity (tested if patient scores 6 in stage V tests)	Tap on biceps, triceps and finger flexor tendons	_NT_ Normal reflex response	0 = ≥2 reflexes are markedly hyperactive 1 = 1 reflex hyperactive or 2 reflexes lively 2 = no more than 1 reflex lively and none hyperactive	NT

Upper Arm Subtotal Score (36 points)   _16 (44%)_

23 (64%)

(continued)

3/15/96

Patient Name __Mrs. G__   Date ____1/27/96____

Wrist

Stage	Instruction	Response	Scoring Criteria	
Wrist stability with elbow flexed	Put the shoulder in 0°, elbow in 90° flexion, and forearm pronated. "Lift your wrist and hold it there."	_1_ Patient extends wrist to 15°. Therapist can hold upper arm in position.	0 = cannot extend 1 = can extend, but not against resistance 2 = can maintain against slight resistance	2
Wrist stability with elbow extended	Put the elbow in 0°. "Lift your wrist and hold it there."	_1_ As above	As above	2
Active motion with elbow flexed and shoulder at 0°	"Move your wrist up and down a few times."	_0_ Patient moves smoothly from full flexion to full extension. Therapist can hold upper arm.	0 = no voluntary movement 1 = moves, but less than full range 2 = faultless	1
Active motion with elbow extended	"Move your wrist up and down a few times."	_0_ As above	As above	1
Circumduction	"Turn your wrist in a circle like this [demonstrate]."	_NT_ Makes a full circle—combining flexion & extension with ulnar & radial deviation.	0 = cannot perform 1 = jerky or incomplete motion 2 = faultless	0
Wrist Subtotal Score (10 points) _2 (20%)_				6 (60%)

Hand

Stage	Instruction	Response	Scoring Criteria	
III: Mass Flexion	"Make a fist"	_2_ Patient flexes fingers.	0 = no flexion 1 = less than full flexion as compared to other hand 2 = full active flexion	2
III: Hook Grasp	"Hold this shopping bag by the handles"	_2_ Grasp involves MCP extension and PIP & DIP flexion.	0 = cannot perform 1 = active grasp, no resistance 2 = maintains grasp against great resistance	2
III – VI: Finger Extension	"Let go of the shopping bag" "Open your hand wide"	_1_ From full active or passive flexion, patient extends all fingers.	0 = no extension 1 = partial extension or able to release grasp 2 = full range of motion as compared to other hand	1
IV: Lateral Prehension	"Take hold of this sheet of paper [or playing card]."	_1_ Patient grasps between thumb & index finger.	0 = cannot perform 1 = can hold paper but not against tug 2 = holds paper well against tug	2
V: Palmar Prehension	"Take hold of this pencil as if you were going to write."	_0_ Therapist holds pencil upright and patient grasps it.	Scoring as above	1
V: Cylindrical Grasp	"Take hold of this paper cup [or pill bottle]."	_0_ Therapist holds the object and patient grasps with 1st & 2nd fingers together.	Scoring as above	0
VI: Spherical Grasp	"Take hold of this tennis ball [or apple]."	_0_ Patient grasps with fingers abducted.	Scoring as above	0
Hand Subtotal Score (14 Points) _6 (43%)_				8 (57%)

(continued)

TABLE 24-1
Fugl-Meyer Assessment of Motor Function: Upper Extremity Subtest *(Continued)*

3/15/96

Patient Name ___Mrs. G_____ Date _____1/27/96_____

Coordination/Speed

Stage	Instruction	Response	Scoring Criteria	
VI: Normal Movement	"Close your eyes. Now, touch your nose with your fingertip. Do that as fast as you can 5 times."	Patient does finger-to-nose test _NT_ Tremor _NT_ Dysmetria _0_ Speed (Compare to unaffected side)	*Tremor:* 0 = marked 1 = slight 2 = none *Dysmetria:* 0 = pronounced or unsystematic 1 = slight and systematic 2 = none *Speed:* 0 = > 6 sec slower 1 = 2 – 5 sec slower 2 = < 2 sec slower	*0* *0* *1*

Speed and Coordination Subtotal Score (6 points) ____0____   *5 (83%)*

TOTAL UPPER EXTREMITY SCORE (66 points) __24 (36%)__   *42 (63%)*

Fugl-Meyer et al., 1975.

Note. The scores pertain to the person described in the case example.

NT, not tested. Because recovery is sequential, more advanced movements are not tested if the patient fails the movements in the earlier stage.

---

percentage of recovery (score obtained divided by total score times 100%) (Duncan et al., 1994).

Both intrarater and interrater reliability of the upper extremity subtest of the *FMA* (33 items) were determined to be strong ($r \geq .96$) (Duncan et al., 1983; Sanford et al., 1993). The *FMA* is more discriminative than the *Motor Assessment Scale* (Malouin et al., 1994). The *FMA* correlates strongly ($r = .97$) with the *Arm Function Test*, which uses tasks for evaluation; however, the *FMA* is more responsive because it does not exhibit the ceiling and floor effects that the *Arm Function Test* does (Berglund & Fugl-Meyer, 1986).

Treatment

Rehabilitation of trunk control precedes treatment of the limbs.

Rehabilitating Trunk Control

Some patients with hemiplegia have poor trunk control and require training to enable them to bend over to retrieve an object from the floor or to dress their lower extremities. To elicit balance responses, the patient is gently pushed forward, backward, and side to side. Reaching for objects in various locations while seated demands dynamic trunk balance responses (Dean & Shepherd, 1997) and seems to be a better, more natural approach to improve balance than simply pushing the patient. Brunnstrom, had she known about the newer research that documents the importance of goal and context on the organization of movement (Trombly & Wu, 1999; van Vliet et al., 1995; Wu et al., 2000), in all likelihood would have incorporated task-oriented movement into her approach.

Brunnstrom emphasized promoting contraction of trunk muscles on the uninvolved side first by pushing the patient off balance toward the involved side (today we would place an object to be touched or grasped on the involved side), while guarding in case of poor response. Then, once it is determined that the person has that skill, recovery from a push toward or reach toward the uninvolved side is sought. This requires contraction of the trunk muscles on the involved side. The patient is pushed or asked to reach only to the point at which he or she can hold the position and regain upright posture. **The patient is guarded throughout**. Training then progresses to promote trunk flexion, extension, and rotation.

Practice in forward flexion of the trunk is assisted. The patient crosses the arms with the uninvolved hand under the involved elbow and the uninvolved forearm

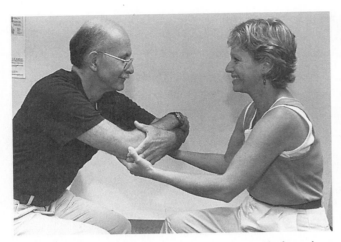

Figure 24-3 Therapist supporting the patient's arms to assist forward flexion of the trunk. The shoulders become more flexed as the patient leans forward.

supporting the involved forearm. The therapist, sitting facing the patient, supports the patient under the elbows and assists in trunk flexion forward, avoiding any pull on the shoulders (Fig. 24-3). Some pain-free shoulder flexion is accomplished during this forward movement. While the patient is concentrating on trunk control, shoulder movement occurs without conscious awareness.

Return from trunk flexion is performed actively by the patient. Then, while sitting without back support and with the involved arm supported as described, the patient is pushed backward and encouraged to regain upright posture actively. Forward flexion in oblique directions is done next, not only to promote regaining balance but also to incorporate more scapular motion with the shoulder flexion already achieved.

Next trunk rotation is practiced with the patient supporting the involved arm and the therapist guiding trunk motion. Trunk rotation can be combined with head movements in the opposite direction of the trunk rotation, so that the tonic neck and tonic lumbar reflexes can be used to begin to elicit the shoulder components of the upper extremity synergies. The arms and trunk move in one direction, and the head turns in the opposite direction (Fig. 24-4). Head and trunk movements are combined with increasing ranges of movement of the shoulder, enabling pain-free shoulder and scapular abduction and adduction during trunk rotation.

Retraining Proximal Upper Extremity Control

The focus of treatment is the recapitulation of normal movement developmentally from its reflexive base to voluntary control of individual motions that can be used functionally. The general format for treatment is listed in

Box 24-5. Because recovery proceeds sequentially, once the stage of recovery is identified, the short-term goal is the next step in the sequence.

Stages I to III

The goal of treatment is to promote voluntary control of the synergies and to encourage their use in functional activities. In these stages, all movements occur in synergy patterns but with increasing voluntary initiation and control of these patterns.

To move the patient from stage I (**flaccidity**) to stage II (beginning synergy), the basic limb synergies are elicited at a reflex level, using as many reflexes, associated reactions, and facilitation procedures as are necessary to elicit a response. The effects of these procedures combine to produce a stronger response. The patient tries to move (willed movement) as these facilitation techniques are used.

The flexor synergy is the first to develop. Elbow flexion, the strongest component of that synergy, is

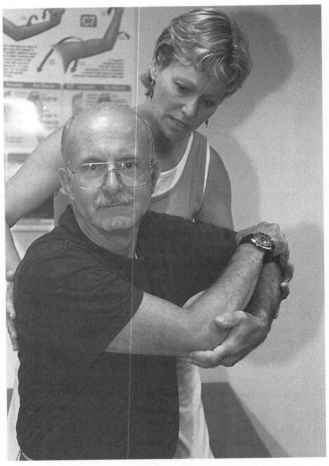

Figure 24-4 Through manual guidance, the therapist helps direct the patient to carry out trunk rotation while keeping the head forward or looking in the opposite direction.

BOX 24-5
PROCEDURES FOR PRACTICE

General Treatment Sequence to Achieve Movement Control Within Brunnstrom's Movement Therapy Approach

1. Gain some movement through sensory facilitation and reflexes, including associated reactions.
2. Resist the movement and ask for a holding (isometric) contraction.
3. If the patient can produce an isometric contraction, ask for a lengthening (eccentric) contraction.
4. If the patient can produce a controlled lengthening contraction, ask for a shortening (isotonic) contraction.
5. Once the patient can voluntarily move the limb to some degree, ask the patient to reverse the movement repeatedly.
6. Provide opportunities for use of the targeted movement and the reversing movement functionally.
7. Provide suggestions of functional situations that would allow practice of the newly acquired movements in daily life.

the first motion to be elicited. Once the elbow flexes, the therapist turns concentration from elbow flexion to the proximal components of the synergy with the goal of enabling the patient to capture the synergy, that is, bring it under voluntary control (stage III). Efforts to achieve voluntary control of the flexor synergy begin with scapular elevation. Lateral flexion of the neck toward the involved side can be used to initiate scapular elevation because the upper trapezius does both motions, although it may have "forgotten" how to elevate the scapula. With the patient's arm supported on a table in shoulder abduction with elbow flexion, the therapist simultaneously gives resistance to the head and shoulder while the patient is asked to hold the head and not let it move away from the shoulder. When the trapezius is felt to respond, both the patient's effort and the therapist's resistance emphasize shoulder elevation when lateral flexion of the neck is repeated. Once elevation begins, active contraction may be promoted by an associated reaction. For example, as the patient attempts bilateral scapular elevation, resistance is given to the uninvolved scapula. If the involved scapula elevates as an associated reaction, resistance is added on the involved side as the patient is asked to hold.

Unilateral scapular elevation of the involved arm is attempted next; it may be achieved as a result of the previous procedures. If the patient cannot do the motion, the therapist supports the patient's arm and assists the patient to elevate the scapula. Percussion or

stroking over the upper trapezius facilitates muscle contraction. The therapist tells the patient to hold and "Don't let me push your shoulder down." After repeated holding with some resistance added, the patient does an eccentric contraction, that is, lets the shoulder down slowly. Then a concentric, or shortening, contraction is attempted when the person is told, "Pull your shoulder up toward your ear."

Active scapular elevation evokes other flexor components and tends to **inhibit** the pectoralis major. The patient repeats scapular elevation and relaxation as the therapist gently abducts the shoulder in increasing increments. Because many patients with hemiplegia have shoulder pain and/or shoulder subluxation, the shoulder is given special care, and the correct scapulohumeral orientation is maintained. Once shoulder elevation and some active abduction have been achieved, external rotation and forearm supination are included in the movement. Reversal of movements to the opposite direction are done from the start, and this begins to develop some components of the extensor synergy.

The extensor synergy tends to follow the flexor synergy but may have to be assisted in its initiation. Contraction of the pectoralis major, a strong component of the extensor synergy, can be elicited by the associated reaction in which the therapist supports the patient's arms in a position between horizontal abduction and adduction, instructs the patient to bring his arms together, and resists the uninvolved arm just proximal to the elbow. As bilateral contraction occurs, the patient is instructed, "Don't let me pull your arms apart." Then the patient attempts to bring the arms together voluntarily.

Because of the predominance of excess tone in the elbow flexors and relative weakness of elbow extensors, elbow extension is usually more difficult to obtain but it can be assisted by the methods in Box 24-6. Other means that may be used to facilitate extension movement include use of supine position (tonic labyrinthine reflex); having the patient watch the extremity, which requires head turning and pulls in the asymmetrical tonic neck reflex; working with the forearm pronated, which is a strong component of the extensor synergy; and rotating the trunk toward the uninvolved side to facilitate extension of the involved arm via the tonic lumbar reflex.

After the patient achieves elbow extension in weight bearing, the goal is to encourage active elbow extension free of weight bearing. Unilateral manual resistance is offered to the patient's attempts to move into an extension synergy pattern. Resistance gives direction to the patient's effort and facilitates a stronger contraction.

As the synergies come under voluntary control, they should be used in functional activities. The extensor synergy can be used to stabilize an object to be worked on by the other arm, to push the arm into the sleeve of a

BOX 24-6
PROCEDURES FOR PRACTICE

Procedures to Develop Elbow Extension

"Rowing"
1. Sit facing the patient.
2. Cross your arms so that your right hand grasps the patient's right hand and your left hand grasps the patient's left hand.
3. Resist as the pronated, uninvolved extremity moves toward the involved knee (Fig. 24-5). This elicits elbow extension in the involved arm through an associated reaction.
4. At the same time, assist the involved arm into extension toward the uninvolved knee.
5. Still holding the patient's hands, guide movements into flexion combined with supination (Fig. 24-6).
6. Repeat steps 3 to 5 until you feel the affected limb actively extending.
7. Then, offer resistance bilaterally.
8. Then, reinforce voluntary effort of the involved extremity by asking the patient to hold against resistance to that limb only.
9. Facilitate the extensors by lightly and repeatedly pushing the involved arm back toward elbow flexion, which causes quick stretches to the triceps.

Weight Bearing
When the extensor synergy is seen to come under some active control, it is further developed through use of bilateral weight bearing.

1. Have the patient lean forward onto extended arms supported by a low stool or cushions placed in front (Fig. 24-7). To make it comfortable for the patient, place a sandbag, pillow, or towel on the stool.
2. Stroke the skin over the triceps vigorously or tap over the triceps tendon while the patient attempts to bear weight on both outstretched arms (Fig. 24-8).
3. Once this is successful, have the patient shift weight so that the involved extremity bears more of the weight of the upper trunk.
4. Again, tap the tendon and apply tactile stimulation to the triceps.
5. In the unilateral weight-bearing position, have the patient do functional tasks such as holding down objects with the affected arm while working on them with the other hand, such as holding a piece of wood while sawing, hammering, or painting it; holding a package steady while opening it, addressing it, or fastening it; supporting body weight while polishing or washing large surfaces with the uninvolved arm.

garment (see Fig. 23-21), to smooth out a sheet on the bed, or to sponge off the kitchen counter. The flexor synergy can be used functionally to assist in carrying items (such as a coat, handbag, or briefcase); feeding oneself; putting on glasses; and combing the hair. Bilateral pushing and pulling reinforce both syner-

gies. Bilateral identical movements performed independently (i.e., no ball or stick connecting the two limbs) were observed to improve movement of the hemiplegic arm when that arm was tested unilaterally. The improvement was limited to the practiced movement patterns but was maintained over time (Mudie & Matyas, 2000). Sanding, weaving, ironing, and polishing use the flexor and extensor synergies alternately and repeatedly.

Stages IV to VI
To promote movement deviating from synergy, motions that begin to combine components of synergies in small increments are encouraged as a transition from stage III to stage IV. For example, as the patient begins to extend the arm consistently in response to the unilateral manual resistance that the therapist provides, the therapist guides the direction of movement away from the exten-

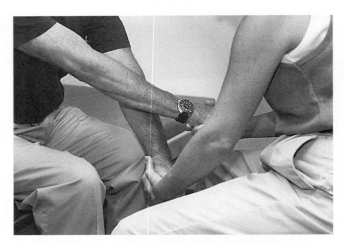

Figure 24-5 "Rowing." The therapist resists the pronated uninvolved (left) extremity while guiding the involved (right) extremity into extensor synergy.

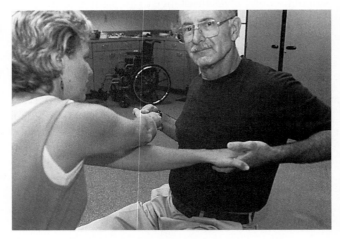

Figure 24-6 "Rowing." The therapist guides the patient into the reverse motion of flexion and supination.

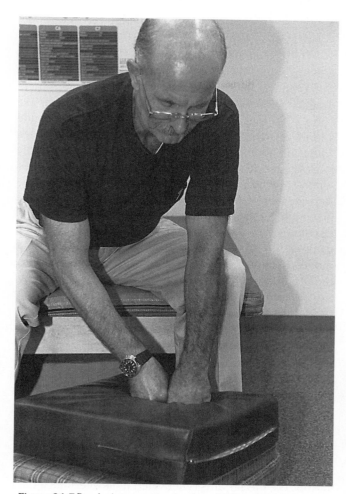

Figure 24-7 Developing arm extension through bilateral weight bearing.

tive shoulder abduction (flexor synergy) with elbow extension and forearm pronation or internal rotation (extensor synergy). This motion requires that the strongest components of each synergy be subdued. A swinging motion of the arm combined with trunk rotation helps to get the hand behind the body. If balance is good, this can be done more easily when standing. As the hand reaches the back of the patient, the patient strokes the dorsum of the hand against the body to complete the sensory awareness of the movement. Stroking the dorsum of the hand on the back is thought to give direction to the attempted voluntary movement. If the patient cannot do the full motion actively, the therapist passively moves the patient's arm into final position and strokes the dorsum of the patient's hand against the sacrum. The patient, while attempting to do the movement independently, is assisted into and out of the pattern, which gradually becomes voluntary with practice. Practice, using functional tasks as much as possible, continues until the motion can be freely accomplished. Examples

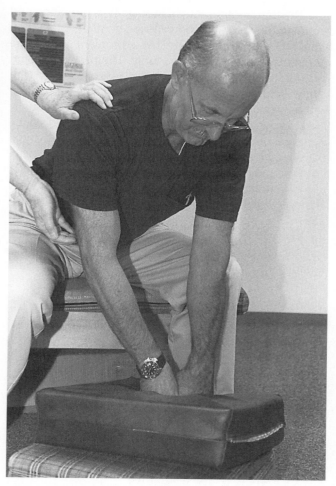

Figure 24-8 The therapist taps on the skin over the triceps to encourage greater muscle contraction and better arm extension while the patient is bearing weight on the outstretched arm.

sor synergy pattern and toward greater shoulder abduction in conjunction with elbow extension. This breaks up the synergistic relationship of shoulder adduction to elbow extension and shoulder abduction to elbow flexion. The therapist directs the patient to push the hand into the therapist's hand and moves the hand in small increments away from the patient's midline. When the triceps and pectoralis major are disassociated, the synergies no longer dominate.

In stages IV and V the goal of treatment is to condition the synergies, that is, to promote voluntary movement combining components of the two synergies into increasingly varied combinations of movements that deviate from synergy. Proprioceptive and exteroceptive stimuli are still used in this phase of training, but tonic reflexes and associated reactions, appropriate in the earlier stages when reflex behavior was desirable, are no longer used. Willed movement with isolated control of muscle groups is the desired goal.

The first out-of-synergy motion of stage IV is hand behind the body (see Box 24-4), which combines rela-

of functional tasks include putting a belt on when the patient is standing, swimming using the crawl stroke, and tucking a shirt into trousers.

The second out-of-synergy motion is shoulder flexion to a forward horizontal position with the elbow extended. If the patient cannot flex the shoulder forward actively, even with the therapist providing local facilitation and guidance of movement, the arm is brought passively into position. While tapping over the anterior and middle deltoid muscles, the therapist asks the patient to hold the position. If the patient can hold after positioning, active motion in small increments is sought, starting with lowering of the arm followed by active shoulder flexion. This continues until the full forward flexion motion can be done. Stroking and rubbing of the triceps are used to help the patient keep the elbow straight as the arm is raised. Repetitive nonresistive activities are used to motivate this action. Raising the arm to forward horizontal is involved in any vertically mounted game, such as tic-tac-toe or checkers (using Velcro tabs to secure the pieces), or painting on an easel, for example.

The third motion sought in stage IV is pronation and supination with the elbow flexed to 90°. Supination would not be expected to be a problem unless the pronators retained some spasticity. The problem would be to combine pronation of the extensor synergy with elbow flexion of the flexor synergy. Initially, pronation can be resisted with the elbow extended, and gradually the elbow can be brought into flexion as the resistance to pronation is repeated. Block printing is an activity to consider when resistance to pronation is wanted. It can be positioned to resist pronation, with gradual changes in the amount of elbow flexion. This motion has been achieved when resistance is no longer required and the patient can supinate and pronate with the elbow near the trunk. Practice should include activities that require turning objects such as a knob, a screwdriver, or a dial to reinforce it. Some games, such as skittles, are knob operated and require rotary motions, as do card games that require turning the cards over and the adapted dice game described by Nelson et al. (1996).

Once the patient is confident of these stage IV movements and performance is fairly consistent, stage V training commences. Movement in stage V entails active attempts by the patient to move in patterns increasingly away from synergy. Excess effort is avoided, however, so that the limbs will not revert to stereotyped movements. The attempts are bolstered by use of quick stretch and tactile stimulation. Each new motion is incorporated into functional activities. Although it is Brunnstrom's approach to regain motion through exercise and then introduce functional activities to practice the motion, recent research indicates that goal is a powerful organizer of movement, including that of stroke patients (Trombly & Wu, 1999; van Vliet et al., 1995; Wu et al.,

2000), so functional activities should be introduced earlier in treatment.

The first motion sought in stage V is arm raised to side horizontal, which combines full shoulder abduction with elbow extension. When this can be accomplished, disassociation of components of the synergies has occurred. No longer will the arm drift toward horizontal adduction when the elbow is extended or the elbow flex when the shoulder is abducted, as it would when the muscles are still under the influence of the synergies. Again, practice with functional tasks assists learning. Activities that have game pieces or materials that can be placed on a high table to the side of the patient to encourage side horizontal movement in order to play the game or do the project are useful in encouraging this motion. The table can be gradually moved to require more and more horizontal abduction and elbow extension. Other activities that could be used to encourage this motion include weaving on a floor loom, table tennis, driving golf balls, and hitting a baseball.

The second motion of stage V is arm overhead. To achieve it, the scapula must upwardly rotate. The serratus anterior must be specifically retrained to do this. If the scapula is bound by spastic retractors, passive mobilization may be necessary before seeking an active protraction response. Passive mobilization of the scapula is done by grasping the vertebral border and repeatedly and *slowly* rotating it as the arm is passively moved into an overhead position. Once the scapula is mobilized, the serratus is activated in its alternative duty of scapula protraction by placing the arm in the forward horizontal position and asking, and assisting, the patient to reach forward. ***Do not put traction on the patient's glenohumeral joint.*** It is helpful to rehearse this motion with the patient using the uninvolved extremity. Apply quick stretches by pushing backward into scapular retraction to activate the serratus. Once the serratus is activated, seek a holding contraction of the serratus. These procedures continue, with the therapist moving the arm incrementally overhead. Once the movement has been achieved, practice with functional activities reinforces it. Sanding on an inclined plane is an example of an activity requiring a forward push with an increasing range of movement in scapular protraction and rotation and shoulder flexion. Bilateral sanding will allow the stronger uninvolved arm to help the weaker one. Table tennis would still be useful, as would shooting baskets and putting on overhead garments every day. Washing a wall or painting it with a roller requires repeated reversal of movement up overhead and down.

The third motion sought in stage V is supination and pronation (external and internal rotation) with the elbow extended. To improve supination, the elbow is at first kept close to the trunk and gradually extended. Brunnstrom had no special treatment recommendations to assist in developing disassociation of supination and elbow flexion. The best way to achieve control of supination and pronation with the elbow extended is to have the patient use both hands in activities of interest that entail supination and pronation in various arm positions. One such activity is grasping a beach ball with the arms outstretched and rotating it so the affected arm is on top (pronated) and the unaffected arm is on the bottom (supinated) and vice versa. The patient can graduate to handling a smaller ball, such as a basketball. Adapted games, such as an adapted dice game, that capture the patient's attention and interest have been found more effective than exercise (Nelson et al., 1996).

Patients who recover comparatively rapidly after a stroke may spontaneously achieve stage VI; however, many patients do not achieve full recovery after stroke. Twitchell (1951) stated that patients who reached stages III and IV within 10 days after stroke recovered completely; however, this observation has never been verified in the literature. In Twitchell's sample, patients who failed to respond to proprioceptive facilitation did not recover willed movement at all. He observed, and it is generally accepted, that the longer the flaccid stage lasts, the less likely recovery will occur. Studies have verified that patients with a severely impaired upper extremity do not regain full voluntary use of that extremity (Duncan et al., 1994).

Retraining Hand and Wrist Control

Training techniques for return of function in the hand are presented separately from the rest of the upper extremity because the hand may be at a different stage of recovery from that of the arm. If the patient cannot initiate active finger flexion (hand stage I) or mass grasp (hand stage II), the traction response in which stretch of the scapular adductors produces reflex finger flexion or an associated reaction of resisted grasp by the unaffected hand may be used in combination with voluntary effort.

In hemiplegia, wrist flexion usually accompanies grasp initially, so stability of the wrist in extension must be developed. It is easier for the patient to stabilize the wrist in extension when the elbow is extended; therefore, training starts with the elbow extended and the wrist supported by the therapist. The wrist extensor muscles are facilitated, and the therapist directs the patient to do a forceful grasp by saying, "Squeeze!" That grasp should promote normal synergistic contraction of the facilitated wrist extensors. This is repeated until the wrist extensors are felt to respond, allowing the therapist to remove support from the wrist with the command, "Hold." Tapping on the wrist extensor muscles facilitates holding. Once wrist extension and grasp with the elbow extended are possible, the process of positioning, percussion, and hold is repeated in increasing amounts of elbow flexion. Emphasis in this stage of training is on wrist stability, although wrist flexion, extension, and circumduction may also be practiced.

To move from hand stage III (flexion) to hand stage IV (semivoluntary mass extension) spasticity of the finger flexors must be relaxed using a series of manipulations listed in Box 24-7. The second motion sought at hand stage IV is lateral prehension and release. The

---

BOX 24-7
PROCEDURES FOR PRACTICE

Procedures to Develop Finger Extension

1. Release the patient's grasp by holding the thumb into extension and abduction.
2. Still holding the thumb, *slowly* and rhythmically supinate and pronate the forearm.
3. Apply cutaneous stimulation over the dorsum of the hand while the forearm is supinated.
4. With the forearm still supinated, apply rapid, repeated stretch to the extensors of the fingers by repeatedly rolling them toward the palm (Fig. 24-9).
5. Continue these manipulations until flexion relaxes.
6. Slowly pronate the forearm and elevate the arm above horizontal to evoke a finger extensor response (Souque's phenomenon).
7. Stroke over the dorsum of the fingers and forearm as the patient attempts extension. To avoid a buildup of flexor tension, do not allow the patient to exert more than minimal effort. Imitation synkinesis, in which the normal

side performs a motion that is difficult for the involved side (Boissy et al., 1997), may be observed when the patient attempts finger extension.
8. After the fingers can be voluntarily extended with the arm raised, gradually lower the arm.
9. If there is a decreased range in extension, repeat all above manipulations to again inhibit flexion and facilitate extension.
10. Provide opportunities for the patient to reach and pick up large, lightweight objects and to release them. Putting bagels, apples, or oranges into a basket is one example of an activity to practice finger extension. The larger the object, the greater the extension required. Other extensor-type activities require the hand to be used flat, such as smoothing out a garment while ironing or a sheet while making the bed.

Case Example

MRS. G.: MOVING FROM BRUNNSTROM'S STAGE III TO STAGE IV

Patient Information

Mrs. G. is a 38-year-old right-hand dominant woman who was employed as a clerk in a local department store prior to her stroke. She was an accomplished amateur artist who did oil portraiture. She lives with her husband, a plumber, and 16-year old son in a ranch-style house.

In January 1996 she had an embolytic stroke of the left middle cerebral artery. After 3 days in acute care, Mrs. G. was transferred to inpatient rehabilitation. At admission, she had no voluntary movement of the right upper extremity, and kinesthesis of that limb was impaired. She was wheelchair dependent. She was discharged after 15 days, independent in walking and in ADL using the unaffected arm. She was referred to outpatient occupational therapy for further rehabilitation.

After evaluation, the occupational therapist concluded that Mrs. G.'s proprioception and tactile localization were intact but that she had limited (about 35%) recovery of the upper extremity (refer to Table 24-1), requiring use of the left upper extremity for self-care and other activities. The therapist noted the following problems concerning motor control:

1. Unable to do extensor synergy movement, although the strongest components were active.
2. Able to maintain wrist extension in any elbow position but could not take resistance.
3. Able to hold a card put between her thumb and index finger but not against resistance; unable to release it actively.
4. Unable to do other types of grasp, other than mass grasp, or to extend the fingers other than release of mass grasp.

Recommendations

Constrained by limited insurance, the therapist recommended outpatient treatment three times weekly for 6 weeks and weekly for an additional 6 weeks. The patient's long-term goals were to use both upper extremities to dress herself, prepare meals, do household tasks and to resume oil painting. She decided to take an extended leave of absence from work because of the continuing excessive effort required for all tasks.

Short-Term Goals

After a discussion of sensorimotor impairments probably preventing achievement of her goals, the patient and therapist set the following goals for therapy:

1. Develop elbow extension (stage III).
2. Develop hand behind back motion (stage IV).

3. Improve wrist stability.
4. Strengthen lateral pinch (stage IV) and develop release.
5. Develop palmar pinch (stage V) to enable use of a paintbrush.
6. Improve dexterity of the unaffected nondominant upper extremity.

The first weeks of therapy focused on developing voluntary control of the extensor synergy. Rowing and weight-bearing maneuvers listed in Box 24-6 were used. Between therapy appointments, Mrs. G. practiced using whatever extensor movement she had to do activities like sponging off the table and kitchen counters after meals, putting her arms into the sleeves of sweaters and jackets, and vacuuming with a self-propelled vacuum cleaner. She interspersed these activities with weight bearing on the affected arm with the elbow extended while working with the other hand. Once the patient was able to do the extensor synergy voluntarily, she was encouraged to continue to do tasks at home that alternated between flexor and extensor synergies. Meanwhile, therapy focused on improving wrist stability and developing the first motion of stage IV, hand behind the back. Wrist stability was encouraged during mass grasp and lift of increasingly heavy shopping bags by tapping the wrist extensors during the lift. After repeated attempts in therapy to swing the hand behind the back, with tactile facilitation of the latissimus dorsi, posterior deltoid and triceps, Mrs. G. was successful in bringing her hand past the anterior superior iliac spine. Encouraged, she continued to practice at home and to use the motion functionally in pulling on her underpants and slacks.

Therapy now focused on developing release of lateral pinch through tapping of the extensor pollicis longus and the abductor pollicis longus tendons. Once release was enabled,

---

CLINICAL REASONING
in OT Practice

Planning Treatment According to Stage of Recovery

List homemaking activities that a patient in stage IV of upper limb recovery and stage V of hand recovery can be expected to do. What are some activities the patient won't be able to do? What treatment may help the patient move from the beginning of stage IV (hand behind the back) to stage V of upper limb recovery?

the resistance was gradually increased and alternated with active release. The patient was given a home program of activities to encourage lateral prehension. She resumed painting with the canvas on the table and used lateral pinch to squeeze the paint tubes and hold the brushes. In the process of using various brushes, she redeveloped palmar prehension without specific treatment. Goal 6 was met by the natural demand to accomplish the tasks of her self-maintenance role.

Revised Goals

Based on the progress made after 6 weeks of therapy (Refer to the column labeled 3/15/96 in Table 24-1) the therapist and patient formulated the following revised goals:

1. Develop arm forward flexion (stage IV) to enable painting on an easel.
2. Develop cylindrical grasp (stage V) to enable use of a toothbrush, broom, mop, large spoons.

---

patient attempts to move the thumb away from the index finger to gain release of lateral prehension while the therapist percusses or strokes over the extensor pollicis longus and abductor pollicis longus tendons to facilitate this motion. Once the patient has some active release, functional use of lateral prehension is encouraged. Activities include holding a book while reading, holding or dealing cards, using a key, and dressing.

Once the patient can extend the fingers voluntarily to release objects, advanced prehensile patterns (hand stage V) are encouraged through activities. As the patient progresses, activities are chosen to reinforce particular prehensions at more precise levels. Holding a pencil or paintbrush encourages palmar prehension. Spherical grasp is used to pick up or hold round objects such as a mayonnaise jar lid or an orange. Cylindrical grasp is used to hold the handles of tools.

Individual finger movements (hand stage VI) may be regained in rare instances. The patient should be given a home program of activities to encourage more and more individual finger use and to increase speed and accuracy of finger movements but should also be cautioned about expecting full recovery. A stroke survivor has recently published a workbook of his exercises for hand recovery that may be incorporated into the home program of a patient with determination to recover hand function (Smits & Smits-Boone, 2000).

Brunnstrom also described gait patterns, principles used in preparation for walking, and training to walk. These procedures are the primary responsibility of the physical therapist.

Effectiveness

The only study of the effectiveness of this approach compared the relative effectiveness of Brunnstrom's movement therapy to Bobath's neurodevelopment treatment (Wagenaar et al., 1990). Seven selected poststroke patients were randomly assigned to one treatment for 5

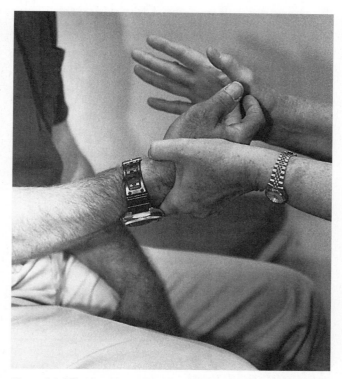

Figure 24-9 The therapist applies rapid repeated stretches to the extensors of the fingers by rolling the fingers toward the palm.

weeks and then to the other for 5 more weeks; this was repeated using a *B-C-B-C* design. Functional recovery of activities of daily living (ADL), upper limb function, and walking ability were assessed weekly. The treatment program included occupational therapy, physical therapy, and nursing. All members of the treatment team adhered strictly to the written protocol for each treatment developed from primary sources. The only significantly different outcome was greater improvement of gait speed by one patient in the Brunnstrom condition compared with the Bobath condition. The lack of difference detected in other subjects and for other assessments may be the result of alternating short periods of each treatment for each subject; that is, no subject received a full treatment program that followed one method. This is an important limitation because these methods have opposite views concerning the use of associated reactions. The recovery graphs for each patient showed steady recovery regardless of treatment, indicating that either (1) both methods were effective or (2) the subjects were recovering spontaneously. The actual interpretation cannot be made, however, because the study did not include a control condition (i.e., no treatment given).

Summary Review Questions

1. What are the assumptions of the Brunnstrom approach?
2. What is an associated reaction and how is it elicited?
3. Describe the flexor synergy of the upper extremity and state which component or components are strongest.
4. Describe the extensor synergy of the upper extremity and state which component or components are strongest.
5. List in order the six recovery stages of the proximal upper extremity.
6. List in order the six stages of hand recovery.
7. Name the treatment principles of the Brunnstrom approach.
8. How is the flexor synergy initiated in the upper extremity when the patient is flaccid?
9. How is elbow extension developed?
10. How is finger extension developed?

Acknowledgment

Photography by Robert Littlefield.

References

Berglund, K., & Fugl-Meyer, A. R. (1986). Upper extremity function in hemiplegia: A cross-validation study of two assessment methods. *Scandinavian Journal of Rehabilitation Medicine, 18,* 155–157.

Boissy, P., Bourbonnais, D., Kaegi, C., Gravel, D., & Arsenault, B. A. (1997). Characterization of global synkineses during hand grip in hemiparetic patients. *Archives of Physical Medicine and Rehabilitation, 78,* 1117–1124.

Brunnstrom, S. (1956). Associated reactions of the upper extremity in adult patients with hemiplegia. *Physical Therapy Review, 36,* 225–236.

Brunnstrom, S. (1966). Motor testing procedures in hemiplegia. *Journal of the American Physical Therapy Association, 46,* 357–375.

Brunnstrom, S. (1970). *Movement Therapy in Hemiplegia.* New York: Harper & Row.

Dean, C. M., & Shepherd, R. B. (1997). Task related training improves performance of seated reaching tasks after stroke. *Stroke, 28,* 722–728.

Duncan, P. W., Propst, M., & Nelson, S. G. (1983). Reliability of the Fugl-Meyer Assessment of sensorimotor recovery following cerebrovascular accident. *Physical Therapy, 63,* 1606–1610.

Duncan, P. W., Goldstein, L. B., Horner, R. D., Landsman, P. B., Samsa, G. P., & Matchar, D. B. (1994). Similar motor recovery of upper and lower extremities after stroke. *Stroke, 25,* 1181–1188.

Fujiwara, T., Hara, Y., & Chino, N. (1999). The influence of nonparetic leg movements on muscle action in the paretic leg of hemiplegic patients. *Scandinavian Journal of Rehabilitation Medicine, 31,* 174–177.

Fugl-Meyer, A. R., Jaasko, L., Leyman, I., Olsson, S., & Steglind, S. (1975). The post-stroke hemiplegic patient. I. A method for evaluation of physical performance. *Scandinavian Journal of Rehabilitation Medicine, 7,* 13–31.

Malouin, F., Pichard, L., Bonneau, C., Durand, A., & Corriveau, D. (1994). Evaluating motor recovery early after stroke: Comparison of the Fugl-Meyer Assessment and the Motor Assessment Scale. *Archives of Physical Medicine and Rehabilitation, 75,* 1206–1212.

Mudie, M. H., & Matyas, T. A. (2000, January 10-20). Can simultaneous bilateral movement involve the undamaged hemisphere in reconstruction of neural networks damaged by stroke? *Disability and Rehabilitation, 22,* 23–27.

Nelson, D. L., Konosky, K., Fleharty, K., Webb, R., Newer, K., Hazboun, V. P., Fontane, C., & Licht, B. C. (1996). The effects of occupationally embedded exercise on bilaterally assisted supination in persons with hemiplegia. *American Journal of Occupational Therapy, 50,* 639–646.

Sanford, J., Moreland, J., Swanson, L. R., Stratford, P. W., & Gowland, C. (1993). Reliability of the Fugl-Meyer Assessment for testing motor performance in patients following stroke. *Physical Therapy, 73,* 447–454.

Smits, J. G., & Smits-Boone, E. C. (2000). *Hand Recovery After Stroke: Exercises and Results Measurements.* Boston: Butterworth Heinemann.

Trombly, C. A., & Wu, C-y. (1999). Effects of rehabilitation tasks on organization of movement after stroke. *American Journal of Occupational Therapy, 53,* 333–344.

Twitchell, T. (1951). The restoration of motor function following hemiplegia in man. *Brain, 74,* 443–480.

van Vliet, P., Sheridan, M., Kerwin, D. G., & Fentem, P. (1995). The influence of functional goals on the kinematics of reaching following stroke. *[American Physical Therapy Association] Neurology Report, 19,* 11–16.

Wagenaar, R. C., Meijer, O. G., van Wieringen, P. C. W., Kuik, D. J., Hazenberg, G. J., Lindeboom, J., Wichers, F., & Rijswijk, H. (1990). The functional recovery of stroke: A comparison between neurodevelopmental treatment and the Brunnstrom method. *Scandinavian Journal of Rehabilitation Medicine, 22,* 1–8.

Wu, C-y., Trombly, C. A., Lin, K-c., & Tickle-Degnen, L. (2000). A kinematic study of contextual effects of reaching performance in persons with and without stroke: Influences of object availability. *Archives of Physical Medicine and Rehabilitation, 81,* 95–101.

25
Optimizing Motor Control Using Biofeedback

Theodore I. King II

Theodore I. King II

LEARNING OBJECTIVES

After studying this chapter, the reader will be able to do the following:

1. Define biofeedback.
2. State the uses of electrogoniometric and electromyographic biofeedback.
3. Organize treatment sessions using biofeedback to recruit or inhibit muscle activity.

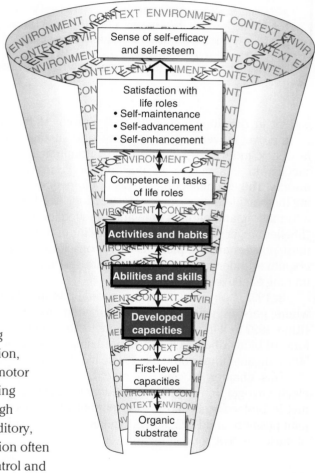

Motor learning requires feedback. (See Chapter 12 for a discussion of motor learning.) Whether a person is acquiring a new skill or modifying a skill because of a physical dysfunction, sensory feedback optimizes motor learning. An intact sensorimotor system provides feedback from many sources to assist in refining movement as it occurs while developing motor learning through repetition. Many systems, including somatosensory, visual, auditory, and vestibular, provide sensory feedback. A physical dysfunction often impairs the sensory feedback necessary to facilitate motor control and learning. Augmented feedback, provided by biofeedback, in a task-oriented occupational therapy treatment session may assist in the relearning of motor skills requisite to occupational functioning.

The term *biofeedback* is used to describe external physiological feedback. It may be defined as the "technique of using equipment (usually electronic) to reveal to human beings some of their internal physiological events, normal and abnormal, in the form of visual and auditory signals in order to teach them to manipulate these otherwise involuntary or unfelt events by manipulating the displayed signals" (Basmajian, 1983, p. 1). Biofeedback may be used by occupational therapists to assist a

---

GLOSSARY

Differential amplifier—Electronic device that enlarges signals of the phenomenon under study while differentially canceling out signals due to artifact. Because EMG signals are so small compared to the ambient electrical signals that the body acts as an antenna for, differential amplifiers are used in electromyography.

Facilitation techniques—Sensory stimulation techniques applied to the skin over the muscle or muscles of interest to encourage recruitment of motor units.

Global aphasia—Overall lack of ability to understand or communicate written or spoken words.

Meta-analysis—Statistical literature review of related studies that summarizes their results quantitatively to yield an overall statistical estimate of the effects of the treatment being studied.

Motor unit—Single lower motor neuron and all the muscle fibers it innervates.

Neuromuscular electrical stimulation (NMES)—Externally applied electrical stimulation to activate motor units.

Quad cane—Walking aid that has four prongs at the end instead of the usual cane with only one. Patients who require greater stability than an ordinary cane provides use it.

Voltmeter—Electronic device that measures the amount of voltage in a circuit. Because the EMG signal is a voltage signal, a voltmeter can be used as a crude EMG biofeedback device.

---

patient in developing specific sensorimotor skills and to improve movement in an occupational task. Biofeedback motivates patients while informing them of success in changing joint position or contracting a muscle. The essential components of biofeedback training include clear goals, proper instructions, feedback of information, and enough time and practice for learning (Shellenberger & Green, 1986). In addition, the patient must possess an adequate level of consciousness and cognitive understanding to participate in biofeedback training effectively.

In 1992, I surveyed 301 occupational therapy clinics where persons with physical dysfunction are treated (King, 1992). Of the clinics, 47% were treating with some form of biofeedback. Of clinics not using biofeedback, 59% indicated they would like to use it in the future.

This chapter focuses on electrogoniometric and electromyographic (EMG) biofeedback. Electrogoniometric biofeedback informs the patient of changes in joint position, and EMG biofeedback informs the patient of muscle activity or contraction.

Electrogoniometry

During attempts to increase range of motion or improve task-oriented movements, electrogoniometry is reported to offer greater success than EMG biofeedback, since the patient's effort is directly linked to movement (Young & Schmidt, 1992). A goniometer is a simple hinged device used to evaluate range of motion by measuring joint angles. An electrogoniometer is a biofeedback device similar to a goniometer but with electronic components that directly inform the patient of joint positions during

movement. Lantz et al. (1999) found that electrogoniometry provides a valid and reliable measure of cervical range of motion. An electrogoniometer was used to measure active and passive cervical range of motion comparing test–retest data between two examiners. The instrument was found to be both reliable and valid when used according to the authors' protocol.

Instruments

Two types of electrogoniometers are commonly used for biofeedback. A static electrogoniometer offers auditory or visual feedback when a target angle is achieved (threshold feedback). The therapist determines the desired angle the patient is to reach and sets the device to offer feedback when that angle is attained. Auditory feedback may simply be a buzzer or similar device that is activated at the desired angle, while visual feedback may be activation of a light when the desired angle is achieved. A dynamic electrogoniometer offers constant visual feedback regarding change in joint angle during movement (motion feedback). The visual feedback is usually offered via a computer monitor on which the patient can view a line graph depicting the angle of the joint, which is constantly traced across the screen.

It is simple to construct a static electrogoniometer from a commercial goniometer adapted to offer a visual or auditory signal when a target angle is achieved. In Figure 25-1, a finger goniometer has been revised by placing metal alligator clips on the movable portion (pointer) of the goniometer and on the immovable dial used to record joint angle. When the patient extends the finger joint to the angle determined by the placement of the alligator clip on the dial, it makes contact with the alligator clip on the movable pointer, closing the circuit. These alligator clips are easily connected by wires to a battery-operated circuit made by the therapist. When the alligator clips touch to complete the circuit, a light for visual feedback or a buzzer for auditory feedback is activated. Several such circuits have been published (Brown et al., 1979; Cohen, 1983).

Koheil and Mandell (1980) demonstrated efficacy in applying threshold electrogoniometric biofeedback for knee joint position during gait training. The biofeedback device allowed for the setting of two boundaries, or limits, so an audible tone would be heard when joint motion exceeded the flexion or extension limit. The researchers presented a single case study of a 53-year-old woman who had had a cerebrovascular accident. By the end of the biofeedback training period, the patient's genu recurvatum had improved, and she was able to progress from a **quad cane** to a standard cane.

A dynamic electrogoniometer must continuously offer feedback as a joint angle changes during movement. To accomplish this, a potentiometer, or variable resistor, is linked to the hinge of a goniometer (Fig. 25-2). A rotary dimmer switch for a light fixture is an example of a commonly used potentiometer. As the dimmer switch is turned, more or less voltage is supplied to the light fixture, causing an increase or decrease in brightness. Similarly, a dynamic electrogoniometer supplies more or less voltage in the circuit based on joint angle. A simple dynamic electrogoniometer can be made by linking a low-voltage potentiometer, available at electronic parts stores, to the hinge of a goniometer and wiring to a battery-operated circuit made by the therapist with a **voltmeter**. The output voltage of the circuit as

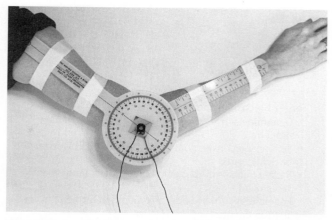

Figure 25-2 Dynamic elbow electrogoniometer made from a standard goniometer.

recorded by the voltmeter is directly proportional to joint angle. When available, a dynamic electrogoniometer displaying a waveform on a computer monitor to indicate joint angle and velocity of change in joint angle is preferred (see Resources).

Treatment Applications

Threshold or target feedback using a static electrogoniometer is used if the goal is to increase range of motion (Box 25-1). The electrogoniometer may be attached to the patient with bandage tape or Velcro straps. After determining a baseline maximum active range of motion for the movement desired using a conventional goniometer, the feedback threshold of the electrogoniometer is initially set at this angle. For example, in Figure 25-1 the alligator clip on the immovable dial portion of the goniometer is positioned to make contact with the alligator clip on the movable pointer of the goniometer when the target angle is achieved. During the treatment session, the target angle is gradually increased as the patient achieves greater motion. Though the patient may be requested simply to move in the desired direction, adding purpose to the movement, such as reaching for objects, is preferable. The therapist should be sure to observe and guide the patient to avoid any substitution movements and to isolate movement at the joint as much as possible. **Facilitation techniques** may also be used to assist movement. Initially, the session should last only 10 to 15 minutes and be self-paced by the patient.

Motion feedback produced by a dynamic electrogoniometer is used to improve speed and direction of movement (Box 25-1). The electrogoniometer may be attached to the patient with bandage tape or Velcro straps. In Figure 25-2 an electrogoniometer has been placed to record movement at the elbow joint. A low-voltage potentiometer has been mounted at the hinge of the goniometer to record movement by measur-

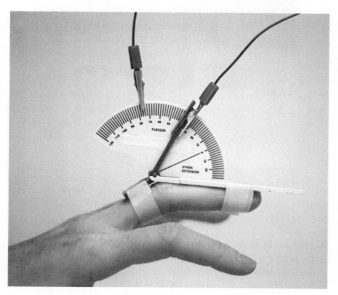

Figure 25-1 Static finger electrogoniometer made by the therapist.

Target Electrogoniometry

► Determine active range of motion goal for movement desired.
► Set up target electrogoniometric device to provide feedback at desired goal.
► Patient initiates movement until feedback from device is obtained.
► Patient repeats movement as prescribed by therapist for 10 to 15 minutes.
► Target angle may be increased during session as the patient improves.

Motion Electrogoniometry

► Set up dynamic electrogoniometric device to record desired joint.
► Passively move patient's limb to record desired waveform on monitor. Pay attention to both the extent and speed of motion. Start at a point where the client can succeed.
► Patient attempts to duplicate waveform produced by therapist's passive movement.
► Patient repeats movement as prescribed by therapist for 10 to 15 minutes.
► As the patient succeeds, change the waveform to upgrade the extent of motion, the speed of motion, or both.

ing change in resistance in a battery-operated circuit, which is displayed as a waveform on a monitor. This type of therapy is especially useful in treating patients with spasticity, ataxia, intention tremors, or loss of proprioception. Usually, the therapist initially moves the patient's limb passively to record a waveform on the monitor for the change in joint angle at the desired speed and direction. Using this display, the patient then repeatedly practices duplicating the same waveform. As with static feedback, it is suggested to begin with a 10- to 15-minute session that is paced by the patient. Greenberg and Fowler (1980) applied motion feedback using a dynamic electrogoniometer to treat elbow range of motion of persons with hemiplegia after stroke and demonstrated ability to increase active range of motion. Twenty subjects were randomly assigned to either the treatment group for kinesthetic (electrogoniometric) biofeedback or the control group for therapy without biofeedback. As subjects in the treatment group attained the desired range, a light would be activated by the electrogoniometer to indicate success. The results indicated that the biofeedback treatment was as effective as the conventional treatment.

Electromyography

EMG is a recording of the electrical activity produced by muscle fibers of activated **motor units** (Herrington, 1996). EMG was developed to assess muscle activity, primarily in cases of polio or stroke. EMG is increasingly widely used in treatment. A typical set-up for treatment is shown in Figure 25-3.

Instruments

When a muscle contracts, the contracting motor units generate an electrical signal. The EMG signal reflects the number and size of motor units contracting. This electrical activity can be measured with needle or surface electrodes. Needle electrodes penetrate the skin and are placed in close proximity to motor units. They are used when the output of a specific, small, or deep muscle is desired. Surface electrodes are placed on the skin overlying the muscle to be measured. Though less sensitive, surface electrodes are more commonly used because of their relative comfort and their noninvasiveness. Typically, an EMG biofeedback unit consists of a central unit to which the electrode wires are connected for signal processing. The central unit has controls to

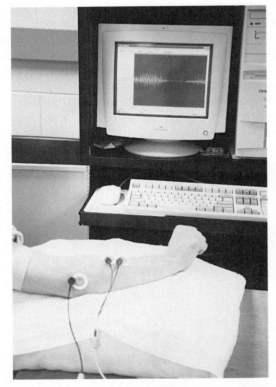

Figure 25-3 EMG biofeedback for wrist extension. Note that the common, or ground, electrode is placed over a nonmuscular area. The feedback the patient is observing is raw signal EMG, which can be seen to vary between full output (full extensor activity) and zero output (no activity).

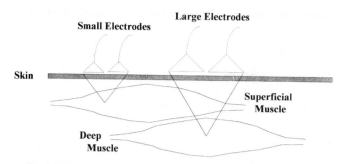

Figure 25-4 Pickup areas of electrodes of various sizes. Adapted from Trombly, C. A., & Tries, J. (1995). Biofeedback. In C. A. Trombly (Ed.), *Occupational Therapy for Physical Dysfunction* (4th ed., pp. 645–657). Baltimore: Williams & Wilkins.

allow the therapist to set parameters such as thresholds and type of output signal. The output signal may emanate from the central unit or from a peripheral device attached to the central unit, such as a computer monitor. An EMG biofeedback unit usually displays readings in microvolts, or millionths of a volt.

Prior to application of electrodes the skin should be cleansed of dirt, oil, makeup, and dead cells, which impede transmission of the electrical signals. At the least an alcohol swab should be used, and some manufacturers recommend use of an abrasive skin cleaner. Several types of reusable or disposable electrodes are available (see Resources). Most are self-adhesive, but some require taping to maintain placement. All electrodes require the use of a conductive gel or cream to establish a uniform connection between the skin and the electrode. Many commercial electrodes come with the gel already applied.

Since size determines the pickup area of the electrode, smaller electrodes should be used for smaller muscles to avoid reception of signals from surrounding muscles (Fig. 25-4). In addition, widely spaced electrodes pick up signals not only from a larger surface but also more deeply, while closely spaced electrodes pick up more specific and superficial electrical signals (Fig. 25-5).

The environment contains electrical energy from many sources, including power lines, lights, and electrical appliances. Human tissue picks up this environmental energy, or noise, and transmits it to EMG electrodes. The EMG signal is very small compared to these noise signals. As a result, EMG devices must be designed to eliminate electrical energy from these environmental sources and display only electrical signals related to motor unit activity. To accomplish this, EMG devices use **differential amplifiers** and electrical filters. Because voltage is the potential difference in electrical charge between two points, two electrodes are used. In addition, to eliminate unwanted environmental electrical

noise, a ground or common electrode is also used. The electrodes to measure muscle activity are placed longitudinally along the belly of the muscle to be measured, and the common electrode may be placed anywhere on the body, though preferably over a bony prominence where muscle activity is not recorded (Trombly & Tries, 1995).

The common electrode picks up the ambient environmental electrical noise but not electrical signals from the muscle. If the muscle underlying the two active electrodes is at rest, only environmental electrical noise is detected by the active electrodes and compared with the common electrode. In this case, the differential amplifier eliminates the environmental signals, since they are sensed as equal to what the common electrode senses, and the resultant EMG reading is zero. If the muscle underlying the two active electrodes is contracting, each electrode receives a slightly different electrical signal because of the difference in the two locations over the muscle belly. As a result, the differential amplifier again eliminates the environmental signals, since they are sensed as equal to what the common electrode senses, but amplifies the difference detected between the two active electrodes, which represents motor unit activity of the muscle (Trombly & Tries, 1995). EMG units also employ electrical filters to eliminate high-frequency electrical noise generated by the circuits of the EMG unit itself and the low-frequency signal generated at the interface of the electrode and the gel (Trombly & Tries, 1995). Therefore, the use of a common electrode and the electrical filters of the EMG unit produce a signal that indicates only the motor unit activity of the muscle. When the muscle is at rest, there is no electrical signal generated, while a greater signal will be generated as more motor units are recruited.

The raw EMG signal received from a contracting muscle is an alternating current (AC) signal. Graphically, this type of signal is represented by an alternation of the signal on either side of the isoelectric line or zero charge

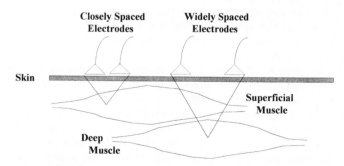

Figure 25-5 Pickup area of variously spaced electrodes. Adapted from Trombly, C. A., & Tries, J. (1995). Biofeedback. In C. A. Trombly (Ed.), *Occupational Therapy for Physical Dysfunction* (4th ed., pp. 645–657). Baltimore: Williams & Wilkins.

Case Example

MRS. K.: REDEVELOPING SHOULDER CONTROL FOLLOWING STROKE

Patient Information

Mrs. K. is a 27-year-old woman 1 month post stroke (occlusion of left middle cerebral artery). She and her husband live alone. She was employed full time as a children's librarian at the local library. Her husband is employed full time as a machinist at a local factory. She participated in an outpatient occupational therapy program, and the following problems were identified during the initial assessment: (1) decreased ability to complete self-care activities; (2) decreased mobility requiring a wheelchair; (3) decreased sitting balance; (4) decreased voluntary control of the right upper extremity, manifested as an inability to voluntarily reach forward or overhead; and (5) **global aphasia**.

Recommendations

The occupational therapist recommended three outpatient treatment sessions per week of 45 minutes' duration for a total of 4 weeks. In collaboration with Mrs. K. and her husband, the occupational therapist established the following long-term treatment goals: (1) Mrs. K. will independently complete light self-care skills, with setup, using the affected upper extremity (i.e., brushing her teeth, washing her face and upper extremities, and upper extremity dressing); (2) Mrs. K. will be able to sit independently and safely in a desk or table chair with arms; and (3) Mrs. K. will be able to control movement in the right shoulder for use in functional tasks.

Short-Term Goal to Control Movement in the Right Shoulder

Mrs. K. will be able to control isolated shoulder flexion to 90 degrees in the affected upper extremity. The decreased voluntary control of the right upper extremity limited Mrs. K.'s ability to use the extremity in functional activities such as self-care. As is commonly seen after stroke, Mrs. K. exhibited flexor synergy pattern of the upper extremity that manifested as increased tone in the upper trapezius and pectoralis major, while the serratus anterior and anterior deltoid were weak. To assist with reacquisition of isolated movement in the shoulder, the therapist incorporated the use of EMG biofeedback in the treatment program. Though the patient had global aphasia, the therapist could communicate with the patient nonverbally to instruct her during the treatment session, and therefore, it did not interfere with the use of EMG biofeedback as a treatment modality. Auditory feedback was used to signal the patient when threshold levels were attained.

Initially, electrodes were placed on the upper trapezius (Fig. 25-7) and pectoralis major using an EMG biofeedback protocol to decrease tone (Box 25-3). Dual EMG channels, monitoring two muscles simultaneously with two separate channels and two sets of electrodes, were used. The biofeedback device received signals from both muscles and processed them so that only when both the upper trapezius and the pectoralis major were relaxing would the patient receive the reinforcement feedback. During the first week of therapy, treatment focused on maintaining relaxation in these muscles while the patient moved the opposite extremity and attempted to flex the shoulder in the affected extremity. During the second week, electrodes were placed on the serratus anterior, which rotates the scapula upward and assists with protraction. The biofeedback program facilitated strengthening of the muscle while engaging the patient in a shoulder protraction activity (moving the upper extremity forward while supported on a table with the shoulder flexed to 90°). In the third weekly session, the anterior deltoid was also encouraged to contract using EMG biofeedback to assist with shoulder flexion. Again, dual-channel EMG was used to encourage simultaneous activity of the serratus anterior and anterior deltoid (shoulder protraction and flexion). Only simultaneous activity above the set thresholds was rewarded with reinforcement feedback. As isolated voluntary movement improved in the third week of treatment, self-care activities were incorporated into the treatment sessions and EMG biofeedback was discontinued. A home program was developed to continue with active exercise with the right upper extremity and use of the extremity in self-care.

Revised Goal

Mrs. K. will use the right upper extremity to complete self-care skills independently.

CLINICAL REASONING
in OT Practice

Biofeedback to Relearn to Combine Shoulder Forward Flexion and Elbow Extension

Although Mrs. K. could voluntarily flex her shoulder, when she attempted to reach forward, her elbow flexed synergistically. How would you structure biofeedback sessions to help her regain the ability to extend her elbow while flexing or abducting the shoulder? Describe a session using EMG biofeedback, including the size and location of electrodes, how the thresholds would be set, whether the feedback would be auditory or visual, and what exercises or activities would be used during the practice. Describe a session using a combination of EMG and electrogoniometric biofeedback.

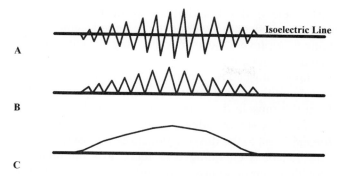

Figure 25-6 EMG signals. **A.** Raw signal. **B.** Rectified signal. **C.** Smoothed signal.

(Fig. 25-6*A*). This is not very useful for biofeedback purposes, so most EMG units rectify and smooth the signal. In rectifying the signal, the EMG unit first transforms the AC signal to a direct current (DC) signal, which is graphically represented as remaining on one side of the isoelectric line (Fig. 25-6*B*). Finally, the EMG unit smoothes the signal through a filter to graph the electrical signal received from the activated motor units as a smooth line whose height is proportional to the level of muscle activity (Fig. 25-6*C*). This signal can be used as visual feedback for the patient and therapist.

Auditory feedback may be incorporated into a treatment session; it is usually used in combination with threshold settings. A threshold may be set to activate audio feedback when EMG readings exceed the threshold value for reeducation or strength training or to deactivate audio feedback when EMG readings fall below the threshold value for relaxation training.

Treatment Applications

Occupational therapists have used EMG to treat patients with a variety of disorders, including low back pain (Strong et al., 1989), cumulative trauma disorder (Reynolds, 1994), traumatic head injury (Lysaght & Bodenhamer, 1990), writer's cramp (O'Neill et al., 1997), shoulder disarticulation (Canelon, 1993), ataxia (Guercio et al., 1997), and stroke (Crow et al., 1989; Wolf et al., 1989). EMG treatment applications discussed in this chapter include muscle reeducation and strengthening, decreasing spasticity, and control of urinary incontinence. The case example illustrates biofeedback used to redevelop shoulder control following stroke.

Muscle Reeducation and Strengthening

EMG biofeedback is used to reeducate weak or flaccid muscles and to strengthen muscles (Asfour et al., 1990; Brucker & Bulaeva, 1996; Morrison, 1988; Reid, Saboe, & Chepeha, 1996) (Box 25-2). At first the electrodes should be large and widely spaced to pick up any signal emitted by the weak muscle. As the patient improves, the electrodes should be smaller and placed closer together. Usually an attainable auditory threshold is set and the patient is encouraged to contract the muscle enough to reach the threshold. The threshold is set by adjusting the microvolt output of the EMG unit to the desired muscle activity required to trigger the auditory or visual feedback. During the treatment session, the threshold is gradually raised to encourage stronger muscle contraction. As soon as possible, the patient should be weaned from EMG biofeedback by incorporating the movement or strength attained into purposeful activities.

Facilitation techniques may also be employed during the EMG biofeedback session to encourage initial motor unit activity or to increase motor unit recruitment. **Neuromuscular electrical stimulation (NMES)** is

BOX 25-2
PROCEDURES FOR PRACTICE

EMG Biofeedback Session for Muscle Reeducation

▸ Begin with large, widely-spaced electrodes over the muscle belly.
▸ Initially set the threshold at an attainable level.
▸ During a 10- to 15-minute treatment session, the patient voluntarily contracts the muscle to reach the threshold level.
▸ When possible, incorporate purposeful activities to facilitate the muscle activity desired.
▸ Gradually raise the threshold during the treatment session to challenge the patient to contract the muscle more strongly.

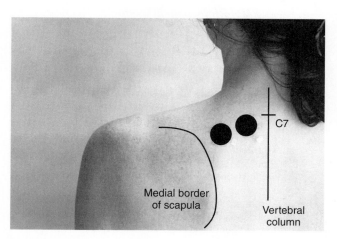

Figure 25-7 Placement of active electrodes for EMG biofeedback of the upper trapezius.

often employed in combination with EMG biofeedback. Dual units (EMG with NMES) are available to allow NMES activation of additional motor units once the patient attains a specific EMG threshold during initial motor unit recruitment. In this way, muscle contraction can be completed to normal levels once initiated by the patient.

In a review of the literature, I found no specific studies indicating that EMG biofeedback elicited greater functional motor return than traditional forms of therapy with patients having hemiplegia after stroke (King, 1994). A **meta-analysis** of literature spanning 1976 to 1992 by Moreland and Thomson (1994) regarding the efficacy of EMG biofeedback compared with conventional therapy for upper extremity function in patients following stroke did not conclusively indicate superiority of either type of therapy, though both were effective. Another meta-analysis of literature between 1976 and 1995 by Moreland et al. (1998) compared the efficacy of EMG biofeedback with that of conventional therapy for lower extremity function in patients following stroke. The results indicated that EMG biofeedback was slightly better than conventional therapy alone, though the findings were not statistically significant. These meta-analyses of the literature indicate efficacy at least equal to that of conventional treatment approaches and indicate the need for further studies.

Decreasing Spasticity

Using EMG biofeedback to decrease spasticity is in many ways the reverse of using it to strengthen (Box 25-3). At first the electrodes should be small and closely spaced to promote success in lowering the recorded signal. As the patient improves, the electrodes may be increased in size and spaced more widely, but not off the margins of the target muscle. An attainable threshold is set to turn off an auditory signal once the electrical signal recorded from the muscle drops below the threshold level. The threshold is set by adjusting the microvolt output of the EMG unit to the desired reduction in muscle activity. The patient is encouraged to relax; it is important to provide a serene atmosphere and have the patient use relaxation techniques. Initially, the patient attempts to maintain relaxation of muscle contraction while remaining still; in later sessions the patient is challenged to maintain relaxation of the spastic muscle during cognitively challenging activities and eventually during contraction of the antagonistic group of muscles. As the patient maintains functional relaxation of the spastic muscle, the use of EMG biofeedback should be decreased and eventually omitted from the treatment program.

Kelly et al. (1979) reported specific procedures they found useful in treating spasticity in upper extremities of patients with hemiparesis after stroke. Their approach was to reduce the hyperactivity in spastic musculature and then to increase activity levels in weak muscles. Crow et al. (1989) reported on the effectiveness of EMG biofeedback to assist in normalizing tone following a stroke (Research Note). EMG biofeedback has also been employed to evaluate spasticity by recording the activity of spastic muscles (Skold et al., 1998). In this study it was found that EMG output was significantly correlated with simultaneous modified Ashworth scale measurements of spasticity in patients with tetraplegia.

Urinary Incontinence

Urinary incontinence is common among older adults. Many therapists have reported success in using EMG biofeedback as a means to control urinary incontinence (Engberg et al., 1997; Jackson et al., 1996; Mathewson-Chapman, 1997; Tries, 1990). As in the use of EMG biofeedback to assist in strengthening muscles as described earlier, urinary incontinence may be treated by assisting a patient to gain control over the pelvic floor muscles. In women, this is usually done with a vaginal EMG sensor to monitor the activity of the periurethral muscles. In men an EMG sensor is inserted rectally to monitor the perineal muscles. Many persons with urinary incontinence need biofeedback training to assist them in improving relaxation of pelvic floor muscles at appropriate times while assisting them to learn to contract these same muscles adequately to prevent premature emptying of the urinary bladder.

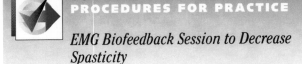

BOX 25-3
PROCEDURES FOR PRACTICE

EMG Biofeedback Session to Decrease Spasticity

- Begin with small, closely spaced electrodes over the muscle belly.
- Initially set the threshold at an attainable level.
- Place the limb in midrange and keep the environment free of distractions.
- During a 10- to 15-minute treatment session, the patient attempts to maintain relaxation of the muscle below the threshold level.
- Gradually decrease the threshold as the patient learns to relax the muscle.
- In subsequent sessions, challenge the patient to maintain relaxation of the spastic muscle while contracting the antagonistic group

RESEARCH NOTE

The Effectiveness of EMG Biofeedback in the Treatment of Arm Function After Stroke

Crow, J. L., Lincoln, N. B., Nouri, F. M., & DeWeerdt, W. (1989). International Disability Studies, 11, 155–160

ABSTRACT

Forty-two patients diagnosed with stroke were studied to determine the efficacy of EMG biofeedback in assisting with the return of upper extremity function. Patients were 2 to 8 weeks post stroke and were randomly placed in a group to receive EMG biofeedback or a control treatment in addition to their routine therapy. For the control group, the EMG unit was switched on but the auditory feedback was switched off and the voltmeter for visual feedback was not visible to the patient. The study reported no significant differences between the groups before treatment, but those who received EMG biofeedback scored significantly higher on tests of arm function after treatment than did the control group. After 6 weeks of treatment, the difference between the two groups was statistically significant ($p < .05$) using a one-tailed *Mann Whitney U Test* in comparing scores on the *Action Research Arm Test*.

IMPLICATIONS FOR PRACTICE

As upper extremity function is important in maximizing functional abilities, occupational therapy practitioners must seek treatment techniques that aid return of upper extremity function following stroke. This study assists in validating the use of EMG biofeedback as a modality to increase upper extremity function.

Summary Review Questions

1. Define biofeedback, electrogoniometric biofeedback, and electromyographic biofeedback.
2. Why would an occupational therapist use biofeedback?
3. Describe an electrogoniometric biofeedback procedure to increase range of motion.
4. What does the EMG signal represent?
5. What factors are important for selecting electrodes for EMG biofeedback? In placing electrodes for EMG biofeedback?
6. What is the function of the third (common) electrode used in EMG biofeedback?
7. Describe an EMG biofeedback procedure used to reeducate a weak muscle.
8. Describe how a treatment session would be organized for a post stroke patient to develop shoulder protraction.

Resources

Distributors for Biofeedback Equipment and Supplies

Aleph One Limited · The Old Courthouse, Bottisham, Cambridge, UK CB5 9BA
www.aleph1.co.uk
(biofeedback devices)

Bio-Medical Instruments, Inc. · 2387 East Eight Mile Rd., Warren, MI 48091-2486
www.bio-medical.com
(biofeedback devices, electrodes)

Biometrics Ltd. · P. O. Box 340, Ladysmith, VA 22501
www.biometricsltd.com
(electrogoniometer devices)

Empi Inc. · 599 Cardigan Road, St. Paul, MN 55126-4099
www.empi.com
(neuromuscular electrical stimulation units, electrodes)

J&J Engineering, Inc. · 22797 Holgar Ct. NE, Poulsbo, WA 98370
www.jjengineering.com
(biofeedback devices)

Masters Medical · 12-18 Victoria Street East, Unit 7, Lidcombe NSW 2141, Sydney, Australia
www.masters.com.au
(biofeedback and neuromuscular electrical stimulation devices, electrodes)

Nexgen Ergonomics Inc. · 3400 de Maisonneuve Blvd. W., Suite 1430, Montreal, Quebec, Canada H3Z 3B8
www.nexgenergo.com
(biofeedback and electrogoniometer devices)

Thought Technology Ltd. · 2180 Belgrave Ave., Montreal, Quebec, Canada H4A 2L8
www.thoughttechnology.com
(biofeedback devices; electrodes)

References

Asfour, S. S., Khalil, T. M., Waly, S. M., Goldberg, M. L., Rosomoff, R. S., & Rosomoff, H. L. (1990). Biofeedback in back muscle strengthening. *Spine, 15*, 510–513.

Basmajian, J. V. (1983). *Biofeedback: Principles and practice for clinicians* (2nd ed.). Baltimore: Williams & Wilkins.

Brown, D. M., DeBacher, G., & Basmajian, J. V. (1979). Feedback goniometers for hand rehabilitation. *American Journal of Occupational Therapy, 33*, 458–463.

Brucker, B. S., & Bulaeva, N. V. (1996). Biofeedback effect on electromyography responses in patients with spinal cord injury. *Archives of Physical Medicine and Rehabilitation, 77*, 133–137.

Canelon, M. F. (1993). Training for a patient with shoulder disarticulation. *American Journal of Occupational Therapy, 47,* 174–178.

Cohen, B. A. (1983). Basic biofeedback electronics for the clinician. In J. V. Basmajian (Ed.), *Biofeedback: Principles and Practice for Clinicians* (2nd ed., pp. 317–329). Baltimore: Williams & Wilkins.

Crow, J. L., Lincoln, N. B., Nouri, F. M., & DeWeerdt, W. (1989). The effectiveness of EMG biofeedback in the treatment of arm function after stroke. *International Disability Studies, 11,* 155–160.

Engberg, S., McDowell, B. J., Donovan, N., Brodak, I., & Weber, E. (1997). Treatment of urinary incontinence in homebound older adults: Interface between research and practice. *Ostomy/Wound Management, 43,* 18–26.

Greenberg, S., & Fowler, R. S. (1980). Kinesthetic biofeedback: A treatment modality for elbow range of motion in hemiplegia. *American Journal of Occupational Therapy, 34,* 738–743.

Guercio, J., Chittum, R., & McMorrow, M. (1997). Self-management in the treatment of ataxia: A case study in reducing ataxic tremor through relaxation and biofeedback. *Brain Injury, 11,* 353–362.

Herrington, L. (1996). EMG biofeedback: What can it actually show? *Physiotherapy, 82,* 581–583.

Jackson, J., Emerson, L., Johnston, B., Wilson, J., & Morales, A. (1996). Biofeedback: A noninvasive treatment for incontinence after radical prostatectomy. *Urologic Nursing, 16,* 50–54.

Kelly, J. L., Baker, M. P., & Wolf, S. L. (1979). Procedures for EMG biofeedback training in involved upper extremities of hemiplegic patients. *Physical Therapy, 59,* 1500–1507.

King, T. I. (1992). Biofeedback: A survey regarding current clinical use and content in occupational therapy educational curricula. *Occupational Therapy Journal of Research, 12,* 51–57.

King, T. I. (1994). Electromyographic biofeedback treatment in hemiplegia. *Critical Reviews in Physical and Rehabilitation Medicine, 6,* 259–272.

Koheil, R., & Mandel, A. R. (1980). Joint position feedback facilitation of physical therapy in gait training. *American Journal of Physical Medicine, 59,* 288–297.

Lantz, C. A., Chen, J., & Buch, D. (1999). Clinical validity and stability of active and passive cervical range of motion with regard to unilateral uniplanar motion. *Spine, 24,* 1082–1089.

Lysaght, R., & Bodenhamer, E. (1990). The use of relaxation training to enhance functional outcomes in adults with traumatic head injuries. *American Journal of Occupational Therapy, 44,* 797–802.

Mathewson-Chapman, M. (1997). Pelvic muscle exercise/biofeedback for urinary incontinence after prostatectomy: An education program. *Journal of Cancer Education, 12,* 218–223.

Morrison, S. A. (1988). Biofeedback to facilitate unassisted ventilation in individuals with high-level quadriplegia. *Physical Therapy, 68,* 1378–1380.

Moreland, J., & Thomson, M. A., (1994). Efficacy of electromyographic biofeedback compared with conventional physical therapy for upper-extremity function in patients following stroke: A research overview and meta-analysis. *Physical Therapy, 74,* 534–543.

Moreland, J. D., Thomson, M. A., & Fuoco, A. R. (1998). Electromyographic biofeedback to improve lower extremity function after stroke: A meta-analysis. *Archives of Physical Medicine and Rehabilitation, 79,* 134–140.

O'Neill, M. E., Gwinn, K. A., & Adler, C. H. (1997). Biofeedback for writer's cramp. *American Journal of Occupational Therapy, 51,* 605–607.

Reid, D. C., Saboe, L. A., & Chepeha, J. C. (1996). Anterior shoulder instability in athletes: Comparison of isokinetic resistance exercises and an electromyographic biofeedback re-education program—a pilot program. *Physiotherapy Canada, 48,* 251–256.

Reynolds, C. (1994). Electromyographic biofeedback evaluation of a computer keyboard operator with cumulative trauma disorder. *Journal of Hand Therapy, 7,* 25–27.

Skold, C., Harms, R. K., Hultling, C., Levi, R., & Seiger, A. (1998). Simultaneous Ashworth measurements and electromyographic recordings in tetraplegic patients. *Archives of Physical Medicine and Rehabilitation, 79,* 959–965.

Shellenberger, R., & Green, J. A. (1986). *From the Ghost in the Box to Successful Biofeedback Training.* Greeley, CO: Health Psychology.

Strong, J., Cramond, T., & Mass, F. (1989). The effectiveness of relaxation techniques with patients who have chronic low back pain. *Occupational Therapy Journal of Research, 9,* 184–192.

Schwartz, M. S. (1987). *Biofeedback: A practitioner's guide.* New York: Guilford.

Tries, J. (1990). Kegel exercises enhanced by biofeedback. *Journal of Enterostomal Therapy, 17,* 67–76.

Trombly, C. A., & Tries, J. (1995). Biofeedback. In C. A. Trombly (Ed.), *Occupational Therapy for Physical Dysfunction* (4th ed., pp. 645–657.) Baltimore: Williams & Wilkins.

Wolf, S. L., LeCraw, D. E., & Barton, L. A. (1989). Comparison of motor copy and targeted biofeedback training techniques for restitution of upper extremity function among patients with neurologic disorders. *Physical Therapy, 69,* 719–735.

Young, D. E., & Schmidt, R. A. (1992). Augmented kinematic feedback for motor learning. *Journal of Motor Behavior, 24,* 261–273.

26

Managing Deficit of First-Level Motor Control Capacities

Catherine A. Trombly

LEARNING OBJECTIVES

After studying this chapter, the reader will be able to do the following:

1. Describe how abnormal tone can affect occupational functioning.
2. List biomechanical problems that develop secondary to abnormal tone and that must be prevented.
3. Describe techniques to facilitate muscle contraction.
4. Describe techniques to inhibit excessive tone.

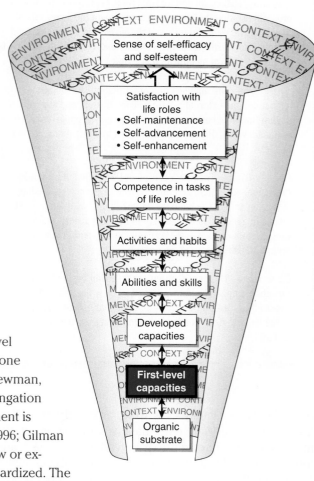

*A*fter central nervous system (CNS) injury, the basic first level capacity of movement, muscle tone, changes (Noth, 1991). Tone is a constant state of mild tension in the muscle (Gilman & Newman, 1992). It is the characteristic of muscle that resists passive elongation or stretching (Gillen, 1998; Gilman & Newman, 1992). Movement is superimposed on normal postural muscle tone (Carpenter, 1996; Gilman Newman, 1992) and is difficult or impossible when tone is low or excessive. Without movement, occupational functioning is jeopardized. The motor relearning treatments described in Chapters 21 to 23 apply to patients with beginning voluntary motion. Although human movement scientists have not yet addressed how to evoke movement in people who cannot move, therapists who developed the neurophysiological treatment approaches in the 1950s and 1960s presented clinical solutions to this question. They used reflex arcs to elicit particular types of motor responses by supplying sensory stimulation in a controlled way. This chapter presents those methods.

For persons with abnormal tone, the goal is **normalization of tone** to enable the patient to engage in, and potentially benefit from, those therapies and to accomplish the activities and tasks of

GLOSSARY

Contracture—Fixed posture secondary to shortening or loss of elasticity of ligaments, joint capsule, tendons, and muscles (Preston & Hecht, 1999).

Controlled sensory stimulation—Concept that the neural component of tone can be affected by sensory stimuli applied in a specific manner to increase or reduce the electrical charge on interneurons or motor neurons, making them more or less likely to fire when they receive additional goal-specific stimulation from supraspinal centers.

D1 extension—The final position of D1 extension is shoulder extension, abduction, and internal rotation; elbow extension; and pronation so that the hand passes the hip on the same side of the body. The wrist, fingers, and thumb extend and fingers and thumb abduct. During range of motion exercises, D1 extension is combined with its reciprocal, D1 flexion.

D1 flexion—The final position of D1 flexion is shoulder flexion, adduction, and external rotation; elbow flexion; and supination so that the hand passes close to the ear on the opposite side of the head. Wrist, fingers, and thumb flex and fingers and thumb adduct.

D2 extension—The final position of D2 extension is shoulder extension, adduction, and internal rotation; elbow extension; and pronation so that the hand moves past the opposite hip. Wrist flexes; fingers flex and adduct; and thumb opposes. During range of motion exercises, D2 extension is combined with its reciprocal, D2 flexion.

D2 flexion—The final position of D2 flexion is shoulder flexion, abduction, and external rotation; elbow flexion; and supination so that the hand comes close to the ear on the same side of the head. Wrist extends and fingers and thumb extend and abduct.

Facilitate—To make easier.

Facilitation—State of readying neurons to depolarize and propagate an impulse or to make contraction of a muscle or a reflex response more likely.

Facilitation techniques—Controlled sensory stimulation used to increase muscle tone and to produce movement responses.

Fight or flight reaction—Sympathetic autonomic nervous system response to a threat (fear, rage, pain, exposure to cold) that mobilizes the body's resources for violent action (Gilman & Newman, 1992). The sympathetic reaction redirects blood flow to areas of intense activity, such as muscles and heart, and away from other functions, such as digestion. Among other reactions, the heart rate and blood pressure increase.

Flaccidity—State of lacking tone; the limb feels limp and falls into place when not supported.

Inhibit—To make more difficult.

Inhibition—State of hyperpolarization of neural cell membrane decreasing likelihood of propagating an impulse or to make contraction of a muscle or a reflex response less likely.

Inhibition techniques—Controlled sensory stimulation used to decrease spasticity.

Normalization of tone—Process of changing excessive tone (hypertonia) or insufficient tone (hypotonia) to a state of normal tone needed for normal motor responses.

Spasticity—State of excessive tone and hyperactive response to stretch. If moderately to severely spastic, the limb feels tight and is difficult to move into position.

---

daily life. Hypotonicity (low tone, or **flaccidity**) is less than normal resistance to passive elongation of the muscle. When a flaccid arm is moved, it feels heavy and the muscles feel soft. If dropped, the arm falls because it cannot hold position against gravity. For persons with low tone, the goal is to increase muscle response through sensory input and blend this with the will to move to accomplish goal-directed actions. Even if movement is not achieved, it is important to increase tone to counteract joint subluxation, overstretching of muscles, edema, pain, and **contracture** (Gillen, 1998).

Hypertonicity, or high tone, is more than normal resistance to passive elongation. An arm that displays high tone requires effort from the therapist to move it in the direction opposite to the high tone, yet it moves easily into the other direction. It was once believed that it was necessary to reduce excessive tone before voluntary movement could develop. Current research indicates that that is not so (Ada et al., 1998; Malouin et al., 1997; O'Dwyer et al., 1996; Teixeira-Salmela et al., 1999). It is possible to improve voluntary movement without affecting **spasticity**. However, it is still important to decrease excessive tone to ease movement, to prevent contractures and deformities, and to improve the ease of accomplishing basic activities of daily living (BADL), such as dressing and washing the axilla of a tight extremity (Gillen).

Tone is normalized through the use of certain appropriately applied sensory stimuli (Rood, 1954, 1962). **Controlled sensory stimulation** is described in terms of **facilitation** and **inhibition** techniques developed primarily by Rood (1954, 1956, 1962).

A conceptual review of the physiology of muscle tone is presented here because an understanding of it is basic to the facilitation and inhibition procedures described later in the chapter.

Spindle Anatomy and Physiology

Muscle spindles are length and velocity detector mechanisms within a muscle. They are normally kept at zero point by impulses from supraspinal control centers. The zero point refers to the exact match of the spindle length to the length of the muscle fibers it is monitoring. CNS dysfunction disturbs this zeroing mechanism. If too few supraspinal impulses are able to reach the spindle via γ-efferents, it goes slack and cannot detect stretch of the muscle. On testing, passive movement of the joint feels mushy or loose. If too many supraspinal impulses are relayed to the spindle, it becomes too taut and overreacts to slight stretches. Movement is curtailed because the muscle automatically contracts reflexively and impedes the opposite movement. On passive movement, the therapist feels a "catch" at the point in the range where the stretch reflex is activated (Levin & Feldman, 1994). Within each spindle are the mechanisms for both the static, or tonic, and the dynamic, or phasic, stretch reflexes.

The muscle spindle is a fusiform encapsulated structure 3 to 4 mm long that is mounted parallel to the extrafusal muscle fibers so it can monitor their length and movement (Gilman & Newman, 1992). Each spindle contains several nuclear chain intrafusal muscle fibers subserving the static or tonic stretch reflex and one to two nuclear bag 1 and bag 2 intrafusal fibers subserving the dynamic or phasic stretch reflex (Gilman & Newman, 1992). These intrafusal muscle fibers have noncontractile midportions and contractile polar regions (Carpenter, 1996). When the contractile portions shorten in response to γ-efferent input, they pull on the midportion of the fiber, which causes that area to be stretched (internal stretch). The midportion is also stretched when the muscle is passively elongated because the ends of the spindle are secured to the ends of the muscle, so the spindle is stretched when the muscle is stretched (external stretch) (Fig. 26-1). When the midportion of an intrafusal fiber is stretched, it generates a neural signal carried back to the spinal cord by afferent neurons.

There are two types of afferent neurons: the primary (Ia) sensory ending that serves the bag and chain intrafusal muscle fibers and the secondary (II) sensory fiber that serves chain fibers. Tentacles of the primary ending coil or clamp around the midportions of both the bag fiber and the chain fibers (Carpenter, 1996; Gilman & Newman, 1992). The primary ending is velocity (rate of

change of stretch) sensitive, so its function is to detect dynamic change of length. It has a low threshold for stretch; that is, it responds to a single brief stretch such as a tap to the tendon (Carpenter, 1996; Gilman & Newman, 1992). The Ia afferent of the bag fiber has a monosynaptic connection to the α-motor neuron of the muscle stretched. Its action facilitates that α-motor neuron and reciprocally inhibits α-motor neurons of the antagonist. The Ia endings around the chain fibers react to repetitive small stretches such as vibration to produce a sustained (tonic) response of the muscle (Carpenter, 1996). The Ia's of the chain fibers connect polysynaptically to the α-motor neurons. Whenever an interneuron is introduced into the chain of activation, there is increased opportunity of influence to the ongoing neural impulse from reverberating circuitry and/or other sources of neural impulses. Therefore, the strength of these reflexes can be altered by other conditions within the CNS, such as an effort to overcome resistance (Braddom, 1996; Carpenter, 1996), emotional stress, urinary tract infection, blocked catheter, and head position (Sloan et al., 1992).

The secondary ending, or II afferent, responds exclusively and proportionately to the amount of static or maintained stretch on the muscle (Carpenter, 1996; Gilman & Newman, 1992). The II afferent excites homonymous α-motor neurons. It is essentially nonadapting and therefore is suited to the static stretch reflex (Carpenter, 1996; Gilman & Newman, 1992).

Regulation of muscle tone requires information about muscle tension as well as muscle length. The Golgi tendon organs (GTOs) are the receptors that sense muscle tension. They lie at the junction between the

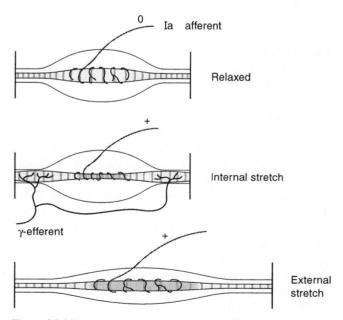

Figure 26-1 Two ways to cause stretch to the midportion of the muscle spindle: internal and external stretch.

muscle fibers and the tendon and along fascial coverings of the muscles. When stimulated by contraction, they inform the CNS about the amount of tension in the extrafusal fibers they monitor. Impulses from the GTOs are transmitted to the spinal cord via Ib fibers, which synapse polysynaptically (Gilman & Newman, 1992) to inhibit the α-motor neurons innervating the agonist muscle and facilitate motor neurons of the antagonist muscle.

Low Tone

Hypotonia is treated by stimulation that affects the γ-motor neurons to increase the sensitivity of the intrafusal muscle fibers and therefore the likelihood they will fire to activate or facilitate agonists and homonymous muscles (Braddom, 1996; Carpenter, 1996). Muscle is facilitated within the context of attempted goal-directed movement or maintained posture (Huss, 1971; Voss, 1967). Application of facilitation techniques alone is inadequate therapy. Even though the patient may not be able to do any activity, the effort to accomplish a simple goal is powerful and should be an integral part of every therapy session. Ayres (1962) noted that activity that directs attention away from the movement aspects of the task and toward a purposeful goal enhances neurological integration. Therefore, facilitation is done within an occupational context.

Facilitation Techniques

Techniques to facilitate muscle activation include application of tactile, thermal, and proprioceptive stimuli and stimuli to the special senses. These various techniques may be combined to produce a greater response.

Tactile Stimuli

Tactile stimulation is done using light touch (A-brushing) or fast brushing (C-brushing).

Light Touch

Light touch or stroking of the skin activates the low threshold A-size sensory fibers to activate a reflex action of the superficial phasic or mobilizing muscles (Rood, 1956, 1962; Stockmeyer, 1967). Light stroking of the dorsum of the webs of the fingers or toes, or of the palms of the hands or the soles of the feet elicits a fast, short-lived withdrawal motion of the stimulated limb (Rood, 1962). The stroking is done at a rate of twice per second for approximately 10 seconds (Rood, 1956). After a rest period this procedure can be repeated 3 to 5 more times. When the reflex response occurs, resistance to the movement is usually given to reinforce it and to help develop voluntary control over it (Stockmeyer, 1967).

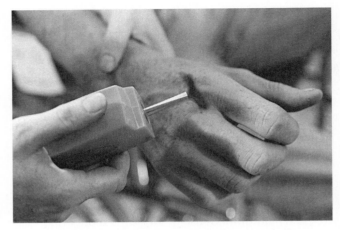

Figure 26-2 Fast brushing with a battery-operated brush to facilitate finger extension.

Brushing

Fast brushing involves brushing the hairs or the skin over a muscle with a soft camel hair paintbrush that has been substituted for the stirrer of a hand-held battery-powered cocktail mixer to produce a high-frequency, high-intensity stimulus (Harris, 1969; Rood, 1962; Stockmeyer, 1967). The revolving brush, held sideways to avoid catching and pulling the hair (Fig. 26-2), is applied on each skin area to be stimulated (Rood, 1956, 1962). Fast brushing is thought to stimulate the C-size sensory fibers, which discharge into polysynaptic pathways that influence the background γ-efferent activity of muscles involved in the maintenance of posture (Harris, 1969; Matyas & Spicer, 1980; Rood, 1962). Spindles so biased respond more readily to added external or internal stretch (Rood, 1962).

Fast brushing over the distribution of the posterior primary rami of the peripheral nerves, which innervate the muscles and skin of the back (Carpenter & Sutin, 1983), facilitates the deep tonic muscles of the back, whereas fast brushing of the skin over the rest of the trunk and extremities, supplied by the anterior primary rami (Carpenter & Sutin, 1983), facilitates a tonic response of the superficial ventrolateral muscles (Rood, 1962).

Brushing is done on the skin of the dermatome (see Fig 6-2) served by the same spinal segment as the muscles whose spindles the therapist is attempting to sensitize (Rood, 1962). For instance, to facilitate the wrist extensors (innervated by C6-8), brushing is applied to the dorsal radial forearm and hand. The skin area often corresponds to the location of the muscle. Brushing is done for 5 seconds for each area (Huss, 1971), followed by a rest period. If there is no response to the brushing after 30 seconds, the brushing of each area should be repeated 3 to 5 times (Rood, 1962).

Rood (1962) proposed that the effect of fast brushing was nonspecific, had a latency of 30 seconds, and reached its maximum facilitative state 30 to 40 minutes after stimulation because of the enhancement of the reticular activating system into which the C-fibers feed. In controlled studies of fast brushing applied to normal and poststroke individuals, however, it was demonstrated that although fast brushing produced a significant immediate facilitatory effect, the effect lasted only 30 to 45 seconds (Mason, 1985; Matyas & Spicer, 1980; Spicer & Matyas, 1980). Moreover, in normal subjects, the facilitatory effect was seen only in the lower extremity, not in the upper extremity. Rider (1971) examined fast brushing, among other stimuli. She found a statistically significant ($p = .01$) increase in the strength of both triceps of eight children with bilateral upper extremity flexor spasticity compared with eight children who had normal upper extremities, following a 2-week period of treatment consisting of brushing, stroking, rubbing, icing, and squeezing of the triceps of one limb.

Some precautions are to be observed in relation to fast brushing. *Fast brushing of the pinna of the ear stimulates the vagal parasympathetic fibers, which influence cardiorespiratory functions (Rood, 1962). Activation of these fibers slows the heart, constricts the smooth muscles of the bronchial tree, and increases bronchial secretions (Gilman & Newman, 1992). Fast brushing or scratching of the skin over the back at the level of S2-4 may cause bladder emptying (Gilman & Newman, 1992).*

Thermal Stimuli

Icing is thought to have similar effects as stroking and brushing through the same neural mechanisms (Harris, 1969; Rood, 1962). Icing, however, has been found to be significantly less effective than fast brushing for recruitment of motor units in hemiplegic patients (Matyas & Spicer, 1980). Two types of icing, A- and C- (referring to the size of the sensory fibers) are used.

A-Icing

A-icing is the application of three quick swipes of an ice cube to evoke a reflex withdrawal, similar to the response to light touch, when the stimulus is applied to the palms or soles or the dorsal webs of the hands or feet (Rood, 1962). The water is blotted up after every swipe. A-icing of the upper right quadrant of the abdomen in the dermatomal representation for T7-9 (along the rib cage) stimulates the diaphragm and inspiration (Rood). Touching the lips with ice opens the mouth (a withdrawal response). But ice applied to the tongue and inside the lips closes the mouth (Rood, 1962). Swiping the ice upward over the skin of the sternal notch promotes swallowing.

C-Icing

C-icing is a high-threshold stimulus used to stimulate postural tonic responses via the C-size sensory fibers (Rood, 1962). Icing to activate the C fibers is done by holding the ice cube in place for 3 to 5 seconds, then wiping away the water. The skin areas to be stimulated are the same as for fast brushing, with one exception: *The distribution of the posterior primary rami along the back is avoided because it may cause a sympathetic nervous system* **fight or flight** *protective response (Rood, 1962; Huss, 1971).* Other precautions about icing are similar to those for brushing. *Icing of the pinna causes vagal responses, including cardiovascular reactions such as low blood pressure (Umphred, 1995). Ice to the back at the level of S2-4 may cause voiding (Rood, 1962).*

Proprioceptive Stimuli

The difference between proprioceptive stimuli and the described tactile and thermal stimuli is that the effect of proprioceptive stimulation lasts only as long as the stimulus is applied, whereas the effects of tactile and thermal stimulation lasts several tens of seconds after the stimulus is removed. There are several types of proprioceptive stimuli, described next.

Quick Stretch

Quick, light stretch of a muscle is a low-threshold stimulus that activates an immediate phasic stretch reflex of the stretched muscle and inhibits its antagonist (Rood, 1962). Stretch is applied in the form of quick movement of the limb or tapping over the muscle or tendon. The therapist uses stiffened fingertips to vigorously tap the skin over a muscle or tendon while the patient is attempting to contract the muscle (see Fig. 24-8). This provides intermittent mechanical stretch to the muscle to evoke a stronger response. Evocation of the stretch reflex without a conjoint attempt to move or hold a position is not therapeutic.

Vibration

High frequency (100–300 Hz, with 100 to 125 Hz preferred) vibration, delivered by an electric personal vibrator that has an excursion of 1 to 2 mm, to the belly or tendon of the slightly stretched muscle is an additional form of stretch (Umphred, 1995) (Fig. 26-3). The action of the vibrator provides a rapidly repeated mechanical stretch to the muscle, which increases the number of motor units recruited. This is the tonic vibratory reflex (TVR). Tension within the muscle in-

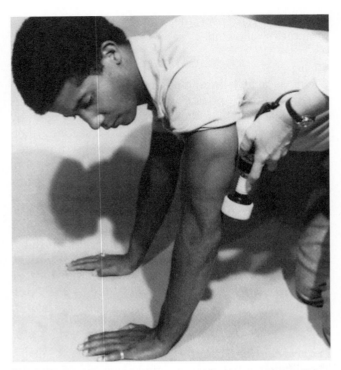

Figure 26-3 An electrical vibrator applied to the triceps tendon to elicit a sustained elbow extensor response while the patient is weight bearing in quadruped.

creases over 30 to 60 seconds and is sustained for the duration of the application of the vibrator (Umphred, 1995). The stronger response is obtained from application over the tendon; however, stimulation applied there can be conducted to adjacent muscles via the bone, and this possibility must be attended to and prevented (Dobkin, 1996; Preston & Hecht, 1999). Vibration evokes a tonic holding contraction and adds to the strength of an already weakly contracting muscle. *Vibration should not be maintained longer than 1 to 2 minutes in any one place because of the heat that develops from the friction and potential for tearing thin skin. Vibration over areas previously immobilized can dislodge a blood clot and cause an embolism (Umphred, 1995).*

Stretch to Finger Intrinsics

Stretch to the intrinsic muscles of the hand is used to facilitate cocontraction, that is, the simultaneous contraction of the muscles around the shoulder joint (Ayres, 1974; Stockmeyer, 1967). Forcefully grasping handles of tools obtains this response, especially if the handles have been modified to be spherical or conical, with the widest part of the cone at the ulnar border of the hand, both of which increase intermetacarpal stretch. This treatment is used for patients who have distal movement but proximal weakness.

Heavy Joint Compression

Heavy joint compression facilitates cocontraction of muscles around a joint. Heavy compression refers to resistance greater than body weight that is applied so that the force is through the longitudinal axes of the bones whose articular surfaces approximate each other (Ayres, 1974; Rood, 1962). Resistance greater than body weight is that which is more than the weight of the body parts usually supported by the joint. Heavy joint compression can be achieved by having the patient, who is in a quadruped position or leaning both arms on a table, lift one limb off the supporting surface. Alternatively, weights can be added to the limb by putting such things as a lead radiography apron on the shoulders or back.

Resistance

Resistance to an ongoing movement or maintained posture is a form of stretch in which many or all of the spindles of a muscle are stimulated (Umphred, 1995). The spindle of course cannot know whether the discrepancy between itself and the extrafusal muscle fibers is due to stretching by a moving force or by resistance that is preventing extrafusal muscle fibers from shortening as the spindle continues to shorten as programmed. The discrepancy causes the spindle to fire. The electrical activity of the interneuronal pool is consequently high, and more and more motor units are more easily recruited to fire, a phenomenon called overflow.

Stimuli for the Special Senses

Rood (1962) used stimulation to the special senses to facilitate or inhibit the skeletal musculature generally. She reasoned that stimuli from all cranial sensory nerves feed into the reticular activating formation, which in turn affects the γ-efferents. Auditory and visual stimuli can be used deliberately. However, auditory and visual stimuli also occur incidental to treatment, a fact of which the therapist needs to be aware. Music with a definite beat is facilitatory. A noisy, raucous clinic is stimulating and may affect the performance of the patient with CNS dysfunction. A colorful, bright multistimulus environment has a general facilitatory effect. The therapist's voice and manner of speech (fast and staccato versus slow and calming) may also affect the patient's performance. A loud, sharp command yields a quick response and recruits more motor units (Voss, 1967). Such a command can overcome the akinesia of Parkinsonism.

Olfactory and gustatory stimuli are facilitating or inhibiting through their influence on the autonomic nervous system. Unpleasant or dangerous stimuli (like ammonia smell) elicit a sympathetic fight or flight reaction, and pleasant stimuli (like vanilla) evoke a parasympathetic response that inhibits the sympathetic response (Rood, 1962). These stimuli, especially olfactory, produce an emotional response as well as a motor response.

Problems Secondary to Low Tone

After a period of therapy, voluntary movement may not develop and tone may remain low. If that is the case, it is important that the patient be taught preventive measures to avoid the problems common to low tone. Those secondary problems include subluxation at joints. One instance of this that is especially prevalent is subluxation of the shoulder after stroke. When the patient sits, gravity pulls down on the heavy, flaccid arm and tips the scapula so the glenoid fossa faces down, allowing the humerus to fall out of the fossa. Positioning devices such as pillows, splints, arm rests, and lap trays for wheelchairs are commonly used. If the patient cannot move the limb, passive range of motion (PROM) must be done at least once per day and positioning changed frequently to prevent contractures that develop when left in one position. ***Scapulohumeral rhythm must be adhered to during PROM to prevent damage to the shoulder muscles and development of pain syndromes.*** The weight of the flaccid arm can throw a hemiplegic patient off balance when he or she attempts to walk or transfer, so the use of an arm sling during these activities may be indicated.

Moving From Muscle Contraction to Movement

As noted earlier, facilitation and inhibition techniques are used in conjunction with attempts at goal-directed action for the purpose of enabling development of movement-related capacities and abilities. Rood (1962) identified a sequence regarding the development of movement that is useful in guiding activity choices. She stated that movement first appears as phasic, reciprocal shortening and lengthening contractions of the muscles that cause movement subserving a protective function. Such movements might be facilitated using A-brushing or A-icing. In these phasic movements, muscles contract to cause movement through range, which according to Sherringtonian physiology, produces reciprocal inhibition of the antagonists (Ayres, 1974; Rood, 1962). The movement of an infant waving his or her extremities back and forth when shown a desired object typifies phasic movement. Movement to touch an object or bat away a lightweight object, such as a balloon or bubble, is the first voluntary movement to aim for in patients beginning to develop tone and movement.

After phasic movements begin, tonic holding contractions are next to develop, according to Rood. Stability is obtained through cocontraction, such as occurs during heavy joint compression (Ayres, 1974; Stockmeyer, 1967). A goal-directed action, such as leaning on the desk with the affected arm while writing with the unaffected hand, is again sought.

Other therapists (e.g., Bobath; see Chapter 23) may choose to seek a stability pattern first in adults with hypotonia, with the idea of normalizing tone through heavy joint compression.

High Tone

Hypertonicity, or increased resistance to passive movement, may be seen in persons after cerebrovascular accident, traumatic brain injury, or spinal cord injury, or in persons with multiple sclerosis, among other diagnoses. Resistance to passive movement can be increased via reflex hyperexcitability (increased stretch reflexes) and/or altered mechanical properties, such as loss of sarcomeres, remodeling of muscle connective tissue, and altered periarticular connective tissue (O'Dwyer et al., 1996). Reflex hyperexcitability is the neural velocity-dependent factor (Braddom, 1996; Noth, 1991) also known as spasticity. Spasticity is defined as an exaggeration of stretch reflexes in both the tonic and phasic reflexes (Ada et al., 1998). The mechanical factor is characterized by velocity-independent resistance to elongation (Gillen, 1998; O'Dwyer et al., 1996).

The mechanism of spasticity is unknown, but many possible explanations have been advanced, giving less credence to the hypothesis of hyperactivity of γ-efferents (Braddom, 1996) for which many of the inhibitory procedures listed later were designed. Hypertonicity develops over days to weeks after ictus (Black-Schaffer et al., 1999; Thilmann et al., 1991). Adaptive changes in muscle tissue are often responsible for the clinical impression of hypertonia. This nonreflexive, viscoelastic component is present by 2 months post stroke and does not change, at least between months 2 to 4, which Malouin et al. (1997) studied.

Spasticity is evaluated using the *Modified Ashworth Scale (MAS)* (see Chapter 5), although this assessment does not distinguish between reflex hyperexcitability and the mechanical aspect of hypertonus (O'Dwyer et al., 1996). Another way to estimate hypertonicity is use of a self-report *Visual Analog Scale (VAS)*. The scale consists of a line 100 mm long with one end marked "no spasticity" and the other, "most imaginable spasticity" (Sköld, 2000). The patient marks a point on the line to correspond to his or her perception of how the limb feels. In one study, the *VAS* correlated significantly, though only moderately, to the *MAS* ($r_s = .44 - .61$) but

Case Example

MS. B.: MANAGEMENT OF HYPOTONICITY

Patient Information

Ms. B. is a 26-year-old woman who had a stroke caused by an aneurysm that ruptured during a recreational basketball game 3 days ago. She is now medically stable. Ms. B. is a domestic relations attorney in a small firm in a midsize town. She lives alone in a one-floor house and treats herself to twice-weekly domestic help for cleaning, laundry, food shopping, and errands. She is learning gourmet cooking, which she enjoys very much. She is engaged to be married in 6 months, and her fiancé thinks he can continue to be supportive despite the possibility that she will have continued paralysis.

Other than this episode, she is in excellent health and has no comorbidities, such as hypertension or diabetes. Her left upper and lower extremities are flaccid (*MAS* = 0). She is receiving PROM twice daily to maintain range of motion, and her left upper extremity (LUE) has been protected during change of position, transfer, and antigravity positions to prevent subluxation at the shoulder. Ms. B. is dependent in all basic activities of daily living (BADL), walking, and transfers. She exhibits neglect of left space but is cognitively sound. She understands what has happened to her and is ready to engage in rehabilitation, starting in the acute stroke unit, although she feels exhausted.

Recommendations

The occupational therapist–physical therapist team recommended six 15-minute treatment sessions, three for occupational therapy and three for physical therapy, spaced throughout each day for the duration of the acute hospitalization (6 days remaining). There will be rest periods of at least 1 hour between each therapy session. The long-term goal for the acute rehabilitation program is that she be independent in BADL at wheelchair level. The goals for the physical therapist are (1) independence in bed mobility, (2) ability to transfer from bed to wheelchair and from wheelchair to toilet, (3) ability to transfer to a bath bench, and (4) wheelchair mobility on level surface. The goals for the occupational therapist are (1) independence in feeding and grooming, (2) independence in adapted dressing of the upper body, (3) moderate assistance with dressing the lower body, (4) independence in toileting, (5) moderate assistance with bathing on a bath bench, and (6) increase the tone of the LUE to develop some movement and/or to prevent shoulder subluxation. Both the occupational therapist and the physical therapist will do a home evaluation by interview of the fiancé and the patient.

Short-Term Goals

▶ **Develop some movement in the LUE.** To counteract the weight of the arm to allow a very weak contraction to manifest a movement, Ms. B.'s LUE was supported in a gravity-eliminated position on an exercise skate that moves easily on the smooth table surface (Fig. 26-7). A balloon was positioned so that if the patient extended her elbow, she would hit it. A target box was set to receive the balloon if the patient "scored." The patient attempted to move to knock the balloon into the target, without effect. The C7-8 dermatome (dorsal and palmar hand from middle finger to ulnar border) was fast-brushed for 5 seconds three times to internally stretch the spindles of the triceps innervated by C7-8. Again, Ms. B. tried to touch or hit the balloon while the therapist tapped the triceps tendon repeatedly during the attempt (external stretch). Dance music was playing on the clinic radio and her fiancé cheered her on. On the best trial, Ms. B.'s hand moved 2 inches toward the balloon. Treatment lasted 15 minutes and was repeated once each day. On the fourth day she moved 6 inches to hit the balloon into the target once. On the sixth and last day she scored five hits.

▶ **Prevent shoulder subluxation.** Although tone had improved (*MAS* = 12) and movement at the elbow was beginning, the arm was not functional, and the shoulder was still in danger of subluxing. The therapist taught Ms. B., her fiancé, and other family members how to position the shoulder and how to handle the LUE during transfers and wheelchair ambulation. W.B.'s left neglect was still present, and sometimes she forgot where the limb was located.

Revised Goals

The staff at the acute stroke unit recommended that Ms. B. be transferred to outpatient rehabilitation care to continue therapy. However, Ms. B. chose to postpone that until after a vacation at her family's mountain cabin to regroup her spiritual resources.

CLINICAL REASONING
in OT Practice

Treatment of Flaccidity

Describe an alternative treatment plan for developing tone and movement in Ms. B.'s upper extremity. Include the details of both controlled sensory stimulation and occupation (goal-directed actions).

was more sensitive than the *MAS* to small changes in spasticity (Sköld, 2000).

Inhibition Techniques

Hypertonicity is treated with general inhibition techniques or by applying tactile, thermal, or proprioceptive stimulation either to the muscle itself or to the antagonists of the spastic muscle in the context of goal-directed activity. It is hypothesized that when stimulation is applied to the antagonist, the relaxation effect in the agonist spastic muscle occurs through reciprocal inhibition. However, the reciprocal inhibition mechanism of persons post stroke has been found to be disturbed and may result in unexpected outcomes. In one study, patients who had marked spasticity exhibited greater Ia inhibition than patients with mild spasticity (Okuma & Lee, 1996). Therefore, responses must be monitored carefully.

Some of the following methods are aimed at the neural component of hypertonicity, and others, such as prolonged stretching, address the viscoelastic component. The therapist should attempt to determine which component needs treatment and choose appropriate techniques.

Tactile Stimuli

Slow stroking over the distribution of the posterior primary rami produces general relaxation. The effect is probably through calming of the output of the sympathetic chain, because the autonomic nervous system is known to affect γ-motor neuron firing via the reticular formation. The person lies prone in a quiet environment. The therapist uses the palm or extended fingers of one hand to apply firm pressure along the vertebral musculature from occiput to coccyx, at which time the therapist's other hand starts at the occiput and progresses likewise to the coccyx. This slow, rhythmical stroking using alternating hands is done until the patient relaxes or for about 3 to 5 minutes (Huss, n.d.; Rood, 1956).

Thermal Stimuli

Both warming and cooling can be inhibitory.

Neutral Warmth

Neutral warmth refers to maintaining body heat by wrapping the specific area to be inhibited—or the area served by the posterior primary rami for a general effect—in a cotton flannel or fleece blanket or a down comforter for 10 to 20 minutes (Ayres, 1974; Huss, 1971). Neutral heat rather than heat greater than body temperature is used to avoid a rebound effect in 2 to 3 hours. The rebound effect manifests as facilitated or even superfacilitated muscles (Rood, 1962). Elastic bandage and air

splints (see Fig. 14-67) can be used also. They not only maintain neutral warmth but also offer sustained pressure, both of which are inhibitory (Preston & Hecht, 1999).

Prolonged Cooling

Sustained cooling of the skin to 10° C decreases the monosynaptic stretch reflex excitability (Preston & Hecht, 1999). A cold pack applied for 20 minutes achieves this effect (Braddom, 1996). ***Do not use prolonged icing for patients with Raynaud's phenomenon or circulatory disorders, including hypertension.***

Proprioceptive Stimuli

Several proprioceptive techniques to inhibit one or both components of hypertonicity are described next.

Prolonged Stretch

Prolonged manual stretch is used to inhibit a specific spastic muscle so that the patient may move more easily (Carey, 1990). The limb is held so that the muscle is *steadily* kept at its greatest length for more than 20 seconds, until letting go is felt as the muscle adjusts to the longer length. As a special case of this inhibitory procedure, prolonged holding of the thumb in abduction and extension relaxes a tight grasp.

Prolonged stretch by splinting or positioning the limb so that the hypertonic muscles are maintained in stretch over several hours to several weeks allows growth of additional sarcomeres and makes the muscle less sensitive to stretch during movement (O'Dwyer et al., 1996). The mechanical lengthening also changes the viscoelastic configuration of muscle by disrupting crossbridges between myosin and actin filaments and/or by reducing the stiffness of periarticular connective tissue (Carey, 1990).

Joint Approximation

Light joint compression, also called joint approximation, can be used to inhibit specific spastic muscles (Ayres, 1974). This procedure is commonly used to relieve shoulder pain due to spastic muscles in hemiplegic patients. The method is to grasp the patient's elbow and while holding the humerus abducted to about 35 to 45°, gently push the head of the humerus into the glenoid fossa and hold it there (Fig. 26-4) until the spastic muscles relax (Ayres, 1963, 1974).

Tendon Pressure

Pressure on the tendinous insertion of a muscle inhibits that muscle through Pacinian corpuscles under the tendinous insertions (Ayres, 1974; Huss, 1971; Stockmeyer, 1967). The extrinsic flexors of the hand may

Case Example

MS. B.: MANAGEMENT OF HYPERTONICITY: THREE MONTHS LATER

Patient Information

When last we heard about Ms. B., she had completed acute rehabilitation and was going for a vacation. Now, 3 months later, she is seeking further occupational therapy on an outpatient basis. She has postponed her marriage for a year to concentrate on reestablishing her exercise and recreational routines, preparing her own meals, returning to work, and resuming gourmet cooking if possible. She wants to swim as part of her exercise and recreational routine, but spasticity is impeding upper and lower extremity use. During her 3-month hiatus, the left neglect cleared spontaneously, but tone increased to an average of 1+ for shoulder motions and an average of 2 to 3 for elbow, wrist, finger, and thumb movements. Total *MAS* score is now 25. The voluntary movement at the elbow improved to flexion against gravity and ability to straighten the elbow to reach forward. She also gained slight voluntary gross grasp and thumb lateral prehension and release but had no voluntary finger extension (release of grasp).

Recommendations

The occupational therapist recommended 1-hour treatments twice a week for 8 weeks. At the same time, Ms. B. will be working on ambulation with the physical therapist. The goals Ms. B. decided on with the occupational therapist:

1. Reestablish an exercise routine of swimming 3 times a week.
2. Prepare breakfast and simple luncheon meals for self using adapted methods for chopping, stirring, spreading, pouring, and opening containers one-handed in the kitchen.
3. Practice physical work skills using the LUE as assistor (one-handed computer use, telephoning, note taking, handling large books).

To accomplish these goals, other goals aimed at normalizing tone and increasing voluntary movement must be accomplished simultaneously:

▶ Decrease spasticity of the elbow, wrist, fingers and thumb.
▶ Increase tone at the shoulder.
▶ Increase active movement of the LUE.
▶ Introduce a routine of inhibitory procedures prior to swimming.

Short-Term Goals

▶ **Decrease spasticity of the elbow, wrist, fingers, and thumb and increase active movement of the LUE.** On the first day of therapy, the therapist wrapped the limb in a warm cotton blanket for 20 minutes while Ms. B. waited for her occupational therapy appointment. When therapy began, the blanket was removed and the wrist and hand appeared relaxed. Ms. B. was eager to focus that day on kitchen activities. The plan was to make muffins from a mix. The left hand held containers: bag of muffin mix and milk container, while they were opened and muffin tin while it was being filled. The left hand also held the mixing bowl with a handle while the mixture was stirred. After this activity, hypertonicity was reappearing. The therapist manually stretched and held the fingers and thumb into full extension with the wrist in neutral position. The tension again reduced. This was repeated throughout the rest of the treatment session as needed, and Ms. B. was taught how to do this for herself at home. The focus of treatment then turned to problem solving and practice of computer use. As therapy concluded that day, the therapist again wrapped the LUE in the cotton blanket and sent Ms. B. to wait for her physical therapy appointment.

▶ **Introduce a routine of inhibitory procedures prior to swimming.** The therapist recommended that Ms. B. come to the pool wearing her bathing suit covered by easily removable pants and top. He recommended that she take a warm shower and then wrap herself in a large, fluffy bath towel for 15 minutes before entering the pool to provide a general inhibition of hypertonic muscles. He further recommended that Ms. B. swim in a pool where the water is kept above 85°F. He recommended that she not try to use both arms and legs at the same time (major effort increases hypertonicity) but to hold on to a float and kick slowly awhile, then, without the float, keep the legs still while trying to do the side stroke with the left arm extending overhead and the right arm providing the power. He further recommended that she stop and float every 5 to 10 minutes to rest.

Revised Goals

1. Teach advanced kitchen techniques requiring ambulatory skill and use of mixer, food processor, oven, and sauté pan for cooking and baking and devices to aid decorative cutting and chopping that Ms. B. liked to do when preparing service of her creations.
2. Return to work half-days to work on cases in the office. The occupational therapist will visit the office when Ms. B. has been back to work for a week to make suggestions for efficient use of office equipment and accomplishment of tasks.

CLINICAL REASONING
in OT Practice

Treatment of Spasticity

Describe the therapy program for day 2 in occupational therapy to decrease spasticity of the elbow, wrist, fingers, and thumb and to increase active movement of the LUE. Include the details of both the controlled sensory stimulation and occupation.

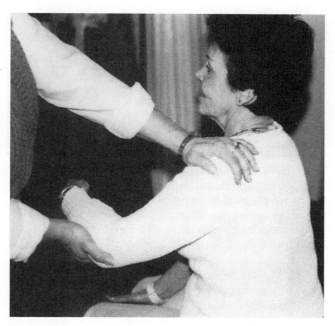

Figure 26-4 Light joint compression, or joint approximation, used to inhibit spastic muscles and to allow range of motion.

be inhibited by applying constant pressure over the length of the long tendons (Stockmeyer) through grasp of enlarged, hard handles of tools or utensils, or via splints.

Activation of GTOs

Another way to inhibit spastic muscles, according to Rood (1962; Stockmeyer, 1967) is to request the patient do a brief, intense contraction before moving the limb into a lengthened position. This is similar to the hold–relax procedure of proprioceptive neuromuscular facilitation (PNF), described next. The brevity and intensity of the contraction are thought to activate a

large number of GTOs all at once, which produces an overriding autoinhibition instead of the facilitation that is seen when resistance is added gradually during an ongoing contraction.

Relaxation techniques of PNF include rhythmic rotation, contract–relax, hold–relax, and slow-reversal-hold–relax (Meyers, 1995). Rhythmic rotation coupled with range of motion is an effective technique used before dressing or splinting a limb in which the muscles are shortened or spastic (Fig. 26-5). The therapist holds the intermediate and distal joints and performs range of

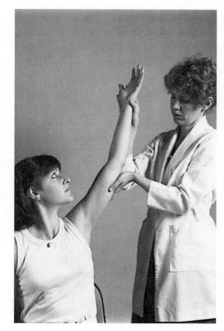

Figure 26-5 Range of motion in D2 flexion. The therapist holds the extensor surface of the limb to facilitate wrist and elbow extension. Manual contact will switch to flexor surfaces as the patient reverses the pattern to D2 extension.

motion within either a **D1 or D2 diagonal pattern**. When the spastic muscle restricts motion, the therapist repeatedly rotates all components of the pattern at the point of limitation, moving slowly and gently. As relaxation is felt, movement may continue through a greater range.

Contract–relax entails an isotonic contraction of the antagonist (stronger) pattern against maximal resistance, then relaxation, after which the therapist passively moves the limb into the agonistic (weaker) pattern. For instance, if the elbow flexors are spastic and no active extension is possible, the patient is directed to move into a D1 or D2 flexion pattern against maximal resistance and relax. Then the therapist moves the limb into the corresponding (D1 or D2) extension pattern (Myers, 1995). Markos (1979) compared the effects of contract–relax with those of passive movement on active hip flexion in 30 able-bodied women. The range of motion increased significantly more in subjects in the contract–relax group than in the passive movement group.

Hold–relax entails an isometric contraction of the tight muscle against maximal resistance, relaxation, then active movement into the agonistic pattern by the patient. For example, if the hamstrings are spastic or tight, the patient is directed to do a forceful holding contraction of these muscles, immediately relax, and then move further into hip flexion with knee extension (Myers, 1995). Tanigawa (1972) compared the effects of hold–relax with those of passive mobilization on tight hamstring muscles. He tested 30 able-bodied men and measured the angle of passive straight leg raising. The results showed that subjects who received the hold–relax procedure increased their range of passive straight

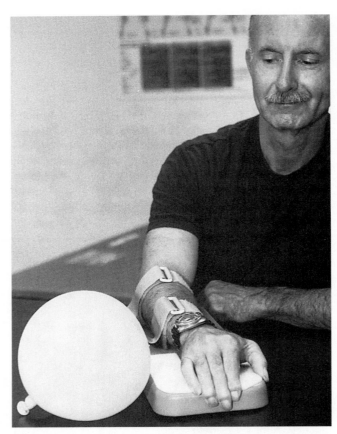

Figure 26-7 Patient's arm supported on a therapeutic skate, a rectangular board supported by easily movable ball-bearing casters at the corners. With the slightest effort, the patient can move the arm at the shoulder and elbow on a smooth surface. The patient should concentrate on an activity goal rather than the movement per se. (Photo by Robert Littlefield. Scientific and Technical Photography, Dorchester, MA.)

leg raising more and faster than the subjects who received passive mobilization.

Slow-reversal-hold–relax begins with an isotonic contraction of the spastic muscle in one of the diagonal patterns against maximal resistance, followed by a maximally resisted isometric contraction, relaxation, then active movement in the direction opposite to the pull of the spastic muscles (Voss et al., 1985).

Vestibular Stimuli

Slow, rhythmical movement is inhibiting (Huss, 1971). Slow rolling is done by the therapist holding the patient at the hip and shoulder and slowly rolling him or her from supine to side-lying (Fig. 26-6). The patient should be lying comfortably with a pillow under the head and between the knees if necessary for comfort. A decrease in hypertonicity should be seen within minutes. Slow rocking in a rocking chair is a variation of this technique. Self-administered rocking must be carefully monitored, however, because if it develops into fast rocking, it facilitates rather than inhibits.

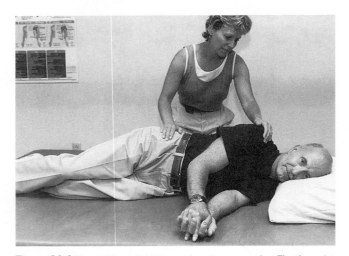

Figure 26-6 Slow rolling to inhibit spastic or tense muscles. The therapist holds the patient at the hip and shoulder and *slowly* rolls him from supine to side-lying and back again. (Photo by Robert Littlefield. Scientific and Technical Photography, Dorchester, MA.)

Stimuli for the Special Senses

Auditory and visual stimuli of a quality opposite to that used for facilitation brings about an inhibitory response whether done deliberately or incidentally during ongoing therapy. Therefore, lullaby music promotes sleep and loss of tone, as does a drab, dull, colorless, and uninteresting environment (Harris, 1969). A soft, low voice command produces a slower response. In the presence of pain, soft commands are always used to avoid stimulating jerky movements and further increasing the pain (Voss, 1967).

Problems Secondary to High Tone

Malalignment of trunk and limbs occurs quickly because of shortening of spastic muscles on one side of a joint (Gillen, 1998). If prolonged malaligned positioning is allowed, the outcome is a contracture with subsequent deformity, interference with BADL, and pain (Gillen, 1998). These should be prevented with daily stretching (Braddom, 1996).

Other Treatments to Decrease Spasticity

The most obvious treatment to decrease spasticity is to remove nociceptive stimuli, such as urinary tract infections, pressure sores, bowel impaction, and bladder distension (Braddom, 1996). Repetitive passive movement has been shown to decrease reflex torque up to 50% of the initial torque (Schmit et al., 2000; Sköld, 2000). Physical agent modalities (Chapter 18) (Preston & Hecht, 1999); splinting (Chapter 14); serial casting, which holds the limb in a position opposite to the contracture and is changed frequently to increase the angle of the contracted joint (Braddom, 1996); EMG biofeedback (Chapter 25); electrical stimulation (Braddom, 1996); medications such as baclofen, dantrolene sodium, diazepam, and clonidine (Black-Schaffer, 1999; Dall et al., 1996; Noth, 1991); nerve blocks (Preston & Hecht, 1999); and botulinum toxin A (Botox) (Dobkin, 1996; Kessler & Benecke, 1997; Pierson et al., 1996) also may reduce spasticity that does not respond to the described inhibition techniques and may help patients in whom there is no recovery of voluntary movement and persistent spasticity is leading to contractures. If persistent contractures interfere with activities of daily living and/or hygiene, surgical release is required. It is better to prevent the contracture than to correct it.

Summary Review Questions

1. Describe the physiology of the dynamic stretch reflex.

2. Describe the physiology of the tonic stretch reflex.
3. What facilitation technique has an immediate effect that lasts only as long as the stimulus is applied?
4. Describe how fast brushing facilitates limb muscles.
5. How does abnormal tone affect occupational functioning?
6. How does flaccidity contribute to contracture development? Spasticity?
7. Describe how general hypertonicity, such as seen in some patients after brain injury, may be inhibited.
8. What does prolonged stretch do and how?

References

Ada, L., Vattanasilp, W., O'Dwyer, N. J., & Crosbie, J. (1998). Does spasticity contribute to walking dysfunction after stroke? *Journal of Neurology, Neurosurgery, and Psychiatry, 64,* 628–635.

Ayres, A. J. (1962). Integration of information. In C. Sattely (Ed.), *Approaches to the Treatment of Patients With Neuromuscular Dysfunction* (Study Course VI, 3rd International Congress WFOT, pp. 49–57). Dubuque, IA: W. C. Brown.

Ayres, A. J. (1963). Occupational therapy directed toward neuromuscular integration. In H. S. Willard & C. S. Spackman (Eds.), *Occupational Therapy* (3rd ed., pp. 358–459). Philadelphia: Lippincott.

Ayres, A. J. (1974). Integration of information. In A. Henderson, L. Llorens, E. Gilfoyle, C. Meyers, & S. Prevel (Eds.), *The Development of Sensory Integrative Theory and Practice: A Collection of the Works of A. Jean Ayers* (pp. 63–82). Dubuque, IA: Kendall-Hunt.

Black-Schaffer, R. M., Kirsteins, A. E., & Harvey, R. L. (1999). Stroke rehabilitation 2. Co-morbidities and complications. *Archives of Physical Medicine and Rehabilitation, 80*(5 Suppl 1), S8–16.

Braddom, R. L. (Ed.). (1996). *Physical Medicine and Rehabilitation.* Philadelphia: Saunders.

Carey, J. R. (1990). Manual stretch: Effect on finger movement control and force control in stroke subjects with spastic extrinsic finger flexor muscles. *Archives of Physical Medicine and Rehabilitation, 71,* 888–894.

Carpenter, M. B., & Sutin, J. (1983). *Human Neuroanatomy* (8th ed.). Baltimore: Williams & Wilkins.

Carpenter, R. H. S. (1996). *Neurophysiology* (3rd ed.). New York: Oxford University.

Dall, J. T., Harmon, R. L., & Quinn, C. M. (1996). Use of clonidine for treatment of spasticity arising from various forms of brain injury: A case series. *Brain Injury, 10,* 453–458.

Dobkin, B. H. (1996). *Neurologic Rehabilitation.* Philadelphia: Davis.

Gillen, G. (1998). Managing abnormal tone after brain injury. *[AOTA] OT Practice, 3*(8), 18–24.

Gilman, S., & Newman, S. W. (1992). *Manter and Gatz's Essentials of Clinical Neuroanatomy and Neurophysiology* (8th ed.). Philadelphia: Davis.

Harris, F. (1969). Control of gamma efferents through the reticular activating system. *American Journal of Occupational Therapy, 23,* 403–408.

Huss, J. (1971). Sensorimotor treatment approaches. In H. S. Willard & C. S. Spackman (Eds.), *Occupational therapy* (4th ed., pp. 373–400). Philadelphia: Lippincott.

Kessler, K. R., & Benecke, R. (1997). Botulinum toxin: From poison to remedy. *Neurotoxicology, 18,* 761–770.

Levin, M. F., & Feldman, A. G. (1994). The role of stretch reflex threshold regulation in normal and impaired motor control. *Brain Research, 657*(1–2), 23–30.

Malouin, F., Bonneau, C., Pichard, L., & Corriveau, D. (1997). Non–reflex mediated changes in plantarflexor muscles early after stroke. *Scandinavian Journal of Rehabilitation Medicine, 29*(3), 147–153.

Markos, P. D. (1979). Ipsilateral and contralateral effects of proprioceptive neuromuscular facilitation techniques on hip motion and electromyographic activity. *Physical Therapy, 59*, 1366–1373.

Mason, C. R. (1985). One method for assessing the effectiveness of fast brushing. *Physical Therapy, 65*, 1197–1202.

Matyas, T. A., & Spicer, S. D. (1980). Facilitation of the tonic vibration reflex (TVR) by cutaneous stimulation in hemiplegics. *American Journal of Physical Medicine, 59*(6), 280–287.

Myers, B. J. (1995). Proprioceptive neuromuscular facilitation (PNF) approach. In C. A. Trombly (Ed.), *Occupational Therapy for Physical Dysfunction*, (4th ed. pp. 474–495). Baltimore: Williams & Wilkins.

Noth, J. (1991). Trends in the pathophysiology and pharmacotherapy of spasticity. *Journal of Neurology, 238*(3), 131–139.

O'Dwyer, N. J., Ada, L., & Neilson, P. D. (1996). Spasticity and muscle contracture following stroke. *Brain, 119*(pt 5), 1737–1749.

Okuma, Y., & Lee, R. G. (1996). Reciprocal inhibition in hemiplegia: Correlation with clinical features and recovery. *Canadian Journal of Neurological Sciences, 23*(1), 15–23.

Pierson, S. H., Katz, D. I., & Tarsy, D. (1996). Botulinum toxin A in the treatment of spasticity: Functional implications and patient selection. *Archives of Physical Medicine and Rehabilitation, 77*, 717–721.

Preston, L. A., & Hecht, J. S. (1999). *Spasticity Management: Rehabilitation Strategies*. Bethesda, MD: American Occupational Therapy Association.

Rider, B. (1971). Effects of neuromuscular facilitation on cross transfer. *American Journal of Occupational Therapy, 25*, 84–89.

Rood, M. S. (1954). Neurophysiological reactions as a basis for physical therapy. *Physical Therapy Review, 34*, 444–449.

Rood, M. S. (1956). Neurophysiological mechanisms utilized in the treatment of neuromuscular dysfunction. *American Journal of Occupational Therapy, 10*, 220–225.

Rood, M. S. (1962). The use of sensory receptors to activate, facilitate, and inhibit motor response, autonomic and somatic, in developmental sequence. In C. Sattely (Ed.), *Approaches to the Treatment of Patients With Neuromuscular Dysfunction* (Study Course VI, 3rd International Congress WFOT, pp. 26–37). Dubuque, IA: W. C. Brown.

Schmit, B. D., DeWald, J. P. A., & Rymer, Z. (2000). Stretch reflex adaptation in elbow flexors during repeated passive movements in unilateral brain-injured patients. *Archives of Physical Medicine and Rehabilitation, 81*, 269–278.

Sköld, C. (2000). Spasticity in spinal cord injury: Self and clinically rated intrinsic fluctuations and intervention in induced changes. *Archives of Physical Medicine and Rehabilitation, 81*(2), 144–149.

Sloan, R. L., Sinclair, E., Thompson, J., Taylor, S., & Pentland, B. (1992). Inter-rater reliability of the modified Ashworth Scale for spasticity in hemiplegic patients. *International Journal of Rehabilitation Research, 15*(2), 158–161.

Spicer, S. D., & Matyas, T. A. (1980). Facilitation of the tonic vibration reflex (TVR) by cutaneous stimulation. *American Journal of Physical Medicine, 59*(5), 223–231.

Stockmeyer, S. (1967). An interpretation of the approach of Rood to the treatment of neuromuscular dysfunction. *American Journal of Physical Medicine, 46*, 900–956.

Tanigawa, M. C. (1972). Comparison of the hold-relax procedure and passive mobilization on increasing muscle length. *Physical Therapy, 52*, 725–735.

Teixeira-Salmela, L. F., Olney, S. J., Nadeau, S., & Brouwer, B. (1999). Muscle strengthening and physical conditioning to reduce impairment and disability in chronic stroke survivors. *Archives of Physical Medicine and Rehabilitation, 80*, 1211–1218.

Thilmann, A. F., Fellows, S. J., & Garms, E. (1991). The mechanism of spastic muscle hypertonus. Variation in reflex gain over the time course of spasticity. *Brain, 114*(Pt 1A), 233–244.

Umphred, D. A. (1995). Classification of treatment techniques based on primary input systems. In D. A. Umphred (Ed.), *Neurological Rehabilitation* (3rd ed., pp. 118–178). St. Louis: Mosby.

Voss, D. E. (1967). Proprioceptive neuromuscular facilitation. *American Journal of Physical Medicine, 46*, 838–898.

Voss, D. E., Ionta, M. K., & Myers, B. J. (1985). *Proprioceptive Neuromuscular Facilitation: Patterns and Techniques* (3rd ed.). New York: Harper & Row.

27

Optimizing Sensory Abilities and Capacities

Karen Bentzel and Lee Ann Quintana

LEARNING OBJECTIVES

After studying this chapter, the reader will be able to do the following:

1. Select appropriate sensory treatment for a patient or description of a patient.
2. Explain the rationale for sensory reeducation and desensitization.
3. Demonstrate a variety of sensory reeducation and desensitization strategies for patients following peripheral nerve injury and stroke.
4. Name several mechanisms of damage to areas of skin with diminished protective sensation and describe related compensatory strategies to prevent injury.

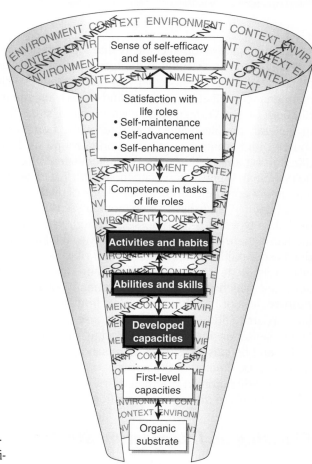

*T*actile sensation is considered by many people to be less important than visual and auditory sensations (Manske, 1999). Most would be surprised to find the extent and number of difficulties resulting from loss of tactile and proprioceptive information. The story of Ian Waterman, who lost all tactile and proprioceptive sensations from the neck down as a result of a rare neurological illness, was introduced in Chapter 6. As Waterman tried to explain to others what was wrong with him, he found that they couldn't begin to understand the severe difficulties he faced as a result of his sensory loss. His family and friends failed to find the connection between his sensory loss and his inability to move and complete activities of daily living. Even many in the medical community didn't comprehend the extent of his difficulties. A detailed account of Waterman's struggle to compensate for his lost sensation is provided in Cole (1991), *Pride and a Daily Marathon.*

GLOSSARY

Decubitus ulcer—Open sore caused by pressure, friction, and moisture. These factors lead to reduced blood flow to the area and consequent tissue death. The most common sites for decubitus ulcers are over bony prominences.

Hypersensitivity, hyperesthesia—Condition in which ordinary stimuli produce an exaggerated or unpleasant sensation.

Learned nonuse—Loss of capacity in an impaired extremity because of the tendency to avoid using that extremity and to use other body parts instead.

Protective sensation—Painful sensation evoked by potentially damaging sensory stimuli, such as excessive temperature, pressure, or tissue stress.

Graphesthesia—The ability to identify numbers or letters traced on the skin.

Touch is a developed capacity that supports abilities and skills such as grasping and releasing objects. These abilities and skills are necessary for competence in self-maintenance, self-enhancement, and self-advancement. Biologist Geerat Vermeij (1999), who is blind, states that in general, people neglect the role of the hand as a source of information about the world around us. Handling and manipulating objects enhances learning and helps human beings appreciate the world. Touch is also a means of communication and a source of pleasure.

Chapter 6 addresses assessment of sensation and describes types of sensory losses. Without sensation in the hand, there is a greater risk of injury to the hand and decreased ability to manipulate small objects. There is also a tendency not to use the hand in functional activities, which adds to the phenomenon of **learned nonuse**, loss of function that results from not using the hand (Carr & Shepherd, 1998). Because of the role of tactile sensation in learning, exploring, and communicating and because loss of hand sensation is particularly disabling, occupational therapists should provide treatment or education in compensatory strategies for patients with lost or diminished sensation.

Choosing an Intervention Strategy

The choice of interventions for sensation is based on the diagnosis, prognosis, and evaluation findings. Diminished or lost **protective sensation**, the inability to feel pain in response to stimuli that are potentially damaging, suggests a need for teaching the patient and/or caregiver compensatory strategies to prevent injury. Findings of discomfort associated with touch (**hypersensitivy**) suggest a need for desensitization. Sensory reeducation is provided for patients who have some sensation and potential for better sensation or better interpretation of sensory information.

All of the sensory interventions described in this chapter are learning experiences for the patient. Strategies of learning (see Chapter 12) should be applied. Dellon (1997) recommends sensory retraining strategies based on learning principles. Each patient should practice within the natural context of activities. The patient needs to attend to provided information and stimuli and perceive them as important and relevant. Tailor training and training materials to the interest and ability of the patient. Grade the activity so that the patient can meet the expectations for improved performance.

Sensory Reeducation

Sensory reeducation is a combination of techniques that helps the patient with a sensory impairment learn to reinterpret sensation (Dellon, 1997). Dellon (1988), a hand surgeon, related his experience in 1970 with nerve-injured patients who could feel fingertip stroking, pinprick, and pressure but could not correctly identify a nickel and a quarter using only touch sensation. These patients could feel a difference between the coins, but they could not identify them, and the coins did not feel the same as before the injury.

Dellon concluded that the sensibility was recovered but that there was a mismatch of the new sensory profile with past profiles in the association cortex. Within a few minutes, he could train patients to tell the difference between the two coins. He gave the patient a nickel, said what it was, and explained that it did not feel the way a nickel used to feel but that what the patient was feeling should thereafter be called a nickel. After repeating the process with a quarter, the patient could correctly identify both coins. The sensation had been reeducated.

Cutaneous information from the fingers, palm, and toes is most important in rehabilitation, because it is generally these skin surfaces that interact with the external environment (Dannenbaum & Dykes, 1988). The focus of sensory reeducation is usually regaining the use of sensation of the hand. Sensory reeducation is an appropriate and commonly used treatment for patients with a variety of peripheral nerve injuries, including nerve lacerations and compressions and injuries resulting in replantation, toe-to-thumb grafting, and skin grafting (Dellon, 1997).

Sensory reeducation is also sometimes used for patients who have had cerebral vascular accidents (CVA). Neistadt and Seymour's (1995) study of occupational therapists treating patients with CVA asked them to rank 10 categories of treatment activities according to frequency of use. Sensory reeducation was ranked ninth, indicating that sensory retraining following CVA has low priority in many clinical settings. Despite evidence that recovery of motor function depends on sensation, the focus of treatment seems to be motor rather than sensory deficits (Dannenbaum & Jones, 1993).

Rationale for Sensory Reeducation Following Peripheral Nerve Injury

Cortical maps have been found to change as a result of peripheral nerve injuries. Loss of sensory input from the peripheral nerve causes the associated areas of the sensory cortex to begin to serve sensory inputs from adjacent areas. After nerve repair, when the peripheral nerve regrowth leads to reinnervation of sensory receptors, the corresponding area of the somatosensory cortex reorganizes to allow interpretation of incoming stimuli from the affected area (Dellon, 1997; Merzenich & Jenkins, 1993). In children, this reorganization is sufficient for return of normal sensory interpretation without sensory retraining. In adults, the neural reorganization may be facilitated by sensory reeducation (Rosén et al., 1994).

The return of sensation following hand injury is an extremely complex event. Recovery is not just a process of altering the cortical representation but also depends on reinnervation. Following nerve laceration and surgical repair, some sensory fibers, given sufficient time, regenerate and reinnervate the tactile receptors. Return of sensation is limited by scar tissue that blocks sensory fiber regrowth and atrophy of sensory receptors prior to reinnervation. Sensory return is also limited by malalignment of axonal sheaths that allows misdirection of regrowing fibers, meaning that fibers do not usually regrow to innervate the same sensory receptors that they did before the injury (Callahan, 1995).

As a result of scar tissue, atrophy of sensory receptors, and the misdirection of fibers, there is an inevitable change in the profile of neural impulses reaching the sensory cortex. A previously well-known stimulus initiates a different set of neural impulses from that elicited by the same stimulus before the injury. When this altered profile reaches the sensory cortex, the patient cannot match it with patterns previously encountered and remembered (Callahan, 1995; Dellon, 1997), hence cannot identify or recognize the stimulus (Fig. 27-1). The purpose of sensory reeducation in patients with peripheral injuries is to help them learn to recognize the distorted cortical impression (Dellon & Jabaley, 1982).

Rationale for Sensory Reeducation Following CVA

Sensory reeducation following CVA is based on the concept of neural plasticity. Carr and Shepherd (1998), in their review of the scientific evidence for the ability of the brain to reorganize following brain lesions, state that reorganization seems to be related to frequency of use.

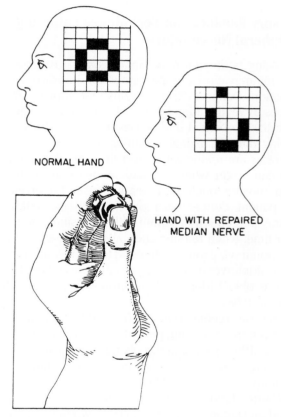

NORMAL HAND

HAND WITH REPAIRED MEDIAN NERVE

Figure 27-1 In the normal hand, a stimulus, such as this gripped bolt, elicits a profile of neural impulses that reaches the sensory cortex and ultimately is perceived, as represented by the checkerboard pattern. After a nerve repair, the same stimulus elicits an altered profile of impulses that reaches the sensory cortex. The new perception, the altered checkerboard pattern, may be so different from the previous one that object recognition is at first impossible. (Reprinted with permission from Dellon, A. [1988]. *Evaluation of Sensibility and Re-education of Sensation in the Hand.* Baltimore: Lucas.)

They suggest that enlargement of sensory receptive areas within the cortex is a result of increased participation of the body part in activities requiring tactile sensations. Therapists may alter the cortical map by directing the sensory experiences of the patient. Therefore, the goal of sensory reeducation following CVA is to gain a larger cortical representation for the areas of skin from which sensory feedback is crucial to performance of daily tasks.

The rationale for sensory reeducation following CVA is also based on the premise that functional use of a body part with reduced sensation is possible but that spontaneous use is limited. Without training, there is a tendency not to use the extremity, and learned nonuse leads to further loss of sensory and motor abilities (Dannenbaum & Dykes, 1988). Sensory reeducation has the potential to facilitate increased functional use of the hand and prevent loss of function due to learned nonuse.

Sensory Reeducation Techniques Following Peripheral Nerve Injury

Following peripheral nerve injury, axonal regeneration and reinnervation are necessary for improvement in sensation. Dellon (1997) cautions that implementation of sensory reeducation before adequate axonal regeneration has no benefit and causes frustration. Because of varying rates of axonal sprouting and growth, sensory receptors are reinnervated over time. Sensory reeducation can begin when the patient first can appreciate deep, moving touch. In the early phase of intervention, the patient concentrates on learning to match the sensory perception of stimuli with the visual perception. After time, when reinnervation allows for perception of light nonmoving touch with good touch localization, the focus of intervention changes to more functional tasks, such as object identification through touch (Fig. 27-2) (Dellon, 1988).

Sensory reeducation protocols differ among facilities, even those treating patients with similar diagnoses. Dellon (1997) shares protocols for sensory reeducation following peripheral injury from five institutions. A summary of the protocol he presents from the Raymond M. Curtis Hand Center of Union Memorial Hospital, based on Dellon's earlier work, is shown in Box 27-1.

Callahan (1995) describes similar procedures. She recommends beginning each moving and constant touch sequence with eyes closed, followed by eyes open, and concluding with eyes closed. She also recommends using a smaller and lighter stimulus as the patient improves, with a goal of localization of a touch that is near the light-touch threshold. She continues touch localization throughout the sensory reeducation and adds

a few more tasks to the training program. Discrimination of similar and different textures using sandpaper, fabrics, and edges of coins are introduced early. Patients practice **graphesthesia**, the ability to identify a letter or number drawn on the skin, and identification of shape or letter blocks. In the later stages of training, patients pick objects from containers filled with sand or rice and practice identification of common objects. Finally, Callahan recommends practice of daily living activities with vision occluded. Callahan states that a variety of tasks, including some that are similar to games or puzzles, are more engaging and therefore more beneficial.

Nakada and Uchida (1997) describe a five-stage sensory reeducation program that was useful for a patient with very limited sensation in her left hand as a result of peripheral neuropathy secondary to leprosy. She also had total impairment of vision, so that sensory feedback was critical to occupational performance. Following reeducation, the patient regained hand function for activities of daily living such as drying dishes, putting on socks, and holding dentures while brushing them. The reeducation program included the following five stages:

Stage 1. Object recognition using feature detection strategies. Objects that vary greatly in shape, material, and weight were used. The patient was encouraged to handle each object and identify the object characteristics.

Stage 2. Prehension of various objects with refinement of prehension patterns. In this stage, grasping objects that vary in size and shape was emphasized. The patient needed to maximize the contact between the object and the hand to develop the ability of the hand to closely contour to objects, which is seen in normal grasp.

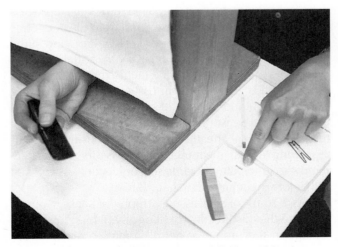

Figure 27-2 Late-phase sensory reeducation following peripheral nerve injury includes identification of various objects by touch.

BOX 27-1
PROCEDURES FOR PRACTICE

Sensory Reeducation

Principles

- Choose a quiet environment that will maximize concentration.
- Sessions should be brief, approximately 5 to 15 minutes.
- Three or four practice or homework sessions per day are recommended.
- Instruct the patient and/or family in techniques to be used during practice.
- Monitor patient's home program and progress during therapy sessions.

Prerequisites for Early-Phase Sensory Reeducation

- Patient must be able to perceive 30 cycles per second vibration and moving touch in the area.
- Patient must be motivated and able to follow through with the program.

Techniques for Early Phase Sensory Reeducation

1. Use the eraser end of a pencil.
2. Apply moving strokes to the area.
3. Use enough pressure for the patient to perceive the stimulus but not so much that it causes pain.
4. Ask the patient to observe what is happening first, then to close the eyes and concentrate on what is being felt.
5. Instruct the patient to put into words (silently) what is being felt.

6. Instruct the patient to observe the stimulus again to confirm the sensory experience with the perception.
7. When perception of constant touch returns to the area, use a similar process for constant touch stimuli.
8. Test the patient by requiring localization of moving and constant touch without seeing the stimulus.

Prerequisites for Late-Phase Sensory Reeducation

- Patient must be able to perceive constant and moving touch at the fingertips.
- Patient must demonstrate good localization of touch.

Techniques for Late-Phase Sensory Reeducation

1. Use a collection of common objects that differ in size and shape.
2. Instruct the patient to grasp and manipulate each item with eyes open, then with eyes closed, then with eyes open for reinforcement.
3. The patient should concentrate on the tactile perception.
4. Test the patient by timing correct identification of each object without vision.
5. Grade the practice by introducing objects of similar size but different texture, then small objects that vary in size and shape but are similar in texture.

Adapted from Dellon, A. L. (1997). *Somatosensory Testing and Rehabilitation.* Bethesda, MD: American Occupational Therapy Association.

Stage 3. Control of prehension force while holding objects. Feedback regarding excessive force that was used to maintain grasp was provided through the use of a strain gauge and therapy putty.

Stage 4. Maintenance of prehension force during transport of objects. While holding an object, the patient moved the shoulder, elbow, and wrist into varying positions of flexion and extension.

Stage 5. Object manipulation. The patient practiced grasp and release of objects and moved objects in the hand into various positions.

Sensory Reeducation Techniques Following CVA

Sensory reeducation following CVA is less well defined than the protocols described for peripheral injuries. Carr and Shepherd, in their *Motor Relearning Program* (1982) and in their more recent work (1998) emphasize the need for sensory learning concurrent with motor learning. They advocate the use of meaningful and relevant sensory and motor experiences very early in rehabilitation. Use of the more involved hand in bimanual tasks such as opening jars and using eating utensils is advocated. They suggest that the patient can be cued to attend to the tactile aspects of the task and that practice of object identification without vision may be helpful.

Dannenbaum and Jones (1993) give detailed goals and proposed methodology for sensory intervention following CVA. They believe that appreciation of some form of tactile stimulation and some basic motor skills are prerequisite to success in sensory reeducation. To establish that a patient with severe sensory loss can perceive some stimuli, they recommend testing and early training using 100-Hz electrical stimulation. Patients identify which finger was stimulated, first with vision, then with eyes closed. Patients with better sensation use a similar process, with textured moving stimuli followed by motionless stimuli.

In addition, Dannenbaum and Jones suggest early incorporation of the hand into functional activities and prevention of abnormal patterns of grasp and movement. Add textures to handle surfaces to increase the friction and support of weak grasping ability. Enlarge or modify handles to facilitate both tactile contact and tactile feedback. Patients should practice modulation of grip forces in response to the objects and maintenance of appropriate grip force during forearm movements.

Yuketiel and Guttman's (1993) research protocol included the following sensory reeducation activities:

► Identification of the number of touches
► Graphesthesia tests
► "Find your thumb" without looking
► Identification of shape, weight, and texture
► Passive drawing and writing: the patient identifies a letter, number, or drawing made by the therapist passively moving the patient's hand while it holds a pencil

These sensory treatment activities are examples of a wide variety of techniques that can be used in clinical treatment for patients following CVA. Therapists working with this population use creativity, patients' interest, and theoretical understanding to develop programs of sensory intervention, since no one protocol has been widely accepted or thoroughly researched.

Effectiveness of Sensory Reeducation Following Peripheral Nerve Injury

Dellon (1997) reviewed a large number of studies of the effectiveness of sensory reeducation following peripheral nerve injury, replantation, and innervated skin graft. Study designs included 1) comparison of patients who today routinely receive sensory reeducation with those in the past before widespread acceptance of the technique, and 2) assessment of the results of sensory reeducation provided long after spontaneous recovery is likely. Dellon concluded that sensory reeducation clearly improves sensory and functional recovery in a shorter period than without training and indicates that the techniques have been globally accepted as necessary following peripheral nerve injury.

The effectiveness of sensory reeducation is confirmed in two studies not included in Dellon's review. Shieh et al. (1995) studied two groups of patients following digit replantation, with only one group receiving sensory reeducation. That group showed significantly lower touch threshold as measured by monofilament testing and better scores on moving two-point discrimination tests. Cheng (2000) divided patients with digital nerve injuries into two groups, with the control group receiving conventional therapy and the experimental group receiving a tactile stimulation program in addition to conventional therapy. Those receiving the tactile program showed significantly greater improvement in two-point discrimination. The authors suggest that sensory reeducation should be included in the protocol for rehabilitation of patients following digital replantation and digital nerve injuries.

Rosén et al. (1994) reported evidence that functional outcome following nerve repair may depend at least to some extent on the individual's cognitive capacities, including learning ability and visuospatial cognition. The role of cognition in sensory reeducation is apparent but has not been tested by scientific research studies.

Effectiveness of Sensory Reeducation Following CVA

The number of research studies of the effectiveness of sensory retraining following CVA is limited, and the results of these studies have not been strong enough for the technique to be recommended in the *Clinical Practice Guideline for Post-Stroke Rehabilitation* (U.S. Department of Health and Human Services, 1995).

Vinograd et al. (1962) documented improvement in sensory measures for a series of three patients with hemiplegia over 1 to 5 months of sensory retraining but also noted that the sensory improvements failed to increase functional use of the hand. In a study comparing sensorimotor integrative treatment with functional treatment following stroke, Jongbloed et al. (1989) found no significant differences in self-care, mobility, or selected sensory test scores. The conclusion was that there was little or no difference in outcomes between the two approaches.

Dannenbaum and Dykes (1988) developed a treatment program based on research findings for patients following sensory stroke and implemented this program in a pilot study. In a description of a single case, they documented improved proprioception and touch localization scores and improved functional use in eating and retrieving a wallet from a pocket following a 13-month, twice-weekly program. They also described improved sensory test scores in five additional subjects after 5 months of intervention, but this improvement did not seem to be related to improved functional use of the hand.

In Yekutiel and Guttman's (1993) study of the effectiveness of sensory reeducation following stroke, 20 experimental subjects received 45-minute sessions of sensory retraining three times a week for 6 weeks. To rule out spontaneous recovery, subjects had to have been diagnosed with stroke more than 2 years prior to the study. Following intervention, the experimental group demonstrated statistically significant improvement in touch localization, static two-point discrimination, proprioception, and stereognosis. A matching control group showed no improvement. Measurements of function were not included in the study.

Carey et al. (1993) documented improvement on proprioceptive and tactile discrimination measures following 10 to 15 sessions of training in a series of eight single-case experiments. The training effect seemed to be modality specific, so that proprioceptive training resulted in improvement on that kind of test but not on the tactile discrimination test. Subjects made spontaneous comments about functional improvements such as improved ability to maintain grasp on objects and improved awareness of hand position, but functional use was not chosen and analyzed as a variable in the study.

This small number of studies of the effectiveness of sensory reeducation following CVA show some evidence, but not conclusive evidence, that the technique may be effective in improving sensation. What is needed to support greater clinical acceptance of sensory retraining following CVA is further documentation that those techniques produce improved sensation and that improved sensation leads to improved occupational performance.

Robertson and Jones (1994) supplied evidence that elevated touch thresholds, as measured by two-point discrimination testing, were correlated with slower object recognition and with decreased ability to control the force used during grasp. The study found no correlation between touch threshold and hand function as measured by the *Jebsen Hand Function Test* in 10 subjects with left-hemisphere CVA. The authors recommend further study with larger samples and modifications in testing measures. Dannenbaum and Jones (1993, p. 136) conclude, "It is not known what level of recovery can be expected following a treatment program, as the treatment for sensory deficits in patients with cortical lesions is still in its infancy."

Desensitization

Desensitization is chosen when the sensory evaluation reveals an area of hypersensitivity, in which ordinary stimuli produce an exaggerated or unpleasant sensation (Yerxa et al., 1983). Desensitization is designed to decrease the discomfort associated with touch in the hypersensitive area. A program of desensitization generally includes contact of the hypersensitive skin with items that provide a variety of sensory experiences, such as textures ranging from soft to coarse.

Rationale for Desensitization

Hypersensitivity is observed in some but not all patients following nerve trauma, crush injuries, scarring, burns, and amputation (Waylett-Rendall, 1995; Yerxa et al., 1983). Patients with hypersensitivity tend to avoid using the affected part in functional activities (Waylett-Rendall) and typically hold the affected part protectively

(Hardy et al., 1982). Hypersensitivity can lead to disability through nonuse of the involved body part (Robinson & McPhee, 1986).

Desensitization is based on the idea that progressive stimulation will allow progressive tolerance. The origin of the concept of desensitization is unknown. Civil War veterans with amputations were known to tap silver spoons on their residual limbs to improve their tolerance of artificial limbs, which in those days were constructed from wood (Hardy et al., 1982). Dellon (1997) considers desensitization a form of sensory retraining during which the patient learns accurate, less painful perception of sensory input. The desensitization program should use principles that enhance learning, such as structured practice within the context of functional activities (Waylett-Rendall, 1995).

Desensitization Techniques

Initially, a patient may have to compensate for hypersensitivity by wearing a splint or padding over the affected area (Anthony, 1993). The patient must be weaned gradually from the protective device as improvement occurs. In treatment, the patient develops progressive tolerance to a hierarchy of sensory stimuli (Waylett-Rendall, 1995). The hierarchy described by Hardy et al. (1982) includes five levels:

Level 1. Tuning fork, paraffin, massage

Level 2. Battery-operated vibrator (Fig. 27-3), deep massage, touch pressure with pencil eraser

Level 3. Electric vibrator, texture identification

Level 4. Electric vibrator, object identification

Level 5. Work and daily activities

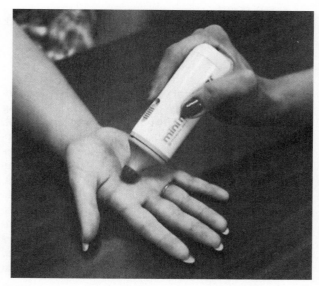

Figure 27-3 The small head of this battery-powered vibrator is useful for desensitization of specific areas of the hand.

Case Example

MR. M.: PROGRESSION IN SENSORY REMEDIATION

Patient Information

Mr. M., a 25-year-old appliance repairman with a laceration of the median nerve, was reassessed approximately 6 weeks after his injury. The outpatient occupational therapy reassessment identified the following sensory problems:

1. Absent and decreased protective sensation in the thumb, index and middle fingers, and radial palm
2. Mislocalization of touch sensations in the radial portion of the palm
3. Hypersensitivity in the area of the scar
4. Decreased ability to pick up and manipulate objects
5. Decreased use of the right hand in functional activities

(See Chapter 6 for description of the assessment process and the patient's background).

Recommendations

At the time of the reassessment, the occupational therapist recommended outpatient occupational therapy twice a week for 6 additional weeks and then reassessment, with reduction to one session per week likely at that time. Mr. M. has demonstrated quick learning of therapy instructions and will be responsible for an intensive home program. Because recovery of the ability to differentiate small objects at the fingertips will probably not occur until 10 to 12 months after the nerve repair, weekly or biweekly therapy will have to continue for that length of time. In collaboration with Mr. M., the occupational therapist established the following long-term goals for sensory intervention:

1. Mr. M. will correctly interpret sensory stimuli throughout the right hand, as demonstrated by correct tactile identification of objects.
2. Mr. M. will demonstrate good use of the right hand in work simulation activities that rely on touch sensation.

Short-Term Goals

1. **Mr. M. will avoid injury to the right hand by demonstrating compensatory protective strategies during functional activities.** The therapist instructed Mr. M. about risk of injury from sharp and hot objects and gripping forces. Mr. M. and the therapist discussed an appropriate routine for skin care and implementation of precautions in his daily routine. By the end of the second session, Mr. M. demonstrated good understanding of these techniques during home and simple work simulation activities.
2. **Mr. M. will tolerate touch of all textures over and around his scar area so that hypersensitivity does not interfere with functional hand use.** Mr. M. ranked the 10 dowel textures from least to most irritating. At that time, he easily tolerated the first four textures as they were rubbed by the therapist over the scar area. He disliked touch from the fifth texture and was unable to tolerate textures 6 through 10. The therapist provided textures for a home desensitization program, beginning with textures 5 and 6. Mr. M. used these textures three or four times a day for scar desensitization. During therapy sessions, massage and vibration were provided around and over the scar area. At the end of 3 weeks, Mr. M. tolerated all textures and no longer reported discomfort from sleeve cuffs or inadvertent touch during functional activities.
3. **Mr. M. will demonstrate touch localization below 10 mm in the right palm to improve interpretation of tactile sensations during work activities.** The therapist initiated a sensory reeducation program for touch localization using moving and static touch stimuli in the palm. Instructions were provided, and Mr. M. faithfully followed through with this program at home, four sessions per day. At the end of 3 weeks, localization in the palm measured 12 to 14 mm. The therapist initiated graphesthesia and texture discrimination activities in the palmar area. After 6 weeks of sensory reeducation, localization measured 9 to 10 mm, and Mr. M. could identify 50% of the letters and shapes drawn in his palm and 40% of the textures.

Revised Goals

To improve interpretation of tactile sensations during work activities:

1. Mr. M. will demonstrate 100% correct graphesthesia and texture identification in his right palm.
2. Mr. M. will demonstrate touch localization below 10 mm in the proximal phalanges of the right thumb, index, and middle fingers.

CLINICAL REASONING
in OT Practice

Transition of Sensory Reeducation Program From Early Phase to Late Phase

Mr. M. will begin the second phase of sensory reeducation at the fingertips approximately 6 to 8 months after his surgery to repair the median nerve. What reassessment findings will indicate the appropriate time for Mr. M. to begin late-phase sensory reeducation? What treatment activities and home program activities would be appropriate for Mr. M. as he begins this phase? What work simulation activities could be incorporated into his therapy program during sensory reeducation?

TABLE 27-1
Hierarchy of Texture and Vibration Used in Desensitization

Level	Dowel Textures	Immersion Textures	Vibration (cps)
1	Moleskin	Cotton	83 cps near area
2	Felt	Terry cloth pieces	83 cps near area, 23 cps near area
3	QuickStick[a]	Dry rice	83 cps near area, 23 cps intermittent
4	Velvet	Popcorn	83 cps intermittent, 23 cps intermittent
5	Semirough cloth	Pinto beans	83 cps intermittent, 23 cps continuous
6	Velcro loop	Macaroni	83 cps continuous, 53 cps intermittent
7	Hard foam	Plastic wire insulation pieces	100 cps intermittent, 53 cps intermittent
8	Burlap	Small BBs, buckshot	100 cps intermittent, 53 cps continuous
9	Rug back	Large BBs, buckshot	100 cps continuous, 53 cps continuous
10	Velcro hook	Plastic squares	No problem with vibration

[a]A closed-cell, firm splint padding material.

Adapted from Barber, L. (1990). Desensitization of the traumatized hand. In J. Hunter, L. Schneider, E. Mackin, & A. Callahan (Eds.), *Rehabilitation of the Hand* (3rd ed., pp. 721–730). St. Louis: Mosby.

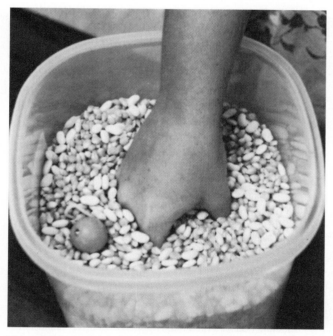

Figure 27-4 Immersion of the hand into a container filled with popcorn kernels and pinto beans facilitates desensitization. Patients use touch to find objects hidden in the immersion particles.

Patients advance to the next level after they demonstrate tolerance of the current level without signs of irritation. Work simulation is believed to be extremely important to ensure that the patient is using the painful site. Activities must be tailored to the patient's interest and occupation.

Table 27-1 shows the Downey Hand Center hierarchy of textures and vibration (Barber, 1990; Yerxa et al., 1983). Commercial dowel and immersion textures (see Resources) are similar to this hierarchy. Patients arrange the dowel textures and immersion textures (Fig. 27-4) in the order that they perceive as least to most irritating. They select the dowel texture, immersion texture, and vibration level that is uncomfortable but tolerable for 10 minutes three or four times daily. Advancing to the next level of treatment depends on tolerance of lower levels (Barber, 1990). Documentation includes the patient's initial hierarchy and progress for each of the three modalities (Waylett-Rendall, 1995).

Other clinical activities thought to decrease hypersensitivity include weight-bearing pressure, massage, transcutaneous electrical stimulation, fluidotherapy, and therapy putty (Anthony, 1993; Dellon, 1997; Waylett-Rendall, 1995). Use of the affected body part in leisure, work, and daily occupations is believed to facilitate desensitization (Anthony; Waylett-Rendall). Activities like typing, hair washing, macramé, and assembling leather link belts can be used to decrease hypersensitivity in the hand or fingers (Anthony; Barber, 1990).

Effectiveness of Desensitization

The success of desensitization in occupational therapy was documented in a case study of a patient with a digital nerve laceration who showed marked improvement following 8 weeks of treatment (Robinson & McPhee, 1986). The patient was seen in the clinic for a total of five sessions, which consisted primarily of reevaluation and home program revision. Initially the patient reported hypersensitivity throughout the tip of the finger and demonstrated very limited use of the finger in functional activities. Following occupational therapy, the patient reported no hypersensitivity and demonstrated full use of the finger in home, work, and leisure. This success was confirmed by measurements of static two-point discrimination, which was initially unmeasurable but had improved to a score within normal limits at discharge.

Hardy et al. (1982) reported on the effect of desensitization in 16 patients following nerve and crush injuries; 13 had successful outcomes and were discharged to their previous occupations. Two-point discrimination improved an average of 19.3 mm for 9 of the patients.

Barber (1990) reported that almost all patients advance at least one level on one modality in the hierarchy of the Downey Hand Center after 2 to 3 weeks of desensitization. Approximately 70% of the patients were able to tolerate all 10 dowel textures within an average of 7 weeks of treatment.

Motivation and psychological status seem to affect the success of desensitization (Barber, 1990). Some diagnostic conditions also seem to limit the success of this treatment. Relatively poor success has been observed clinically for patients with diagnoses of cumulative trauma (Waylett-Rendall, 1995) and reflex sympathetic dystrophy (Dellon, 1997).

Compensation for Impaired or Absent Protective Sensation

Protective sensations are sensations of pain and temperature extremes that signal the threat of tissue damage. When the brain receives this message, the normal response is to move the body part away from the source of the stimulus. Without this message, tissue damage can quickly occur. The goal of treatment for the patient with diminished or absent protective sensation is to avoid injury. Treatment consists of teaching the patient and/or the caregiver precautions necessary to prevent injury.

Rationale for Compensation

In a classic 1969 article in the *American Journal of Occupational Therapy*, Helen Wood described the role of the occupational therapist in preventing injury and deformity in hands that lacked sensitivity. She stated that when hands are used in activities without protective sensory feedback, there is a high frequency of burns, cuts, lacerations, and bruises. Damage or injury to an insensitive limb is the result of external forces that are normally avoided by people who are able to feel pain, which acts as a warning mechanism. Therefore, pain has been considered the most valuable sensation that humans have (Brand, 1979).

Brand (1979) described five mechanisms of damage to insensitive limbs: continuous low pressure, concentrated high pressure, excessive heat or cold, repetitive mechanical stress, and pressure on infected tissue (Box 27-2). Prevention principles evolve from an understanding of these mechanisms of damage.

Compensation Techniques

Brand (1979), Callahan (1995), and Eggers (1984) recommend the following content for patient education sessions, based on the five mechanisms of damage to insensitive skin. Frequent position changes are necessary for patients with decreased or absent protective sensation to avoid damage due to continuous low pressure. Cushions for seating and shoe insoles help to distribute forces over larger areas. Skin areas over bony prominences are particularly prone to pressure ulcers because the cutaneous tissue is trapped between the unyielding bone and the external pressure.

Patients are instructed to avoid concentrated high pressure by careful handling of sharp tools and by using enlarged handles on suitcases, drawers, and keys. Patients may need to become consciously aware to use only as much force as necessary to grasp objects. High pressure can result from splint straps that are too narrow and splints that are too tight; therefore, therapists must carefully construct splints to prevent injury.

Patients are also taught to increase their awareness of potential sources of extreme heat or cold and to

---

BOX 27-2
Mechanisms of Damage Secondary to Loss of Protective Sensation

- Continuous low pressure: With sustained pressure as light as 1 pound per square inch, capillary flow is blocked; this can cause tissue necrosis, leading to pressure sores (decubitus ulcers).
- Concentrated high pressure: Sudden high force that is accidental and/or a high force applied over a very small area, so that the force is inadequately distributed. This may result in tearing of skin and/or soft tissue or tissue necrosis as a result of insufficient blood supply.
- Excessive heat or cold: Temperature extremes that lead to burn or frostbite injuries.
- Repetitive mechanical stress: Repetitive motions or shearing of skin against clothing or objects that causes inflammation of the tendons or skin. Blistering of skin can also occur.
- Pressure on infected tissue: Continued use and pressure on infected tissue can hinder or prevent the natural healing process.

Adapted from Brand, P. (1979). Management of the insensitive limb. *Physical Therapy, 59*, 8–12.

protect themselves from contact with them. Insulated coffee mugs are recommended. Oven mitts or quality pot holders are necessary for cooking. Utensils with wooden or plastic handles are better than metal ones. Patients using wheelchairs should insulate exposed hot water pipes under sinks. In cold weather, gloves or mittens are necessary protection for insensate hands.

Patients need to be taught to avoid repetitive motions and friction between skin and objects. Methods to reduce friction include wearing gloves and using enlarged or padded handles on tools. They can decrease repetitions by working for shorter periods, resting, using a variety of tools, or alternating hands or type of grip.

Patients who have lost protective sensation should be instructed to give special care to blisters, cuts, and bruises to avoid infection if possible. If infection occurs, the infected part should be completely rested to keep it free from pressure and overuse, allowing healing to occur.

In addition, techniques of compensating for absent sensation include reliance on other senses. For example, vision may be used to prevent contact with sharp objects. Using a body part with intact sensation to test water temperature before immersion of any body part without sensation is recommended. Auditory cues may also help to prevent injury. For instance, a person with paraplegia may hear the rubbing of the wheelchair caster against the foot if it slips from its proper position on the leg rest.

Finally, patients should be instructed in good skin care. Applying lotion or oil daily enhances skin hydration. Skin needs to be visually inspected daily. A warm or reddened area indicates a possible site of tissue breakdown, which will lead to a **decubitus ulcer**, and extreme care must be taken to relieve pressure totally from this area until the color returns to normal. *If the time for the skin to recover its normal color exceeds 20 minutes, it is absolutely essential to discover the cause of the skin irritation and correct it. Modification of position, schedule, procedure, equipment, or orthotics is necessary.* If the patient cannot inspect and care for the skin properly, a care provider should be instructed to perform these tasks every day.

Effectiveness of Compensatory Techniques

A review of the literature reveals no research studies that confirm the effectiveness of instructing patients to avoid injury. These compensatory techniques have some face validity in that they evolved out of evidence that patients lacking protective sensation had received injuries, many of which could have been prevented. Anecdotal evidence of effectiveness includes Wood's (1969) description of a patient who had a series of hand injuries prior to occupational therapy and none following instruction and fitting of gloves to be worn in his electronics repair work.

Widespread acceptance of compensatory techniques is further evidence of reliance on their effectiveness. The American Diabetes Association (1999) recommends sensory testing of the feet of all people with diabetes so that foot ulcers and amputations can be prevented in those with sensory loss. Techniques of testing and education for patients with diabetes appear in the nursing and physical therapy literature (May, 1996; Sloan & Abel, 1998).

Summary Review Questions

1. What is the rationale for sensory reeducation following peripheral nerve injury and CVA?
2. What are the differences and similarities between early-phase and late-phase sensory reeducation for patients with peripheral nerve injury?
3. Describe or demonstrate intervention techniques for a patient with hypersensitivity following a fingertip amputation.
4. List five mechanisms of injury for skin areas with absent or diminished protective sensation. For each of the five mechanisms of injury, describe appropriate preventive education and/or adaptive strategies.
5. What should be done if a patient with sensory loss develops an area of skin redness?

Acknowledgment

I extend my appreciation to Paul Petersen and Melanie Seltzer for their assistance with some of the photography for this chapter.

Resources

Sensory Treatment Equipment Suppliers

North Coast Medical (three-phase desensitization kit, portable desensitization kit, vibrators) • 187 Stauffer Boulevard, San Jose, CA 95125-1042. 800-821-9319. Fax 408-283-1950
www.ncmedical.com

Sammons Preston (tactile activity kit, vibrators) • P. O. Box 5071, Bolingbrook, IL 60440-5071. 800-323-5547. Fax 800-547-4333

Smith & Nephew, Inc. (reeducation wands and home program kit, multiphase desensitization kit, stereognosis kit, vibrators) • One Quality Drive, P. O. Box 1005, Germantown, WI 53022-8205. 800-558-8633. Fax 800-545-7758
www.easy-living.com

References

American Diabetes Association (1999). Position statement: Preventive foot care in people with diabetes. Available: www.diabetes.org.

Anthony, M. (1993). Desensitization. In G. Clark, E. Shaw Wilgis, B. Aiello, D. Eckhaus, & L. Eddington (Eds.), *Hand Rehabilitation* (pp. 73–79). New York: Churchill Livingstone.

Barber, L. (1990). Desensitization of the traumatized hand. In J. Hunter, L. Schneider, E. Mackin, & A. Callahan (Eds.), *Rehabilitation of the Hand* (3rd ed., pp. 721–730). St. Louis: Mosby.

Brand, P. (1979). Management of the insensitive limb. *Physical Therapy, 59,* 8–12.

Callahan, A. D. (1995). Methods of compensation and reeducation for sensory dysfunction. In J. M. Hunter, E. J. Mackin, & A. D. Callahan (Eds.), *Rehabilitation of the Hand: Surgery and Therapy* (4th ed., pp. 701–713). St. Louis: Mosby.

Carey, L. M., Matyas, T. A., & Oke, L. E. (1993). Sensory loss in stroke patients: Effective training of tactile and proprioceptive discrimination. *Archives of Physical Medicine and Rehabilitation, 74,* 602–611.

Carr, J. H., & Shepherd, R. B. (1982). *A Motor Relearning Programme for Stroke.* Oxford: Butterworth-Heinemann.

Carr, J., & Shepherd, R. (1998). *Neurological Rehabilitation: Optimizing Motor Performance.* Oxford: Butterworth-Heinemann.

Cheng, A. S. (2000). Use of early tactile stimulation in rehabilitation of digital nerve injuries. *American Journal of Occupational Therapy, 54,* 159–165.

Cole, J. (1991). *Pride and a Daily Marathon.* Cambridge: MIT.

Dannenbaum, R., & Dykes, R. (1988). Sensory loss in the hand after sensory stroke: Therapeutic rationale. *Archives of Physical Medicine and Rehabilitation, 69,* 833–839.

Dannenbaum, R. M., & Jones, L. A. (1993). The assessment and treatment of patients who have sensory loss following cortical lesions. *Journal of Hand Therapy, 6,* 130–138.

Dellon, A. (1988). *Evaluation of Sensibility and Re-education of Sensation in the Hand.* Baltimore: Lucas.

Dellon, A. L. (1997). *Somatosensory Testing and Rehabilitation.* Bethesda, MD: American Occupational Therapy Association.

Dellon, A., & Jabaley, M. (1982). Reeducation of sensation in the hand following nerve suture. *Clinical Orthopedics, 163,* 75–79.

Eggers, O. (1984). *Occupational Therapy in the Treatment of Adult Hemiplegia.* Rockville, CO: Aspen.

Hardy, M., Moran, C., & Merritt, W. (1982). Desensitization of the traumatized hand. *Virginia Medical Journal, 109,* 134–137.

Jongbloed, L., Stacey, S., & Brighton, C. (1989). Stroke rehabilitation: Sensorimotor integrative treatment versus functional treatment. *American Journal of Occupational Therapy, 43,* 391–397.

Manske, P. R. (1999). The sense of touch. *Journal of Hand Surgery, 24A,* 213–214 (editorial).

May, B. J. (1996). *Amputations and Prosthetics: A Case Study Approach.* Philadelphia: Davis.

Merzenich, M. M., & Jenkins, W. M. (1993). Reorganization of cortical representations of the hand following alterations of skin inputs induced by nerve injury, skin island transfers, and experience. *Journal of Hand Therapy, 6,* 89–104.

Nakada, M., & Uchida, H. (1997). Case study of a five-stage sensory reeducation program. *Journal of Hand Therapy, 10,* 232–239.

Neistadt, M. E., & Seymour, S. G. (1995). Treatment activity preferences of occupational therapists in adult physical dysfunction settings. *American Journal of Occupational Therapy, 49,* 437–443.

Robertson, S. L., & Jones, L. A. (1994). Tactile sensory impairments and prehensile function in subjects with left-hemisphere cerebral lesions. *Archives of Physical Medicine and Rehabilitation, 75,* 1108–1117.

Robinson, S., & McPhee, S. (1986). Case report: Treating the patient with digital hypersensitivity. *American Journal of Occupational Therapy, 40,* 285–287.

Rosén, B., Lundborg, G., Dahlin, L. B., Holmberg, J., & Karlson, B. (1994). Nerve repair: Correlation of restitution of functional sensibility with specific cognitive capacities. *Journal of Hand Surgery (British), 19B,* 452–458.

Shieh, S.-J., Chiu, H.-Y., Lee, J.-W., & Hsu, H.-Y. (1995). Evaluation of the effectiveness of sensory reeducation following digital replantation and revascularization. *Micorsurgery, 16,* 578–582.

Sloan, H. L., & Abel, R. J. (1998). Getting in touch with impaired foot sensibility. *Nursing, 28(11),* 50–51.

U.S. Dept. of Health and Human Services (1995). *Clinical Practice Guideline: Post-Stroke Rehabilitation* (AHCPR Publication 95-0662). Rockville, MD: Author.

Vermeij, G. J. (1999). The world according to the hand: Observation, art, and learning through the sense of touch. *Journal of Hand Surgery, 24A,* 215–218.

Vinograd, A., Taylor, E., & Grossman, S. (1962). Sensory retraining of the hemiplegic hand. *American Journal of Occupational Therapy, 16,* 246–250.

Waylett-Rendall, J. (1995). Desensitization of the traumatized hand. In J. M. Hunter, E. J. Mackin, & A. D. Callahan (Eds.), *Rehabilitation of the Hand: Surgery and Therapy* (4th ed., pp. 693–700). St. Louis: Mosby.

Wood, H. (1969). Prevention of deformity in the insensitive hand: The role of the therapist. *American Journal of Occupational Therapy, 23,* 488–489.

Yekutiel, M., & Guttman, E. (1993). A controlled trial of the retraining of the sensory function of the hand in stroke patients. *Journal of Neurology, Neurosurgery, and Psychiatry, 56,* 241–244.

Yerxa, E., Barber, L., Diaz, O., Black, W., & Azen, S. (1983). Development of a hand sensitivity test for the hypersensitive hand. *American Journal of Occupational Therapy, 37,* 176–181.

28

Optimizing Vision, Visual Perception, and Praxis Abilities

Lee Ann Quintana

LEARNING OBJECTIVES

After studying this chapter, the reader will be able to do the following:

1. Identify and describe specific treatments for **low vision** and oculomotor dysfunction.
2. Identify and describe five treatment approaches for unilateral neglect.
3. Identify and describe specific treatment for apraxia, including limb, constructional and dressing apraxia.

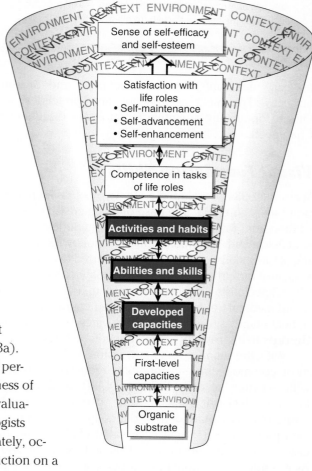

*O*ccupational therapists working with adults with brain injury have traditionally emphasized evaluation and treatment of perceptual dysfunction (Abreu & Toglia, 1987; Warren, 1993a). Although the literature on the identification and evaluation of perceptual dysfunction is extensive, information on the effectiveness of treatment is limited. Much of the research on diagnosis and evaluation has been carried out by psychologists and neuropsychologists who have only recently begun to focus on function. Unfortunately, occupational therapists, who see the effects of perceptual dysfunction on a person's daily living skills, have been slow to generate research, hence support for their treatment.

Remediation of perceptual deficits generally falls under the realm of cognitive rehabilitation, which is provided by occupational therapists, speech and language pathologists, neuropsychologists, and psychologists (Harley et al., 1992). Historically, occupational therapists have emphasized the area of perception, whereas speech and language pathologists and psychologists have emphasized cognition.

Rather than focus on higher-level perceptual skills, this chapter discusses specific treatment for visual foundation skills including low vision, and ocular motor dysfunction, unilateral neglect and

---

GLOSSARY

Anchoring—Method of providing a cue on the side contralateral to the brain damage in the presence of unilateral neglect.

Chaining—Method by which a task is broken down into steps. Patients learn the first step, then the next, and then put the two together, after which they learn the third step and put them all together, and so on. In backward chaining, the therapist completes the task except for the last step, which the patient does; then the therapist completes all except the last two steps, which the patient does; and so on.

Extinction—Phenomenon of neglect that occurs when stimuli are presented in both visual fields or both sides of space at one time and only one stimulus is reported, whereas if presented to either side individually the patient reports the stimulus.

Fresnel prism—Temporary prism used with a patient with hemianopsia or unilateral neglect; applied to the patient's glasses, it shifts the visual field toward the intact side.

Low vision—Any condition in which a person's vision is not adequate for his or her needs.

Occlusion—Covering of part or all of the visual field of the eye.

Prism—Type of lens that is thicker on one side than the other; purpose is to bend light and move the image coming onto the fovea.

Vision therapy—Intervention generally prescribed and carried out by or under the supervision of the eye care professional.

---

apraxia, including limb, constructional, and dressing apraxias. Treatment approaches and principles specific to optimizing cognitive function are discussed in Chapter 29.

Visual Foundation Skills

Warren (1993a) developed a hierarchy of visual perception (see Figure 7-1). The base of this hierarchy consists of the visual foundation skills, which include acuity, visual fields, and oculomotor function. Following a screening of these skills, patients may be referred to an eye care specialist for further evaluation and diagnosis of deficits. These specialists diagnose the problem and may recommend medical treatment, such as medication or surgery; optical changes; use of assistive devices; and/or **vision therapy** to improve the visual function of the patient.

With the aging population, vision loss is the third most common chronic condition requiring assistance with activities of daily living (ADL) (Colenbrander & Fletcher, 1995). At the same time, people may not be aware of or complain of their difficulty, just accepting it as a part of aging. Some age-related changes and diseases increase the likelihood of vision loss (Table 28-1). As a result, occupational therapists work with many patients who have vision loss of one kind or another and who may or may not be labeled as having low vision.

Low Vision

"Low vision can be considered any condition in which a person's visual function is not adequate for his or her visual needs" (Kern & Miller, 1997, p. 495). Based on acuity, low vision (LV) covers anywhere from 20/80 to

TABLE 28-1 Age-Related Changes in Vision	
Cataracts	Acuity can be good, but decreased contrast sensitivity with clouding of the lenses occurs. Surgical treatment is typically successful.
Glaucoma	Results in decreased peripheral vision; generally controlled medically.
Diabetic neuropathy	Bleeding from small blood vessels in retina leads to serious vision loss.
Age-related macular degeneration	Results in loss of central vision; no effective medical or surgical treatment.
Lens tends to yellow	Changes color perception; glare may be a problem.

total blindness, which denotes **no** residual vision at all (Box 28-1) (Colenbrander & Fletcher, 1995; Kern & Miller, 1997).

The focus of occupational therapy in LV rehabilitation is "training the patient to use remaining vision as efficiently and effectively as possible to complete daily activities and includes training in use of optical devices" (Warren, 1995, p. 877). Occupational therapy treatment includes environmental adaptation, compensatory techniques, assistive devices, and patient and family education (Warren, 1999b).

Most occupational therapists do not specialize in treating LV per se but rather encounter LV as a complication in patients with other functional impairments and medical conditions (Kern & Miller, 1997). They are in a unique position to aid LV specialists (Box 28-1) by

BOX 28-1
Low Vision Definitions

Normal Vision

▶ Normal: 20/12, 20/16, 20/20, 20/25; able to read a standard letter size at a standard distance (e.g., approximately 8-point print at a 40 cm)

▶ Near normal: 20/30 to 20/60; generally able to read newsprint by bringing the print closer (may need stronger reading prescription)

Low Vision

▶ Moderately low vision: 20/80 to 20/160; must bring the print very close, which isn't comfortable for prolonged use, but can maintain nearly normal reading speeds with assistive devices (i.e., base in prisms, reading glasses, magnifiers).

▶ Severely low vision: 20/200 to 20/400; must bring print so close that binocularity is no longer possible and person must use the best eye to read; as a result, reading is slower than normal and vision substitution (i.e., listening to the radio rather than reading) comes into use.

▶ Profoundly low vision: 20/500 to 20/1000; must bring print to within less than 2 inches, so reading is limited to essential materials; use of video magnification may be mandatory as well as use of vision substitution.

Blindness

▶ Near blindness: 20/1250 to 20/2500; vision is unreliable and is used as an adjunct to other senses; emphasis is on vision substitution techniques and devices.

▶ Total blindness: no residual vision at all.

Reference: Colenbrander, A., & Fletcher, D. C. (1995). Basic concepts and terms for low vision rehabilitation. *American Journal of Occupational Therapy, 49,* 865–869.

Low Vision Specialists

Rehabilitation Teacher

Emphasis on effect of visual impairment on ADL, patient and family. Teach techniques, technology, and use of devices for persons with low vision or blindness.

Orientation and Mobility (O & M) Specialist

Teach orientation techniques (use of sensory information to determine position in space relative to the environment) and mobility skills (use of canes, sighted guides, travel aids, dog guides) for safe and independent travel.

Rehabilitation Counselor

Provide counseling related to occupation and employment; provide career guidance; assist with job placement (from teaching interviewing skills to adjusting to the workplace).

Low Vision Assistant

Demonstrate and teach patient use of and maintenance of prescribed optical and nonoptical devices.

Reference: Kern, T., & Miller, N. W. (1997). Occupational therapy and collaborative interventions for adults with low vision. In M. Gentile (Ed.), *Functional Visual Behavior: A Therapist's Guide to Evaluation and Treatment Options* (pp. 493–536). Bethesda, MD: American Occupational Therapy Association.

TABLE 28-2
Environmental Factors and Adaptations

Lighting	Care must be taken not to increase glare. Move closer to task. Increase lighting.
Contrast	Change the background to increase contrast. Use different colors (e.g., blue plates on a white place mat).
Pattern	Keep the environment uncluttered and simple.
Task demands	Break it down, start with something simple, and gradually increase the demands.
Print size	Enlarge print, increase contrast, increase print quality.
Working distance	Important for both near and far activities, especially with bifocal and trifocal lenses, which are distance specific. Normal working distance is about 16 inches.

providing input on the patient's functional impairment and how it may affect the selection and use of assistive devices. For example, the patient with tremors may not benefit from a hand-held magnifier or may require certain positioning before using the device. Occupational therapists should have supervision and/or specialized training to recommend and train patients in use of prescribed LV aids (Kern & Miller, 1997).

Many basic self-care activities can be completed with minimal vision, but LV becomes more of a problem with such ADL as meal preparation, managing finances, and community activities. Generally, when working with patients who have LV, we should consider both the functional implications and environmental factors involved (Lampert & Lapolice, 1995). For example, patients with poor contrast sensitivity require increased contrast and lighting and have difficulty with curbs, stairs, and finding objects in low light, while a person with visual field loss has more difficulty in a busy, moving environment. Environmental factors (Table 28-2) can be manipulated to improve the person's ability to perform the task. For example, with the patient who is having difficulty with meal preparation, consider changing the lighting, marking the controls with bright contrasting colors, organizing the kitchen and keeping items in their assigned places, and marking containers with large-print labels.

In addition to manipulation of the environment, compensatory techniques include use of optical devices, such as lenses and telescopes, and nonoptical devices, such as large print, contrasting tape to mark stair steps, felt-tip pen, and a computer (Beaver & Mann, 1995). The patient and family should be taught what the limitations are and how to compensate and manipulate the environment so that they can transfer the techniques to new situations as they arise.

Ocular Motor Dysfunction

Ocular motor dysfunction typically results in diplopia, or double vision. Treatment includes lenses, **prisms**, or **occlusion**. Lenses are used to treat a variety of refractive, accommodative, and binocular disorders. In most cases, they are used as a means of compensation to allow the person to function in spite of the disorder (Scheiman, 1997). A prism is a type of lens that is thicker on one side than the other. Its purpose is to bend the light coming into the eye, moving the image onto the fovea, allowing single vision. Lenses and prisms are recommended by the eye care professional, who is responsible for strength of the lenses and prisms and any exercise programs. The occupational therapist assists the patient with follow-through of the eye care professional's recommendations and encourages compliance with the wearing schedule.

Occlusion should be carried out in consultation with the eye care professional. It may be either total or partial. Total occlusion is achieved by means of a patch or opaque tape on the patient's glasses (Fig. 28-1). Compliance with this method is often poor for these reasons: (1) Total occlusion can cause patients to feel off balance because of loss of peripheral and central vision input to the central nervous system, and it reduces depth perception. (2) Monocularity can cause discomfort, especially when the dominant eye is occluded (Warren, 1999a). The recommendation is to avoid total occlusion if at all possible (Hellerstein & Fishman, 1997) and if it is necessary, to alternate occlusion between the eyes every hour (Warren, 1999a). Partial occlusion appears to have better compliance. In this case, an opaque material added to the patient's glasses blocks input to the central visual field, leaving the peripheral field unobstructed (Fig. 28-2). Since diplopia in the central visual field is the most bothersome, the tape is applied to the nasal portion, of the glasses of the nondominant eye (Warren, 1999a). As the patient focuses on a target, the tape is applied as far centrally as the patient reports diplopia. As the muscles get stronger, the occluded area is decreased. When using occlusion, the patient should do range of

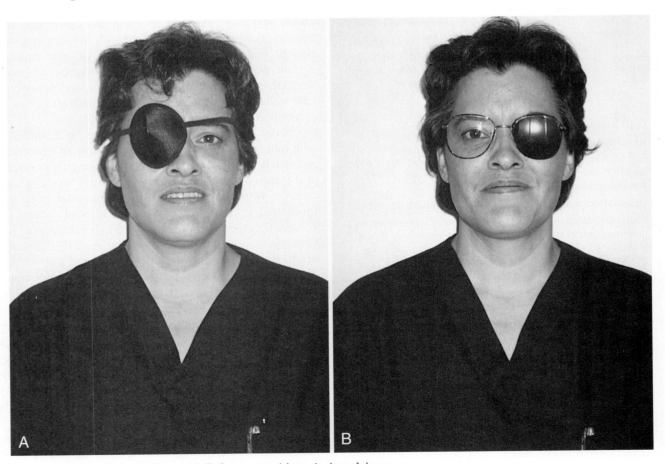

Figure 28-1 Total occlusion. **A.** Pirate patch. **B.** Opaque material covering lens of glasses.

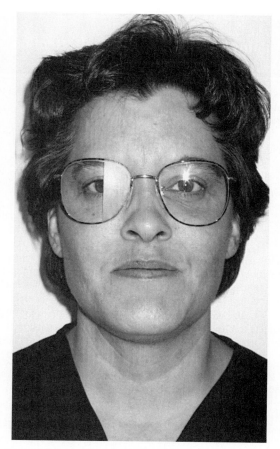

Figure 28-2 A method of partial occlusion to alleviate diplopia.

motion exercises to prevent contractures to the unaffected eye. Warren (1999a) recommends that exercises first be done with the unaffected eye covered and then with both eyes together.

Vision therapy "is an organized regimen utilized to treat a number of neuromuscular, neurophysiological, and neurosensory conditions that interfere with visual function" (Scheiman, 1997, p. 171). It is generally used to treat disorders of binocular vision, accommodation, ocular motility, strabismus, and visual information processing (Scheiman, 1999). The occupational therapist should provide vision therapy, especially involving lenses, prisms, and occlusion, only under the supervision of an eye care professional (Hellerstein & Fishman, 1999).

Unilateral Neglect

Unilateral neglect (UN) has a variety of names, including hemi-inattention, hemispatial neglect, and unilateral spatial agnosia. It is manifested by a failure to respond or orient to stimuli presented contralateral to a brain lesion (Heilman et al., 1993). It is observed functionally in the patient who eats the food on only half of the plate,

shaves only one side of the face, and walks into objects on the side contralateral to the brain lesion.

The treatment of unilateral neglect can be approached in any of several ways. First, the patient must be aware of the problem. If aware that they have a problem, many of these patients can voluntarily orient, even though they have difficulty with automatic orienting (Ladavas et al., 1994). If they are unaware and unable to orient voluntarily or automatically, the only recourse is to modify and simplify the environment (Warren, 1999a).

Some of the early work on the treatment of neglect was done by Weinberg et al. (1977), who developed a training program that included reading, writing, and calculation. It was expanded to include sensory awareness and spatial organization and tasks to increase complex visual perception (Weinberg, et al., 1979, 1982). Unfortunately, while improvement was seen, it tended to be task specific, with little generalization to other tasks or areas of self-care. It is therefore important to train persons in a functional setting using objects readily available in the environment.

The areas of treatment for neglect include sensory manipulation, attention training, scanning, spatiomotor cueing, patching, prisms, and compensation. Documentation of the effectiveness of these approaches is scarce; even more so is documentation of the influence of treatment on a person's functional ability. Since sensory manipulation, including caloric stimulation, optokinetic stimulation, and use of medication, are not within the scope of occupational therapy practice and the effects so far are transitory and without carryover, this area is not addressed.

Attention Training

One theory of UN is that it is due to a deficit in attention. If this is the case, a treatment program aimed at increasing attention and general level of alertness should improve UN. Robertson et al. (1995) trained eight right-brain-damaged (RBD) patients with UN to self-alert during activities. With 5 hours of training, they could mentally tell themselves to pay attention frequently during tasks. Improvement in UN and sustained attention lasted 1 to 14 days.

In another study, Robertson et al. (1998) found that providing a warning tone as a means of alerting the patient that something was going to happen prior to a task increased perceptual processing and shifting of spatial attention to the left. Another method of self-activation is the patient's use of the contralateral extremity as a cue (e.g., to mark the left side of the page while reading or to move the extremity while walking to increase attention to that side). Robertson et al. (1994)

found that patients who moved their contralateral hand when walking through a doorway exhibited a decrease in neglect.

Scanning

Visual scanning training is frequently used in treatment for UN. This can include paper-and-pencil tasks; computer programs; scanning in a functional setting, such as a grocery store; and use of the Dynavision (Fig. 28-3). Research supports improvement on visual perceptual tasks, reading, and academic work with this type of training, but it does not generalize to gross motor tasks (Wagenaar et al., 1992). The literature indicates that the effects of scanning training are specific to the situation. If the goal is to improve the patient's ability to read or scan at tabletop, tabletop scanning training is appropriate; but if the therapist wants to improve a patient's ability to scan in the community, practice in the community is needed. Warren (1993b) provided guidelines for selection of treatment activities for patients with deficits in visual attention and visual scanning (Table 28-3).

Patients who are being trained to scan must learn to take in the information in an organized manner, such as left to right. **Anchoring** (supplying a cue on the impaired side to indicate starting position) can be used to help the patient bring attention back to the neglected side (Table 28-4). During practice of scanning using cancellation tasks, a structured array (symbols arranged in neat, straight rows across the page) should be used at first, because patients with RBD have difficulty with organized search (Weintraub & Mesulam, 1988). This array can be made increasingly complex (e.g., requesting two target letters, decreasing the spacing between letters, or decreasing the size of the letters) as the patient progresses (Cooke, 1992). Scanning tasks must be practiced in a variety of settings, because patients can

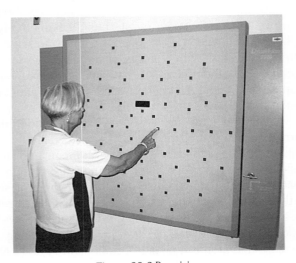

Figure 28-3 Dynavision.

TABLE 28-3
Training Guidelines for Visual Attention and Visual Scanning

Train patients to reorganize their scanning strategy.	Use of anchoring techniques and scanning devices (Weinberg et al., 1979).
Broaden visual field that patient must scan.	Use of activities that require the patient to turn the head or change body positions to complete the task (e.g., scanning items on a kitchen shelf).
Reinforce visual experience with sensorimotor experiences.	Use of activities in which the patient is required to manipulate what is seen (e.g., reach for or touch items scanned).
Emphasize conscious attention to detail and careful inspection of objects.	Use of matching tasks in which the patient may be encouraged to slow down and double-check interpretation of what is seen.
Practice the skill in context to ensure carryover.	Treatment may begin in the clinic, but strategies must be practiced in a variety of real-life situations.

Reference: Warren, M. (1993b). A hierarchical model for evaluation and treatment of visual perceptual dysfunction in adult acquired brain injury, part 2. *American Journal of Occupational Therapy, 47*, 55–66.

improve on a task without an improvement in neglect. An excellent therapeutic intervention is the use of Toglia's (1991) multicontext treatment approach. An example of levels of transfer for a letter, consisting of crossing out a specific letter on a page of four rows of random letters, can be seen in Table 28-5.

Spatiomotor Cueing

If there are two types of neglect, as has been suggested (Bisiach et al., 1990; Coslett et al., 1990; Tegner & Levander, 1991), it is reasonable to expect that each has its own form of treatment. For a patient with primarily a motor or output neglect, encouragement of left-hand activation may reduce neglect to a greater extent than visual perceptual cueing. An example might be having the patient move the left hand (whatever movement is available) while performing a scanning task instead of using a visual anchoring technique (supplying a visual cue on the impaired side to indicate starting position). Robertson and North (1992) found that left motor activation in left hemispace reduced neglect more than did left motor activation in right hemispace, right motor activation in left hemispace, or visual cueing. Robertson (1992) further reported that (1) left lower extremity activation reduced neglect, (2) passive movement of the left extremity had no effect on neglect, (3) bilateral movements produced no effect, and (4) there was no effect if the movement became automatic. In a further study, Robertson and North (1994) found that simultaneous activation of right and left hands produces a phenomenon similar to **extinction**, such that the advantage gained by activating the left hand is lost. Only single left hand movement produced a large reduction in neglect. This may have implications for use of bilateral activities, such as those used in the Bobath technique. Opportunity for unilateral activation of the hemiplegic arm should be provided along with bilateral activation (Robertson & North, 1994).

If the patient has more of a perceptual or input neglect, he or she may benefit from visual cueing such as anchoring (Table 28-4) or reminders to look to the left. Training the patient to use the left upper extremity as an

TABLE 28-5
Levels of Transfer for a Letter Cancellation Task

Transfer Distance	Task
Near	Patient is instructed to cross out the number 5 (number cancellation task)
Intermediate	Four horizontal rows of various coins are presented. Patient is instructed to place a marker over all the nickels (tabletop task)
Far	Patient is presented with a spice rack and is asked to pick out all of the jars that need to be refilled (standing and reaching at kitchen cabinets)
Very far	Patient is evaluated on the ability to initiate spontaneously left-to-right scanning in the context of simple, everyday life tasks (reading four lines in a large-print magazine or locating an item in the medicine cabinet or on a shelf)

TABLE 28-4
Anchoring Technique

Sequence of Cueing	Task Demand
1. A vertical anchoring line is used on the left side; the beginning and ending of the line are sequentially numbered	Patient uses the vertical line to find the beginning and the numbers to avoid skipping lines.
Example: 1 The law was passed to allow the 1 / 2 state to conduct a national FBI 2 / 3 criminal records check before 3 / 4 certifying teachers. 4	
2. A vertical anchoring line is used on the left side; only the beginning of the line is sequentially numbered	Patient uses the vertical line and numbers on the left; the number cue on the right has been eliminated
Example: 1 Family members, followed by / 2 coworkers, are the most / 3 frequent targets of / 4 anger.	
3. A vertical anchoring line is used on the left side	Patient uses only the vertical line to find left side
Example: Environmental groups hope to minimize the divisiveness and avoid mistakes made in the Pacific Northwest.	
4. No cues are provided	Patient must read without any cues
Example: The state distributes its lottery proceeds without regard to which communities generate the revenue.	

Reference: Quintana, L. A. (1995). Remediating perceptual impairments. In C. A. Trombly (Ed.), *Occupational Therapy for Physical Dysfunction* (4th ed., pp. 529–537).

anchor during functional activities provides both a perceptual anchor and a means of left-limb activation (Robertson et al., 1992).

Patching

Eye patching techniques for UN include single-eye patching (Fig. 28-1) and half-field patching (Fig. 28-4). The patient with neglect has covered either the entire eye ipsilateral to the lesion or the hemifield of both eyes (i.e., in the case of left UN, the right eye or right hemifields of both eyes). Patching one eye is believed to influence the central nervous system by way of the superior colliculus (Posner & Rafal, 1987), increasing eye movements to the contralateral side and decreasing neglect. Patching the ipsilateral hemifield is felt to increase activation of the involved hemisphere, resulting in increased attention to the contralateral side.

Butter and Kirsch (1992) found that patching the right eye of patients with left neglect decreased the patients' left neglect score. When lateralized visual stimulation was added, the relative benefits were larger. However, the beneficial effects were present only when the eye patch was on, and the study did not include generalization to functional tasks.

Beis et al. (1999) followed 22 patients with UN: 7 wore glasses with patches covering the right eye, 7 wore glasses with right half-field patches, and 8 controls had no patching. The patches were worn up to 12 hours a day for 3 months. The patients with the right half-field glasses were significantly different from the controls and exhibited an increase in total *Functional Independence*

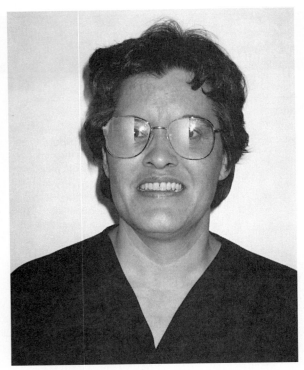

Figure 28-4 Right hemifield patching for left visual neglect.

Measure score (Uniform Data System for Medical Rehabilitation, 1997), and increased time looking to the left.

Arai et al. (1997) also looked at the effects of half-field patching with 10 RBD patients. They found a decrease in neglect, improvement on pencil-and-paper tasks, and good functional return in one patient. Harrell et al. (1995) also found an improvement of neglect in patients wearing goggles with half-field glasses.

In summary, patching has many benefits. It can be used throughout the day during a variety of functional activities and does not rely on memory or training. Patching is simple, inexpensive, and usable in a variety of disciplines.

Prisms

In the case of UN or hemianopsia the prisms are called yoked because the base of the prisms are on the same side of each eye (Scheiman, 1997). They function by shifting the visual field toward the intact side and thereby providing the patient with the ability to see things on the involved side. These prisms may involve the whole visual field or a partial field. They can be the temporary **Fresnel prism**, a flexible plastic sheet with small ridges that can be cut to shape and stuck to the patient's glasses or a permanent prism, part of the patient's prescription. Advantages of the Fresnel prism is that it is inexpensive and temporary, and it can be

applied and removed easily. The disadvantage is that it may distort visual acuity (Hellerstein & Fishman, 1997).

Gianutsos and Suchoff (1997) recommend the use of Fresnel prisms as a temporary or diagnostic device. They have found that partial Fresnel prisms (covering half of the patient's glasses) are not as beneficial as yoked prisms ground into the patient's prescription.

Rossetti et al. (1998) used prisms to shift the visual field (VF) to the right in 16 RBD patients with left UN. Initially the patients exhibited a shift to the left when pointing straight ahead. Following adaptation, patients were given tasks including line bisection, line cancellation, copying, drawing from memory, and reading. Patients in the experimental group exhibited an improvement in neglect that was maintained for 2 hours. Rossi et al. (1990) found that the use of Fresnel prisms improved visual perception in stroke patients with homonymous hemianopsia or unilateral visual neglect.

Compensation

Compensation can be environmental or cognitive. Adaptation of the environment includes such things as arranging the patient's bed so that the uninvolved side is toward the activity in the room and always interacting with the patient on the uninvolved side. While this may be a good idea initially to evaluate patients and to keep them from harming themselves, it does nothing to help patients overcome the deficit. It is recommended that both the remedial and adaptive approaches be used.

Cognitive compensation includes metacognitive training (Toglia, 1991), use of videotaped feedback (Söderback et al., 1992), or sometimes teaching the patient a routine to complete a specific activity (i.e., donning a shirt) with patients cognitively cueing themselves through each step. Patients must be aware that there is a problem before they can use compensatory techniques (Crosson et al., 1989; Tham et al., 2000). These techniques must be practiced, and eventually, if the patient becomes an active problem solver, the techniques can be generalized to new situations.

Apraxia

Apraxia is the inability to carry out purposeful movement in the presence of intact sensation, movement, and coordination (Heilman & Rothi, 1993). Three types of apraxia are addressed: limb, constructional, and dressing.

Limb Apraxia

Whereas there are volumes of literature describing apraxia, little is written on treatment. Treatment recommendations are usually based on neurobiological principles, but they have not been tested in controlled research to determine outcome (Farber, 1993). The lack of research on treatment is most likely a result of the following (Maher & Ochipa, 1997):

▶ Many patients are unaware of the deficit (involvement of the nondominant extremity) or don't complain (often associated with aphasia).

▶ Many treatment personnel believe that patients will recover spontaneously.

▶ The method of identification of apraxia is usually by pantomime (which we do not use on a day-to-day basis) and praxis usually improves with tool use. Therefore, many believe that it will have little effect on the patient's life.

The therapist should ask whether the patient's clumsiness and/or difficulty with gestures interferes with daily living skills. If so, this area should be addressed. In the case of the patient who has difficulty with actual tool use, the need for treatment is more obvious. Manipulation of patients' environments or their interaction with the environment is one means of managing apraxia. Usually these changes are related to tool use and/or clumsiness (Table 28-6).

Suggested treatment activities include gross motor activities involving interpretation and use of tactile, kinesthetic, and proprioceptive stimulation to influence motor patterns; manual contact or guiding of the apraxic extremity through the task; and **chaining** (Farber, 1993; Zoltan, 1996). The therapist should keep verbal commands to a minimum and ask the patient to perform activities in the environment in which they would normally be done. Furthermore, the patient can be asked to visualize the movement before attempting to carry it out (Zoltan, 1996). The therapist may have to break down the activity into component parts and teach each part separately; then, as each is learned, the parts are integrated into more complex activities.

In a study using physical manipulation and verbalization of task elements, improvement was noted in areas trained but did not generalize to other tasks (Pilgrim & Humphreys, 1994). Maher & Ochipa (1997) looked at the effects of treatment (verbal instructions, practice, feedback) on specific error types (external configuration, movement, internal configuration) and found that the treatment was task specific. An improvement in one error type did not generalize to another error type, nor did treatment of a specific error type improve across gestures.

Smania et al. (2000) developed a training program consisting of gesture production exercises. Experimental subjects were trained in production of transitive gestures (those involving objects), intransitive symbolic gestures (wave good-bye), and intransitive nonsymbolic gestures (put your hand under your chin). The control subjects received an equal amount of aphasia training. They found a significant improvement on tests of ideational apraxia and ideomotor apraxia that indicated a generalization of the training to untrained tasks. It was thought that their positive results were possibly due to the extensive training, which was aimed at a wide range of gestures and error types. How this training generalized to daily life was not addressed in this study and should be researched further.

Further research on the efficacy and outcome of treatment for apraxia should be carried out. Until then, it appears that while apraxia can be treated, treatment is task specific, should be based on functional relevance of the task, and should take place in its natural environment.

Constructional Apraxia

Patients with constructional apraxia (CA) cannot "correctly draw or assemble parts to form a unitary structure" (Sunderland et al., 1994, p. 916). Difficulty drawing and constructing designs in two and three dimensions may be caused by any number of problems (e.g., executive, perceptual). There is little in the literature on the treatment of CA, possibly because treatment should be based on function and focus on the underlying cause.

Neistadt (1992) compared the effects of adaptive training (preparing snacks and beverages) and remedial training (using parquetry blocks) on head-injured patients' performance. She found that patients who received training with parquetry blocks improved most on the parquetry block test and least on the food preparation task, whereas those who received the functional

---

TABLE 28-6
Management of Apraxic Deficits

If tool use is a problem:
▶ May have to limit patient's access to tools that may be dangerous (e.g., power tools).
▶ Have patient involved in tasks requiring no tools, or a minimum of tools.
▶ Limit the number of tools used for a given task.
▶ Avoid series of tasks.
▶ Have patients perform tasks with which they are most familiar.

If clumsiness, accuracy of production is an issue:
▶ Use proximal movement where ever possible.
▶ Decrease the complexity of the required movement.

Data from Maher, L. M., and Ochipa, C. (1997). Management and treatment of limb apraxia. L. J. G. Rothi and K. M. Heilman (Eds.), *Apraxia: The Neuropsychology of Action* (pp. 75–92). Hove, UK: Psychology.

Case Example

MR. D.: TREATMENT OF VISUAL PROBLEMS AFTER STROKE

Patient Information

Mr. D., a 21-year-old man 15 months post right CVA, participated in an outpatient occupational therapy assessment. These problems were identified: (1) apparent field cut on the left; (2) decreased ocular motor skills, including decreased convergence, decreased accommodation, and inefficient saccades and smooth pursuits; (3) left visual neglect. (Chapter 7 describes the assessment and patient's background.)

Recommendations

The occupational therapist recommended weekly 1-hour treatment sessions for a total of 12 to 16 sessions. In collaboration with Mr. D., the occupational therapist established the following long-term goals: (1) Mr. D. will read his homework with accuracy and good speed. (2) Mr. D. will demonstrate the ability to maneuver throughout familiar and unfamiliar environments independently. (3) Mr. D. will independently use appropriate compensatory strategies for visual field deficit and neglect as needed during functional activities.

Short-Term Goals and Intervention

► **Mr. D. will demonstrate the ability to copy information from 5 feet away to a sheet of paper with 80% accuracy.** Mr. D. is having difficulty with accommodation, which interferes with participation in his college classes, as he cannot copy information from the chalkboard. The task was varied by the size and location of the information on the board, by the density of the information, and by organization of the information. (Mr. D. was a math major, and math problems do not tend to be presented in a well-organized manner on the board). Goal of 80% was met.

► **Mr. D. will maneuver his wheelchair through an unfamiliar environment with minimal verbal cues.**

Since Mr. D. was having difficulty both maneuvering his wheelchair without running into objects on the left side and locating items in the kitchen, it was decided to work on a task that involved both. That is, he was asked to maneuver down a hallway or in a room while being asked to locate items and numbers placed at various heights and locations around the room. Upon recommendation of the optometrist, partial occlusion was used as one means of compensation for the left neglect. Although he was usually able to find 90% to 100% of the objects, it took him a long time to do so. Therefore, he was encouraged to use an organized scanning strategy. He met the goal, requiring minimal verbal cues to locate items on the floor to his left side, and his scanning strategy improved, as evidenced by increased speed of locating objects.

Revised Short-Term Goals

► Mr. D. will copy information from 5 feet away to a sheet of paper with 95% accuracy.
► Mr. D. will copy words from one sheet of paper to another with 90% accuracy.
► Mr. D. will maneuver his wheelchair in unfamiliar environments with two or three verbal cues and independently in familiar environments.

CLINICAL REASONING
in OT Practice

Extending the Benefits of Treatment

After completion of the initial phase of his treatment for decreased ocular motor skills, Mr. D. continued to have occasional problems copying information from the blackboard (approximately 20% of the time). What additional recommendations might the therapist offer to help Mr. D. compensate for these problems in the classroom?

---

training improved more on the food preparation task. The results suggested that learning in adult head-injured men at least 6 months after injury is task specific; this supports the use of the functional approach.

There is information in the literature on how to improve performance on drawing and construction tasks (Hecaen & Assal, 1970; Neistadt, 1989; Warrington et al., 1966; Zoltan, 1996), but as these are not based on function, they appear not to be useful in today's health care market. Some of the ideas, such as practice, use of a

model, use of cues and landmarks, and progressing from simple to complex, can be applied to functional tasks.

Dressing Apraxia

Dressing apraxia refers to inability to dress oneself. Little is written specifically regarding treatment. Treatment generally consists of teaching the patient a pattern of dressing. Cognitive cues, such as using the label to tell front from back and talking through the steps of putting on each item of clothing, are used, and the patient eventually learns through practice (Zoltan, 1996). Cook et al. (1991) described the use of an audiotape and a specific method of stacking (sequencing) clothing to improve dressing in an elderly woman with cognitive and perceptual impairments. If the basis for the dressing apraxia is found to be constructional apraxia, unilateral neglect, or body scheme disturbances, treatment is aimed at ameliorating those deficits.

Summary Review Questions

1. List three compensatory techniques for use with patients with low vision and give two examples of each.
2. You have a patient with double vision. What should you do first?
3. Based on an optometrist's report, your patient's best corrected acuity is 20/160. He has a cataract in the right eye and glaucoma in both eyes, for which he is receiving medication. How may his low vision affect his ability to do self-care, meal preparation, and money management?
4. Summarize the guidelines for visual scanning training.
5. How does the use of occlusion for diplopia differ from that used for unilateral neglect?
6. Your patient with left unilateral neglect is having difficulty finding things in the kitchen cabinets during meal preparation. What activities might you plan for your therapy session?
7. Describe four activities to use with limb apraxia.
8. Your patient is a 40-year-old dentist who has apraxia. He can use tools but is clumsy. How would your treatment of this patient differ from that for the 70-year-old retired man with the same clumsiness?
9. What deficits can cause dressing apraxia? Indicate how intervention may differ according to the hypothesized underlying cause of this problem.
10. Why is it important for occupational therapists to become involved in research?

Acknowledgments

Thanks to Liz Stuewe, MS, OTR, for her input and assistance with preparation of the case study and to Janette Rodriguez, OTR, her assistance with the photographs.

References

Abreu, B. C., & Toglia, J. P. (1987). Cognitive rehabilitation: A model for occupational therapy. *American Journal of Occupational Therapy, 41,* 439–448.

Arai, T., Ohi, H., Sasaki, H., Nobuto, H., & Tanaka, H. (1997). Hemispatial sunglasses: Effect on unilateral spatial neglect. *Archives of Physical Medicine and Rehabilitation, 78,* 230–232.

Beaver, K. A., & Mann, W. C. (1995). Overview of techniques for low vision. *American Journal of Occupational Therapy, 49,* 913–921.

Beis, J.-M., Andre, J.-M., Baumgarten, A., & Challier, B. (1999). Eye patching in unilateral spatial neglect: Efficacy of two methods. *Archives of Physical Medicine and Rehabilitation, 80,* 71–76.

Bisiach, E., Geminiani, G., Berti, A., & Rusconi, M. L. (1990). Perceptual and premotor factors of unilateral neglect. *Neurology, 40,* 1278–1281.

Butter, C. M., & Kirsch, N. (1992). Combined and separate effects of eye patching and visual stimulation on unilateral neglect following stroke. *Archives of Physical Medicine & Rehabilitation, 73,* 1133–1139.

Colenbrander, A., & Fletcher, D. C. (1995). Basic concepts and terms for low vision rehabilitation. *American Journal of Occupational Therapy, 49,* 865–869.

Cook, E. A., Luschen, L., & Sikes, S. (1991). Dressing training for an elderly woman with cognitive and perceptual impairments. *American Journal of Occupational Therapy, 45,* 652–654.

Cooke, D. (1992). Remediation of unilateral neglect: What do we know? *Australian Occupational Therapy Journal, 39,* 19–25.

Coslett, H. B., Bowers, D., Fitzpatrick, E., Haws, B., & Heilman, K. M. (1990). Directional hypokinesia and hemispatial inattention in neglect. *Brain, 113,* 475–486.

Crosson, B., Barco, P. P., Velozo, C. A., Bolesta, M. M., Cooper, P. V., Werts, d., & Brobeck, T. C. (1989). Awareness and compensation in post acute head injury rehabilitation. *Journal of Head Trauma Rehabilitation, 4(3),* 46–54.

Farber, S. (1993, March). *OT Intervention for Individuals With Limb Apraxia.* Paper presented at the AOTA Neuroscience Institute, Baltimore, MD.

Gianutsos, R., & Suchoff, I. B. (1997). Visual fields after brain injury: Management issues for the occupational therapist. In M. Scheiman, (Ed.), *Understanding and Managing Vision Deficits: A Guide for Occupational Therapists* (pp. 333–358). Thorofare, NJ: Slack.

Harley, J. P., Allen, C., Braciszeski, T. L., Cicerone, D. K., Dahlberg, C., Evans, S., Foto, M., Gordon, W. A., Harrington, D., Levin, W., Malec, J. F., Millis, S., Morris, J., Muir, C., Richert, J., Salazar, E., Schiavone, D. A., & Smigielski, J. S. (1992). Guidelines for cognitive rehabilitation. *Neurological Rehabilitation, 2(3),* 62–67.

Harrell, E. H., Kramer-Stutts, T., & Zolten, A. J. (1995). Performance of subjects with left visual neglect after removal of the right visual field using hemifield goggles. *Journal of Rehabilitation, 61(4),* 46–49.

Hecaen, H., & Assal, G. (1970). A comparison of constructive deficits following right and left hemispheric lesions. *Neuropsychologia, 8,* 289–303.

Heilman, K. M., & Rothi, L. J. G. (1993). Apraxia. In K. M. Heilman & E. Valenstein (Eds.), *Clinical Neuropsychology* (3rd ed., pp. 141–163). New York: Oxford University.

Heilman, K. M., Watson, R. T., & Valenstein, E. (1993). Neglect and related disorders. In K. M. Heilman & E. Valenstein (Eds.), *Clinical Neuropsychology* (3rd ed., pp. 279–336). New York: Oxford University.

Hellerstein, L. F., & Fishman, B. I. (1997). Visual rehabilitation for patients with brain injury. In M. Scheiman (Ed.), *Understanding and Managing Vision Deficits: A Guide for Occupational Therapists* (pp. 249–281). Thorofare, NJ: Slack.

Hellerstein, L., & Fishman, B. I. (1999). Collaboration between occupational therapists and optometrists. *Occupational Therapy Practice, 4,* 22–30.

Kern, T., & Miller, N. W. (1997). Occupational therapy and collaborative interventions for adults with low vision. In M. Gentile (Ed.), *Functional Visual Behavior: A Therapist's Guide to Evaluation and Treatment Options* (pp. 493–536). Bethesda, MD: American Occupational Therapy Association.

Ladavas, E., Carletti, M., & Gori, G. (1994). Automatic and voluntary orientating of attention in patients with visual neglect: Horizontal and vertical dimensions. *Neuropsychologia, 32,* 1195-1208.

Lampert, J., & Lapolice, D. J. (1995). Functional considerations in evaluation and treatment of the client with low vision. *American Journal of Occupational Therapy, 49,* 885–890.

Maher, L. M., & Ochipa, C. (1997). Management and treatment of limb apraxia. In L. J. G. Rothi & K. M. Heilman (Eds.), *Apraxia: The Neuropsychology of Action* (pp. 75–92). Hove, U.K.: Psychology.

Neistadt, M. E. (1989). Normal adult performance on constructional praxis training tasks. *American Journal of Occupational Therapy, 43,* 448–455.

Neistadt, M. E. (1992). Occupational therapy treatments for constructional deficits. *American Journal of Occupational Therapy, 46,* 141–148.

Pilgrim, E., & Humphreys, G. W. (1994). Rehabilitation of a case of ideomotor apraxia. In M. J. Riddoch & G. W. Humphreys (Eds.), *Cognitive Neuropsychology and Cognitive Rehabilitation* (pp. 271–285). Hove, UK: Lawrence Erlbaum.

Posner, M. I., & Rafal, R. D. (1987). Cognitive theories of attention and the rehabilitation of attentional deficits. In M. J. Meier, A. L. Benton, & L. Diller (Eds.), *Neuropsychological Rehabilitation After Brain Injury* (pp. 182–201). New York: Churchill Livingston.

Robertson, I. (1992, October). *Treatment of Neglect.* Paper presented at the conference for Evaluation and Treatment of Disorders of Memory, Attention and Visual Neglect, Philadelphia.

Robertson, I. H., Mattingley, J. B., Rorden, C., & Driver, J. (1998). Phasic alerting of neglect patients overcomes their spatial deficit in visual awareness. *Nature, 395,* 169–172.

Robertson, I. H., & North, N. (1992). Spatio-motor cueing in unilateral left neglect: The role of hemispace, hand and motor activation. *Neuropsychologia, 30,* 553–563.

Robertson, I. H., & North, N. T. (1994). One hand is better than two: Motor extinction of left hand advantage in unilateral neglect. *Neuropsychologia, 32,* 1–11.

Robertson, I. H., North, N. T., & Geggie, C. (1992). Spatiomotor cueing in unilateral left neglect: Three case studies of its therapeutic effects. *Journal of Neurology, Neurosurgery, and Psychiatry, 55,* 799–805.

Robertson, I. H., Tegner, R., Goodrich, S. J., & Wilson, C. (1994). Walking trajectory and hand movements in unilateral left neglect: A vestibular hypothesis. *Neuropsychologia, 32,* 1495–1502.

Robertson, I. H., Tegner, R., Tham, K., Lo, A., & Nimmo-Smith, I. (1995). Sustained attention training for unilateral neglect: Theoretical and rehabilitation implications. *Journal of Clinical and Experimental Neuropsychology, 17,* 416–430.

Rossetti, Y., Rode, G., Pisella, L., Farne, A., Li, L., Boisson, D., & Perenin, M. T. (1998). Prism adaptation to a rightward optical deviation rehabilitates left hemispatial neglect. *Nature, 395,* 166–169.

Rossi, P. W., Kheyfets, S., & Reding, M. J. (1990). Fresnel prisms improve visual perception in stroke patients with homonymous hemianopsia or unilateral visual neglect. *Neurology, 40,* 1597–1599.

Scheiman, M. (1997). *Understanding and Managing Vision Deficits: A Guide for Occupational Therapists.* New Jersey: Slack.

Scheiman, M. (1999, March). *Understanding and Managing Visual Deficits: Theory, Screening, Procedures, Intervention Techniques.* Conference of Vision Education Seminars, Jacksonville, FL.

Smania, N., Girardi, F., Domenicali, C., Lora, E., & Aglioti, S. (2000). The rehabilitation of limb apraxia: A study in left-brain-damaged patients. *Archives of Physical Medicine and Rehabilitation, 81,* 379–388.

Söderback, I., Begtsson, I., Ginsburg, E., & Eleholm, J. (1992). Video-feedback in occupational therapy: Its effect in patients with neglect syndrome. *Archives of Physical Medicine and Rehabilitation, 73,* 1140–1146.

Sunderland, A., Tinson, D. & Bradley, L. (1994). Differences in recovery from constructional apraxia after right and left hemisphere stroke? *Journal of Clinical and Experimental Neuropsychology, 16,* 916–920.

Tegner, R., & Levander, M. (1991). Through a looking glass: A new technique to demonstrate directional hypokinesia in unilateral neglect. *Brain, 114,* 1943–1951.

Tham, K., Borell, L., & Gustavsson, A. (2000). The discovery of disability: A phenomenological study of unilateral neglect. *American Journal of Occupational Therapy, 54,* 398–405.

Toglia, J. P. (1991). Generalization of treatment: A multicontext approach to cognitive perceptual impairment in adults with brain injury. *American Journal of Occupational Therapy, 45,* 505–516.

Uniform Data System for Medical Rehabilitation (1997). *Guide for the Uniform Data Set for Medical Rehabilitation.* Buffalo, NY: State University of New York.

Wagenaar, R. C., Van Wierignen, P. C. W., Netelenbos, J. B., Meijer, O. G., & Kuik, D. J. (1992). The transfer of scanning training effects in visual inattention after stroke: Five single-case studies. *Disability and Rehabilitation, 14,* 51–60.

Warren, M. (1993a). A hierarchical model for evaluation and treatment of visual perceptual dysfunction in adult acquired brain injury, part 1. *American Journal of Occupational Therapy, 47,* 42–54.

Warren, M. (1993b). A hierarchical model for evaluation and treatment of visual perceptual dysfunction in adult acquired brain injury, part 2. *American Journal of Occupational Therapy, 47,* 55–66.

Warren, M. (1995). Providing low vision rehabilitation services with occupational therapy and ophthalmology: A program description. *American Journal of Occupational Therapy, 49,* 877–883.

Warren, M. (1999a). *Evaluation and Treatment of Visual Perceptual Dysfunction in Adult Brain Injury, Part 1.* Conference of visABILI-TIES Rehabilitation Services, Nashville, TN.

Warren, M. (1999b). *Occupational Therapy Practice Guidelines for Adults With Low Vision.* Bethesda MD: American Occupational Therapy Association.

Warrington, E. K., James, M., & Kinsbourne, M. (1966). Drawing disability in relation to laterality of cerebral lesion. *Brain, 89,* 53–82.

Weinberg, J., Diller, L., Gordon, W. A., Gerstman, L. J., Liberman, A., Lakin, P., Hodges, G., & Ezrachi, O. (1977). Visual scanning training effect on reading-related tasks in acquired right brain damage. *Archives of Physical Medicine & Rehabilitation, 58,* 479–486.

Weinberg, J., Diller, L., Gordon, W. A., Gerstman, L. J., Liberman, A., Lakin, P., Hodges, G., & Ezrachi, O. (1979). Training sensory awareness and spatial organization in people with right brain damage. *Archives of Physical Medicine & Rehabilitation, 60,* 491–496.

Weinberg, J., Pcasetsky, E., Diller, L., & Gordon, W. (1982). Treating perceptual organization deficits in nonneglecting RBD stroke patients. *Journal of Clinical Psychology, 4,* 59–75.

Weintraub, S., & Mesulam, M. M. (1988). Visual hemispatial inattention: Stimulus parameters and exploratory strategies. *Journal of Neurology, Neurosurgery and Psychiatry, 51,* 1481–1488.

Zoltan, B. (1996). *Vision, Perception and Cognition: A Manual for the Evaluation and Treatment of Neurologically Impaired Adult* (3rd ed.). Thorofare, NJ: Slack.

29

Optimizing Cognitive Abilities

Mary Vining Radomski and Elin Schold Davis

LEARNING OBJECTIVES

After studying this chapter, the reader will be able to do the following:

1. Compare and contrast remedial and adaptive therapy specific to optimizing patients' cognitive abilities.
2. Describe how remedial cognitive retraining can be incorporated into an occupational therapy treatment plan.
3. Analyze how changes in the physical or social context contribute to improved cognitive function.
4. Outline methods for helping patients reestablish routines and habit sequences.
5. Discuss how various compensatory cognitive strategies can be used to override cognitive impairments and inefficiencies.

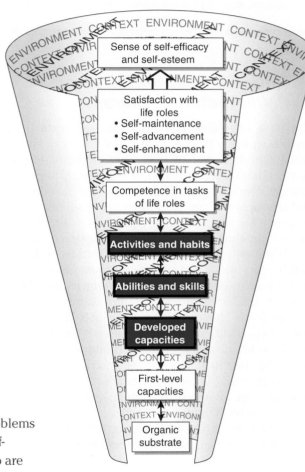

A person's ability to concentrate, remember, and solve problems are central to the ability to fulfill valued self-maintenance, self-advancement, and self-enhancement roles. Many people who are referred to occupational therapy services have organic cognitive impairments or short-term cognitive inefficiencies related to illness, injury, pain, or emotional distress. These impairments and inefficiencies are often the primary barriers to occupational functioning and therefore are the primary targets of occupational intervention. This chapter presents a working definition of cognitive rehabilitation, discusses linkage with occupational therapy, and describes specific approaches used in occupational therapy to optimize cognitive abilities.

GLOSSARY

Cognitive compensatory strategies—Array of techniques, devices, and aids that people use to circumvent cognitive limitations.

Cognitive rehabilitation—Multidisciplinary field and a broad category of intervention methods aimed at improving cognitive function.

Cognitive retraining—Remedial therapy aimed at restoring cognitive capacities through practice, exercise, and stimulation.

Habits—Automatic motor sequences and behaviors that people perform with little or no conscious awareness.

Routines—Semiautomatic clusters of activities that are prompted by physical context and fairly consistent for each individual on a day-to-day basis.

Cognitive Rehabilitation and Links With Occupational Therapy

The term **cognitive rehabilitation** describes both a multidisciplinary field and a broad category of intervention methods aimed at improving cognitive function. Many rehabilitation disciplines, including occupational therapy, speech–language pathology, special education, and neuropsychology, attempt to help patients optimize cognitive abilities. With many parallels to occupational therapy treatment planning, contemporary cognitive rehabilitation practice places less emphasis on the drill and practice models of its beginnings and more emphasis on human cognition and its interfaces with health, emotion, individual differences, and context (American Occupational Therapy Association, 1999; Wilson, 1997). For occupational therapists, a patient's problems with cognition are always incorporated into a broader treatment plan that may also address motor, perceptual, or emotional issues. Whether occupational therapists characterize their efforts to optimize cognitive function as cognitive rehabilitation, occupational therapy, or both, the aim is the same: to help patients fulfill their own role aspirations with minimal interference from cognitive limitations.

The development of cognitive rehabilitation has been and continues to be plagued by the lack of standard, agreed-upon operational definitions (Carney et al., 1999). However, the Commission on Accreditation of Rehabilitation Facilities (CARF) provides a useful working definition for this chapter. Cognitive rehabilitation is a "functionally oriented service of therapeutic activities . . .[that] are directed to achieve functional changes by reinforcing, strengthening, or reestablishing previously learned patterns of behavior or establishing new patterns of cognitive activity or mechanisms to compensate for impaired neurological systems" (CARF, 1999, p. 359).

Treatment Approaches in Occupational Therapy to Optimize Cognitive Function

Occupational therapists use the same broad approaches described in Chapters 1 and 19 to optimize patients' cognitive abilities: remedial therapy and adaptive therapy, further characterized as changing the context, establishing habits and behavioral routines, and acquiring compensatory skills and strategies. In selecting a primary treatment approach to optimize cognitive abilities, therapists ask themselves a number of questions about the patient and the anticipated outcomes of therapy including these:

► Are the patient's problems attributed to organic impairments in primary cognitive abilities or characterized as a shorter-term cognitive inefficiency?
► How are other systems, such as motor, visual, and perceptual systems, functioning? (Schwartz, 1995)
► Who is considered the primary recipient of treatment: the patient, the patient–family team, or the significant other?
► Is the patient aware of the cognitive problems and motivated to improve function in this area?
► Does the patient appear to have the capacity to transfer skills learned in therapy to new situations? Does the patient have the resources (e.g., time, financial, emotional) to participate in therapy for the length of time necessary to achieve transfer of training?

Each approach to improving cognitive function is described in detail (Table 29-1). However, in practice it is almost impossible to separate these approaches (Ben-Yishay & Diller, 1993). Consider a patient who is learning to use a day planner to compensate for memory impairment. While the primary treatment approach centers on acquiring compensatory skills and strategies, successful outcome depends on teaching the patient's family to provide the right prompts and reinforcement (changing the social context) and creating a daily planning routine in which the person reviews and adds notes to the planner (establishing behavioral routines). Furthermore, it is possible that the learning process challenges the attentional and memory systems in such a way as to stimulate neuroanatomical and physiological changes (remediation).

Remediate Deficits

Remedial therapy for cognitive problems, or **cognitive retraining**, is the therapeutic effort to restore cognitive capacities through practice, exercise, and stimulation (Wilson, 1997) in the hope that these gains will translate to improvements in the tasks and activities to which these capacities and abilities relate (Radomski, 1994). In this approach, the therapist identifies impaired cognitive domains, such as attention or memory, and provides graded activities that challenge the weakened process. Cognitive exercises, typically pencil-and-paper, tabletop, or computer-based, are a means of attacking the deficient cognitive capacity but may have little inherent value in and of themselves (Sohlberg & Mateer, 1989). The therapist collects data on the patient's performance, such as percent correct and speed of performance. As

the patient masters therapy tasks or meets criterion levels, the therapist raises the complexity or difficulty of the cognitive exercises, still challenging the original weakened process or capacity (Sohlberg & Mateer, 1989). This progression culminates with rehearsal of a naturalistic activity supported by the previously weakened cognitive capacity (Sohlberg & Mateer, 1989). This intervention sequence is founded on the premise that one cognitive capacity may be treated in isolation from other dimensions of cognition and is predicated on the therapist's ability to select the foundational skills that actually respond to therapy.

Graded Cognitive Exercises

To optimize cognitive capacities, Abreu and Toglia (1987) recommended that therapists present targeted exercises and activities that "gradually increase demands on the information processing system" (p. 443). They described three phases of activity presentation in an effort to illustrate the progression from simple to complex and automatic to effortful and the ability to respond to the external environment versus the ability to manipulate the internal environment. Blundon and Smits (2000) surveyed Canadian occupational therapy programs and found the most common cognitive rehabilitation activities to be pencil-and-paper tasks, such as mazes and work sheets; computer-based activities; and board games.

TABLE 29-1

Use of Multiple Treatment Approaches to Help a Brain Injury Survivor Optimize Cognitive Abilities

Treatment Approaches[a]	Remedial Therapy	Adaptive Therapy		
Intervention	Remediate impairment	Change context	Establish behavioral routines, habits	Learn cognitive compensatory strategies
Treatment fraction[b]	10%	25%	35%	30%
Example	Given recency of injury and Mr. B.'s interest in repairing his memory, therapist used paper-and-pencil activities as part of his homework geared to challenging and improving his attentional system.	Therapist helped Mr. B. determine how to change physical environment to optimize attention and concentration. Therapist also attempted to change social context by teaching Mr. B.'s brother appropriate ways to provide cues.	Developed checklists specific to key self-maintenance tasks (initially ADL and use of the planner) in hope that with enough consistent repetition, Mr. B. would maintain habits and routines without cues.	Assisted Mr. B. to select a number of memory prostheses, including day planner, alarm watch, and medication container; provided numerous opportunities to use these strategies in increasingly novel situations.

[a]See Chapter 1.
[b]See Chapter 19.
ADL, activities of daily living.

Pencil-and-Paper and Tabletop Activities

Therapists often use mazes, math, or seek-and-find work sheets to challenge weakened cognitive capacities. Here is an example of using a worksheet to address attention and concentration: The patient is presented with a worksheet consisting of random symbols and letters spread across the page in rows. The patient is instructed to find and circle a specific target, such as a triangle. The therapist encourages the patient to work as quickly as possible while maintaining accurate performance. The therapist times the activity and episodes of off-task behavior, and together the patient and therapist score the worksheet for accuracy (Fig. 29-1). Because a remediation approach requires a great deal of repetition and rehearsal to be effective (Chen et al., 1997), the patient performs attention-challenging exercises and activities at home as well as at subsequent sessions. Table 29-2 has other examples of using work sheets and tabletop tasks to improve attention.

Computer-Based Exercises

Computer-based cognitive remediation optimizes the ability to provide repetition and consistency of administration of cognitive stimuli (Fig. 29-2) (Goldstein et al., 1996). Specialized cognitive remediation software, such as *Captains Log* and the *NeuroXercise System* (see

Resources), are evaluation and treatment modules that target underlying cognitive capacities, such as attention and memory. They use a combination of graded game-style attention-friendly activities. One activity, for example, requires the patient to scan the screen from left to right and top to bottom and respond each time a target that is the same color as the border appears. The speed and length of presentation progress as the patient improves task performance. Commercial computer games also stimulate attention, memory, and processing speed at a more affordable price. Specialized cognitive rehabilitation software, however, collects data on patient performance, such as speed of response and accuracy over trials, a feature not available with commercial computer games. It is advisable to select software (specialized modules or computer games) that include disks the patients can use on their own for independent practice.

Effectiveness of Cognitive Remediation

Proponents of this approach suggest that remediation that targets specific cognitive deficits enhances the biological recovery mechanisms during acute recovery from brain injury and facilitates functional reorganization of the brain regardless of the time post injury (Sohlberg & Mateer, 1989). Unfortunately, neither claim

Task description: Check writing worksheets		
Session date: 10/20 Time of day: 10 a.m. Location: O.T. clinic		
Target behavior	**Tally:** The frequency of behaviors	**Comments/observations:** Describe performance antecedents or patterns
◆ **Off Task – a break in ability to maintain attention (internal)**	3	Occasionally D.B. simply stopped working + didn't restart until therapist offered specific cues
◆ **Off Task – in response to an interruption (external source)**	5	Pt chose to sit near entrance to clinic — looked away from work every time someone entered
◆ **Accuracy rate**	62 %	Accuracy improved mid-task p̄ therapist reinstruction
◆ **Performance time**	Total work time – 18 minutes	

Figure 29-1 A work sheet is used to record observations during performance of cognitive retraining activities.

TABLE 29-2 Treatment Activities for Attention	
Type	**Activity**
Sustained attention (tasks that require consistent response to either visually or auditorily presented stimuli)	The therapist reads a list of letters; the patient indicates hearing the letter *b*; then every time he or she hears a *b* or an *h*; then every time he or she hears each of those letters come just after the one before it in the alphabet (e.g., *k, q, g, **h**, m, l, v, a, **b***)
Selective attention (tasks that incorporate distracting or irrelevant information)	While patient is performing a task (e.g., math exercises, pegboard designs) a tape is played that may distract the patient (e.g., conversations, news broadcast, music); the tape used is determined individually, depending on the patient's interests.
Alternating attention (tasks that require flexibility, redirection, and reallocation of attention)	Big-little task: the words *big* and *little* are written in big and little letters; the patient is to read what is written as words or size (e.g., *BIG, little, LITTLE, big* when read as words is "big, little, little, big" but when read as size is "big, little, big, little"). The patient is given a sheet with numbers on it and is asked to cross out the even numbers; at some point while doing this he or she is asked to change and cross out the odd numbers
Divided attention (tasks with multiple kinds of information or those that involve simultaneous use of two or more tasks)	The patient is asked to sort cards by suit and specific cards (e.g., those that contain the letter *e*: 1s, 3s, 5s, 8s) must also be turned as they are sorted

(Sohlberg & Mateer, 1989.)

has been well supported empirically, nor has a definite link been established between improvements in specific cognitive capacities and functional performance (Carney et al., 1999; Malec & Basford, 1996). However, there is some evidence that drill and practice in areas of attention and memory are correlated with improvement in these areas on neuropsychological testing (Carney et al.).

Based on their review of studies of outcomes post acute brain injury, Malec and Basford (1996) suggested that there may be secondary benefits from a remedial approach. They posited that it may facilitate the patient's initial acceptance that a problem exists and promote improved awareness of deficits (Box 29-1). Similarly, Gianutsos (1992) suggested that therapy should begin with remediation as the goal "even if that goal is remote" (p. 27), because if the patient is satisfied that every attempt was made to restore function, he or she may be more inclined to work on compensating for the deficit.

In summary, when planning treatment aimed at optimizing cognitive function, occupational therapists consider the likelihood that a patient's cognitive capacities are expected to be restored to premorbid status through time, natural healing, and/or structured therapeutic stimulation. Because research regarding intervention to remediate cognitive capacities is inconclusive, if not discouraging, therapists should always incorporate adaptive therapy into their treatment fractions (see Chapter 19). In cognitive rehabilitation, adaptive therapy is generally believed to be more efficacious in improving patients' functioning than remedial therapy (Carney et al., 1999; Salazar et al., 2000).

Adaptive Therapy

As previously mentioned, adaptive therapy is characterized as intervention aimed at circumventing impairments and inefficiencies through changes in context, habits and routines, and strategies. These three synergistic focuses of intervention are based on what we describe as cognitive ergonomics, that is, use of human information processing principles to decrease the demands on working memory.

Change the Context
When intervention centers on changing the context, the therapist or family makes changes that lower the cognitive demands placed on the patient to optimize his or her

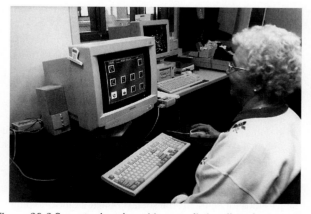

Figure 29-2 Computer-based cognitive remediation allows for extensive rehearsal and repetition.

BOX 29-1
PROCEDURES FOR PRACTICE

Helping Patients Improve Self-Awareness

Occupational therapists use a variety of techniques to help patients become more aware of their cognitive strengths and weaknesses:

- Appreciate the different contributions of organically based unawareness and adjustment-based denial. Anticipate that sometimes as patients become more aware of impairments, they may feel emotional distress, including depression and anxiety (Fleming & Strong, 1995).
- Recognize levels of awareness and focus intervention on helping the patient move up the hierarchy (see Chapter 8). For example, therapists try to help patients who are unaware of their cognitive impairments first to develop intellectual awareness of the problem and then to progress toward emergent or anticipatory awareness (Crosson et al., 1989).
- Create opportunities for the patient to monitor and judge his or her own performance, analyze the results, and determine what to continue or do differently next time. Dougherty and Radomski (1993) recommended a graded approach to performance analysis that consisted of three levels: (1) using an answer key to self-correct, (2) answering multiple choice questions about various aspects of performance after performing the task, (3) making predictions about performance ahead of time, comparing actual performance to predictions, and determining how to modify performance in the future.
- Introduce therapeutic structured failure when appropriate. That is, do not interfere with the natural consequences of the cognitive impairment during selected supervised activities. For example, if the patient fails to initiate a cognitive compensatory strategy in response to general or specific cues, do not provide further instruction but rather create an opportunity for the patient to observe what happens when the strategy is not used.
- Collaborate with family members to provide feedback. Some family members should focus on maintaining harmony in the household and appropriately prefer that the therapist assume the responsibility of providing any negative feedback to the patient. In other cases, family members or coworkers are so afraid of offending or discouraging the patient that they insulate the patient from any and all challenges or avoid mentioning errors and as a result deprive him or her of information that might improve self-awareness.
- Respect the patient's readiness to participate in therapy. Avoid badgering the patient into improved awareness of deficits by maintaining a therapeutic partnership so that he or she will want to return for services in the future.

BOX 29-2
PROCEDURES FOR PRACTICE

Changing the Context

Suggestions for changing the physical context include the following:

- Place the notebook open to today's page in a consistent spot on the counter.
- Use a large wall calendar so all family members can check for needed information.
- Place items in consistent places by using hooks or baskets as receptacles.
- Install a Rangetimer set at a 30-minute delay. The stove will automatically turn off after 30 minutes, eliminating the risk of forgetting to turn a burner off.
- Remove clutter to minimize the stimulus arousal properties of work space.

Suggestions for changing the social context include helping family members do the following:

- Shift roles. The spouse may fill out the schedule each day before leaving for work. The patient's responsibility may beto refer to the schedule regularly and retrieve the information at the correct time. The expectation that the patient will record information on the schedule has been eliminated.
- Simplify tasks so that the patient can participate. For example, setting out supplies for an activity decreases the memory and problem solving demands on the patient.
- Wait to pass on schedule or to-do information until the patient is seated with paper and pen in hand to maximize the opportunity for the patient to initiate note taking. Sometimes family members benefit from recognizing their contribution to a forgetting error, such as passing on the time of an appointment to the patient who is cooking dinner.

success in carrying out tasks (Box 29-2). That is, the patient is not expected to change, but the physical properties of the context or social expectations do.

Physical Context

In manipulating the physical context, the therapist looks for ways to use the physical properties of the space to provide information or cues. For example, needed items are strategically placed so as to attract the patient's attention. Drawers can be labeled to help the patient locate items, or important information is positioned so that the patient will see it often (Fig. 29-3). The physical space may also be altered to minimize its stimulus-arousal properties. Items that provoke distraction or worry, such as the mail or unpaid bills, are stored so that the patient will not see them when attempting to concentrate on other tasks. Finally, demands of the physical context can be lowered through use of tools and appliances that eliminate memory requirements by, for example, turning themselves off.

Social Context

Therapists also focus on teaching the patient's family to set the stage for the patient's success. This may mean temporarily or permanently changing roles and responsibilities in the family and learning to capitalize on the patient's strengths. Consider the patient who loves to cook but whose memory and judgment problems make this an unsafe activity. As the family members understand the patient's limitations, they adapt their approach to cover what is difficult, such as remembering to gather the correct ingredients, but facilitate what the patient can do, such as measure and mix. The patient's cognitive abilities are also optimized as families learn appropriate ways to offer prompts and cues (Box 29-3).

Establish Behavioral Routines and Habit Sequences

People's everyday lives are composed of activities that have been repeated with such frequency and consistency that they are performed accurately with little or no

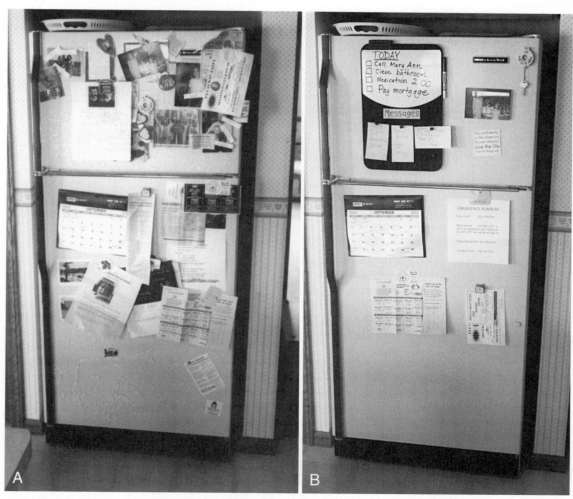

Figure 29-3 A and **B.** Simple changes in the kitchen let a person with cognitive limitations easily find important information.

Case Example

MR. B.: USING MULTIPLE APPROACHES TO OPTIMIZE COGNITIVE ABILITIES AFTER TRAUMATIC BRAIN INJURY

Patient Information

Mr. B., a 26-year-old man 3 months post traumatic brain injury, participated in an outpatient occupational therapy assessment and these problems were identified: (1) decreased initiation of activities of daily living and instrumental activities of daily living, (2) decreased productivity as a result of poor stamina and limited appropriate avocational outlets, (3) memory impairment and inadequate repertoire of memory compensation strategies, (4) decreased awareness of cognitive deficits interfering with compensatory strategy use. (Chapter 8 describes the assessment process and patient's background.)

Recommendations

The occupational therapist recommended two or three treatment sessions each week for 8 weeks. In collaboration with Mr. B. and his brother, the occupational therapist established the following long-term treatment goals: (1) Mr. B. will independently initiate and carry out all self-care and selected light housekeeping tasks through use of external memory aids. (2) Mr. B. will increase his level of productive activity at home such that he initiates avocational activities at least 3 times per week. (3) Mr. B. will follow through on intended tasks at least 85% of the time through use of external memory aids and strategies.

Short-Term Goals

Here is a summary of short-term goals and progress during the first month of treatment.

▶ **Mr. B. will independently begin note taking when presented with occupational therapy homework at least 60% of the time and thereby improve his follow-through on intended tasks.** The therapist ascertained that Mr. B. would be most likely to carry a memory aid if it was highly portable. Therefore, she assisted Mr. B. in selecting a pocket-sized week-at-a-glance planner. The therapist created opportunities for Mr. B. to practice filing and finding information in function-specific planner sections. The therapist used an event record to log each of the three or four homework assignments she presented to Mr. B. during all treatment sessions, taking note of the extent to which Mr. B. required cues to initiate note taking. Any level of note taking initiation was verbally reinforced. Progress in this realm was reviewed at each session, graphing both note taking initiation and homework completion as reinforcement and to improve insight. During the last week of this period, Mr. B. averaged a 65% independent note taking rate and a 70% homework completion rate.

▶ **Mr. B. will initiate and employ consistent routines for self-care tasks, including medication management, through use of checklists and alarm cueing devices.** Following the therapist's recommendation, Mr. B. purchased a container for medications taken each week and an alarm watch. The therapist set the alarm to sound at 6:00 P.M. as a prompt to refer to his medication checklist and take medications. Mr. B. required cueing and supervision with this system for 2 weeks, but by the end of the month he took medications on schedule, once his brother filled the medication container. A morning checklist (Mr. B.'s hygiene sequence) was posted in Mr. B.'s bathroom, and after 1 month he progressed to the point that he required his brother's cueing to initiate these activities only once or twice a week.

▶ **Mr. B. will improve his attention to detail such that he has an error rate of less than 10% on pencil-and-paper tasks.** Mr. B. was highly motivated to fix his memory and eager to carry out any exercises that might help. To that end, he agreed to work on various attention–concentration work sheets as part of his homework while experimenting with various strategies that might help him focus on the task. For example, he tracked and compared his performance in various conditions: while watching television versus sitting in a quiet room; in the morning when rested versus after dinner; working in space crowded with many papers and belongings versus a corner of his bedroom from which his personal paperwork was not visible.

Revised Short-Term Goals: 1 Month

▶ Mr. B. will use his daily planner and planning checklists to schedule and carry out at least two housekeeping tasks and three avocational activities each week.

▶ Mr. B. will demonstrate improved awareness of his problems with memory by independently initiating note taking upon presentation of homework at least 85% of the time and at least 75% of the time when his brother provides instructions.

CLINICAL REASONING
in OT Practice

Mr. B. appeared to have limited awareness of cognitive deficits and implications of these problems on his functioning and future. How might the treatment fraction (Table 29-1) have been different if Mr. B. were keenly aware of cognitive impairments and highly motivated to minimize their influence on his life?

Graded or vanishing cues are used in cognitive rehabilitation to enable the patient to perform tasks with the least amount of cueing (Dougherty & Radomski, 1993). The following terms (from Sohlberg & Mateer, 1989) are useful when writing goals and documenting progress.

► A general or nonspecific cue alerts the patient to monitor performance. It usually takes the form of a statement such as "You'll need to make sure you remember to do this before our next session." The therapist or family offers a general cue if the patient fails to recognize situational or environmental conditions that might otherwise prompt use of a compensatory strategy or behavior.

► A specific cue, presented if the patient does not respond to a general cue, reminds the patient he or she must act. It often takes the form of a question, such as "What do you need to do to make sure you remember to do your homework before our next session?"

► An explicit instruction, the most directive of the graded cues, is sometimes provided if the patient does not initiate the desired strategy or behavior upon first receiving a general cue and then a specific cue. For example, the patient may be asked to take out the planner and record the assignment to ensure follow-through before the next session.

attention to the component steps. Normal daily living requires not just proficiency with skills or motor sequences but efficiency that allows people to focus on matters of greater interest and reward than whether or not they brushed their teeth, locked the house, watered the plants, took medication, or turned off the coffee maker. However, many persons who have cognitive impairments or cognitive inefficiencies complain of daily life problems associated with disintegrated routines and habit sequences. Sudden onset of illness or disability disrupts well-established procedures, giving way to effortful and error-laden performance.

Terminology: Routines and Habits

Routines and habits have long been central to occupational therapy practice (Reed & Sanderson, 1999; Zemke, 1994), but the profession has no apparent consensus regarding language to describe these constructs. We suggest that routines and habits are exemplars of the same phenomenon: human behavior that with repetition is increasingly under automatic control. Similar to Kielhofner (1995), we define **routines** as elements of the context-specific scaffolding that provides order and consistency to the typical flow of tasks and activities in a person's daily life. Once triggered, behavioral routines minimize the demands on decision making and are performed semiautomatically (Kielhofner). The establishment of behavioral routines is facilitated by consistent physical and temporal context, and these activities

become more conscious, effortful, and inefficient when performed under different circumstances. Our workday mornings, for example, are clearly routinized, following predictable courses of events with relatively mindless transitions from self-care activities to departure and transportation activities and then activities to jump-start the work day. On Saturdays, however, most people do not have a default routine, and therefore must deliberately plan the course of the day.

Habits are automatic motor sequences and behaviors that under some conditions combine to constitute larger daily routines. We view habits as motor acts that people perform with virtually no conscious awareness. In fact, the automaticity of some habits is so profound that people often have only retrospective awareness of their occurrence. For clarity, we propose two types of habits: (1) automatic motor sequences that are specific to physical context, which we call habit sequences, and (2) automatic behaviors prompted by personal context that occur in many environments and become linked with personal identity, style, even character, which we call habit patterns (Andersen, 1992; Stephens & Marlatt, 1987; Webster's New Collegiate Dictionary, 1970).

Consider the distinction between these two types of habits, beginning with an example of a habit sequence. Mr. R. always hangs his car keys on a hook near the door as he enters his home, doing so with no conscious awareness whatsoever. Even if the hook is temporarily removed, Mr. R. reaches for the hook upon entering the home despite his best intention to set the keys elsewhere. This habit sequence is embedded in his coming home from work routine, a sequence of semiautomatic tasks comprising letting out the dog, checking the answering machine, and thumbing through the mail. On the other hand, Mr. D. has a habit pattern of biting his nails. Stress seems to catalyze this motor behavior at work and at home. He has every intention of stopping but is often not aware he is biting his nails until he catches himself in the act. Stephens and Marlatt (1987) suggested that all habits are adaptive, beginning as behaviors that are reinforced because they satisfy an innate need or acquired desire. Both habit sequences and habit patterns seem to fit that description—initially satisfying an internally or externally generated need and increasingly under stimulus control rather than conscious control. Because of the link to routines, this chapter addresses intervention specific to habit sequences but not habit patterns.

We suggest that with enough consistency of repetition and context, some new skills can become automatic habit sequences and that strings of habit sequences can link to create semiautomatic routines (Stephens & Marlatt, 1987). For example, in occupational therapy, Ms. S. learns to use a checklist system to ensure that she takes her morning medication (new skill). Over time, Ms. S. becomes so used to this procedure that she sets out the medication, marks the checklist, and takes the pills with little or no attention to what she is doing (habit sequence). Her pill taking procedure is part of the sequence of activities she performs each morning to get ready for work (routine).

Cognitive Basis for the Development of Automatic Behavior

There is no consensus regarding which cognitive capacity subserves our ability to perform tasks and activities automatically. Bachevalier (1990) and Palmeri (1997) suggested that automaticity is a function of the memory system. Consistent with the distinctions between procedural memory (knowing how) and declarative memory (knowing that), Bachevalier defended the notion of two independent memory systems. One system supports gradual or incremental learning as in the acquisition of habits and skills and the other is for rapid one-trial learning that is necessary for forming memories for specific situations and episodes. Zanetti et al. (1997) studied procedural memory stimulation for persons with Alzheimer's disease (AD), and that research seems to support this hypothesis. Adults with mild to moderate AD improved their speed of performance of activities of daily living and instrumental activities of daily living tasks with 3 weeks of training despite no change on neuropsychological measures of cognition. Palmeri's (1997) conceptions of memory's role in automaticity are somewhat different. He suggested that as task repetition occurs, instances are stored in memory, which results in a decreased amount of time for retrieval. He emphasized the importance of consistency of repetition in developing automaticity, with fast-action retrieval occurring only as the catalysts for the behavioral sequence match particular instances of skilled action that have been experienced and stored in memory.

Based on Shiffrin and Schneider's (1977) early models of information processing, Montgomery (1995) emphasized the attentional system in the development of routines and habit sequences, distinguishing automatic from controlled operations. He suggested that the frontal lobes have a central role in active, effortful control of arousal activation, attention, and new learning. He posited that with practice, action sequences become increasingly autonomous at a subcortical or posterior level, and the management role of the frontal brain diminishes. After injury, diffuse cortical or subcortical lesions in the brain may interrupt the efficient and automatic activation of neural pathways and routines, again requiring involvement from the frontal lobes and resulting in less efficiency and greater effort and fatigue.

Similar to Montgomery (1995), Tofil and Clinchot (1996) suggested that the unraveling of automatic behavior occurs after brain injury because of damage to neural pathways. Furthermore, survivors with changed motor abilities are not likely to be able to employ premorbid

habits and routines that are predicated on abilities they no longer possess. Individuals whose problems are less clearly linked to neurological damage, such as those with fibromyalgia, also describe effort and errors in carrying out daily activities that they previously performed with ease (Fransen & Russell, 1996). People with fibromyalgia typically have pain and fatigue that vary unpredictably throughout the day and week. Their variable symptoms interfere with consistent management of time and activities and ultimately erode daily routines and habit sequences. The net effect is similar to that of persons with brain injury: tasks that were once automatic become disrupted, requiring the person to approach many self-care activities as if they were new events each time they are performed (Radomski, 1994).

Guidelines for Establishing Routines and Habit Sequences

Numerous case examples and single-subject research studies in the rehabilitation literature describe the use of applied behavioral analysis to establish or reestablish self-care and/or home management routines and habit sequences for persons with cognitive impairment (Giles & Clark-Wilson, 1988; Giles & Shore, 1989a; Giles et al., 1997; Katzmann & Mix, 1994; Kime et al., 1996; O'Reilly et al., 1990; Schwartz, 1995; Zanetti et al., 1997). The following principles of applied behavioral analysis frame occupational therapy intervention to establish routines and habit sequences.

► With input from the patient and caregiver, the therapist selects a key behavioral sequence that becomes the target of intervention (Giles, 1998). Giles emphasized the importance of selecting behaviors and prospective routines with clinical and personal significance.

► The therapist analyzes the physical and social context in which the routine or sequence is expected to occur to identify built-in cues or determine where to create them (Schwartz, 1995). At a minimum, significant others participate in the selection of target behavioral sequences and appreciate the methods and benefits of intervention. As routines and habit sequences are thought to be context specific, training is most effective if it occurs in the environment in which they will ultimately be performed (Giles).

► A task analysis is performed on the target behavioral routine or sequence (Giles; O'Reilly et al., 1990). Task analysis involves examining each step of the task as well as the setting, stimulus events, and consequences (Gelfand & Hartmann, 1984).

► The therapist and patient decide on an optimal sequence of steps and use chaining, prompting, and reinforcement each time the sequence is performed (Giles et al., 1997). They suggested that "[routine] tasks can be thought of as complex-stimulus-response chains in which the completion of each activity acts as the stimulus for the next step in the chain" (Giles et al., 1997, p. 257). They recommended the use of the whole-task method, in which each step of the chain is trained on each presentation. The therapist often creates a checklist that outlines each component of the task so that the desired sequence of steps remains invariant (Davis & Radomski, 1989) (Fig. 29-4).

For some patients, prompts and reinforcers are established. The checklist itself may be both a prompt if placed in an obtrusive location and a reinforcer as the

Morning planning checklist

Directions: Check-off each step after it is completed.

	M	T	W	Th	F	Sa	Su
1) After breakfast, open planner to yesterday's page.							
2) Check off all of the tasks you completed yesterday.							
3) Draw an arrow in front of undone or incomplete tasks							
4) Re-write these tasks on today's page.							
5) Move the bookmark to today's planner page.							
6) Review your schedule.							
7) Ask your wife if there are any tasks or appointments that you should write down for today.							
8) Write down at least 3 tasks you intend to complete today.							

Wind-down routine

Directions: Check-off each step after it is completed.

	M	T	W	Th	F	Sa	Su
1) When your MotivAider vibrates at 9:00 p.m, discontinue your current activity.							
2) Make notes where you left off on your project.							
3) Put on your pajamas.							
4) Brush your teeth.							
5) Wash your face.							
6) Gather your magazines and go to your recliner.							
7) Set the MotivAider for 30 minutes and peruse your reading material.							
8) When cued by the MotivAider, retire to bed.							

Figure 29-4 Checklists like these are used to help patients reestablish routines and habit sequences.

patient checks each completed step. Technology may also be employed. Schwartz (1995) reported use of a daily tape-recorded message activated by an automatic timer that prompted initiation of a self-care routine. Wilson et al. (1997) described how NeuroPage, a time- and task-specific vibrating prompt that is described in the next section, appeared to facilitate establishing routines related to taking medication and checklist use. Family members may also be enlisted to provide prompts and reinforcement, typically social praise. In our practice, the final step on many patients' checklists requires that they call and leave a voice mail message stating they completed the sequence as an incentive and a reinforcer of the routine.

The therapist facilitates consistent repetition of the behavioral routine or sequence beyond mastery to promote overlearning (Giles, 1998). As discussed in Chapter 12, full automaticity requires at least 200 trials of a task but begins with as few as 10 consistent repetitions (Sternberg, 1986). As the patient frequently and consistently performs the behavioral sequence, steps begin to prompt one another and may be removed from the checklist (Katzman & Mix, 1994). The therapist tracks ongoing compliance with the target behavioral sequence, monitors the patient's perceptions of ease, accuracy, and speed (evidence of increasing automaticity), and, with the patient, determines when applied behavioral analysis methods should be employed to routinize another important task.

Whether because of damage to neural pathways or as a consequence of lack of daily consistency, many persons with cognitive impairment or inefficiency benefit from intervention focused on establishing behavioral routines or habit sequences. However, most adults are embarrassed to admit that they make frequent errors on tasks that are supposed to be easy and may be reluctant to bring these problems to the attention of the therapist. In our clinical practice, patients are often relieved that these errors in everyday tasks can not only be explained but also treated.

In summary, the goal of establishing automatic behavior is to return frequently performed self-management tasks to their status as background activities in everyday life, as described so eloquently by a man with brain injury:

> "Routine is a constant reference as to when and where I am. . . . Routine allows me to compensate for my lack of initiative. I may not notice that the house needs vacuuming, but I know that on Mondays I vacuum. . . . Many people view routine as boring. 'Boring as compared to what?' I ask. 'Boring as compared to being confused and inactive?' . . . I get my variety because routine keeps the distractions at bay."

> (Strand, 2000, p. 9)

Learn Compensatory Strategies

In addition to context-specific habits and routines, many recipients of occupational therapy services need new strategies that allow them to compensate for cognitive impairments or inefficiencies in a variety of settings. Implicit in this approach is the expectation that the patient will use **compensatory cognitive strategies**, such as aids, devices, and thinking techniques, in multiple contexts, and so intervention is designed to promote the likelihood of generalization. Toglia's multicontext approach (1998) informs the intervention model adapted from Sohlberg and Mateer's (1989) memory notebook training protocol.

Multicontext Approach

Based on Toglia's (1998) Dynamic Interactional Model of Cognition, in which cognitive dysfunction is viewed as a mismatch among the person's capabilities, task, and environment, a multicontext approach involves the therapeutic manipulation of performance variables to optimize an individual's function. This approach emphasizes the acquisition of new information-processing strategies, establishment of outcome and transfer criteria, and practice in multiple environments (Table 29-3). Patient-specific processing strategies are selected or designed and then practiced in a variety of tasks and settings. The therapist guides the transfer of learning by

---

TABLE 29-3
Components of the Multicontext Treatment Approach

Component	Definition	Example
Processing strategies	Situational strategies: effective in specific tasks and environments.	Rehearsal, visual imagery, left-to-right scanning.
	Nonsituational strategies: effective in a wide range of tasks and environments.	Planning ahead, organizing information by priority before beginning task, use of self-monitoring.
Task analysis and establishment of criteria for transfer	Identify series of tasks that decrease in degrees of physical and conceptual similarity to the original task.	Task: donning a pullover T-shirt in the therapy area.
	Near transfer: only one or two surface characteristics changed.	Donning a pullover sweater (color and texture different from T-shirt).
	Intermediate transfer: three to six surface characteristics change; tasks share some physical similarities.	Donning a button-down silk blouse in the patient's room (type of clothing, color and texture, movement requirements, and environment changed).
	Far transfer: tasks are conceptually similar; surface characteristics are different or only one surface characteristic is similar.	Donning pants or socks (strategy of dressing affected side first remains the same, while almost everything else changes).
	Very far transfer: generalization, spontaneous application of what is learned to everyday functioning.	Use of an external aid within everyday activity such as reading a checklist posted on the closet door before dressing.
Use of multiple environments	The patient is asked to practice a strategy in multiple situations or environments to facilitate generalization.	Left-to-right scanning is practiced on cancellation tasks and then used to locate items in a medicine cabinet or to count books on a shelf.
Relation of new knowledge to previously learned knowledge or skill	Information is learned and retained better when the patient can relate it to previously learned skills or knowledge.	Choose treatment tasks with the patient's personality, interests, and experiences in mind; connect each new treatment task with prior tasks and experience.
Metacognitive training	Metacognitive skills include task evaluation, prediction of consequences, formulation of goals, plan, self-monitoring performance, self-control, and self-initiation.	Self-estimation (e.g., of task difficulty, time required, and number of cues needed); self-questioning ("How am I doing?"); focus on the process rather than the end product of the task; role reversal (the therapist performs the task and the patient identifies the therapist's errors)

(Toglia, 1991, 1993)

asking the patient to employ the new strategy first on similar tasks and then in the context of those that are increasingly dissimilar (Toglia, 1991).

A General Model for Learning Compensatory Cognitive Strategies

Schmitter-Edgecombe et al. (1995) adapted Sohlberg and Mateer's schema for memory notebook training (1989), and this model applies to helping patients acquire and employ any compensatory cognitive strategy. Intervention is organized around four training phases, anticipation, acquisition, application, and adaptation, and in addition to learning new skills, intervention is typically aimed at improving self-awareness (Box 29-1).

▶ Anticipation—Through the use of homework, feedback, and possible structured failure, patients with low insight experience the consequences of cognitive deficits to heighten motivation for treatment. Patients receive information about human information processing and possible solutions for cognitive problems.

▶ Acquisition—Through drill and practice exercises, patients learn the mechanics of using the compensatory tool or strategy. For example, with coaching and written instructions from the therapist, patients rehearse setting their alarm watches or practice filing and finding information in function-specific sections of their planners.

▶ Application—Patients use the compensatory strategy during clinic-based simulated work tasks. These tasks are designed to require use of the targeted strategy. In our practice, they consist of clerical or clinic maintenance projects or crafts. With guidance from the therapist, patients also directly apply the compensatory strategy to real-life problems at home or work.

▶ Adaptation—Once he or she has experience with the strategy in simulations and real-life tasks, the strategy may be further adapted to the patient's personal preferences and the demands of additional areas of application in daily life.

An exhaustive review of all possible methods to circumvent cognitive impairments or inefficiencies is beyond the scope of this chapter. However, we do provide an overview of three categories of compensatory cognitive strategies: internal information processing strategies, memory prostheses, and problem-solving schemas.

Internal Information-Processing Strategies

Occasionally occupational therapists teach patients to use mental strategies that facilitate the encoding and

---

TABLE 29-4
Internal Compensatory Strategies

Technique	Description
Rehearsal	Patient repeats out loud or to self the information to be remembered
Visual imagery	Patient consolidates information to be remembered by making a mental picture that includes the information (e.g., to remember the name *Barbara*, the patient pictures a barber holding the letter A)
Semantic elaboration	Patient consolidates information by making up a simple story (e.g., patient who is to remember the words *lawyer*, *game*, and *hat* develops a sentence such as "The lawyer wore a hat to the game").
First letter mnemonics	Patient consolidates information to be remembered by using the first letter of each word to make up a word or phrase to be remembered (e.g., to remember a shopping list of salt, ham, olives, peanut butter, pickles, ice cream, napkins, and grapes, use of the word *SHOPPING*).
PSQRT rehearsal method	Patient (1) previews (skims the material for general content), (2) questions (asks questions about the content), (3) reads (actively reads to answer the questions), (4) states (rehearses or repeats the information read), and (5) tests (tests self by answering the questions)

(Glasgow et al., 1977; Malec & Questad, 1983; Milton, 1985; Wilson, 1982)

---

storage of information (Parenté & DiCesare, 1991). Theoretically, the techniques outlined in Table 29-4 enable the patient to keep information in working memory and thereby facilitate encoding. Because of the extensive rehearsal involved in learning these techniques, intervention based on internal information processing strategies has similar features to a remedial approach. Most people find internal information processing strategies time-consuming to learn and inconvenient to employ. Rather than concocting a first-letter mnemonic to make sure that one purchases everything one needs at the grocery store, one simply makes a list.

Memory Prostheses: Day Planners

Many persons with and without memory problems use day planners to help them keep track of information. Routine use of prosthetic memory aids such as day planners, also known as diaries or memory notebooks, is frequently cited in the rehabilitation literature as a means of circumventing memory impairments and inefficiencies. For example, in a small study in which persons with severe brain injury were randomly assigned to one of two conditions, patients receiving memory notebook training reported significantly fewer observed everyday memory failures at discharge than those receiving supportive treatment (Schmitter-Edgecombe et al., 1995). Some 75% of the patients in the notebook condition were using the notebooks at 6 months of follow-up (Schmitter-Edgecombe et al.). Zenicus et al. (1990) compared the effectiveness of three memory strategies (written rehearsal, verbal rehearsal, acronym) with notebook use in terms of clients' assignment completion rates. They found the notebook condition the clearly superior technique for assignment completion. In another multiple-baseline study, Zenicus et al. (1991) examined the effectiveness of memory notebook training on the ability to remember assignments and appointments with four survivors of severe brain injury. The results suggested that all four participants demonstrated improved follow-through on assignments with notebook use compared to baseline.

To use a day planner effectively to compensate for cognitive impairment or inefficiency, the user must religiously record important information in the appropriate notebook sections, carry the planner about, and look at it regularly during the day. Despite the appearance of an easy, straightforward method to compensate for memory problems, successful intervention is often time-consuming. Schmitter-Edgecombe et al. (1995) described an 8-week protocol of 16 sessions, and Donaghy and Williams (1998) used a 9-week protocol of 27 sessions for patients with brain injury to learn to use memory aids of this nature. Good outcome also appears to be linked to patients' characteristics, such as strong motivation, some degree of insight, and absence of

aphasia and motor deficits that interfere with handwriting (Donaghy and Williams).

Patients may purchase commercial day planners or obtain them from clinicians who create computer-generated forms and calendars (Fig. 29-5). Day planners are composed of a limited number of function-specific sections such as daily log, assignments and appointments, current work, and long-term information (Dougherty & Radomski, 1987). Table 29-5 summarizes the treatment protocol used at the Brain Injury Clinic at Sister Kenny Rehabilitation Services in Minneapolis. Treatment addresses only learning objectives that are appropriate for the individual and incorporates other compensatory cognitive strategies, such as use of alarm cueing devices, checklists, and problem-solving schemas.

Memory Prostheses: Devices
Alarm watches, pagers, and palm-top computers are often used in conjunction with or as an alternative to day planners (Lynch, 1995). A variety of devices may also be used to minimize cognitive burden, including those that help individuals manage their medications (Fig. 29-6). Giles and Shore (1989b) described the successful use of a Psion Organizer, a palm-top computer, by a woman with acquired brain injury. Among other features, this device provides time-specific prompts for information related to schedule, appointments, and tasks. With 4 hours of therapy and 6 hours of supervised practice with family, this patient with memory impairment but normal intelligence could independently program the device, and she preferred it to a day planner because of its alarm functions. Kim et al. (1999) also used a Psion Organizer, but with an inpatient with severe cognitive impairments. Staff programmed the schedule and alarms into the device; it improved the patient's punctuality at therapy sessions and after 5 days, was effective in prompting the patient to take medications. Finally, Wilson et al. (1997) conducted a study using NeuroPage, more recently called LifeMinder, with 15 neurologically impaired subjects, all of whom had significant everyday memory impairment or problems with planning and organization. NeuroPage is a simple portable paging system with a screen that can be attached to a belt (Hersh & Treadgold, 1994). It uses microcomputers linked to conventional computer memory and a paging company. Information about the patient's schedule is entered into the computer, and on the appropriate date and time, NeuroPage accesses the user's data files, determines the reminder to be delivered, and transmits the information (Wilson et al., 1997). These researchers reported that all 15 subjects benefited from the pager and showed significant improvement on task follow-through. Furthermore, even when the pager was removed after 3 months, some subjects were able to maintain the routines initially

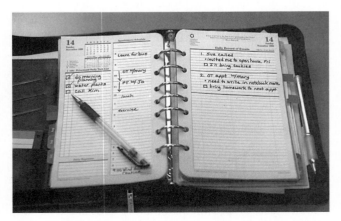

Figure 29-5 Use of function-specific portions of the planner page helps the patient organize notes about the day.

TABLE 29-5
Compensatory Strategy Training Protocol Used in the Brain Injury Clinic at Sister Kenny Rehabilitation Services

Sample Long-Term Goals

The patient will be able to accurately and efficiently file and locate information in the planner.

The patient will be able to get to appointments and complete intended tasks on time through use of compensatory cognitive strategies, such as planner, daily and weekly planning checklists, alarm watch.

The patient will be able to use compensatory cognitive strategies to carry out routine personal, household, and work tasks accurately and efficiently without omissions or repetitions.

The patient will take notes at such times and in such ways that information stored in and retrieved from the planner is accurate and useful for later reference.

The patient will be able to carry out novel multistep tasks through employment of compensatory cognitive strategies.

Training Hierarchy and Sample Short-Term Goals

Learning Objective	Patient Learns To
Information retrieval	Select and obtain an appropriate planner with assistance of therapist.
	Locate information in function-specific notebook sections.
	Use written instructions to set alarm watch.
	Refer to time-specific entries in planner in response to alarm.
	Use asterisk recorded by therapist to prompt reference to other sections of planner.
Basic planning	Use a checklist to engage in regular daily and weekly planning.
	Create daily to-do lists that reflect realistic scheduling and priorities.
	Recognize situations in which time-specific prompts would be helpful and make alarm settings that are pertinent to daily schedule.
Basic information entry	Record appointments, to-do items, and lists in correct sections of planner.
	Initiate use of asterisk on daily planner to cross-reference to other sections.
	Routinely employ these note-taking mechanics: inclusion of date and topic, organize notes by steps or points, check-off completed steps or tasks, oral verification of accuracy after recording notes.
Complex information entry	Use people logs to record information pertaining to conversations with significant people.
	Employ main idea–example mnemonic to keep track of what to say during discussion.
	Use tape recorder with note taking and identify situations when use of this combination would be most appropriate.
	Use customized forms to record information pertaining to specific work or household situations.
Complex planning	Analyze long-term projects or tasks in terms of breakdown of steps.
	Incorporate project plans and goals into weekly planning.

prompted by the device, such as taking medication on time and using checklists.

Giles and Shore (1989b) offered suggestions for determining who might profit from using an electronic aid. They recommended that good candidates have average or nearly average intelligence, retained or mildly impaired reasoning skills, insight into deficits, adequate ability to initiate behavior, and some form of functional disorder resulting from significant memory impairment. When caregivers or family members assume responsibility for programming the device, however, persons with more severe impairment appear to benefit as well.

Problem-Solving and Decision-Making Schemas
The enterprise of human problem solving is thought to be comprised of the situation (a conglomeration of task, environment, and person variables) and process

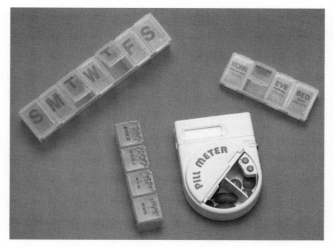

Figure 29-6 A variety of medication containers facilitate compliance with medication regimens.

Project title: <u>Clean the garage</u>

ORDER	STEPS	COMPLETION DATES

Remove the debris

4	Collect items for recycling	9/4
5	Bring to recycling center	9/4
2	Collect trash	9/1
1	Purchase large trash bags	9/1
6	Bring unwanted items to thrift store	9/4

Clean the floor

12	Get everything off the floor	9/10
13	Sweep	9/10
14	Rinse down the floor	9/10
15	Put everything back	9/10

Organize storage

3	List the items I plan to store	9/1
7	Decide on what add'l storage is needed	9/5
8	List supplies needed + measurements	9/5
9	Purchase supplies	9/5
10	Install	9/5
11	Put items away	9/5

Figure 29-7 Means–ends analysis (also known as divide and conquer) helps patients break large, unstructured projects into a sequence of steps: (1) List major task components (shaded boxes). (2) Write down substeps under each task component in no particular order. (3) Number the substeps. (4) Set completion dates if desired.

(problem definition, evaluation of alternative solutions, determining and implementing a plan, evaluating the results) (Radomski, 1998). The demands on problem solving can sometimes be minimized by changing the environment, establishing consistent routines, or employing problem solving schemas. Means–ends analysis and the IDEAL Problem Solver (Bransford & Stein, 1984) are examples of these schemas.

Means–ends analysis, known to our patients as divide and conquer, is used to organize multistep, unstructured projects—those that have no obvious first steps and that can be carried out in any number of ways. It entails a four-step process: (1) List the major task components. (2) Under each component, write down all the substeps you can think of (in no particular order). (3) Number the substeps. (4) Decide on deadlines if desired (Fig. 29-7).

The IDEAL Problem Solver was developed for a college course in which students learned problem-solving techniques, learned about the process of solving problems, and uncovered their own strengths and weaknesses in this realm (Bransford & Stein, 1984). This acronym stands for the 5 steps of problem solving: I, Identify the problem; D, Define the problem; E, Evaluate all possible solutions; A, Act; L, Look back.

While problem solving schemas are useful because they are applicable to a wide range of situations, they place much greater demands on patients' metaprocessing abilities (executive functions and metacognition) and require much more training time than simply changing the environment or establishing a routine (Radomski, 1998). Sternberg (1987) questioned whether a program of less than a semester would be adequate for teaching college students to learn and employ problem-solving schemas, and therefore, occupational therapists are advised to be selective in using this approach in treatment.

Summary Review Questions

1. Describe diagnoses of patients who are likely to have organically based cognitive impairments. What types of circumstances or conditions result in cognitive inefficiency?
2. Analyze the relative costs and benefits of a remedial approach to cognitive problems versus an adaptive approach.
3. How would your efforts to optimize cognitive function be different for a person with Alzheimer's Disease compared with a patient in acute recovery from a traumatic brain injury?
4. Write down the steps to one of your daily routines or habit sequences. Now change the order of steps and next time, try to follow this revised sequence. How do the attentional requirements change? How do these changes impact your speed of performance?
5. Describe three changes you could make to your own living environment to decrease its cognitive demands.
6. What cognitive compensatory strategies, if any, are a part of your information processing repertoire? Consider practices or habits that optimize your memory performance, ability to concentrate, plan, or problem solve. How might these same strategies be used by an individual with cognitive impairment?

Resources

Remediate the Deficit

Captain's Log (Computer-based cognitive retraining programs)
www.braintrain.com

NeurXercise System
www.neurx.com

Brainwave (comprehensive pen-and-paper-based cognitive rehabilitation program divided into five hierarchically graded modules: attention, visual processing, memory, information processing, and executive functions)
www.proedinc.com

Attention Processing Training-II (APT-II)
Sohlberg, Johnson, Paule, Raskin and Mateer (1993)
Association for Neuropsychogical Research and Development · 1420 S. Meridian, Suite A, Puyallup, WA 98371

Board games, such as Master Mind, Simon, Connect Four; a deck of cards.

Change the Physical Context

Rangetimer (shuts off stove automatically)
Logan Powell Company · 2415-A Old Gettysburg Road, Camp Hill, PA 17011. 717-730-2671
www.seaside.org/9505.html

Appliances With Automatic Shutoff (coffee pots, curling irons)

Exit alarms can be a standard feature on security systems.

Learn Compensatory Cognitive Strategies
Day Planners (essential features are predated pages and defined notebook sections)

- ▶ FranklinCovey
  www.franklincovey.com
- ▶ Daytimer
  www.daytimer.com

Alarms and Cueing Devices That Support Scheduling and Time Management

- ▶ Timex (Beepwear pager watch, a pager, a watch, and an organizer all in one from Timex and Motorola)
  www.timex.com
- ▶ Data Link watches (alarms, text messages, phone numbers; allows wireless download from computer scheduling program)
- ▶ Casio alarm watches (can set multiple alarms for daily routine such as meals or medications)
  www.casio.com
- ▶ MotivAider System (vibrates at preset intervals)
  http://l_barron.tripod.com/motelec.htm
- ▶ IQ Voice Organizer (can record message to be played at prompt of alarm, letting client receive audible reminder in familiar voice and with explicit detail)
  www.sparkus.com/voice/model.htm
- ▶ Palm Pilot (computer scheduling device)
  www.palm.com
- ▶ Psion hand-held computer
  www.psionusa.com
- ▶ LifeMinder (Formerly NeuroPage)
  www.ticklebox.com

Medication boxes with or without alarms

Available from medication aisle in the pharmacy section of stores such as Walgreen's, Kmart, or specialized equipment vendors
www.sammonspreston.com
www.abledata.com.

Resources for Professionals

Brain Injury Association
www.biausa.org

Society for Cognitive Rehabilitation(education, certification, and annual membership includes *Journal of Cognitive Technology*)
www.cognitive-rehab.org.uk

References

Abreu, B. C., & Toglia, J. P. (1987). Cognitive rehabilitation: A model for occupational therapy. *American Journal of Occupational Therapy, 41*, 439–448.

American Occupational Therapy Association (1999). Management of occupational therapy services for persons with cognitive impairments. *American Journal of Occupational Therapy, 53*, 601–607.

Andersen, H. J. (1992). Habits and rituals. *Danish Medical Bulletin, 39,* 273–274.

Bachevalier, J. (1990). Ontogenetic development of habit and memory formation in primates. *Annals of the New York Academy of Sciences, 608,* 457–484.

Ben-Yishay, Y., & Diller, L. (1993). Cognitive remediation in traumatic brain injury: Update and issues. *Archives of Physical Medicine and Rehabilitation, 74,* 204–213.

Blundon, G., & Smits, E. (2000). Cognitive rehabilitation: Pilot survey of therapeutic modalities used by Canadian occupational therapists with survivors of traumatic brain injury. *Canadian Journal of Occupational Therapy, 67,* 184–196.

Bransford, J. D., & Stein, B. S. (1984). *The IDEAL Problem Solver: A Guide for Improving Thinking, Learning, and Creativity.* New York: W. H. Freeman.

CARF (1999). *1999 Medical Rehabilitation Standards Manual.* Tucson, AZ: Author.

Carney, N., Chestnut, R. M., Maynard, H., Mann, N. C., Patterson, P., & Helfand, M. (1999). Effect of cognitive rehabilitation on outcomes for persons with traumatic brain injury: A systematic review. *Journal of Head Trauma Rehabilitation, 14,* 277–307.

Chen S. H. A., Thomas J. D., Glueckauf R. L. & Bracy O. L. (1997). The effectiveness of computer-assisted cognitive rehabilitation for persons with traumatic brain injury. *Brain Injury, 11,* 197–209.

Crosson, B., Barco, P. P., Velozo, C. A., Bolesta, M. M., Cooper, P. V., Werts, D., & Brobeck, T. C. (1989). Awareness and compensation in postacute head injury rehabilitation. *Journal of Head Trauma Rehabilitation, 4,* 46–54.

Davis, E. S., & Radomski, M. V. (1989). Domain-specific training to reinstate habit sequences. *Occupational Therapy Practice, 1,* 79–88.

Donaghy, S., & Williams, W. (1998). A new protocol for training severely impaired patients in the usage of memory journals. *Brain Injury, 12,* 1061–1076.

Dougherty, P. M., & Radomski, M. V. (1987). *The Cognitive Rehabilitation Workbook.* Rockville, MD: Aspen.

Dougherty, P. M., & Radomski, M. V. (1993). *The Cognitive Rehabilitation Workbook* (2nd ed) Gaithersburg, MD: Aspen.

Fleming, J., & Strong, J. (1995). Self-awareness of deficits following acquired brain injury: Considerations for rehabilitation. *British Journal of Occupational Therapy, 58,* 55–60.

Fransen, J., & Russell, I. J. (1996). *The Fibromyalgia Help Book.* St. Paul, MN: Smith House.

Gelfand, D. M., & Hartmann, D. P. (1984). *Child Behavioral Analysis and Therapy.* Needham Heights, MA: Allyn & Bacon.

Gianutsos, R. (1992). The computer in cognitive rehabilitation: It's not just a tool anymore. *Journal of Head Trauma Rehabilitation, 7,* 26–35.

Giles, G. M. (1998). A neurofunctional approach to rehabilitation following severe brain injury. In N. Katz (Ed.) *Cognition and Occupation In Rehabilitation* (pp. 125–147). Bethesda, MD: American Occupational Therapy Association.

Giles, G. M., & Clark-Wilson, J. (1988). The use of behavioral techniques in functional skills training after severe brain injury. *American Journal of Occupational Therapy, 42,* 658–665.

Giles, G. M., Ridley, J. E., Dill, A., & Frye, S. (1997). A consecutive series of adults with brain injury treated with a washing and dressing retraining program. *American Journal of Occupational Therapy, 51,* 256-266.

Giles, G. M., & Shore, M. (1989a). A rapid method for teaching severely brain injured adults how to wash and dress. *Archives of Physical Medicine and Rehabilitation, 70,* 156–158.

Giles, G. M., & Shore, M. (1989b). The effectiveness of an electronic memory aid for a memory-impaired adult of normal intelligence. *American Journal of Occupational Therapy, 43,* 409–411.

Glasgow, R. E., Zeiss, R. A., Barrera, M., & Lewisohn, P. M. (1977). Case studies on remediating memory deficits in brain-damaged individuals. *Journal of Clinical Psychology, 33,* 1049–1054.

Goldstein, G., Beers, S. R., Longmore, S., & McCue, M. (1996). Efficacy of memory training: A technical extension and replication. *Clinical Neurologist, 10,* 66–72.

Hersh, N., & Treadgold, L. (1994). NeuroPage: The rehabilitation of memory dysfunction by prosthetic memory aid cueing. *Neurorehabilitation, 4,* 187–197.

Katzmann, S., & Mix, C. (1994). Improving functional independence in a patient with encephalitis through behavior modification shaping techniques. *American Journal of Occupational Therapy, 48,* 259–262.

Kielhofner, G. (1995). Habituation. In G. Kielhofner (Ed.), *A Model of Human Occupation: Theory and Application* (2nd ed., pp. 63–82). Baltimore: Williams & Wilkins.

Kim, H. J., Burke, D. T., Dowds, M. M., & Georges, J. (1999). Utility of a microcomputer as an external memory aid for a memory-impaired head injury patient during inpatient rehabilitation. *Brain Injury, 13,* 147–150.

Kime, S. K., Lamb, D. G., & Wilson, B. A. (1996). Use of a comprehensive programme of external cueing to enhance procedural memory in a patient with dense amnesia. *Brain Injury, 10,* 17–25.

Lynch, W. J. (1995). You must remember this: Assistive devices for memory impairment. *Journal of Head Trauma Rehabilitation, 10,* 94–97.

Malec, J., & Basford, J. (1996). Postacute brain injury rehabilitation. *Archives of Physical Medicine and Rehabilitation, 77,* 198–207.

Malec, J., & Questad, K. (1983). Rehabilitation of memory after craniocerebral trauma: Case report. *Archives of Physical Medicine and Rehabilitation, 64,* 436–438.

Milton, S. B. (1985). Compensatory memory strategy training: A practical approach for managing persistent memory problems. *Cognitive Rehabilitation, 3,* 8–15.

Montgomery, G. K. (1995). A multi-factor account of disability after brain injury: Implications for neuropsychological counselling. *Brain Injury, 9,* 453–469.

O'Reilly, M. F., Green, G., & Braunling-McMorrow, D. (1990). Self-administered written prompts to teach home accident prevention skills to adults with brain injuries. *Journal of Applied Behavior Analysis, 23,* 431–446.

Palmeri, T. J. (1997). Exemplar similarity and the development of automaticity. *Journal of Experimental Psychology: Learning, Memory, and Cognition, 23,* 324–354.

Parenté, R., & DiCesare, A. (1991) Retraining memory theory, evaluation and applications. In J. S. Kreutzer & P. H. Wehman (Eds.), *Cognitive Rehabilitation for Persons With Traumatic Brain Injury: A Functional Approach* (pp.147–162). Baltimore: Paul H. Brooks.

Quintana, L. A. (1995). Remediating cognitive impairments. In C.A. Trombly (Ed.), *Occupational Therapy for Physical Dysfunction* (4th ed., pp. 539–548). Baltimore: Williams & Wilkins.

Radomski, M. V. (1994). Cognitive rehabilitation: Advancing the stature of occupational therapy. *American Journal of Occupational Therapy, 48,* 271–273.

Radomski, M. V. (1998). Problem solving deficits: Using a multi-dimensional definition to select a treatment approach. *Physical Disabilities Special Interest Section Quarterly, 21,* 1–4.

Reed, K. L., & Sanderson, S. N. (1999). *Concepts of Occupational Therapy,* (4th ed.). Baltimore: Lippincott Williams & Wilkins.

Salazar, A. M., Warden, D. L., Schwab, K., Spector, J., Braverman, S., Walter, J., Cole, R., Rosner, M. M., Martin, E. M., Ecklund, J., & Ellenbogen, R. G. (2000). Cognitive rehabilitation for traumatic brain injury: A randomized trial. *Journal of the American Medical Association, 283,* 3075–3081.

Schmitter-Edgecombe, M., Fahy, J. F., Whelan, J. P., & Long, C. J. (1995). Memory remediation after severe closed head injury: notebook training over supportive therapy. *Journal of Consulting and Clinical Psychology, 63,* 484–489.

Schwartz, S. M. (1995). Adults with traumatic brain injury: Three case studies of cognitive rehabilitation in the home setting. *American Journal of Occupational Therapy, 49,* 655–667.

Shiffrin, R. M., & Schneider, W. (1977). Controlled and automatic human information processing: II. Perceptual learning, automatic attending, and a general theory. *Psychological Review, 84,* 127–190.

Sohlberg, M. M., & Mateer, C. A. (1989). *Introduction to Cognitive Rehabilitation.* New York: Guilford.

Stephens, R. S., & Marlatt, G. A. (1987). Creatures of habit: Loss of control over addictive and non-addictive behaviors. *Drugs and Society, 1,* 85–103.

Sternberg, R. J. (1986). *Intelligence Applied: Understanding and Increasing Your Intellectual Skills.* New York: Harcourt Brace Jovanovich.

Sternberg, R. J. (1987). Questions and answers about the nature and teaching of thinking skills. In J. B. Baron & R. J. Sternberg (Eds.), *Teaching Thinking Skills: Theory and Practice* (pp. 251–259). New York: W.H. Freeman.

Strand, M. (2000, Winter). A routine gift. *Headlines* (Brain Injury Association of Minnesota), 1–14.

Tofil, S., & Clinchot, D. M. (1996). Recovery of automatic and cognitive functions in traumatic brain injury using the Functional Independence Measure. *Brain Injury, 10,* 901–910.

Toglia, J. (1993, March 19). *OT intervention for individuals with constructional apraxia.* Paper presented at the AOTA Neurosciences Institute, Baltimore.

Toglia, J. P. (1991). Generalization of treatment: A multi-contextual approach to cognitive perceptual impairment in the brain injured adult. *American Journal of Occupational Therapy, 45,* 505–516.

Toglia, J. P. (1998). A dynamic interactional model to cognitive rehabilitation. In N. Katz (Ed.), *Cognition and Occupation In Rehabilitation* (pp. 5–50). Bethesda, MD: American Occupational Therapy Association.

Webster's New Collegiate Dictionary (7th ed). (1970). Springfield, MA: G. & C. Merriam.

Wilson, B. (1982). Success and failure in memory training following a cerebral vascular accident. *Cortex, 18,* 581–594.

Wilson, B. A. (1997). Cognitive rehabilitation: How it is and how it might be. *Journal of the International Neuropsychological Society, 3,* 487–496.

Wilson, B. A., Evans, J. J., Emslie, H., & Malinek, V. (1997). Evaluation of NeuroPage: A new memory aid. *Journal of Neurology, Neurosurgery, and Psychiatry, 63,* 113–115.

Zanetti, O., Binetti, G., Magni, E., Rozzini, L., Bianchetti, A., & Trabucchi, M. (1997). Procedural memory stimulation in Alzheimer's disease: impact of a training programme. *Acta Neurologica Scandinavica, 95,* 152–157.

Zemke, R. (1994). Habits. In C.B. Royeen (Ed.), *The Practice of the Future: Putting Occupation Back into Therapy* (pp. 1–24). Bethesda, MD: American Occupational Therapy Association.

Zenicus, A., Wesolowski, M. D., & Burke, W. H. (1990). A comparison of 4 memory strategies with traumatically brain injured clients. *Brain Injury, 4,* 33–38.

Zenicus, A., Wesolowski, M. D., Krankowski, T., & Burke, W.H. (1991). Memory notebook training with traumatically brain injured clients. *Brain Injury, 5,* 321–325.

30
Restoring the Role of Independent Person

Catherine A. Trombly

LEARNING OBJECTIVES

After studying this chapter, the reader will be able to do the following:

1. Describe the use of occupation-as-end as a therapeutic medium.
2. Distinguish between basic activities of daily living and instrumental activities of daily living.
3. State principles to restore adapted function to persons with various functional limitations.
4. Modify tasks and the environment to promote independence.
5. Prescribe and evaluate the use of assistive devices to promote safe independence.
6. Guide problem solving and implementation of solutions to unique situations for persons with a variety of functional limitations.

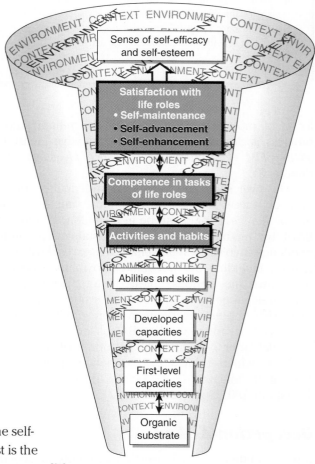

*A*ctivities of daily living (ADL) are a major component of the self-maintenance role (Trombly, 1995). The occupational therapist is the rehabilitation specialist responsible for teaching the patient to accomplish these tasks. The assumption is that people want to care for themselves to the best of their ability. This may include directing and/or delegating to others tasks that are beyond the person's capabilities.

The term *basic activities of daily living* (BADL) is synonymous with self-care. BADL include feeding, grooming, dressing, bathing, toileting, and mobility. These universal tasks are necessary to maintain health. The first five BADL are included in this chapter. Mobility, from turning over in bed to transferring to driving, is addressed in Chapter 31. While every human does these BADL to some degree, the way that each is done and the importance attached to each differ culturally. BADL is the

---

GLOSSARY

Adaptation—Process of learning to function in an environment. Occupational therapists enable that process by modifying a task, the method of accomplishing the task, and/or the environment to promote independence in occupational functioning.

Blocked practice—Practice that consists of drills of many repetitions of the same task in the same way (Schmidt & Lee, 2000).

External compensatory techniques—Use of help from sources other than the self. For example, the use of assistive devices, such as pictures of the steps of a task (van Heugten et al., 1998).

Internal compensatory techniques—Use of cognitive functions other than the distorted ones, such as visual or verbal functions. For example, the patient verbalizes the proper sequence of steps in an activity while performing the activity (van Heugten et al., 1998).

Random practice—Practice of several related tasks within one session; sequence of tasks varies randomly (Schmidt & Lee, 2000).

Shaping—A behavior modification technique in which at first any approximation of the desired behavior is rewarded. As the person is able to produce the behavior consistently, only the next higher level of performance is rewarded, and so forth until the desired behavior is performed consistently well. Rewarding feedback is then faded.

---

focus of most insurance coverage for rehabilitation; progress is documented by such evaluative measures as the *FIM* (*Functional Independence Measure*) (see Chapter 3).

However, stating that a person is independent based only on these activities gives a false impression of independence. People can be independent in these six BADL but unable to live without assistance. True independence involves *instrumental activities of daily living* (IADL), including but not limited to management of one's own medications, food, shelter, finances, and communications for safety, personal business, and sociability. IADL require greater interaction with the physical and social environments than BADL. There is no developmental order to the ability to perform IADL in contrast to BADL, which follow an ontogenetic sequence from feeding to toileting (Katz et al., 1963; Norström & Thorslund, 1991; Spector et al., 1987).

Occupation-As-End

If remedial therapy can correct impairments, no special therapy is needed to teach ADL; the patient does important tasks as able. Intervention is necessary for those who do not regain full capabilities or prefer not to engage in remedial therapy. Occupation-as-end, that is, relearning how to accomplish the activities and tasks that constitute roles in an adapted way, is the intervention (Trombly, 1995). If possible, the therapist helps the patient reestablish his or her habits and daily routines to restore a sense of normalcy and meaning. Habits are a powerful reminder to the patient of who he or she is (Hasselkus, 2000). However, if the person cannot rees-

tablish habits, the therapist teaches adaptive strategies—new ways of doing tasks—or prescribes assistive equipment that will enable the person to be independent of the caregiver for the task or a major aspect of the task. The therapist suggests environmental adaptations to promote independence and safety for both the patient and the caregiver (Chen et al., 2000).

The extent of services offered to a particular patient depends on the person's motivation and the level of independence he or she needs. The patients' perceptions of ADL capabilities may differ from those of staff (Atwood et al., 1994) and affect investment in treatment. Use of an instrument such as the *COPM* (*Canadian Occupational Performance Measure*) or the *Link-Nelson Self-Identified Goals Assessment* (www.mco.edu/allh/OT/link-nelson.html) can identify patients' perceptions, values, and goals. Independence in BADL may be sufficient for a person returning to a sheltered and supportive living situation in which IADL needs are few and willingly assumed by others, but it is never enough for a person who expects to reintegrate into community life. This person not only must learn solutions to BADL and common IADL tasks but also must learn to identify and solve problems that prevent accomplishment of unique tasks. On the other hand, independence in only one activity, such as transferring or toileting, may determine whether discharge is to home or institution. Therefore, full effort should concentrate on achievement of this goal for a person who has otherwise limited potential for full independence.

Intervention by occupation-as-end, then, is a compensatory approach that uses education of adaptive techniques and assistive technology, and adaptation of environment and context to enable patients to live with a permanent or temporary disability.

Education

In the compensatory, or rehabilitative, approach, the therapist is teacher, and patient and family are learners. Both teaching and learning are active processes. The patient must be motivated to learn and must be able to learn. Motivation is sparked by values; that is, values guide actions and efforts (Trombly, 1995). Therefore, the therapist must plan which aspects of ADL to concentrate on, guided not only by knowledge of the tasks that will be within the person's capabilities but also by the patient's values and goals.

Some patients are unable to learn or have difficulty learning. Learning is prevented by loss of recent or short-term memory, severe receptive aphasia, disorientation to person and place, or ideational apraxia (see Chapters 8 and 29). Persons with ideomotor apraxia have difficulty but are able to learn new procedures, even those involving hand position sequences such as the one-handed shoe tie (Poole, 1998). A person who cannot follow directions imparted through his or her most receptive channels or who cannot remember is not a candidate for ADL training. The family should be taught to care for the patient and told to seek reevaluation if the patient's cognitive status improves.

Other barriers to learning include depression, anxiety, pain, different language, and low literacy. Therapy to reduce anxiety that includes low-challenge activities at first may allow learning to take place. Patients who speak a language not known to the therapist and who do not understand demonstration must be taught through the help of an interpreter. See Chapters 9 and 12 concerning ways to reduce the effects of low literacy.

BOX 30-1
PROCEDURES FOR PRACTICE

Effective Teaching

1. Determine what the learner knows.
2. Establish the learning objective.
3. Choose teaching techniques congruent with what is to be taught.
4. Adapt the presentation to the learner's capabilities.
5. Provide opportunities for practice, considering context and schedule.
6. Offer useful feedback at the right time.
7. Test the learner in the appropriate context or contexts to confirm that learning has occurred.
8. Discuss progress toward goals and revise teaching strategy or goal as indicated.

Points of effective teaching are noted below and summarized in Box 30-1.

1. Determine what routines and skills the learner has retained and whether he or she does them safely. Determine whether the learner figures out adapted methods independently.
2. Find out what the learner needs to know, the patient's goals (Shotwell & Schell, 1999). These become learning objectives. A learning objective is a goal expressed in behavioral terms, such as "The patient will be able to brush his teeth, without assistance or supervision, in less than 5 minutes."
3. Present the material in a way that is congruent with the objective. If the patient needs to learn some principles of energy conservation, the teaching method includes auditory and visual methods, such as discussion perhaps with slides or videotaped examples, problem solving, and application of ideas to the patient's own situation. If the patient needs to learn a motor task, such as putting on a shirt with one arm paralyzed, the teaching is guided by motor learning principles (see Chapter 12), in which the person first understands the task, then visually pays attention to the steps of the task, then begins to pay attention to the proprioceptive feedback while doing the task, and finally does the task skillfully.

   When first learning an activity, the challenge should be kept low to avoid anxiety and to promote success (Law, 1991). The lessons should be structured so that the patient has early success. For example, if the patient must learn to eat with adapted utensils, the training starts with sticky foods that do not easily slide off of the spoon and progresses to difficult foods, such as spaghetti and sliced peaches.
4. Adapt the presentation to the particular learner, given his or her abilities and deficits. For patients without brain damage and with average intelligence and literacy, the teaching methods can be discussion, demonstration, printed instructions (Schemm & Gitlin, 1998), or simply describing methods that others have found helpful. Printed materials should be written simply and directly, because about 50% of the U. S. population has difficulty with the written word, although this is not detectable through conversation (Thomas, 1999). Non–brain-damaged persons should be taught strategies and trained in various contextual situations so that they become independent problem solvers. They need to learn to identify the problem, to understand the principle involved, and to be able to match a solution from a repertoire of solutions that have been found helpful in the past or that others have used. The patient may have suggestions about how a task might be accom-

plished, and those ideas should be respected and encouraged. Many techniques commonly in use have been developed by therapist–patient collaboration.

Patients with brain damage require more attention to the actual teaching process, which is guided by the patient's particular problem. If the patient cannot do the task automatically using old habit programs, he will be learning a new skill. Behavior modification, including a step-by-step structure, **shaping**, verbal cues, physical cues, and social praise after completion of the whole task, was found effective (Giles et al., 1997; Katzman & Mix, 1994). A step-by-step program that subjects had to memorize and verbalize was also found effective for patients with Parkinson's disease (Kamsma et al., 1995). For instruction, use short, concise verbal cues. Brain-damaged patients often have difficulty processing abstract information or large chunks of information at a time, and they need the instructions reduced to one- or two-word concrete cues. Given consistently over the course of practice sessions, these key word cues help the patient chain the task from beginning to end. It may be necessary to practice one step at a time; steps may be combined as learning progresses. Some patients, however, can do a task only if the whole chain is completed (Brodal, 1973). Use a variety of contexts for practice (Katzman & Mix, 1994). Even with this kind of practice, the learning may or may not transfer to other tasks or contexts; therefore, the patient must practice each task until it is learned within all the contexts in which it will be required.

Brain-damaged patients may not become problem solvers, and their prognosis for independence outside of a sheltered or familiar environment may be limited. ADL tasks that may result in injury if precautions are not practiced, such as cutting with a sharp knife or standing to pull up trousers, require supervision for as long as judgment is impaired.

Some profoundly brain-damaged yet teachable patients benefit from backward chaining, an adaptation of Skinner's (1938) Law of Chaining: One step acts as the stimulus for another. In backward chaining of dressing skills, for example, assistance is given to do the task until the last step of the process is reached. The patient performs this one step independently and gets the satisfaction of having completed the task. Once the patient has mastered the final step, the therapist assists only to the next to the last step, and the patient completes the two remaining steps. This process continues until the patient can do the entire task from start to finish independently. Progress in learning ADL for those

with brain damage is slow, with regressions (Diller et al., 1972). Given the economic constraints, it is unrealistic to expect to teach such patients in the brief period of treatment authorized. The therapist should teach the caregiver how to help the patient learn some ADL skills at home.

Patients with damage to their dominant hemispheres usually have difficulty processing verbal or written language but may benefit from demonstrated or pictorial instruction (Diller et al., 1972). Those with damage to their nondominant hemisphere may have difficulty with spatial relationships that make it difficult to interpret pictures and demonstrations but be able to process step-by-step verbal instruction.

5. Arrange appropriate practice schedules. Motor skills are learned only through practice. Motor skills learned with contextual interference (**random practice**) were retained better than when practiced in repetitive drill (**blocked practice**) (Hanlon, 1996). Chapter 12 has a discussion of practice schedules.

6. Provide appropriate feedback. Motivational feedback ("Great!" "Looks good!" "Keep trying!") does have some benefit, but specific feedback about what was correct and what was not correct during a particular trial has more definitive benefit. Occasional feedback concerning the performance (keep your elbow straighter next time) offered immediately after a trial is helpful. If the person is not aware of the outcome of his or her efforts, call attention to it so that he or she gains knowledge of the results, a requirement for learning (Schmidt & Lee, 2000).

7. Test whether the learner has acquired the knowledge or skill by requiring that it be done independently at the appropriate time and place.

8. Discuss progress toward goals and revise teaching strategy or goal as indicated (Shotwell & Schell, 1999).

Adaptation

Adaptation is the process by which a person maintains a useful relationship to the environment (Thorén Jönsson et al., 1999). It is a cumulative process that evolves over time (Spencer et al., 1999). Older people therefore have a rich repertoire of adaptive strategies based on personal experience that may be helpful in dealing with disability.

Adaptive therapy refers to modifying the task, the method of accomplishing the task, and/or the environment to promote independence in occupational functioning. Examples of modifying the task are to switch to loafers instead of tie shoes or to order from catalogs instead of going to the shops. Adapted methods of dressing for persons with loss of the use of one side of the body or weakness of all four extremities (discussed later) are examples of modifying the method of accomplishing a task. Installation of grab bars in the bathroom to enable safe transfers and storing often-used items within easy reach are examples of modifying the physical environment. Teaching a wheelchair user ways of interacting with nondisabled individuals so that he presents himself as a self-assured, capable person is an example of adapting the social environment.

Prescription of and training in the use of assistive devices or adapted tools and utensils to enable occupational functioning by the physically disabled is a primary function of occupational therapy. Examples are use of a buttonhook to button a shirt and adding extensions to keys and door handles to extend the force arm and reduce the force required to turn the key or knob (Figs. 30-1, 30-2). Grasp, a problem for many patients, can be helped by using enlarged handles (Fig. 30-3). A therapist may experiment with adaptations to utensils by wrapping a washcloth, foam rubber, or other material

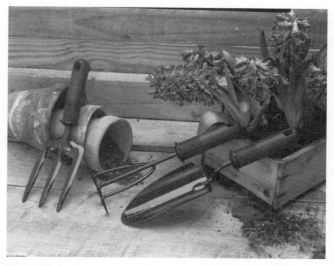

Figure 30-3 Good Grips garden tools with large handles. (Courtesy of SammonsPreston, Bolingbrook, IL.)

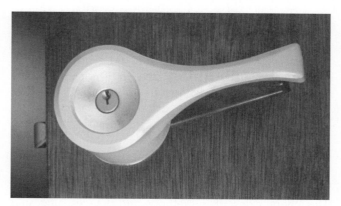

Figure 30-1 Doorknob extension. (Courtesy of SammonsPreston, Bolingbrook, IL.)

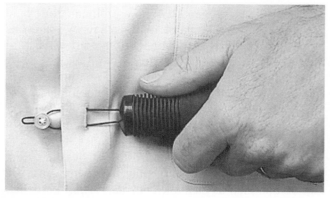

Figure 30-2 Good Grips button hook. (Courtesy of North Coast Medical, Morgan Hill, CA.)

around the handle and securing it with a rubber band. If enlarging the handle improves performance, permanent adaptation is prescribed and purchased or if necessary, custom built. Low-temperature thermoplastic materials that bond to themselves can be used for this purpose (see Chapter 15). Patients accept with satisfaction devices that allow them to accomplish valued activities (Mann et al., 1995).

Adaptation entails the following seven aspects, summarized in Box 30-2:

1. Analyze the task. Determine the essential demands of the task. The task demands are a combination of the performance requirements of a task, such as lifting, reaching, bending, and pulling, and the environmental requirements, such as counter height, location of faucets in the bathtub, and type of carpeting. Performance requirements must be quantified: What is the weight to be lifted? How high must it be lifted? and so on. Examination of these objective dimensions of the tasks suggests how the environment and equipment can be adapted to meet the capabilities of the person (Clark et al., 1990). Studies are beginning to appear that evaluate specific performance requirements of particular ADL tasks, such as the minimal wrist ranges of motion needed to accomplish ADL (Ryu et al., 1991) and pinch and grasp strength requirements to open containers (Rice et al., 1998).
2. Identify the problem. Why can't the person do what the task demands? The reason will identify his or her functional limitations, such as inability to reach above shoulder height, precaution against bending

BOX 30-2
PROCEDURES FOR PRACTICE

Adaptation Process

1. Analyze task and environmental demands.
2. Identify the problem: what limitation prevents the person from accomplishing the task in that environment?
3. Know principles of compensation for the given limitation.
4. Creatively apply principles of compensation to solve the problem.
5. Select appropriate assistive devices and specify methods for adapting the environment to implement the solution.
6. Check out all modifications to verify that they solve the problem.
7. Train in safe use of the assistive devices or modified environment.

over, inability to lift an object weighing more than a given amount.

3. Know the principles of compensation. Principles of compensation for representative functional limitations are presented in Box 30-3.

4. Propose solutions. Creatively consider ways that the principles of compensation can be applied to a particular task to enable the particular person to do it. Collaboration with the patient or a group of similarly involved patients often generates solutions.

5. Know the resources for implementing the solution. For example, it is important to know what reliable and safe equipment is available to solve the problem. Sources of equipment are rehabilitation supply stores, mail-order businesses, and gadget stores (see Resources). The occupational therapist needs to know and evaluate each piece of equipment being recommended. The fact that a piece of equipment is sold does not mean that it is effective or safe (Conine & Hershler, 1991). The therapist must know construction techniques needed to implement the solution when environmental modification is needed. The therapist also needs to know which contractors reliably provide quality home modifications.

6. Check it out. The assistive device or environmental modification should be checked out for reliability (always works as it should), durability (can withstand repeated use at the force levels the person will apply to it), safety, effectiveness, and patient satisfaction.

7. Train the person. The person must understand and be able to implement the safe use of the assistive device, environment, or method. Gitlin and Burgh

(1995) suggest five aspects to device training: develop an activity in which to introduce the device; choose a site for instruction; determine the best time in the rehabilitation process to introduce the device; provide instruction, including verbal instruction, demonstration, role modeling of others, inclusion of family members, and group training depending on the patient and the device; and reinforce device use with the patient and caregivers.

It is important to some people that assistive devices be transparent (McCuaig & Frank, 1991), that is, not call attention to the person as disabled or reveal the extent of disability. Use of conventional devices or gadgets that are sold to the general public qualify as transparent. Examples are felt-tipped pens, slip-on shoes, lightweight pots and pans, and magnifying makeup mirrors. They become adaptive because of their specific application. This perception of transparency and its importance are unique to the individual. Transparency is becoming easier because the principles of universal design have been found profitable by manufacturers of personal care and home products (One Shape Serves All, 1998).

Beyond transparency is the issue of gadget tolerance. Transparent or not, some people do not want to use special tools to do a task most people do without such a tool. However, the person will value the device if the task is important and cannot be done any other way (Bynum & Rogers, 1987; Parker & Thorslund, 1991; Rogers & Holm, 1992; Tyson & Strong, 1990). The number of devices prescribed should be reasonable and should enable important tasks. Otherwise the device ends up in the closet.

Activities of Daily Living

This chapter describes methods and devices suggested by occupational therapy practitioners and former patients to enable independence in BADL and IADL. These suggestions are presented according to the problem. Many patients have more than one problem. For example, persons with rheumatoid arthritis have weakness as well as limited range of motion. Persons with spinal cord injury have decreased sensation as well as weakness. The therapist will have to use information from pertinent sections for a patient with particular combinations of impairments. Procedures to enable BADL are presented. The need to do these activities and the task demands of each are fairly universal. However, because each person has unique constellations of IADL that describe their roles (Trombly, 1993, 1995), only representative IADL can be included as examples of solutions for particular problems.

All tasks that the patient expects to perform independently after discharge must be practiced as they will be done. For example, if a patient will bathe in a tub at home, it is inadequate to practice only sponge bathing while he or she is hospitalized. It is also inadequate to eliminate from practice the IADL of self-care, such as nail care, ear care, menstrual care, handling catheters, hair care, and contact lens care, or to assume that all self-care

tasks that a particular person may need to learn are listed on an evaluation checklist.

Techniques and equipment for self-care presented in this chapter are not the only methods of accomplishing these particular tasks. This presentation is meant to provide the student therapist with a repertoire of basic

---

BOX 30-3
Compensation Principles for Particular Impairments

Weakness
- Use lightweight objects, utensils, and tools.
- Let gravity assist.
- Use assistive devices or methods to replace lost functions such as grasp.
- Use power tools and utensils.
- Use biomechanical principles of levers (e.g., lengthen the force arm in relation to the resistance arm) and friction (e.g., increase friction to decrease power required for pinch or grasp).
- Use two hands for tasks ordinarily done one-handed.

Low Endurance
- Use energy conservation methods (see Box 30-4).
- Pace work to prevent fatigue.
- Use principles listed for weakness that reduce workload, such as lightweight utensils and power equipment.
- Match activity demands to ability.
- Avoid stressful positions and environmental stressors.

Limited Range of Motion
- Use long-handled tools and utensils to increase reach and/or eliminate the need for bending over.
- Build up handles to compensate for limited grasp.
- Store frequently used things within easy reach.
- Use joint protection techniques for rheumatoid arthritis (see Chapter 44).

Incoordination
- Stabilize the object being worked on.
- Stabilize proximal body parts so that need to control is reduced to the distal body parts.
- Use assistive devices that reduce slipperiness or provide stability.
- Use heavy utensils, cooking equipment, tools, and so on.
- Use adaptations that substitute for lack of fine skill.

Loss of the Use of One Side
- Provide assistive devices that substitute for the stabilizing or holding function of the involved upper extremity.
- Teach one-handed methods for activities ordinarily done two-handed.
- Provide assistive devices that change the few truly bilateral tasks into unilateral tasks.
- Improve dexterity of the uninvolved upper extremity if the dominant arm is the involved one.

Limited Vision
Blindness
- Organize the living space so that there is a place for everything and stress the importance of putting everything in its place after use (e.g., in the pantry cabinets, on refrigerator shelves, and in the medicine cabinet).

- Use Braille labels or optical scanners to distinguish canned goods, medications, clothing colors, and so on.
- Use devices that operate through voice commands.
- Use assistive devices that provide auditory, tactile, or kinesthetic feedback to compensate for low vision and blindness.
- Eliminate environmental clutter.
- Expect tasks to require extra time.

Low Vision
Some of the above principles are useful for those with low vision. Others:
- Provide high color contrast (e.g., white mug for coffee, colored towels in a white bathroom)
- Increase the light on a task by bringing the light closer, adding more lights, changing the background to increase contrast (Lampert & Lapolice, 1995).
- Use techniques and devices that magnify type or images.
- Reduce visual clutter.
- Use organized scanning techniques (e.g., left to right, top to bottom) when functioning in a stationary environment.

Decreased or Absent Sensation
- Protect the anesthetic part from abrasions, bruises, cuts, burns, and decubiti.
- Substitute vision for poor awareness of limb position and limb movement or to detect texture.
- Develop habits of directing attention to the affected part.

Poor Memory and/or Organizational Skills
- Use assistive devices that substitute for memory or poor organizational skills (e.g., pill minders, day books, electronic reminder devices, sticky notes, watches with programmable multiple alarm systems, palm-size computers and organizers).
- Teach strategies such as writing memos to self, making to-do and other lists, placing objects together and at the point needed ahead of time.
- Develop habits regarding time use and how activities are to be accomplished.

Low Back Pain
- Teach body mechanics for moving and lifting (e.g., hold objects close to the body, squat to lower the body rather than bending over).
- Use long-handled or bent-handled equipment or sit to substitute for bending over.
- Change position frequently.
- When standing, put one foot up on a step to rotate the pelvis.
- Rest before fatigue results in awkward, careless movements.
- Avoid twisting the trunk.

skills with which to approach patients with confidence. The principles of compensation for each problem are key pieces of information that allow the student to evaluate other techniques or equipment to meet the needs of the patient. For many tasks not mentioned here, either no adaptation is required or the adaptation can be extrapolated from the examples cited.

As each task is taught, all equipment should be close at hand. For early training in dressing, clothing that is a size too large should be used, because it can be managed more easily. The patient's attention should be called to design details of clothing, as persons with certain disabilities find it difficult to don some designs. The details to be considered are the cut of the garment, sleeve style, type of fabric, and type of closure or fasteners (Dallas & White, 1982). Clothing especially designed for the handicapped can now be purchased (see Resources).

Weakness (Box 30-3)

For other information and suggestions see Chapters 17, 40, and 43.

Suggestions for BADL

When muscle weakness affects all four extremities, the techniques and devices are extensive; therefore, this section focuses on compensation for involvement of all four extremities. If the patient is paralyzed in the lower extremities but has normal upper extremities, many of the techniques or devices are unnecessary. Some of the principles apply as well to limited weakness, such as weak pinch secondary to osteoarthritis of the carpometacarpal joint.

When paralysis is extensive, a personal care attendant (PCA) is needed to carry out BADL. The patient must learn to hire, supervise, instruct, compensate, set limits for, and terminate personnel (DeGraff, 1989).

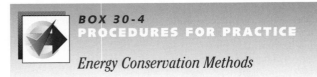

BOX 30-4
PROCEDURES FOR PRACTICE

Energy Conservation Methods

- ▸ Plan ahead. Organize work.
- ▸ Eliminate unnecessary tasks.
- ▸ Sit to work when possible.
- ▸ Have all required equipment and supplies ready before starting the task.
- ▸ Combine tasks to eliminate extra work.
- ▸ Use electrical appliances to conserve personal energy.
- ▸ Use lightweight utensils and tools.
- ▸ Work with gravity assisting, not resisting.
- ▸ Rest before fatiguing.

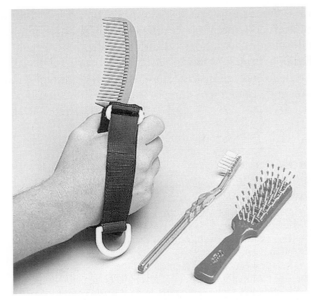

Figure 30-4 Universal cuff. (Courtesy of North Coast Medical, Morgan Hill, CA.)

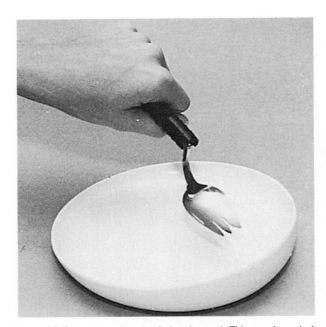

Figure 30-5 Spork (combination fork and spoon). This one also swivels.

Feeding

The problem with feeding is the inability to grasp and/or bring the hand to the mouth. A universal cuff can be used to hold the utensil if grasp is absent (Fig. 30-4). This cuff fits around the palm and has a pocket for insertion of the handle of a utensil. Alternatively, the handle can be woven through the fingers, that is, index and ring fingers on top and middle and little fingers under, and held in place passively. A spork, a utensil that combines the bowl of a spoon with the tines of a fork (Fig. 30-5), can be used with the cuff to eliminate the need to change utensils. Some of these have a swivel feature to substitute for the inability to supinate. Gravity and weight of the food keep the bowl level on the way to the mouth. If the patient has weak grasp, lightweight enlarged handles can be used. The patient may use a wrist-driven wrist–hand orthosis to increase the strength of grasp (see Chapter 14). For cutting, a sharp serrated knife is used, because less force is needed and it is less likely to slip.

An attachable open-bottomed handle can be added to a glass or soft drink can to permit picking it up in the

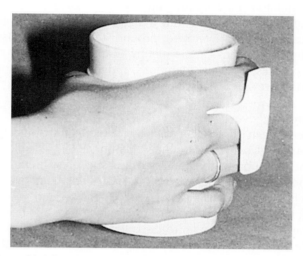

Figure 30-6 Cup with T-shaped handle assists drinking when grasp is weak.

absence of grasp. A mug with a T-shaped handle (Fig. 30-6) or a handle that allows all four fingers to be inserted provides leverage and stabilizes the fingers around the mug, allowing pick-up with tenodesis grasp. A foam can insulator can be used for a glass to provide friction to assist weak grasp. A mobile arm support or suspension sling (see Chapter 14) may be required to allow reaching and bringing the hand to the mouth. A table placed at axilla height offers support for the arm and eliminates the pull of gravity, allowing the patient with elbow flexors graded 3 or 3+ to bring the food to the mouth. As strength increases, the surface can be lowered.

Grooming

The inability to grasp and pinch must be dealt with to enable grooming. Adaptations for makeup jars, tubes, and applicators have been suggested (Hage, 1988). A universal cuff or a splint can be used to hold a rattail comb, toothbrush, lipstick tube, or safety razor if grasp is absent. A handcuff can be constructed to hold an electric razor. If grasp is weak, lightweight enlarged handles may be enough. Applying friction material to the utensil or tool can provide added assistance. A small plastic brush with a cuff attachment may be used to assist in shampooing hair. Lengthening the force arm relative to the resistance arm may allow use of spray deodorant (Fig. 30-7) or nail care (Fig. 30-8).

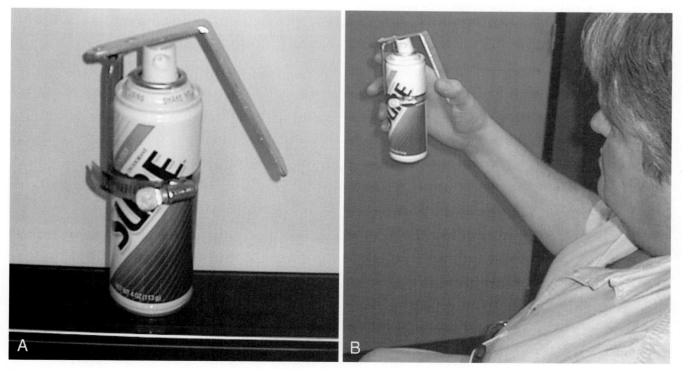

Figure 30-7 A. Aerosol can adapter that reduces the force needed to operate the spray. **B.** Operation of the adapter.

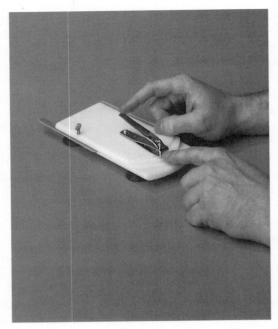

Figure 30-8 Nail clipper and emery boards stabilized to allow one-handed use, and with elongated handle to reduce force required. (Courtesy of SammonsPreston, Bolingbrook, IL.)

Toileting

Transfers, the handling of the body to lower and raise the clothing, and weak pinch and grasp are problems. For patients with spinal cord injury, concomitant loss of bowel and bladder control requires special procedures, including bladder irrigation, use of a catheter, or intermittent catheterization (Lewis, 1993). Generally the patient can push down the pants while in the wheelchair by leaning from side to side. If the patient cannot stand or has precarious standing balance, it is necessary to transfer back to the wheelchair before raising the clothing after toileting. If the patient uses an indwelling catheter or external drainage device, the collection bag can be emptied into the toilet without transfer or removal of clothing. Usually nurses or enterostomal therapists teach clean intermittent self-catheterization, but the occupational therapist should be aware of the process of this activity of daily living: (1) The person washes hands with soap and water. (2) Males lubricate the catheter tip with water-soluble lubricant, hold penis at sides, and insert catheter with firm, gentle pressure. Females separate labia, palpate meatus, and insert catheter into the bladder. (3) The patient pushes catheter in 2.5 cm (1 inch) after urine starts to flow. (4) The person allows urine to flow until it stops and then slowly removes the catheter, holding catheter tip as it is removed to prevent spilling. (5) The catheter is washed with soap and water, rinsed, dried, and stored in a plastic bag. (6) The person washes hands with soap and water (Clarkson, 1982).

Those who need a bowel program use a style of raised toilet seat that creates a space between the seat and toilet bowl rim to allow for insertion of a suppository. Suppository inserters for those with weak or absent pinch are commercially available. Cuffs are attached to these devices so that patients who lack good grasp can manipulate them using leverage. They may have a spring ejector that releases the suppository after it is properly positioned in the rectum. An inspection mirror is needed if the patient lacks anal sensation. Digit stimulators may be the method of choice for some patients. For patients with weak grasp and pinch, toilet tissue can be wrapped around the hand for use. Menstrual needs can be met by adaptations to positioning, pants, pad versus tampons, and aids such as mirrors and knee spreaders (Duckworth, 1986).

Dressing

Dressing in less than an hour is considered functional for tetraplegics (Weingarden & Martin, 1989). Problems include moving the paralyzed limbs to dress them and the need to compensate for the lack of pinch and grasp. While in bed, using the wrist extensors and elbow flexors, patients with spinal cord injuries at C6 and below can pull the knees up to dress the lower extremities. A dressing stick (Fig. 30-9) with a loop that goes around the wrist attached to the end opposite the hook can help. The person pulls against the loop, using wrist extension and leverage, to stabilize tenodesis grasp of the stick. Loops of twill tape can be added to the cuffs of socks to

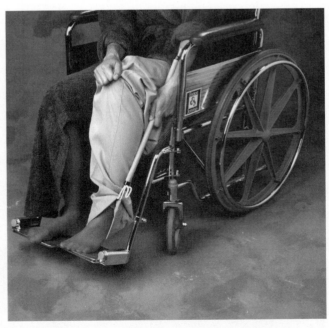

Figure 30-9 Dressing stick. (Courtesy of The Rehabilitation Division of Smith & Nephew, Germantown, WI.)

facilitate pulling them on by hooking the thumb in the loop when pinch is absent.

A buttonhook attached to a cuff or with a built-up handle is used when fingers are unable to manipulate buttons (Fig. 30-2). The hook is inserted through the buttonhole to hook the button and pull it through the buttonhole. The other hand is used to hold the garment near the buttonhole. A loop of string or leather lacing may be attached to the zipper pull of trousers or other garments so that in the absence of pinch, the thumb can be hooked in the loop to close the zipper. A zipper hook can also be used.

Also to be considered is adaptation of clothes to facilitate dressing, undressing, toileting, and moving about, to regulate temperature, to increase comfort, and to increase feelings of self-confidence (Kratz et al., 1997). For business people confined to wheelchairs, suit jackets, trousers, and skirts tailored to accommodate the sitting position look better than off-the-rack suits.

Runge (1967) described the following methods of tetraplegic dressing.

Trousers and Undershorts

1. While the patient is sitting in a hospital bed with side rails up, the trousers are positioned with the front up and legs over the bottom of the bed. The trousers are positioned by tossing them or using a dressing stick with a wrist loop.
2. One leg is lifted by hooking the opposite wrist or forearm under the knee, and the foot is put into the pants leg. The thumb of the other hand hooks a belt loop or pocket to hold the trousers open. Working in a cross-body position aids stability for those with poor balance.
3. The other foot is inserted.
4. The palms of the hands are used to pat and slide the trousers onto the calves and to get the trouser cuffs over the feet. The wrist or wrists are hooked under the waistband or in the pockets to pull the trousers up over the knees.
5. The patient continues to pull on the waistband or pockets while returning to supine position to pull the trousers up onto the thighs. This may have to be repeated. Hooking the wrist or thumbs in the crotch helps pull up the trousers.
6. In a side-lying position, the thumb of the top arm is hooked in the back belt loop, and the pants are pulled over the buttocks. Then the patient rolls to the other side and repeats the process until the trousers are on.
7. In a supine position, the trousers can be fastened using a zipper pull loop and Velcro tab closing or buttonhook.

8. The trousers are removed by reversing the procedures and pushing the pants off.

Socks. While sitting in the wheelchair, the patient crosses one leg over the other and uses tenodesis grasp to put on the sock and the palms of the hands to help pull it on. If the patient cannot cross his or her legs, the foot can be placed on a stool or chair. If trunk balance is poor, one arm can be hooked around the wheelchair upright while reaching with the other hand, or the socks can be put on while sitting in bed by crossing first one leg and then the other. Socks are removed by pushing them off with a dressing stick, long shoehorn, or the thumb hooked over the sock edge.

Knee–Ankle–Foot Orthosis for Paraplegics

1. While the patient is sitting in bed, the orthosis is positioned beside the leg, and the patient lifts his or her leg over into it.
2. If the shoe is attached to the orthosis, the foot is first put into the shoe. It is helpful to unlock and flex the knee of the orthosis to press the shoe against the bed and pull on the uprights to get the heel into the shoe.
3. With the knee still flexed, the shoe can be tied.
4. The knee is straightened and the straps are fastened.

For an orthosis to be worn under trousers, it must be detachable from the shoe. In this instance the patient puts on socks, the orthosis, trousers, then shoes and finally attaches the orthosis to the shoe. Once the patient is in the wheelchair, other garments are put on.

Shoes. Loafers are most practical for patients who cannot walk. Shoes are put on by crossing one leg at a time as for putting on socks. The shoe is pulled onto the foot by balancing the sole of the shoe in the palm of the hand. Then with the foot on the floor or on the foot pedal of the wheelchair, the foot is pushed down into the shoe by pushing on the knee. A long shoehorn may be helpful for getting the heel into the shoe. Shoes can be removed by pushing them off with the shoehorn.

Cardigan Garments: Shirts and Blouses

1. The shirt is positioned with the brand label of the shirt facing down and the collar toward the knees.
2. The patient puts his or her arms under the shirt and into the sleeves.
3. The shirt is pushed on until the sleeves are over the elbows.
4. The shirt is gathered up by using wrist extension and by hooking the thumbs under the shirt back.
5. The shirt is placed over the head.

6. The patient shrugs to get the shirt down across the shoulders and hooks the wrists into the sleeves to free the axillae.
7. The patient leans forward and reaches back with one hand to rub on the shirt back to pull it down.
8. The shirt fronts are lined up, and buttoning begins from the bottom button up, using a buttonhook.

A cardigan garment is removed by pushing first one side and then the other off the shoulders and then alternately elevating and depressing the shoulders to allow gravity to assist in lowering the shirt down the arms. Then, one thumb is hooked into the opposite sleeve to pull the shirt over the elbow, and the arm is removed from the shirt.

With the exception of buttons, an overhead garment is put on in a similar manner and removed by hooking one thumb in the back of the neckline and pulling the shirt over the head. The sleeves are pushed off each arm.

Bra. Either a front- or back-closure bra can be used. Velcro can replace hooks for fastening, but some patients can manage the standard hook fastener if it is hooked in front at waist level. After the bra is hooked, it is positioned with the cups in front, and the arms are placed through the shoulder straps. Then, by hooking the opposite thumb under a strap, one strap at a time is pulled over the shoulder.

Bathing

The problems with bathing include the transfer, dynamic sitting balance, lack of lower extremity movement (Shillam et al., 1983), and lack of pinch and grasp. Transfer tub seats (Fig, 30-10), which have two legs in the tub and two legs outside the tub, provide a safe means to transfer from the wheelchair to tub. Patients prone to

decubiti need padded seats. Each patient's requirements should be evaluated and a seat selected to fit them. The bath seat must be placed so that the faucets are within reach. Grab bars help during the transfer and while the patient is seated (Box 30-5). Nonslip material is used in the bottom of the tub. The faucets must have lever handles for ease in tapping them off and on with the fist. A hand-held shower that is adapted with a hook handle is used. No-scald faucets and shower heads should be used, but if they are unavailable, water temperature should be regulated by turning on the cold water first and then adding the hot, which prevents scalding desensitized skin. Soap on a string or in a dispenser is helpful. A bath mitt is used if grasp is weak or absent. The person dries off before transferring back to the wheelchair. Bathing and drying the feet and legs are particular problems for patients with poor trunk balance; such patients may prefer to do foot hygiene while in bed (Shillam et al., 1983).

A custom-made shower stall provides the best solution for a patient confined to a wheelchair. The shower area should have a raised slope to prevent the water from running out but allow the person to enter the shower on a shower wheelchair. Plans for such bath enclosures are shown in books on the Resources list.

Suggestions for Selected IADL

For the severely paralyzed, high-tech adaptations as described in Chapter 17 offer opportunities to engage in communication, leisure, and work activities. Some low-tech adaptations are suggested here.

Handling a Book

The tetraplegic patient encounters problems with holding a book and turning the pages, with writing or recording notes in business or school, and possibly in telephoning. Some book holders support a book on a table, whereas others are designed to hold a book when reading supine in bed. If a person is reading while supine and the book is not held directly above, prism glasses are needed to direct the vision to a 90° angle so that the book may be seen.

To turn pages, some solutions are as follows: (1) when wearing a splint, the patient can use a rubber thimble or finger cot on the posted thumb. (2) A pencil with the eraser end down can be used in a universal cuff (typing stick) or hand splint. (3) Electric page turners automatically turn pages when activated by a micro-switch or other means of control. (4) A mouthstick with a friction tip end may be useful (Fig. 30-11). Mouthsticks with flat mouthpieces can be purchased commercially. However, for long sessions of use, a mouthstick with a molded mouthpiece that conforms to the patient's dentition is preferred (Smith, 1989). The mouthpiece has a lightweight plastic or aluminum rod to which an eraser

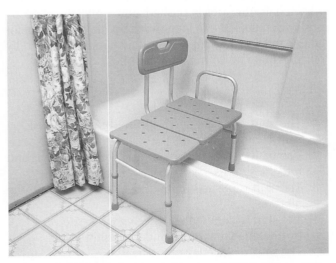

Figure 30-10 Transfer bath bench. (Courtesy of S&S, Colchester, CT.)

BOX 30-5
PROCEDURES FOR PRACTICE
Grab Bars

Selection

Grab bars can be purchased from rehabilitation supply houses and some plumbing supply centers. ***Towel bars are NOT safe for use as a grab bar.*** Grab bars must be able to accept 200 to 250 pounds of force, more if patient weighs more.

Horizontal bars are for pushing up; vertical bars are for pulling up (Garee, 1992). An L-shaped grab bar that includes both vertical and horizontal legs is a good choice for the bathtub or shower enclosure.

A clamp-on bathtub-mounted safety grab rail cannot be used on fiberglass tubs because those tubs cannot tolerate the stress (Burke, 1989).

The optimum diameter for grab bars is 1.25 to 1.5 inches for adults. The distance between the wall and the bar should be 1.5 inches. A wider space is dangerous because if the arm slips, it may get caught between the wall and the bar and/or the person may fall (Salmen, 2000).

Placement

Locate bathtub grab bars where a person may be off balance, such as going into or out of the tub, turning in the tub or shower, or standing up from or sitting down on a bench or seat. One vertical bar outside the tub and one horizontal or diagonal bar on the wall along the length of the tub is recommended as a basic installation. An L-shaped bar can be substituted for the bar on the wall along the length of the tub. If an L-shaped bar is used, locate the horizontal bar 16 inches above the tub rim and the vertical bar approximately 32 inches from the corner of the tub or as the placement suits the height and transfer and bathing process of the user.

Although the most common site for grab bars is in or near the bathtub enclosure, bars near the toilet (Fig. 30-15) are often necessary. Bars that look like armrests attach to the toilet; those that have legs that extend to the floor are most stable and safe.

Installation

Grab bars must be mounted to the wall with 2-inch stainless steel screws driven into the wall studs. Use a stud finder to locate the studs. It may be necessary to locate the studs from the other side of the wall if the bathroom walls are tiled. The typical mounting flange has three holes for three screws. Use an eighth-inch masonry bit to drill three holes in the ceramic tile for the mounting screws. Only two screws will actually fit into the stud. Therefore, use a toggle bolt for the third screw. Grab bars from Invacare (see Resource Box) have two screws that can be oriented so that both line up with the stud.

In new construction, double the studs where grab bars are to be fastened so there will be a 3-inch place to fasten the screws rather than the 1.5 inches offered by only one stud. For horizontal bars, add a 2 × 4 between the studs as a screwing surface; some people cut into existing walls to add the horizontal 2 × 4 and then replace the wall board.

---

or other type of end piece, such as pencil, pen, or paintbrush, can be added.

An alternative is talking books, or books on tape, which can be obtained from libraries and bookstores. The Library of Congress has a large collection of tapes, including many current issues of magazines, and tape players that are available to the blind and the physically disabled. They are free (see Resources).

Writing

Extensive writing is usually done with computerized word processing and typing sticks or a mouthstick for hitting the keys. If speed is important, as in taking notes in the classroom or in business, a tape recorder can be used.

Handwriting is important for legal documents and personalizing cards and typed notes. Splints that provide pinch can be used to hold a writing instrument. If pinch is absent and the patient does not use a splint, a pencil holder (Fig. 30-12) that encircles the pencil, thumb, and index finger can be made of thermoplastic materials. Pens with textured grips provide friction to make a weak grip more effective. Felt-tipped pens require little pres-

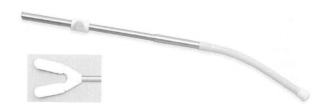

Figure 30-11 Mouthstick. (Courtesy of North Coast Medical, Morgan Hill, CA.)

sure and are therefore easier to use than other types of pens. If the arms cannot be used, with practice a mouthstick with pencil attached can become an effective writing tool.

Telephoning

A person whose spinal cord was injured at C6 or below can pick up a traditional telephone receiver and bring it to his or her ear. An executive shoulder rest attached to the receiver holds it there until the conversation is finished. If the person has an injury at a higher level, uses the phone often, or has a cordless phone, he or she can

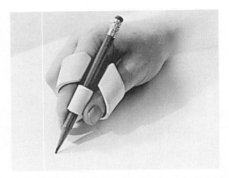

Figure 30-12 Pencil holder made of thermoplastic material.

wear a headset or use a speaker phone that precludes the need to hold the phone.

Push buttons can be depressed with a mouthstick or typing stick. Speed dial or memory dial reduces the number of buttons to depress. For persons unable to press any buttons, high-tech solutions are possible.

Turning Electrical Appliances On and Off

The burgeoning field of electronic aids to daily living (EADLs), formerly known as environmental control units, includes remote control devices for TV, entertainment centers, VCRs, lights, door openers, electric beds, and appliances. See Chapter 17 for a discussion of high-tech assistive devices that are useful for persons with severe weakness or paralysis resulting from a spinal cord injury or degenerative disease such as amyotrophic lateral sclerosis.

Sexual Activities

Most persons have concerns about their sexuality early after spinal cord injury, although they are not ready to learn about the particulars concerning resuming sexual activities or procreation. Early on they appreciate acknowledgment of their concerns and sources of information for when they are ready (McAlonan, 1996).

In a pioneering book, *Sexual Options for Paraplegics and Quadriplegics*, Mooney et al. (1975) explicitly described methods of sexual expression for persons with spinal cord injury. They pictured the process of getting ready for sex (emptying the bladder, washing). They addressed how to handle a catheter that is left in place during sex (bend the catheter and fold it over along the shaft of the penis where it will be out of the way, but do not anchor it until the erection has taken place to avoid pulling out the balloon of the Foley catheter; be sure the tubing and collection bag are not leaned on to prevent the flow of urine). They presented positions for genital and orogenital sexual expression, alternative means of sexual expression (vibrators, touch, talking), and how to achieve and maintain a reflex erection of the penis. They discussed fertility of men: ability to ejaculate depends on the level of the lesion, and production of sperm depends on healthy testicles. They pointed out that women remain fertile and therefore pregnancy is as possible as for able-bodied women. Although this book is out of print, it is still worth obtaining from the library. Also, other books have become available as sexuality for the disabled is fully acknowledged (see Resources).

Low Endurance (Box 30-3)

For other information and suggestions, see Chapter 47.

Suggestions for BADL

Patients of various diagnoses and circumstances (e.g., post bed rest) have low endurance, at least temporarily. Patients with cardiac or pulmonary disease have a more or less permanent reduction of endurance to which they must adapt. These patients have reduced ability to use oxygen needed for muscle, including cardiac muscle, and brain functions. If oxygen deprivation is severe enough, neuropsychological changes involving memory, perception, and information processing occur. These affect the effectiveness of the teaching and learning process as well as performance.

Adaptations for BADL and IADL involve awareness and reduction of the metabolic cost of activities and working within limits of cardiac and pulmonary capacity. Cardiac patients are cautioned to stop activity when they have angina or shortness of breath (SOB). Patients with chronic obstructive pulmonary disease are taught to work slowly, pacing themselves and taking resting pauses during tasks. Both types of patients are taught to take rest periods throughout the day and use other energy-conserving techniques. Energy conservation methods are listed in Box 30-4 and elaborated on in Chapter 32.

Some activities require higher levels of energy than do others. One way to guide activity selection is to use metabolic equivalent (MET) tables. Most self-care activities require less than 3 METs; however, showering, tub bathing, toileting, and washing and setting hair require higher levels. It should be remembered that MET charts are averages, and do not account for particular circumstances, and therefore cannot be used without also monitoring the patient's breathing or heart rate. Dyspnea (SOB) signals the patient that the activity he or she is doing is beyond his or her capacity. Angina or excessive increase in heart rate (20 beats over resting rate) signals the cardiac patient that he or she has reached his or her limit. Stressful positions and circumstances, including the following, are to be avoided (Berzins, 1970; Cristy & Sarafconn, 1990; Pomerantz et al., 1975):

▶ Bending over. Slip-on shoes, sock aids, reachers, and long-handled sponges can be used to assist ADL independence without bending over.

► Reaching overhead. Store clothes and utensils within easy reach; rest arms on something when reaching or repeatedly lower arms to rest if reaching up is necessary.

► Isometric contractions, including pushing, pulling, and maintained grasp. Patients should exhale or count while they do these actions, if the actions cannot be avoided.

► Hot, humid environment. Such conditions increase shortness of breath and reduce the patient's aerobic capacity.

► Overexertion.

Suggestions offered for persons with low endurance (Cristy & Sarafconn, 1990):

► Get sufficient sleep. Strategies for the patient who is having trouble sleeping include developing a bed-time routine and schedule; practicing relaxation techniques, such as visualization, listening to soothing music, progressive relaxation technique, and meditation; and avoiding upsetting or exciting activities just before bedtime.

► Consider your energy budget. Identify essential tasks and eliminate nonessential ones. Spread the performance of tasks that must be done throughout the day or week and delegate the rest to others.

► Do preventive maintenance and cleaning. A small chore left undone becomes an energy-consuming one later on.

► Organize working space. Organize to allow sitting without reaching, stretching, or bending while working.

► Use labor-saving products and techniques. Examples of ways to save energy include soaking dishes before washing them and using a computer program that writes checks and maintains household accounts simultaneously.

► Organize work and errands. Organize to eliminate backtracking, extra steps or trips, and to allow planned rest periods. Keep commitments within manageable limits.

► Emotions, good and bad, use energy, too. Consider the emotions when budgeting energy.

Sexual Activities

The American Heart Association (1999) booklet *Sex and Heart Disease* discusses the cardiovascular changes that occur during sexual intercourse, when the patient can resume sex after myocardial infarction or heart surgery, how other factors affect sex interest and capacity, guidelines for resuming sex, what to do if symptoms arise during sex, Viagra, and myths and misconceptions. The booklet can be helpful to both the patient and the health professional.

Limited or Restricted Range of Motion (Box 30-3)

For other information and suggestions see Chapters 41, 42, 44, and 45.

Suggestions for BADL
Feeding

The problem with feeding may be inability to close the hand enough to grasp the utensil or inability to bring the hand to the mouth. Enlarged or elongated handles can be added to spoons or forks. The elongated handle may have to be angled to enable the patient to reach the mouth. Remember that the longer the handle (resistance arm), the heavier and less stable the device; therefore, the handle should be only as long as is necessary and made of lightweight material.

A universal cuff, or utensil holder, can be used when grasp is not possible (Fig. 30-4). For some patients, such as those with arthrogryposis, independent eating may be impossible. An electric device can be used to give a sense of self-reliance. However, the device must be set up and cleaned up by an assistant, and some insurance carriers will not pay for both device and assistant. Another factor to be considered when prescribing this device: for an institutionalized person, being fed by another may be an opportunity for social contact that the device would eliminate (Hermann et al., 1999).

Grooming

The problems with grooming are the same as for feeding. Enlarged or extended handles can be attached to a comb (Fig. 30-13), brush, toothbrush, shampoo brush,

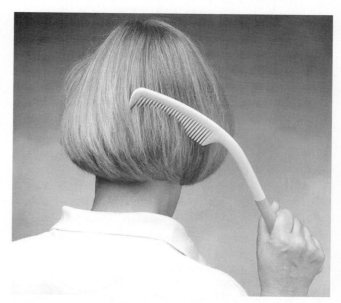

Figure 30-13 Long-handled comb. (Courtesy of North Coast Medical, Morgan Hill, CA.)

Case Example

MRS. L.: EDUCATION AND ADAPTATION TO RESTORE ROLE OF INDEPENDENT PERSON

Patient Information

Mrs. L. was admitted to hospital via ambulance from home suffering from a suspected heart attack. On examination, the physician confirmed the myocardial infarction and, in addition, found her to be anemic and depressed. On query, she revealed that she rarely prepared meals.

Mrs. L. is a 70-year-old widow who lives alone in a small house. She retired 5 years ago from her position as administrative assistant to the president of a major bank. Until her husband died 2 years ago, they were active in a weekly couples bridge club and a drama club. They took one 3-week tour yearly. She was a volunteer at the American Red Cross blood bank. Since her husband's death, she has limited her activities to grocery shopping and Sunday church. Her daughter and son-in-law visit once a week for dinner and to do heavy chores for her such as washing the floors and mowing the lawn.

Her long-term goal is to return home. After treatment at the acute care center, she was discharged to a skilled nursing facility (SNF) because she was unready to return home and her daughter was unavailable to be at home with her because of work responsibilities. Mrs. L. was referred to occupational therapy to prepare to return home.

Recommendations

Evaluation revealed that Mrs. L. could complete tasks at a 2-MET level. In response to questions generated from the *COPM*, Mrs. L. identified the following problems preventing her from returning home: (1) inability to shower because of fatigue and unmotivated to dress in street clothes, (2) lack of motivation to prepare meals for self because of fatigue and sadness, (3) anticipated problem caring for the house because of fatigue, and (4) anticipated problem doing laundry because of fatigue and fear of overexertion, since the washer and dryer are in the basement.

The occupational therapist recommended treatment 1 hour a day 5 days a week for 3 weeks. Physical therapy was scheduled in the morning, so the occupational therapist scheduled Mrs. L. for occupational therapy at 3 PM, after her after-lunch rest.

Short-Term Goals

Goals that the occupational therapist and Mrs. L. agreed on for the 3-week period:

1. Mrs. L. will regenerate motivation to engage in social and other activities.
2. Mrs. L. will learn to use the energy she was recovering in physical therapy to do BADL and IADL.
3. Mrs. L. will learn to apply energy conservation techniques to, and how to select assistive devices for, self-care, meal preparation, and basic home care.

Therapy started with developing rapport over card games. This developed into interest by Mrs. L. in joining card games in the activity room "while I am waiting to go home." Her spirits brightened in resuming this set-aside hobby. Rapport was easily established, leaving Mrs. L. open to therapy. The therapist discussed energy conservation methods with her, gave her a written work sheet with some of the methods listed, and assigned her "homework" using these methods for showering. The **night before**, she was to **gather all supplies, clothing, and towels needed** for a shower the following morning. The next day she was **to sit on a bench** in the shower in tepid (not hot) water, taking **rest breaks** between washing each section of her body. She used a **lightweight bath sponge** to wash her back and lower extremities to eliminate the need for bending over. She dried **with a terry robe rather than rubbing**. She then **rested before** dressing. Pleased with her accomplishment, Mrs. L. discussed how she would use liquid soap next time to use even less energy in soaping herself.

Mrs. L. felt somewhat in control of her fatigue and was ready to try new tasks. In collaboration with the occupational therapist, she applied energy conservation techniques to dusting, tidying, and dry-mopping her room. The occupational therapist reviewed the energy conservation methods with her again, and they discussed which applied to each task. Successful with that, Mrs. L. chose to prepare supper in the occupational therapy kitchen for herself and her bridge partner. The occupational therapist suggested that Mrs. L. plan the menu, the shopping list, and the procedures to be used over the several days before the day of the meal. Again, Mrs. L. and the occupational therapist discussed the energy conservation methods that applied to each task. On the day of the meal, Mrs. L. started 2 hours ahead to ensure enough time for rest breaks and cooking. Some devices and methods she used included a spike board to hold vegetables while cutting with a very sharp knife; an oven-to-table dish, which she transported from the counter to the oven and from the oven to the table on a wheeled cart; prepared foods for dessert, including store-bought cake, frozen berries, and frozen dairy whip.

Revised Goals

The patient was discharged at the end of the 3 weeks with these goals to achieve before follow-up:

1. Mrs. L. will keep a journal and record at least once a day how she used energy conservation methods and/or adapted methods to resume care of the home.
2. Mrs. L. will resume volunteering, starting with one morning a week.
3. Mrs. L. will visit the senior center regularly on card game afternoons.

lipstick tube, or safety razor. Aerosol deodorant, hair spray, powder, and perfume can be used by those with limited range. Another person may be needed to wash thoroughly and style hair; if the person can reach the head to do it independently, a simple hairstyle is recommended. For patients who have had hand surgery and are prohibited from getting the incision wet, a waterproof plastic mitten allows the patient to use the hand as much as possible during self-care and kitchen activities (Fig. 30-14).

Toileting

The problem with toileting is the inability to reach. The toilet tissue dispenser should be within reach. Wiping tongs can extend reach when using toilet tissue. If grasp is poor, the tissue can be wrapped around the hand. A bidet eliminates the need for wiping by hand. A bidet accessory is available to retrofit regular toilets. Gravity assists in pulling clothes down; loose clothes slide off easily. A dressing stick can be used to pull up the clothing (Fig. 30-9). Sanitary napkins with adhesive strips can be used more easily than tampons; the protective paper can be removed with the teeth. If the patient is not able to sit and arise from a low commode, a raised toilet seat may solve the problem (Fig. 30-15).

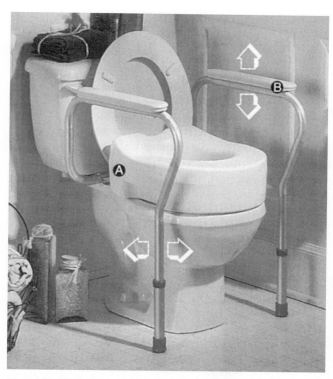

Figure 30-15 The Invacare Toilet Safety Frame and CareGuard by Invacare Raised Toilet Seat make the bathroom a safer environment for those with special needs. These products are recommended for combined use. (Courtesy of Invacare.)

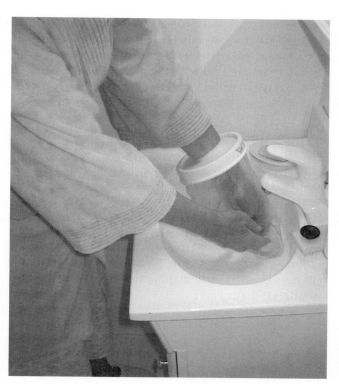

Figure 30-14 Plastic glove prevents operated hand from getting wet during washing of the other hand.

Dressing

Lack of ability to reach and grasp and limited shoulder, back, hip, or knee range of motion are problems encountered in dressing. For 3 months following hip replacement, patients are restricted from flexing the hip past 90°, adducting the leg past midline, externally rotating the leg, or bearing full weight on the leg (Seeger & Fisher, 1982); therefore, they need to use the suggestions in this section temporarily (see also Chapter 41).

A dressing stick can be used to pull clothing over the feet or to reach hangers in the closet. Reachers can be used to remove clothes from shelves, to start clothes over parts of the body, and to pick up objects from the floor (Fig. 30-16).

Dressing the lower extremities is a particular problem. People who cannot reach their feet or who are not allowed to flex the hip can dress the lower extremities using a sock or stocking aid (Fig. 30-17). To use, the cone is inserted into the foot of the stocking; the top of the stocking is pushed down below the top edge of the cone. While the strings are held, the stocking aid with stocking in place is tossed over the toes, and the person's foot is moved into the foot of the stocking. The cone is then removed by pulling the strings, bringing it out of the stocking behind the heel. This brings the stocking within reach and can be pulled up the leg. One study found that patients identified the sock aid as the most useful device at the 2-week follow up interview at home, but it was the most rejected aid at the time of dispensing in the hospital (Finlayson & Havixbeck, 1992).

An alternative method is to place a piece of foam rubber on the floor to help get the stocking onto the foot after it is placed on the toe with a reacher. This method consists of pushing the foot forward across the foam rubber, which provides friction and holds the stocking as the foot slides into it. As this method can be done standing up or sitting on a high stool, it may be particularly helpful to post-hip replacement patients, who are not allowed to flex the hip.

A long shoehorn assists in putting on shoes when the feet cannot be reached (Seeger & Fisher, 1982). Some long shoehorns have a hook on the opposite end that may be used as a dressing stick. Slip-on shoes and elastic shoelaces avoid the need to tie shoelaces. The reacher and/or dressing stick may be used to pull up slacks.

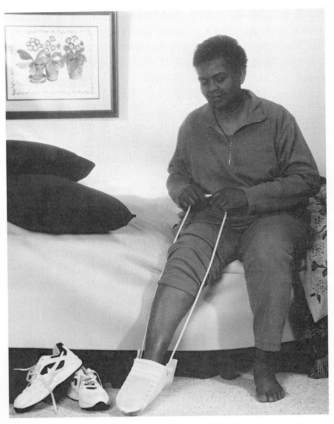

Figure 30-17 Stocking aid in use. (Courtesy of The Rehabilitation Division of Smith & Nephew, Germantown, WI.)

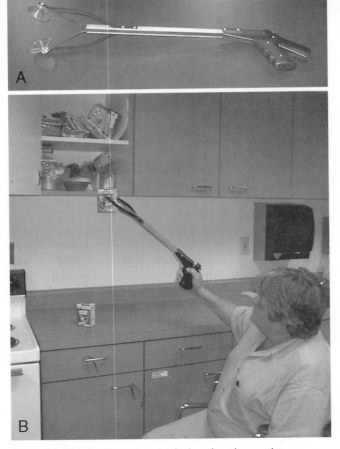

Figure 30-16 A. Reacher with a pistol grip and suction cup tips. **B.** Reacher in use.

Dressing the upper body can be accomplished by using button- or zipper-front garments instead of over-the-head garments. A dressing stick or reacher is used to bring the garment around the shoulders. Fasteners are particularly difficult, especially if limitation in the range of motion is accompanied by weakness. In a study of ability of 97 arthritic women to use clothing fasteners, zippers, especially easy-sliding, large-toothed plastic ones, were found to be easiest. Snaps and buttons were rated as difficult, although vertical buttonholes made buttoning easier (Dallas & White, 1982). Velcro tabs can replace buttons, snaps, or hooks if limited mobility in the fingers prevents buttoning or fastening. Because few clothes come with this type of fastener, the patient's clothing must be adapted. To preserve the look of a buttoned garment, the buttonhole is sewn closed and the button is attached over the hole. The hook and pile Velcro tabs are sewn to replace the buttons (Reich & Otten, 1980).

Bathing
The transfer into the tub is facilitated by grab bars (Box 30-5). Nonslip material should be placed on the bottom of the tub. A tub seat is used when the patient is unable

or not allowed to get down into the tub or up from the bottom of the tub (Mann et al., 1996; Seeger & Fisher, 1982). Different heights and styles of tub benches are available, and it is important to select the right one for each patient in terms of stability, ease of transfer, and position of hips and knees (Fig. 30-10). A hand-held shower hose is used for rinsing if a tub seat is required. It is essential to provide practice of strategies to bathe the back, feet, and private area when bathing on a tub seat. Lever handles on faucets are recommended because they do not require grasp and they allow better leverage for turning on and off. It is helpful if the soap is on a string. The soap is either worn around the neck or hung within easy reach.

The same problems of reach and grasp encountered in dressing are seen to interfere with bathing. When grasp is limited, a sponge or terry cloth bath mitt works well. A long-handled bath sponge can be used to reach the feet or back; some are designed to hold the soap inside the sponge and others are designed especially for cleaning feet. A terry cloth bathrobe is effective for drying.

See Chapter 41 for transfer into the tub for patients after unilateral total hip replacement. The following is the procedure for unilateral total knee replacement when the knee cannot be bent and less than full weight bearing is allowed (Platt et al., 1992):

1. The patient walks to the side of the tub using the walker or crutches and turns to face away from the tub.
2. The patient reaches for the back of the tub bench with one hand while the other hand remains at the center of the top rail of the walker.
3. The patient sits down on the tub bench and lifts both legs into the tub, turning to face the faucet. The operated leg should be held in extension.

Suggestions for Selected IADL
Writing
Use roller ball pens that glide easily. If pinch is limited, the size of the writing instrument can be increased by using sponge rubber, passing it through the holes in a practice golf ball, using commercially available grips that slip on the instrument, or using a comfort-grip pen (Peterman Schwarz, 1997).

Telephoning
Cordless phones near where the person is sitting or working are useful, as is one-button automatic dialing.

Shopping
Shop-at-home services by phone or computer are becoming more common, convenient, and economical. If the patient goes to the shops, he or she should go at off-hours so that clerks are available to get out-of-reach items too heavy to be obtained by use of a reacher.

Opening Containers
Jar openers, including rubber sheets, clamp style, and mounted style, or pliers can be used to open jars, bottles, and pill bottles. Pliers are also useful in other tasks that require pinch, such as weeding or sewing thick fabric. In one study, a pop-off lid was found to require approximately 13 pounds of force to open and medicine bottles required 2 to 6 pounds (Rice et al., 1998). To avoid struggling with pill bottles, medications should be received from the pharmacy in easy-open, not childproof, containers.

Gardening
Choose low-maintenance perennial plants. Use seedlings rather than seeds. Wear a carpenter's apron with pockets for tools. Use tools with ergonomic grips (Fig. 30-3). Use a rolling or stationary stool to sit while working. Wear gloves to protect the skin and joints. Keep pruners sharp to make cutting easier. Use a sprinkler rather than a watering can (Arthritis Foundation, 1997).

Sexual Activities
Intercourse should be planned for the time of day of highest energy level, and the patient should time pain relief medication so its effects are greatest during intercourse. A warm bath is relaxing as well as serving as a part of foreplay. Satisfying sex includes romance and intimacy, even though engaging in intercourse may be too exhausting or painful. Skin-to-skin contact is important but does not have to cause pain. If holding hands is painful, the partner can touch or rub the patient's body with a light, open hand. The patient and partner can use a trial-and-error process of working out new, comfortable positions for intercourse. For example, both partners may lie on their sides with the man entering from behind for a woman with hip problems; both partners may lie on their sides facing each other with the woman providing most of the hip movement, which is good for a man with back problems (Houtchens, 1998).

Sexual activities such as touching, holding hands, and caressing can be resumed immediately after total joint replacement. Patients with total hip replacement can generally resume intercourse 8 weeks postoperatively or according to the surgeon's guidance. The patient should position the affected joint appropriately by avoiding extremes of range of motion, which are flexion less than 90°, external rotation less than 45°, and abduction less than 30°. Whether male or female, the patient should take the passive position. After 4 to 6 weeks, patients with unilateral knee replacement no longer have restrictions on resumption of sexual activities except to avoid kneeling positions (Spica & Schwab, 1996).

Incoordination and Poor Dexterity (Box 30-3)

For more information and suggestions, see Chapter 40.

Suggestions for BADL

The patient is taught to use the body in as stable a posture as is possible, to sit when possible, and to stabilize the upper extremities by bearing weight on them against a surface or by holding the upper arms close to the body, or both. Stabilizing the head may improve a person's ability to control the upper extremities. Friction surfaces, weighted utensils, or weighted cuffs (see Fig. 11-16) added to the distal segments of the extremities and the use of larger and/or less precise fasteners all contribute to increasing independence by lessening the effects of the incoordination.

Feeding

The plate can be stabilized on a friction surface, such as a wet towel, wet sponge cloth, or nonskid mat. A plate guard or scoop dish can be used to prevent the food from being pushed off the plate. The utensil may be weighted for stability, may have an enlarged handle to facilitate grasp, and may be plastic coated to protect the person's teeth. Sharp utensils are to be avoided. A weight cuff on the wrist is often chosen rather than a weighted utensil because the cuff can be heavier; also the cuff makes it unnecessary to weight each item that the patient will use. The person may successfully drink from a covered glass or cup with a sipping spout. An ordinary cup can be so adapted by using plastic food wrap as a cover, with a straw poked through it. Some may use a long plastic straw that is held to the side of the cup or glass by a straw holder attachment; the patient moves the head to the straw but does not touch it or the cup or glass with the hand.

Grooming

Weighted cuffs on the wrists may help some patients gain greater accuracy while grooming. Large lipstick tubes are easier to use than small ones. The arms must be stabilized to use lipstick. A simple hairstyle is the best choice. For a patient who has difficulty holding a large comb, a military-style brush with a strap can be used. Roll-on or stick deodorant is preferred to spray because these types eliminate the risk of accidentally spraying the substance into the eyes. An electric razor is preferred to a safety razor both because it is more easily held and because a safety razor can cut if it is moved sideways over the skin. Patients with fairly good head control improve their accuracy by holding the electric razor

steady and moving the face over the cutting surface. An electric toothbrush is also useful both because it is heavier and because it can be held steady while the head is moved. This same principle can be employed when filing the nails: fasten the emery board to a flat surface and move each nail over the emery board. Cutting the nails may be unsafe for incoordinated patients, so filing is recommended. Sanitary napkins with adhesive strips to hold them in place may be easier to use than tampons.

Dressing

Clothes that facilitate independent dressing are front-opening, loosely fitting garments with large buttons, Velcro tape closures, or zippers. Wrinkle-resistant and stain-shedding materials enable the person to look well groomed throughout the day. To overcome difficulty with buttoning, a buttonhook with an enlarged and/or weighted handle, if necessary, can be used. A loop of ribbon, leather, or chain can be attached to the zipper pull so that the person can hook it with a finger instead of pinching the zipper pull. Velcro can be substituted to eliminate the need to fasten hooks on a bra. To don the bra, it is easier for the patient to put it around her waist, which is thinner and puts less tension on the garment, then fasten it in front where she can see what she is doing, turn it around, put her arms in, and pull it up into place. Elastic straps or elastic inserts sewn into the straps make this relatively easy.

Shoe style should eliminate tying. Tie shoes can be adapted using zipper shoelaces or Velcro. If a man wears a tie, he may choose to slide the knot down and pull the tie off over his head without undoing the knot or to use clip ties if the degree of dexterity allows that.

Bathing

The patient may bathe independently but must adhere closely to safety precautions. Nonslip material is used in the bottom of the tub and a nonskid mat is placed outside the tub to stand on while transferring. Safety grab bars should be placed where they would be most useful to the particular person's needs. A tub bench or seat can eliminate the difficulty of sitting in and getting up from the bottom of the tub and provides a stable position for the patient who is washing the feet. If a seat is used, a hand-held shower spray is necessary.

If the patient chooses to shower instead of bathe, the nonslip material, grab bars, and seat also must be provided. In either case, the water should be drawn once the patient has transferred in and is seated; a mixer tap is ideal, but if it is unavailable, the cool water should be turned on first and the hot water added to prevent scalding. Soap on a string keeps the soap retrievable, or a bath mitt with a pocket to hold the soap is useful. The water should be drained before the person attempts to

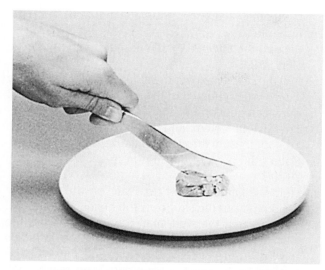

Figure 30-18 Rocker knife for one-handed cutting.

stand to transfer out of the tub. An extra large towel or large terry wrap-around robe facilitates drying.

Suggestions for Selected IADL

Communication

Writing and speech are problems for some incoordinated persons. See Chapter 17 for alternative communication systems and adaptations for computers that are appropriate for incoordinated patients. If the patient speaks understandably, the use of large-button phones reduces the fine motor requirements of dialing the telephone.

Playing Games

Board game pieces can be weighted or turned into pegs for stability. Game boards can be reproduced to enlarge the squares. Card holders and card shufflers are useful. Computer games that use keyboarding or switches rather than a mouse or joystick are appropriate.

Loss of Use of One Side of the Body or One Upper Extremity (Box 30-3)

For other information and suggestions, see Chapters 38, 42, and 46.

Suggestions for BADL

The methods described here pertain to the hemiplegic patient who has lost the use of one side of the body. Most stroke patients can be independent in their BADL. However, some are prevented from developing independence, especially of the less automatic tasks, such as one-handed upper extremity dressing, by cognitive-perceptual impairments (Edmans & Lincoln, 1990; Walker & Lincoln, 1991).

The methods and equipment described here may also be used by the unilateral upper extremity amputee. However, the amputee needs less adaptation because he or she has normal trunk and lower extremity function and normal perception and cognition. Persons with temporary casts or restrictions of use of one upper extremity after surgery can also benefit from these ideas.

Feeding

Feeding is essentially a one-handed task, except for cutting meat and spreading bread, and these tasks can be done with assistive devices. Food can be simultaneously stabilized and cut by use of a rocker knife, a knife with a sharp curved blade that cuts when rocked over the food (Fig. 30-18). Bread can be spread if stabilized on a nonslip surface or trapped in the corner of a spike board and spread toward the corner (Fig. 32-2). Soft spreads facilitate this process.

Grooming

The problems with grooming are the care of the unaffected extremity and finding substitutions for two-handed activities. Spray deodorant for the unaffected arm is easier to use than other types of applicators. Fingernails of the unaffected hand are cleaned by rubbing them on a small suction cup brush attached to the basin (Fig. 30-19). Fingernails of the affected hand can be trimmed with a stabilized nail clipper (Fig. 30-8), and those of the unaffected hand, with an emery board fastened down to stabilize it. The fingernail is moved back and forth over the emery board.

Using another suction cup brush fastened to the inside of the basin, the person can scrub dentures by rubbing them over the brush. Partially filling the basin with water and laying a face cloth in the bottom cushions the dentures if they are dropped. An electric razor is recommended for shaving for a poststroke

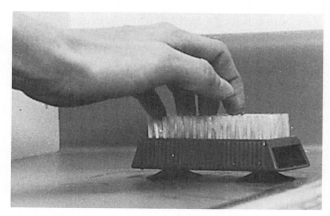

Figure 30-19 Suction cup brush for cleaning nails or dentures one-handed.

patient because accidents are possible with a safety razor.

Toileting

The problem with toileting is arranging the clothing, which is normally a two-handed activity. There should be a grab bar mounted on the wall beside the toilet and/or a frame mounted on the toilet (Fig. 30-15) to assist transfers. Once standing, anyone wearing trousers unfastens them and gravity takes them down. If the patient's balance is precarious and will interfere with retrieving them after using the toilet, the person can put the affected hand in the pocket, which prevents the trousers from sliding below the knees. A woman with a dress can lean her affected side against the adjacent wall, if available, for balance; she can then raise her dress on the affected side and tuck it between her body and the affected arm. Then she lowers her underpants to knee level and pulls the dress up on the unaffected side. A dress or skirt that wraps around facilitates this process by allowing the woman to reach across her front and pull the material forward to anchor it between her body and the affected arm; then she lowers her underpants and holds the remaining material aside while seating herself using the grab bar. The toilet tissue should be mounted conveniently to the unaffected side. The patient can manage menstrual needs by use of tampons or adhesive sanitary napkins.

Dressing

Certain prerequisite abilities are considered important for successful dressing. These are ability to reach each foot, stand unsupported for 10 seconds, and maintain sitting balance when reaching down. The most difficult tasks for both men and women were found to be pulling trousers up, putting the shoe on the affected foot, and lacing shoes (Walker & Lincoln, 1990, 1991).

The following methods are taken from material prepared by the occupational therapy staff of the former Highland View Cuyahoga County Hospital (Cleveland, Ohio) and published by Brett (1960). As a general rule, the affected limb is dressed first and undressed last.

Shirt or Cardigan Garment: Overhead Method. The overhead method for putting on and removing front-opening tops is least confusing for a patient with sensory and perceptual impairment. But this method is cumbersome for dresses and is not suitable for coats.

1. To keep the shirt from twisting, hold the collar and shake.
2. Put the shirt on the lap, label facing up, and the collar next to the abdomen; drape the shirttail over the knees (Fig. 30-20A).

3. Open the sleeve for the affected arm from the armhole to the cuff.
4. Pick up the affected hand and put it into the sleeve (Fig. 30-20B).
5. Pull the sleeve up over the elbow (Fig. 30-20C). If the sleeve is not pulled past the elbow, the hand will fall out when continuing.
6. Put the unaffected hand into the armhole. Raise the arm and push it through the sleeve (Fig. 30-20D).
7. Gather the back of the shirt from tail to collar (Fig. 30-20E).
8. Hold the gathered shirt up, lean forward, duck the head, and put the shirt over the head (Fig. 30-20F).
9. To straighten the shirt, lean forward and work the shirt down over the shoulders. Often the shirt gets caught on the affected shoulder and must first be pushed back over the shoulder. Then reach back and pull the tail down (Fig. 30-20G).
10. To button, line up the shirt fronts and match each button with the correct buttonhole, starting with the bottom button. Velcro tape is the better fastener both for ease of use and patient preference (Huck & Bonhotal, 1997); however, this adaptation requires someone to replace the buttons with Velcro tabs.

To remove the shirt, the patient unbuttons it, leans forward, and uses the unaffected hand to gather the shirt up in back of the neck. He or she ducks the head, pulls the shirt over the head, then takes the shirt off the unaffected arm first.

Shirt or Cardigan Garment: Over-the-Shoulder Method. Some patients do better with the over-the-shoulder method, especially if they have some voluntary control of the affected extremity and can place it in the garment, because it is similar to the customary method. This method is also used for coats.

1. To keep the shirt from twisting, hold the collar and shake.
2. Put the shirt on the lap, label facing up, and the collar next to the abdomen with the shirttail draped over the knees (Fig. 30-20A).
3. Put the affected hand into one sleeve. (Fig. 30-20B).
4. Pull the sleeve up over the elbow (Fig. 30-20C).
5. Grasp the collar at the point closest to the unaffected side (Fig. 30-21A).
6. Hold tightly to the collar, lean forward, and bring the collar and shirt around the affected side and behind the neck to the unaffected side (Fig. 30-21B).
7. Put the unaffected hand into the other armhole. Raise the arm out and up to push it through the sleeve (Fig. 30-21C).
8. To straighten the shirt, lean forward, work the shirt down over the shoulders, reach back and pull the

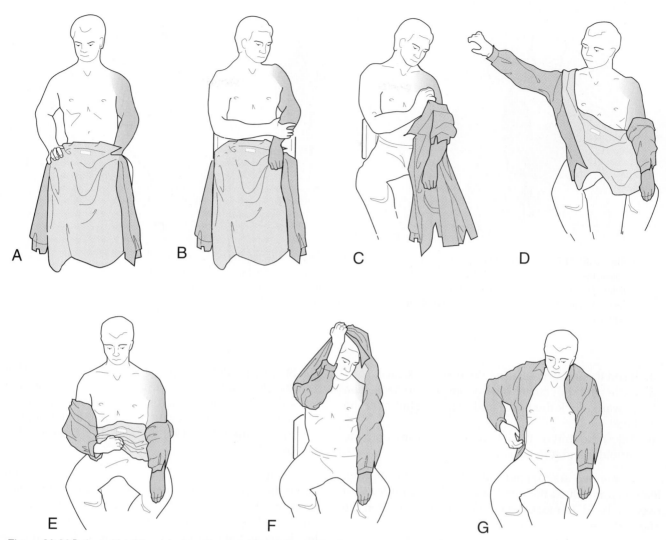

Figure 30-20 Patient with left hemiplegia putting on a shirt, overhead method. **A.** Put shirt on the lap, label facing up, collar next to abdomen, shirttail draped over knees. **B.** Pick up the affected arm and put it into the armhole. **C.** Pull the sleeve well over the elbow. **D.** Put the unaffected hand into the armhole and raise the arm to push it through the sleeve. **E.** Gather the back of the shirt from the tail to the collar. **F.** Hold the gathered shirt up. Lean forward and duck the head to put the shirt overhead. **G.** To straighten the shirt, lean forward and work the shirt over the shoulders. Reach back and pull the tail down and the front sides forward. Button it.

tail down, and then straighten the sleeve under the affected axilla (Fig. 30-20*G*).

9. To button, line up shirt fronts and match each button with the correct buttonhole, starting with the bottom button.

To remove the shirt, unbutton it and use the unaffected hand to throw the shirt back off the unaffected shoulder. Work the shirt sleeve off the unaffected arm. Press the shirt cuff against the leg and pull the arm out. Lean forward. Use the unaffected hand to pull the shirt across the back. Take the shirt off of the affected arm.

Pullover Garment. The following steps are used for putting on a pullover garment.

1. Position the garment on the lap, bottom toward chest and label facing down.
2. Using the unaffected hand, roll up the bottom edge of the shirt back, all the way up to the sleeve on the affected side.
3. Spread the armhole opening as large as possible. Using the unaffected hand, place the affected arm into the armhole and pull the sleeve up onto the arm past the elbow.

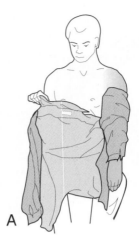 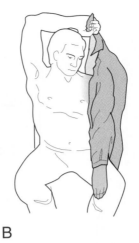 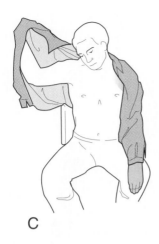

A   B   C

Figure 30-21 Patient with left hemiplegia putting on a shirt. **A.** After putting the affected arm in the armhole and pulling the sleeve up above the elbow, grasp the collar at the point nearest the unaffected side. **B.** Hold the collar tightly. Lean forward and bring the shirt up, around, and behind toward the unaffected arm. **C.** Put the unaffected arm into the armhole. Extend the arm out and up to push it through the sleeve. Straighten the shirt and button it.

4. Insert the unaffected arm into the other sleeve.
5. Gather the shirt back from bottom edge to neck, lean forward, duck the head, and pass the shirt over the head.
6. Adjust the shirt on the involved side up and onto the shoulder and remove twists.

To remove, starting at top back, gather the shirt up, lean forward, duck the head, and pull the shirt forward over the head. Remove the unaffected arm and then the affected arm.

Trousers. The following steps describe how to put on trousers. Modifications of the following method are used for men's and women's underclothing and pantyhose.

1. Sit. ***If a wheelchair is used, the brakes should be locked and the footrests should be up and/or swung out of the way.*** Move the unaffected leg beyond the midline of the body for balance (Fig. 30-22*A*).
2. Grasp the ankle or calf of the affected leg. Lift and cross the affected leg over the unaffected leg (Fig. 30-22*B*).
3. Pull the trousers onto the affected leg up to but not above the knee (Fig. 30-22*C*).
4. Uncross the legs.
5. Put the unaffected leg into the other pant leg.
6. Remain sitting. Pull the pants up above the knees (Fig. 30-22*D*).
7. To prevent the pants from dropping when standing, put the affected hand into the pant pocket or the thumb into a belt loop (Fig. 30-22*E*).

8. Stand up. Pull the pants up over the hips (Fig. 30-22*F*); button and zip pants while standing. Persons with poor balance should remain seated and pull the pants up over the hips by shifting from side to side; they should button and zip the pants while seated.

To remove, unfasten the trousers and work them down the hips as far as possible. Stand. Let the trousers drop past the knees. Sit. Remove the trousers from the unaffected leg. Cross the affected leg over the unaffected leg. Remove the trousers from the affected leg. Uncross the legs.

Persons with poor balance should use this method: Place locked wheelchair or chair against a wall. Sit. Unfasten the trousers. Work the trousers down on the hips as far as possible. Put the wheelchair footrests up and/or swing them out of the way. Lean back against the chair and press down with the unaffected leg to raise the buttocks slightly. Lean from side to side in the chair. Use the uninvolved arm to work the trousers down past the hips. Remove the trousers from the unaffected leg. Cross the affected leg over the unaffected leg. Remove the trousers from the affected leg. Uncross the legs.

Socks or Stockings. The following method is used to put on socks or stockings.

1. The person sits in a straight chair (with arms if balance is questionable) or in a locked wheelchair with footrests in the up position.
2. The unaffected leg is placed slightly beyond midline of body toward the affected side, and the affected

leg is crossed over it by grasping the ankle. If the person has difficulty in maintaining the leg in this position, a small stool under the unaffected leg increases hip flexion angle and holds the affected leg more securely. The patient who cannot cross the legs can rest the heel on a small stool and uses a reacher to put the sock onto the toe and pull it up.

3. The top of the sock is opened by inserting the fist into the cuff area and then opening the fist and spreading the fingers.
4. The sock is put on the foot by slipping the toes into the cuff opening made under the spread hand. The sock is then pulled into place, and wrinkles are eliminated.

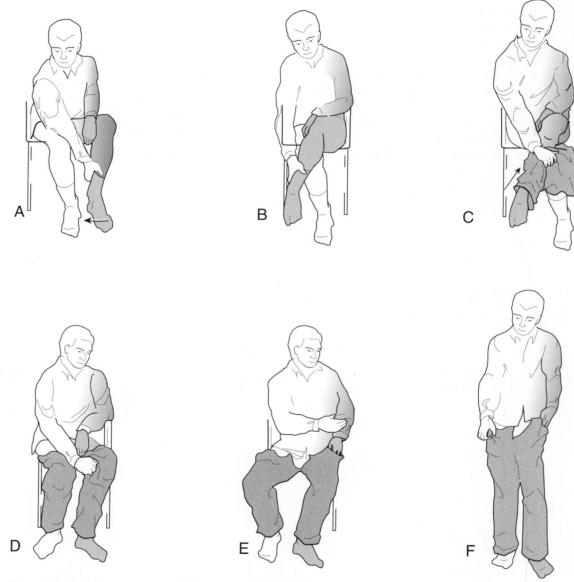

Figure 30-22 Patient with left hemiplegia putting on trousers while sitting. **A.** With knees bent, move the unaffected foot across the midline of the body toward the unaffected side. **B.** Grasp the ankle of the affected leg, lift it, and cross it over the unaffected leg. **C.** Pull the trousers onto the affected leg up to but not above the knee. **D.** Uncross the legs, put the unaffected leg into the trousers, and pull them up above the knees. **E.** To prevent the trousers from dropping when the person stands up, put the affected hand into the pocket. **F.** Stand up. Pull the trousers over the hips and fasten, or sit to fasten if balance is not good enough to do it while standing.

To remove, the leg is positioned as for putting the sock on. The sock is pushed off with the unaffected hand.

Shoes. A loafer is put on the affected foot with the shoe on the floor. The foot is started into the shoe, and a shoehorn is used to help ease the foot into the shoe. A tie shoe is put onto the affected foot after the leg is crossed over the unaffected one to bring the foot closer. If the laces have been thoroughly loosened, the person often can work the shoe on while the leg is crossed over by grasping the heel of the shoe with the unaffected hand and working it back and forth over the heel until it goes on completely. Sometimes it is necessary to insert a shoehorn while the leg is crossed over and then carefully lower the foot with the shoe half on and shoehorn in the shoe and finish putting on the shoe by repeatedly pushing down on the knee and adjusting the shoehorn.

Tying the shoes is a problem. It is possible to tie a conventional bow one-handed, but it requires fine dexterity and normal perception. The amputee may prefer to do this or use loafers. The hemiplegic patient can use adapted shoe closures or learn a simple, effective one-handed shoe tie as illustrated in Figure 30-23. Putting the lace through the last hole from the outside of the shoe toward the tongue lets the tension of the foot against the shoe hold the lace tight while the bow is being tied. One-hand shoe tying is especially difficult for patients with cognitive-perceptual deficits.

Ankle–Foot Orthosis. The posterior shell or molded ankle–foot orthosis (AFO) is put on the leg, and the strap is fastened before the shoe is put on. It may be necessary to add a temporary strap near the ankle to hold the orthosis on the foot while attempting to put on the shoe. The shoe is put on as described for the unaffected foot. It is difficult to put the shoe on with the posterior shell in place. Plans for a shoe donner for those who wear an AFO have been published (Bobco, 1988). If all else fails (as this method could bend or break the orthosis, check with the orthotist first), the plastic AFO can be placed in the shoe before the patient puts the foot in. The important thing to remember is to have the laces quite

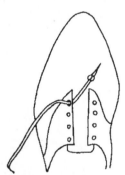

1. Tie a knot in one end of the shoelace. Thread the unknotted end up through the hole nearest the toe of the shoe on the left.

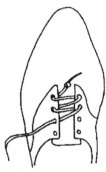

2. Take the lace across the tongue of the shoe and up under the flap on the opposite side of the shoe.

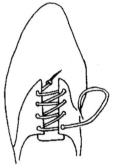

3. Continue to go across the tongue and up under the flap on the next highest hole on the opposite side until you reach the top (or go down through the last hole so the tension will be maintained for tying.)

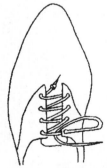

4. Circle around toward the toe of the shoe and go under the part of the lace that is going across the tongue to the last hole.

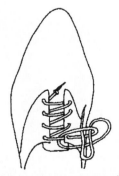

5. Circle aroung toward the top of the shoe. Pull free lace through the loop down toward the ankle and out to the left side.

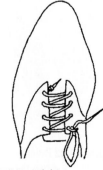

6. Pull loop tight

Figure 30-23 One-handed shoe tie for a left hemiplegic. For a right hemiplegic, start the lace on the right side of the shoe so that the lace ends on the left side at the top.

loose to allow the maximum room possible for getting the foot into the orthosis and shoe.

Bra. The bra is placed around the waist and hooked in front, where the patient can see what she is doing. One end can be tucked into the waistband of panties until the other end is brought around. It is fastened and rotated to the proper position; the affected arm is placed through the shoulder strap; and the unaffected arm is placed through the other shoulder strap. The bra is pulled up into place. It is removed by reversing the process.

A plump patient may need an adapted front-closing bra if she cannot approximate the two edges of the bra to fasten it. The bra is adapted by belt keepers attached on the side of the bra opening on the involved side and cotton twill straps opposite these keepers on the other side of the bra opening. After the bra is around the waist, the straps are threaded through the keepers and pulled to bring the two ends of the bra together. The straps are secured with Velcro.

Bathing

The bathing arrangements described for patients with incoordination apply to hemiplegic persons also. In addition, these patients find a long-handled bath sponge with a pocket to hold the soap useful to allow bathing of the unaffected upper arm and the back. The lower arm of the unaffected side is bathed by putting the soapy washcloth across the knees and rubbing the arm back and forth over it, unless the patient has some return of function and can use a bath mitt on the affected hand. Pump bottles of liquid soap and shampoo are useful, as is putting the soap in a nylon stocking and tying the end of it to the grab bar for easy retrieval (American Heart Association, 1994). If sensory impairment exists, extra precautions should be taken to be certain of water temperature.

The hemiplegic patient should dry off as much as possible while still seated on the bath seat before transferring out of the tub. The water should be completely drained from the tub before the transfer is attempted. The patient may need assistance with the transfer if there is not enough room near the tub to position the wheelchair so that the uninvolved side leads. A unilateral amputee can bathe as usual, but a rubber mat or nonskid strips in the tub, a grab bar, and letting the water drain before exiting are worthwhile safety measures.

Suggestions for Selected IADL
Writing

Persons with only one functional arm have to stabilize the paper when writing with the unaffected hand. The paper can be secured using masking tape, a clipboard, a weight, the affected extremity, or other similar means. If

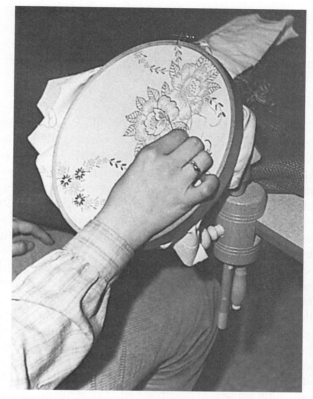

Figure 30-24 Frame for one-handed embroidery and sewing.

the dominant hand is the affected one, writing practice, especially for the signature, is usually required.

Leisure Activities

Devices can be made to allow doing two-handed leisure tasks unilaterally. One example is a frame that holds cloth for embroidering (Fig. 30-24). A temporary card-holder can be made out of an upended scrub brush or a slotted piece of wood and a commercial one purchased for more permanent use. Many helpful suggestions, such as buying scissors for the left hand if that is the strong hand, have been published by the American Heart Association (1994) and other references listed in the Resources.

Sexual Activities

A helpful booklet, *Sex After Stroke* (American Heart Association, 2000), is available on-line (www.american-heart.org/Patient_Information/SexStroke/read.html) or in print from the local affiliate of the American Heart Association. It discusses sexuality and body image (coping with bodily changes, dressing and grooming), fears about resuming sex (intercourse with mate is unlikely to cause another stroke, energy required is equal to the energy needed to walk up two flights of stairs, impotence and depression), specifics of sexual intimacy after stroke (bowel and bladder control, change of position to accommodate paralysis, birth control, pregnancy, ways to make love other than intercourse), and suggestions for further reading for stroke survivors and their mates or health professionals.

Limited Vision (Box 30-3)

The suggestions listed here pertain to blindness (20/1250 to worse than 20/2500) and to low vision (20/80 to 20/1000) (Colenbrander & Fletcher, 1995). The person with low vision may find some of these useful and others unnecessary. Organization and consistency in the placement of objects is necessary for the blind person to locate things efficiently. Memory training may be necessary for the newly blinded individual. He or she must develop increased awareness of the information received from the senses of smell, touch, hearing, and taste. This awareness does not automatically occur but must be developed through training. Full concentration, the need for which increases as more stimuli are added (e.g., traffic, people, noise, objects) requires energy, and therefore it is important to incorporate energy conservation techniques into treatment (Rosenthal, 1995). Orientation to the environment is achieved through all remaining senses, although a verbal description of the surroundings by someone else is extremely valuable.

The American Foundation for the Blind is a major source for obtaining information and assistive devices for blind persons (see Resources). For other information, see Chapter 28.

Suggestions for BADL
Feeding
The patient explores the placement of dishes, glasses, and utensils. If dining alone, he or she explores the location and identifies the food by feel, using the fork and taste. If dining with a companion, the companion can report locations using a clock method of description, such as "Meat is at 3 o'clock." When pouring liquid, the correct amount is determined by the weight of the cup when it is full or by inserting a clean finger over the rim to feel when the liquid is near the top. Salt is distinguished from pepper by taste or use of differently shaped shakers. Food is cut by finding the edge of the food with the fork, moving the fork a bite-size amount onto the meat, and then cutting the food, keeping the knife in contact with the fork. For those with low vision, the plate, glass, and utensils should be a color that contrasts with both the table covering and the food.

Grooming
A major problem is identification of objects. This can be done through the use of taste, touch (size, shape, and texture), location, and Braille or bar code labels. The application of cosmetics or toiletries is another problem; fingers of the assistive hand can be guides, such as when shaving sideburns or applying eyebrow pencil. Aerosol sprays are a poor choice because the blind person cannot determine the extent of the spray.

Dressing
Limited vision creates no difficulty with the physical aspects of dressing. The only problems that arise relate to appearance and appropriateness. The blind person needs a system to coordinate colors of clothes and compatibility of style. One system is to store clothes of like color together. Hems, buttons, seams, and socks should be checked for mending. Colorless wax polishes can be used to shine shoes. Clothes should always be hung properly to prevent wrinkles. Wrinkle-free, stain-resistant, no-iron fabrics are desirable. Listening to the weather report guides the person's selection of appropriate clothing, as for anyone. Clothing selection should be done with the assistance of a sighted person who can describe colors and style. Purchase of garments of the same style in different colors should be avoided because color identification is often done by remembering which style is a certain color.

Suggestions for Selected IADL
Writing and Reading
The blind person can use a signature or writing guide to stay within boundaries while writing in longhand. The person with low vision can use a black felt-tipped pen for good contrast. Braille can be written by hand using a stylus and plate or on a Braille writer. For reading, besides Braille and talking books and magazines, computerized optical scanning devices convert the ordinary printed word into spoken word or Braille displays. For those with moderately low vision, books, popular magazines, and *The New York Times* come in large-print versions. There are hand-held computerized devices (www.envisionamerica.com) that scan bar codes and identify products, which can be useful in the household and at work, and others that scan medicine bottles and inform the person of the medicine in the bottle and the dosage schedule.

Telephoning
Using a telephone is no problem for the blind person as soon as he or she memorizes the dial or location of touch buttons. A phone with one-button automatic dialing is very useful.

Time
The person can tell time using a Braille watch. Sounds of the day, the radio, or television can provide a general

orientation to time. Clocks that announce the time are sold in gadget catalogs.

Shopping

Much shopping by persons with low vision can be done through catalogs, read by use of closed-circuit television (CCTV) and talking computer (Rosenthal, 1995).

Handling Money

Tactile discrimination enables the person to identify coins. Paper money is discriminated by the way it is folded after its denomination has been identified previously by someone else or viewed by use of a CCTV. Consistency is important here as in all aspects of the blind person's life. Some countries use paper money of different sizes for different denominations, but unfortunately that is not so in the United States.

Playing Games

Braille versions of popular games, such as Monopoly, Bingo, and playing cards, are available. Large-numbered cards are also available for those with low vision.

Computer Usage

Many people need to use computers for work as well as personal organization and entertainment. Persons with low vision need not be denied employment that requires computer usage; these persons can use computers. The adapted computer is a reasonable accommodation available through the Americans with Disabilities Act. Macintosh computers can be equipped with software that translates information displayed on the monitor into synthesized speech. This is used in conjunction with a page scanner and optical character recognition software to convert the scanned images of printed text into computer documents. Macintosh is the only computer system with a GUI (graphical user interface) that is accessible to persons with visual impairments because it does not require pointing, clicking, or dragging. Instead, the user can direct the mouse with keystrokes and listen to a spoken narrative of the graphics-based menus, windows, and icons (Buning & Hanzlik, 1993). See Chapter 17 for further discussion of high-tech adaptations.

Decreased Sensation (Box 30-3)

For other information, see Chapter 27.

Suggestions for BADL

Problems of absent, decreased, or disturbed sensation affect performance of ADL whenever a possibly dangerous situation is encountered and because the automatic knowledge of the performance of limbs may be missing.

Dressing

Wrinkles and pressure are potential problems. For example, wrinkled socks pressing against the skin inside the shoe and tight elastic cuffs and waistbands can cause decubitus ulcers within a short time and therefore should be eliminated. Persons with insensitive skin must be careful to dress warmly in cold weather to prevent frostbite.

Bathing

With bathing, there is danger of scalding. When turning water on, the cold is turned on first, then the hot added gradually. Mixer valves should be installed to compensate when decreased sensation is a permanent condition.

Suggestions for Selected IADL

Poor sensation does not allow graduated pinch and grip on tools and utensils to meet the demands of the task. The person grips with excessive pressure (Johansson & Westling, 1984). Prolonged, excessive grip or pinch can cause bruising and decubiti. Poor sensation also results in letting go, when the attention is directed away from the object being held. The person's attention must be directed to maintain the grip of an object.

Activities that involve heat, such as using a riding mower or cooking at an outdoor barbecue, pose a threat because anesthetic lower extremities can be burned if allowed to rest against the hot engine cover or bottom of the barbecue.

Cognitive-Perceptual Impairments (Box 30-3)

See Chapters 28 and 29 for information concerning methods to compensate for cognitive or perceptual impairments in activities of daily living.

Pain, Including Low Back Pain (Box 30-3)

See Chapters 32 and 41 for information concerning body mechanics to be used during occupational functioning for persons with low back pain.

Continued Independence

Studies have reported that patients lose some of their independence when discharged home (Andrews & Stewart, 1979; Egan et al., 1992; Strub & Levine, 1987; Weingarden & Martin, 1989). No studies identify the reasons for this. I will suggest a few hypotheses and propose counteractions.

First, adjustment to living on a day-to-day basis with a permanent disability is overwhelming and confusing.

Full education of the patient and family in preparation for the return home, including weekend passes and community reintegration preparation, may help (Strub & Levine, 1987). Home care follow-up to facilitate the adjustment may be helpful. Rehabilitation in the home may prevent this reaction.

Second, the patient who expects everything will be okay when he or she gets home encounters reality and undergoes reactive depression and reduced activity. Attention to the emotional aspects of disability during inpatient rehabilitation, community reintegration practice, community follow-up, and support groups may be effective interventions.

Third, the family provides more care than they did before the disability and more than is needed. Family education about the person's abilities and the importance of activity for health may prevent this. Community follow-up and support groups may also be beneficial. Family dynamics and family values may resist a change toward independence for the former patient.

Fourth, the person sees independence as "too much time and too much work." Persons with new or severe disabilities have limited energy. They may choose to use their time and energy for activities of greater value to them than BADL. That may be a healthy choice for them. They still need to learn the techniques because they have to instruct personal care attendants.

Fifth, failure to perform at home what was learned in the rehabilitation center may reflect inability to transfer skills from one context to another. Use of actual objects and real contexts, such as Easy Street Environments, within the rehabilitation center may facilitate carryover, as will practice in varied contexts. Home-based therapy is probably best to overcome this problem for patients with limited problem-solving abilities.

Effectiveness of Therapy to Restore the Role of Independent Person

The following studies show accumulating evidence that occupational therapy, in the form of teaching adapted strategies or methods and prescribing assistive devices, is effective.

Assistive devices and adapted methods reduced by 42% the difficulty in doing daily activities among women aged 29 to 54 years who have rheumatoid arthritis. The range of items that the women found difficult reduced from 13 to 99 items to 6 to 57 items. Some 91% of the devices issued were still in use 6 to 12 months after issuance (Nordenskiöld et al., 1998), presumably because they were helpful. The researchers found that eating, cooking, and toileting were most improved, and dressing, clothes care, cleaning, outdoor mobility, and shopping were least improved by assistive devices or methods. They concluded that better devices or methods are needed for the latter categories of activities.

Gibson and Schkade (1997) tested the effect of individualized patient-centered intervention (Occupational Adaptation, or OA) as compared with standardized occupational therapy intervention on improved independence in ADL and the restrictiveness of the discharge environment. The standard occupational therapy group was an historical cohort. Both groups improved significantly, but the OA group reached a significantly higher level of independence than the traditional group. Significantly more patients in the OA group were discharged to less restrictive environments.

A pretest–posttest study addressed an occupational therapy program of 12 weeks in which 33 patients in 16 occupational therapy departments were taught strategies to compensate for apraxia. Patients were taught **external compensatory techniques** and **internal compensatory techniques**. After statistically controlling for the apraxia score, motor functioning score, and spontaneous recovery, the results indicated large improvements in ADL. Effect sizes were large: .86 on the Barthel Index; .92 on ADL observation, and 1.06 on ADL questionnaire (patient perception) (van Heugten et al., 1998).

Some 19 patients completed bathing training administered by occupational therapists over 2 to 12 sessions (Shillam et al., 1983). Bathing was defined as either showering or tub bathing according to the patient's preference. Treatment consisted of evaluation of status and skill level in bathing, training in techniques likely to improve those skills, and prescription of appropriate equipment (bathtub bench or seat or shower wheelchair, grab bars, flexible-hose shower head, nonskid bath surface, soap on a rope, long-handled sponge, bath mitt, soap holder, shampoo dispenser). Using the bathing portion of the *Klein-Bell ADL Scale*, the 19 patients improved significantly from pretest to posttest (average of 14 points). Four patients went from dependent to full independence. The greatest barrier to full independence for the others was the wheelchair to tub transfer; however, they did improve from maximal assist to contact guarding. Washing and drying the feet and legs were also problems for many due to limited sitting balance.

Walker et al. (1999) randomly assigned 185 community-dwelling patients who had had a stroke to one of two groups: occupational therapy or control. The occupational therapy goal was independence in personal ADL (bathing, feeding, dressing, and stair mobility) and IADL (outdoor mobility, driving a car, use of public transportation, household chores, and leisure activities). At 6 months' follow-up, patients who received occupational therapy scored significantly higher than controls on the extended (instrumental) ADL scale and the *Barthel Index* (BADL). The conclusion was that occupational therapy significantly reduced disability and handicap in patients with stroke who were treated in the community.

In a randomized crossover design 15 subjects who had trouble dressing at home for 6 months after discharge from hospital post stroke received 3 months of dressing training in the home followed by 3 months of no treatment. Another 15 similar subjects first received no treatment, then dressing training. Both groups showed significant improvement during the treatment phase, but neither group improved during the no-treatment phase. The group that received treatment during the first 3 months maintained their gains. Walker et al. (1996) concluded that "dressing practice given at home to patients who have residual problems in dressing 6 months after acute stroke leads to sustained reduction in their problems" (p. 23).

In a randomized controlled trial, a 12-week rehabilitation program for 22 patients with chronic obstructive pulmonary disease that included occupational therapy (2 lessons of techniques to overcome problems with everyday tasks for groups of 4 to 5 patients, grouped because of similar ADL scores) and physical therapy (individualized therapy delivered in a group 1 hour three times a week for 12 weeks, including strength training, walking and running in various directions to improve balance, and stair climbing for endurance training) was found to significantly improve BADL and IADL, which was maintained 12 weeks later. However, the authors attributed the improved ADL scores to increased exercise tolerance achieved in physical therapy, not occupational therapy (Bendstrup et al., 1997). Continued study is needed by occupational therapists.

Summary Review Questions

1. How is occupation-as-end used to improve occupational functioning?
2. What conditions interfere with the patient's ability to benefit from instruction in ADL methods?
3. What principle of compensation is implemented when a patient with limited or restricted range of motion uses a stocking aid?
4. What device can enable use of utensils when a patient lacks grasp?
5. What modifications may be necessary to enable a C6 tetraplegic college student majoring in journalism to do tasks required of that role?
6. What principles of compensation are used for problems of incoordination?
7. State the steps a stroke patient can use to put on and remove a cardigan-type garment.
8. Name five energy conservation techniques and give an example of each that could be used by a cardiac patient.
9. Describe how a person with low vision can decorate and arrange the bathroom to facilitate efficient independence.
10. Define and contrast IADL and BADL.

Resources

Resources for Promoting the Role of Independent Person

Books, Articles, and Web Sites

Some of these publications describe strategies, technology, and environmental modifications found helpful by persons with disabilities and by professionals. Others provide sources for assistive devices.

Accent on Living · Quarterly magazine that addresses all aspects of living a full life with a disability and makes good suggestions for solving problems of persons with physical disabilities.
www.blvd.com/accent

Accent on Living yearly buyer's guide · Accent on Living, P.O. Box 700, Bloomington, IL 61702-0700. 800-787-8444.
www.accentonliving.com

American Occupational Therapy Association · AOTA's Occupational Therapy Buyer's Guide, *OTPRACTICE*, yearly supplement.
www.aota.org

Anson, D. K. (1996) · *Alternative Computer Access: A Guide to Selection*, Philadelphia: F. A. Davis.
www.fadavis.com

Cheever, R., & Elmer, C. D. (1975) · *Bowel Management: A Manual of Ideas and Techniques*, Bloomington, IL: Accent Special Publications, Cheever Publishing, Inc. 800-787-8444.

Cornacchio, D., & Howard, A. (Eds.). (1996) · *Fodor's Great American Vacations for Travelers With Disabilities* (2nd ed.), New York: Fodor's Travel.
www.amazon.com

DuCharme, S. H., & Gill, K. M. (1997) · *Sexuality After Spinal Cord Injury: Answers to Your Questions*. Baltimore: Paul H. Brookes.
www.barnesandnoble.com

Ford, J. R., & Duckworth, B. (1987) · *Physical management for the quadriplegic patient* (2nd ed.), Philadelphia: F. A. Davis.
www.fadavis.com

Garee, B. (Ed.). (1988) · *Single-handed: Devices and aids for one handers and sources of these devices*, Bloomington, IL: Accent Special Publications, Cheever Publishing, Inc. 800-787-8444.

Greenstein, D. B. (1997) · *Easy things to make things easy: Simple do-it-yourself home modifications for older people and others with physical limitations*, Cambridge, MA: Brookline Books. 617-868-0360.
www.brooklinebooks.com

Karp, G., & Lamb. L. (1999) · *Life on wheels: A guide for the active wheelchair user*, Cambridge, MA: O'Reilly & Associates. 617-354-5800. 800-775-7731.
www.oreilly.com

Krantz, G. C., Christenson, M. A., & Lindquist, A. (Eds.). *Assistive products: An illustrated guide to terminology*. Bethesda, MD: American Occupational Therapy Association, Inc. 800-SAY-AOTA (members). 301-652-2682 (nonmembers).
www.aota.org

Kroll, K., & Levy Klein, E. (1992). *Enabling romance*, Bethesda, MD. Woodbine House, Inc, 6510 Bells Mill Rd, Bethesda, MD 20817. 800-843-7323.
www.barnesandnoble.com

Mayer, T-K. (2000). *One-handed in a two-handed world* (2nd ed.). Boston: Prince-Gallison, P. O. Box 23, Hanover Station, Boston, MA 02113-0001. 617-367-5815.
www.gis.net/princeg

Neistadt, M. E., & Freda, M. (1987) · *Choices: A Guide to Sex Counseling With Physically Disabled Adults*, Melbourne, FL: Krieger Publishing.
www.barnesandnoble.com

Richardson, N. K. (n.d.) · *Type With One Hand*, North Coast Medical, Inc., 18305 Sutter Blvd, Morgan Hill, CA 95037-2845. 800-821-9319.
www.ncmedical.com

Schwarz, S. P. (1997) · *Dressing Tips and Clothing Resources for Making Life Easier* (3rd ed.), Madison, WI: AJ Press.
www.amazon.com

Sipski, M., & Alexander, C. (1997) · *Sexual function in people with disabilities and chronic illness: A health professional's guide*, Gaithersburg, MD: Aspen.
www.aspenpub.com

Woy, J. (1997) · *Accessible Gardening: Tips and Techniques for Seniors and the Disabled*, Mechanicsburg, PA: Stackpole. 800-732-3669. 717-796-0411.
www.stackpolebooks.co

Selection of Assistive Devices

Information services that list all assistive devices help in the selection of assistive devices, as do the catalogs of rehabilitation supply houses.

Information

ABLEDATA · Database funded by the U. S. Department of Education National Institute on Disability and Rehabilitation Research. It lists 17,000 products from 2,000 companies and 8,000 items no longer commercially available, customized devices, and noncommercial prototypes.
www.abledata.com

National Library Service for the Blind and Physically Handicapped · Library of Congress, Washington, DC 20542. 800-424-9100.
Has talking books, popular magazines, and playback machines (adapted to needs) free to the blind, learning disabled, and physically disabled. The materials are returned to the National Library postage free, but there is also a network of cooperating libraries.
www.lcweb.loc.gov/nls

REHABDATA · A bibliographical database of documents on rehabilitation that includes journals, unpublished documents, audiovisual materials, commercial publications, and government reports.
NARIC · 1010 Wayne Ave., Suite 800, Silver Springs, MD 20910. 800-34-NARIC.
Material written between 1956 and 1992 (38,000 documents):
www.naric.com/search/rhab/rhabback.html
Material from 1993 to present (12,000 documents):
www.naric.com/search/rhab/index.html

AARP Connections for Independent Living. (1997) · *Home Modification, Independent Living Kit*, Washington: Author, 601 E Street NW, Washington, DC 20049.
www.aarp.org

AARP Independent Living. (1999) · *How Well Does Your Home Meet Your Needs?* Washington: Author.
www.aarp.org
A checklist to identify problems.

Tools and gadgets for independent living (for seeing, hearing, remembering, getting around).
www.aarp.org/gadgets

The Adaptive Environments Center (1995) · *A Consumer's Guide to Home Adaptation*, Boston: Author, 374 Congress St., Suite 301, Boston, MA 02210. 617-695-1225.
In addition to suggestions for devices and choice of appliances and fixtures, directions for common modifications such as grab bars, ramps, doorways are provided.

Canine Companions for Independence · There are six regional centers in the United States; they supply service dogs to perform helpful tasks, signal dogs to alert owners, social dogs to provide pet-facilitated therapy for persons with developmental disability, specialty dogs for persons with multiple handicaps and unique needs. P.O. Box 446, Santa Rosa, CA 95402-0446. 800-572-BARK.
www.caninecompanions.org

Consumer Information Catalogue · U. S. Government Publications, Pueblo, CO 81009.
www.pueblo.gsa.gov

Rehabilitation Equipment Suppliers

Access-USA · 800-263-2750.
www.access-usa.com
Supplier of Braille stickers (salt, pepper, food, beverage, spice tags) and other Braille products, such as menus and maps.

Easy Street Environments · Customized real-life settings for evaluation and training in IADL, 6031 South Maple Drive, Tempe, AZ 85283. 800-733-8442.
www.easystreetenvironments.com

FashionAble for better living · Catalog of clothing for the disabled, 5 Crescent Ave., Box 5, Rocky Hill, NJ 08553. 609-921-2563.

Invacare · One Invacare Way, Elyria, OH 44036-4028. 800-333-6900. Personal Care Products catalog. Also a source for bathroom and other equipment for people weighing over 200 pounds.
www.invacare.com

Journey Forth Inclusive Apparel Line · Clothing that looks ordinary but is easy to put on and take off. 800-510-7170.

North Coast Medical, Inc. Rehabilitation catalog · 18305 Sutter Blvd, Morgan Hill, CA 95037-2845. 800-821-9319.
www.ncmedical.com

Optelec (on-screen magnifier for low vision) · 6 Lyberty Way, Westford, MA 01886. 800-828-1056.
www.optelec.com

S & S Worldwide · Opportunities catalog, P. O. Box 513, Colchester, CT 06415-0513. 800-266-8856.
www.snswwide.com

Sammons® Preston · Enrichments catalog, P. O. Box 5071, Bolingbrook, IL 60440-5071. 800-323-5547.
www.sammonspreston.com

Smith + Nephew, Inc. Rehabilitative Care catalog · Rehabilitation Division, One Quality Drive, P.O. Box 1005, Germantown, WI 53022-8205. 800-558-8633.
www.easy-living.com

Techni-Flair · 2nd & Dalton Street, Cotter, AR 72626. 800-643-5656.
Adapted clothing catalog

The Left Hand · Electronic catalog only
www.thelefthand.com

The Lighthouse Catalogue · 111 East 59th St., New York, NY 10022-1202. 800-829-0500.
www.lighthouse.org
Equipment for the blind

Vermont Country Store Catalog · P. O. Box 3000, Manchester Center, VT 05255-3000. 800-362-8440. Clothing and devices.

Organizations

These organizations provide information for regaining independence for the professional and consumer and offer support groups and free brochures.

American Foundation for the Blind · 15 West 16th St., New York, NY 10011.

www.afb.org

American Heart Association

www.americanheart.org

American Stroke Association

www.strokeassociation.org

Arthritis Foundation

www.arthritis.org

National Head Injury Foundation · 1776 Massachusetts Avenue NW, Suite 100, Washington, DC 20366.

National Multiple Sclerosis Society · 733 Third Ave., New York, NY 10017. 800-344-4867.

www.nmss.org

National Parkinson Foundation, Inc. · Bob Hope Parkinson Research Center, 1501 N. W. 9th Ave., Bob Hope Road, Miami, FL 33136-1494. 800-327-4545.

www.parkinson.org

National Spinal Cord Injury Association · 8701 Georgia Ave., Suite 500, Silver Springs, MD 20851. 301-588-6959. 800-962-9629.

www.spinalcord.org

National Stroke Association

www.stroke.org

References

American Heart Association (1994). *The One-Handed Way: Living With the Use of One Hand.* Dallas: Author.

American Heart Association (1999). *Sex and Heart Disease.* Dallas: Author.

American Heart Association (2000). *Sex After Stroke.* Dallas: Author.

Andrews, K., & Stewart, J. (1979). Stroke recovery: He can but does he? *Rheumatology and Rehabilitation, 18* (1) 43–48.

Arthritis Foundation. (1997). *Gardening and Arthritis.* Atlanta: Author (brochure).

Atwood, S. M., Holm, M. B., & James, A. (1994). Activities of daily living capabilities and values of long-term care facility residents. *American Journal of Occupational Therapy, 48* (8), 710–716.

Bendstrup, K. E., Ingemann Jensen, J., Holm, S., & Bengtsson, B. (1997). Out-patient rehabilitation improves activities of daily living, quality of life and exercise tolerance in chronic obstructive pulmonary disease. *European Respiratory Journal, 10,* 2801–2806.

Berzins, G. F. (1970). An occupational therapy program for the chronic obstructive pulmonary disease patient. *American Journal of Occupational Therapy, 24,* 181–186.

Bobco, J. M. (1988). Shoe donner. *American Journal of Occupational Therapy, 42* (12), 811–813.

Brett, G. (1960). Dressing techniques for the severely involved hemiplegic patient. *American Journal of Occupational Therapy, 14* (5), 262–264.

Brodal, A. (1973). Self-observations and neuro-anatomical considerations after a stroke. *Brain, 96,* 675–694.

Buning, M. E., & Hanzlik, J. R. (1993). Adaptive computer use for a person with visual impairment. *American Journal of Occupational Therapy, 47,* 998–1008.

Burke, D. A. (1989). *Bathroom Aids.* Newton Square, PA: Universal Management Systems (brochure).

Bynum, H. S., & Rogers, J. C. (1987). The use and effectiveness of assistive devices possessed by patients seen in home care. *Occupational Therapy Journal of Research, 7* (3), 181–191.

Chen, T.-Y., Mann, W. C., Tomita, M., & Nochajski, S. (2000). Caregiver involvement in the use of assistive devices by frail older persons. *Occupational Therapy Journal of Research, 20* (3), 179–199.

Clark, M. C., Czaja, S. J., & Weber, R. A. (1990). Older adults and daily living task profiles. *Human Factors, 32,* 537–549.

Clarkson, J. D. (1982). Self-catheterization training of a child with myelomeningocele. *American Journal of Occupational Therapy, 36,* 95–98.

Colenbrander, A., & Fletcher, D. C. (1995). Basic concepts and terms for low vision rehabilitation. *American Journal of Occupational Therapy, 49,* 865–869.

Conine, T. A., & Hershler, C. (1991). Effectiveness: A neglected dimension in the assessment of rehabilitation devices and equipment. *International Journal of Rehabilitation Research, 14,* 117–122.

Cristy, D., & Sarafconn, C. A. (1990). *Pacing Yourself: Steps to Help Save Your Energy.* Bloomington, IL: Cheever.

Dallas, M. J., & White, L. W. (1982). Clothing fasteners for women with arthritis. *American Journal of Occupational Therapy, 36,* 515–518.

DeGraff, A. H. (1989). Managing your own care. *Accent on Living, 34* (2), 42–47.

Diller, L., Buxbaum, J., & Chiotelis, S. (1972). Relearning motor skills in hemiplegia: Error analysis. *Genetic Psychology Monographs, 85,* 249–286.

Duckworth, B. (1986). Overview of menstrual management for disabled women. *Canadian Journal of Occupational Therapy, 53* (1), 25–29.

Edmans, J. A., & Lincoln, N. B. (1990). The relationship between perceptual deficits after stroke and independence in activities of daily living. *British Journal of Occupational Therapy, 33* (4), 139–142.

Egan, M., Warren, S. A., Hessel, R. A., & Gilewich, G. (1992). Activities of daily living after hip fracture: Pre- and post-discharge. *Occupational Therapy Journal of Research, 12,* 342–356.

Finlayson, M., & Havixbeck, K. (1992). A post-discharge study on the use of assistive devices. *Canadian Journal of Occupational Therapy, 59* (4), 201–207.

Garee, B. (1992). *Ideas for Making Your Home Accessible.* Bloomington, IL: Cheever.

Gibson, J. W., & Schkade, J. K. (1997). Occupational adaptation intervention with patients with cerebrovascular accident: A clinical study. *American Journal of Occupational Therapy, 51,* 523–529.

Giles, G. M., Ridley, J. E., Dill, A., & Frye, S. (1997). A consecutive series of adults with brain injury treated with a washing and dressing retraining program. *American Journal of Occupational Therapy, 51,* 256–266.

Gitlin, L. N., & Burgh, D. (1995). Issuing assistive devices to older patients in rehabilitation: An exploratory study. *American Journal of Occupational Therapy, 49,* 994–1000.

Hage, G. (1988). Makeup board for women with quadriplegia. *American Journal of Occupational Therapy, 42,* 253–255.

Hanlon, R. E. (1996). Motor learning following unilateral stroke. *Archives of Physical Medicine and Rehabilitation, 77,* 811–815.

Hasselkus, B. R. (2000). Habits of the heart. *American Journal of Occupational Therapy, 54,* 247–248.

Hermann, R. P., Phalangas, A. C., Mahoney, R. M., & Alexander, M. A. (1999). Powered feeding devices: An evaluation of three models. *Archives of Physical Medicine and Rehabilitation, 80,* 1237–1242.

Houtchens, C. J. (1998). A guide to intimacy with arthritis. *Arthritis Today.* Atlanta: Arthritis Foundation (reprint).

Huck, J., & Bonhotal, B. H. (1997). Fastener systems on apparel for hemiplegic stroke victims. *Applied Ergonomics, 28* (4), 277–282.

Johansson, R. S., & Westling, G. (1984). Roles of glabrous skin receptors and sensorimotor memory in automatic control of precision grip when lifting rougher or more slippery objects. *Experimental Brain Research, 56,* 550–564.

Kamsma, Y. P. T., Brouwer, W. H., & Lakke, J. P. W. F. (1995). Training of compensational strategies for impaired gross motor skills in Parkinson's disease. *Physiotherapy Theory and Practice, 11,* 209–229.

Katz, S., Ford, A. B., Moskowitz, R. W., Jackson, B. A., & Jaffee, M. W. (1963). Studies of illness in the aged: The Index of ADL: A standardized measure of biological and psychosocial function. *Journal of the American Medical Association, 185,* 914–919.

Katzmann, S., & Mix, C. (1994). Case report: Improving functional independence in a patient with encephalitis through behavior modification shaping techniques. *American Journal of Occupational Therapy, 4,* 259–262.

Kratz, G., Söderback, I., Guidetti, S., Hultling, C., Rykatkin, T., & Söderström, M. (1997). Wheelchair users' experience of non-adapted and adapted clothes during sailing, quad rugby, or wheel walking. *Disability and Rehabilitation, 19* (1), 26–34.

Lampert, J., & Lapolice, D. J. (1995). Functional considerations in evaluation and treatment of the client with low vision. *American Journal of Occupational Therapy, 49,* 885–890.

Law, M. (1991). Muriel Driver Lecture: The environment: A focus for occupational therapy. *Canadian Journal of Occupational Therapy, 58* (4), 171–180.

Lewis, R. I. (1993). Catheter choice if needed. *Accent on Living, 38* (1), 44–48.

Mann, W. C., Hurren, D., & Tomita, M. (1995). Assistive devices used by home-based elderly persons with arthritis. *American Journal of Occupational Therapy, 49,* 810–820.

Mann, W. C., Hurren, D., Tomita, M., & Charvat, B. (1996). Use of assistive devices for bathing by elderly who are not institutional-ized. *Occupational Therapy Journal of Research, 16,* 261–286.

McAlonan, S. (1996). Improving sexual rehabilitation services: The patient's perspective. *American Journal of Occupational Therapy, 50,* 826–834.

McCuaig, M., & Frank, G. (1991). The able self: Adaptive patterns and choices in independent living for a person with cerebral palsy. *American Journal of Occupational Therapy, 45,* 224–234.

Mooney, T. G., Cole, T. M., & Chilgren, R. A. (1975). *Sexual Options for Paraplegics and Quadriplegics.* Boston: Little, Brown.

Nordenskiöld, U., Grimby, G., & Dahlin-Ivanoff, S. (1998). Question-naire to evaluate the effects of assistive devices and altered working methods in women with rheumatoid arthritis. *Clinical Rheumatology, 17* (1), 6–16.

Nordström, T. & Thorslund, M. (1991). The structure of IADL and ADL measures: Some findings from a Swedish study. *Age and Ageing, 20,* 23–28.

One Shape Serves All (1998). *Modern Maturity, 41* (1), 28.

Parker, M. G., & Thorslund, M. (1991). Use of technical aids among community-based elderly. *American Journal of Occupational Therapy, 45,* 712–718.

Peterman Schwarz, S. (1997). *250 Tips for Making Life With Arthritis Easier.* Atlanta: Longstreet Press (Arthritis Foundation).

Platt, J. V., Begun, R., & Murphy, E. D. (1992). *Daily Activities After Your Knee Replacement.* Bethesda: American Occupational Therapy Association.

Pomerantz, P., Flannery, E. L., & Findling, P. K. (1975). Occupational therapy for chronic obstructive lung disease. *American Journal of Occupational Therapy, 29,* 407–411.

Poole, J. (1998). Effect of apraxia on the ability to learn one-handed shoe tying. *Occupational Therapy Journal of Research, 18* (3), 99–104.

Reich, N., & Otten, P. (1980). Are buttons and zippers confidence trippers? *Accent on Living, 25* (3), 98–99.

Rice, M. S., Leonard, C., & Carter, M. (1998). Grip strengths and required forces in accessing everyday containers in a normal population. *American Journal of Occupational Therapy, 52,* 621–626.

Rogers, J. C., & Holm, M. B. (1992). Assistive technology device use in patients with rheumatic disease: A literature review. *American Journal of Occupational Therapy, 46,* 120–127.

Rosenthal, S. B. (1995). Living with low vision: A personal and professional perspective. *American Journal of Occupational Therapy, 49,* 861–864.

Runge, M. (1967). Self dressing techniques for patients with spinal cord injury. *American Journal of Occupational Therapy, 21,* 367–375.

Ryu, J., Cooney, W. P., Askew, L. J., An, K.-N., & Chao, E. Y. S. (1991). Functional ranges of motion of the wrist joint. *Journal of Hand Surgery, 16A,* 409–419.

Salmen, J. P. S. (2000). *The Do-able Renewable Home: Making Your Home Fit Your Needs.* Washington: American Association of Retired Persons.

Schemm, R. L., & Gitlin, L. N. (1998). How occupational therapists teach older patients to use bathing and dressing devices in rehabilitation. *American Journal of Occupational Therapy, 52,* 276–282.

Schmidt, R. A., & Lee, T. (2000). *Motor Control and Learning: A Behavioral Emphasis* (3rd. ed.). Champaign, IL: Human Kinetics.

Seeger, M. S., & Fisher, L. A. (1982). Adaptive equipment used in the rehabilitation of hip arthroplasty patients. *American Journal of Occupational Therapy, 36,* 515–518.

Shillam, L. L., Beeman, C., & Loshin, P. M. (1983). Effect of occupa-tional therapy intervention on bathing independence of disabled persons. *American Journal of Occupational Therapy, 37,* 744–748.

Shotwell, M. P, & Schell, B. A. (1999). Occupational therapy practi-tioner as health educator: A framework for active learning. [AOTA] *Physical Disabilities Special Interest Section Quarterly, 22* (4), 1–3.

Skinner, B. F. (1938). *The Behavior of Organisms.* New York: Appleton-Century-Crofts.

Smith, R. (1989). Mouthstick design for the client with spinal cord injury. *American Journal of Occupational Therapy, 43,* 251–255.

Spector, W. D., Katz, S., Murphy, J. B., & Fulton, J. P. (1987). The hierarchical relationship between activities of daily living and instrumental activities of daily living. *Journal of Chronic Disease, 40* (6), 481–489.

Spencer, J., Hersch, G., Eschenfelder, V., Fournet, J., & Murray-Gerzik, M. (1999). Outcomes of protocol-based and adaptation-based occupational therapy interventions for low-income elderly per-sons on a transitional unit. *American Journal of Occupational Therapy, 53,* 159–170.

Spica, M. M., & Schwab, M. D. (1996). Sexual expression after total joint replacement. *Orthopaedic Nursing, 15* (5), 41–44.

Strub, N., & Levine, R. E. (1987). Self care: A comparison of patients' institutional and home performance. *Occupational Therapy Jour-nal of Research, 7* (1), 53–56.

Thorén Jönsson, A.-L., Möller, A., & Grimby, G. (1999). Managing occupations in everyday life to achieve adaptation. *American Journal of Occupational Therapy, 53,* 353–362.

Thomas, J. J. (1999). Enhancing patient education: Addressing the issue of literacy. [AOTA] *Physical Disabilities Special Interest Section Quarterly, 22* (4), 3–4.

Trombly, C. A. (1993). Anticipating the future: Assessment of occupa-tional function. *American Journal of Occupational Therapy, 47,* 253–259.

Trombly, C. A. (1995). Occupation: Purposefulness and meaning-fulness as therapeutic mechanisms: 1995 Eleanor Clarke Slagle Lecture. *American Journal of Occupational Therapy, 49,* 960–972.

Tyson, R., & Strong, J. (1990). Adaptive equipment: Its effectiveness for people with chronic lower back pain. *Occupational Therapy Journal of Research, 10* (2), 111–121.

van Heugten, C. M., Dekker, J., Deelman, B. G., vanDijk, A. J., Stehmann-Saris, J. C., & Kinebanian, A. (1998). Outcome of strategy training in stroke patients with apraxia: A phase II study. *Clinical Rehabilitation, 12,* 294–303.

Walker, M. F., Drummond, A. E. R., & Lincoln, N. B. (1996). Evaluation of dressing practice for stroke patients after discharge from hospital: A crossover design study. *Clinical Rehabilitation, 10,* 23–31.

Walker, M. F., Gladman, J. R. F., Lincoln, N. B., Siemonsma, P., &

Whiteley, T. (1999). Occupational therapy for stroke patients not admitted to hospital: A randomised controlled trial. *Lancet, 354,* 278–280.

Walker, M. F., & Lincoln, N. B. (1990). Reacquisition of dressing skills after stroke. *International Disability Studies, 12,* 41–43.

Walker, M. F., & Lincoln, N. B. (1991). Factors influencing dressing performance after stroke. *Journal of Neurology, Neurosurgery, and Psychiatry, 54,* 699–701.

Weingarden, S. I., & Martin, C. (1989). Independent dressing after spinal cord injury: A functional time evaluation. *Archives of Physical Medicine & Rehabilitation, 70,* 518–519.

31
Restoring Competence in Mobility

Susan Pierce

LEARNING OBJECTIVES

After studying this chapter, the reader will be able to do the following:

1. Identify areas of mobility that an occupational therapy treatment plan should include.
2. Identify aids and devices used to restore mobility.
3. State the hierarchy of mobility skills used to plan treatment.
4. Describe various transfer techniques and strategies for achieving mobility for persons with physical dysfunction.
5. Describe the role of the driver rehabilitation therapist in assisting with community mobility goals.

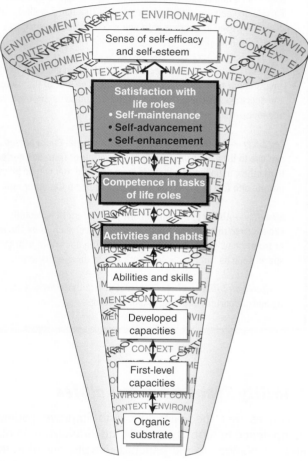

Sense of self-efficacy and self-esteem

Satisfaction with life roles
• Self-maintenance
• Self-advancement
• Self-enhancement

Competence in tasks of life roles

Activities and habits

Abilities and skills

Developed capacities

First-level capacities

Organic substrate

*R*estoring competence in **mobility** in the home and community is a key goal of rehabilitation. For persons to participate in the activities and tasks of their life roles, they must be able to move about in their surroundings. This may entail moving around in bed to dress or moving out of bed to go into the bathroom to use the sink or toilet, or moving about the community to a workplace, grocery store, theater, or church. The occupational therapist assesses mobility as it relates to each occupational role. After remedial treatment to restore sensory, perceptual, cognitive and motor components of occupational performance, the occupational therapist must reassess these areas in terms of residual deficits and how they will affect a person's ability to be mobile. Understanding the patient's overall functioning is crucial to structuring a treatment program for each person's particular mobility independence.

GLOSSARY

Driver rehabilitation therapist—Allied health professional with specialized training, experience, and credentials in driver rehabilitation services, including evaluating and training persons with disabilities in driving or safe transportation.

Ecological validity—Treatment that reflects a person's actual home and living environment.

Hemiwalker—A one-handed walker with four legs and a wider base than a quad cane. It is held by the strong upper extremity. This device gets its name because it looks like half a walker and is typically used by persons with one-sided weakness, such as those with hemiplegia.

In-home assessment—Objective evaluation of a patient's living environment that takes place at the home. The size of the rooms and doorways, placement of the furniture, and so on are observed and measured (see Chapter 10).

Leg lifter—Device usually made of soft material that a person can use to lift a leg from one place to another or from one surface to another; usually has a large loop on one end that can be placed around one foot or thigh and a loop or handle on the other end.

Mobility—Ability to move from one place to another. Mobility ranges from moving one's body in close space, such as on the bed or from the wheelchair to the bed, to moving oneself in a larger space, such as from home to a work site or the grocery store.

Orthotic mobility device—External device that provides stability and support for standing and/or walking.

Quad cane—Straight cane with four short legs in a wide base for stability.

Rope ladder—Ladder device with two long parallel pieces of strapping connected by "rungs." One end of the rope ladder is attached to the foot of the bed. A person pulls up gradually to a sitting position by pulling on the rungs in progression.

Transfer—Movement of one's body from one surface to an adjacent surface. A transfer may be performed independently or with the assistance of one or two persons.

Transfer belt—Wide belt with handles that is wrapped snugly around a client's waist to provide a handhold for another person to pull the client to a standing position and/or to assist the client's balance during transfers or walking.

Transfer board—Device made of hard material, such as wood or fiberglass; placed under the buttocks to bridge the space between two surfaces during transfer.

Wheelchair and occupant restraint system—Crash-tested passive or active restraint system that secures a wheelchair and the occupant separately and appropriately.

Wheelchair wheelie—Maneuvering of a manual wheelchair onto its rear tires and balancing in this position to raise the front casters off the ground.

Mobility Treatment Principles

Principles that therapists follow to improve patients' competence in mobility include individualizing training and adaptations to the patient's deficits, ensuring that the training is ecologically valid, following a hierarchy of skills, and coplanning with other disciplines, especially physical therapy.

Mobility Training Is Individualized

The therapist must keep in mind that each patient has unique problems and ways of doing activities of daily living (ADL); therefore, customization of techniques and equipment is often necessary. The patient must have input into the strategies and problem solving. The therapist must be an active listener to the patient's thoughts and opinions and be willing to modify techniques as needed.

Every mobility task requires a certain amount of strength, coordination, and range of motion. Many patients have more than one area of deficit. A person with rheumatoid arthritis may have range of motion deficits as well as weakness and problems with fatigue. A person with spinal cord injury may have decreased sensation as well as paralysis or weakness. A person who has deficits in any or all areas of physical or sensory functioning may have to be evaluated for orthotic or assistive devices and for compensatory techniques to achieve independence. Deficits may affect mobility differently in different environments, so the therapist must consider the patient's functional mobility and activities in all relevant environments. For example, a person who has had a stroke may require a wheelchair outside the home but be able to get around at home with the assistance of a **quad cane** or **hemiwalker**.

Strive for Ecological Validity

The first phase of training in mobility independence takes place in the accessible environment of the rehabilitation facility or hospital. The second phase addresses mobility independence at home and in the community. The occupational therapist should strive for **ecological validity**, which simply means that the training takes into consideration the actual environment that the patient comes from and will be returning to. The environment includes home, yard, neighborhood, and community— where the person works, plays, and/or goes to school.

Assessment of patients' personal environments must be made so that training in the second phase can take place realistically. This training can first use the mock environment of the therapy clinic or custom clinical environments that simulate real indoor and outdoor environments. Once the therapist is familiar with the home and community to which the person will be returning, the therapist can seek environments in or around the treatment facility that best simulate the patient's home. A questionnaire for the family on the patient's home and community can be useful in early planning, but a comprehensive **in-home assessment** is crucial for discharge planning (see Chapter 10). Even if the patient will be discharged to a nursing home or assisted-living environment, maximum independence for that environment should be sought.

The occupational therapist and physical therapist should make a home visit together to see the patient's own world. His or her world may not consist of level floors, low-pile carpet, easy curb cuts, or nicely ramped entrances, as found in hospitals and rehabilitation facilities. The outdoor terrain may be soft dirt, sand, or bumpy grass. Wheelchair maneuverability in the home may be through narrow hallways and doorways. The patient may have to transfer onto a waterbed or soft mattress rather than the adjustable-height surface of a firm hospital bed. There may not be a roll-in shower or money or room to have one built, so the patient may have to learn to use a regular tub with a tub bench. Whether the patient can walk or must use a wheelchair, has the ideal situation or not, the home assessment is necessary so that the treatment plan and discharge recommendations take into consideration the environment to which he or she will be returning.

Today, with shorter periods of inpatient rehabilitation, the level of mobility an inpatient achieves on discharge may not be the same level that the person can achieve 6 or 8 months post discharge. The therapist should plan long-term postdischarge goals for mobility with the patient so that he or she can work on continued goals of maximum independence and mobility after discharge.

Follow the Hierarchy of Skills for Mobility

Each area of mobility requires a certain skill level in occupational performance. A hierarchy of skills dictates the order in which each area is addressed. Mobility in basic activities of daily living (BADL) is first, followed by mobility in instrumental activities of daily living (IADL) (Fig. 31-1). Some occupational therapy goals for motor, sensory, perceptual, and cognitive functioning must be achieved prior to ADL training and specifically mobility training. The person with quadriplegia secondary to a spinal cord injury must be able to sit on a hard surface

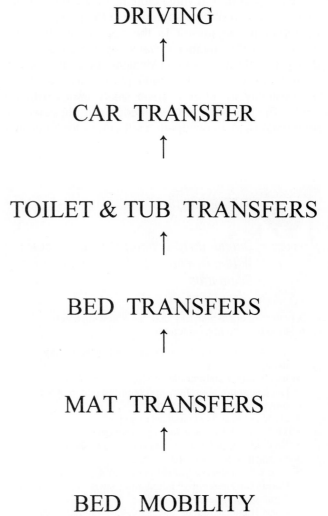

DRIVING
↑
CAR TRANSFER
↑
TOILET & TUB TRANSFERS
↑
BED TRANSFERS
↑
MAT TRANSFERS
↑
BED MOBILITY

Figure 31-1 Hierarchy of mobility skills illustrates the order of accomplishing mobility skills.

without support, such as a mat, before sitting on a soft surface, such as a bed. This accomplishment precedes learning to dress in bed or in a wheelchair.

Transfers to bed must be mastered before transfers to a car. A car transfer is more complicated and difficult because the wheelchair seat height is different from the car seat height and the distance between the two is greater than for other transfers. The person must also handle his or her legs through the cramped space of a car door. Since the task demands for driving are higher than for any other IADL, driving should be the last IADL the occupational therapist addresses. Driving is the most complex IADL for most persons, as it requires good physical, visual, perceptual, psychological, and cognitive skills. Consequently, most patients are not ready for a driving evaluation before discharge from the inpatient facility. Box 31-1 has guidelines to determine when a person with a disability is ready for a driving evaluation.

If the patient is driving before he or she is ready, the therapist has an obligation to protect the public welfare by reporting the person to the appropriate licensing authority in the manner dictated by the state of residency. In 1999 the American Medical Association passed a landmark decision to assign physicians the ethical responsibility to address driver safety issues with patients. The decision further encourages physicians to refer patients to an occupational therapist for an evalua-

tion. Every occupational therapist should know the procedure for reporting impaired drivers in his or her state and which functions a therapist is authorized, obligated, or responsible to perform (Kaplan, 1999). The occupational therapist should also know the **driver rehabilitation therapists** in the community or state who can be used for referral when this service is needed.

During the inpatient stay, the client may be allowed home visits on the weekends in preparation for discharge. it is important to work on mobility early in rehabilitation so that the patient will not develop feelings of isolation upon returning home during these visits or after discharge. Transportation needs, particularly for the wheelchair user, may have to be addressed long before driving, as the person may not be ready for a driving evaluation until 8 to 12 months after discharge. A referral to the driver rehabilitation therapist for transportation only may be appropriate before discharge so that the patient, family, and funding source can be guided toward the appropriate vehicle and modifications. If the driver rehabilitation therapist can determine that the patient may be able to drive later, vehicle selection and modifications for transportation can be made with future driving needs taken into consideration.

Interdisciplinary Team Approach

Teamwork between occupational therapy and physical therapy is important so that the two coordinate treatment and share a vision of how this treatment relates to future goal planning in IADL and mobility. Communication between team members eliminates unnecessary duplication and promotes carryover of skills. The direction the occupational therapist takes in pursuing IADL should be influenced by the patient's achievements in physical therapy and basic mobility activities. Achievement of the physical therapy goals may take several weeks, so the occupational therapist uses this time to work on BADL that do not demand a high level of strength and endurance. A patient who will walk at some time first learns to brush his or her teeth, wash hair, and don a shirt sitting down. When the patient has achieved standing tolerance and balance in physical therapy, the occupational therapist can incorporate standing in activities such as brushing teeth and washing dishes while standing at a sink. If the patient will be using a wheelchair for all mobility, the occupational therapist works on upper extremity strengthening as it relates to propelling a wheelchair and performing activities from the chair, such as dressing and grooming. If the patient will be a functional but limited walker with an orthotic device, the occupational therapist must incorporate these devices into the IADL and BADL training. For example, a person who uses a cane or walker has to learn to maneuver in the kitchen with these devices while cooking.

BOX 31-1
PROCEDURES FOR PRACTICE

Guidelines to Determine When a Person With a Disability Is Ready for a Driving Evaluation

A patient or client who has all of the following can be referred for a driving evaluation:

- Maximum independence in basic activities of daily living
- Independent ambulation or wheelchair mobility
- Good strength, sensation, and coordination in at least one or ideally two extremities
- 20/40 visual acuity in at least one eye*
- 140° of total field of vision with both eyes*
- No double vision with or without compensation*
- No seizures for 6 months*
- Spasticity under control with or without medication
- Good visual-perceptual functioning, such as depth and figure ground perception
- Good cognitive functioning; short-term memory can be minimally to moderately affected
- Valid driver's license or learner's permit

*Specifications vary among states.

Mobility Training

This section discusses bed mobility; wheelchair mobility, including transfer methods; functional ambulation with or without orthotic devices; and vehicle mobility. It also describes strategies, methods, and equipment suggested by therapists and former patients that can be used in restoring mobility for persons with a variety of physical disabilities.

Bed Mobility

The ability to roll over and to sit up in bed is necessary for dressing and transferring. Gillen and Burkhardt (1998) suggest that one of the most common movement strategies in rolling from supine to prone is a lift-and-reach pattern. To begin rolling over, the person throws the arms in the direction he or she wants the body to go. The upper trunk, hips, and legs follow with the momentum.

A person with weakness or paralysis in the lower extremities and trunk may need a device to pull on, to turn over. Examples are a rope ladder, a leg lifter, an overhead trapeze, a bed rail, and a portable half bed rail (Fig. 31-2). A person who uses a wheelchair can pull against it if it is close to the bed with the brakes locked. A person with upper extremity weakness or weak grasp can use the same devices by hooking the forearm or extended wrist around the railing or a part of the wheelchair, such as the push handle. The person first holds the bedrail or wheelchair part with the arm closest to the side of the bed toward which he or she is rolling. The momentum for rolling the upper trunk is gained by flinging the other arm across the body. Pulling with both arms should turn the hips and legs. If not, he or she can use an extended wrist of the arm on top to push the thigh or use a **leg lifter** to pull the leg over.

Figure 31-3 illustrates the sequence a person with quadriplegia may use in coming from a supine to a seated position in a regular bed. If the person cannot independently pull the trunk to a sitting position, he or she may be able to do so using an overhead trapeze bar, a **rope ladder**, or bed loops. Good scapular, shoulder, and elbow strength is the minimum requirement for using these devices. The rope ladder or bed loops are attached to the foot of the bed, and the person loops the arms in the first rung, then in the next one, and so forth.

A person who cannot perform this task requires one or two persons to assist with rolling the upper and lower body in the proper sequence or using a log roll technique that moves the entire body at once. Figure 31-4 shows a spouse assisting her husband, who has incomplete quadriplegia with proximal weakness in the shoulders and hips, in bed mobility. Figure 31-5 shows mechanical and powered devices that assist the caregiver in moving a dependent person in bed or out of bed,

over a toilet or shower chair, or into a tub. The mechanical and hydraulic lifts can be on a movable frame, on a freestanding frame that hangs over the bed, or on a moving track that runs on the ceiling. Some lifts can move the person from one room to another.

The occupational therapist must assess sitting balance in order to pursue other bed activities. Balance in long- and short-leg sitting should be assessed. Long-leg sitting is the posture in which the legs are extended straight out in front of the person on a flat surface and the hips are flexed to at least 90°. A position beyond 90° of hip flexion must be achieved to maintain balance in a long-leg sitting position when trunk and hip musculature are weak. Short-leg sitting is the posture in which a person sits with the hips flexed at least to 90° and the knees flexed over the edge of the surface. The feet may or may not touch the floor, but stability is aided if they do.

Achieving sitting balance on a flat, hard mat precedes working on balance on a soft bed mattress. Upper extremity activities, such as throwing and catching a large ball, can be used to challenge the patient's balance. Balance improves either because weak trunk muscles get stronger or because the patient learns to balance by lowering the center of gravity and using the neck muscles to right the body. *While the person is working on improving balance, the therapist must maintain close supervision and contact and be ready to catch the person if balance is lost in any direction.*

A person who has good trunk balance may wish to dress while sitting on the edge of the bed. If the lower extremities are paralyzed, the person must manually move the legs over the side of the bed. Patients who have hip flexion limitations, so that they cannot reach their legs, or have balance difficulties in a long-leg sitting position can use a leg lifter. For the dependent person, another individual swings the person's legs off the edge of the bed. *When working with a dependent person or a person with poor sitting balance, the therapist must provide close supervision or constant manual contact to aid the person in sitting upright and prevent falling in any direction.*

A person who will dress in bed but who cannot reach his or her feet must flex the hip and knee to bring the foot closer to the hands for preparing to don pants, socks, and/or shoes. If a person has balance problems due to ataxia or trunk weakness or paralysis, a powered hospital bed that raises and lowers the upper body and knees can help with the task demands of lower extremity dressing, self-catheterization, and a bowel regulation program. The top and bottom of the bed can be elevated so that the upper trunk and knees are raised and the person's hands are freed from maintaining balance to perform these activities.

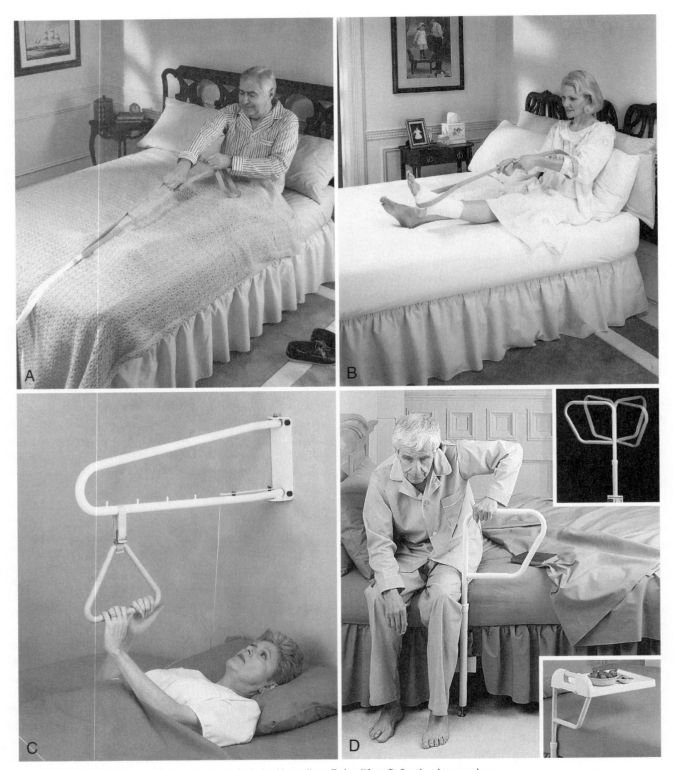

Figure 31-2 Devices that assist with bed mobility. **A.** Bed ladder pull-up. **B.** Leg lifter. **C.** Overhead trapeze bar. **D.** Bed rail assist. (Courtesy of Sammons Preston, Bolingbrook, IL.)

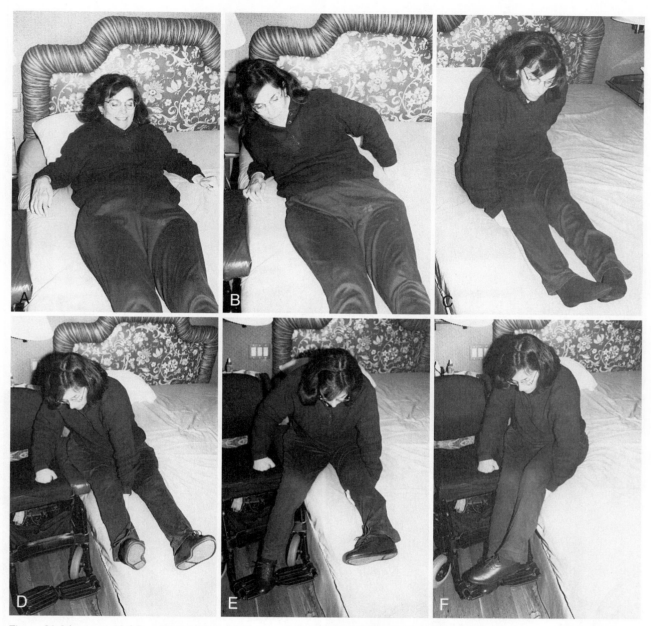

Figure 31-3 A person with C-7 quadriplegia illustrates the steps for coming to sitting position in bed without use of assistive devices. **A.** The person uses shoulder and scapula muscles to move to resting on elbows. **B.** She uses the triceps in one arm to lift her upper trunk while balancing on the other bent elbow. Using the triceps in the bent arm, she pushes the whole trunk upright until she is in long-sitting position. **C.** She can hold her balance with one arm behind her while using the other arm to reposition the legs as needed. **D.** Once she is close to the edge of the bed, she can lean on one arm that is pressing into the wheelchair seat to hold her balance while she moves the outside leg off the side of the bed. **E.** She then moves the inside leg off the side of the bed. **F.** Now in a short-legged sitting position, she can prepare for a sliding transfer into her wheelchair.

Wheelchair Mobility

For a person who cannot walk or has limited walking ability, a wheelchair provides mobility. A manual wheelchair is appropriate for a person who can propel the wheelchair using two arms, one arm, the feet, or a foot and an arm. A powered wheelchair or motorized scooter is appropriate for the person who does not have the physical capability to propel a manual chair or has low physical endurance. A scooter can be used by a person who is limited in walking because of low endurance or lower extremity weakness but who can transfer, has

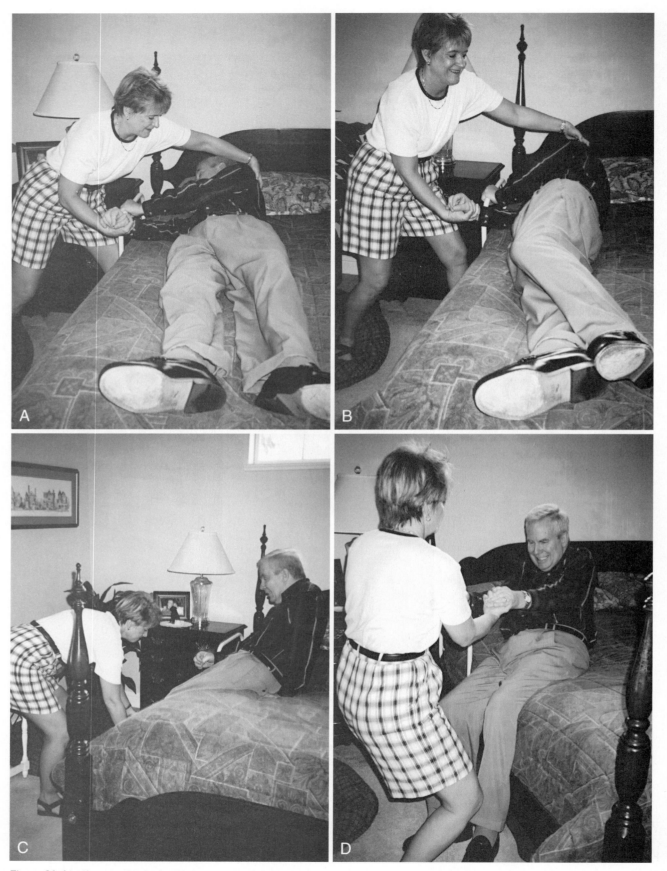

Figure 31-4 A wife assists her husband in bed mobility. **A.** Using proper body mechanics, the wife assists her husband to roll over by first pulling his left shoulder toward her. **B.** The husband can assist by using his hip and knee flexors and pulling against the half bed rail. **C.** The wife swings his legs off the bed and lowers his feet to the floor while the husband uses the stronger left arm to push against the bed to hold his balance in a half-sitting position. **D.** Again using proper body mechanics and allowing her legs and arms to do the work, the wife helps her husband come to a full sitting position.

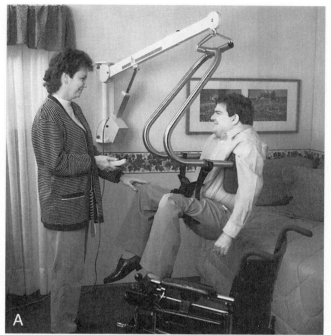

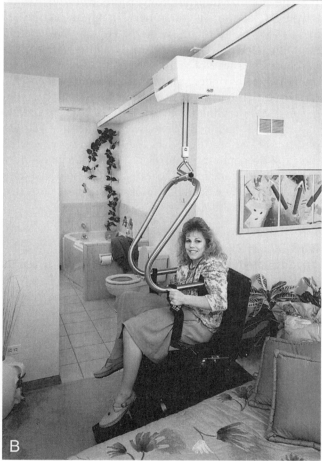

Figure 31-5 Powered and mechanical lifting systems. **A.** Mechanical unit attached to the wall. **B.** Ceiling-mounted powered track to carry a person from room to room. (Courtesy of SureHands Lift & Care Systems, Pine Island, New York.)

good trunk balance, and can maintain an upright posture. There are many styles and types of chairs and scooters from which to choose (see Chapter 16).

The patient's home and community must be considered when assisting him or her in choosing the most appropriate wheelchair. For example, a person who lives in a rural environment with sandy or grassy terrain may require a four-wheel scooter or a more powerful motor on a powered wheelchair. Also, the means of vehicle transportation is a factor to consider when choosing the type of wheelchair or scooter. A manual or powered wheelchair can be properly restrained, however a scooter cannot. The occupant of the scooter will have to transfer into a vehicle seat for safe transportation. The rehabilitation team should consult a driver rehabilitation therapist before prescribing a wheelchair or scooter for a patient to ensure that the chair is suitable for the person's vehicle and driving or transportation needs.

President George Bush signed into law the Americans with Disabilities Act (ADA) in July 1990. The law prohibits discrimination in employment, public accommodations, and transportation (Americans with Disabilities Act, 1990; O'Shea & Murphy, 1991). Public places, such as restaurants, private schools, shopping centers, banks, exercise facilities, transportation terminals, and prisons, must be accessible, as required by the law. The effect of the ADA has been to enhance the environment for accessibility, but there is not complete accessibility in all environments, particularly old buildings. Therefore, architectural barriers will most likely affect a person's wheelchair mobility at some point, and he or she should be taught to deal with such barriers.

When a patient receives a new wheelchair, indoor and outdoor mobility training is important so that he or she learns to handle and maneuver the chair in whatever circumstances he or she may encounter, such as tight spaces, up a curb or a ramp, and over rough and uneven terrain. A program graded toward independent mobility should be a team effort among the physical, occupational, and recreational therapists, with the practice of skills incorporated into other rehabilitation activities. For example, the occupational therapist may take the person to the grocery store to shop for food in preparation for cooking a meal during therapy. This experience gives the person an opportunity to explore wheelchair mobility in this environment while also carrying items or pushing a shopping cart.

The initial stages of wheelchair training take place inside the rehabilitation facility. In the first phase, the patient learns how to propel the wheelchair on a smooth, uncluttered surface. The patient learns to manipulate the wheelchair and its parts and to transfer in and out of the wheelchair. The second phase is learning to use the wheelchair outside. The patient learns to maneuver on various terrains, such as uneven sidewalks, gravel, and sand. Then the patient learns to negotiate obstacles such as curbs and steps. Once the patient can traverse outdoor surfaces, public buildings, such as grocery stores and shopping malls, can be used to teach the person to handle the wheelchair in crowded, narrow spaces.

Negotiating Ramps

A ramp enables a person to overcome a height discrepancy in a doorway, entrance, or step. Ramps come in many shapes, sizes, and dimensions. Ramps can be custom built or purchased and assembled from a kit. Factors that influence how a wheelchair user negotiates a ramp include his or her strength and balance, length and slope of the ramp, and the stability of the wheelchair. The ADA specifies how ramps in public places should be constructed in terms of length, slope, texture, and so on. For example, for every inch of rise, the ramp must have 12 inches of length (1:12 slope). If there is a 4-inch step, the ramp must be 48 inches long. A ramp in a public place must have a surface with a detectable texture for persons with visual impairments. It must have sides that are not vertical but slope at 1:10 maximum. There must be 4 feet of level landing at the top of the ramp. For private construction, a ramp that is longer and therefore has less slope (1:20) is more satisfactory for a person who uses a manual wheelchair and has upper extremity weakness because it is easier for that person to propel up the ramp.

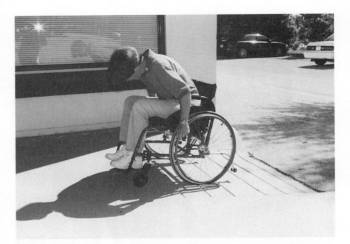

Figure 31-7 A therapist demonstrates how a person with good arm and trunk strength can safely negotiate a steep ramp by moving backward down the ramp. Leaning forward to shift the center of gravity prevents the chair from tipping backward.

The popular minivan conversions with the 10-inch lowered floor modifications have ramps measuring 53 inches long by 29 inches wide for entering and exiting the vehicle. Before a person in a manual wheelchair purchases this type of vehicle, particularly for independent driving, his or her ability to ascend and descend the ramp safely should be evaluated (Fig. 31-6).

One safe technique to use in descending a steep ramp is to orient the chair backward and lean forward to place most of the weight over the front caster wheels as the chair descends the ramp (Fig. 31-7). If the wheelchair has a tendency to tip backward easily, a helper should stand behind the wheelchair and walk with the person to catch the chair should it begin to tip backward.

Wheelchair Wheelies

An advanced wheelchair skill called a **wheelchair wheelie** can be used to elevate the caster wheels so that objects on the floor, sidewalk, or ground can be cleared or a curb or step can be managed. The person must have good upper extremity strength, coordination, and the ability to maintain balance when performing this activity (Pierson, 1999).

Because of the complexity of this task and the danger of losing balance and falling backward, the therapist must practice wheelchair wheelies with the patient many times on level surfaces before attempting curbs and steps. In the clinic a mat can be placed behind the wheelchair or the therapist can stand behind the chair ready to catch the wheelchair should it tip too far backward. A length of rope attached to the push handles and running through a ceiling pulley can also be used to protect the person

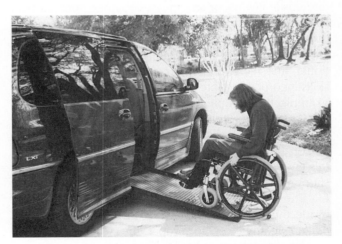

Figure 31-6 A person with quadriplegia in a manual wheelchair attempts to push up the ramp into a minivan whose floor has been lowered 10 inches. This task is easy in a powered wheelchair, but difficult in a manual wheelchair.

from falling and allow him or her to practice without a person behind him (Nixon, 1985).

The first step in performing a wheelie is to grasp the front portion of the wheel rims and quickly pull back equally on both hand rims. This places the hands in a rearward position on the hand rims. Another quick forward thrust on the wheels and then an abrupt stop rotates the chair frame backward with the rear axle acting as a fulcrum. The caster wheels rise, and the wheelchair balances on the rear wheels only. Small movements of the rear wheels control the balance of the chair (Deusterhaus-Minor & Deusterhaus-Minor, 1999).

Negotiating Curbs

In today's world and particularly since passage of the ADA in 1990, curbs on sidewalks at street intersections are becoming less of a problem as curb cuts proliferate. However, sometimes the wheelchair user still has to negotiate a curb. Ascending and descending a curb or step can be done independently by a manual wheelchair user who can perform a wheelie. First the person approaches the curb or step, facing it. Once the wheelie position has been obtained, the casters are placed on the curb. The person leans forward to balance the chair and redistribute the weight and propels the large rear wheels up the curb or step with a hearty push. A person must have good balance and hand function to perform this maneuver.

To go down a curb or a step, the person approaches it backward, leans forward in the chair, and rolls the rear wheels over the step or curb. An alternative method for going down a curb is to approach the curb facing it, move into the wheelie position and roll off the curb using the back wheels. The person must have an excellent sense of balance and control to perform this technique safely.

If a wheelchair user cannot move up or down a curb or step or roll through grass or over uneven surfaces, another person can provide assistance. In an assisted wheelchair wheelie, the helper pushes the wheelchair once the wheelchair is in the wheelie position (Fig. 31-8).

Negotiating Steps

Ascending or descending steps in a scooter or power wheelchair is impossible except for a few powered chairs that are designed to jump curbs of 6 inches. A strong manual wheelchair user may be able to descend a few steps safely by performing a wheelie, but ascending is impossible. A person who can perform a wheelchair-to-floor transfer may be able in an emergency to get out of the wheelchair and "bump" up or down the steps while pulling the chair along. ***Training to do this should occur before the emergency.***

Moving a wheelchair and its dependent occupant up and down steps safely requires the assistance of two people. The back of the wheelchair should be positioned against the steps with one person standing behind the chair and the other person in front of it. The chair is tipped backward, with one person holding the push handles and the other person holding the front of the chair by its frame or leg rests. While the person in front maintains balance of the chair, the person behind pulls the chair up step by step. That person should take care to keep his or her back straight and use leg strength to move the chair. To take a person down the steps, approach the steps forward with the wheelchair tipped and balanced. The procedure is reversed, with the person in front of the chair holding onto the chair while guiding and controlling the speed of the chair down each step.

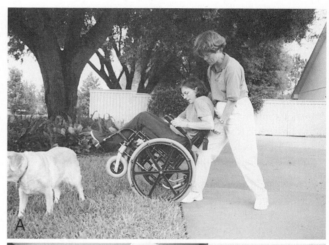

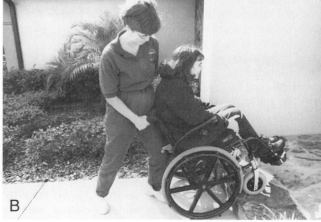

Figure 31-8 A. A therapist performs an assisted wheelchair wheelie so the wheelchair can easily be moved through grass and uneven terrain. **B.** An assisted wheelie is also used to move a person in a manual wheelchair up a step or curb.

Case Example

MR. J.: MOBILITY TRAINING AFTER STROKE

Patient Information

Mr. J., a 67-year-old man with right hemiplegia and expressive aphasia resulting from a left cerebral vascular accident, was assessed in an outpatient rehabilitation center. These problems were identified by the occupational therapist:

▶ Client can roll over and sit up in bed but has difficulty moving his right leg off the bed in preparation for transferring and dressing.

▶ Client cannot complete a stand–pivot transfer independently, as he needs assistance coming to standing.

▶ Client can propel his manual wheelchair with a one-arm drive on level surfaces but cannot negotiate a ramp or uneven terrain.

▶ Client cannot perform bathroom activities at home because his bathroom is inaccessible to his wheelchair.

▶ Client cannot drive and cannot load or unload his wheelchair to and from the car.

Recommendations

The occupational therapist recommended two treatment sessions per week for 8 weeks in outpatient therapy. In collaboration with the patient and his wife, the occupational therapist established the following long-term treatment goals:

▶ Mr. J. will be independent in bed mobility and sitting on the edge of the bed.

▶ Mr. J. will be able to perform a stand–pivot transfer independently.

▶ Mr. J. will improve his ability to negotiate outdoor terrain and ramps with his manual wheelchair and be advised on motorized scooters for use in independent long-distance mobility in the community.

▶ In collaboration with physical therapy, Mr. J. will be instructed in using his hemiwalker to walk into the bathroom and perform sink activities while standing.

▶ Mr. J. will be referred to a driver rehabilitation therapist for a driving evaluation once he can transfer in and out of the car.

Short-Term Goals

▶ **Mr. J. will be able to move his weak leg off the edge of a bed and come to a seated position with or without orthotic devices.** The therapist ascertained after a week of occupational therapy that Mr. J. could move his weak leg off the bed using his stronger left leg but that he would require a device to use to pull against to come into a sitting position on the edge of the bed. In the second week various techniques and assistive devices were demonstrated to him, and it was determined that a portable half bed rail worked best. By the fourth week, Mr. J. could come to a sitting position on the bed independently. He was also shown how to use the bed rail to help him stand up and ready himself for the stand–pivot transfer.

▶ **Mr. J. will become independent in sink activities in the bathroom.** The first week of occupational therapy revealed that the patient's standing tolerance and balance were not sufficient to perform sink activities while standing even though he can walk short distances. In the second week he was taught to stand up from his wheelchair outside the bathroom door, walk into the bathroom using his hemiwalker and short leg brace, and sit on a tall-legged stool at the sink. The occupational therapist determined that a higher seat helped him come to standing and that he could pull on the sink for assistance in standing up when ready to leave.

▶ **Mr. J. will be able to transfer into the passenger and driver side of his car independently.** By the third week, Mr. J. could handle his leg on and off the bed and could stand up independently. In the fourth week, Mr. J. was instructed in steps for getting in and out of the passenger side of a car. After he could perform this transfer, he was taught how to transfer into the driver's side of the car, maneuvering his legs under the steering wheel. In the sixth week, he was referred to a driver rehabilitation therapist, who instructed Mr. J. in the use of a left-foot gas pedal and spinner knob. In collaboration with the driver rehabilitation therapist, the occupational therapist determined that Mr. J. could not independently load or unload his manual wheelchair in his four-door sedan. He did not have the standing balance or endurance to use a wheelchair loader, either bumper mounted or mounted in the trunk. Instead, he required a motorized chair loader, such as the Braun Chair Topper to use for effortless loading of his folding wheelchair on top of the car. By his discharge date, the client had received all necessary in-vehicle training by the driver rehabilitation therapist and had had all driving equipment and the car topper installed on his car for independent driving.

Transfers

A **transfer** is a method that a person with any physical deficit uses to move from one surface to another. There are various techniques and methods for performing a transfer. The type chosen depends upon the patient's disability, upper and lower extremity strength, trunk balance, body type, orthotic devices, and/or wheelchair style (Box 31-2). A graded training program for transfers may be necessary as a patient progresses through rehabilitation. The complexity of the transfer the patient is taught must reflect his or her physical and functional status at the time. A dependent transfer may be necessary until the person can begin learning assisted or independent transfers.

The treatment program should include family training so that a family member also learns to perform each step of the transfer. The family member should practice with the therapist and patient in a protected, supervised environment. It is important to practice proper body mechanics throughout any transfer to protect the helper as well as the person being transferred. ***To prevent back injury, the helper should keep the back and spine straight so that the physical lift or rotation of the transfer is done using the stronger muscles of the arms and legs.***

Dependent Transfer

A person who is too weak to move requires another person or persons to lift or move him or her in a dependent transfer. A one-person technique entails standing in front of the patient and placing him or her in a forward flexed position with the chest lying on the thighs. This method cannot be used for the patient with limited hip flexion, for example, those with hip fracture or heterotopic ossificans. This position shifts the patient's

body weight over the knees and ankles rather than on the buttocks, which allows the buttocks to be picked up and moved more easily. This method has proven worthy to teach family members, as it enables the helper to control the movement of the patient's body while lessening the probability of hurting his or her own back (Fig. 31-9).

For the patient with limited hip flexion, this technique can be modified to sliding the buttocks toward the edge of the wheelchair and placing the patient's knees between the assistant's knees. Using proper body mechanics, the assistant squeezes the knees of the patient with his or her own knees while rocking the patient forward slightly and simultaneously pulling on the patient's pants or belt and rotating the hips to the surface being moved to.

For a two-person dependent transfer using a similar method, the second person stands behind the patient and moves the buttocks to the transfer surface while the first person moves the legs. A sliding board can be used to bridge the gap if the buttocks cannot easily be picked up. A mechanical-hydraulic, or powered body lifter can be used by one or two persons to transfer a dependent person (Fig. 31-5).

Sliding Board Transfers

A person who cannot stand can use a **transfer board** to slide the buttocks and bridge the gap between the two transfer surfaces. The therapist should be familiar with the variety of shapes, lengths, weights, and styles of transfer boards available from various manufacturers (Fig. 31-10). A long transfer board may be needed to bridge the gap between a wheelchair and a car seat, but a smaller board can be used for transfer to the toilet or bed. A cutout on one end of the board may be needed to allow someone with weak grasp to pick up the board. An angled or notched board may be best for maneuvering around the rear wheel of the wheelchair while transferring. A board made of high-density polished polyethylene plastic provides a slippery surface for bare skin, and a board with a moving center disc may allow easy sliding of the body. Off-the-shelf boards do not always meet specific needs of clients. Figure 31-11 shows a variety of custom transfer boards made by an occupational therapist to meet clients' needs when off-the-shelf boards were not useful.

Most transfer boards are positioned with one end under the patient's buttocks and thighs and the other end on the surface to which the person is transferring. Level surfaces greatly aid in the transfer, although one can use gravity to assist when sliding to a lower surface. For an independent transfer, the patient performs shoulder depression with the elbows extended and locked to raise and/or slide the buttocks along the surface of the

---

BOX 31-2
Various Levels of Transfers

Dependent Transfer
Person requires maximum assistance of one or more persons using a special technique or device to assist in moving from one surface to another.

Sliding Board Transfer
Person cannot bridge the gap between two surfaces without the use of a sliding board.

Standing Pivot Transfer
Person can stand up, then pivot the feet and turn the trunk, then sit down on the transferring surface.

Independent Transfer
Person can perform all steps of a transfer with no physical assistance of another person. A device may or may not be used.

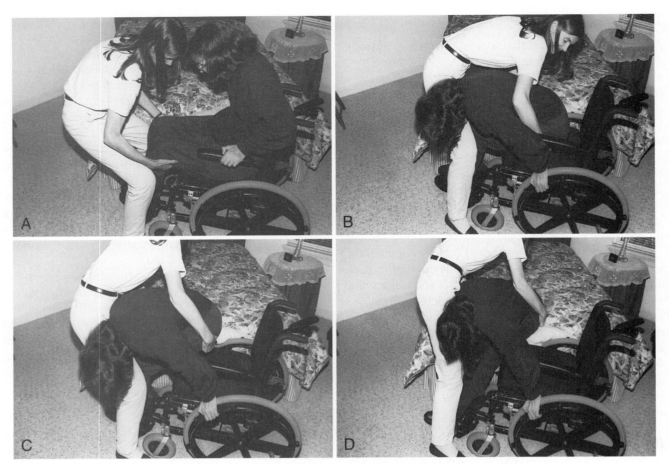

Figure 31-9 A therapist demonstrates one type of dependent wheelchair to bed transfer that can be performed by one person. **A.** The therapist readies the patient by sliding the buttocks forward in the seat to avoid bumping into the rear wheel during the transfer. **B.** The patient is leaned forward onto the therapist's right thigh. If able, the patient can assist with the left hand on the wheelchair tire. The therapist has her legs around the patient's legs and readies herself with proper body alignment. **C.** The therapist uses the strength in her arms and legs to rock the client forward, lift the patient's buttocks, and rotate the patient to the bed. **D.** Since the patient's weight was shifted forward, there is little weight to pick up.

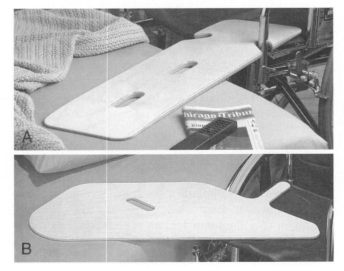

Figure 31-10 Two styles and shapes of transfer boards available through suppliers. **A.** Transfer board with hand holes and notches allows transfers from either side. **B.** Offset transfer board fits around the wheel of the wheelchair when the armrest is removed. (Courtesy of Sammons-Preston, Bolingbrook, IL.)

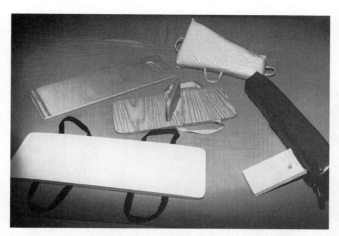

Figure 31-11 An occupational therapist designed and built these specialized transfer boards to meet various clients' needs.

board (Fig. 31-12). The person must also be able to handle his or her own legs to put them in place after the transfer. Factors that impede this type of transfer include poor trunk balance, spasticity, excessive body weight in relation to strength, joint tightness, and a high ratio of trunk length to arm length.

The same principles apply to tub or shower and toilet transfers. Equipment such as grab bars, a raised toilet seat, and tub bench make these transfers easier and safer. Car transfers are difficult because of the large gap between the car seat and wheelchair and the seat height discrepancy. A person may require a transfer board for this transfer but not for other transfers in the home (Fig. 31-13).

Stand–Pivot Transfer

A person with lower extremity deficits who can support his or her weight on one or both legs may be able to perform an independent or assisted stand–pivot transfer. An assisted stand–pivot transfer is performed with the helper standing in front of the patient and the transfer surface as close as possible. Generally it is best to transfer the patient toward his or her stronger side. The patient should first be slid toward the edge of the surface from which the transfer is taking place, with care to protect the person from slipping off the edge completely, especially if there is lower extremity or trunk spasticity. The patient is assisted to stand (Fig. 31-14). The helper places his or her knees in front of one or both of the knees of the patient to prevent the patient's knees from buckling upon standing. The patient wraps his or her arms around the helper's body or neck, but only for support, not to pull up. The helper bends his or her knees, keeps the back straight, and grabs the waist or belt of the patient's pants or a **transfer belt**. The helper rocks the person back and forth several times and then, using momentum, pulls the person to a standing posi-

tion. A patient who can assist uses leg strength to stand or upper body strength to push off the wheelchair armrest or bed rail to come to standing. By pressing against the weak knee or knees, the helper assists the patient to swivel or slide the heels toward the transfer surface while standing. The helper can then guide the patient's hips over and down to the transfer surface. A transfer disk or a rotating pole can be used if needed for moving the person's feet.

Independent Transfers

Patients with adequate strength to push up and move the trunk and to handle the lower extremities can transfer without assistive equipment. Figure 31-15 illustrates an independent transfer from wheelchair to bed by a person with C7 quadriplegia.

Independent Walking With Orthotic Devices

A person with balance difficulties or weakness in one or both lower extremities may require some type of **orthotic mobility device** for stability and support for walking. Canes and walkers come in various styles and shapes (Fig. 31-16). The type of cane chosen by the physical therapist depends on the person's balance and gripping ability, with personal preference considered. A straight cane is selected for a person with good strength, coordination, and balance who nevertheless requires a device for support. The four-prong or quad cane is chosen for a person who is weak or has increased muscle tone or ataxia and needs a more stable base than is

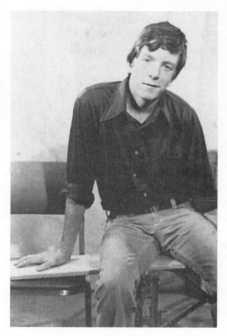

Figure 31-12 Independent sliding board depression transfer.

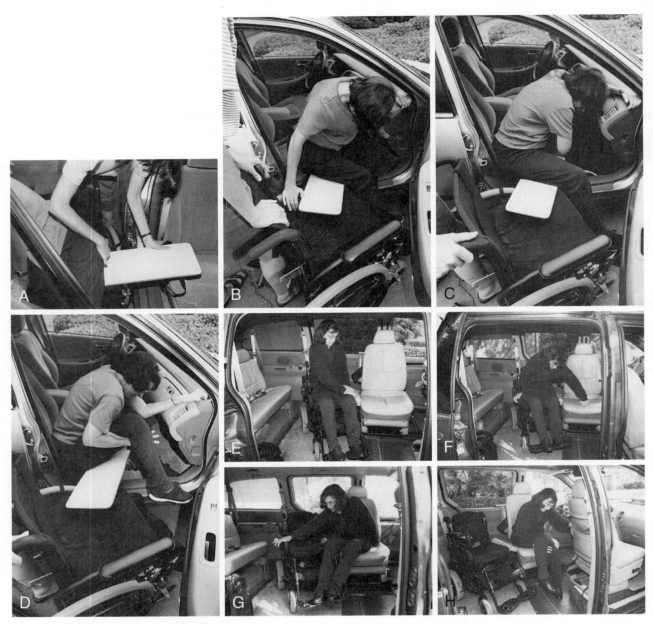

Figure 31-13 Steps for transfer from wheelchair to car (**A–D**) and an independent transfer from wheelchair to van driver's seat (**E–H**). **A.** The person leans to the outside of the wheelchair while the helper places the transfer board under the person's buttocks and on the car seat. The sliding board is necessary to bridge the large gap between the wheelchair and the car seat. **B.** The person slides onto the board by pushing off the wheelchair and maintains balance by leaning against the dashboard of the car. The legs remain outside the car until the person is situated on the car seat. **C, D.** The legs are separately lifted into the car and the sliding board is removed. **E.** The person rolls into the van backward and aligns her wheelchair with the van seat. **F.** She prepares to do a depression transfer. **G.** She lifts her body to the driver's seat. **H.** She positions her legs. The seat is then swivelled and moved under the steering wheel.

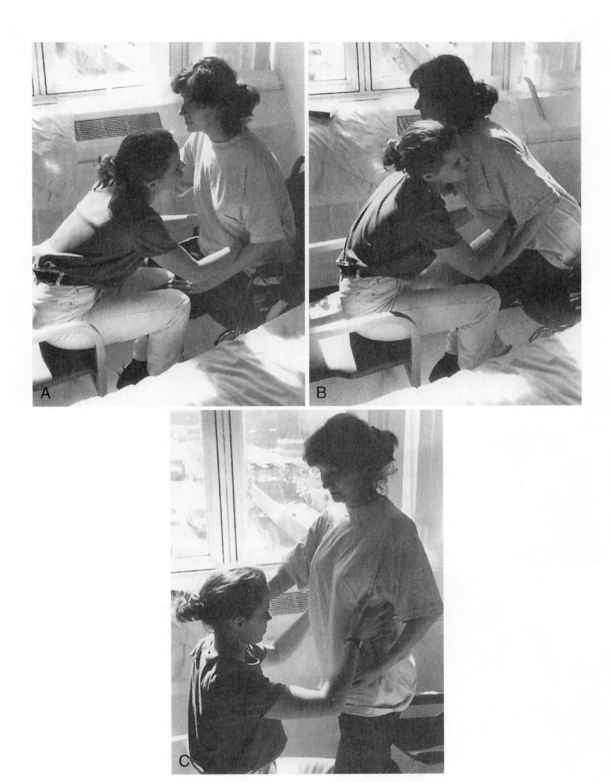

Figure 31-14 A patient with left hemiplegia is assisted in a sit-to-stand position. **A.** The patient places her unaffected hand on the therapist's shoulder for support. The therapist supports the patient's weak left knee by placing her knee against the patient's knee. **B.** The patient leans forward to move the center of gravity forward. **C.** The patient uses the strength of the unaffected side, with the help of the therapist, to stand. (Reprinted with permission from Gillen, G., & Burkhardt, A. [Eds.] [1998]. *Stroke Rehabilitation: A Function-Based Approach* [p. 231]. St. Louis: Mosby.)

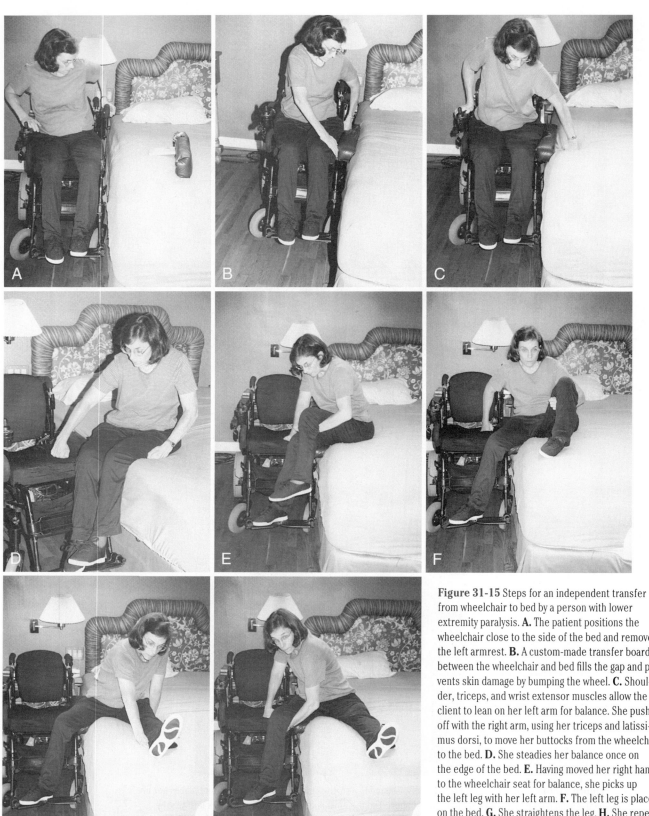

Figure 31-15 Steps for an independent transfer from wheelchair to bed by a person with lower extremity paralysis. **A.** The patient positions the wheelchair close to the side of the bed and removes the left armrest. **B.** A custom-made transfer board between the wheelchair and bed fills the gap and prevents skin damage by bumping the wheel. **C.** Shoulder, triceps, and wrist extensor muscles allow the client to lean on her left arm for balance. She pushes off with the right arm, using her triceps and latissimus dorsi, to move her buttocks from the wheelchair to the bed. **D.** She steadies her balance once on the edge of the bed. **E.** Having moved her right hand to the wheelchair seat for balance, she picks up the left leg with her left arm. **F.** The left leg is placed on the bed. **G.** She straightens the leg. **H.** She repeats the process to move the other leg up onto the bed. Maintaining balance is the key to performing this move independently and without assistive devices.

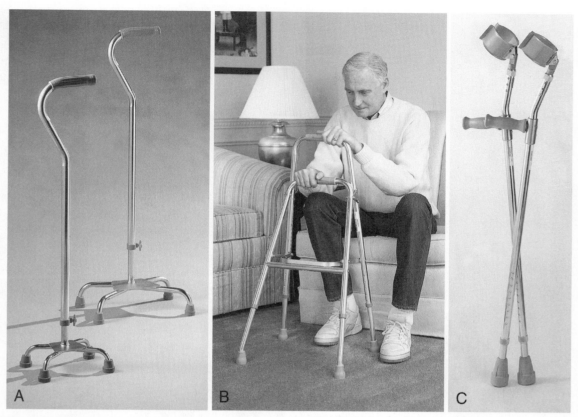

Figure 31-16 Various orthotic devices for walking. **A.** Quad cane has wide base with four points of contact to the ground to provide stability. **B.** Sidestepper Cane/Walker is typically used by a person with hemiplegia who requires more stability than the quad cane supplies. **C.** Forearm crutches allow a wide base of support for those who have leg weakness but good balance. (Courtesy of Sammons-Preston, Bolingbrook, IL.)

offered by a straight cane. The hemiwalker, so called because it is often used by persons with hemiplegia, provides the greatest stability for a one-handed orthotic device.

Some patients have the strength and balance to stand without these devices while performing light ADL. Patients who do not have the standing balance or strength to stand at a work surface and use both hands may have to sit or perform ADL one-handed while standing. These individuals have limited ability to carry things while walking. Small carrying bags can be strapped to a hemiwalker or quad cane, but these devices cannot carry a heavy item without throwing off the person's balance (Fig. 31-17). A stable pushcart can substitute nicely for a cane or walker for carrying items.

A walker gives the person bilateral support for balance and stability while walking (Fig. 31-18). A regular or rolling walker requires the partial use of both upper extremities. The rolling walker is often used by individuals with an ataxic gait, such as is seen in cerebral palsy or Frederick's ataxia, since it is easier to push the walker than to pick it up for each step. It can be difficult

for the person using a rolling walker to pivot to turn corners or prepare to sit down. With the standard walker, the user can simply rotate around the axis of the body and carry the walker during the turn. The standard walker can be fitted with a fold-down seat for resting or a pouch or basket for carrying items. Folding-frame walkers are easy to store in a car's back seat or trunk or on the back of a scooter. Also, simple, lightweight devices can be attached to a walker and provide a handle for a person to push down on to assist in standing from a bed, chair, or a car.

A three-wheel walker has the advantage of larger pneumatic wheels for a more stable base and hand brakes for safety. This type of walker can carry heavier items and can have a fold-down seat for individuals who fatigue easily, such as those with multiple sclerosis or arthritis. This type of walker is not indicated for a person who leans on the walker for support. The width and turning radius of these walkers is greater than those of standard walkers and may affect the user's maneuverability where space is limited. The problem of loading the device into a vehicle must be solved if it is to be used in the community.

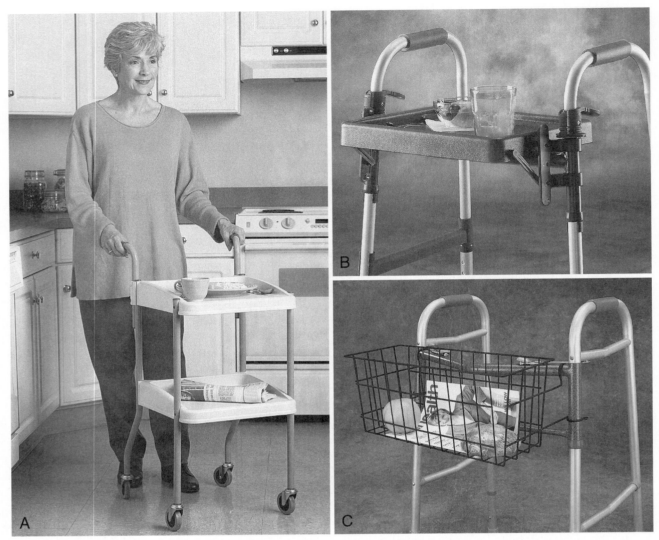

Figure 31-17 Carrying items on orthotic walking devices. **A.** Rolling cart with push handles for carrying many or heavy items. **B.** Tray for walker. **C.** Basket attached to walker. (Courtesy of Sammons Preston, Bolingbrook, IL.)

Patients who can walk only short distances with or without an orthotic device may also require the use of a manual wheelchair or scooter for longer distances. Using the wheelchair may be a more practical solution to enable performing ADL that require two hands, balance, and/or stability. By sitting in a wheelchair, the person frees up both hands for activities. A person who has good trunk balance may be able to use a stool for working at counter surfaces. Some persons can use a powered up–down seat on a wheelchair or scooter to reach high work surfaces or tall cabinets (Fig. 31-19).

Figure 31-20 illustrates various mechanical and electric devices to assist a person in standing up or rotating and swiveling preparatory to standing. The lift chair (Fig. 31-21) is popular for persons with a variety of disabilities because the chair raises the person totally supported to a partial standing position. Also, some devices, such as the swivel disk or lift seat, can be placed in a vehicle seat to help the person move his or her legs or start the momentum for standing upright (Fig. 31-20 A & C). Electric seats for vans and cars similarly assist a person (Fig. 31-20 B & D).

Standing improves circulation, renal and bowel functions, reduces spasticity, and prevents many of the effects of prolonged immobilization. If a person has good upper extremity strength and a job that requires standing, such as a beautician or a schoolteacher, a stand-up manual or power wheelchair is a great means of mobility and of meeting the task demands of the job. These wheelchairs hold a person upright while freeing

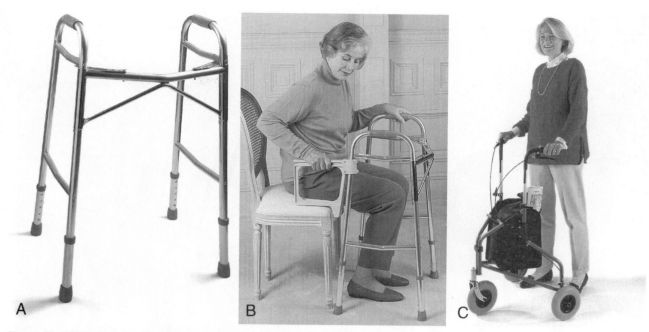

Figure 31-18 Walkers. **A.** Standard walker for child or adult. Small roller wheels can be provided on the front legs to assist with moving the walker. **B.** Easy-Up™ handle for walkers provides leverage for persons who can rise unassisted. The lightweight handle folds into the walker frame when not in use. **C.** Rolling three- or four-wheel walker can be used by child or adult who needs support to walk but has good balance. The large wheels travel over outdoor terrain easily. Hand brakes allow for safe slowing. A pack can be added to transport things. (Courtesy of Sammons-Preston, Bolingbrook, IL.)

both hands. The person using a powered chair that has this capability can move around in a standing or seated position (Fig. 31-22). The manual chairs with this capability are heavier than standard manual wheelchairs and may not be conducive to outdoor mobility. An active person therefore may need a second lighter-weight wheelchair to use away from work.

Community Mobility

Today most people go into the community for almost everything they need. Although the Internet and mail order provide extensive resources for persons to purchase drugs, supplies, clothes, and other personal items without store shopping, these resources are inaccessible to some and can be unsatisfying in terms of social interaction. Therefore, community mobility is a goal for most patients in occupational therapy. Community mobility includes moving about as a pedestrian, driving a vehicle, or using public transportation. The feasibility, safety, and personal control of mobility are affected by (1) the socioeconomic status of the person (income may limit the type of transportation available), (2) physical characteristics of the site, and (3) transportation technology (Carp, 1988).

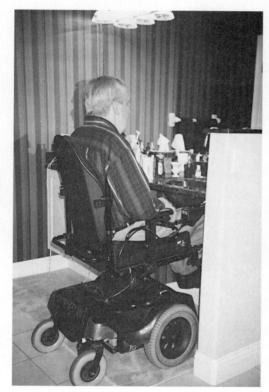

Figure 31-19 Use of a powered vertical up-and-down seat on a powered wheelchair to allow near approach to the sink for grooming.

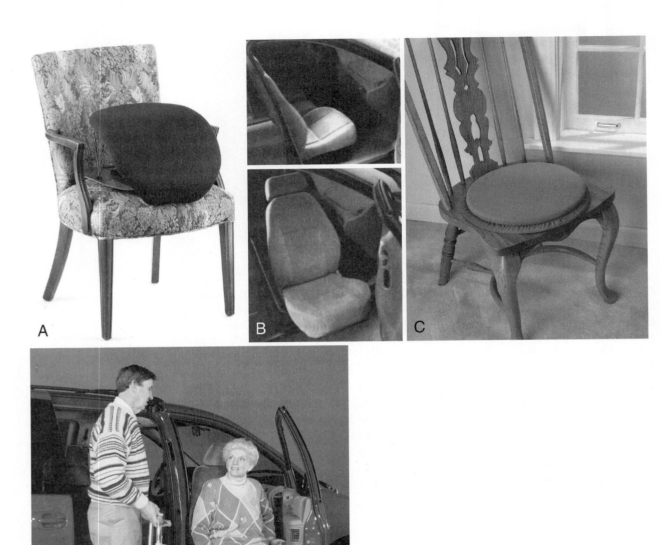

Figure 31-20 Mechanical devices to assist in standing up. **A.** Hydraulic action in this portable seat lift assists the person in rising. **B.** Car swivel seat. **C.** Cushioned seat that swivels 360°. **D.** Braun Companion seat. (Photos A and C courtesy of Sammons Preston, Bolingbrook, IL. Photos B and D courtesy of Braun Corporation, Winamac, IN.)

Pedestrian Mobility

Accident rates for elderly pedestrians resemble those for elderly drivers; that is, the rate is higher than for any other age group. Elderly pedestrians are often hit in crosswalks or when crossing intersections. They are generally hit when they have almost finished crossing. They are usually observing the law and not behaving danger-

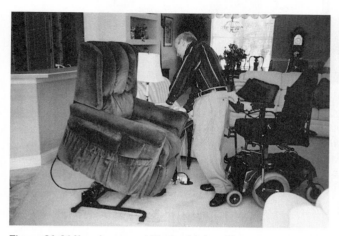

Figure 31-21 Use of a powered lift wheelchair and lounge chair to stand from and sit in both chairs.

ously. Many do not see the vehicle that hit them, and when they do see the vehicle, they usually believe that the driver has seen them and will avoid them. Given the number of accidents occurring in crosswalks, experts have questioned the role of traffic signal timing in accidents involving elderly pedestrians (Rosenbloom, 1988). It follows that persons with walking impairments and those in wheelchairs may encounter the same dangers at intersections or crosswalks as the elderly do. A wheelchair user is considered a pedestrian. McKnight (1988) suggested that training persons of all ages could play a vital role in decreasing the problems that affect the safety of drivers and pedestrians. The occupational therapist should include some of this information when training a person to be mobile in the community via a wheelchair, cane, walker, scooter, personal vehicle, or public bus.

Driving

In restoring community mobility, driving can be key for a person to be independent in leisure and employment and to feel a sense of personal well-being and satisfaction. Development of driving technology over the past 25 years has allowed persons with a variety of disabilities to drive. If there is funding available , a person with a severe physical disability can drive. Driving technology can cost

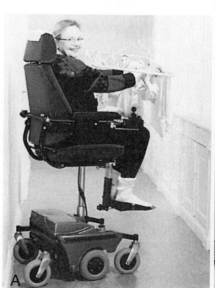
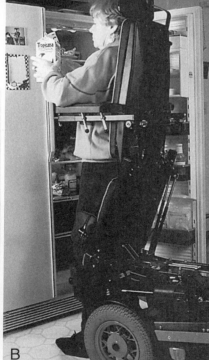
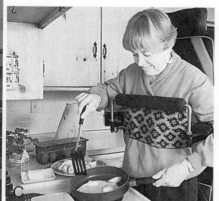

Figure 31-22 Permobil wheelchair options allow for many adjustable sitting and standing positions for activities and tasks at work and at home. (Courtesy of Permobil Company, Woburn, MA.)

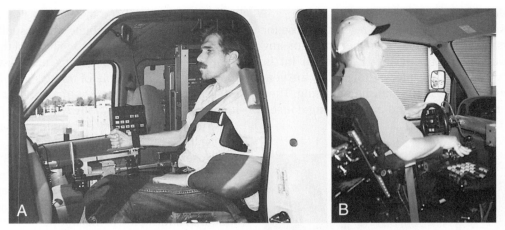

Figure 31-23 The Scott System allows many persons with polio, muscular dystrophy, C4-5 quadriplegia, and triplegia to drive independently. **A.** Person with C5 quadriplegia drives with the right hand in a tri-pin device. He pushes forward for gas and pulls back for braking and supinates his forearm for turning right and pronates for turning left. **B.** One-handed steering with a small wheel by this person who uses his normal left extremity to push and pull the wheel for gas and brake; the wheel rotates 90° right or left for turning. (Courtesy of Driving Systems Inc., Van Nuys, CA.)

as little as $75 for a steering device or as much as $55,000 for a modified van with a sensitive steering, gas, and brake system (Fig. 31-23). For some persons, need for special driving equipment may be minimal, but they require specialized and lengthy training in a vehicle.

Because of its complexity, driving should be one of the last ADL resumed during rehabilitation (Pierce, 1996). Driver rehabilitation programs throughout the United States are housed in hospitals, rehabilitation facilities, private practices, and state agencies. According to the Association of Driver Rehabilitation Specialists (ADED), 350 of their 500 members are occupational therapists (See Resources). When looking for the right driver rehabilitation specialist to assist your patient, consider the diagnosis of the patient and the background and experience of the specialist. A driver rehabilitation therapist is an allied health professional, such as an occupational therapist, physical therapist, recreational therapist, or speech therapist, with specialized training and experience in driver education and driver rehabilitation for persons with disabilities.

I recommend that therapists seek a driver rehabilitation therapist who meets the following criteria: (1) is an allied health professional, (2) is certified by ADED, and (3) has a minimum of 3 years of experience doing driver rehabilitation with persons with disabilities. The occupational therapist is well equipped to perform holistic driving evaluations and assessments (Monga et al., 1997). An occupational therapist–driver rehabilitation specialist can perform a formal clinical evaluation of a person's physical, visual, perceptual, cognitive, and psychological functioning as it relates to driving (Gillen & Burkhardt, 1998) as well as assess driving performance.

Following a clinical assessment of function, a driver assessment is necessary. An appropriate evaluation vehicle is used to assess the person's driving abilities on the road and in traffic. By knowing the exact deficits of the person, the driver rehabilitation therapist can plan a route to challenge the client and can determine whether the identified deficits interfere with safe driving.

Vehicle Assessment

The vehicle that will be used to transport a person is the foundation for the modifications. A driver rehabilitation therapist must evaluate the client's vehicle to assess its appropriateness. The client must be able to enter and exit the vehicle and store the wheelchair, scooter, or other orthotic device as needed (Fig. 31-24). The necessary adaptive equipment for driving must be compatible with the client's personal vehicle or specific recommendations must be given regarding purchase of a more appropriate vehicle.

In past decades the automobile industry produced many two-door cars from which disabled drivers could choose. The two-door cars allowed for easy loading of a folding-frame manual wheelchair behind the driver or passenger seat. Today few two-door cars exist that can accommodate loading the popular rigid-frame wheelchairs. There are more four-door cars, minivans, and trucks that allow easier loading of the rigid-frame wheelchair, either manually or electrically. Wheelchair loading devices have particular vehicle and wheelchair requirements. A driver rehabilitation therapist should evaluate the client, the wheelchair, and the personal vehicle for appropriateness along with the client's ability to operate the device safely and efficiently.

A van can be set up for a person to drive from the wheelchair or to enable the person to make an independent transfer from the wheelchair to the driver's seat (Fig. 31-13 E–H). A van can be adapted with a device such as a wheelchair lift or a motorized ramp so that the person can ride the wheelchair into the vehicle. Structural modifications, such as a raised roof or lowered floor, are generally necessary to give the wheelchair user additional headroom, doorway clearance, and front windshield visibility.

A person who can afford a van, its modifications, and the insurance can have a vehicle built to specifications. The person should be an informed consumer before buying any adapted van. The driver rehabilitation therapist can advise the person on the available options, what specific modifications and assistive technology are needed, and finally what it will cost.

Driving Aids

Persons with physical deficits or mobility challenges may require special driving devices or aids to assist them with particular driving tasks. Turning the ignition key can be difficult for a person with severe arthritis. Turning the head to check for cars prior to changing lanes can be impossible for persons with fused necks without adaptations. Dynamic balance in the driver's seat may be difficult for a person with quadriplegia or ataxia. The driver rehabilitation therapist analyzes each driving task for the person and determines the client's needs and desires and what specific aids are necessary for safe driving (Monga et al., 1997). According to Koppa (1990), the driver who is physically disabled requires provisions for the following:

- ▶ Ability to enter and exit
- ▶ Ability to operate primary and secondary controls
- ▶ Ability to secure himself or herself, along with any mobility equipment that cannot be separated from the driver's body

To assist with steering, add-on devices for the steering wheel include the spinner knob for one-handed steering and the tri-pin device, which compensates for lack of hand grip for persons with quadriplegia. Various levels of sensitized steering in combination with varying steering wheel diameter and placement are available to compensate for upper extremity range of motion and strength deficits. For example, a 6-inch steering wheel can be placed in a horizontal plane directly in front of the client's arm.

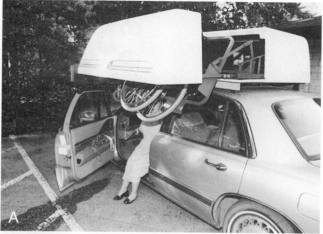
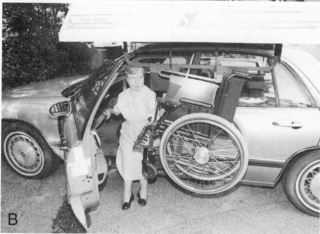
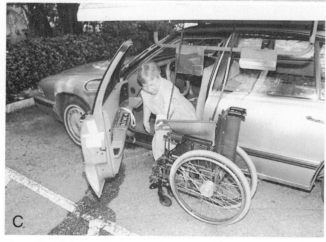

Figure 31-24 A woman with rheumatoid arthritis illustrates how she uses a Braun Chair Topper, a mechanical device, to unload her manual wheelchair.

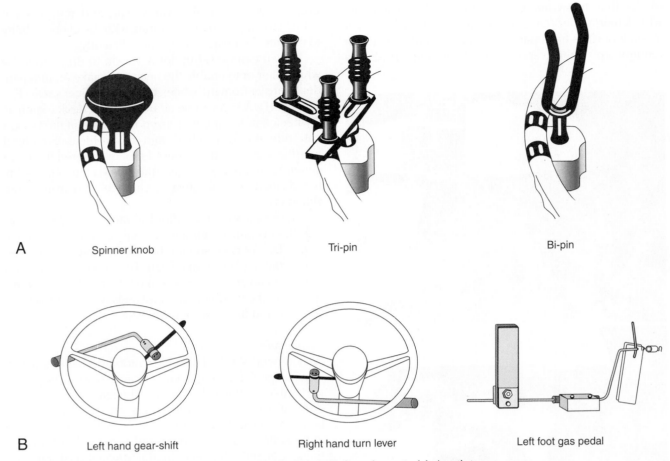

A
Spinner knob   Tri-pin   Bi-pin

B
Left hand gear-shift   Right hand turn lever   Left foot gas pedal

Figure 31-25 Various add-on assistive driving devices. **A.** Steering devices. **B.** Secondary control devices that cross over the functions of the gearshift (*left*), turn signal (*middle*), or gas pedal (*right*) that would be required by some persons after stroke.

Pedal extensions ranging from 1 to 10 inches can be used by persons of short stature. A left-foot gas pedal can be installed for a person with right hemiplegia. A turn signal crossover can benefit a person with left hemiplegia to allow safe use of the turn signal with the right hand (Fig. 31-25).

A variety of mechanical hand controls are available for persons with normal or weak upper extremities but no use of the lower extremities. The driver rehabilitation therapist must consider the person's strength, range of motion, sensation, coordination, balance, and posture in determining which style of hand control is best for the individual. Electronic hand controls are available for a person with no use of the legs and limited range of motion and strength in the arms and hands. A handle on the control box moves 4 to 6 inches from full brake to full acceleration and operates with only 2 ounces of pressure. A person with muscular dystrophy or polio with proximal weakness but distal strength in the hands can use this control easily for gas and brake operation (Fig. 31-26).

Driver Assessment

After a successful vehicle assessment, driver training and education ensure that the person can safely operate the vehicle controls and adaptive driving aids. Persons who have had a traumatic brain injury or stroke should be evaluated not only for their physical control of the vehicle but also their reaction time, judgment, decision-making and problem-solving skills, selective and divided attention, and dynamic visual skills.

Driving simulators are available, but expensive, and their contribution to the full assessment of a person's driving abilities is limited. A few simulators are relatively cost effective to a therapy program and are designed to give more pertinent information on the person with a disability. An example is the Elemental Driving Simulator by Life Sciences has face validity and provides feedback on more visual and cognitive skills than other typical driving simulators (Gianutsos, 1997). Research indicated that the strongest independent predictors of crash-involved drivers was failure of the *Useful Field of Vision* test, which addresses several visual and cognitive processing domains, including visual sensory function, visual processing speed, and divided and selective attention (Sims et al., 1998).

A necessary evaluation tool for a driving program is a dual-controlled vehicle that can be used to assess a person's driving abilities on the road. In the evaluation vehicle a real driving test can be given with a route established by the driver rehabilitation therapist to bring out the known deficits of the patient and evaluate whether the deficits permit safe driving.

There is little to no research on the safety of disabled drivers of any age. Age, however, does affect safe driving. The Transportation Research Board's special report, *Transportation in an Aging Society*, noted that in terms of rate per vehicle mile, the elderly have more accidents than any other age group except the youngest (Carp, 1988). When in accidents, older drivers have much greater physical vulnerability than their younger counter-

parts and are much more likely to be injured or die (Carp, 1988). Research concerning safety statistics of disabled drivers is needed.

Public Transportation

A person using a powered wheelchair who cannot drive a car generally needs a van for transportation. Although the ADA mandated wheelchair accessibility for public buses, inaccessible bus and train stops make it difficult for some wheelchair users to use accessible public vehicles. These stops can also be inaccessible because of distance to a person's home, the terrain around the stop, or height of the landing in relation to the height of the vehicle floor. Large cities offer door-to-door service for persons who cannot use public transportation.

A **wheelchair and occupant restraint system** is necessary to transport a person in a wheelchair safely (Fig. 31-27). As of 2000, wheelchair manufacturers must address the standards for restraining a wheelchair and the occupant in transit. The American National Standards Institute and the Rehabilitation Engineering Society of North America have contributed in an important way to the development of these standards (Box 31-3; see Resources).

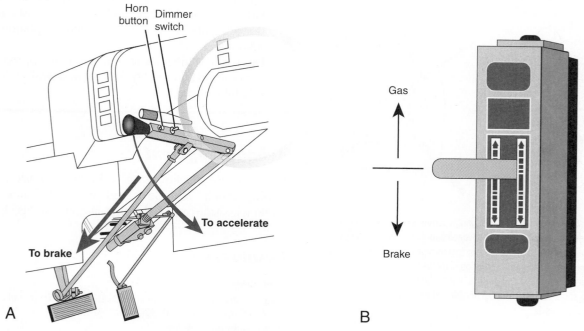

Figure 31-26 Mechanical hand controls or more expensive electromechanical hand controls aid in safe operation of gas and brake. **A.** Push right-angle mechanical hand controls. Requires scapular stabilization and 4− (good minus) strength of shoulder flexion, internal rotation, and elbow extension. **B.** Electroserver hand control requires 3 (fair) strength within a 4-inch range. Can be operated by weak fingers or shoulder flexion and extension.

Viewed from above

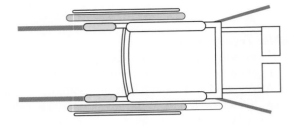

Viewed from the side

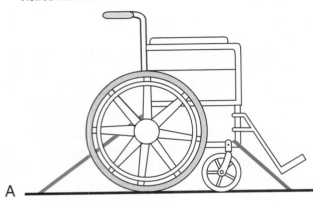

A

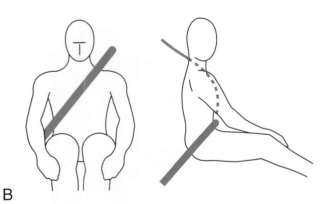

B

Figure 31-27 Wheelchair and occupant restraint system. **A.** Four points of attachment of tie-downs onto the wheelchair frame. **B.** An effective shoulder and lap belt restraint system requires proper belt angles. Incorrect belt placement can limit protection in a crash or load the occupant so as to cause injury. One end of the shoulder belt should be anchored higher than shoulder level. The lap belt should lie low across the bony structure of the pelvis.

Summary Review Questions

1. Describe the hierarchy of mobility skills.
2. Describe how therapists can protect their own back when assisting a patient in a dependent transfer.

> **BOX 31-3**
> *Basic Criteria for Proper Wheelchair Restraint*
>
> ► There must be four points of attachment to the wheelchair.
> ► The attachment points must not be to any part of the wheelchair that is movable or removable, such as the armrests, footrests or wheels.
> ► Proper strapping material and hardware must be used to withstand the forces generated by the wheelchair and the occupant in case of a collision.
> ► The occupant must be in a forward or rear-facing position, never a sideways or diagonal position.
> ► Occupant safety belts must be provided on the wheelchair.
>
> Data from Bertocci, Hobson, & Digges, 2000; Schneider, 1981, 1997.

3. Plan a treatment session to train a patient on outdoor mobility in a manual wheelchair.
4. Describe mobility aids that assist in bathroom activities, walking, and with community mobility.
5. What precursor abilities and skills must a patient with paraplegia have accomplished before learning to transfer into a wheelchair?
6. What are the options available in teaching this patient how to negotiate a curb?
7. What are the qualifications of a driver rehabilitation therapist, and how can you find one in your area?
8. How does the driver rehabilitation therapist assist the occupational therapist in treatment planning for mobility?
9. Discuss why the interdisciplinary team approach is important with mobility training and goal setting in rehabilitation.

Acknowledgment

I thank Carol Blackburn, OTR, Brenda Johnston, OTR, Daphne Cronin, Joan Bova, and Linda and Chuck Green for their assistance with the photography for this chapter.

Resources

Associations

Adaptive Mobility Services, Inc. · 1000 Delaney Avenue, Orlando, FL 32806. 407-426-8020. Fax 407-426-8690.
www.adaptivemobility.com

American National Standards Institute · 11 West 42nd St., Floor 13, New York, NY 10036. 212-642-4900.
www.ansi.org

Association of Driver Rehabilitation Specialists · 109 West St., Edgerton, WI 53534. 608-884-8833. Fax 608-884-4851.
www.driver-ed.org

National Highway Traffic Safety Administration · Office of the Chief Counsel, 400 7th St., SW, Washington, DC 20590. Fax 202-336-3820. www.nhtsa.dot.gov/

Rehabilitation Engineering and Assistive Technology Society of North America (RESNA) · 1700 North Moore St., Suite 1540, Arlington, VA 22209-1903. 703-524-6686. Fax 703-524-6630.
info@resna.org

Society of Automotive Engineering World Headquarters · 400 Commonwealth Dr., Warrendale, PA 15096-0001. 724-776-4841. Fax 724-776-5760.
www.sae.org

Sources for Ramps

Accessible Housing Design · Van Nostrand Reinhold, 7625 Empire Dr., Florence, KY 41042. 800-842-3636.

AlumiRamp, Inc. · 855 Chicago Rd., Quincy, MI 49082. Phone 800-800-3864. 517-639-8777. Fax 800-753-7267.

Center for Universal Design · Center for Accessible Housing, North Carolina State University, P. O. Box 8613, Raleigh, NC 27695-8613. 800-647-6777 V/TTY.
www.ncsu.edu/ncsu/design/cud

EZ-Access Ramps · 15824 SE 296th St., Kent, WA 98042. 800-451-1903.

Travel Ramp, Inc. · P. O. Box 2015, Alachua, FL 32615. 904-462-5267. 904-462-7744.

Sources for Mobility Aids

Braun Corporation · 1014 South Monticello, Winamac, IN 46996. 219-946-6157.

Bruno Independent Living Aids · 430 Armour Court, Oconomowoc, WI 53066. 414-567-4990. 800-882-8183.

Drivemaster Corporation · 9 Spielman Rd., Fairfield, NJ. 201-808-9709. 800-826-7368.

Driving Systems Incorporated · 16139 Runnymede Street, Van Nuys, CA 91406. 818-782-7693. Fax 818-782-6485.

Electronic Mobility Controls, Inc. · 6141 Crestmount Dr., Baton Rouge, LA 70809. 225-927-5558. Fax 225-924-5556
www.emc-digi.com

Q-Straint (w/c restraint) · 5553 Ravenswood, Bldg 104, Ft. Lauderdale, FL 33312. 800-987-9987.

Ricon Corporation · 7900 Nelson, Panorama City, CA 91402. 800-322-2884.

References

Americans with Disabilities Act of 1990. Public Law 101-336, 42 U. S. C. A. § 12101.

Bertocci, G. E., Hobson, D. A., & Digges, K. H. (2000). Development of a wheelchair occupant injury risk assessment method and its application in the investigation of wheelchair securement point influence on frontal crash safety. *IEEE Transactions of Rehabilitation Engineering, 8* (1), 126–139.

Carp, F. M. (1988). Significance of mobility for the well-being of the elderly. In National Research Council Committee for the Study on Improving Mobility and Safety for Older Persons. Transportation in an aging society: Improving mobility and safety for older persons. (Vol.1, pp. 1–20). Washington: Transportation Research Board.

Deusterhaus-Minor, M. A., & Deusterhaus-Minor, S. (1999). Patient Care Skills (4th ed.). Stamford, CT: Appleton & Lange.

Gillen, G., & Burkhardt, A. (1998). Stroke rehabilitation: A function-based approach. St. Louis: Mosby–Year Book.

Gianutsos, R. (1997). Driving and visual information processing in cognitively at risk and older drivers. In M. Gentile (Ed.), *Functional Visual Behavior: A Therapist's Guide to Evaluation and Treatment Options* (pp. 321–342). Bethesda, MD: American Occupational Therapy Association.

Kaplan, W. (1999). The occupation of driving: Legal and ethical issues. *American Occupational Therapy Association Physical Disabilities Special Interest Section Quarterly, 23* (3), 1–3.

Koppa, R. J. (1990). State of the art in automotive adaptive equipment. *Human Factors, 32,* 439–455.

McKnight, A. J. (1988). Driver and pedestrian training. In National Research Council Committee for the Study on Improving Mobility and Safety for Older Persons. *Transportation in an Aging Society: Improving Mobility and Safety for Older Persons* (Vol. 1, pp. 101–133). Washington: Transportation Research Board.

Monga, T., Ostermann, H., & Kerrigan, A. (1997). Driving: A clinical perspective on rehabilitation technology. *Physical Medicine and Rehabilitation: State of the Art Reviews, 11* (1), 69–92. Philadelphia: Hanley & Belfus.

Nixon, V. (1985). Spinal cord injury: A guide to functional outcomes in physical therapy management. Gaithersburg, MD: Aspen.

O'Shea, R., & Murphy, E. (1991). Americans with Disabilities Act of 1990. *Business Review for Central Florida, 2* (10), 1.

Pierce. S. (1996). A roadmap for driver rehabilitation. *OT Practice, 10* (1), 30–38.

Pierson, F. M. (1999). Principles and techniques of patient care (2nd ed.). Philadelphia: Saunders.

Rosenbloom, S. (1988). The mobility needs of the elderly. In National Research Council Committee for the Study on Improving Mobility and Safety for Older Persons. *Transportation in an Aging Society: Improving Mobility and Safety for Older Persons* (Vol. 1, pp. 21–71). Washington: Transportation Research Board.

Schneider, L. W. (1981). Dynamic testing of restraint system and tie-downs for use with vehicle occupants seated in powered wheelchairs. UM-HSRI Report 81-18. Ann Arbor, MI: University of Michigan Transportation Research Institute.

Schneider, L. W. (1997). Transportation of severely disabled children. In H. M. Wallace, J. C. McQueen, R. F. Biehl, & J. A. Blackman (Eds.), Children With Disabilities and Chronic Illness (pp. 421–434). St. Louis: Mosby.

Sims, R., Owsley, C., Allman, R., Ball, K., & Smoot, T. (1998). A preliminary assessment of the medical and functional factors associated with vehicle crashes by older adults. *Journal of the American Geriatrics Society, 46,* 556–561.

32

Restoring Competence for Homemaker and Parent Roles

Susan E. Fasoli

LEARNING OBJECTIVES

After studying this chapter the reader will be able to do the following:

1. State the principles of compensation and adaptation.
2. State the principles of work simplification.
3. Identify adapted methods and equipment that enable persons with varied physical challenges and diagnoses to regain competence in homemaking roles.
4. Identify adapted methods and equipment that enable persons with varied physical challenges and diagnoses to regain competence in parenting roles.
5. Describe and teach proper body mechanics for homemaking and parenting tasks and activities.

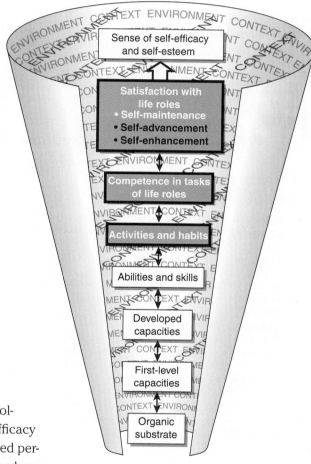

*R*estoring competence in homemaker and parenting roles following a disabling event can greatly enhance one's sense of efficacy and feelings of self-esteem. Therapists typically address impaired performance of these life roles after a patient has regained independence in basic activities of daily living (e.g., self-care). However, home management and parenting tasks can be incorporated into the rehabilitation process at any time, depending on the individual's own priorities and needs.

Homemaking and parenting tasks may be used as both occupation-as-means and occupation-as-end, depending on the client's rehabilitation potential and desired goals. This chapter focuses on the use of occupation-as-end to restore a client's competence and participation in homemaker and parent roles. This treatment approach allows for addressing significant impairments in occupational performance components (e.g., incoordination or visual impairments) via the principles for compensation and adaptation highlighted in Box 32-1.

Principles of work simplification and energy conservation can be taught to clients with physical impairments who lack sufficient endurance to accomplish daily life tasks. Work simplification and energy conservation principles are commonsense ideas to improve task efficiency and reduce energy expenditure during all occupational tasks and roles, including those related to homemaking and parenting (Box 32-1).

Homemaker Roles and Tasks: Treatment Principles and Methods

Many factors, including psychosocial adjustment, cognitive or perceptual impairments, and physical limitations, can influence a client's ability to take part in homemaker roles and tasks.

Psychosocial Adjustment

When faced with the onset or progression of physical disability, a client and family may have a variety of psychological responses. These reactions may be characterized by lack of motivation and refusal to participate in therapy, expressed feelings of hopelessness or anger, and denial (American Occupational Therapy Association, 1997). The family's expectations and reactions must also be considered when occupational therapists are setting intervention goals and establishing plans for treatment. These psychological reactions must be acknowledged and addressed by the occupational therapist if identified goals are to be achieved.

BOX 32-1
PROCEDURES FOR PRACTICE

Principles of Adaptation to Compensate for Functional Limitations

Principles for Compensation and Adaptation

▸ Limited ROM—Increase the person's reach via extended handles and organize needed items within a compact work space.
▸ Weakness and low endurance—Use lightweight and/or powered equipment and allow gravity to assist. Employ work simplification and energy conservation techniques.
▸ Chronic pain—Reinforce use of proper body mechanics and pacing during physical tasks.
▸ Unilateral loss of motor control and limb function—Use affected limb to stabilize objects when possible. Use adapted methods and/or assistive equipment to perform bilateral activities with one hand.
▸ Incoordination—Stabilize at proximal joints (e.g., elbow) to reduce degrees of freedom necessary for control. Use weighted objects to minimize distal incoordination.
▸ Visual impairments—Use senses of smell, touch, and hearing to substitute for low vision. Enhance performance of visual tasks by improving lighting, reducing glare, or increasing contrast.
▸ Cognitive limitations—Employ visual and auditory aids to enhance memory and organization. Plan steps prior to beginning task. Work in familiar environment (e.g., home kitchen) to enhance cognitive performance during homemaking tasks.

Principles of Work Simplification and Energy Conservation

▸ Limit the amount of work. When possible, avoid overfatigue by assigning heavy homemaking tasks (e.g., vacuuming, cleaning bathrooms) to family members or a housekeeper.
▸ Help the client explore ways to reduce homemaking demands and expectations, such as using packaged mixes or frozen foods to decrease time and energy for meal preparation.
▸ Plan ahead. Schedule homemaking, child care tasks (e.g., changing bed linens, giving tub baths), and community outings (e.g., shopping, doctor visits) to distribute energy-demanding tasks throughout the week. Prioritize, to complete important tasks before fatigue sets in.
▸ Use efficient methods. Organize work areas and store frequently used supplies in a convenient location. Avoid standing when it is possible to sit while doing the task (e.g., ironing). Slide objects across a counter or table rather than lift them. Identify needed items at the beginning of a task to avoid extra trips. Use a utility cart to transport items.
▸ Use correct equipment and techniques. Use assistive equipment (e.g., long-handled reachers) to decrease bending and stooping. Avoid prolonged holding by stabilizing items with nonskid mats. Adjust work height and use tools most appropriate for the job. When physical limitations are present, choose equipment that does not promote further deformity.
▸ Balance daily tasks with rest breaks. Clients should perform energy-demanding tasks early in the day, when they are most rested. Encourage self-pacing of tasks (don't rush!) to avoid fatigue. Frequent rest periods of 5 to 10 minutes can greatly enhance functional endurance during homemaking and parenting tasks.

Barriers to Effectiveness

During rehabilitation, the occupational therapist must identify factors in addition to psychosocial concerns that may interfere with the effectiveness of intervention and inhibit performance during homemaking tasks. These factors include, but are not limited to, cognitive and perceptual impairments, poor vision, and environmental constraints including lack of family support.

Persons with cognitive impairments as a result of central nervous system disorders may have more difficulty learning compensatory techniques than persons with musculoskeletal or peripheral nervous system disorders. The client needs good memory, judgment, and problem solving abilities to learn how an assistive device is used, when it is needed, and how it can safely enhance task performance (Moyers, 1999). Cognitive demands are increased when the adapted methods greatly alter the way the task is performed (e.g., ordering groceries on-line or learning to use a utility cart to transport items).

In the absence of intact cognitive abilities, clients may be able to learn new task methods, such as how to operate a microwave oven for meal preparation, if they can follow visual cues or instructions. The occupational therapist must ensure that the client can safely perform the task with the prescribed adaptations and meet unexpected challenges encountered during task performance.

Perceptual impairments, including poor figure ground skills, spatial orientation, and visual neglect, can also interfere with one's ability to manage homemaking tasks independently. Limitations in perceptual processing can interfere with one's ability to find needed items in the cupboard, decrease safety of pouring hot coffee into a cup, and increase the likelihood of falls when vacuuming or sweeping floors. In addition, poor visual processing, such as loss of central vision or decreased contrast sensitivity, can inhibit safety during homemaking tasks. Environmental changes, such as increasing available lighting throughout the home and enhancing contrast (e.g., pouring coffee into a light-colored mug) can improve performance (Lampert & Lapolice, 1995).

Support of family or friends can be instrumental for carrying out recommended adaptations, reinforcing the use of assistive devices, and identifying additional concerns in need of intervention. When family assistance is not available, other support services (e.g., homemaker, companion) may be employed to ensure safety in homemaking tasks.

Preventing Decline in Homemaker Role and Tasks

Occupational therapists are often involved with preventing disability in persons who are at risk for developing impairments, activity limitations, and restrictions in the performance of life tasks and roles (Moyers, 1999). Prevention programs for elderly persons include exercise classes to reduce physical limitations in balance, range of motion and strength, in addition to group activities that exercise cognitive abilities, such as judgment and problem solving (Jackson et al., 1998). Homemakers may be instructed in home safety tips directed toward reducing clutter, removing loose rugs, and arranging furniture to clear walkways and allow access to electrical plugs and windows. Environmental modifications, such as the installation of grab bars and railings, can significantly decrease the occurrence of falls (Plautz et al., 1996).

Occupational therapists can be instrumental in identifying hazards in the home and providing ideas that may enhance a person's safety and continued independence. Many limitations encountered by well elderly persons during homemaking tasks may be prevented or alleviated by relatively simple and inexpensive solutions.

Homemaking: Techniques and Therapeutic Aids

Competence in the role of homemaker can be attained in either of two ways, depending on the client's level of physical and cognitive ability: by managing and directing others to perform homemaking tasks or by direct participation.

Although persons with severe physical disabilities may not be able to perform many homemaking tasks without assistance, they can be effective home managers. For instance, individuals with high-level spinal cord injuries can independently manage household tasks by directing family members or paid housekeepers, managing finances, and overseeing shopping. Computerized banking systems and shopping services are accessible to those with Internet access and are relatively easy to use. Occupational therapy at this level may focus on organizing how household tasks may be scheduled, instructing the client in computer use, or identifying service resources in the community. Homemaker services, home health aides, and Meals on Wheels may provide the support necessary for a person with limited abilities to remain at home.

Persons who can physically participate in homemaking tasks can benefit from a variety of interventions that maximize role performance. The following sections discuss equipment and adapted methods for homemaking.

Equipment Considerations

A number of factors contribute to the selection and use of assistive devices and adapted equipment for homemaking. Simple modifications in the way a task is performed sometimes eliminate the need for an assistive device, and this is the preferable solution. When equipment is recommended, a primary concern is that the assistive device satisfies the needs of the client and enables the person to accomplish tasks that are otherwise impossible or difficult (Axtell & Yasuda, 1993). The person must be comfortable with the idea of using an assistive device and satisfied with its appearance.

When making equipment recommendations, the occupational therapist must consider both the immediate and long-term needs of the patient. Individuals with a progressive disease, such as rheumatoid arthritis or multiple sclerosis, benefit from equipment that can enhance current functional performance and provide for anticipated changes in physical status. In contrast, persons with nonprogressive conditions, such as acquired brain injury or spinal cord injury, often use fewer assistive devices as they regain physical abilities or learn alternate ways to accomplish their tasks without equipment.

Generally, assistive devices should be simple to use and maintain, as lightweight as possible, and dependable (Axtell & Yasuda, 1993). If a client has mild cognitive impairments that interfere with equipment use, family members may be taught ways to enhance carryover at home. Insurance providers generally do not pay for assistive devices and adapted equipment. For those who cannot afford to purchase such items, loaner equipment may be available from local organizations, including disability support groups and senior citizen centers.

Meal Preparation, Service, and Cleanup

Efficient work areas, adapted techniques, and assistive devices can greatly enhance a client's safety and participation in meal preparation tasks.

Kitchen Storage and Work Area

Kitchens should be organized so that frequently used items are within easy reach of the place they are most often used. On average, persons who use a wheelchair can reach to retrieve items between 15 inches (low reach) and 48 inches (high reach) from the floor. Those who are ambulatory, but have difficulty bending generally can reach 30 inches (low reach) to 60 inches (high reach) from the floor, depending on the person's height (Anderson, 1981).

Pull-out shelves and turntables in cabinets can compensate for limited reach and maximize usable storage space. Pans, dishes, and so on may be stored vertically to alleviate the need to move unwanted items to obtain the one underneath. Pegboards with hooks can be attached to the back of closet doors to hold pots, pans, and utensils for easy access. Shelves attached to the inside of cabinet doors are handy for holding assorted wraps, canned goods, and cleaning supplies.

Items that are seldom used should be removed to eliminate unnecessary clutter.

Safety and independence in the kitchen can be enhanced by the availability of clear and accessible work spaces. For persons in wheelchairs, work counters should be 30 to 35 inches from the floor and have a depth clearance of 24 inches underneath to allow room for wheelchair leg rests. A work area that is at least 30 inches wide is recommended to provide sufficient space for needed items during meal preparation (Eberhardt, 1998).

Gathering and Transporting Items

An important role of the occupational therapist is to help the client solve problems about gathering and transporting items at home by using work simplification principles and proper body mechanics (Boxes 32-1 and 32-2). Long-handled reachers can be helpful but should be used primarily for retrieving lightweight unbreakable items.

The wide range of assistive devices for transporting items around the home includes cup holders and walker or wheelchair bags. Homemakers who use a wheelchair may benefit from using a lap tray that easily slides on and

---

BOX 32-2
PROCEDURES FOR PRACTICE

Principles of Correct Body Mechanics

Principles of correct body mechanics that should be used during homemaking and parenting tasks (Melnik, 1994; Saunders, 1992):

► Keep the shoulders and hips parallel and facing the task. Do not twist the trunk when lifting.
► Maintain good balance by positioning the feet shoulder distance apart with one foot forward.
► When standing for long periods, reduce pressure on the lower back by placing one foot on a low stool and changing positions frequently.
► When sitting or standing, maintain a neutral position in the lower back by tilting the pelvis slightly forward to maintain the natural curve of the spine. Use this neutral back position when lifting as well.
► Use the strongest or largest muscles and joints when lifting (e.g., use legs rather than back, palms rather than fingers).
► Keep the back upright and bend at the hips and knees rather than bending forward at the waist when reaching for low items.
► Push before pulling and pull before lifting.
► While lifting or carrying, keep the object close to the body.
► Avoid rushing. Proper body mechanics are more effectively used when working at a comfortable pace.

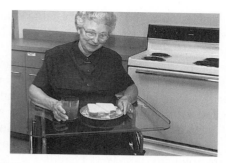

Figure 32-1 Woman eating her lunch on a clear acrylic wheelchair lap tray that allows her to observe her lower body. (Photo by Robert Littlefield.)

off the wheelchair arms (Fig. 32-1). A variety of wire baskets and trays that attach to a standard walker are available for purchase, but many of these devices accommodate only a few things at a time, such as a sandwich and covered beverage. Individuals who perform homemaking tasks either from a wheelchair or ambulatory level may prefer to use a wheeled utility cart because of its larger carrying capacity. The therapist can help clients learn to maneuver the cart efficiently. Homemakers who use an assistive device or adapted methods to transport hot foods and beverages must follow strict safety precautions to avoid burns.

When limited income inhibits a client's ability to purchase assistive aids, the creative therapist can work with the patient to identify inexpensive workable alternatives. No-cost solutions, such as attaching a plastic grocery bag or used bike basket to a walker, can add to independence in transporting certain items.

Food Preparation

The use of assistive devices and adapted equipment can make food preparation easier and more enjoyable. Homemakers who have lost the use of one arm following stroke or fracture find an adapted cutting board extremely useful when peeling or cutting vegetables, fruit, or meat. A raised edge along one corner of the board can stabilize a slice of bread for spreading butter or jam (Fig. 32-2).

The occupational therapist helps clients with physical limitations to solve problems such as the safest way to open cereal boxes and juice cartons. Some persons can open packaged food with one-handed techniques, while others prefer to use adapted scissors with a looped handle (Fig. 32-3). Homemakers with weakness and impaired hand function may find it easier to open plastic milk jugs than cartons. Smaller containers are generally easier to manage than large ones. Nonslip mats or suction holders may be used under jars or bottles to hold them steady for opening with one hand and to reduce sliding or turning of bowls when mixing.

Knives, vegetable peelers, and other kitchen tools are available in many shapes and sizes. Clients with rheumatoid arthritis benefit from using utensils with ergonomically designed handles that require less hand strength and reduce ulnar drift (Fig. 32-4). Incoordination due to ataxia may be somewhat alleviated by the use of weighted utensils and tools. Freestanding or mounted jar openers can be helpful to persons with a variety of physical limitations. Homemakers can be taught adapted methods for cracking eggs (Fig. 32-5 and Box 32-3).

Electric equipment, such as food processors, blenders, can openers, and electric knives, can conserve energy by reducing the physical demands and time needed for meal preparation. However, to be truly beneficial, this equipment must be easy to use and maintain and suited to the person's disability. For example, most one-handed cordless can openers are available only in right-handed models and therefore are not convenient for persons with significant right hemiparesis after stroke.

Homemakers with limited mobility or reach find a side-by-side refrigerator more accessible than other models. Loops of webbing or rope can be attached to the door handles to enable clients with limited hand function to pull the doors open. Heavy items should be stored

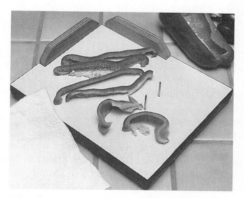

Figure 32-2 Spiked cutting board with corner guards. (Photo courtesy of North Coast Medical, Inc. Morgan Hill, CA.)

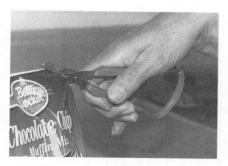

Figure 32-3 Looped scissors. (Photo by Robert Littlefield.)

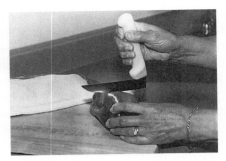

Figure 32-4 Ergonomic right-angled knife. (Photo by Robert Littlefield.)

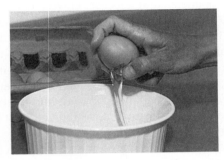

Figure 32-5 One-handed egg crack. (Photo by Robert Littlefield.)

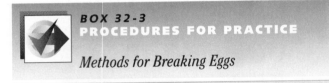

BOX 32-3
PROCEDURES FOR PRACTICE

Methods for Breaking Eggs

► Individuals with weak grasp can grossly hold the egg, throw it sharply into the bottom of an empty glass or metal bowl, where it will split in two, and then remove the shell.
► Clients with functional use of only one hand may prefer to use the chef's method, as follows. Place the egg in the palm with one end held by the index and middle fingers and the other end held by the thumb to form a C around the egg. Sharply crack the egg on the side of a bowl, then in one motion pull the thumb down and the fingers up to pull the two halves apart (Fig. 32-5).

---

casserole dishes, pots, and pans can enable joint protection by evenly distributing the weight of the pan between both hands.

Ambulatory clients with back or lower extremity pain or limited endurance can save energy by sitting whenever possible while preparing meals. Individuals who prepare food in a wheelchair can use a mirror mounted at an angle over the stove to keep an eye on cooking foods. Persons with hemiparesis may use a suction cup holder to stabilize pot handles while stirring. Homemakers can conserve energy when straining vegetables or pasta by placing a french-fry basket in the pot before cooking or by using a slotted spoon. This practice eliminates the need to carry a hot pot to the sink to drain it. Those who can safely transport and drain hot foods at the sink can reduce the need for lifting and holding and enhance stability by resting the pot on the sink's edge when pouring. An adjustable strainer that clamps onto the top of a pot or pan can also be used.

Homemakers who prepare meals from a wheelchair will find a self-cleaning stove with front-operated controls and a low wall oven (30–42 inches from the floor)

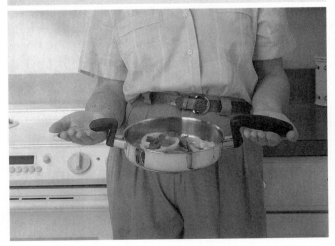

Figure 32-6 Ergonomic cookware with easy-grip handles. (Photo provided by Sammons Preston.)

on a shelf that is level with a lapboard or wheeled cart so they can be moved in and out with minimal lifting.

Cooking

Most persons with physical impairments find lightweight nonstick pots and pans to be the easiest to handle and maintain. Ergonomically designed cookware with easy-to-grip handles can be ideal for persons with limited distal strength (Fig. 32-6). The use of double-handled

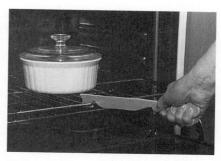

Figure 32-7 Oven push–pull stick. (Photo by Robert Littlefield.)

the most practical to use and operate (Eberhardt, 1998). *Individuals with limited proximal arm strength or grasp should not remove hot items from a wall oven higher than waist level without supervision because of the potential for burns due to spilling or dropping.* An oven push-pull stick may be used to manage oven racks or reposition hot dishes safely during baking (Fig. 32-7). If a client is planning to buy a new stove, the therapist may recommend a gas rather than electric range to reduce the risk of burns (Eberhardt, 1998), because the gas flames provide a visual cue that the burner is on.

Microwave ovens provide a cost-effective and safe alternative to conventional ovens and stoves. Elderly persons with arthritis, visual impairments, and limited endurance can be taught to use a microwave instead of a conventional stove to cook meals more easily and in less time (Kondo et al., 1997).

Dishwashing

Dishwashing can be made easier for individuals working in a wheelchair by placing a removable wooden rack in the bottom of a standard sink to reduce its depth to approximately 5 inches. The under-sink cabinet can be removed to allow persons in a wheelchair to face the sink head-on. However, any exposed piping should be insulated to protect lower extremities from burns. A swing-away faucet with a single control lever can enhance the ability of a person with limited hand function to adjust water flow (Eberhardt, 1998). Installing this faucet beside rather than at the back of the sink further increases accessibility for persons in wheelchairs (Eberhardt, 1998).

Dishwashing in a double sink should be organized to allow the person to work from one direction to the other: dirty dishes, wash water, rinse water, and drying rack. Homemakers with hemiparesis may wash dishes with greater ease when the rinse water and dish rack are on their unaffected side. Suction bottle brushes and scrub brushes can be attached to the sink to allow for cleaning glasses or silverware with one hand. A rubber

mat at the bottom of the sink prevents plates from sliding when they are washed and reduces breakage. Persons with limited grasp may prefer to use a terry cloth mitt or sponge mitt when washing dishes.

Work simplification includes air drying versus towel drying dishes and reusing them directly from the dish rack or dishwasher. Use of an electric dishwasher aids energy conservation, particularly when little prerinsing of soiled dishes is required.

Whenever possible, the homemaker can eliminate unnecessary cleaning by using oven-to-table ware or by serving directly from the pot. Pans can be lined with foil to reduce washing after baking or broiling. It is recommended that individuals clean as they prepare the meal and soak hard-to-clean dishes while eating to reduce the amount of cleanup required when the meal is over.

Grocery Shopping

Persons with physical impairments or limited endurance can more easily participate in grocery shopping with a few task modifications or assistive devices. When transportation is readily available, individuals may find that frequent visits to the market are more manageable because they can purchase and carry smaller quantities of food items at one time. Shopping at a small local market, although sometimes more expensive, can be easier and less energy consuming than shopping at a superstore. Grocery shopping can become a social event when done with a friend. Shopping together may provide an additional advantage if the friend can assist with reaching items on high and low shelves or carrying the bags.

Planning

A well-organized shopping list is necessary to make the most efficient use of time and conserve energy at the store. Individuals should keep the list in a convenient location at home, so that needed items can easily be added between shopping trips. Store maps, available at the customer service desk of many large grocery stores, can be used to organize the list. The homemaker or occupational therapist can arrange the items on the list (e.g., produce, dairy, meats) according to the store layout, aisle by aisle. Copies of this list can be used between store visits to record the items needed under each category.

The person should plan ahead and shop during off-peak hours, when the store is not crowded. Once at the store, a client can use the grocery list and signs above the aisles to find needed items.

Carts

Ambulatory persons with mild balance impairments can use a standard grocery cart when shopping; however, they should not use it for support when bending to reach items on low shelves. Individuals who use a wheelchair may find that adapted shopping carts that attach to the wheelchair are more convenient than a standard cart. However, some have found that these attached carts interfere with their ability to reach items. When this is the case, homemakers who are independent with wheelchair mobility may prefer to leave a standard cart at the end of an aisle, gather needed items in a small lap basket, and transfer them into the cart before proceeding to the next aisle.

Large stores have motorized carts for shoppers with limited endurance and mobility. These carts are handy for getting around the store, but it may be necessary to call the store in advance to reserve one. The baskets on these carts are generally small, which may be problematic if the person is planning to purchase a large order. The client may need help to figure out the safest and most effective ways to obtain items from high or low shelves from a motorized cart.

Selecting and Retrieving Items

It is wise to shop for items that are easy to open and require little preparation. Persons with limited endurance can increase the ease of meal preparation by selecting frozen rather than fresh vegetables and skinless or boneless meats.

Individuals who have limited upper extremity range of motion or who use a wheelchair find it difficult or impossible to reach items on high shelves. A reacher can be used to retrieve lightweight unbreakable items, but assistance may be needed for heavier objects. Most stores provide an employee to assist with shopping if asked. However, outgoing persons may prefer to ask people in the aisle for occasional help to increase opportunities for socialization.

Some individuals with traumatic brain injury or cerebrovascular accident have visual perceptual problems that interfere with their ability to locate items (e.g., hemianopsia or impaired figure ground skills). These persons can be taught to find objects more easily by scanning shelves in an organized manner, top to bottom and left to right. A person with severe visual impairments needs assistance to ensure safety and effectiveness while shopping.

Transporting Items Home

Generally, plastic grocery bags are easier to manage than paper. Foam tubing can be placed around the bag handles to reduce joint stress. At the checkout counter, the client should ask the clerk to keep grocery bags as light as possible and to bag refrigerated foods separately. Several half-filled bags are easier to manage than one or two full ones. Most stores provide assistance for transferring groceries into the car, but store workers should be instructed to place them within easy reach.

At home, a wheeled cart can be used to transport groceries into the house (Fig. 32-8). Persons with limited endurance can leave nonrefrigerated items in the car until later, when the person has rested or a family member is available to bring them into the house.

Computerized Shopping

Clients with physical limitations and limited endurance may find computer shopping to be a wonderful, energy-efficient alternative to conventional shopping. Persons with Internet access find that grocery orders can be easily placed on-line. Deliveries are made directly to the home, eliminating transportation and accessibility issues that may arise at the grocery store. The occupational therapist can help the client identify which method of shopping is most practical, based on the individual's priorities, physical limitations, knowledge of computer use, and financial situation.

Clothing Care

When a homemaker identifies clothing care as an important goal, the occupational therapist can help the

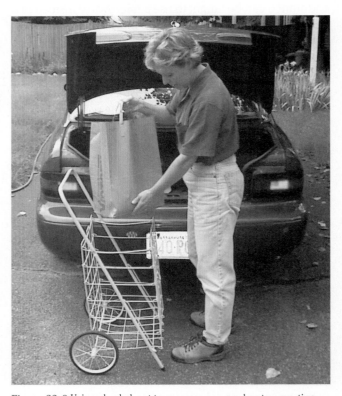

Figure 32-8 Using wheeled cart to conserve energy when transporting items.

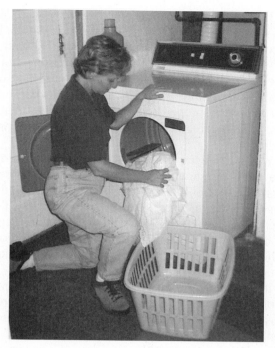

Figure 32-9 Kneeling to keep back straight when removing laundry from dryer.

person modify the way laundry tasks are performed. Even persons with severe physical impairments can engage in some aspect of clothing care (e.g., sitting at table to fold clothes).

In-Home Appliances Versus Self-Service Commercial Laundries

Although top-loading washers decrease the amount of bending required to load and unload clothing for persons who are ambulatory, they provide an additional challenge for persons in a wheelchair. Front-loading laundry machines are easier for seated individuals to access, but persons who are ambulatory may need training in body mechanics, particularly when loading or unloading wet clothes. For example, it is recommended that ambulatory clients with low back pain kneel on one knee, bending at the hips and knees and keeping the back upright, when loading or removing clothes from a front-loading machine (Fig. 32-9) (Saunders, 1992). Homemakers with limited hand function due to spinal cord injury or rheumatoid arthritis find it easier to use knob turners to set machine dials (Fig. 32-10).

Individuals who use a self-service commercial laundry for clothing care should bring needed coins and premeasured packages of soap for each load. Many such laundries have rolling carts available for carrying wet clothes from washer to dryer. If possible, persons with physical impairments should choose a staffed laundry.

These individuals can be called on for assistance if problems arise.

Collecting and Transporting Clothing

Ideally, the home laundry room should be on the same floor as the bedrooms to minimize the need to carry clothes up and down stairs. When this is not an option, family members can assist as needed to transport clothing to and from the laundry area.

Soiled clothing can be placed in a hamper lined with a plastic or cloth bag with handles. Seated individuals with good upper body strength can transport clothes to the washer by lifting the bag out of the hamper and either carrying it on their lap or hooking the drawstrings on the wheelchair handles. If the person is ambulating but has difficulty bending, a clothes basket can be kept on a waist-high table or shelf to collect soiled laundry. A wheeled cart is handy for transporting clothes for persons at an ambulatory level.

Washing and Folding

Laundry detergents and bleaches should be kept within easy reach of the washing machine. Hand washing can be eliminated by laundering delicate clothing in a mesh laundry bag in the machine. Persons with visual impairments can fasten paired socks with pins when they are taken off so they don't have to be sorted when clean.

A person in a wheelchair can use a hand-held mirror and reacher to remove clothes from the bottom of a top-loading washer. Homemakers with very limited grasp due to spinal cord injury have found that stubborn items can be more easily removed from the washer tub after a wet towel or shirt is put back into the washer and the spin cycle is restarted. Movement of the wet towel inside the spinning washer can loosen clothes that are stuck to the tub.

Clothes can be folded while the person sits or stands at a table. An adjustable rod 42–60 inches high is convenient for hanging permanent-press items as they are removed from the dryer. Large items, like sheets and bath towels, can be reused immediately after cleaning so

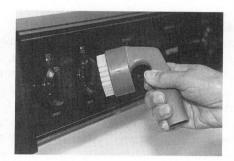

Figure 32-10 Knob turner. (Photo by Robert Littlefield.)

they don't have to be folded. Those who choose to fold sheets may find the task easier if they use the bed as a work surface.

Ironing

One challenging task for homemakers with physical impairments is to fold and unfold an ironing board. When possible, it is best to leave the ironing board set up in a convenient, out-of-the-way place. The board surface should be at waist level for persons who stand when ironing to reinforce good posture and body mechanics. Persons who iron while seated in a wheelchair generally find a work surface 30 to 35 inches high comfortable (Eberhardt, 1998). A heat-resistant pad can be placed at the end of the ironing board to eliminate the need to stand the iron up while arranging clothes on the board.

When buying a new iron, individuals should select a lightweight model with an automatic shut-off switch. A cord holder can reduce effort and keep the iron cord from getting in the way. Permanent press clothing requires less care than cotton or linen fabrics and thus reduces ironing needs. Persons who iron only occasionally may prefer to use a small tabletop ironing board if they have sufficient upper body strength to store and retrieve it from a closet easily.

Sewing

Homemakers may enjoy sewing as a hobby or may only make occasional alterations or repairs. Persons who have hemiparesis after a stroke can still sew with an electric machine by using the unaffected leg to operate foot or knee controls. Persons who do not have use of their lower extremities can place the foot pedal of an electric sewing machine on the table and use one hand or elbow to depress it. Sewing is generally most successful when there is an adequate work space and adapted methods to stabilize materials when cutting or stitching.

Persons with limited use of an affected arm can hand-sew by using an embroidery hoop attached to the edge of a table or counter with a C-clamp. To minimize sewing needs, sticky iron-on tape or fabric glue can be used for hems and small repairs. Rotary cutters instead of scissors make cutting fabric easier.

Indoor Household Maintenance

The occupational therapist helps clients identify effective ways to do household maintenance tasks, such as bed making and floor care. Adapted techniques and assistive devices can help the client to safely perform necessary chores without assistance.

Bed Making

Bed making can be simplified by straightening the sheets and blankets as much as possible before rising in the morning. Homemakers with limited mobility or impaired upper extremity function find it easier to make the bed by completing one corner at a time, starting with the head of the bed. If the individual is working from a wheelchair, the bed should be positioned so that both sides are accessible. Persons with chronic back pain must adhere to proper body mechanics when making beds, being careful to eliminate excessive forward bending.

When changing the sheets, a person can reduce extra work by carefully pulling blankets and spreads toward the foot of the bed, trying not to dislodge them from under the mattress. In this way the person will not have to expend unnecessary energy to find and reposition the top edge of the blankets or bedspread. Although the bottom sheet should be fitted, it should also be loose enough to be easily applied.

If the client or a friend is handy at sewing, several adaptations can be made to standard sheets to increase the ease of bed making. Fitted sheets can be adapted by opening the two fitted corners at the bottom end and sewing Velcro straps onto each side. When fastened, these straps securely hold the bottom corners together. Another adaptation is sewing the bottom edge of a top sheet to the bottom edge of a fitted sheet. Although this large sheet is more difficult to launder, this can eliminate the need to lift the mattress to tuck under the top sheet. Persons with limited upper body strength or hemiparesis may find lightweight blankets and spreads and satin pillowcases easier to manage.

Dusting

Physically challenged homemakers can dust hard-to-reach places with assistive devices. Persons with limited upper extremity reach because of orthopaedic or neurological changes can use a long-handled duster that is lightweight and easily extended to reach high places. Individuals with good hand strength may prefer to hold a dust rag with a long-handled reacher or use a vacuum cleaner attachment to clean hard-to-reach places. Persons who cannot afford assistive devices may find that a dust cloth secured to the end of a yardstick with a rubber band meets their needs. Clients with limited grasp or fine motor control may find that an adapted spray handle attached to the furniture polish can and an old sock or duster mitten significantly enhance their independence in dusting.

Floor Care

Heavy homemaking tasks, such as floor care, are often the first activities that elderly persons or individuals with physical impairments find difficult because of the amount of strength and endurance required (Axtell &

Yasuda, 1993). When the client's goal is independence in floor care, the occupational therapist must determine how this can be safely and efficiently accomplished.

Cleaning supplies can be conveniently stored and transported in a handled bin or canvas bag with a shoulder strap. When feasible, duplicate sets of equipment can be kept around the home to reduce the need to carry items. A dolly with large casters can reduce the physical demands of transporting heavy pails of water for mopping. Individuals should only partially fill cleaning pails to lessen their weight. A sponge mop with the squeeze lever on the handle minimizes bending and can be used with one hand. Individuals with limited hand function but adequate proximal arm strength can use a grasping cuff to hold mop or broom handles. Persons working from a wheelchair may find it best to start at the farthest corner and work backward out of the room. Furniture should be fitted with casters if moved regularly.

Lightweight upright vacuums provide a good alternative to using heavier canister-style models because they work well and are easier to manage for both ambulatory and wheelchair-bound persons. A lightweight carpet sweeper is another good choice because it is maneuverable, is relatively inexpensive, and does not have to be plugged in to an electrical outlet. Although the carpet sweeper is easier to push, more repetitions are generally needed to clean the same area. Long-handled dustpans and brushes can ease cleanup because they

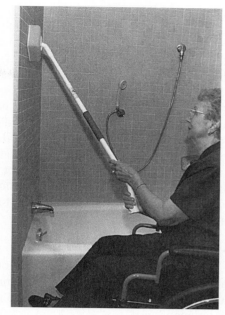

Figure 32-12 Cleaning bathroom tile using a long-handled cleaner. (Photo by Robert Littlefield.)

eliminate the need for bending and stooping (Fig. 32-11). If the client has good hand function, cordless handheld vacuum cleaners are handy for cleaning up small messes within easy reach.

Bathrooms

After a disabling event, a homemaker who cannot afford a housekeeper or does not have family members to assist may have to learn adapted ways to clean the bathroom. Cleaning needs can be reduced by rinsing the sink or tub immediately after use to wash away soap residue. Toilet cleaning tablets can be dropped into the toilet tank to reduce the growth of bacteria between thorough cleanings. A long-handled mop with a small head is useful for cleaning inaccessible areas behind the toilet.

Many homemakers with physical impairments find that cleaning the bathtub is difficult or impossible. These suggestions may make it possible. Persons with limited endurance or balance concerns should sit to clean the tub. A long-handled bathroom cleaner with a nonscratch scrubbing sponge can enable persons with limited reach to clean tubs and shower enclosures without assistance (Fig. 32-12). Replacing sliding doors with a plastic shower curtain can make the bathtub more accessible for bathing and cleaning. The plastic curtain can be laundered in the washing machine or inexpensively replaced when it becomes soiled.

Hard-to-Manage Tasks

No matter how creative the occupational therapist and client are, some household tasks may be impossible for

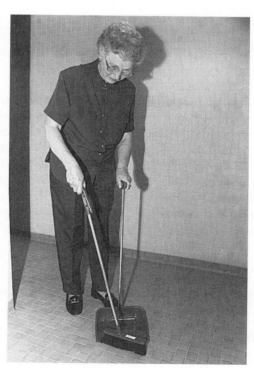

Figure 32-11 Use of a long-handled brush with dustpan. (Photo by Robert Littlefield.)

persons with physical impairments. However, a large number of assistive devices have recently entered the marketplace to ease the physical requirements of previously difficult tasks. Electric outlet extensions can be plugged into existing baseboard outlets and secured to the wall to eliminate the need to bend when inserting or removing a plug. New devices that make it easier to replace hard-to-reach light bulbs are also available. The adaptive therapist is well able to analyze task demands and identify modifications or assistive devices that promote independence. When a client cannot accomplish household tasks despite adapted methods, the occupational therapist can initiate a referral to homemaker services.

Outdoor Household Maintenance

When a client's goal is to do outdoor household maintenance, such as yard work or gardening, the occupational therapist can offer suggestions to increase safety and independence.

Yard Maintenance

Persons with mild physical impairments can return to some level of outdoor home maintenance if desired. Individuals with good endurance can mow with a self-propelled lawn mower and accomplish small projects, such as maintaining a patio area. When mowing, individuals should avoid stopping and turning the mower in order to reduce the risk of back injury. For this reason, a lawn with rounded rather than angled corners is easier to mow (Yeomans, 1992). Rechargeable battery-operated edgers are more convenient than models that must be connected to an electric cord when operated. Numerous ergonomically designed products have recently been developed to reduce injury during outdoor work. For example, bent-handled shovels reduce excessive back strain and forward bending by altering the fulcrum of movement (Fig. 32-13).

Gardening

Homemakers who are physically challenged need not give up the joy of gardening. Tools can be adapted, flower and vegetable beds raised, and wider walkways or wheelways created to increase a person's access to the garden. Container gardening is also feasible for persons with limited mobility.

Gardeners with limited hand function can adapt ordinary hand tools with foam pipe insulation, available at most building supply stores (Yeomans, 1992). This foam, presplit for easy application, can significantly enhance the comfort of grasping and holding the tool. Individuals who garden from a wheelchair can increase their reach by using long-handled spades, shovels, and pruners. Persons with limited trunk mobility or balance

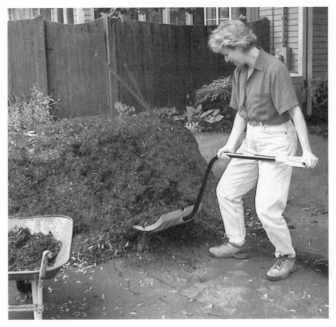

Figure 32-13 Protecting the back while shoveling by using an ergonomically designed shovel with bent handle and lifting with the legs, not the back.

may increase their safety by sitting on a garden stool and using long-handled tools. Gardeners who are fairly mobile can use a kneeling bench, with handles that assist them in getting up and down. Tools can be transported around the yard in apron pockets, a backpack, or a child's wagon, depending on the person's needs and available options. Tools with brightly colored handles are easy to see and therefore not likely to be lost in the garden (Yeomans, 1992).

Homemakers who return to gardening need to take care of themselves while caring for their flowers. Stretching exercises before gardening can reduce muscle stiffness and prevent injuries (Adil, 1994; Yeomans, 1992). Work simplification, energy conservation, and proper body mechanics are essential. Gardeners should keep themselves safe by using sun and insect protection, drinking plenty of fluids, and carrying a whistle around their neck in case they encounter unexpected problems when alone in the garden (Yeomans, 1992).

Tasks and Activities of the Parenting Role: Treatment Principles and Methods

The occupational therapist and client work closely to identify adapted methods and equipment that enhance participation and independence in parenting tasks. A holistic approach addresses parent and family needs within the home and community.

Psychosocial Adjustment

Parents whose physical limitations are due to an acute event, such as spinal cord injury or cerebrovascular accident, may initially lack a sense of competence, not only in their ability to care for themselves but also in their ability to care for their children. The occupational therapist must be sensitive to the client's psychosocial concerns. The impact of the client's impairments on family responsibilities and expectations must be considered when establishing a treatment plan. Restoration of parenting roles can be challenging for the client, the family, and the therapist.

Parents with diminished physical abilities following an acute event (e.g., spinal cord injury) are likely to have different intervention needs than parents with a chronic or progressive disease or disorder (e.g., rheumatoid arthritis or multiple sclerosis). Persons subjected to the acute onset of physical or cognitive impairments are confronted by sudden and sometimes drastic changes in the ways they can participate in important life roles and tasks. In contrast, individuals with progressive conditions and their families can gradually learn adapted ways to cope with changing abilities and levels of role participation over time.

During the evaluation, the occupational therapist should ask clients to identify which parenting tasks they highly value (e.g., play time, nursing, or bottle feeding) and which tasks are necessary for them to resume their parenting role. The client should then prioritize parenting goals in a way that addresses both valued and necessary tasks in a balanced way.

Barriers to Effectiveness

Barriers to a client's ability to return to parenting tasks and roles are similar to those for homemaker responsibilities. In addition, factors such as the child's age, activity level, and obedience greatly influence the challenges encountered by the parent with physical impairments. The occupational therapist works to identify the barriers that interfere with a client's ability to accomplish important parenting tasks, devise adapted methods that reduce or remove these constraints, and assist the individual in regaining competence in his or her parenting role.

Child Care: Techniques and Therapeutic Aids

Parents with rheumatoid arthritis, spinal cord injury, and stroke have reported that child care tasks that require lifting and carrying are the most challenging, followed by tasks that demand fine motor dexterity and/or grip strength (Joe, 1997; Ostensen & Rugelsjoen, 1992). A national survey of parents with physical disabilities revealed that parenting tasks such as traveling outside the home with a child, recreational activities, and chasing and retrieving children require the greatest assistance from others (Barker & Maralani, 1997). Funding for adapted parenting equipment and personal assistance services to help with child care is extremely limited. Therefore, the parent and therapist must work together to identify adapted methods and inexpensive solutions that best address parenting needs.

Equipment Considerations

The occupational therapist and client should initially explore whether simple adaptations to the way child care tasks are performed can enhance performance. When these simple solutions do not work, the client and therapist should evaluate whether commercially available child care equipment can feasibly meet the needs of the parent and child. If not, more creative solutions and adaptations should be devised.

The occupational therapist must consider the cost of the adapted equipment and whether it is acceptable to the client in terms of appearance and ease of use. In addition, the therapist must understand that the appropriateness of any equipment changes over time as the child grows and develops (DeMoss et al., 1995).

Bathing

Parents need to be sure that all necessary equipment and clothes have been gathered and are within easy reach before they begin bathing their infant or young child. A terry cloth apron worn during bathing can protect clothing and dry the baby after the bath.

Persons who are ambulatory may find that bathing the infant in a portable plastic tub in or near the kitchen sink is a good option, because the height of the sink or counter minimizes bending and the tub can be easily filled and drained at the sink. However, parents who use wheelchairs may find this arrangement inconvenient because it is too high for safely lifting the baby in and out of the tub. Persons in wheelchairs also find it difficult to bathe the infant if the baby tub is in a regular bathtub, because it is too low (DeMoss et al., 1995). An alternative is to secure the baby bathtub to a sturdy table or serving cart near a sink. A portable dishwasher hose can be connected to the sink faucet for filling the tub, and a separate hose can be used to drain the bath water (DeMoss et al., 1995). It may be easier for the parent to use this arrangement to bathe the older infant until the child is mobile enough to help with getting in and out of a regular bathtub. This diminishes the parent's need to lift a wet, slippery child from a low tub.

Diapering and Dressing

Commercially available changing tables are usually inaccessible for persons who use a wheelchair because the wheelchair does not fit under the table for diapering or dressing the child. In addition, the surface may be too high for a seated parent to lift and transfer the baby safely, particularly as the infant grows (DeMoss et al., 1995). The client and therapist should work together to determine the changing surface that most effectively and safely meets the individual's needs.

Safety straps should always be used to secure the active baby and prevent falls. These straps are particu-

---

Case Example

MRS. M.: HOMEMAKING AND CHILD CARE

Patient Information

Mrs. M. is a 54-year-old widow referred for a home occupational therapy assessment following recent exacerbation of rheumatoid arthritis (RA). She lives alone in a ranch house and ordinarily cares for her 6-month-old granddaughter 3 days a week while her daughter works. Prior to her exacerbation, she was fairly active and able to manage all household and child care tasks independently with the exception of yard work. An avid gardener, she spent a good deal of time in her greenhouse prior to her exacerbation. She is able to use joint protection principles (e.g., avoiding positions of deformity, such as ulnar deviation) during functional tasks.

As a result of this exacerbation, she has decreased strength and dexterity in her hands and wrists, increased pain during activity, and a significant decrease in overall endurance. The occupational therapy evaluation identified the following problems: (1) moderately decreased ability to perform the household management tasks needed to maintain her independence at home, with fatigue after 30 minutes of activity; (2) moderate impairments in her ability to care for her granddaughter secondary to decreased strength and pain during resistive activities, such as opening baby food jars and attempting to lift the child; and (3) poor use of body mechanics and a tendency to rush through tasks when fatigued.

Recommendations

The occupational therapist recommended three treatment sessions each week for 4 weeks. In collaboration with Mrs. M. and her daughter, the therapist established the following long-term treatment goals: (1) Mrs. M. will independently perform all indoor homemaking tasks except floor care with only occasional complaints of fatigue, using energy conservation and work simplification techniques. (2) Mrs. M. will independently care for her granddaughter for 4-hour periods with only occasional complaints of pain, demonstrating appropriate use of assistive devices to protect joints during resistive activities. (3) Mrs. M. will use proper body mechanics when lifting and carrying her granddaughter and performing household tasks, such as meal preparation and laundry.

Short-Term Goals

▶ **Mrs. M. will independently and safely prepare a light meal for herself without complaints of fatigue, using work simplification and energy conservation principles after initial instruction.** The therapist and Mrs. M. first reviewed work simplification principles in the context of preparing a hot beverage, taking the opportunity to organize work areas in the kitchen so frequently used items were easily accessible. They identified ways Mrs. M. could conserve energy during meal preparation, such as by retrieving all items needed at one location (e.g., refrigerator) before moving on to the next and sitting when possible to prepare foods. After instruction in self-pacing, Mrs. M. was more willing to take brief rests during meal preparation *before* fatigue or pain began to worsen. After practicing proper body mechanics, she was better able to obtain and carry items safely around the kitchen without increasing pain. In addition, use of a jar opener significantly reduced the discomfort in her hands. To reduce preparation time and effort, Mrs. M. decided to use frozen rather than fresh vegetables until her endurance improved. Mrs. M. found that these strategies greatly reduced her level of fatigue during meal preparation, and she began to apply these techniques to other tasks around the house.

▶ **Mrs. M. will safely and independently transfer her granddaughter from the infant seat to changing pad on the kitchen table with good body mechanics and safety and no complaints of discomfort.** Mrs. M., her daughter, and the occupational therapist determined that the need for lifting and carrying the infant could be minimized by organizing essential child care materials, such as the infant seat, changing pad with straps, diapers, and toys, on one side of the oversized kitchen table and nearby hutch. Mrs. M. found that bilateral wrist supports greatly reduced pain in her wrists when she lifted the baby.

Proper body mechanics were reinforced and practiced, such as standing close to the child with feet staggered and placed shoulder distance apart and using stronger muscles (legs rather than back) when lifting. Mrs. M. progressed from requiring minimal assistance to lift and transfer the baby safely to performing the task independently. As she gained confidence in her abilities, her body mechanics improved and complaints of discomfort decreased.

Revised Goals

▶ Mrs. M. will use work simplification techniques and proper body mechanics to do laundry independently.

▶ Mrs. M. will safely and independently lift and transfer her granddaughter from a stroller to the infant seat with good body mechanics and will prepare and feed the child a warm meal without assistance.

CLINICAL REASONING
in OT Practice

Effects of Arthritic Changes in the Wrists and Hands and Impaired Endurance During Gardening Tasks

Although Mrs. M. was diagnosed with rheumatoid arthritis 15 years prior to this OT assessment, she managed homemaking and gardening tasks with little adapted equipment until this exacerbation. While Mrs. M. worked in her greenhouse, the occupational therapist observed her bending from the waist to pick up a bag of potting soil and watering can from the floor. In addition, Mrs. M. complained of wrist and hand pain and fatigue while standing at her work counter to transplant seedlings into a window box for her deck.

How could the therapist help Mrs. M. to problem solve ways to use compensatory strategies and adapted equipment to decrease pain and improve her safety while gardening? How might the therapist reinforce use of proper body mechanics? Consider what work simplification and energy conservation techniques might be useful, in addition to addressing her joint protection needs.

---

larly helpful when the parent needs extra time to manipulate diaper or clothing fasteners because of diminished fine motor control. A mobile attached to the changing table and assorted toys can keep the baby distracted during changing.

Although adapted fasteners for diapers and baby clothing can require initial assistance from family or friends, they can greatly enhance one's independence in child care during the day. For example, loops made of packing tape can be attached to disposable diaper tabs to reduce fine motor demands (DeMoss et al., 1995). Wraps that hold either cloth or disposable diapers can be adapted by attaching metal key rings to small holes made in the Velcro tabs (DeMoss et al., 1995). Small pieces of Velcro can also be sewn onto a variety of infant and baby clothes. Ideally, clothing should have full-length openings with closures that the parent can manage. Zippers are easier to manipulate than snaps when a zipper pull is used.

Feeding

Mothers with physical challenges may choose to nurse or bottle-feed their baby. After an initial adjustment period, breast-feeding can be easier than bottle-feeding because it eliminates formula preparation. However, if the mother is taking medications, it is important that she check with her physician before deciding to breast-feed to be sure that the medication will not harm the nursing infant. The mother should sit in a relaxed, comfortable position, using pillows to support the holding arm and baby while nursing.

Some parents find bottle-feeding easier and more convenient with the older infant in a child seat, while others prefer to hold the child close to them when feeding (Fig. 32-14). Individuals with limited grasp may be able to hold a bottle and feed their infant after slipping their hand through a loop of webbing material attached to the bottle (DeMoss et al., 1995). Lightweight plastic bottles with screw-on lids are recommended over glass bottles.

Older babies can be spoon-fed by a person with tetraplegia when the parent's wrist cock-up splint is adapted by attaching Velcro loop to the palmar surface. The spoon is inserted into a utensil pocket made of Velcro hook and attached to the splint at the best angle for feeding (DeMoss et al., 1995). An insulated baby dish can be used to keep food warm throughout the meal. Spoons should be rubber coated to protect the baby's gums and teeth if bumped while feeding.

Parents with impaired grasp and arm strength may not be able to attach or remove the tray on commercial high chairs (DeMoss et al., 1995). In addition, it may be

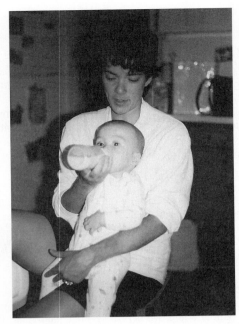

Figure 32-14 Alternative feeding position for mother with mild left hemiparesis following CVA.

difficult for the parent to lift the child in and out of a standard high chair. Options to make high chairs more accessible for parents with physical limitations include altering the chair height, designing swing-away trays, and adding a climbing ladder to encourage the older infant to climb into the seat with supervision only (DeMoss et al., 1995).

Lifting and Carrying

Adapted equipment that provides alternative ways of carrying the infant or young child or reduces the need for multiple transfers can greatly enhance the parent's satisfaction and ability to care for the child. Parents with distal weakness and pain, as seen with rheumatoid arthritis, benefit from wearing wrist supports to reduce joint stress when lifting and carrying their child (Nordenskiold et al., 1998). Many clients prefer to practice lifting and carrying techniques with a weighted doll before trying to manage an active child.

A variety of cloth infant carriers and child front packs are available. Although these carriers allow the parent to transport a small child while leaving hands free, they may be contraindicated for persons with chronic back pain because the shoulders and back carry the weight of the child. Individuals who use wheelchairs may find child front packs handy for holding the infant while performing other homemaking tasks. Ease of use is important: adaptations may be needed to enable the parent with physical impairments to get the baby into and out of the infant carrier. The straps can be modified to reduce the parent's coordination needs (DeMoss

et al., 1995). Older babies with good neck and trunk control can safely ride on their parent's lap with only a safety belt attached to the wheelchair (Fig. 32-15).

Play

Parents with physical impairments may find that their ability to play with their young children is hindered because they cannot sit on the floor or bend to reach into standard playpens. Although infants can be entertained while they are sitting in a bouncy seat, older babies need a larger safe area to play in order to develop gross motor skills. If cost is not an issue, a play care center, essentially a raised playpen that allows wheelchair access, can be built in the corner of a room (DeMoss et al., 1995). If the center is equipped with swing-away doors, the parent can wheel up to the play center and easily reach into it to play with the baby. This play area can also be used for the child's naps during the day, eliminating extra transfers in and out of the crib (DeMoss et al., 1995). Walking toddlers and their parents may find that a child's table approximately 18 inches high is a convenient place to play while the parent is sitting in a wheelchair or standard chair.

Cribs

Standard cribs are inaccessible for parents who use wheelchairs, and they require ambulatory parents to bend forward when putting the baby in or out of bed. A standard drop-side crib can be adapted in several ways, depending on the parent's physical needs.

Persons who are ambulatory but have difficulty bending because of chronic back pain can raise the crib

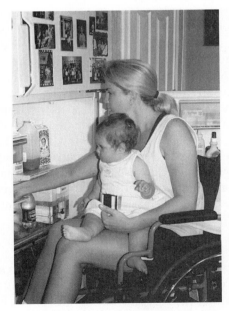

Figure 32-15 A mother confined to a wheelchair using a safety strap for an older baby while gathering items from the refrigerator.

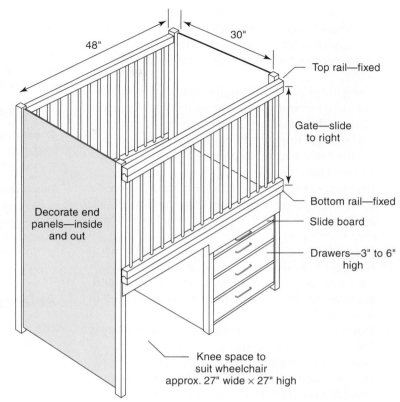

Figure 32-16 Crib with storage area, sliding gate side rails, and knee space to accommodate a wheelchair. (Designed by Lee Heintzman and Gordon Heintzman. Adapted from Dunn, V. M. [1978]. Tips on raising children from a wheelchair. *Accent on Living, 22,* 78–83.)

by inserting leg extenders or blocks of wood under the crib legs. The crib mattress can also be raised to the highest setting but should not remain in this position once the baby is old enough to sit or to climb over the crib rail.

Parents who use a wheelchair find it easier to transfer the baby in and out of the crib if the rail is adapted. One modification is cutting the rail in half to form two gates. These gates are attached with hinges to the head and foot of the crib. Center latches that are inaccessible to the child secure the gate when the baby is sleeping (DeMoss et al., 1995). Another option is to adapt the crib rail so that it slides along a horizontal channel (DeMoss et al., 1995; Dunn, 1978) (Fig. 32-16). Whatever crib design is used, the release mechanism for the crib rail must be child resistant yet manageable for the parent to manipulate with one hand or with limited coordination and dexterity.

Efficacy and Outcomes Research

Empirical evidence supporting the effectiveness of occupational therapy and the benefits of adapted techniques and equipment is growing. Training in the use of assistive devices, environmental modifications, and instruction of adapted methods (e.g., energy conservation principles) can significantly improve performance dur-

ing homemaking and parenting tasks. These benefits have been reported for persons with rheumatoid arthritis (Nordenskiold et al., 1998), stroke (Walker et al., 1999), spinal cord injury (Barker & Maralani, 1997; Eberhardt, 1998), multiple sclerosis (Fernie et al., 1994), and the elderly (Axtell & Yasuda, 1993; Fox, 1995; Kondo et al., 1997). More research is needed to examine the degree to which adapted methods and equipment (i.e., occupation-as-end) contribute to one's satisfaction and competence in homemaker and parenting roles after a disabling event. Empirical support for the cost-effectiveness of adapted equipment and supportive services may lead to improved reimbursement from third-party payers.

Summary Review Questions

1. Describe how work simplification and energy conservation techniques can help persons with low endurance and shortness of breath due to chronic obstructive pulmonary disease with meal preparation and household maintenance tasks.
2. Identify at least three principles of correct body mechanics that a person with chronic back pain should use when doing laundry and transporting groceries from the store.

3. Describe how a homemaker who has pain and weakness in her hands and wrists due to rheumatoid arthritis can use adapted methods or assistive equipment when preparing brownies from a mix.

4. Using the principles of compensation and adaptation, what recommendations would you make to a client with limited upper extremity coordination and strength due to multiple sclerosis when gathering the items needed to prepare breakfast from a wheelchair?

5. Give two examples of adaptations that may assist a paraplegic parent with spinal cord injury at T4 to lift and carry an 11-month-old infant from the crib to the changing area.

6. Describe how a mother with upper extremity weakness and limited hand function in her right arm after a stroke can use one-handed techniques and assistive equipment to prepare a bottle and feed her 5-month-old infant.

7. How would you recommend that a parent set up a baby bathtub and needed supplies to bathe a 2-month-old infant from a wheelchair?

8. Discuss proper body mechanics for a person with general pain related to fibromyalgia who is playing with a 10-month-old baby and putting the baby to bed.

Acknowledgments

Many thanks to Robert Littlefield, photographer, and to Sammons Preston for the assistive devices pictured in this chapter. Special thanks to the individuals who shared their ideas about adapted techniques with me, based on their personal experience with physical challenges.

Resources

Sources of Information for Homemaking and Parenting for Persons with Physical Disabilities

Books

Klinger, J. L. (1997) · *Meal Preparation and Training: The Health Care Professional's Guide*. Thorofare, NJ: Slack.

Mayer, T. K. (2000) · *One-Handed in a Two-Handed World: Your Personal Guide to Managing Single Handedly* (2nd ed.). Boston: Prince Gallison.

Organizations, Associations, and Services

The Internet offers a wealth of information concerning resources for specific disabilities. Some organizations that listed information specific to home management or parenting at the time of publication:

The Arthritis Foundation · Atlanta, GA. 800-283-7800.
www.arthritis.org

National Multiple Sclerosis Society · New York, NY. 800-624-8236.
www.nmss.org

National Stroke Association · Englewood, CO. 800-STROKES.
www.stroke.org

Through the Looking Glass (addresses the needs of parents with disabilities and parents of disabled children) · Berkeley, CA. 800-644-2666.
www.lookingglass.org

Computerized Information Services for Persons with Disabilities

ABLEDATA · Silver Springs, MD. 800-227-0216.
www.abledata.com

Manufacturers and Distributors of Adaptive Devices

North Coast Medical · Morgan Hill, CA. 800-235-7054.
www.ncmedical.com

Sammons Preston · Bolingbrook, IL. 800-323-5547.
www.sammonspreston.com

References

Adil, J. R. (1994). *Accessible Gardening for People With Physical Disabilities: A Guide to Methods, Tools, and Plants*. Bethesda, MD: Woodbine House.

American Occupational Therapy Association (1997). The psychosocial core of occupational therapy. Position paper. *American Journal of Occupational Therapy, 51*, 868–869.

Anderson, H. (1981). *The Disabled Homemaker*. Springfield, IL: Charles C. Thomas.

Axtell, L. A., & Yasuda, Y. L. (1993). Assistive devices and home modifications in geriatric rehabilitation. *Clinics in Geriatric Medicine, 9*, 803–821.

Barker, L. T., & Maralani, V. (1997). *Challenges and Strategies of Disabled Parents: Findings From a National Survey of Parents With Disabilities: Final Report*. Oakland, CA: Berkeley Planning Associates.

DeMoss, A., Rogers, A., Tuleja, C., & Kirshbaum, M. (1995). *Adaptive Parenting Equipment: Idea Book I*. Berkeley, CA: Through the Looking Glass.

Dunn, V. M. (1978). Tips on raising children from a wheelchair. *Accent on Living, 22* (4), 78–83.

Eberhardt, K. (1998). Home modifications for persons with spinal cord injury. *OT Practice, 3*(10), 24–27.

Fernie, G. R., Griggs, G. T., Holliday, P. J., & Topper, A. (1994). Increasing the accessibility of a conventional cooking range for wheelchair users. *American Journal of Occupational Therapy, 48*, 463–466.

Fox, P. L. (1995). Environmental modifications in the homes of elderly Canadians with disabilities. *Disability and Rehabilitation, 17*, 43–49.

Jackson, J., Carlson, M., Mandel, D., Zemke, R., & Clark, F. (1998). Occupational lifestyle redesign: The well-elderly study occupational therapy program. *American Journal of Occupational Therapy, 52*, 326–336.

Joe, B. E. (1997, January 30). Small changes: Big differences. *OT Week*, 16–17.

Kondo, T., Mann, W. C., Tomita, M., & Ottenbacher, K. J. (1997). The use of microwave ovens by elderly persons with disabilities. *American Journal of Occupational Therapy, 51*, 739–747.

Lampert, J., & Lapolice, D. J. (1995). Functional considerations in evaluation and treatment of the client with low vision. *American Journal of Occupational Therapy, 49*, 885–890.

Melnik, M. (1994). *Understanding Your Back Injury*. Rockville, MD: American Occupational Therapy Association.

Moyers, P. A. (1999). The guide to occupational therapy practice. *American Journal of Occupational Therapy, 53*, 247–322.

Nordenskiold, U., Grimby, G., & Dahlin-Ivanoff, S. (1998). Questionnaire to evaluate the effects of assistive devices and altered working methods in women with rheumatoid arthritis. *Clinical Rheumatology, 17*, 6–16.

Ostensen, M., & Rugelsjoen, A. (1992). Problem areas of the rheumatic mother. *American Journal of Reproductive Immunology, 28*, 254–255.

Plautz, B., Beck, D. E., Selmar, C., & Radetsky, M. (1996). Modifying the environment: A community-based injury-reduction program for elderly residents. *American Journal of Preventive Medicine, 12* (Suppl. 4), 33–38.

Saunders, H. D. (1992). *For Your Back*. Eden Prairie, MN: Viking.

Walker, M. F., Gladman, J. R., Lincoln, N. B., Siemonsma, P., & Whitley, T. (1999). Occupational therapy for stroke patients not admitted to hospital: A randomised controlled trial. *Lancet, 354* (9175), 278–280.

Yeomans, K. (1992). *The Able Gardener: Overcoming Barriers of Age and Physical Limitations*. Pownal, VT: Storey.

33

Restoring Competence for the Worker Role

Valerie J. Rice and Stephen Luster

LEARNING OBJECTIVES

After studying this chapter, the reader will be able to do the following:

1. Understand and articulate the reasons people work.
2. Recognize and verbalize the unique role of occupational therapy in the return-to-work process.
3. Describe job analysis, how it is used in the return-to-work process, and other possible applications for the results of job analysis.
4. Describe functional capacity evaluations and considerations in selecting appropriate evaluations for clients.
5. Recognize how return-to-work evaluation tools can be used as treatment tools.

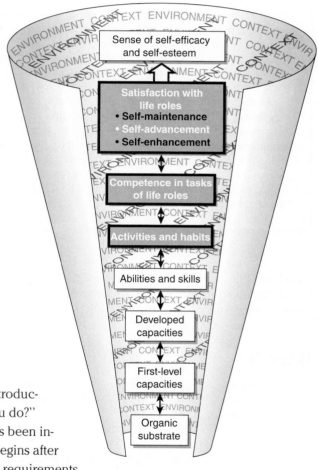

*T*wo people meet for the first time at a social event. After introducing themselves, the inevitable question is asked: "What do you do?"

The focus of this chapter is on returning a worker who has been incapacitated in some way to the workforce. The intervention begins after an individual has been identified as being unable to meet the requirements of his or her job. Thus, the primary roles for the clinician are *evaluating* the individual's functional performance, strengths, and impairments as compared with the job requirements, *treating* the client, *matching* the client–worker with the job (enabling and integration process), and *reevaluation*. To understand the progression, it is first necessary to understand why people work, recognize how occupational therapists view work and their role in work rehabilitation, understand how the work role can be interrupted, and become acquainted with a few work-related assessments. An extensive explanation of the evaluation process is provided to enable a thorough understanding of the process and permit tailoring of the intervention to both the individual and the context in which the

---

GLOSSARY

Functional Capacity Evaluation (FCE)—Systematic process designed to assess a client's functional abilities. Functional abilities may include all physical and pyschosocial abilities required in a work setting, such as physical, cognitive, emotional, and communication abilities. The two performance categories include a general evaluation of physical abilities and an evaluation of job-specific capabilities.

Functional work assessment—Entire return-to-work evaluation process, including evaluations of (1) the individual client (occupational therapy and FCEs) and (2) the requirements of the job or potential jobs (job analysis).

Job analysis—Systematic evaluation of a job. A physical evaluation of the job site, observing workers performing their tasks, measuring equipment and equipment placement, reviewing work-related documents such as job descriptions, and interviewing those who perform the job and their supervisors.

Task component testing, training—Functional capacity testing that identifies criterion tasks based on the most difficult, essential components of a job and develops specific evaluations or training programs based on those components. It is assumed that evaluating or training using task components critical to job success is a valid approach to determining work performance, as the content requirements of the job are used to develop the evaluation or training.

Work conditioning—Treatment program focused on functional requirements of a job or employment setting; incorporates basic physical conditioning such as restoration of flexibility, strength, coordination, and endurance. Work conditioning is conducted after completion of acute care and before work hardening.

Work hardening—Multidisciplinary structured, graded return-to-work treatment program that progressively introduces greater rehabilitation requirements on the client–worker to achieve full capability of the worker to meet the demands of a job. Work hardening includes all aspects required for the client to return to full function in employment, such as psychosocial, communication, physical, and vocational needs, and typically incorporates work simulation as part of the treatment process.

Work-related musculoskeletal disorder (WRMD)—Wide range of health problems arising from repeated stress to the body encountered in the workplace; may affect the musculoskeletal, nervous, and neurovascular systems and include the various occupationally induced cumulative trauma disorders, cumulative stress injuries, and repetitive motion disorders.

---

individual will work. With this knowledge, the occupational therapy process can be understood within the appropriate context.[1]

What Is Work?

"He who complains against his work knoweth not life; work is an uplifting force by which all things may be moved. Repose is death, and work is life!"
(Jastrzebowski, 1857, p. 1)

Although we may not all agree with Jastrzebowski's enthusiastic assertion that work is uplifting and *life itself*, there is some merit in his declaration. Used in the broadest sense of the term, everyone must work. It is part of life. For work, as seen in the first definition in Box 33-1, consists of any physical or mental effort or activity directed toward the purposeful production or accomplishment of something. This means that work occurs in the home, in schools, as part of one's employment, and as part of one's leisure. To work is *to do*, to accomplish. With this definition, returning the worker to work encompasses occupational therapy as a whole, as clinicians assist their clients to achieve their fullest capacity in all aspects of life. In this chapter, however, returning the worker to work refers to helping a client reenter the workforce, go to a place of employment or job, and/or develop a means to earn a livelihood.

Motivations for Work

Why would an individual want to reenter the labor force? Why do people work in the first place? Obviously, for most people, it is an economic necessity. In earlier times, people traded their wares and their abilities to attain the goods they needed. Although this still exists in some small communities, most residents of industrialized countries have distinct employment and pay for their goods and services with money earned at their jobs.

---

[1]With the focal point being on returning workers to work, prevention is considered as a separate entity, to be conducted before injuries or illness occur. In this context, prevention techniques are employed only in the respect of trying to prevent reinjury.

Self-Creation and Self-Identity Through Work

We work to finance lives, homes, families, education, and fun. However, especially in industrial societies, we do not have to work from dawn to dusk to earn a living, nor are we required to enter jobs dictated by our birth or heritage. Instead, for the most part, we have choices. We can choose our line of work according to our own value systems. Christiansen (1999) asserts that occupations are key not just to being a person but to being a particular person and to creating and maintaining an identity. He explains that the use of one's time during the day within various contexts provides one with a sense of purpose and structure, as well as building an identity. We create ourselves through our actions. For some people, then, the choice of a job or vocation is a step in self-creation.

Since a full 30% of our lives are spent at the labor that pays the bills and since this 30% is the world's greatest insight into our lives, it would seem that most of our self-respect and whatever respect is to be garnered from the rest of the world emanates from our workaday lives (Raven, 1999, p. 2).

While we may define ourselves daily through our work, we may also fulfill other needs. Although our values and the meaning of our lives may be derived during other parts of life, such as leisure, home, self-care, and family, they may also arise from our work. Work can fulfill our primary motivations (needs), as defined by some of the great psychologists and psychiatrists of our time. Work can fulfill the need to find meaning in life as asserted by Frankl's (1984) logotherapy. Work can fulfill the need to find pleasure, on which Freudian psychology is based. Work can also fulfill the need for power or striving for superiority stressed by Adlerian psychology (Frankl). Obviously, the point is that work can answer a number of needs. For some, work provides financial achievement, a sense of accomplishment and competence, socialization and status within society, pleasure and gratification, a sense of meaning and purpose, self-respect and an identity. For others, work also answers a singular need, leaving them to meet other needs elsewhere in their lives.

BOX 33-1
Work-Related Definitions

Work (noun)
1. Physical or mental effort or activity directed toward the purposeful production or accomplishment of something: Labor. **2.** Employment: job <out of work> **3.** The means by which one earns one's livelihood. **4.** a. Something that one is doing, making, or performing, esp. as part of one's occupation: a duty or task. b. The amount of effort required or done.

Work (verb)
1. To exert one's efforts for the purpose of doing or making something: LABOR. **2.** To be employed. **3.** To perform a function or act: OPERATE.

Work (synonyms)
Business, employment, job, occupation. Core meaning: what one does to earn a living. Work, the most general of these terms, can refer to the mere fact of employment or to a specific activity.

Career
1. Chosen profession or occupation. **2.** The general progression of one's life, especially in one's profession.

Job
1. An action that needs to be done: TASK. **2.** An activity performed regularly for payment, especially a trade, occupation, or profession. **3.** A specific piece of work to be done for a set fee. **4.** A position in which one is employed.

Occupation
1. a. An activity serving as one's regular employment: VOCATION. **1.** b. An activity engaged in, especially as a means of passing time.

Vocation
A regular occupation or profession, especially one for which an individual is particularly suited or qualified.

Matching Personal Values With Work Requirements

If our work forces us to behave in ways that directly conflict with our view of ourselves, we feel discomfort and are motivated to change our line of work. This is because people try to maintain positive views of themselves and refute or avoid feedback that is negative or disagrees with their ideal self (Swann, 1987; Swann and Hill, 1982). As an example, Enid DuBois worked as a telephone solicitor for a newspaper. Often, the solicitors were told to tell the potential customers that a portion of their money would go to a particular cause to encourage people to subscribe. "[A]fter a while, I didn't care. Surely I could have fast-talked people. Just to continually lie to them. But it just wasn't in me. The disgust was growing in me every minute. I would pray and pray to hold on a little longer" (Terkel, 1974, pp. 94–97).

We have seen a change in the desires of the workforce. Besides emphasis on pay and security, workers value and expect their work to be psychologically meaningful. They also expect to participate in decisions that affect their work lives (Hendrick, 1998). Our better-educated workforce in industrialized nations seeks challenges, advancement, and a voice in their work lives.

Interruptions in the Ability to Work

People's ability to work may be interrupted by changes in physical, psychosocial, or sociocultural status.

Physical Status

Mr. L. worked in a collision repair shop. His brother was fond on saying that he "banged on cars" for a living. The job required him to stand and manually remove the dents from car fenders using specialized tools. He was physically strong because his job demanded it. He wasn't prepared for what happened after he broke his leg. It never seemed to heal correctly. He developed what they called reflex sympathetic dystrophy. The term didn't matter. All he knew was it hurt all the time and he couldn't stand or even sit for long periods. He received workers compensation and wondered if he'd ever work again (Rice, D., personal communication, 2000).

The direct result of injury or illness may be inability to resume work activities permanently or temporarily, as the worker cannot fulfill the physical, cognitive, or emotional demands of the job. This mismatch between requirements and performance has been traditionally addressed by retraining the individual. The focus was on improving the deficits; thus the therapist worked to diminish individual shortfalls in strength, dexterity, coordination, range of motion, endurance, or memory. Whatever interrupted the client's ability to resume normal activities was addressed. More recently, the focus has broadened to include altering or redesigning the job to realign its requirements to the individual's residual abilities.

Nontraumatic injuries may also interfere with a person's ability to work. Nontraumatic injuries thought to be related to workplace demands are called **work-related musculoskeletal disorders (WRMDs)**. These injuries are typically thought of as transient, although they can result in permanent disability. WRMDs include a wide range of health problems arising from repeated stress to the body encountered in the workplace. These health problems, which may affect the musculoskeletal, nervous, and neurovascular systems, include the various occupation-induced cumulative trauma disorders (CTDs), cumulative stress injuries, and repetitive motion disorders. Examples include damage to tendons and tendon sheaths and synovial lubrication of the tendon sheaths, bones, muscles, and nerves of the hands, wrists, elbows, shoulders, neck, back, and legs. Specific diagnoses include chronic back pain, carpal tunnel syndrome, de Quervain's disease, epicondylitis (tennis elbow), Raynaud's syndrome (white finger), synovitis, stenosing tenosynovitis crepitans (trigger finger), tendinitis, and tenosynovitis. (For a thorough review of WRMDs, see Kuorinka et al. [1995] and Sanders [1997].) Once again, the reason for not being able to return to work is the person's inability to fulfill the requirements of the job tasks, such as the administrative assistant with severe, chronic carpal tunnel symptoms who cannot use a keyboard without pain.

Traumatic injury, aging, or progressive disability may also alter self-perception and personal identity. When a person loses his or her sense of identity, life becomes less meaningful and can become meaningless (Debats et al., 1995; Moore, 1997; van Selm & Dittmann-Kohli, 1998), leading to depression so severe that it can interfere with a person's ability to carry out daily work. Thus, it is not always the initial injury that prevents a return to work: the resulting psychological adjustments can also interfere. Unless both the physical and psychological problems are addressed, the individual may not develop the skills needed to return to work.

Psychological and Behavioral Status

Psychosocial events may interrupt a person's ability to work, either temporarily or permanently. Divorce, severe illness, death of a family member, or change in job status sometimes triggers underlying psychopathology such as a mood or anxiety disorder. The disruption may be due not to underlying psychopathology but also to the expression or manifestation of a normal reaction to a difficult situation. Each individual reacts differently to life situations, and adaptation may come more quickly for some than for others. Examples of an individual's inability to meet work requirements include disruptions in the ability to concentrate and follow complex directions, to react quickly to emergencies (psychomotor retardation), to attend to detail, or to handle the pressures and anxieties associated with the work environment. Although there is relatively little information on individuals returning to work after a psychological disorder, this is no less a problem than is a physical injury. In fact, it may be more difficult to return to work because of the attitudes and lack of knowledge and empathy of employers and coworkers, in addition to fears and concerns of the workers themselves.

In 1990, mental illness cost the United States $150 billion, including $67 billion for treatment and another $75 billion for decreases in productivity or premature death (National Commission for Disease Control and Prevention, 2000). Depression is predicted to be one of the fastest-growing maladies of the 21st century. Although treatment for depression and other psychological and emotional disturbances has vastly improved, there remain definite implications for the individual's ability to work. For example, in an occupational therapy case study of work-related issues for someone with bipolar affective disorder, the person had long periods of relative work and life stability punctuated by mania and depression severe enough to keep the client from working (Samson et al., 1999).

Sociocultural Status

Recently, President Clinton signed a bill that will allow millions of disabled Americans to keep their government-funded health coverage when they take a job (Ross, 1999), as it is believed that many disabled individuals do not seek employment for fear of losing Medicare and Medicaid benefits. Fewer than 1% of those who receive government disability ever leave that system. The new law should remove some of that fear, and up to 550,000 disabled persons will receive rehabilitation and training in preparation for return to the workforce (Ross, 1999).

Aging and age discrimination may also prevent workers from continuing to work or from returning to work following physical or psychological problems or following a downsizing. This problem may become more evident as the proportion of workers aged 45 to 54 years increases, to be followed in the next 10 years by a substantial increase in the proportion of workers 55 years of age and older (Yelin, 1999).

Work and Occupational Therapy

Adolph Meyer advocated a "freer conception of work, a concept of free and pleasant and profitable occupation—including recreation and any form of helpful enjoyment as the leading principle." He said the "whole of human organization has its shape in a kind of rhythm" and through structured use of time, people could achieve well-being (Meyer, 1922, pp. 1–2). By assisting the client to achieve a balanced lifestyle in work, play, rest, and sleep, early occupational therapists helped clients achieve a sense of homeostasis and health. Meyer broadly defined the term *occupation* as purposeful activity within the full spectrum of a person's life.

Occupational therapy is soundly based on the concept of returning the injured worker to work, as it was founded on the belief that merely eliminating the disease or providing immediate treatment for traumatic injury was insufficient for the full recovery of ill or injured clients. Instead, a client should be guided through a strengthening and training process, both physically and mentally, to prepare him or her to resume occupational status in society (Committee on Installations and Advice, 1928; Rice, 1999b). Therapists used "crafts" in their treatment. What were once called crafts are today considered jobs. The term *craft* included activities such as carpentry, metal work, and bookbinding, all of which

could be full-time employment. Initially, a wide variety of crafts or jobs were used in occupational therapy clinics. Occupational therapists realized, however, that carefully chosen occupation-based activities resulted in a transfer of training to almost any occupation the recovered client chose to pursue. This is opposite the current trend of **work hardening**, which simulates specific job tasks that will be required of the client upon return to work. The latter certainly has greater face validity, but to date no published outcome research clearly supports one approach as superior to the other.

Occupational Therapists' Unique Contributions

Occupational therapists, with their solid background in the full spectrum of human performance (physiological, biomechanical, psychosocial, and behavioral) are uniquely qualified to help clients return to work. A fundamental goal of occupational therapy is to facilitate the client's highest level of functional status in all occupations and all contexts of life, including physical, emotional, social, cognitive, and communicative dimensions. Occupational therapists recognize that successful return to work is likely to depend on adequate function in many aspects of life, not solely task performance at the work site. For example, occupational therapists use their knowledge of human performance and the human mind to determine whether the impediments to returning to work are physical, psychosocial, or both. Therapists also use their knowledge of human psychology to discern possible motivations for the client to achieve well being.

With some clients, the urge toward competence is obvious, and they work quickly to master their environment (White, 1971). Therapists can motivate others by having them visualize what they want to be able to do or the type of person they want to be and by working with them to achieve their *possible selves* (Markus & Nurius, 1986). Those who value work or for whom we can find the motivational factors in work are most inclined to participate fully in rehabilitation. They are also the most likely to return to the workforce. Providing small successes along the way does much to encourage the process, but without work that has intrinsic value for the individual, the return to work is likely to be unsuccessful. The application of the full spectrum of human performance elucidates the unique contributions of occupational therapists in returning the injured worker to the workforce.

Burwash Model

One model depicting the knowledge and intervention necessary for occupational therapists to evaluate and intervene in work practices is that presented by Burwash (1999), shown in Figure 33-1 and further described in Table 33-1. Although returning to work is seen as one of the triangles representing concerns of clients, to facilitate a return to work, the therapist may be involved in each of the eight areas. For example, the client may be leaving one line of work because of disease or disability and need to reevaluate his or her values to explore and choose another career. While building the requisite physical and cognitive skills for the chosen job or career field, the client may also need to develop skills in searching for work along with the work habits needed to sustain a successful career.

The therapist must understand the client's value of work and self-perception as related to work (such as self-definition and self-esteem), so as to design the rehabilitation process and identify short-term goals and techniques to motivate the client. This client-centered approach to evaluation and treatment involves joint identification of goals and priorities by the therapist and the client (Law et al., 1994; Mattingly, 1991; Neistadt, 1995). For example, therapists can help clients ascertain whether they want their work to be a job rather than a career (Box 33-1) by examining where they fulfill their social, emotional, and achievement needs.

The Return-to-Work Process

Returning to work entails three main procedures: evaluation, intervention, and reevaluation.

Functional Work Assessments

Functional work assessments include evaluation of both the individual client and the work requirements the client will encounter. Individual evaluations incorporate the standard occupational therapy assessment, a delineation of the conditions preventing the client from returning to work, and a **functional capacity evaluation (FCE)**. The evaluation of the work requirements is often referred to as a functional job analysis or simply **job analysis**.

Job Analysis

A job analysis is a systematic evaluation of the job that identifies its physical, cognitive, social, and psychological requirements. Conducting a job analysis entails going to the job site, observing workers performing their tasks, measuring equipment and equipment placement, and interviewing those who perform the job and their supervisors. Some of the tools employed in the job

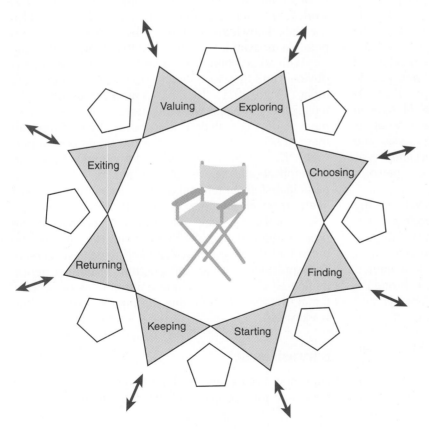

Figure 33-1 Work Practice Model (Burwash, 1999). The circular shape suggests many entry and exit points; intervention may progress in a linear fashion around the circle, or only one or two areas of concern may be addressed. The director's chair in the center is a reminder that focus is on the individual and his or her values, and the individual, rather than diagnosis or age, should be the director. The eight triangles represent concerns expressed by clients and are part of occupational therapy's professional heritage and within therapists' competencies. The pentagons suggest artists' palettes as a reminder that the intervention requires both art and science in dealing with productivity issues. The double-headed arrows represent environmental factors that influence and can be influenced by the client and therapist; they include social, cultural, and political factors, among others.

TABLE 33-1
Examples Using the Burwash Model (1999)

Model Segment	Client Concerns	Therapist Resources: Assessment Tools, Techniques, Programs	Environmental Considerations
Valuing	"Why work?" "How does work fit into my life?" "What are my personal values and what types of work fit?" "Why am I not happy in this work?" "Is working worth it?"	*Work Values Inventory, Life Roles Inventory,* work values auction, spirituality of work questionnaire, *Occupational Performance History Interview*	Family and social group attitudes toward work; economic considerations for persons on disability pensions; religious beliefs about work; work and gender issues
Exploring	"I don't know what I'm physically capable of." "Are there any occupations that match my interests?" "What am I good at?"	*Functional Capacity Evaluation, Self-Directed Search,* work samples, computerized career exploration systems	Role definition of OT vs. other team members (career counselors, vocational rehabilitation counselor, teachers); family expectations
Keeping	"How is this health problem going to affect my work?" "I hurt so much after a day at work!" "I'm about to take stress leave; all of these changes are really getting to me." "I can't figure out how to get ahead at work; I'm really feeling stuck."	Ergonomic interventions, stress management and relaxation techniques, energy conservation and work simplification techniques, goal setting, injury prevention and health promotion programs, advocacy	Family and friends' expectations; public laws on disability and workplace, ergonomic standards; employer, coworker, public attitudes toward persons with disabilities; client's support system; funding issues; job market; physical accessibility; access to transportation
Returning	"Will I be able to work again?" "How do I prevent reinjury?" "How do I deal with coworkers' comments about my illness?" "If I'm hurting at work, how do I cope with the pain?"	*Work Environment Impact Scale, Worker Role Interview,* graduated RTW programs, work-hardening and chronic pain programs, assertiveness skills, *Loma Linda Activity Sort,* other resources in Exploring section	Laws on injured workers and employers' responsibilities to them, job market, funding for retraining, family responsibilities, possible financial settlements, advice from lawyers and others, employer–employee relations

BOX 33-2
PROCEDURES FOR PRACTICE

Ways to Use Job Analysis Data

- Develop FCE
- Match injured workers' capabilities to job task requirements
- Place workers on light duty
- Return previously injured workers to work
- Identify risk factors associated with work-related musculoskeletal disorders
- Develop preplacement, postjob offer screenings
- Write job description (possibly using ADA terminology)
- Describe and advertise jobs

analysis are video cameras, tape measures, scales, goniometers, stopwatches, dynamometers, still cameras, and strain gauges. The results of a job analysis can be used in several ways, as seen in Box 33-2.

Basic Components of Job Analysis

Components of any job analysis include the job title, basic description or objectives of the job, number of employees performing the job, the work and break schedule, a description of any rotation or enrichment program, and output requirements for the workers. A description of the environment should include temperature, available space, a list of fixed and movable equipment, personal protective equipment, and a sketch of the area. A sequential description of each task (essential function) and the component steps to complete it is also necessary. This should include measurements such as heights, weights, duration, distances, and so on.

Rationale for Conducting Job Analysis

The reason for conducting the job analysis dictates its questions and procedures. Purposes of conducting a job analysis include returning a disabled person to work, identifying musculoskeletal risk factors, matching a rehabilitated or new worker with job demands, and developing assessments such as FCEs and preplacement screening tests.

For example, if the results are to be used to return to his or her work an individual classified as disabled according to the Americans with Disabilities Act (ADA) (Federal Register, 1991), the job must be described in terms of its **essential functions** (Box 33-3). Therapists whose responsibilities include industrial rehabilitation and returning injured or disabled workers to the workforce or helping employers to advertise jobs should be well versed in Title I of the ADA. Several excellent book chapters for therapists are available (Bloswick et al., 1998; Isernhagen, 1995; Kornblau, 1998a), and therapists should also refer to the regulations and guides themselves (ADA Title I Regulations, 1991; Americans with Disabilities Act, 1990; Equal Employment Opportunity Commission, 1992).

If the reason for performing the job analysis is to identify risk factors that may predispose a person to musculoskeletal disorders, listing the essential functions is not compulsory. A job analysis primarily geared to injury prevention, such as work-related musculoskeletal disorders, should include descriptions of observed risk factors, such as repetitive motions, force, static postures, awkward postures, mechanical compressions, vibration, and the acceleration and velocity of dynamic motions, noted for each body part and quantified. For example, the duration of static hold using a pinch grip is noted in seconds. Literature on job analysis related to injury prevention can be found in several excellent sources (Alexander, 1999; Ellexson, 1997; Isernhagen, 1995; Karwowski & Marras, 1999; Pulat & Alexander, 1992; Rice, 1998; Rogers, 1983, 1992; Sanders, 1997).

For matching workers' capabilities with the job requirements, placing workers on light duty, or returning previously injured workers to work, tasks (i.e., essential functions) are broken into their component steps and quantitatively described in enough detail to permit them to be matched with the worker's residual capabilities (Box 33-4). The therapist who only occasionally participates in returning injured workers to the workforce may prepare a unique job analysis for each client. However, therapists who work full time in industrial rehabilitation generally keep a file of job descriptions that let them quickly determine whether a client can return by comparing the results of the FCE with the job description (Isernhagen, 1995b). One benefit of having occupational therapists involved in job analysis is the ability to combine these purposes for conducting job analysis and develop a comprehensive database for an industry's use.

Use of Job Analysis in Developing and Selecting a Functional Capacity Evaluation

A job analysis should be conducted *prior to development or selection of an FCE*. An FCE consists of two parts: a general evaluation of physical abilities and a job-specific evaluation. Before one can decide whether to use solely the general evaluation versus the job-specific evaluation, the therapist must know whether the client intends to return to a specific job or type of job. If so, the information from the job analysis can be used to develop one of two types of FCE using criterion-referenced tasks. The first uses task components, while the second uses work simulations (both discussed later in the chapter). In both cases, the initial information is gathered during the job analysis.

Predicting Work Performance

The results of job analysis can also be used to predict performance. A review of 21 research studies designed to predict work performance, found static, dynamic, and combined strength tests and simulations predicted job performance. The most successful predictions, those that accounted for 60% of the variance or more, demonstrated several consistencies. A major one was a well-constructed job analysis, with a breakdown of job tasks into component parts. (An example of component tests and a work simulation can be seen in Box 33-5.) Successful predictions also used multiple assessment techniques, such as interviews with ratings of key tasks for frequency, duration, and difficulty; direct observation; videotaping; measurements of masses moved and forces exerted; and identification of pace and frequency. The fidelity of the evaluative tool depends on use of the multiple constructs identified during the job analysis and accurately translating the description into the development of the FCE.

Job Analysis Conclusion

The ability to conduct a thorough job analysis is an essential skill for an occupational therapist working in an

---

BOX 33-3
ADA Terminology

Essential Functions
Fundamental, not marginal job duties. Some considerations in determining whether a function is essential:

▶ Whether the position exists to perform that function
▶ The number of other employees available to perform the function or among whom the function can be distributed
▶ The degree of expertise required
▶ Whether past and/or present employees in the job have performed the function
▶ The time spent performing the function
▶ The consequences of not performing the function

Reasonable Accommodations
Modifications of the work environment, such as job restructuring, providing adaptive or adaptable equipment, and similar modifications to enable equal opportunities for employment by individuals with disabilities.

BOX 33-4
PROCEDURES FOR PRACTICE

Matching Job Analysis With Functional Capacity Evaluation

Job Title: Meat grinder (ground beef, chicken, pork, turkey)
Job Analysis

Tasks	Physical Requirements
1. Load grinder 2. Grind and load meat tubs	Standing, walking, climbing stairs, carrying, lifting, stooping, handling, reaching, grasping
STEPS for task 1	
Remove top from tub of meat	0.5 lb
Place top of tub to the side	Turn and place
Lift tub from stack	Lift 70 lb
Carry tub up stairs	Carry 70 lb 5 ft, climb 3 stairs
Empty meat from tub into grinder	Lift to height of 4.5 ft
Walk down stairs	Climb down 3 stairs
Place empty tub on stack behind grinder	Walk 3 ft
STEPS for task 2	
Retrieve empty tub	Walk 6 ft, weight 1.5 lb
Place tub beneath grinder spigot	Stoop
Turn on grinder	Turn handle, 0.8 lb resistance
Visually supervise grinding	Stand
Guide beef from spigot	Use, handle large metal spoon
Spread beef in tub	Use, handle large metal spoon
Turn off grinder	Turn handle, 0.8 lb resistance
Lift tub	Lift 5 tubs at 28 lb each
Carry tub either up the stairs to reload grinder (repeat steps 4–6 task 1) or to packaging area	See steps 4–6 Carry 5 tubs at 28 lb each 15 ft

Functional Capacity Evaluation Results	FCE Results Match Job Requirements
No limitations standing, walking, climbing, and descending stairs	Yes
Vision: 20/20 with glasses	Yes
Upper extremity reach and manual dexterity within normal limits as measured by Purdue pegboard Grasp: 50 lb	Yes

Lifts
   Single lift to 4-ft height 29 kg
   Repetitive lift to 4 ft height
   One lift every 8 min 20 kg	

From Pentikis, personal communication, December 10, 1993.

industrial setting. However, the prudent therapist conducts a similarly comprehensive analysis of the job of a homemaker, athlete, or child. The instruction received during entry-level training for occupational therapy in task analysis provides an excellent basis for building expertise in job analysis. The one area of job analysis that neither is well-defined nor has a large number of case studies available for guidance is the cognitive, psychological, and social requirements of work.

One important concept is that while the job analysis is part of the evaluation, the results are used to develop the treatment intervention and establish the end goals. In traditional occupational therapy, the treatment intervention and goals are based solely on the evaluation of the client and his or her desires, not on evaluation of the work site and the job demands.

Functional Capacity Assessments

A variety of assessments are available for evaluating work performance, with the majority coming under the classification of an FCE. An FCE is a systematic process designed to assess a client's physical capacities and

Example of Component Tests and Work Simulation for Military Medic Task—Stretcher Carrying

Job Title: Military Medic

Task: Carrying stretcher containing a wounded soldier to and from medical transport vehicles as part of a two-person team

Task Description: Maximal height a stretcher must be lifted is 135 cm, based on ground and air ambulance loading platform heights. Literature review revealed weight of 50th percentile male U.S. army soldier as 78.5 ± 11 kg (Gordon et al., 1989). The stretcher weighed 6.8 kg. When unloading air ambulances, patients must be carried to a ground ambulance, typically approximately 50 m.

Task Components for Functional Capacity Evaluation
1. Lift and lower a box approximately 71 kg to and from a 135-cm height.
2. Perform isometric grip strength test.
3. Run 1 mile in 10 min or perform aerobic treadmill testing.
4. Carry hand-held weights approximately 35.5 kg for 50 m.

Work Simulation for Functional Capacity Evaluation: Soldier walks or runs 50 m on treadmill carrying stretcher holding 88.6-kg mannequin. Soldier dismounts treadmill and walks or runs 5 m to a weight stack machine adjacent to treadmill and lifts weight equal to the patient's load to 135 cm to simulate loading patient into ground or air ambulance. Soldier gets back on treadmill and walks or runs 50 m to retrieve next patient. Treadmill speed is self-paced using toggle switch attached to stretcher handle.

Most FCEs include a review of the client's medical record, an interview that includes a work and educational history and sometimes a self-administered questionnaire, a basic musculoskeletal evaluation, performance evaluations, and a comparison of the findings with the job requirements (Isernhagen, 1995a). As mentioned previously, the two performance categories are a general evaluation of physical abilities and a set of job-specific evaluations. Some therapists include psychosocial aspects; however, this remains more of an exception than the rule unless the individual has specific mental health or neurological concerns. Both the psychosocial and cognitive aspects of FCEs are ripe for exploration, implementation, and research.

General Evaluation of Physical and Cognitive Abilities

Physical and cognitive abilities are evaluated to examine basic functional abilities thought to be common to a number of jobs. The evaluation is conducted to give baseline information and is a special concern when the job to which the individual will return is unknown. The general evaluation of physical abilities may include measures of flexibility, strength, balance, coordination, cardiovascular condition, and body mechanics. It should also include the individual's ability to sit, stand, walk, lift, carry, bend, squat, crawl, climb, reach, stoop, and kneel and any limitations with those activities. Work-related musculoskeletal disorders have become prevalent; therefore, the individual's ability to do particular types of repetitive motions should also be noted. Documentation should specify weight limits, duration of activity tolerance, unambiguous environmental restrictions, and exact side effects of medications. Subjective findings, such as reported degree and frequency of pain, along with any observations (grimacing), should be noted.

Job-Specific Evaluations

The second part of an FCE is job specific. This means that specific work tasks are designed to simulate the critical tasks associated with a specific job or set of jobs (described previously in the job analysis section as either task components or simulations). For example, the city of Calgary, Alberta, has developed a two-part FCE for its firefighters (Calgary Fire Department, 1999). The first portion is a physical fitness evaluation that includes cardiovascular respiratory fitness, muscular endurance, and flexibility. The second portion comprises job-specific tasks, including a tower rope pull, hose line extension, victim drag, ventilation exercise, equipment carry, smoke mask haze, and aerial ladder climb.

Identifying Task Components. **Task component testing** means that the most difficult and important functions of the job are identified and an evaluation or treatment plan is developed using the task components. An

functional abilities. Identification of an individual's capabilities also reveals his or her limitations. The FCE uses information available from traditional occupational therapy and medical evaluations along with performance-based evaluations.

The information gained from an FCE can be used to match the individual's residual capacities with the demands of a specific job, as a basis for establishing work or work site modifications or accommodations, as evidence in the determination of disability or compensation status, and/or as a baseline for noting the physical capabilities of new employees. FCEs can be used in a variety of circumstances, including industrial settings for preemployment and postoffer screenings, clinical settings for setting goal and treatment regimens, and for determining a worker's ability to resume his or her job duties. According to Crowe and Shannon (1997), an FCE can be an essential tool in determining whether a claimant is eligible for Social Security disability benefits.

example of selecting the most difficult essential task is when a person must lift tools weighing 10 pounds and a 50-pound toolbox. The criterion task includes the more difficult of the two tasks on the assumption that a worker who can accomplish the more difficult task is also competent for the lesser one. The criterion tasks, in the form of task components or work simulations, are used because they are believed to predict job performance. It is assumed that testing applicants on single aspects of job performance that are critical to job success is a valid approach to determining work performance, as the content requirements are used (Wigdor & Green, 1991). An example of the development of criterion-referenced tasks using both the task component and work simulation techniques can be seen in Box 33-5.

Work Simulations. **Work simulations** differ from task components in that they replicate essential series of tasks required on a job. For example, a firefighter's task of removing a hose, attaching it to a nozzle, and holding the hose during spraying is one task simulation. The same task series analyzed according to its task components might include only two portions, lifting an item that weighs the same as the hose and pushing a sled whose weight equals the amount of hose pressure. Work simulations frequently involve multiple constructs, such as strength, balance, and agility, and they have more face validity.

Psychosocial Behaviors

Some evaluations include the individual's psychosocial behaviors as they apply to work habits and motivation; however, this is not consistently part of the process. This part of the FCE should describe the client's limitations in comprehension, recall, and ability to follow instructions. Other psychosocial issues, such as ability to handle work pressures, respond to supervision, and relate to coworkers or customers, should also be noted.

Many FCEs use an evaluation called the detection of sincerity of effort, said to be an indication of a client's motivation to perform optimally during an FCE. The belief is that a client who is not sincere may have a less successful recovery or prolonged recovery, overuse treatment, have increased costs of care, and receive unwarranted disability payments (Lechner et al., 1998). In their excellent review article, Lechner et al. reviewed several sincerity-of-effort evaluation methods for reliability and validity. They also examined the concept of using the coefficient of variation in muscle performance tests, the correlation between musculoskeletal evaluations and FCEs. They concluded, "To date, none of the previously discussed methods for detecting sincerity of effort have been adequately studied for its use with clients with LBP" (low back pain). They further state, "Therapists also are advised to avoid reporting

test results as 'valid' or 'invalid' based on perceived levels of cooperation and to avoid using the terms 'symptom magnification' and 'exaggerated pain behavior' to describe client behavior" (Lechner et al., pp. 884, 885).

Since alterations in mood and affect commonly coexist with and exacerbate physical problems, these issues should be included in the assessment. A brief screening tool can be used in conjunction with clinical observations to determine the influence of any psychosocial problems. The *Generalized Contentment Scale* is a quick 25-item paper-and-pencil measure of nonpsychotic depression that is useful in determining the extent of mood alterations associated with loss of the work role (Dorsey Press, 1982). If significant test results are obtained, assistance from psychological services may be indicated.

Selecting a Functional Capacity Evaluation

More than 55 FCEs are available, and selection of an appropriate one can be difficult. They differ in the physical and psychological factors they assess and the way the measures are administered. They also differ in the training required for competency in administration and interpretation. Some use a battery of tests that may or may not be based on a specific task analysis of the job in question. Such a battery may include strength, flexibility, and endurance tests. Others use actual simulations of the tasks required of the job. Few have undergone rigorous examination to determine whether the evaluation predicts actual job performance (Innes & Straker, 1999; Rice, 1999c). Although it may seem easy to select an FCE based on availability of workshops and products or repute, these are unacceptable methods of selecting a tool. However, some good review articles assist with selecting FCEs (Innes & Straker, 1999; King et al., 1998) and preplacement tests (Rice, 1999c). King et al. (1999) reviewed 10 FCEs for their years of availability, format, length of assessment and report, validity and reliability, availability of peer-reviewed published research, standardization of instruction, whether the FCE is norm or criterion referenced, and costs. Innes and Straker (1999) reviewed the test–retest, interrater, intratest, and instrument precision reliability of 28 evaluations. Both articles contain charts that are well worth having as references for selection of evaluations. No single evaluation is likely to suffice in all cases for all clients. Therefore, clinicians should be familiar with various evaluations and select those most suitable for their setting and their clients.

Functional Work Assessments Conclusion

Knowledge of the two primary means of assessment in industrial rehabilitation, job analysis and functional capacity assessment, sets the stage for intervention. Individual clients' goals, work site design alterations, and bringing the capabilities of the worker closer into alignment with the demands of the job are all built on a well-done set of assessments. The practitioner must integrate into the intervention process the detail the assessments provide, and the results of the FCE should be used to indicate a client's potential to work. This information should be clearly communicated to the employer and to the client.

Intervention

Intervention that is specific for returning the individual to the workforce builds upon traditional occupational therapy intervention, taking it a few steps further into the daily work requirements of the client. Throughout intervention, the therapist should maintain communication with the client's work supervisor and iteratively determine the potential for work site modification to match the levels of performance being discovered during the evaluation. These modifications may continue throughout the process, permitting the client to return to a work setting much earlier and encouraging personal identification as a contributing, competent worker.

Work Conditioning

Work conditioning generally follows acute care and precedes work hardening. Like traditional occupational therapy intervention, work conditioning focuses on remediation of underlying physical or cognitive deficits to improve function. The difference between traditional rehabilitation and work conditioning is that the intervention is focused on functional requirements of a job or employment setting rather than on life skills required at home or for recreational activities. Restoration of flexibility, strength, coordination, and endurance may be addressed. Work conditioning should increase physical abilities, engineer successful performance, and provide realistic feedback regarding the client's capabilities (Fig. 33-2). The client's day may include a regimen of warm-up exercises tailored to the activities planned for the day, conditioning exercises based on job requirements, and job-related tasks using work samples that replicate essential task components of a job. A program may begin with sessions of an hour or two and progress as the client–worker's condition improves to 8 hours per day.

Work Hardening

Work hardening is a multidisciplinary structured treatment designed to maximize a client's ability to return to employment. Work hardening includes all aspects required for the client to return to full employment function, such as psychosocial, communication, physical, and vocational needs. While general physical abili-

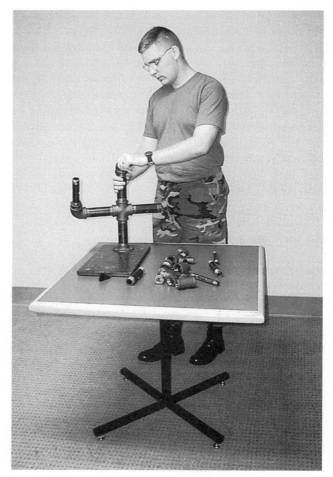

Figure 33-2 Work conditioning using a simulated work task. This is an initial simulation, as the requirements for bending and stooping have not yet been added.

ties are addressed in work conditioning, work hardening is aimed more specifically at a particular job or classification of jobs, so it tends to use work simulation. Considerations added during work hardening include productivity (speed, accuracy, efficiency), safety (ability to adhere to safety principles, use of safety equipment and algorithms), physical tolerances for specific tasks (endurance, ability to carry out the repetitive task requirements), organizational skills, and decision making. The key differences are the use of real or simulated work activities in a graded fashion, building to work over periods comparable with those in actual work settings; the full spectrum of work-related intervention, and the use of a multidisciplinary approach (Isernhagen, 1988). Disciplines included in a work-hardening program can include occupational and physical therapy, psychology, vocational rehabilitation, social work, and social services. Other professionals that may participate full time or as needed include drug and alcohol counselors, nutritionists, and educators (special education or educational evaluators).

Work-hardening environments should replicate the workplace as closely as possible. Sufficient space is needed for both traditional equipment for work conditioning and specialized equipment that may be brought from a job site. Also, the behaviors and interactions required of the clients should replicate a work setting, such as arriving and leaving on a set schedule, working with fixed breaks, having supervisors who give positive and negative feedback on performance, performance standards, and so on. Returning a client to a part-time or full-time light duty assignment during rehabilitation may help the client feel part of the team. It may also assist employers by building their confidence in the process and by letting them observe first-hand the capabilities of the client–worker.

All involved parties should be kept informed of the process. This includes employers, supervisors, insurance representatives, occupational health nurses, and the physician.

Reevaluation of the Client and Program Evaluation

Two types of evaluation should be conducted, and they are intertwined. Individual clients should be reevaluated, and the program as a whole should be evaluated. Monitoring clients' progress and annotating whether they have achieved functional goals should occur as in traditional occupational therapy during clinic-based treatment. However, follow-up evaluations with the client and the client's supervisor are suggested so that in case of a problem the therapist can intervene before reinjury or exacerbation of the injury occurs. In addition, it is important to combine this information (having removed individual identifiers) with that of other clients to determine whether overall program goals are being met. It is important to know whether the program is meeting the needs of individual clients as well as those of the referral sources (employers). Tracking information such as the rate of successful return to work, the length of limited-duty time, and the subjective responses of past clients and their supervisors enables the therapist to improve the program. This information is important for showing the cost–benefit value of the services and should be available if reimbursement questions arise. The same information can be used in marketing strategies.

A Clinical Implementation of the Return-to-Work Process: Brook Army Medical Center

This chapter contains basic information about work-related assessment, intervention through work condi-

tioning and work hardening, and reevaluation of both the individual and the program, along with background information on work motivation, interruption of work, and ways occupational therapists can intervene. Still, the application of this knowledge can be confusing without a framework. Therefore, this section describes a decision pathway and an example of an FCE (Appendix 33-A) in use at Brook Army Medical Center (BAMC), Fort Sam Houston, Texas.

The return-to-work decision pathway shown in Figure 33-3 presents work rehabilitation processes in the larger context of injury, medical management, and acute rehabilitation. As cost containment is a paramount issue in any health care organization, the decision pathway encourages a logical process to return the client to the workforce in a time-efficient manner. As can be seen in Figure 33-3, the decision pathway begins with an interruption of the work process, includes medical and rehabilitative intervention, incorporates the return-to-work process of evaluation and intervention, and offers several junctures at which the client may return to work.

The FCE in Appendix 33-A is composed of measures that are routinely available in most clinical settings (see Resources). Additional tests can be added as available and desired. As the many available off-the-shelf FCEs all have some limitations as well as merits, therapists should be broad-minded in their selection of tools for the FCE. It may be most efficacious for therapists first to develop an understanding of the return-to-work evaluation and intervention process, then develop a structured evaluation system composed of available components that are specific to individual patients and the specific environmental context to which they must return.

The first page of information seen on the BAMC FCE (Appendix 33-A) contains the evaluation of the findings, an explanation of the discrepancies between the job requirements and work performance, and recommendations. This arrangement seems to put the end (the results) at the beginning, before permitting the reader to follow and understand the evaluative process. The format is designed so the "bottom line" is immediately available for the employer and/or client to read. Background information in the form of the evaluative process is then provided as substantiation of the findings.

Each section of the BAMC decision pathway and FCE is explained in the next section. Also refer to the case example, which further demonstrates the use of the BAMC FCE.

Medical Management and Acute Rehabilitation

The return-to-work process begins as soon as a patient enters the medical system for treatment. Medical management (Fig. 33-3) concerns the use of medical and surgical treatment to control and remedy acute medical

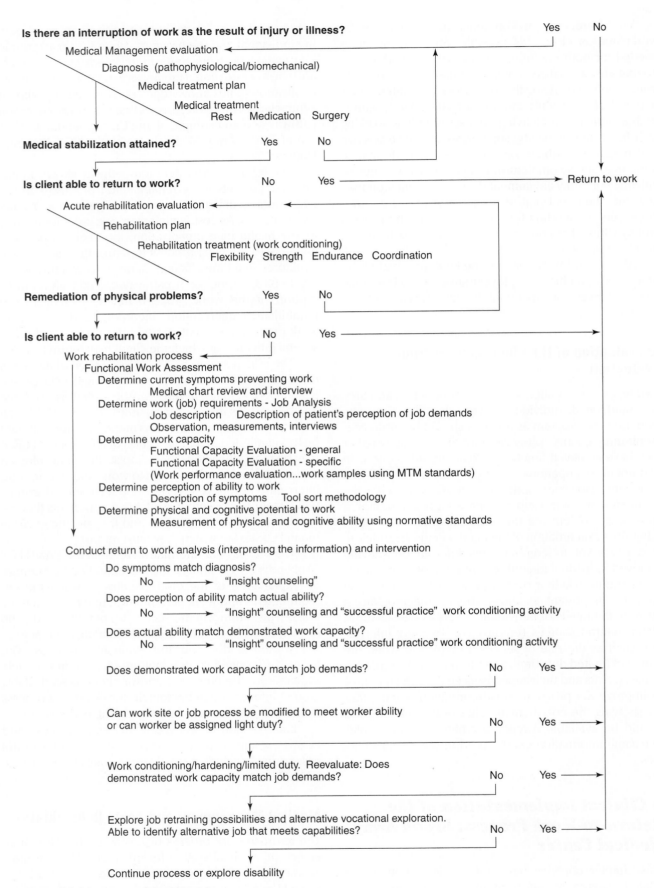

Figure 33-3 Return-to-work decision pathway.

problems that have interrupted the work role. Acute rehabilitation naturally follows medical management when medical problems and their treatments have caused physical debilitation, muscle weakness, impaired joint motion, decreased flexibility and/or coordination, or other limitations. Acute rehabilitation for physical injuries can involve the use of physical agents, exercise, and education to restore abilities impaired by injury, illness, surgery, or enforced inactivity. Both medical management and acute rehabilitation entail evaluation, diagnosis, and procedures to remedy pathological conditions. At the end of each of these processes, a decision as to the potential for the client to return to work must be made. If the client is able and willing to return to work at these junctures, intervention is discontinued. Many clients with minimal residue of injury or illness and high internal motivation return to work without further intervention.

Work Rehabilitation

If medical management and acute rehabilitation do not result in a return-to-work status, efforts focus on the feasibility of returning the client to work. The method to determine return-to-work feasibility is the functional work assessment, which includes general medical information, a job analysis (if the job or type of job is known), an FCE, and an assessment of the client's perceptions of his or her abilities.

In addition to being evaluative, the functional work assessment forms the framework within which the therapist builds intervention strategies to bring about the return to work. The FCE used here can be carried out in seven steps.

Step 1: Preevaluation Information
As indicated in Appendix 33-A, information is recorded about the client's job, along with demographics and information regarding the client's medical condition and symptoms. Details about the job can be obtained though the client's self-report, a written job description, interviews with the employer, and/or an on-site job analysis.

Job Demands
The evaluator seeks to determine the specifics of the job in terms of physical, cognitive, and social demands. Careful review of the job description and interviews with client and supervisor allow the therapist to form a picture of the demands of the job. The therapist may also choose to conduct a job site analysis so that objective measurements and observations can further elucidate the demands. These job demands are key in setting up work samples later in the evaluation.

Medical History and Current Symptoms
In addition to a complete review of the medical record, the client is asked to describe the medical history, including medical treatment, surgery, rehabilitation and time off work. Information about the client's current symptoms is gathered. The grid "Current symptoms relating to work situation" allows the client to describe symptoms and rate them on intensity. Clients are encouraged to state their desired resolutions to the current work-disability situation so as to enable the therapist and client to establish goals jointly. Even though the evaluation is in the early stages, at this point there is usually sufficient information to initiate treatment that can coincide with the continuing evaluation.

The therapist should determine whether the cluster of symptoms presented by the patient matches those usually associated with the diagnosis or disorder. Significant variances between diagnosis and expected symptoms can be a sign of a client being overwhelmed by the situation. At this point the evaluation changes to an intervention called **insight counseling**, a process by which the client is assisted in explaining the discrepancies between conflicting findings. Although a disconnect between diagnosis and symptoms may not be at the client's conscious level, it should be addressed at once. During this intervention it is appropriate to provide the client with additional information about the medical condition and its usual presentation and course in rehabilitation. It is important during this type of low-level confrontation to allow the client a face-saving way out, such as the opportunity to restate or discuss symptoms. The purpose of insight counseling is to help the patient either clarify information or adjust behavior according to new information presented by the therapist. Alignment of symptoms may also help to delineate those who have a well-defined WRMD versus those who may have signs and symptoms of overuse that are not yet at a stage of clinical diagnosis. This process may also assist the client to accept and understand his or her symptoms.

Step 2: Work Performance Measurement
In accordance with the job demands identified in step 1, the therapist determines which of the available work performance measures best simulates the demands of the current or target job. While testing of ability components can be fairly general and applied to many jobs and tasks, if the job to which the client will return is known, the evaluation should be tailored to it. Appendix 33-A has a reporting format for selected work performance measures, including the following:

► Valpar 1: Small tools; fine motor dexterity
► Valpar 4: Upper extremity range of motion; prolonged use of both hands in confined space with awkward angles (Fig. 33-4).

Case Example

SGT. B.: FACILITATING RETURN TO WORK FOR A MAN WITH CHRONIC FIRST DORSAL WRIST COMPARTMENT STENOSING TENOSYNOVITIS

Patient Information

Sgt. B. is a 37-year-old married active-duty soldier. He works as an audiovisual support assistant and has a 2-year history of right-dominant hand radial wrist pain. Sgt. B. was intermittently treated for stenosing tenosynovitis of the first dorsal wrist compartment (de Quervain's disease) during the previous year. Conservative treatment, including activity limitations, limiting wrist motion with a thermoplastic thumb spica-type splint, superficial heat and cold, deep heat using ultrasound, and trials of transcutaneous and percutaneous corticosteroid medication via phonophoresis, iontophoresis, and injection, did not relieve symptoms to a level allowing Sgt. B. to work at full capacity. About 6 weeks prior to referral for FCE, Sgt. B. underwent a surgical procedure to release the right first dorsal wrist compartment. The surgery and postoperative recovery period were unremarkable. By postoperative week 6, however, Sgt. B. could not return to work because of continued pain in the radial wrist during job-specific tasks. His superior officer referred Sgt. B. to occupational health services, and Sgt. B. was subsequently referred to occupational therapy for FCE and recommendations for return to duty.

Description of Assessment

The task for the occupational therapist was to discover the reason this medical condition continued to limit Sgt. B.'s ability to return to full duty and whether remediation of symptoms could permit Sgt. B. to return to work. Necessary information included Sgt. B.'s medical history, continuing symptoms, and the requirements of the target job. This information would be combined with observations of sample job performance, queries of Sgt. B.'s perception of his ability to work, and measurement of physical and cognitive abilities.

A review of Sgt. B.'s medical record and results of an initial interview revealed that he was in reasonable health and excluding de Quervain's tendonitis, was without significant pathological medical history. Sgt. B. had not been working for a total of 8 weeks, including the postoperative phase of his treatment. He was now back to work and on unofficial light duty status administered by the good graces of his supervisor.

Sgt. B. gave the therapist a specific listing of job tasks that included infrequent lifting and carrying of 50-pound items and fairly frequent lifting of approximately 25-pound objects. As part of his additional duties, Sgt. B. was required to lift with one hand and carry a flagpole base weighing 17 pounds. The lift and carry were usually done with the right wrist slightly flexed and in radial deviation. Aspects of Sgt. B.'s job description were verified by review of his written job description, an interview with his supervisor, and on-site observation.

Sgt. B. stated that any use of his right hand caused wrist pain. He could perform all basic and instrumental activities of daily living but could not perform his job except for answering the phone and doing paperwork. He stated that it had taken "the doctors" 2 years to figure out his problem and the surgery had not fixed it. When asked about his desired outcome, he replied that he needed either to be trained for another kind of job or receive disability for this work-related injury.

Based on his job demands, the occupational therapist decided to use the Valpar 1 (small tools), Valpar 9 (whole-body range of motion), and Valpar 19 (dynamic physical capacity) to sample Sgt. B.'s actual work performance. Sgt. B. performed at the MTM rate of 95% on the Valpar 1, 90% on the Valpar 9, and 78% on the Valpar 19. Work performance on the Valpar 1 and 9 met competitive work standards; performance on the Valpar19 was below competitive work standards.

The occupational therapist gathered subjective and objective data about Sgt. B.'s abilities to examine the possible causes of the discrepancy between his abilities and the test and job demands. The *Loma Linda Activity Sort (LLAS)* and the *West Tool Sort (WTS)* allowed Sgt. B. to express his perceptions of his ability to use common tools in work and leisure. Results of these two sorts revealed that he perceived he could use 77% of the tool tasks in the *LLAS* at normal or subnormal rates and intensity (categories A, B and C); 33% of the *LLAS* tool tasks were rated as unusable in his present condition. Also, 84% of the *WTS* tools tasks were reported in the A, B and C categories, with 16% in the unusable category. (The *LLAS* consists of leisure, lighter, and less strenuous use tools, while the *WTS* represents heavier and industrial tool tasks.) Many of the tools in both categories reported as not usable did not fall into the work domains usually associated with hand and wrist pain.

Measurement of physical abilities revealed the following results. Body range of motion and ability to maintain static postures were within normal range. Hand sensation was normal. Three of the seven subtests on the *Jebsen Taylor Hand Test* were greater than two standard deviations below the mean. Static isometric strength testing using the *BTE* indicated that the right arm was below the first percentile, while the left arm showed average strength ratings at the 60th percentile. Lifting, pushing, and pulling ability of both arms using the *BTE* dynamic lift tests was below the first percentile. The general contentment scale score was 62; scores above 60 are significant for possible depression. Cognitive performance as measured by the decision-making test was at the 10th percentile. Physical endurance using the step test was three standard deviations below the mean for age group, indicating debilitation, possibly secondary to inactivity.

At no time during the evaluation did Sgt. B. appear to be exerting himself to the full extent of his ability, as would be evidenced in concentrated facial expression, sweating, or grimacing with effort. At no time did he express pain or appear to be in pain.

Analysis of Results

The severity of Sgt. B.'s symptoms did not match the expected response to surgical treatment and recovery for de Quervain's disease. Sgt. B.'s perception of his performance ability did not match the severity of his reported symptoms but did match measurement of physical and cognitive abilities. Work sample performance was greater than would be expected from the evaluation of his physical abilities. Finally, sample work performance did not fully meet target job requirements.

The occupational therapist's interpretation of evaluation findings was that the mismatches between diagnosis and symptoms, symptoms and abilities, and abilities and performance fit a pattern of psychological overlay that limited the application of ability to work performance. Combined with this situation was a general physical debilitation from several months of inactivity. The duration of his symptoms and perceived slow postoperative recovery were no doubt influencing symptom intensity and were limiting his willingness to exert full effort during ability testing. At the time of testing he did not appear ready or willing to return to full duty.

Recommendations

The occupational therapist interpreted his potential for return to work as moderate and recommended that Sgt. B. participate in a work rehabilitation program. Skillful application of physical and psychosocial therapeutic interventions would be required to meet the long-term goal of return to full-time work, and Sgt. B.'s perceptions regarding his ability and performance would probably have to change to restore Sgt. B.'s work role competency.

Short-Term Goals

In 1 month, Sgt. B. will be able to do the following:

▶ Use principles of body mechanics, energy conservation, and work simplification to perform work simulations
▶ Improve his endurance and work tolerance so that he can use his right hand and wrist during work activities
▶ Problem-solve with the therapist regarding necessary adaptations to work task and work area

Occupational Therapy Intervention

Here is a summary of Sgt. B.'s formal work rehabilitation.

▶ The results of the test data were reviewed with Sgt. B. and he was encouraged to explore and explain the variances in the data. Selective retesting (requested by Sgt. B. and agreed upon by the therapist) allowed Sgt. B. to clarify conflicts in data and demonstrate higher performance levels.
▶ The therapist provided several lessons on anatomy, pathophysiology, and wound healing, which related to Sgt. B.'s surgical procedure. A focal point was that wound healing is a multiple-month process and that some pain during that process is normal.

▶ Based on recommendations from the FCE, the referring physician assigned Sgt. B. to an official light-duty status that specified physical demand limitations with Sgt. B. participating in work in accordance with FCE results.
▶ Sgt. B. participated in daily 1-hour work conditioning treatment activities with emphasis on regaining physical endurance and progressive use of the right hand and wrist during work activities. A secondary purpose was to arrange for progressive successful work experiences so Sgt. B. began to habituate a positive work role.
▶ Sgt. B. was provided training in body mechanics, energy conservation, and work simplification, especially as they related to his FCE results and the demands of his job.
▶ A formal work site and job analysis provided the work site supervisor with sufficient information to modify task and pace to match Sgt. B.'s abilities.
▶ The occupational therapist fabricated an ergonomic tool adaptation to correct the identified injury-producing task. This modification corrected the extreme hand posture of radial deviation, allowing a more neutral posture. The device was adopted shopwide in Sgt. B.'s work area.
▶ Following 1 month of work conditioning, Sgt. B. completed a partial FCE. Testing with the Valpar work samples indicated ability to work at target job standards. Sgt. B. subsequently returned to full duty.

Addendum

At no time during the evaluation or intervention phases of Sgt. B.'s participation in the return-to-work process was there any attempt to confront, catch, or expose his psychological issues. The therapist was careful to remain neutral and request only that he try to explain the variances in the data. Sgt. B. was always given wiggle room and face-saving avenues in all interactions. Over the course of the rehabilitation, the combination of education, nonjudgmental interactions, and successful repetitive work experience encouraged Sgt. B. to choose to alter his perceptions of ability and performance and regain work role competency.

CLINICAL REASONING in Work Rehabilitation

Wrist pain was the dominant feature in Sgt. B.'s inability to return to work. At the time of the evaluation, Sgt. B. was 6 weeks post surgery from a right first dorsal wrist compartment release and still complaining of significant wrist pain with work-related activities. At that time, Sgt. B.'s surgical wound was most probably at the end of the second stage of healing (proliferation) or early in the third stage (scar maturation). Conventional wisdom regarding soft tissue wound healing holds that the third and last phase may continue 9 months or longer.

▶ How should the therapist interpret Sgt. B.'s emphasis on wrist pain? Is it real or enhanced?
▶ Should Sgt. B. have been given a longer period of protection from work stressors following the surgery?
▶ What is a possible consequence of an extended recuperation period?

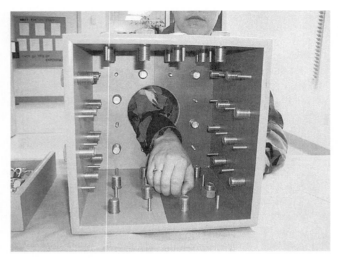

Figure 33-4 Valpar 4. Upper extremity range of motion work sample.

▶ Valpar 9: Whole-body range of motion; reaching, bending, and stooping while using hands
▶ Valpar 19: Dynamic physical capacities; reaching, lifting, reading, decision making, following directions (Fig. 33-5)

Methods Time Measurement (MTM) scoring criteria are used with all of these work performance measurements (Valpar International Corp., 1992). MTM compares work sample performance against an engineered standard that relates to competitive performance rather than to normative data. The standards were developed by an engineering company and are designed to mimic the real pace of work rather than the burst activity common to testing. MTM grades performance in a percent rate of work from 0 to 150%. The percent rate of work is scaled against the following competitive work standards:

▶ Performance exceeding work standards
▶ Performance meeting work standards
▶ Performance below work standards with potential to meet standard
▶ Performance below work standard with minimal potential to reach standard

MTM can at first be confusing to clinicians accustomed to using only standard normative data, but it is essential for the therapist to understand it for proper analysis of work performance measurement data and to explain the results to the client and employer.

In the event that the client's work sample performance falls below competitive standards, steps 3 and 4 of the evaluation are used to discover the deficits responsible for the impaired work performance. Deficient work performance is generally the result of disconnects between job demands, internal motivation based on perception of ability, and/or performance and ability levels. If, however, demonstrated work performance on job-specific work samples meets the competitive standards, steps 3 and 4 can be omitted and the therapist can proceed to data analysis and recommendations.

Step 3: Client's Perception of Ability to Work

Appendix 33-A shows two methods for gathering information regarding clients' perception of their abilities. The West Tool Sort (Fig. 33-6) and the Loma Linda Activity Sort (Work Evaluation Systems Technology, 1984) use card sorting. The client views 65 picture cards of tools and activities and sorts them into four categories based on his or her perception of ability to use the tools or perform the activities. The categories:

▶ "I would have no change in the speed at which I work."
▶ "I would have a decrease in the speed at which I work."
▶ "I would be unable to continue work without an extra break."
▶ "I would be unable to work."

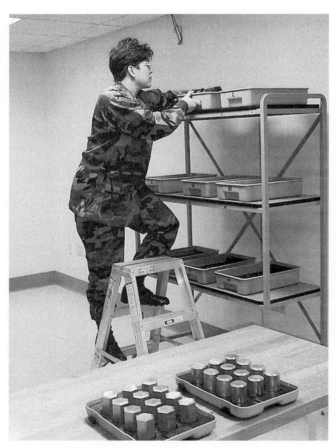

Figure 33-5 Valpar 19. Work dynamic physical capacities sample.

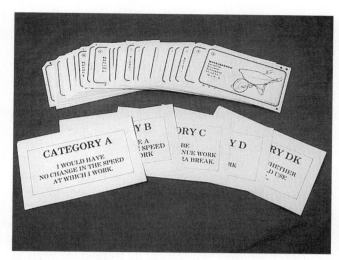

Figure 33-6 West Tool Sort Evaluation of patient's perception of ability to perform work tasks.

Card sort results can be analyzed in depth and compared with 28 work category domains as an aid in determining the match of symptoms to perceived performance. The second method of gaining the client's perception of ability is a self-rating of performance on a variety of common work tasks. Careful analysis of card sort results and self-reports of ability give important information about the client's perception of his or her ability and how this may either hinder or help with the return-to-work process.

Step 4: Ability Measurement

Appendix 33-A incorporates tests and measures of ability, including body range of motion; static posture tolerance; hand sensation and dexterity; extremity strength; lifting, pushing, and pulling strength; physical endurance; mood and affect; and cognitive problem solving. These are tests of general abilities that may affect an individual's capabilities at a number of jobs, rather than being tailored to any particular job or set of tasks. Examples:

▶ Body range of motion, assessed by observing functional movements of the trunk and extremities to include reaching, touching hands to back of neck and middle of back, and bending or stooping toward the floor.
▶ Tolerance to the static postures of sitting and standing, observed and documented as the client performs other components of testing that require sitting or standing for extended periods.
▶ Physical strength, documented using both static strength and dynamic lift tests. A device such as the work simulator (Baltimore Therapeutic Equipment Co., 1992) can accomplish both static and dynamic

lifting tests and allow comparison of strength between body sides and comparison against normative standards (Fig. 33-7).
▶ Physical endurance, using either a step test (Tuxworth & Shanawaz, 1977) or treadmill testing if available. Before any strength or physical endurance testing, it is essential to ensure that the patient's medical record has been reviewed and the referring physician has given clearance for physical testing.
▶ Hand dexterity and function, using any of a number of tests. The *Jebsen-Taylor Hand Function Test* is a standard in most clinical settings and can rapidly gather information on hand function using common objects rather than pegs or pins (Jebsen et al., 1969).
▶ Mood and affect; alterations can exacerbate physical problems. This aspect of function should therefore be included in the assessment. A brief screening tool can be used in conjunction with clinical observations to determine any potential psychosocial problems. (See previous discussion of the *Generalized Contentment Scale.*) If significant findings are obtained, assistance from psychological services may be indicated.
▶ Cognition, tested to determine whether difficulties with attention, memory, vision, reading skills, and problem solving are contributing to work deficits. The *Allen Cognitive Level Screening* (Allen et al., 1992) is a leatherwork completion task that can provide a wealth of information regarding cognitive functioning. In addition, the *PSI Decision Making Test* is a 5-minute standardized paper-and-pencil test measuring attention, immediate memory, reading, and judgment (Ruch et al., 1981). Either or both of these tests can give the evaluator a general idea of cognitive function and help in determining whether further specialized testing is indicated.

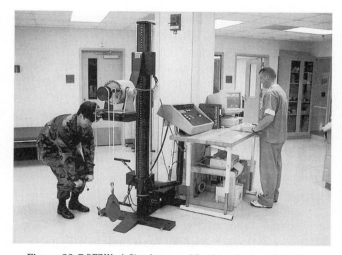

Figure 33-7 *BTE* Work Simulator used for dynamic strength testing.

Step 5: Summarize Test Data

The complexity of work demands and human behavior requires that therapists approach evaluation and intervention in a structured manner. If a structured approach is not used, there is a risk of being overwhelmed by the sheer amount of data or by the difficulties inherent in multifaceted behavioral interventions. To help manage information and use it as the basis for analysis, treatment, and recommendations, the BAMC FCE uses grids for summarizing and recording perception of ability, actual ability, and performance and work data. The evaluator summarizes observations from the tests and converts raw data to standard scores using either normative or MTM criteria. Completion of this section begins to paint a comprehensive picture of the patient's perceptions, abilities, and demonstrated performance in sample work situations. This information is the basis for the analysis in step 6.

Step 6: Analyze Findings

Under Assessment of Evaluation Findings, Appendix 33-A shows the variables to be considered in analyzing the results of test data. The first opinion relates to the quality of the FCE. Was this an incomplete or invalid evaluation, and if so, why did the therapist perceive it as such? The therapist annotates the client's demonstrated work performance to the job requirements on the Department of Labor Physical Demand Characteristics chart (United States Employment Service Dictionary of Occupational Titles). If work performance in sample testing does not meet competitive standards of job requirements, the therapist explains the difference in terms of the client's abilities and/or motivation. In essence, this is a return-to-work equation involving several variables. The therapist must look for matches and disconnects in the data collected during the evaluation to present a meaningful analysis and recommendations.

1. The first match is between the diagnosis and symptoms. A given diagnosis usually results in a constellation of symptoms. The therapist must decide whether the symptoms match the diagnosis.
2. The next match is the agreement between the symptoms and the client's perception of his or her ability to work as expressed in the card sort. An example of a disconnect is for the client to report hand paresthesias but not to indicate problems with precision tools on the card sort.
3. Next is assessment of the degree of agreement between the client's perception of ability to work and his or her demonstrated physical and cognitive abilities (potential to work). Examples of disconnects include the client who indicates inability to use heavy tools on the card sort but shows above-normal strength and endurance during physical testing.
4. The therapist compares the client's physical and cognitive abilities (potential to work) with actual work performance demonstrated during work simulations or task component testing to determine the level of agreement. Demonstrated physical and cognitive abilities should be close to those demonstrated during performance of work samples.

The analysis in this section is the basis for flowing the evaluation process seamlessly into treatment. Problems in incorrect perception can be addressed through insight counseling and education about the pathophysiological aspects of the injury or disorder and expected course of recovery. Education in techniques such as joint protection, energy conservation, and body mechanics can increase the patient's ability to deal with symptoms and limitations. Instruction in movement and stretching exercises can provide further skills for managing symptoms and limitations. Work conditioning can be initiated. Work conditioning using work samples can increase physical abilities, engineer successful performance, help the client to recognize his or her abilities, and assist the client to develop realistic goals.

Step 7: Recommendations

Appendix 33-A incorporates recommendation statements that can be supported from the information gathered in steps 1 to 4, summarized in step 5, and analyzed in step 6. The first section of recommendations concerns the client who can return to either full duty or limited or light duty. The referring physician may well use evaluation recommendations to determine the parameters of light duty, so it is important to base the definition of the limits of light duty on the results of test data and to include what the individual can do as well as what he or she cannot do. The recommendations section also addresses clients who are not ready to return to work but who may be brought to work standards with interventions such as education or work conditioning and hardening. Finally, for clients who do not appear to have the potential to return to target-level work or the preinjury job, the practitioner may recommend prevocational testing and vocational exploration of jobs within the client's physical demand capability.

Specialized Occupational Therapy Practice

Return-to-work evaluation and therapeutic intervention are complicated yet fascinating and rewarding. Work-oriented therapy, also known as industrial therapy, pushes the envelope of professional practice by demanding the blending of expert skill in assessment and data gathering with clinical reasoning and behavioral treatment. Applying occupational therapy skills and knowledge to the process is equally challenging because of the necessity of using physical and biomechanical knowledge along with cognitive and psychosocial knowledge. One particular benefit of practicing in the return-to-work field is being able to see the results of therapeutic efforts beyond those seen when practicing exclusively within the confines of a clinic.

Although the core of occupational therapy practice can be used as a basis for work rehabilitation and following step-by-step procedures should greatly increase the probability of seamlessly moving clients through the return-to-work process, this is considered to be a practice area that requires specialization. Therapists who specialize in return-to-work rehabilitation must develop observational and communication skills that are clearly understood by the client–worker, the supervisor, the insurance representative, and medical professionals. They must become comfortable in the work settings of their clients, just as they are comfortable in clinic settings.

Return-to-work rehabilitation programs that use a comprehensive multidisciplinary approach provide an improved service to clients, as guiding clients through the medical and rehabilitation processes without abandoning them along the way to fend for themselves in their quest to return to meaningful employment. Instead, the needs of both client and employer are addressed, one by one, until the client is a client no more, having once again become a worker and a valued contributing member of the workforce and of society.

Summary Review Questions

1. List four reasons people work and explain how each might affect their ability to return to work.
2. Describe the unique contributions of occupational therapy to the return-to-work process.
3. Describe how job analysis is used in both the evaluation and treatment phases of the return-to-work process.
4. Describe other potential uses for the results gained from a job analysis.
5. Compare and contrast the two types of performance evaluation suggested in a FCE.
6. Using the job grocery store clerk and scanning, keying, and bagging as the essential tasks, write a brief description of a treatment program based on task components and a description of a treatment program based on work simulation.

7. Use the return-to-work decision pathway to develop an evaluation plan for a 42-year-old diabetic who has intermittent retinal bleeding (loss of sight) and who has recently lost his job as a computer systems analyst.

Resources

Work Evaluation Equipment · Baltimore Therapeutic Equipment Co., 7455-L New Ridge Road, Hanover, MD 21076. 410-850-0333. www.bteco.com

Valpar International Corporation · P. O. Box 5767, Tucson, AZ 85703. 800-528-7070. www.valparint.com

References

Alexander, D. (Ed.) (1999). *Applied Ergonomics Case Studies*. Atlanta: Engineering and Management.

Allen, C., Earhart, C., & Blue, T. (1992). *Occupational Therapy Treatment Goals for the Physically and Cognitively Disabled*. Rockville, MD: American Occupational Therapy Association.

Americans with Disabilities Act (July 26, 1990). Public Law 101–336.

ADA Title I Regulations (1991). 29 CFR §1630.01 et seq. and appendix.

Baltimore Therapeutic Equipment Co. (1992). *BTE Work Simulator Operator's Manual*. Hanover, MD: Author.

Bloswick, D. S., Jefferies, D. C., Brakefield, S., & Dumas, M. (1998). Industrial setting case study: Ergonomics and Title I of the Americans with Disabilities Act. In V. Rice (Ed.) *Ergonomics in Health Care and Rehabilitation* (pp 307–334). Boston: Butterworth-Heinneman.

Burwash, S. C. (1999). A teaching model for work practice in occupational therapy. *Work, 12*, 133–137.

Calgary Fire Department (1999). http://www.gov.calgary.ab.ca/fire/.

Christiansen, C. H. (1999). Defining lives: Occupation as identity: An essay on competence, coherence, and the creation of meaning. 1999 Eleanor Clarke Slagle lecture. *American Journal of Occupational Therapy, 52*, 547–558.

Committee on Installations and Advice (1928). Analysis of crafts. *Archives of Occupational Therapy, 6*, 417–421.

Crowe & Shannon Social Security Law Group (1997). *The Nuts and Bolts of Functional Capacity Evaluations*. http://www.crowe-shanahan.com/capacity2.html.

Debats, D. L., Drost, J., & Hansen, P. (1995). Experiences of meaning in life: A combined qualitative and quantitative approach. *British Journal of Psychology, 86* (3), 359–375.

Dorsey Press (1982). The Generalized Contentment Scale. In *The Clinical Measurement Package*. Homewood, IL: Author.

Ellexson, M. (1997). Job analysis and work-site assessment. In M. Sanders (Ed.) *Management of Cumulative Trauma Disorders* (pp 195–213). Boston: Butterworth-Heinneman.

Equal Employment Opportunity Commission. (1992). *A Technical Assistance Manual on the Employment Provisions (Title I) of the Americans with Disabilities Act*. Washington: Author.

Federal Register (July 26, 1991). Part V: Equal Employment Opportunity Commission 29 CFR part 1630, *Equal Employment Opportunity for Individuals with Disabilities*; Final Rule (p 357336).

Frankl, V. (1984). *Man's Search for Meaning*. New York: Touchstone.

Hendrick, H. (1998). Macroergonomics: A systems approach for dramatically improving occupational health, safety and productivity. In S. Kumar (Ed.), *Advances in Occupational Ergonomics and Safety* (p. 26). Philadelphia: Taylor & Francis.

Innes, E., & Straker, L. (1999). Reliability of work-related assessments. *Work, 13*, 102–124.

Isernhagen, S. J. (1988). *Work Injury*. Rockville, MD: Aspen.

Isernhagen, S. J. (Ed.). (1995a). *The Comprehensive Guide to Work Injury Management*. Gaithersburg, MD: Aspen.

Isernhagen, S. J. (1995b). Job analysis. In S. J. Isernhagen (Ed.), *The Comprehensive Guide to Work Injury Management* (pp. 70–85). Gaithersburg, MD: Aspen.

Jastrzebowski, W. (1857). *An Outline of Ergonomics, or the Science of Work Based Upon the Truths Drawn From the Science of Nature.* Warsaw: Central Institute for Labor Protection, 1997. T Baluk-Ulewiczowa (trans).

Jebsen, R. H., Taylor, N., Trotter, M. J., & Howard, L. A. (1969). An objective and standardized test of hand function. *Archives of Physical Medicine and Rehabilitation, 50*, 311.

Karwowski, W., & Marras, W. S. (Eds.). (1999). *The Occupational Ergonomics Handbook*. New York: CRC.

King, P. M., Tuckwell, N., & Barrett, T. E. (1998). A critical review of functional capacity evaluations. *Physical Therapy, 78* (8), 852–866.

Kornblau, B. (1998a). Health care ergonomics and the Americans with Disabilities Act: An introduction. In V. Rice (Ed.). *Ergonomics in Health Care and Rehabilitation* (pp 287–294). Boston: Butterworth-Heinneman.

Kornblau, B. (1998b). The Americans with Disabilities Act: Legal ramifications of ADA consultation. In V. Rice (Ed.) *Ergonomics in Health Care and Rehabilitation* (pp 295–306). Boston: Butterworth-Heinneman.

Kuorinka, I., Hagberg, M., Silverstein, B., Smith, M., Forcier, L., Perusse, M., Welb, R., & Hendrick, H. (Eds.). (1995). *Work Related Musculoskeletal Disorders (WMSDs): A Reference Book for Prevention*. Philadelphia: Taylor & Francis.

Law, M., Baptiste, S., Carswell, A., McColl, M. A., Polatajko, H., & Pollock, N. (1994). *Canadian Occupational Performance Measure (2nd ed.).* Toronto: Canadian Association of Occupational Therapists.

Lechner, D. E., Bradbury, S. F., & Bradley, L. A. (1998). Detecting sincerity of effort: A summary of methods and approaches. *Physical Therapy, 78*(8), 867–888.

Marcus, H., & Nurius, P. S. (1986). Possible selves. *American Psychologist, 41*, 954–969.

Mattingly, C. (1991). The narrative nature of clinical reasoning. *American Journal of Occupational Therapy, 45*, 998–1005.

Meyer, A. (1922). The philosophy of occupational therapy. *Archives of Occupational Therapy, 1*, 1–10.

Moore, S. L. (1997). A phenomenological study of meaning in life in suicidal older adults. *Archives of Psychiatric Nursing, 11* (1), 29–36.

National Commission for Disease Control and Prevention (2000). Healthy People 2000 Review 1997. Summary: Public Health Service, National Center for Health Statistics, Center for Disease Control and Prevention, Hyattsville, Md. http://www.cdc.gov/nchs/data/hp2k97/pdf.

Neistadt, M. E. (1995). Methods of assessing clients' priorities: A survey of adult physical dysfunction settings. *American Journal of Occupational Therapy, 49*, 428–436.

Pulat, B. M., & Alexander, D. C. (Eds.) (1992). *Industrial Ergonomics: Case Studies*. New York: McGraw-Hill.

Raven, M. (1999). http://www.artrans.com/rmsg/megsed/3rd.htm.

Committee on Installations and Advice (1928). Analysis of crafts. *Archives of Occupational Therapy, 6*, 417–421.

Rice, V. (Ed.) (1998). *Ergonomics in Health Care and Rehabilitation*. Boston: Butterworth-Heinemann.

Rice, V. (1999a). Ergonomics and therapy: An introduction. In K. Jacobs (Ed) *Ergonomics for Therapists* (pp. 4–19). Boston: Butterworth-Heinemann.

Rice, V. (1999b). Preplacement strength testing. In W. Karwowski & W. S. Marras (Eds.), *Occupational Ergonomics* (1299–1319). Washington: CRC.

Rice, V. J. (1999c). Pre-placement strength screening. In W. Karwowski & W. Marras (Eds.). *The Industrial Ergonomics Handbook* (pp. 1299–1319). Washington, DC: CRC Press.

Rogers, S. (Ed.) (1983). *Ergonomic Design for People at Work* (Vol. I and II). New York: Van Nostrand.

Rogers, S. (1992). A functional job analysis technique in ergonomics. In J. S. Moore & A. Garg (Eds.), *State of the Art Review* (Vol 7, no. 4, pp. 679–711). Philadelphia: Hunley & Belfus.

Ross, S. (December 17, 1999). HistoryChannel.Com, Associated Press. 10:26 AM Eastern Standard Time.

Ruch, W. W., Shub, S. M., Moinat, & Dye, D. A. (1981) Decision Making (part of) PSI Basic Skills Test for Business, Industry and Government. Glendale, CA: Psychological Services.

Samson, S. T., Yeats, M., & Walsh, A. E. (1999). A single case study: Striving for stability and work: "It's a real bastard of a disease." *Work, 12*, 151–157.

Sanders, M. (Ed.) (1997). *Management of Cumulative Trauma Disorders*. Boston: Butterworth-Heinemann.

Swann, W. B. (1987). Identity negotiation: Where two roads meet. *Journal of Personality and Social Psychology, 53*, 1038–1051.

Swann, W. B., & Hill, C. A. (1982). When our identities are mistaken: Reaffirming self-conceptions through social interaction. *Journal of Personality and Social Psychology, 43*, 59–66.

Terkel, S. (1984). *Working: People Talk About What They Do All Day and How They Feel About What They Do*. New York: Pantheon.

Tuxworth, W., & Shanawaz, H. (1977). The design and evaluation of a step test for the rapid prediction of physical work capacity in an unsophisticated industrial work force. *Ergonomics, 20* (2), 181–191.

Valpar International Corp. (1992). Valpar Work Sample Administration Manual (pp. 2–3). Tucson: Author.

Van Selm, M., & Dittmann-Hohli, F. (1998). Meaninglessness in the second half of life: The development of a construct. *International Journal of Aging and Human Development, 47* (2), 81–104.

Work Evaluation Systems Technology. (1984). 1950 Freeman Avenue, Long Beach, California 90804.

White, R. W. (1971). The urge toward competence. *American Journal of Occupational Therapy, 25*, 271–274.

Wigdor, A. K., & Green, B. F. (1991). *Performance Assessment for the Workplace*. Washington: National Academy.

Yelin, E. (1999). Measuring functional capacity of persons with disabilities in light of emerging demands in the workplace. In *Summary of a Workshop: Measuring Functional Capacity and Work Requirements*. Division of Health Care Services, Institute of Medicine and Committee on National Statistics, Commission on Behavioral and Social Sciences and Education, National Research Council. http://stills.nap.edu/readingroom/books/mfc/.

Appendix: Functional Capacity Evaluation Used at Brook Army Medical Center (Fort Sam Houston, Texas)

FUNCTIONAL CAPACITY EVALUATION
OCCUPATIONAL THERAPY SERVICE

Note: Patient has been medically evaluated and cleared for Functional Capacity Evaluation by _____

- **Evaluation Initiated (Date)** _____   **Completed (Date)** _____
- **Evaluation Conducted by:** _____

Patient/Client Name _____

ASSESSMENT of EVALUATION FINDINGS

____ **Incomplete and/or invalid evaluation**

____ Insufficient information to determine physical and/or work capacity
____ Patient refused to participate or complete evaluation process
____ Patient's symptoms prevented active participation in complete evaluation process

____ **Successful demonstration of work performance**

Department of Labor Physical Demands of Work Level

Job requirement		Demonstrated performance
	Less than sedentary—Infrequent lifting <2 lb, minimal walking, no carrying	
	Sedentary—Infrequent lifting of 10 lb or less, no sustained walking or carrying	
	Sedentary-Light—Infrequent lifting of 15 lb, frequent lifting of 10 lb or less, intermittent self-paced no-load walking	
	Light—Infrequent lifting of 20 lb, frequent lifting of 10 lb or less, no grade slow speed 10-lb load carry/walking	
	Light-Medium—Infrequent lifting of 35 lb, frequent lifting of 20 lb or less, no grade slow speed 20-lb load carry/walking	
	Medium—Infrequent lifting of 50 lb, frequent lifting of 25 lb or less, no grade slow speed 25-lb load carry/walking	
	Medium-Heavy—Infrequent lifting of 75 lb, frequent lifting of 35 lb or less, no grade slow speed 35-lb load carry/walking	
	Heavy—Infrequent lifting of 100 lb, frequent lifting of 50 lb or less, slow speed 50-lb load carry/walking	
	Verv-Heavy—Infrequent lifting in excess of 100 lb, frequent lifting of 50 to 100 lb, slow speed 50-lb load carry/walking	

Factors explaining discrepancies between job requirements and work performance

____ Suboptimal voluntary effort in testing
____ Discrepancies between diagnosis and symptoms presented
____ Discrepancies between patient's perception of ability and actual ability

____ Limited physical abilities
____ Joint motion/flexibility   ____ Strength
____ Physical endurance
____ Hand sensation   ____ Hand dexterity
____ Limitations in psychosocial abilities
            ____ Mood/affect   ____ Cognition   ____ Pain tolerance

Additional comments and explanations _____

RECOMMENDATIONS

____ **Perform target job at full capacity**
____ **Demonstrated work capacity matches job requirements**
____ **Perform target job with limits or light duty**
    ____ Full time
    ____ Part time ____ hr/day ____ days/week

Current "Safe" performance recommendations
    • Maximum infrequent (<1 lift/hr in optimal position/conditions) limitations calculated
    at 60% of maximum demonstrated lift

Two hand floor to thigh level	____#
Two hand thigh to shoulder level	____#
Two hand shoulder to overhead	____#
Push (waist level)	____#
Pull (waist level)	____#
Overhead pull	____#

• Sit	____Unlimited	____ Limit to _____
• Stand	____Unlimited	____ Limit to _____
• Walk	____Unlimited	____ Limit to _____
• Bend/stoop	____Unlimited	____ Limit to _____
• Reach overhead	____Unlimited	____ Limit to _____
• Precision tools	____Unlimited	____ Limit to _____
• Hand/power tools	____Unlimited	____ Limit to _____

Other _____

_____

_____

____ **Work Site Modification**—Ergonomic work site evaluation with recommendations for job
pace/process or equipment modification
____ **Work Conditioning**—Structured, supervised work activity

____ **Retest Functional Capacity** _____

BACKGROUND INFORMATION

Age _____ **Sex** _____ **Hand dominance** _____

Current Employment ____ Full time ____ Part time ____ Days/week

____ Hr/day ____ Full duty ____ Light duty ____ Not employed

Job Title _____

Essential tasks of current or target job (Key physical and cognitive tasks)

Mark "best fit" rating of current job physical demands

	Less than sedentary—Infrequent lifting <2 lb, minimal walking, no carrying
	Sedentary—Infrequent lifting of 10 lb or less, no sustained walking or carrying
	Sedentary-Light—Infrequent lifting of 15 lb, frequent lifting of 10 lb or less, intermittent self-paced no-load walking
	Light—Infrequent lifting of 20 lb, frequent lifting of 10 lb or less, no grade slow speed 10-lb load carry/walking
	Light-Medium—Infrequent lifting of 35 lb, frequent lifting of 20 lb or less, no grade slow speed 20-lb load carry/walking
	Medium—Infrequent lifting of 50 lb, frequent lifting of 25 lb or less, no grade slow speed 25-lb load carry/walking
	Medium-Heavy—Infrequent lifting of 75 lb, frequent lifting of 35 lb or less, no grade slow speed 35-lb load carry/walking
	Heavy—Infrequent lifting of 100 lb, frequent lifting of 50 lb or less, slow speed 50-lb load carry/walking
	Very-Heavy—Infrequent lifting in excess of 100 lb, frequent lifting of 50 to 100 lb, slow speed 50-lb load carry/walking

Medical Condition

Diagnosis related to work deficit _____

Concurrent medical conditions _____

Time off work _____

Surgery and medical treatment _____

Current symptoms relating to work situation
Rated by severity: Mild Moderate Severe

Symptom	Min Mod Sv	Symptom	Min Mod Sv

(Patient) Desired resolution of current work situation: _____

EVALUATION DATA

DEMONSTRATED WORK CAPACITY USING SELECTED WORK SAMPLES

VALPAR Standardized Work Samples Rate quality of work performance (1 poor to 5 excellent) during testing situation	Time in Seconds	MTM Rate
1 Small tools 1 2 3 4 5 **Follows instructions** 1 2 3 4 5 **Maintains physical stamina** 1 2 3 4 5 **Maintains motivation** 1 2 3 4 5 **Communicates** 1 2 3 4 5 **Shows self-confidence**		
4 Upper extremity range of motion 1 2 3 4 5 **Follows instructions** 1 2 3 4 5 **Maintains physical stamina** 1 2 3 4 5 **Maintains motivation** 1 2 3 4 5 **Communicates** 1 2 3 4 5 **Shows self-confidence**		
9 Whole-body range of motion and endurance 1 2 3 4 5 **Follows instructions** 1 2 3 4 5 **Maintains physical stamina** 1 2 3 4 5 **Maintains motivation** 1 2 3 4 5 **Communicates** 1 2 3 4 5 **Shows self-confidence**		

19 Dynamic physical capacity
    (Endurance test at PDC level set by BTE
    strength testing and actual job demand)
 	
PDC test level _____
 	
1 2 3 4 5 **Follows instructions**
1 2 3 4 5 **Maintains physical stamina**
1 2 3 4 5 **Maintains motivation**
1 2 3 4 5 **Communicates**
1 2 3 4 5 **Shows self-confidence**
	Number of completed tasks	

PERCEPTION OF ABILITY TO PERFORM WORK

<u>**Loma Linda Activity and West Tools Sorts:**</u> Perceived ability to use 65 common home environment–related hand tools/utensils (LLAS) and 65 industrial work–related tools (WTS)

	LLAS % of total	WTS % of total
Can use normally		
Can use but would be slower than "normal"		
Can use but would need extra rest breaks		
Would be unable to use		
Don't know		

<u>Client Description of Role Demands and Perceived Performance</u>

	Required	Perform Well	Perform Poorly	Unable
Standing =>50% of work day				
Sitting =>50% of work day				
Frequent walking =>30 min/hr				
Frequent/prolonged bending or stooping				
Occasional (1–2/day) max lift Circle "best fit" 100# 50# 20# 10#				
Frequent (1/hour) lift/carry Circle "best fit" 50# 20# 10# <10#				
Frequent overhead reach =>10 times/hr				
Frequent/prolonged computer use =>45 min/hr				
Frequent/prolonged use of hand tools with tight prolonged grasp				
Frequent/prolonged use of vibrating power tools				
Frequent/prolonged use of precision instruments				
Analytical decision making				
Personnel supervision				

<u>Abilities</u> (potential to work)

- Body range of motion (check all motions accomplished successfully) ___ Touch hand to back of neck ___ Touch hands to middle of back   ___ Reach overhead   ___ Bend to touch floor   ___ Kneel on floor

- Static postures (time in minutes maintaining posture before onset of symptoms):   ___ Sitting   ___ Standing ___ Reaching above shoulder level

- Hand sensation (Moving two-point discrimination at digit tips)

	Thumb	Index	Middle	Ring	Small
Right hand					
Left hand					

Abilities (continued)

- Jebsen-Taylor Hand Function Test (Time in seconds)(Benchmark score = 2 SD below mean)

Item	Writing	Turning Cards	Pick Up Small Objects	Feeding	Placing Checkers	Stacking Light Cans	Stacking Heavy Cans
Raw score Right hand							
Raw score Left hand							
Male dom hand	19.2	5.8	7.9	8.2	4.7	3.8	4.0
Male nondom hand	55.9	6.3	8	10.5	5.0	4.4	3.9
Female dom hand	15.9	7.1	7.1	8.9	4.5	4.1	4.2
Female nondom hand	47.4	7.0	8.0	11.2	5.2	4.5	4.3

- Static isometric strength BTE work simulator testing

	Right			Left		
	Mean In #	Percentile rank	CV	In #	Percentile rank	CV
Grip (6-second test; see attached graphs)						
3-jaw pinch						
Wrist extension						
Directional strength trial						
Pronation						
Supination						
Elbow flexion						
Shoulder flexion						

- Dynamic isotonic lifting, pushing, and pulling (BTE testing)

Perform to fatigue, initial onset of symptoms, or evidence of deteriorating technique

	Tool	Weight Lifted	Percentile Rank
Floor to knuckle	191#		
Knuckle to shoulder	191$		
Shoulder to overhead	191+		
Push (waist level)	191@		
Pull (waist level)	191		
Overhead pull	191%		

Abilities (continued)

	Prelift	Postlift
• Pulse	_____	_____
• Blood pressure	_____	_____

- Generalized contentment scale
  Range 25–125 (lower score suggests greater life contentment)

☐

- Decision making test   Percentile rank

☐

- Allen Cognitive Level Screening   Level (1 low–6 high)

☐

- Physical endurance

(Tuxworth Step Test) 5 min (25 steps/min rate) 16 in (40 cm) step

Formula = cumulative resting heart rates (HR)/body weight

HR 0.5–1 min × 2 _____ + HR 1.5–2 min × 2 _____ + HR 2.5–3 min × 2 _____

- Body weight _____ kg (1 lb = 2.2 kg)

  Mean = 5.40   SD = 1.145   z score =

SUMMARY OF FINDINGS

- **Average symptom severity:**   Mild   Moderate   Severe

- **Patient's description/perception of job requirements**
  ___ Less than sedentary   ___ Sedentary   ___ Sedentary light   ___ Light   ___ Light medium

  ___ Medium   ___ Medium heavy   ___ Heavy   ___ Very heavy

- **Client's perception of performance ability**

  Light activities/tools   % able to perform   Match diagnostic expectations   Y   N

  Heavy activities/tools   % able to perform   Match diagnostic expectations   Y   N

- **Mood, affect, cognition**

- **Body range of motion**

  Limitations: ___ Shoulders   ___ Arms   ___ Hands   ___ Back   ___ Legs   ___ None

---

- **Static posture tolerance:**   ___ Standing   ___ Sitting
                                    ___ Bending   ___ Reaching

---

- **U/E strength percentile ranking (average)   Right   Coefficient of variance**
- **U/E strength percentile ranking (average)   Left   Coefficient of variance**
- **6-second grip test profiles**   Right   Flat/low   Excessive variations   Normal peak & decline
                                      Left   Flat/low   Excessive variations   Normal peak & decline
- **Lifting pushing pulling percentile ranking**   Coefficient of variance

---

- **Physical endurance**

  Less than 2 standard deviations below mean (within normal limits)

  Greater than 2 standard deviations below mean

  Resting to post activity Pulse and BP differential

- **Hand dexterity**

  Less than 2 standard deviations below mean (within normal limits)

  Greater than 2 standard deviations below mean

Work Performance **VALPAR Work Samples**	**Worker Qualification Profile** Indicate level based on MTM percent rate of work

Valpar 1 Small Tools
   (Hand tool use in awkward and confined space)
	Not tested
	Exceeds work standard
	Meets work standard
	Does not meet work standard
	   (good potential to meet standard)
	Does not meet work standard
	   (minimal potential to meet standard)

Valpar 4 Upper extremity range of motion in function
   (Finger/hand dexterity in
   awkward and confined space)
	Not tested
	Exceeds work standard
	Meets work standard
	Does not meet work standard
	   (good potential to meet standard)
	Does not meet work standard
	   (minimal potential to meet standard)

Valpar 9 Whole body range of motion
   (Hand function in combination
   with reaching and bending)
	Not tested
	Exceeds work standard
	Meets work standard
	Does not meet work standard
	   (good potential to meet standard)
	Does not meet work standard
	   (minimal potential to meet standard)

Valpar 19 Dynamic physical capacity
   (manual materials
   handling)
	Not tested
	Exceeds work standard
	Meets work standard
	Does not meet work standard
	   (good potential to meet standard)
	Does not meet work standard
	   (minimal potential to meet standard)

34

Restoring Competence in Leisure Pursuits

Carolyn Hanson and Douglas Jones

LEARNING OBJECTIVES

After studying this chapter, the reader will be able to do the following:

1. Define leisure in a conceptual and pragmatic fashion.
2. Evaluate the physiological and psychological benefits of engagement in active and passive leisure.
3. Describe how leisure can be integrated into occupational therapy practice.
4. Identify various leisure assessments and describe how they are used.
5. Discuss barriers and challenges for clients and therapists engaging in leisure activities.

Sense of self-efficacy and self-esteem

Satisfaction with life roles
- **Self-maintenance**
- **Self-advancement**
- **Self-enhancement**

Competence in tasks of life roles

Activities and habits

Abilities and skills

Developed capacities

First-level capacities

Organic substrate

A ctivities of daily living, work and play–leisure are core aspects of occupational therapy with the ultimate goal of promoting self-efficacy and self-esteem (Trombly, 1995). A central tenet of our profession is the balance of these core areas (Primeau, 1996). Information concerning the use of play in occupational therapy is scarce in comparison with our core areas of activities of daily living (ADL) and work. Most of our profession's efforts in research and treatment have focused on play with children, commonly viewed as a child's work. However, the use and study of play should not be confined to children but should encompass the entire lifespan (Bundy, 1993). Play and **leisure** have commonly been considered a luxury, which has resulted in a paradox: "If we cannot think seriously about play, we cannot be serious about assessing, implementing, or promoting it. If we cannot assess, implement, and promote play, we do not take it seriously" (Florey, 1971, p. 218).

GLOSSARY

Chat room—Internet site where people communicate with each other in real time during a certain period on specific topics.

Electronic mail (E-mail)—Correspondence with people via the computer; sending a letter electronically.

Free time—Time other than that spent in work or self-care activities.

Horticulture therapy—Gardening as a therapeutic intervention.

Leisure—Freely chosen activity that requires control and commitment. Active leisure involves mental and physical exertion (e.g., wheelchair sports), whereas quiet leisure involves activities, such as reading and crafts, that require less physical effort. Socialization entails contact with others via telecommunication, computer, and/or in person.

Internet surfing—Using the Internet to access information.

Occupational imbalance—Excessive time spent in one area, usually work, at the expense of another, usually leisure. May aggravate health and quality of life.

Recreation—Time that is not spent in work or self-care and may or may not result in observable activity; similar to free time.

Therapeutic recreation—Professional use of recreational activities as primary form of treatment with patients; sometimes called recreational therapy.

Therapeutic recreation specialist—Trained professional who uses recreational activities as a therapeutic intervention with patients.

Recreation is also often used to describe how we occupy time that is not devoted to work or self-care. Recreational activity has been used as a therapeutic intervention throughout most of the 20th century. **Therapeutic recreation specialists**, professionals who are trained to use recreational activities to improve the quality of life for patients, have played a major role in developing leisure programs in medical settings. The profession of **therapeutic recreation (TR)** gained prominence and became more formalized after World War II, as recreational activities were used in the treatment of disabled war veterans. The history of TR is similar to the history of occupational therapy, as our profession was launched after working with veterans from World War I. The distinguishing difference between the two professions is that treatment protocols for TR always use recreational activity as the primary form of treatment. Occupational therapists concentrate on the overall functioning of the individual, of which recreation is one component.

Terms such as *play*, *leisure*, and *recreation* are often used interchangeably in conversation. Play, like leisure and recreation, has been difficult to define precisely but is the "purest expression of who we are as persons" (Bundy, 1993, p. 217). Leisure can be viewed as the adult version of play, as many similarities are present. Also, leisure is viewed as a more encompassing concept than play or recreation and is the term most frequently used in the occupational therapy literature. The purpose of this chapter is to review briefly the use of leisure with those with disabilities; to highlight particular leisure assessments; to recommend the development of specific leisure programs and activities for adults with physical disabilities; to discuss barriers for both therapists and clients; to present case studies regarding the use of leisure in occupational therapy; and to provide leisure resources.

Defining Leisure

Leisure is conceptualized as a self-enhancement role that is under control of and chosen by the individual (Trombly, 1995). There are four conditions of leisure: it is "freely chosen, intrinsically satisfying, optimally arousing, and requiring a sense of commitment" (Tinsley et al., 1993, p. 447). Leisure has been viewed in three principal ways: (1) leisure as time, or how we spend our time when not involved in work or self-care (**free time**); (2) leisure as activity, or what types of things we choose to do during our free time; (3) leisure as an experience or state of mind, or qualities inherent in the chosen activity that appeal to us, such as stimulating, invigorating, or relaxing (Gunter & Stanley, 1985). Leisure has also been separated into three major categories: **active leisure**, which consists of recreational activities incorporating physical exertion, such as wheelchair sports and travel; **quiet leisure**, which incorporates activities such as watching television, reading the newspaper, and crafts; and **socialization**, which consists of visiting and correspondence (Law et al., 1994).

Defining leisure in a precise manner is a difficult task, as our selection of leisure activities may change as we age. For example, jogging and tennis early in life may be replaced by activities with our children as we become parents. Culture affects the selection of leisure; some activities may be considered appropriate, while others are discarded on account of traditional beliefs about appropriate ways to use one's time. The categorization of leisure may be problematic as well, since attitude toward the activity plays a part in our perception of leisure. For example, sewing may be leisure for one person but considered work by another, which makes differentiation between the two complicated. Work and play, however, should not be viewed as dichotomous experiences, since they are often blended (Primeau, 1996). Balancing work and leisure is crucial for mental and physical health. Excessive time spent in work at the expense of leisure or vice verse may lead to **occupational imbalance** (Wilcock, 1998). Occupational imbalance may aggravate health and quality of life, resulting in injury or illness. For avoidance of occupational imbalance, leisure opportunities must be available and accessible to all people, including those with disabilities.

Engagement in leisure activity is important to a balanced life and satisfaction with life. Fines & Nichols (1994) commented that satisfaction with leisure was a chief factor in predicting psychological well-being, as it provides opportunities to develop social networks (Hanson, 1998). Leisure goals for clients vary according to the type of leisure selected and the individual's culture but may include the following:

- ▶ Using free time in a meaningful way
- ▶ Developing or improving socialization skills
- ▶ Increasing physical components such as strength, range of motion, coordination, and endurance
- ▶ Facilitating emotional components such as self-esteem, confidence, relaxation
- ▶ Improving cognitive components such as maintaining attention, and following instructions

Impact of Leisure on Occupational Balance

Both quiet and active leisure activities appear to contribute to occupational balance, self-esteem, and wellness for persons with disabilities.

Quiet Leisure

Needlecrafts, such as knitting, crochet, and embroidery, are examples of popular quiet leisure activities (Fig. 34-1). In a study conducted by an occupational therapist in the United Kingdom, narratives were obtained from 35 women with rheumatoid arthritis who all shared needlecraft as a leisure activity and responded to a research project announcement in a needlecraft magazine (Reynolds, 1997). Respondents mentioned three major ways in which they became involved in needlecraft: knowledge as a child, a way of coping with their disease (hospitalization, recuperation), or by chance. None of the respondents mentioned that an occupational therapist introduced or reintroduced needlecraft to them. The gradual demise of using arts and crafts in physical disability settings was mentioned as partially explaining the lack of occupational therapy intervention in this area (Taylor & Manguno, 1991). Comments from the respondents about the value of needlecraft included improved competence and self-esteem; a way to cope with anxiety, depression, and pain; a way to meet people; and a way to contribute to others, such as by gifts and items for charity sales. Reynolds (1997) recommended that leisure counseling be conducted for individuals with new diagnoses and chronic illness to encourage "constructive use of leisure time to improve quality of life" (p. 352).

Horticulture therapy (HT) entails gardening for therapeutic reasons. Occupational therapists have traditionally used HT to facilitate leisure and occupational skills in diverse populations. The nonthreatening environment of the garden assists in enhancing the emotional well-being of patients (Brenda Jesse, COTA, per-

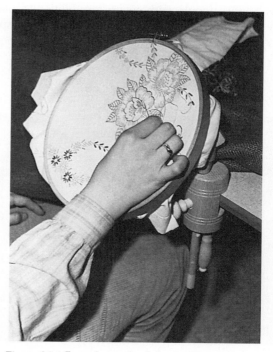

Figure 34-1 Frame for one-handed embroidery and sewing.

sonal communication, November 3, 1999). Personnel in rehabilitation facilities have developed butterfly gardens with raised flower boxes to enable wheelchair users to employ gardening skills while improving functional, emotional, cognitive, and physical skills (Wendy Alexander, OTR, personal communication, November 2, 1999). Various tools are designed to allow people with arthritis and upper extremity weakness to garden (see Resources).

Active Leisure

Historically, sports for those with disabilities have been connected to rehabilitation and occupational therapy (Jackson & Davis, 1983). In 1948, rehabilitation personnel at Stoke Mandeville Hospital in England used archery as therapy for their paraplegic war veterans. This program was successful and repeated for years, as it was seen as instrumental in promoting social and community integration. Over the past 50 years, wheelchair sports have continued to grow.

Well-established sports, such as wheelchair basketball, tennis, and racing, are attracting more participants (Fig. 34-2). Quad rugby, a popular recently recognized sport, includes team players who have quadriplegia, or tetraplegia, and overall extremity weakness. Quad rugby is played on a basketball court with two teams of four players. The purpose of the game is to cross the court and make a goal with a volleyball. Players use their bodies and wheelchairs to block shots and gain advantage in taking the ball down the court. Though quad rugby allows people with severe disabilities to play a team sport, it is not for the weak spirited. Other sports that require less bodily contact and use adaptive equipment and adaptive techniques range from water skiing and snow skiing to track and field to scuba diving.

Efficacy and Outcomes Research Specific to Leisure

Several studies demonstrate the contribution of active and quiet leisure to health and life satisfaction for persons with disabilities and the elderly.

Persons With Physical Dysfunction

A 12-week kayaking program consisting of weekly 60- to 90-minute sessions was designed to explore satisfaction with and attitude about leisure in a group of eight adults who had had a traumatic brain injury (TBI), been discharged from rehabilitation for at least a year, and mentioned an interest in kayaking. The *Leisure Satisfaction Measure* and the *Leisure Assessment Measurement*, used before and after the kayaking program, showed a significant improvement in both attitude and satisfaction (Fines & Nichols, 1994). Researchers commented that not only were programs of this nature beneficial for their therapeutic value, but opportunities were provided for individuals to use the skills they had learned in therapy. Active leisure participation in kayaking helped "refine the self to a) develop a sense of mastery; b) develop a view of self as productive; and c) enhance body image perceptions" (p. 10). In a qualitative study regarding sea kayaking, Taylor and McGruder (1996) interviewed three individuals with spinal cord injury. Kayaking was viewed as being a meaningful use of time and allowed these individuals to be seen as "able in the eyes of others" (p. 39).

In testing physically active and inactive individuals who were blind, had cerebral palsy, had amputations, or used a wheelchair for mobility, researchers found that the athletic groups had higher self-esteem and were better educated and better satisfied with life than their disabled nonathletic counterparts (Valliant et al., 1985). Physiological benefits identified in this study included increased cardiorespiratory endurance and muscular strength. In addition, the amputee population demonstrated improved proprioception and proficiency in using prosthetic devices.

Researchers surveyed 160 persons with spinal cord injury regarding their postdischarge activities (Hoffmann et al., 1995). On the basis of their activity level, respondents were placed in an active or an inactive group. The mean number of hours spent in daily sitting for the active group was 11.2 hours versus 8.6 hours for the inactive. Over a one-year period, the active individuals spent on average 3.2 days in the hospital compared to 10.7 days for the inactive. Inactive individuals were more than 2.5 times as likely to have pressure sores as the active ones.

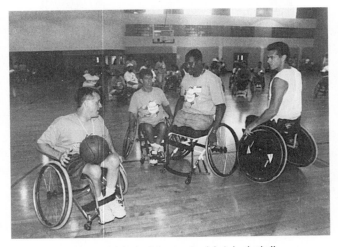

Figure 34-2 Active leisure: wheelchair basketball.

Results of this study underscore the cost-saving benefits of being physically active.

Elders

More than 1,000 elders were followed for 30 months in the Northern Manhattan Stroke study. Stroke studies generally follow individuals who have sustained a stroke over time to determine the effects of stroke and to monitor mortality rates. In the Northern Manhattan Stroke study, individuals who engaged in physically active leisure were found to have a decreased incidence of ischemic stroke (Sacco et al., 1998). Researchers have stressed that physically active leisure be emphasized in stroke prevention campaigns (Sacco et al., 1998). As elders constitute more of our population, it behooves us to create and promote leisure opportunities in assistive living facilities and retirement homes. In addition to a variety of sports, physically active leisure such as walking, armchair or wheelchair aerobics (exercising the upper extremities while seated), swimming, and weight training (using light weights or machines; using resistive bands) are all ideal for increasing endurance and tone in elders.

Potential Contributions From Occupational Therapy

Retirement was identified as being one of the top 10 most stressful life events for well elders. In retirees who had adapted well to retirement, Oakley and Pratt (1997) found a high correlation between life satisfaction and high activity levels. These researchers emphasized that the number and type of activities may be more important than the frequency of activity. Activities with both social and physical components had the strongest effect on life satisfaction. As occupational therapists value and understand the power of occupation, we can facilitate role change in elders and encourage adaptation to a new lifestyle through engagement in leisure (Fig. 34-3). To facilitate role change, we must be knowledgeable about appropriate leisure activities for our patients, discuss leisure interests, and provide opportunities for exploration.

Insufficient physical activity has been identified as the major factor in the deteriorating health of people with disabilities (Coyle & Santiago, 1995). Despite the increased growth of wheelchair sports, many people with disabilities lead sedentary lives. Investigations regarding sports and disability are lagging behind research on the benefits of sports for the able-bodied. Research data on the activity patterns of those with disabilities are scarce. Occupational therapists can create sports programs or provide physically active leisure opportunities for people with disabilities, and they have the

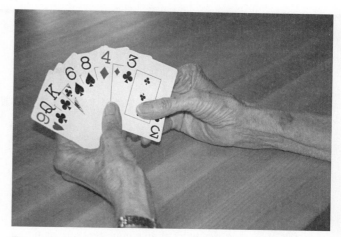

Figure 34-3 Large-print playing cards typify leisure adaptations available to elders. (Photo by Laurie Manuel.)

responsibility to inform patients about active, quiet, and socialization activities within their communities. Incorporating leisure activity into our assessment and treatment encourages the individual to take risks and be exposed to activities that they might not have attempted on their own.

Assessment Tools

Before recommending specific leisure activities or using leisure as an intervention, one should assess the patient's interest in leisure. The following are instruments that identify the types of activities that are meaningful to patients. Though not an exhaustive list of the leisure assessments available in the fields of occupational therapy and therapeutic recreation, it presents some of the better-known instruments.

The *Canadian Occupational Performance Measure*

Designed by occupational therapists, the *Canadian Occupational Performance Measure (COPM)* detects self-perceived change in occupational performance over time (Law et al., 1994). The *COPM* contains three sections: self-care, productivity, and leisure. The leisure section is divided into quiet recreation, such as hobbies, crafts, and reading; active recreation, such as sports, outings, and travel; and socialization, such as visiting, phone calls, and correspondence. Individuals are requested to identify any problems in the three sections and to rate the importance of each activity on a scale of 1 to 10. Then five of the most important problems are identified and individuals rate their performance and satisfaction with performance on these five problems (Table 34-1 and case example).

Case Example

MR. C.: USING THE COPM TO ASSESS LEISURE

Patient Information

Mr. C. was a 62-year-old janitor who had a right cerebrovascular accident (CVA). Problems identified included (1) decreased ability to engage in instrumental activities of daily living because of paresis on left side; (2) periodic incontinence; (3) lack of exposure to leisure activities. Mr. C.'s past occupations consisted of his janitorial work at an elementary school, home maintenance, and church attendance.

Description of Assessment

The *COPM* was used to create a client-identified list of the top five most important problems for Mr. C. These included (1) transportation—inability to drive; (2) home maintenance—inability to mow lawn, repair roof, and paint walls; (3) quiet recreation—no past interests other than watching television; (4) active recreation—past interest in sports and travel; con-cern about not being able to use two hands; (5) socialization—limited by embarrassment about incontinence. On a scale of 1 to 10, the client ranked the importance of these activities, his ability (performance), and his satisfaction in how he could now engage in these activities (Table 34-1).

Analysis of Results

The *COPM* indicated that transportation and active recreation were the most important problems Mr. C. identified. Intervention such as driver training using adaptive devices, leisure counseling, sports exploration, use of adaptive equipment, bladder training for continence, and teaching one-handed techniques will help Mr. C. to participate in desired activities.

Adapted from Jongbloed and Ernest-Conibear (1995).

TABLE 34-1
COPM Scores

Problems	Importance	Performance	Satisfaction
Transportation	10	1	1
Home maintenance	5	5	4
Quiet recreation	5	2	3
Active recreation	9	2	1
Socialization	7	2	3

Interest Checklists

Occupational therapists have developed and used many interest checklists. The *Nottingham Leisure Question-naire*, developed in England for stroke patients, is a 38-item list of activities ranging from watching television to doing sporting activities (Drummond & Walker, 1994). A five-point scale is used to describe frequency of doing the activity, ranging from regularly (every day) to never. Though developed for stroke patients residing in England, all activities are culturally relevant to us except "going out to pubs." Test–retest reliability has been discovered to be good for most items, and it has satisfactory interrater reliability.

The *Interest Checklist* (Matsutsuyu, 1967) consists of 80 items grouped into the following categories: ADL, manual skills, cultural–educational, physical sports, and social recreation. The rating given to each item ranges from no interest to casual interest to strong interest.

Another interest checklist with similar categories plus categories such as games, organizational activities, and entertainment has been designed specifically for those with arthritis. This instrument consists of 64 items rated according to their importance, ranging from none to high and their relevance to the person with arthritis (importance of activity and whether a priority for further development) (Kautzmann, 1984).

Finally, the *Lin Interest Check List (LICL)*, developed in 1991, contains 151 interests and activities within 6 categories: sports, physical activities, and nature; crafts; games; sociocultural and entertainment activities; community and education; and hobbies and miscellaneous. Level of interest, frequency, and history of participation are to be identified for each item. The *LICL* has high content validity and good test–retest reliability (Lin, S. Content validity and test–retest reliability of the *Lin Interest Check List.* Unpublished thesis, Virginia Commonwealth University [Richmond], 1991).

Occupational Therapy Assessment of Leisure Time

The *Occupational Therapy Assessment of Leisure Time (OTALT)* was based on a review of the leisure literature in occupational therapy and provides a frame of reference specifically for leisure (Soderback & Hammarlund, 1993). The purpose of the *OTALT* is to enable the patient to use leisure time more effectively and to improve satisfaction with leisure activities. Using open-ended questions, the therapist interviews the patient on the dimensional concepts of time, intrinsic motivation, free choice of leisure activity; capability; structure of social and cultural environment; engagement in leisure activity; pleasure for pleasure's sake; goal self-fulfillment, goal diversion, recreation, and relaxation; leisure role; leisure behavior; and influence on his or her leisure role and leisure behavior. Though multiple questions are provided for each dimension, therapists are encouraged to structure the interview the best way they see fit and to add and delete questions as needed.

Leisure Questionnaires From Therapeutic Recreation

Beard and Ragheb (1980) have developed four leisure questionnaires that are commonly used by therapeutic recreation specialists in medical settings. The *Leisure Satisfaction Measure (LSM)* contains 51 statements about how patients perceive their needs being met through leisure. The *Leisure Attitude Measurement (LAM)* contains 36 items that quantify the patient's attitude in 3 areas, cognitive, affective, and behavioral (Ragheb & Beard, 1982). The *Leisure Interest Measure (LIM)* identifies patients' interest in the following eight domains: physical, outdoor, mechanical, artistic, service, social, cultural, and reading (Beard & Ragheb, 1990). The *Leisure Motivation Scale (LMS)* contains 48 items regard-

ing motivation to engage in leisure activities and reflects four areas: intellectual, social, competence–mastery, and stimulus avoidance (Beard & Ragheb, 1983). As a whole, reliability and validity are good for these measures as items, and domains have been analyzed extensively.

Arenas for Leisure Intervention

Occupational therapists help clients resume premorbid leisure interests and explore new options. Table 34-3 describes leisure activities that persons with various diagnoses are commonly able to perform. The discussion that follows highlights two other broad areas of leisure intervention: information technology and sports camps.

Information Technology

Computers can provide leisure interests, such as accessing information on activities and organizations and developing intellectual and creative abilities. Computer activities such as communicating with people in **chat rooms**, using **electronic mail (E-mail)**, **Internet surfing**, and playing video games are becoming more popular and accessible. Providing information on the use of computers to people with disabilities allows them to compete on even ground with the able-bodied (Curtin, 1994). If there is interest, therapists ensure a proper match between the person and the hardware and software. A structured training program is recommended to allow experimentation with appropriate equipment before purchase. With the right match, the computer can provide educational and social opportunities. (See Chapter 17 for a detailed discussion of computer access adaptations for persons with disabilities.) Though distinctly having many advantages, computers may encourage individuals to be sedentary, remaining indoors and in one position for extended periods. As with any activity, moderation is the key. Frequent breaks and repositioning are especially important for engaging in computer activities.

Sports Camps

Camps have been developed to introduce sports and leisure activities to people with disabilities to facilitate engagement in physically active leisure and to promote health (Hanson, 1998). Focus may be on one particular sport, such as with wheelchair tennis camp, or an introduction to a variety of sports. For example, during its annual 2-day GatorSport Exploration Camp, the Department of Occupational Therapy at the University of Florida offers weight training, swimming, quad rugby,

Case Example

MS. C.: USING THE LICL TO ASSESS LEISURE

Patient Information

Ms. C. is a 20-year-old college student who sustained severe fractures of the tibia and fibula from a motorcycle accident resulting in amputation of her left leg below the knee. Problems included (1) inability to transfer independently and walk; (2) inability to engage in premorbid activities such as marching band, karate, running, and hiking; (3) time needed for healing of stump before any attempt at weight bearing on prosthesis.

Description of Assessment

During Ms. C.'s training to walk and fitting for a prosthesis, the focus was on identifying past activities with possible recommendations for adaptations. The *LICL* was used to determine Ms. C.'s level of interest in crafts, community, education, hobbies, games, sociocultural and entertainment activities, sports and physical activities, and nature. Ms. C. was directed to scan the list of activities and mark her level of interest (like a little, moderately like, like very much), the frequency of

performing the activity (occasionally, regularly, frequently), and the history of participation (active in past, present, or future). In reference to the largest category of sports, physical activities, and nature, Ms. C. was to specify whether she typically watched or performed these activities.

Analysis of Findings

Ms. C. selected few activities in crafts and community and education, with embroidery being one in which she currently participated. She identified numerous hobbies and games ranging from cooking and reading to card games and pinball. In sociocultural and entertainment, Ms. C. checked activities that she liked very much: going to restaurants, movies, museums, and musicals. The area that primarily interested Ms. C. was sports, physical activities, and nature. A list of the activities she liked very much is presented in Table 34-2. As can be seen, Ms. C. was determined early in rehabilitation to return to her past leisure activities, acknowledging that an excellent prosthetic fit and training were essential.

TABLE 34-2
LICL: Sports, Physical Activities, Nature Category

Activity	Status	Frequency	History
Biking	Perform	Occasionally	Past, future
Camping	Perform	Frequently	Past, future
Canoeing	Perform	Occasionally	Past, future
Dancing	Perform	Occasionally	Past
Hiking	Perform	Occasionally	Past, future
Karate, judo	Watch	Occasionally	Past, present, future
Rock climbing	Perform	Occasionally	Past, future
Rowing	Perform	Occasionally	Past, future
Walking	Perform	Occasionally	Past, future
Weight lifting	Perform	Occasionally	Past, future
Marching band	Perform	Occasionally	Past

and wheelchair tennis, basketball, and racing for adults with spinal cord injury and lower extremity amputation. Adaptations for these sports include gloves with Velcro strapping to allow individuals with tetraplegia to grasp a tennis racket and pool floats to facilitate buoyancy in those with limited muscle use. Sports such as wheelchair basketball, tennis, and quad rugby require sport-specific

wheelchairs, known as sports chairs, that are easily maneuverable. Leisure activities such as table tennis, billiards and bowling, with a bowling ball ramp, which is a descending platform that guides the ball down the lane, are available for individuals with limited upper and lower extremity use.

Camps may be specialized for individuals with

particular diagnoses or may include anyone with a mental or physical disability (David Jones, Florida Disabled Outdoors Association, personal communication, July, 1999). Because of the focused nature of the camp and the time invested—camps may last from several days to several weeks—participants have the chance to socialize and learn specific sport skills. In addition, camp participants often learn techniques and

TABLE 34-3
Leisure Activity Chart

Activity Level	Paraplegia, Lower Extremity Amputation[a]	Tetraplegia[b]	Cerebrovascular Accident[c]	Traumatic Brain Injury[d]	Dementia[e]
Sedentary	Cards Board games Puzzles Painting, drawing Music listening Reading Computer activities Video games Needlecrafts Movies	Cards Board games Puzzles Painting, drawing Music listening Reading Computer activities Video games Movies	Cards Board games Puzzles Painting, drawing Music listening Mirror games Needlecrafts Computer activities Photo albums, scrapbooks Movies	Cards Board games Puzzles Painting, art, drawing Music listening Mirror games Needlecrafts Computer activities Photo albums, scrapbooks Movies	Matching games Sequencing games Sing-alongs Show and tell
Mild	Archery Bowling Target shooting Billiards Flying Camping Fishing Photography Gardening Travel	Archery Target shooting Fishing Photography Gardening Travel	Paved nature walks Pet therapy Bowling Gardening	Paved nature walks Pet therapy Bowling Gardening	Putt putt Bowling Fishing Parties Gardening
Moderate	Sailing Swimming Weight training Horseback riding Scuba diving Golf Table Tennis Dance	Sailing Swimming Weight training Creative movement, dance	Weight training Assisted swimming Creative movement, dance	Weight training Assisted swimming Creative movement, dance	Walking groups Creative movement, dance Weight training Swimming Table tennis
Vigorous	Wheelchair basketball Racing, track Tennis Softball Snow skiing Water skiing Rowing, kayaking Hand cycling Sled hockey	Quad rugby Racing Tennis	Stationary bicycle Rowing, kayaking Other activities depending on degree of paralysis or paresis	Stationary bicycle Rowing, kayaking Other activities depending on degree of paralysis or paresis	Speed walking, jogging Bicycling, tricycling Tennis Rowing

This table provides suggested activities for persons with disabilities. The appropriateness of any activity is greatly influenced by the individual's functional level. Specific adaptive equipment and special assistance may be required.

[a] Treatment should emphasize activities that reinforce functional independence and physical fitness.

[b] Specialized adaptive equipment is required for most activities. Functional independence is possible in many of these activities with proper planning and practice.

[c] Treatment should emphasize visual–perceptual and one-handed activities. Activities that improve range of motion and visual field on the impaired side are valuable.

[d] Activities should focus on cognitive challenges and games to strengthen fine and gross motor skills without complex rules or higher-order thinking.

[e] Activities to improve socialization, cognitive orientation, and recollection are important.

Case Example

MS. J.: USING LEISURE TO ENHANCE MOTIVATION AND FUNCTION AFTER NONTRAUMATIC SPINAL CORD INJURY

Patient Information

Ms. J. is a 42-year-old woman who developed a fever and leg weakness after abdominal surgery. She was diagnosed as having an inflammation of the spinal cord of unknown cause. Evaluation in a subacute nursing facility revealed the following problems: (1) weak upper and lower extremity strength, (2) inability to groom and dress, and (3) sadness and hopelessness because of the loss of her previous lifestyle.

Recommendations

The occupational therapist recommended daily treatments for 4 weeks and established these long-term treatment goals: (1) Ms. J. will have increased upper extremity strength (increase by one muscle grade), (2) Ms. J. will be able to carry out all grooming and dressing needs with minimal assistance, and (3) Ms. J. will be encouraged to engage in her past leisure interests of basketball, driving her sports car, and dining in restaurants.

Short-Term Goals

As psychosocial issues were interfering with the patient's progress, the therapist arranged for a professional wheelchair basketball athlete to visit the patient to demonstrate skills at the basketball hoop in the facility courtyard and to instill hope about returning to former interests. Goals: (1) Ms. J. will be exposed to wheelchair basketball. (2) Ms. J. will interact with a person similar in age who also has a disability. (3) Ms. J. will have the opportunity to ask specific questions about how to play wheelchair basketball and about driving with adaptive equipment.

Ms. J. enjoyed the interaction with the wheelchair athlete and became animated when talking about the possibility of driving again. Though she viewed playing basketball as being too difficult for her, she was hopeful about driving because she had seen an adapted car driven by the wheelchair athlete who had no lower extremity use. This positive experience improved the patient's mood and outlook on life.

Revised Goals

▶ Ms. J. will be able to groom and dress independently with adaptive equipment.
▶ Ms. J. will be able to access information on adaptive equipment for driving.
▶ Ms. J. will be able to dine in public with her friend and her therapist.

CLINICAL REASONING
in OT Practice

Promotion of Leisure Exploration

Before her abdominal surgery Ms. J. found meaning in her life through engagement in leisure activities. In what ways did providing her with experiences to reengage in interests motivate her to participate in her rehabilitation more fully?

---

obtain tips from each other on daily living skills such as transferring and catheterization. Follow-up interviews of the 1998 GatorSport participants revealed that the most important benefit of attending the camp was making friends and acquaintances. Affiliation with others is a strong motivating factor in promoting leisure activities.

Occupational therapists realize the many benefits of directing a camp, which range from raising the awareness of the able-bodied to providing the disabled with opportunities to explore sport. Additional benefits may include training for students and staff who serve as camp volunteers. Volunteers assist in monitoring participants for heat exhaustion and any untoward effects of exercise (Box 34-1) and assist with coaching. Volunteers may also provide valuable service to campers by helping with their personal care. Continuing education units may be a by-product of the camp, since students and staff receive hands-on training as volunteers which can be combined with lectures, small group projects, and discussion about sports program implementation for people with disabilities. It is also possible to conduct research in camp, such as collecting outcome data on patients who do and do not participate in sports and their functional abilities and the incidence of secondary medical complications in those who are active and inactive on a regular basis. A wide range of other research projects can also enable us to promote wellness and sports opportunities for individuals with disabilities. It is not enough to give anecdotal accounts of our successful interventions with clients; we must back up our statements with research data.

Barriers to Leisure Engagement

A number of factors interfere with ensuring that persons with disabilities ultimately can engage in leisure activities that maintain a satisfactory occupational balance. Some factors stem from contemporary trends in occupational therapy, other interfering factors have to do with client access.

Barriers for Therapists

Barriers must be overcome before we regain our foothold in leisure. Occupational therapists were surveyed regarding their use of treatment activities (Taylor & Manguno, 1991). Physical dysfunction therapists used crafts less and physical modalities, defined in the study as employment of a therapeutic agent, more than therapists in mental health or developmental disabilities. Therapists in physical dysfunction may consider their background limited in suggesting leisure activities to

BOX 34-2
PROCEDURES FOR PRACTICE

Strategies to Promote Leisure

- Elicit enthusiasm and support from health professionals through in-service education that links leisure, health, and quality of life.
- Elicit support from family and friends.
- Identify interest and enjoyment in activity via leisure assessments and interviewing techniques.
- Evaluate for special needs and assist in choosing an appropriate activity based on current abilities.
- Provide exposure to activity and establish a schedule to learn.
- Set basic goals for activity that can be mastered early, and establish more challenging goals with progress.
- Follow up to evaluate success and to make possible adjustments.
- Create opportunities to reinforce engaging in activity that may be external or internal (longer-lasting effect).

BOX 34-1
SAFETY BOX

Spinal Cord Injury

Individuals with spinal cord injury (lesion at T6 and above) are at risk for autonomic dysreflexia, which is brought on by being overheated or having an obstructed fecal mass, a kink in a catheter tube, or pain. Symptoms and signs include hypertension, pounding headache, profuse sweating, flushing, pupil constriction, and nasal congestion. This is a MEDICAL EMERGENCY. Obtain medical help while removing restrictive binders or clothing, elevating head, checking leg bag for obstruction, and monitoring blood pressure (Hollar, 1995).

Engagement in Physically Active Leisure Pursuits

The new participant requires supervision from a therapist, with subsequent monitoring by the participant. Environmental conditions with extreme heat (outdoor wheelchair racing in Florida in July) or cold (snow skiing in Colorado) should be cautiously considered and consistently evaluated for potential ill effects. Terminate activity if safety is questionable.

- Monitor body temperature.
- Monitor sweating and color of skin.
- Observe for signs of fatigue.
- Check for incontinence.
- Encourage skin inspection.
- Encourage fluid intake.
- Recommend pressure relief.
- Evaluate positioning, cushioning and strapping during activity.
- Consider special training for activity.

patients and thus rely on providing medical intervention. In some areas of practice, modality use potentially preempts therapy time that might otherwise be devoted to providing leisure experience, whether crafts or other activities. Asking about leisure interests and desires allows us to provide exploratory experiences in a monitored and controlled setting and offer the "just right" challenge to our patients. Moreover, we can follow up by forging relationships with community and recreational centers to encourage continued participation upon discharge (Box 34-2).

Barriers for Clients

Access to recreational and leisure pursuits may be difficult for persons with disabilities. Though more opportunities are becoming available, our communities offer a narrow range of activities to those with physical disabilities (Hanson, 1998). Architectural barriers in parking lots and sidewalks without curb cuts may prevent access. A recreational facility may have outdated, inaccessible bathrooms. Transportation to a facility or center may also pose problems, as may the financial requirements for specialized equipment such as wheelchairs designed for specific sports and adapted sports equipment. It may be difficult to find coaches and other personnel who understand the needs of those with disabilities. In spite of these possible barriers, it is vital that people with disabilities have support and encouragement from their family and friends to participate in leisure activities that interest them and are within their capabilities.

Case Example

MR. M.: USING LEISURE TO ENHANCE ADAPTATION AFTER STROKE

Patient Information

Mr. M. is a 78-year-old man with a history of multiple strokes, emphysema, and heart disease. Mr. M. recently had a right ischemic stroke and was treated in a hospital for several days and discharged to his son's home. A home health evaluation visit revealed the following problems: (1) dependence in all ADL and meal preparation as a result of left-side paresis, (2) lack of endurance in performing ADL, (3) slow and unbalanced gait (used quad cane to walk), and (4) sadness because of health problems and limited activity. Prior to his stroke, Mr. M. enjoyed playing bridge once a week and golfing and/or swimming about once a month. He had also assumed primary responsibilities for meal preparation since his retirement, and this role had come to inspire pride and kudos from friends and family.

Recommendations

Patient was to have occupational therapy three times a week for 4 weeks in his son's home. In collaboration with the patient's wife, the following long-term goals were established: (1) Mr. M. will be independent in feeding, dressing, grooming, toileting, and bathing. (2) Mr. M. will improve his endurance to the point that he tolerates sustained activity for at least 15 minutes. (3) Mr. M. will engage in meaningful leisure activity to stimulate interest and enjoyment in life.

Short-Term Goals

▶ Using energy conservation techniques, Mr. M. will be able to dress himself in the morning independently, requiring no more than two short breaks to rest.

▶ Mr. M. will improve his endurance enough to walk safely in the kitchen with his quad cane while preparing a cold meal.

▶ Mr. M. will be able to don his swim trunks independently and, with supervision, attempt to enter his home outdoor pool to float and swim (a goal of primary importance to Mr. M.).

Over a 2-week period, Mr. M. tolerated 10 minutes of walking indoors and outdoors and progressed to needing only verbal cues to perform his ADL independently, including donning swim trunks. He showed great interest in entering the pool, though the pool had deep steps and no handrail. On the appointed day, Mr. M. changed into his swim trunks and tentatively began to step into the pool; a thick piece of wood was placed on the first step to make it less steep. Mr. M. was not confident in his ability to manage the steps, and the activity was discontinued. It seemed that having attempted this activity of such personal significance, Mr. M. was now ready to focus on leisure outlets that more closely matched his current abilities.

Revised Goals

▶ Mr. M. will be able to incorporate his involved left upper extremity into bilateral tasks such as moving and holding playing cards, holding and swinging a golf club.

▶ Mr. M. will increase his sustained activity tolerance to 20 minutes, enabling him to carry out light kitchen tasks daily.

▶ Mr. M. will attempt to enter the pool when he is stronger and feels more capable.

CLINICAL REASONING
in OT

Trial Experience in Engaging in Leisure Activity

Mr. M. lacked confidence in his ability to enter his pool, though he was making good progress during therapy. How can confidence be restored? What types of activities could be used to instill in Mr. M. confidence and belief in his skills? What types of leisure activities could be proposed as interim goals?

Attitudinal barriers are often more disabling than any physical barriers. Individuals with disabilities such as tetraplegia and bilateral upper or lower extremity amputations may not believe that they are capable of participating in a variety of activities because of the attitudes of others. Advances in technology have allowed people with spinal cord injury and neuromuscular diseases to water ski using a sit ski; people with hand amputations can wind surf using sport-specific prostheses; wheelchair users can rock-climb with special equipment (Fig. 34-4). Wheelchairs designed specifically for use on the beach have been developed in addition to numerous models for various sports. With developing technology, opportunities to engage in numerous activities are possible if there is interest and motivation on the part of the therapist and the individual.

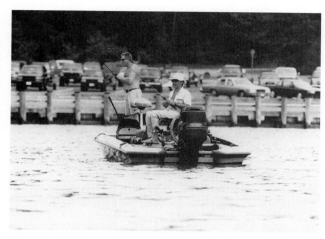

Figure 34-4 Technology to allow independent fishing from a wheelchair. (Photo by Gary Rudolph.)

In conclusion, human occupation is commonly taken for granted, and its health benefits are not acknowledged (Wilcock, 1998). This is even more pronounced in leisure. Engagement in leisure promotes health and decreases medical costs. Efforts to provide leisure opportunities for adults with disabilities are gradually increasing as we shift from hospital- to community-based treatment and from care and cure to prevention and promotion (Finlayson & Edwards, 1997). Our renewed interest in community-based intervention supports our efforts to encourage leisure exploration and develop leisure programs for all people, including those with disabilities. Occupational therapists can become more aware of existing leisure opportunities and integrate leisure activities into assessment and treatment. By forming partnerships with others to develop and promote leisure options in new areas for people with disabilities, we can provide better quality of life for our patients.

Summary Review Questions

1. How would you define leisure to a patient?
2. What are the benefits of engaging in quiet leisure? Active leisure? Socialization?
3. How might leisure goals be different for someone with a stroke? Spinal cord injury? Lower extremity amputation?
4. Why has leisure not been as fully studied or implemented as our other core areas of work and ADL?
5. Describe specific ways that occupational therapists can integrate leisure into evaluation and treatment.
6. What kinds of barriers limit leisure introduction and exploration? How would you remove those barriers in your own practice?

7. Describe the ways in which leisure activities enhance health and wellness for all people, including individuals with disabilities.
8. Discuss the advantages and disadvantages of the 4 types of leisure assessments described in this chapter.
9. What leisure activities would you recommend for people with no lower extremity use? No use of one side of the body? Overall general weakness?

Acknowledgments

We thank Pat Dasler for her case study contribution and Laurie Manuel and Gary Rudolph for the photographs.

Resources

Sport organizations

Disabled Sports USA · Provides sports opportunities to people with disabilities. Listing of summer and winter sports, methods to contact existing chapters.
http://www.dsusa.org/

Adaptive Sports Association · Offers snow skiing instruction and summer sports options to physically and developmentally disabled persons of all ages.
http://www.frontier.net/~asa

Mesa Association for the Disabled · Nonprofit organization providing sports and recreational opportunities to people with disabilities. Other links to sports organizations.
http://www.geocities.com/HotSprings/5896/

National Wheelchair Basketball Association · Provides rules, team registration, and divisions of wheelchair basketball. Additional links.
www.nwba.org

Paralyzed Veterans of America · Research and education, sports and recreation, resources for professionals, publications and products.
http://www.pva.org/

U.S. Cerebral Palsy Athletic Association · Player classification for sports; information for those with cerebral palsy, traumatic brain injury, and stroke.
http://www.uscpaa.org/

Wheelchair Sports USA · Qualifying standards and rules for sports. Links to various organizations.
http://www.wsusa.org/

Specific Sports and Leisure Activities

Paddle sports information · Canoeing, kayaking, rafting.
http://www.aca-paddler.org/

American Horticulture Therapy Association · Membership information, conferences and educational opportunities, publications and information packets, and other HT sites.
www.ahta.org/

Travel options focusing on accessible services and transportation. Excellent source of links to sports and other disability sources.
http://www.access-able.com/

Snow skiing in Canada · Additional skiing links.
http://www.canuck.com/cads/index.html

Travel information for individuals with disabilities.
http://www.disabilitytravel.com/

Wheelchair racing resource page · Additional links.
http://www.execpc.com/~birzer/

Texas Adaptive Aquatics program · Provides water skiing instruction to individuals with disabilities.
http://www.neosoft.com/~txadaqua/

Quad rugby home page · History of the sport, rules, U.S. teams, classification of players.
http://www.quadrugby.com

Sled hockey rules and regulations (using a sled instead of ice skates to play hockey).
http://www.sledhockey.org/

Skiing, horseback riding, camping, canoeing and sailing. Additional links.
http://www.sover.net/~vass/

Inclusive sporting events emphasizing involvement of people with disabilities.
http://www.worldteamsports.org/

Miscellaneous Resources

Disability sport organizations, sport offerings, classification systems, major competitions for athletes with a disability, summaries of research papers on disability sport topics, and more. A scholarly approach to sports for the disabled.
http://ed-web3.educ.msu.edu/KIN866/contents.htm

Information and referral service for sports, recreation and physical activity programs. Additional links.
http://education.gsu.edu/blazenet

GatorSport Adult Exploration Camp · Camp designed for adults with spinal cord injury and lower extremity amputation. Resources and organizations for a variety of sports.
http://www.gatorsport.org

Equipment

Scuba equipment touted as the future of scuba.
http://www.aquadyn.com/

Information on disability and medical products. Categories of sports and recreational products and services; travel and tours; recreational vehicles. Additional sites and more.
http://www.coast-resources.com

Cycles for the physically challenged: hand cycles, tandem tricycles, tandem bicycles, seats, backrests, footrests, and accessories.
http://www.haverich.com

TRS · Prosthetic hands for sports and other leisure activities, such as photography and playing musical instruments.
http://www.oandp.com/trs

KY Enterprises · Adaptive recreational equipment and controllers for video games for those without use of their hands.
http://www.quadcontrol.com

Adaptive recreation and sporting equipment for people with disabilities and the aged. Leisure activities range from crafts and gardening to motorcycling and sailing.
http://www.achievableconcepts.com.au/

References

Beard, J. G., & Ragheb, M. G. (1980). Measuring leisure satisfaction. *Journal of Leisure Research, 12,* 20–33.

Beard, J. G., & Ragheb, M. G. (1983). Measuring leisure motivation. *Journal of Leisure Research, 15,* 219–228.

Beard, J. G., & Ragheb, M. G. (1990). Leisure Interest Measure. Paper presented at the meeting of the National Recreation and Park Association Symposium on Leisure Research, Phoenix, Arizona.

Bundy, A. C. (1993). Assessment of play and leisure: Delineation of the problem. *American Journal of Occupational Therapy, 47,* 217–222.

Coyle, C. P., & Santiago, M. C. (1995). Aerobic exercise training and depressive symptomatology in adults with physical disabilities. *Archives of Physical Medicine and Rehabilitation, 76,* 647–652.

Curtin, M. (1994). Technology for people with tetraplegia, part 1: Accessing computers. *British Journal of Occupational Therapy, 57,* 376–380.

Drummond, A., & Walker, M. (1994). The Nottingham leisure questionnaire for stroke patients. *British Journal of Occupational Therapy, 57,* 414–418.

Finlayson, M., & Edwards, J. (1997). Evolving health environments and occupational therapy: Definitions, descriptions and opportunities. *British Journal of Occupational Therapy, 60,* 456–460.

Fines, L., & Nichols, D. (1994). An evaluation of a 12 week recreational kayak program: Effects on self-concept, leisure satisfaction, and leisure attitude of adults with traumatic brain injuries. *Journal of Cognitive Rehabilitation, 12,* 10–15.

Florey, L. (1971). An approach to play and play development. *American Journal of Occupational Therapy, 25,* 275–280.

Gunter, B. G., & Stanley, J. (1985). Theoretical issues in leisure study. In B. G. Gunter, J. Stanley, & R. St. Clair (Eds.), *Transition to Leisure: Conceptual and Human Issues* (pp. 35–51). Lanham, MD: University Press of America.

Hanson, C. S. (1998). A sports exploration camp for adults with disabilities. *OT Practice, 3,* 35–38.

Hoffmann, L., Williford, R., Mooney, B., Brown, C., & Davis, C. (1995). Leisure activities provide rehab potential. *Case Management Advisor, 6,* p. 71.

Hollar, L. D. (1995). Spinal cord injury. In C. A. Trombly (Ed.), *Occupational Therapy for physical dysfunction* (4th ed., pp. 795–813). Baltimore: Williams & Wilkins.

Jackson, R. W., & Davis, G. M. (1983). The value of sports and recreation for the physically disabled. *Orthopaedic Clinics of North America, 14,* 301–315.

Jongbloed, L., & Ernest-Conibear, M. (1995). Regaining participation in leisure-time activities. In C. A. Trombly (Ed.), *Occupational Therapy for Physical Dysfunction* (4th ed., pp. 351–359). Baltimore: Williams & Wilkins.

Kautzmann, L. (1984). Identifying leisure interests: A self-assessment approach for adults with arthritis. *Occupational Therapy in Health Care, 2,* 45–51.

Law, M., Polatajko, H., Pollock, N., McColl, M. A., Carswell, A., & Baptiste, S. (1994). Pilot testing of the Canadian Occupational Performance Measure: Clinical and measurement issues. *Canadian Journal of Occupational Therapy, 61,* 191–197.

Matsutsuyu, J. (1967). The Interest Checklist. *American Journal of Occupational Therapy, 11,* 170–181.

Oakley, C., & Pratt, J. (1997). Voluntary work in the lives of post-retirement adults. *British Journal of Occupational Therapy, 60,* 273–276.

Primeau, L. A. (1996). Work and leisure: Transcending the dichotomy. *American Journal of Occupational Therapy, 50,* 569–577.

Ragheb, M. G., & Beard, J. G. (1982). Measuring leisure attitude. *Journal of Leisure Research, 14,* 155–167.

Reynolds, F. (1997). Coping with chronic illness and disability through creative needlecraft. *British Journal of Occupational Therapy, 60,* 352–356.

Sacco, R. L., Gan, R., Boden-Albala, B., Lin, I. F., Kargman, D. E, Hauser, W. A., Shea, S., & Paik, M. C. (1998). Leisure-time physical activity and ischemic stroke risk: The Northern Manhattan Stroke Study. *Stroke, 29,* 380–387.

Soderback, I., & Hammarlund, C. (1993). A leisure-time frame of reference based on a literature analysis. *Occupational Therapy in Health Care, 8,* 105–133.

Taylor, E., & Manguno, J. (1991). Use of treatment activities in occupational therapy. *American Journal of Occupational Therapy, 45,* 317–322.

Taylor, L. P., & McGruder, J. E. (1996). The meaning of sea kayaking for persons with spinal cord injuries. *American Journal of Occupational Therapy, 50,* 39–46.

Tinsley, H. E., Hinson, J. A., Tinsley, D. J., & Holt, M. S. (1993). Attributes of leisure and work experiences. *Journal of Counseling Psychology, 40,* 447–455.

Trombly, C. A. (1995). Theoretical foundations for practice. In C. A. Trombly (Ed.), *Occupational Therapy for Physical Dysfunction* (4th ed., pp 15–27). Baltimore: Williams & Wilkins.

Valliant, P., Bezzubyk, I., Daley, L., & Asu, M. (1985). Psychological impact of sport on disabled athletes. *Psychological Reports, 56,* 923–929.

Wilcock, A. A. (1998). Occupation for health. *British Journal of Occupational Therapy, 61,* 340–345.

35

Optimizing Personal and Social Adaptation

Jo M. Solet

LEARNING OBJECTIVES

After studying this chapter, the reader will begin to do the following:

1. Integrate the psychosocial perspective in formulating a rehabilitation program.
2. Consider alternative practice models and value their application within the therapeutic relationship.
3. Place patients within life cycle and family contexts and recognize the implications of this placement for occupations and life roles.
4. Understand the impact of history and course of disability on psychosocial adaptation.
5. Appreciate existential issues raised by illness, injury, and disability; describe ways individuals construct meaning from these experiences.
6. Be alert for psychiatric complications and recognize indications for referral.

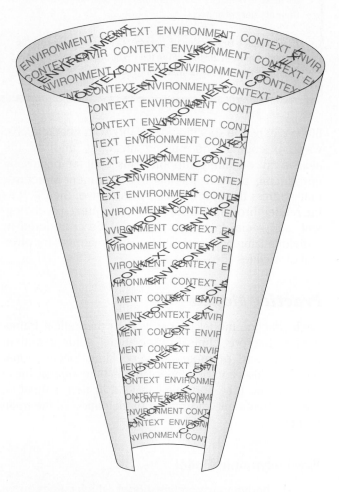

> "Man's origin is dust and his end is dust. He spends his life earning bread. He is a clay vessel, easily broken, like withering grass, a fading flower, a passing shadow, a fugitive cloud, a fleeting breeze, a scattering dust, a vanishing dream."
>
> *Mazor for Rosh Hashanah and Yom Kippur: A Prayer Book for the Days of Awe* (1972)

*T*he immediate change in physical functioning that an individual undergoes as a result of illness or injury is not alone a sufficient predictor of the capacity to benefit from treatment or of the future quality of life. While the **adaptation** process may follow a general outline of stages, it is unique for each person and is influenced by the circumstances of onset and course, by the age and place in the

GLOSSARY

Adaptation—Alteration or adjustment by which an individual or species improves its condition in relation to its situation or environment.

Attribution—Assigned cause or the process by which an individual assigns cause.

Continuity—The quality of persisting over time in an uninterrupted way.

Coping—Cognitive, emotional, and behavioral efforts individuals make to manage external and internal challenges that tax their ordinary resources.

Existential—Description of a perspective that emphasizes the human condition, including the felt necessity to create meaning in a universe that seems indifferent.

Pathography—Written personal story of illness or injury.

Posttraumatic stress disorder (PTSD)—Lasting psychological response to witnessing or experiencing traumatic events, especially when helpless to prevent them.

Relaxation response—Inborn human capacity to enter a special physiological state characterized by slowed brain waves, lowered heart and respiratory rates, and lowered blood pressure, believed to be health enhancing.

Retribution—That which is given or demanded as repayment or punishment for transgression; penance.

Termination—Period of closing a therapeutic relationship at the end of treatment.

---

life cycle, by the specific personality with characteristic ways of coping and finding meaning, and by the availability of family support. This chapter begins by introducing practice models and treatment structures that address the psychosocial perspective, then guides the reader through each of these life context, psychological, and social factors, which must be considered in individualizing occupational therapy treatment for physical disabilities (Box 35-1).

Practice Models

Each practice model uses a its own theoretical framework to interpret clinical observations, guide treatment planning, and promote recovery. Many occupational therapists use components of more than one of these models, and they find this can lead to rich, empathic, creative treatment and fruitful participation of the treatment team.

Psychodynamic Model

The psychodynamic practice model, which had its origin in Freud's theories, emphasizes the relationship with the therapist as providing a safe, empathic, and consistent environment in which healing may take place (Rowe & MacIsaac, 1991). It considers patients' internal experiences, conscious and unconscious longings for wholeness, love, and protection, and conflicts about dependency and helplessness. Motivation is conceived as the critical element for successful rehabilitation. The psychodynamic model both values the symbolic nature of

BOX 35-1
PROCEDURES FOR PRACTICE

Attending to Psychosocial Aspects of Physical Disabilities

In attending to the psychosocial aspects of physical disabilities, the occupational therapist works in partnership with patients to develop, reorganize, or restore occupational performance and life roles.

► The occupational therapist serves as a caring, consistent guide in patients' efforts to find meaning and as a resource for knowledge, skills, and competencies in personal, interpersonal, social, and vocational arenas.
► The occupational therapist, through both group and individual treatment, acknowledges and addresses patients' feelings, personal and social histories, and the contexts within which they live and work.
► The occupational therapist identifies strengths, assets, and possibilities with the goal of mobilizing patients' motivation and coping abilities and encouraging full participation in rehabilitation.
► The occupational therapist serves as an interface with patients' families.
► The occupational therapist directs focus of the treatment team to the recognition and integration of the multiple dimensions of patients' life roles and relates the effect of altered capacities upon these life roles.

activities and mandates that they be selected for intrinsic meaning and relevance for the patient. It advises special care in the ending of treatment, known as **termination**.

Cognitive-Behavioral Model

The cognitive-behavioral practice model focuses therapeutic efforts on the development of patterns of thinking and specific behaviors (Burns, 1990). Therapists who use a cognitive-behavioral model are careful observers and recorders who look for patients' reactions to their environment and for interactions between their ways of thinking and ways of behaving. These therapists enhance motivation through planned rewarding of successive graded goals, called reinforcement; they shape thoughts and behaviors that indicate successful adaptation and extinguish those that are maladaptive. For example, they reinforce treatment adherence and good self-care, such as wearing a splint or taking medication, and extinguish health-damaging habits, such as smoking, and socially isolating behaviors, such as aggressive outbursts. Skills for self-regulation, such as the **relaxation response** and assertive communication, are also often components of cognitive-behavioral treatment (Basco, 1993).

Model of Human Occupation

While the cognitive-behavioral and psychodynamic models are also applied by psychologists, social workers, and psychiatrists, the Model of Human Occupation (Kielhofner, 1992) evolved in the context of occupational therapy. This model focuses on purposeful activities and their central place in the experience of living. Human activities are recognized as multidimensional—physical, social, spiritual, and symbolic—and as embedded within each individual's specific physical and cultural environment. Assessment in this model considers strengths and difficulties in occupational behaviors that are necessary to the fulfillment of life roles such as worker, parent, or friend. Treatment seeks to develop, remediate, or enhance performance. Success in occupational performance is inherently organizing to the personality and is importantly related to feelings of mastery, competence, group acceptance, and sense of identity (AOTA, 1995a, 1995b).

Wellness Model

Research over the past decade confirms that we function as integrated organisms, with changes in one bodily system felt throughout. Separation of the mind from the body is increasingly understood to be an academic exercise rather than a true reflection of the functioning of the human organism. For example, mainstream medicine now recognizes important relationships between immune functioning and psychological health first proposed in the early 1980s (Ader, 1981). Psychological states such as depression (Denollet, 1998) and anxiety (Kubzansky et al., 1998) are now routinely assessed as risk factors for heart disease, not just as reactions to it. In addition, the growing preventive perspective in health care has begun to define the behaviors and habits related to sleep (Edinger & Erwin, 1992), nutrition (Buning, 1999), and exercise (Thoren et al., 1990) that through multiple interconnected channels are likely to extend life and lead to greater physical and psychological well-being. Health behaviors may be particularly difficult to address and psychological well-being especially difficult to achieve in the face of the stresses of physical disability; these often include pain and limited mobility, compromised social integration, and altered sleep and appetite. The occupational therapist works with other members of the clinical team to ensure that treatment addresses a foundation of health-promoting behaviors that can be maintained after discharge (Johnson, 1986).

Practice Structures

Occupational therapists work with patients individually and in groups. Group participation is often an adjunct to or follow-up for individual treatment.

Individual Treatment

Individual treatment is framed by the therapeutic relationship, the alliance between a patient and therapist, which begins during the assessment period. As the relationship develops, the occupational therapist learns not only about the physical capacities of the patient, such as strength and range of motion, but about the type and degree of explanation the patient will find helpful during the course of treatment.

Patients who retain the capacity may wish to tell their story, describing to the occupational therapist how the illness or injury came to pass, their reactions to it, their losses, and their expectations of recovery. Listening attentively to patients' stories, even when their histories are available in some form in the charts, develops trust and tells patients they are unique and their feelings and experiences are valued. Listening also supplies important information about communication ability, mood states such as depression or anxiety, ways of **coping**, and family and cultural contexts. All of these are critical to formulating social and psychological goals for ongoing treatment.

Group Treatment

Group treatment supplies a practice environment for patients' social participation, a therapeutic envelope or safe holding environment, broader than that of individual treatment. Group treatment interrupts isolation and provides a context within which to identify and solve common problems (Ziegler, R. G. [1999]. *Individual and Group Psychotherapy: Principles for an Epilepsy Practice*, unpublished manuscript. Seizure Unit, Children's Hospital, Boston, MA). Groups may be organized to address goals related to specific disabilities, to promote mastery of skills, to practice leisure or creative activities, or to facilitate transitions. Even though the primary focus of the group may not be to address psychological or social needs, treatment components influence patients' total well-being and provide a shared space for creating dignity, responsibility, meaning, and pleasure (Ziegler, [1999]. *Individual and Group Psychotherapy: Principles for an Epilepsy Practice*, unpublished manuscript, Seizure Unit, Children's Hospital, Boston, MA).

As groups evolve beyond parallel participation into interaction among members, patients support and learn from each other and begin to value themselves more highly. A group can also serve as a magnifying glass in which difficult behavior can be brought under the observation of others. When supportive confrontation is used to address and modify this behavior, it improves an individual's opportunities outside the treatment setting. When group discussions deepen, they provide for disclosure of grief and fears, for voicing **existential** concerns, and for engendering shared hopes (Alonso & Swiller, 1993; Weber, R. L. [1993]. *Group Therapy Training Materials*, unpublished documents, Cambridge Health Alliance and Harvard Medical School). Occupational therapists include these social and psychological goals in all group planning, treatment, and documentation (Box 35-2).

The Adaptation Process

There are substantial variations in psychological and social adaptation to disability that are related to its onset and course, the patient's age and place in the life cycle, and individual differences in personality, ways of coping, and attributing meaning to experience.

Stage Theories

Viewing adaptation to disability as a natural course of stages such as shock, denial, anger, depression, and acceptance can be a useful way to conceptualize the psychological reorganization associated with an illness or injury (Miner, 1999). However, clinicians may unconsciously protect themselves from recognizing the realities of living with a disability by assuming that all patients are passing through a natural series of stages that will eventually lead to a satisfying outcome; not all disabled individuals reach a stage of acceptance or well-being.

The four stages from acute injury through rehabilitation described by Morse and O'Brien (1995) constitute a template, summarized next, that may help therapists to recognize changing psychological states and anticipate the needs of their patients. The empirical study of traumatic injury and hospitalization upon which the stages are based demonstrates the special challenges of traumatic onset and offers illustrations of each stage using the language of patients' own recollections.

The first stage, "vigilance: becoming engulfed," is overwhelming physiological insult in which extraordinary cognitive efforts and heightened senses are recruited to preserve life. During this period immediately following traumatic injury, some patients in the study recalled detachment, a sense of being both observer and participant, as they began to direct the helpers who had arrived to care for them.

The second stage, "disruption: taking time out," begins when the individual relinquishes responsibility to caregivers or becomes unconscious. Patients remembered this part of their experience as a fog in which they were lost between nightmares and intolerable wakefulness. Patients in critical condition could not distinguish

---

BOX 35-2
PROCEDURES FOR PRACTICE

Planning Group Treatment

Choosing Goals for Group Participation

- Practicing social behaviors
- Following rules and recognizing group needs
- Identifying and solving common problems
- Learning specific skills and activities
- Accepting supportive confrontation and modifying behavior
- Disclosing feelings, existential concerns, and shared hopes
- Enhancing self-esteem through supporting others

Considerations for Choosing Group Members

- Cognitive and social capacities
- Readiness for broader interaction
- Congruence with other members
- Attention and memory
- Psychosis and dangerousness
- Communication ability
- Cultural background
- Energy limits

reality or focus beyond themselves. They were disoriented, heavily sedated, and not in control of their reactions. Patients at this stage sometimes perceived their caregivers as dangerous and the environment as hostile. Recognizing that during this stage many patients are afraid to be alone, the occupational therapist in the acute setting facilitates the continuous presence of friends and family members, enlisting their help in orienting the patient.

The third stage, "enduring the self: confronting and regrouping," starts as the patient becomes more aware of his or her surroundings and begins to recognize the extent of the injuries. This is a time of focus on the present in which the conscious decision to carry on and rejoin the world must be made, even as growing awareness intensifies the psychological pain. Patients in the study described fear, panic over complete dependence, dread of painful treatments, and desperate efforts at control. During this stage, patients expressed shock at the loss of their former selves and began to anchor to staff and others for support and assistance. Some expressed an idealized view of their past selves as competent and attractive and their lives before the disablement as fully satisfying. Often they believed full recovery would occur in weeks or months, even with severe spinal cord injuries; the smallest gains were very important.

This is a time when the sensitivity of caregivers is critical for supporting hope. The occupational therapist is careful not to break the patient's denial prematurely because this defense serves as protection against psychologically overwhelming losses. The therapist should also avoid making promises about the expected degree of recovery, since it may later prove to be unattainable, compromising the therapeutic relationship and leaving the patient feeling cheated, angry, resentful, and depressed (Davidhizer, 1997). An early intervention for certain patients during this stage is training in diaphragmatic breathing to induce the relaxation response. Breathing may provide the first avenue for perceived self-control. In addition, the relaxation response is associated with reduced pain and anxiety (Kabat-Zinn, 1991).

The last stage, "striving to regain the self: merging the old and new reality," is the period of physical and psychological challenge in which active rehabilitation takes place. The goals of active rehabilitation include making sense of the event, getting to know the altered body, and accepting the consequences of the experience, including the possibility of continued dependency. This is the stage at which patients may begin to revise and reformulate expectations. The occupational therapy treatment plan integrates these psychological goals and addresses them in concert with activities of daily living, strengthening, endurance, mobility, and prevocational training. As preparation for the social

situations that may be encountered after discharge from the protective rehabilitation environment, treatment anticipates and addresses fears of inadequacy and of rejection by others (Gardner, 1999). Participation in group treatment, including role-playing specific situations, such as facing direct questions about the disability or about altered appearance, may be a component of this social preparation.

Onset and Course

The circumstances of onset and the course of the specific disability are important factors influencing the adaptation process.

Early Acquisition

When an individual is born with a disability such as spina bifida or has an injury in early childhood, the sense of self develops continuously with the disability, typically within the framework of the family and often with the support of therapy mandated through school programs. The challenge for the individual born with a disability or disabled in early childhood is to grow into each life stage encountering new developmental challenges, physical, psychological, and social. A disability that does not have major effects in childhood may later become significant as cognitive, emotional, and behavioral demands change and expectations for independence increase (King et al., 1993; Simkins, 1999).

Degenerative Illness

When disability has a slow onset and course, as is the case with degenerative illnesses such as rheumatoid arthritis and multiple sclerosis, increasing disability is expected. Degenerative illnesses are not fully predictable; the course may be slow or rapid. Each loss can feel like a reminder, a new insult. There may be plateaus or even periods when symptoms remit but later recur (Mairs, 1996). Postpoliomyelitis syndrome occurs in a related pattern. Individuals who had a primary polio infection years before develop new symptoms, such as fatigue, pain, and atrophy, that require them to revisit struggles from their past (Jonsson et al., 1998). Maintenance of a hopeful attitude can be difficult when stabilization or recovery cannot be anticipated. The challenge is to reorganize life roles, maintain internal resources, and evolve concrete supports continually in the face of impending decline.

Traumatic Injury and Illness of Rapid Onset

Traumatic injuries, such as spinal cord injury, and disease processes with extremely rapid onset, such as Guillain-Barré syndrome, do not allow for psychological preparation. The dramatic nature of the onset may quickly exhaust the reserves of friends and family.

Affected individuals may undergo not only an immediate change in ability to function but also a discontinuity in time and sense of self, a loss of personal identity, and a shift in confidence about the world as safe and just (Gardner, 1999; Morse & O'Brien, 1995). The occupational therapist considers each of these in treatment planning.

Disability and the Life Cycle

The developmental tasks of each period of life are biologically, socially, and culturally determined, and they build upon those that have preceded them (Franz & White, 1985). Therefore, the point in a person's life at which he or she becomes disabled helps to determine what adaptation will entail. The occupational therapist must keep in mind the normal demands of patients' period of life and consider ways these demands may be met within the context of the disability.

Adolescence

Adolescent or young adults who have begun to acquire some independence from their parents may find a disability that throws them back into childhood dependence especially painful. Psychological distress in adult rehabilitation inpatients has been reported to be greatest among these younger patients, decreasing with age (Laatsch & Shahani, 1996). The emphasis on peer acceptance, athletic ability, physical appearance, and emerging sexuality at this time of life puts the disabled young adult at special risk for rejection and social isolation; development of social competence is an especially important contributor to successful adaptation (King et al., 1993). In addition, as they reach the age that society presumes coincides with independence, young adults who were disabled earlier in their development no longer qualify for the mandated instruction and therapy available through the public schools. Each year 300,000 of the disabled students who depart the secondary schools in the United States do not go on to live independently; rather, they watch from the sidelines as their peers move on without them (Betz, 1998).

Adulthood

The developmental tasks of adulthood generally include career choice, finding a partner, and parenting small children. When an adult at this point in the life cycle becomes disabled, plans and conceptions about the future, which may already have been the focus of substantial effort, require reorganizing. A disability at this stage may require altering vocational course, finding different leisure activities, redesigning an intimate partnership, and rebalancing parenting roles—just when some sense of confidence and direction was newly reached (Rena et al., 1996).

Midlife

A disability that strikes in midlife may find the individual at the peak of his or her career mastery and earning capacity, sometimes with adolescent children or aging parents as dependents. While there may already be a history of successful coping with multiple life roles, this may be a difficult time to adapt and reorganize responsibilities (Quigly, 1995). There may be limited available resources, especially when the disabled person is the head of the household. A person disabled at midlife may feel prematurely aged, deprived of enjoying the anticipated leisure activity of healthy retirement and the hard-earned relief that follows discharge of career and parenting duties. In addition, marriage or intimate partnership may be at risk, as some nondisabled partners choose to avoid additional demands or to seek a different mate.

Later Life

Disability in later life, even at a time when health decline may be anticipated, threatens the individual's ability to participate in the community in which he or she may have a long history and feel an important identification. Isolation is common. The elderly person may be realistically worried about losing his or her home or may already be institutionalized. He or she may be concerned about being a financial or care burden to an aging partner or to children who are stressed by their own responsibilities. Interests and leisure activities developed over a lifetime may have to be abandoned and efforts made to find other satisfactions (Hasselkus, 1991). Anticipated generative roles such as grandparent or mentor, with the opportunity to offer wisdom and nurturance, may be altered. An elderly disabled person may already have lost his or her social cohort and main supporting relationships. When a disability is imposed on an already frail system, accommodation can be extremely difficult. Furthermore, the devaluation of the elderly in our society, commonly combined with limited financial resources, can compromise care and undermine motivation (Kemp, 1993). With recognition of limited remaining time before death, some elderly disabled people feel an urgent need to undertake a life review, drawing together the strands of meaning from their past.

Individual Differences

The occupational therapist will find it helpful to remember that patients come to treatment with formed personalities and ways of interacting with the world that may or may not have been healthy or effective even before the injury or illness. In addition, patients may regress during hospitalization when deprived of their usual roles, relationships, and areas of control, which served as supports to their personal and cultural identities. Some must deal with lost bowel or bladder function or inability to walk, capacities that they developed as babies. Others may have brain damage, altering memory or the ability to make plans or follow directions. Some patients have been hospitalized following traumatizing events that compromise psychological functioning.

Some patients seem easy to treat; others are recalcitrant, uncooperative, or resistant. Some become increasingly demanding, asking for special treatment, breaking rules and exhausting all efforts (Main, 1957). Some appeal to the therapist's wish to rescue them; others, in their failure to improve, stir feelings of disappointment, shame, and helplessness in the therapist (Groves, 1978; Kahana & Bibring, 1964). It is some comfort for the new occupational therapist to recognize that these are all part of the normal experience of being a clinician. Collegial support and knowledgeable supervision help with the treatment of difficult patients and the management of the therapist's feelings.

Personality

Individual differences in personality, along with variations in cultural context and personal history, contribute to the uniqueness of responses to illness and injury. For example, it is often said about head injury that it is not just the injury but the head that matters. Serious stresses may intensify normal fears, longings, and relationship demands. Ongoing pain, with the attendant loss of sleep and degraded sense of mastery, can further alter functioning. Psychiatric illness and character problems can be exacerbated by threats to physical health and the integrity of the body (Zegans, 1991). While each individual must be treated as unique, the occupational therapist should be prepared to recognize and address distinctions among an array of personality styles (Kahana & Bibring, 1964) and ways of coping (Solet, 1991), some of which are summarized next.

Personality characteristics that have driven an individual's career choices and have helped defined his or her relationships may be a mismatch for the requirements of hospitalization. Patients who are orderly, punctual, and conscientious may find that perceived loss of control distorts their self-esteem. They may react by becoming demanding, inflexible, and obstinate; if they become openly angry, they may feel ashamed and conscience-stricken (Kahana & Bibring, 1964). A clinical approach that is congenial, efficient, predictable, and routine and that includes explanations as well as inclusion in decision making is most reassuring for these individuals. The occupational therapist takes special care in pacing and grading challenges to provide for periods of control and success.

Patients who have a history of loss, helplessness, abuse, or abandonment may react to illness or injury

with fears that no one will take care of them. They may make intense, urgent demands, seem overdependent, easily disappointed, occasionally impulsive, and insatiable in their need for reassurance. Some, feeling unlovable, may expect abandonment and may withdraw rather than cling (Kahana & Bibring, 1964). A successful clinical approach for these individuals includes readiness to give care and to show concern along with limit setting that is consistent and not punitive. Good coordination between team members is especially important for these patients, who sometimes compare team members or complain about one team member to another.

Some individuals act guarded or suspicious when hospitalized (Kahana & Bibring, 1964). These characteristics may be an intensified part of their usual personality, but may also arise from the disorientation and lost **continuity** accompanying illness or injury. Neurological and sensory changes can make relatively ordinary events difficult for patients to interpret; a right hemisphere lesion or even the loss of one's eyeglasses or hearing aid may have important ramifications. The occupational therapist is alert to the variety of conditions and diagnoses that may relate to such behavior. Wary, suspicious patients may need continual orienting and often benefit from the reassurance and company of friends or family. The occupational therapist uses language patients can understand to acknowledge their worries, answer questions, and address complaints without arguing or reinforcing false observations. Especially if suspiciousness evolves or becomes more elaborate, the occupational therapist seeks neurological or psychiatric consultation.

Patients may react to their helpless state by asserting their importance, being smug or grandiose, or demanding that only the most esteemed clinicians be involved in their care. When they are deprived of the surroundings, belongings, and roles from which they derive status and identity, patients need confirmation that these are recognized. The occupational therapist uses history taking as a time to begin offering this recognition and acknowledgment. Repeatedly feeling forced to confront their impairments can provoke some patients to make compensatory claims of superiority. The therapist resists the urge to put these difficult patients in their place, because such expressions of entitlement are often a sign of deep vulnerability (Groves, 1978). The occupational therapist is hopeful and points out areas of strength and strategies for ongoing effort (Keith, B. [1999]. "Notes from the rehabilitation center: Psychological aspects of recovery from brain surgery," unpublished manuscript).

Some patients seem to reject caregivers' efforts to reduce their suffering. They may appear self-sacrificing, have a history of bad luck, or even seem to revel in their misery (Kahana & Bibring, 1965). When patients do not seem to wish to recover, their symptoms may be serving a hidden purpose, such as penance or atonement. The occupational therapist may have to refer a patient who appears excessively guilt-ridden for psychotherapy. Alternatively, illness or injury sometimes returns isolated or lonely people to a caring social environment from which they do not wish to be separated by recovery. Treatment planning should recognize needs for social stimulation and companionship. In collaboration with the patient, the occupational therapist organizes in advance for appropriate social contact after discharge.

Ways of Coping

Coping can be defined broadly as the cognitive, emotional, and behavioral efforts individuals make to manage external and internal challenges that tax their ordinary resources. Coping includes what people think, feel, and do in response to stress. Ways of coping can be understood as organized between three sets of poles: seeking versus withdrawing from social connections; seeking versus avoiding information and control; and expressing or repressing emotional reactions. Coping efforts contribute to health because they help define capacity for perceiving and reporting symptoms, for decision making, for complying with treatment demands, and for accepting comforting and support, all of which affect physiological processes and the sense of well-being (Stone & Porter, 1995).

While individuals may have characteristic ways of coping that align with their personalities, the demands of any particular situation, including the length of time the challenge has lasted, are also important in determining ways of coping. For example, the period before surgery that provides the opportunity for active coping by seeking information and making decisions is situationally very different from the postsurgical period, in which little control can be exercised and detachment or distraction may be most useful. In parallel fashion, coping with an acute health crisis may draw on different coping capacities from a patient and family from those required for an ongoing disability. As coping requirements change or become more clear, the patient and family may reappraise their situation, recognizing new possibilities and drawing on additional resources.

In the clinical setting, ways of coping are assessed by self-report questionnaires, clinical observation checklists, and interviewing (Lazarus & Folkman, 1984; Solet, 1991). The occupational therapist can ask the patient or family members about prior challenges or crises and the coping efforts that were made. Treatment draws on past coping successes, for example, by making arrangements for continued religious participation during treatment when this has been an important source of strength in the past (Larson & Milano, 1995). Treatment can also

include active teaching to broaden patients' range of coping alternatives. For example, keeping a journal may encourage emotional expression (Pennebaker, 1995); group treatment may enhance social connection (Weber, R. L. [1993]. *Group Therapy Training Materials*, unpublished documents, *Cambridge Health Alliance and Harvard Medical School*); a pet or animal assistant may offer direct help, companionship, and comfort (Gal, 1999). Training in assertive communication empowers patients to ask questions and participate in treatment decisions; relaxation response training may decrease perceived pain and anxiety (Kabat-Zinn, 1991).

No particular way of coping is in itself good or bad; it must suit the individual in the specific circumstances. For example, coping by denial and withdrawal may serve important protective purposes early after an injury, when recognition of the extent of losses would overwhelm the individual. The occupational therapist is cautious about fracturing patients' protective ways of coping. However, denial or withdrawal persisting over an extended period may prevent full participation in treatment and limit emotional expression and social reintegration. Continued denial or withdrawal may indicate cognitive impairments, overwhelming fears, guilt, or self-loathing and is cause for seeking psychiatric or neurological consultation.

The Search for Meaning

Occupational therapists are confronted daily with illness and injury. We grapple with ways to make sense of the suffering we witness. Our patients, facing these same questions of meaning, look to us not just for help in physical recovery but for our wisdom to guide them in interpreting their experiences. Their confrontation with the fragile nature of life may bring their deepest longings to the surface: they wish for vanished loved ones, protection, belonging, vigor, significance, and relief.

Existential Questions

"What is really important for a life to be worth living? What is it others will say about me when I die? What will my life say? Those are the kinds of questions my brain was filled with after the accident. It's no wonder I couldn't focus on details when the questions of life were asking to be answered."

Alice Lowenstein, *Alice's Story*, 1999

Our patients ask us to recognize and acknowledge these questions and longings. They offer us the privilege of helping them to claim personal continuity and to create meaningful life narratives, which integrate their experiences of illness or injury (Helfrich et al., 1994). They challenge us to seek and reinforce their motivation

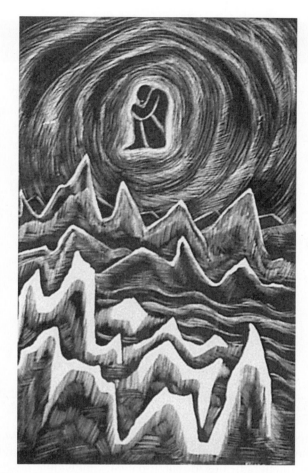

Figure 35-1 The Self in Danger. (Pen and ink by Margaret Rusciano Tolksdorf.) Pelham, NY. See www.virtualeasel.com.

to heal and to nurture their well-being even in the face of what for some will be lasting physical compromise. They need us to join with them in celebrating the presence of interior life, personal connection, and the mystery of existence despite ambiguity, painful loss, and the final certainty of death (Fig. 35-1).

Attributions

Meaning and belief systems are fundamentally woven into the human organism and human society. The way we make sense of experience not only describes but actually affects our reality (Kleinman, 1988). Most people with an illness, injury, or traumatic life event eventually ask "Why me?" and try to make an attribution about or create an explanation for their experience. Clinical research has demonstrated the range and character of these attributions (Solet, 1991) (Table 35-1). Dangoor and Florian (1994) have established sense of coherence, a measure of ability to construct meaning from experience, as more important than actual degree

of disability in contributing to well-being among chronically disabled women.

Retribution

Some individuals see their illness or injury as a punishment, penance, or **retribution**. Because as children we are taught that when we break rules, we will be punished, it may be natural on some deep level to believe that a painful event indicates badness or unworthiness deserving punishment. There may be no realistic connection between patients' behavior and their injury, or they may be accurate in describing a connection, such as a history of drunk driving or unsafe sexual practices. In either case, attributions of retribution can render individuals immobilized by guilt, unable to seek information or emotional support or to participate actively in their own recovery (Solet, 1991). They may require support to forgive themselves; some also need to focus on altering their dangerous behaviors. The opportunity to be heard and the reality of being accepted by the occupational therapist can help them begin to value themselves, feel worthy of treatment, and invest in the future.

Victimization

Again, either through a realistic analysis or based on deep feelings alone, some patients see themselves as victims. Especially when facts support the construction, such as in an assault or an accident from a faulty product, the occupational therapist validates the attribution and acknowledges the loss of trust that accompanies such an experience. The risk for patients who make attributions of victimization is that they may take on the role of victim more broadly as a lasting self-characterization. They may be unable because of fear, anger, or sense of helplessness to see the world as a place that is safe to rejoin. The occupational therapist helps by showing the realistic boundaries of these beliefs and by being a reliable and trustworthy caregiver.

Chance

Chance or luck is sometimes invoked by patients to explain illness or injury. Such an arbitrary universe as these patients perceive may be seen as dangerous and out of control, a form of impersonal victimization. Alternatively, an arbitrary universe may be benign and open to individual willingness to accept not just loss but opportunity. The occupational therapist encourages patients who endorse chance to see hopeful possibilities.

Faith

Many patients demonstrate faith that their experience of illness or injury will in the end have meaning and purpose. These attributions based on faith need not exist

TABLE 35-1
Patient Attributions

Type of Attribution	Description of Individual and Situation	Quotation Showing Explanation for Illness or Injury
Retribution	Salesman drinking and driving, now a paraplegic following an accident.	"I don't believe God could be persuaded to forgive me for killing a child in the accident."
Faith	Computer expert, mother, hit by an electronic garage door when dropping off her car for repair.	"I have learned to live one level higher. Life requires a leap of faith when you no longer understand or validate in the same way. The intuitive comes to the forefront; before it stood behind."
Personal responsibility	Poet, mother, rode as a passenger on an icy day in a car she knew to be in poor repair.	"I never thought about what I was doing then, but since my injury I think about that choice all the time."
Victimization	College student, former swim champ, attacked when skinny dipping by hoods offended by his exposure in front of their girlfriends.	"I am afraid the possibilities for my future are diminished. It is so hard to see friends and younger sibs going through school, finishing, moving on with their lives. I am NOT an evil guy, what is this for? When this happened I was sure I had died and gone to purgatory."
Acceptance	Biochemist hit by a bus crossing the street.	"Is there any *reason* the owl eats the bunny and not the other way around? Injury and death are part of all nature. I am different now: I have lost my arrogance."
Chance	Engaged woman following an accident that disabled her and killed her boyfriend.	"People like to take credit for the good things and blame others for the bad things, but really an awful lot happens by chance. The important thing is to be ready for the good things—*and I am ready*."

only within the context of formal religion to engender optimism and encourage adaptation (Benson, 1995). They may convey a deep conviction that there is a plan for the universe in which good will ultimately prevail, a plan beyond ordinary human understanding (Rankin, 1985). Attributions of faith may be especially poignant for those who are isolated and have few relationships because of their disability (Solet, 1991); recent research points to the healing nature of deep self-disclosure such as takes place in prayer (Pennebaker, 1995). Occupational therapists are open to hearing about patients' spiritual lives and practices as elements of culture and daily life that can support healing.

Narratives and Metaphors

Patients want to tell their stories, and they need to be heard. The process of constructing and sharing a narrative of illness or injury organizes experience, shapes continuing perceptions, and breaks isolation. Through narrative, patients connect the present to the past, forming continuity in their lives and identities (Spencer et al., 1995).

Occupational therapists use several narrative structures to collaborate with patients in interpreting their lives, including life charts, assisted autobiographies, and occupational storytelling (Frank, 1996). Through attentive listening, occupational therapists not only validate their patients' experiences but also enhance their own clinical reasoning, tailoring empathic language and treatment activities to match patients' individual needs and motivations (Kautzman, 1992).

A common characteristic of these narratives is the use of certain metaphors that connect individuals' experiences to universal themes of culture and help to place their suffering in a meaningful context. Hawkins (1993) described five metaphors that frequently serve as frames for interpreting illness or injury; each can be understood as coordinating with role expectations for the therapist and with specific risks for patient adaptation (Solet, J. M. [1994]. Narratives: Empathic listening and therapist role expectations. *Training Program Lectures*. Cambridge Health Alliance and Harvard Medical School).

Rebirth

The metaphor of rebirth is a central religious and mythological theme. Through it, illness, injury, and the closeness of death are seen as transformative and regenerative (Hawkins, 1993). It is common for patients to reevaluate their lives around their illness or injury and to describe a profound altering of values and priorities. The old self dies and a new and different self is born through suffering. The change brought about through this confrontation can be experienced like a religious conversion; wisdom and spiritual renewal can become the gift and compensation for suffering. Part of the role of the occupational therapist is to bear witness to these changes. Sometimes, as described earlier, the illness is equated with a life of sinfulness: drugs, unsafe sex, smoking, bad diet, aggressive treatment of others. The patient may wish the therapist to serve in a priest's role, to grant absolution and confirm goodness and worthiness for care. The risk to patients using this metaphor is its association with attributions of deserved punishment, described earlier. Patients may become passive in penance, feel undeserving of health, and be unable to mobilize for the rigors of treatment (Solet, 1991).

Battle

The metaphor of battle is also common and is the most congruent with the Western system of medical care (Hawkins, 1993). The battle metaphor is frequently used by clinicians and politicians, not only by patients. We hear often of "the war on cancer." In this metaphor the patient is the hero doing battle with a monstrous foe; the therapist is the ally in "fighting disease." The illness or disease is seen as exogenous, from the outside, and a crusade is launched to attack it. This metaphor combines aggression with social optimism and dignifies the active, courageous stance known colloquially as fighting spirit (Walker, 1999). While some patients may relate easily to this aggressive stance, others by personality or beliefs are a poor match and find the metaphor disturbing. Furthermore, the battle metaphor of attack on the invader may not be fully suitable for some illnesses. Cancer cells are, in fact, not an external threat, like plague or tuberculosis, but parts of the self turned unruly. Pain can also be difficult to conceptualize as an invading adversary with which to do battle, since it may be experienced as from within the patient. In treating rheumatoid arthritis and other autoimmune diseases, the goal is to help the patient's body to stop fighting itself.

Athlete

Somewhat related to the battle metaphor is that of the athlete. The patient deals with illness as a game or sport in which the central issues are courage, stamina, and endurance (Hawkins, 1993). The therapist is the coach; the patient is in training; new skills are learned through practice. This is particularly effective for individuals who have a history of sports participation or are sports fans. The risk to patients of this metaphor is in its implications regarding performance. There is an audience in sports; there is competition for who is best; there are rules and standards that must be followed, and trespass may lead to shame, as if the game were lost. The requirement to be courageous and strong throughout the ordeal so as not to lose or disappoint may prevent real communion with others over the reality of suffering and the inevitability of

death. It may be helpful to emphasize that patients, caregivers, and family are all part of the team.

Journey

Illness as journey is a common metaphor found in narratives in which the patient travels to the kingdom of the sick, returning with the gift of wisdom. Susan Sontag (1988), writing about cancer, describes the disease as granting "a more onerous citizenship (p. 3)." Within this metaphor, the therapist serves as a guide, having traveled with others in this same land. The journey of illness or injury may be a rite of passage involving degradation, humiliation, and depersonalization (Hawkins, 1993). This metaphor of the journey fits especially well with the loss of vision (Hull, 1990) or with traumatic brain injury and the subsequent period of rehabilitation (Keith, B. [1999]; Lowenstein, A. [1999]. "Alice's Story," unpublished manuscript; "Notes from the rehabilitation center: Psychological aspects of recovery from brain surgery," unpublished manuscript). The individual leaves the world of ordinary sensations and consciousness and finds that expectations must be redefined; roles and relationships are changed and activities that were once taken for granted must be relearned or abandoned (Pasciewicz, 1987). One risk to patients of the journey metaphor is that it can lead to a perception of exile; injury, illness, and disability can be isolating, sometimes permanently. In a real sense, withdrawal from society may be the result when the individual cannot cope with alterations in appearance, personality, mastery, or ability to communicate. Historically, exile has been forced when behavior or appearances ranged far from society's accepted norms or when the spread of infectious diseases threatened, as with AIDS or leprosy. Group participation with fellow travelers may help limit isolation.

Nature

In contrast to the four metaphors described above, the New Age, or nature, metaphor places faith in the healing powers of nature, especially the efficacy of positive emotions. This metaphor may be construed as a reaction to aspects of modern medical care, which defines the patient as the passive focus of technology, subject to external treatment forces, rather than as a vessel filled with self-healing resources. The therapist's role here is as caring partner. The disease or injury may be described in narrative as presenting an opportunity to improve quality of life, to alter values, or to recognize and integrate hidden powers of the self. The risk to patients is the sense of bafflement, failure, and shame they may feel if the anticipated level of recovery is not achieved. Because this construction emphasizes the requirement to be "positive," individuals may develop guilt about their own normal feelings of grief, fear, or anger, believing that they are hindering their own recovery. They may be deprived of legitimate ownership of their authentic feelings. This metaphor works best when the occupational therapist demonstrates belief in the goodness of the full spectrum of human feelings and in the whole cycle of nature, which includes not only spring but also winter.

Pathography

Occupational therapists may prepare themselves to respond with empathy to their patients' narratives by exploring published accounts of illness or injury known as **pathographies** (see suggested reading list). These authors have many motivations for writing, including trying to find meaning in their own experience, consolidating a changed identity, breaking isolation, validating others, offering hope or counsel, exposing inhumane care, and giving specific information about treatment alternatives. Some pathographies are inspiring tales of recovery or of transcendence over pain or disability (Hull, 1990), even over imminent death (Bauby, 1997; Broyard, 1992). Some are written by family members as a testimonial to a loved one or a journal of the shared ordeal (Wiltshire, 1994), while others aim to elevate natural healing capacities and transform our health care system (Barasch, 1993). For some patients or their families the occupational therapist selects readings as an educational component of treatment.

The Healing Context

Though health care policy makers assume families will provide a healing context for their disabled members, very little formal structure is in place to support their efforts (Levine, 1999). As our population ages and as advances in medical technology extend lives, the burden on family members is expected to grow. Idealizing or romanticizing the position of disabled individuals and their families avoids confronting the real deprivations many suffer and camouflages important ethical questions regarding responsibility for the allocation of societal resources (Saetersdal, 1997).

Family Caregiving

There are 25 million unpaid informal caregivers in the United States, providing an estimated $196 billion worth of labor; the overwhelming majority are family members (Rolland, 1993). Evidence as to stress on partners of disabled spouses suggests they carry a level of responsibility that can damage their own health and well-being.

Loss of disabled persons' income often places these families in financial jeopardy. Dangoor and Florian (1994) identify socioeconomic status as one of the criteria that are more important than actual degree of disability in contributing to adaptation among chronically disabled women. In 1997, one-third of adults with disabilities lived in households with an annual income less than $15,000, compared with only 12% of the nondisabled; Americans with disabilities spent four times as much on medical care, services, and equipment as their nondisabled counterparts (Kilborn, 1999).

Family Reorganization and Identity

Along with added financial burdens, the family with a newly disabled member experiences grief, increased demands, and changes in routines, roles, structures, and expectations (Lynch, Kaplan, & Shema, 1997). Additional stresses may exacerbate preexisting marital discord or substance abuse. Such problems are reflected in the divorce rate, which is higher than normal among couples, one of whom is disabled, with men leaving their wives more frequently than the reverse (Kilborn, 1999). Adaptation requires learning and transformation within the family unit parallel to that of the disabled person. Through ongoing interactions, families learn to construct ways of coping with specific problems and to forge new identities among themselves and within their communities.

Engaging with Family Members

The occupational therapist, often working in concert with a nurse or social worker, may be the major preparatory interface with the formal health care system for a family planning to receive a disabled member at home. To initiate collaboration with the family, the occupational therapist assesses readiness and does not force premature instruction that could frighten, anger, or alienate the family (Levine, 1999). In all contacts with the family, the occupational therapist remains aware of and respects the rights and wishes of the patient with regard to privacy and confidentiality (Box 35-3).

Important differences between what occupational therapists and family members value as treatment and support are common (Humphrey et al., 1992). Hasselkus (1991, 1994) found that occupational therapists focused treatment planning on disabled individuals' level of independence, while family members were more likely to express concern that their returning member be safely cared for with a sense of maintained identity. Ongoing life satisfaction rather than level of self-care is becoming recognized as the most valuable measure of rehabilitation success and one that may be more congruent with patient and family needs and expectations (Levine, 1987).

Engaging With Family Members

Goals of Interaction With Patients' Families

- Seeking information about family medical and social history
- Offering specific information about disability and treatment
- Collaborating and fostering inclusion in decision making
- Validating feelings
- Acknowledging experiences
- Fostering hope and successful coping
- Guiding reconnection with patient
- Instructing in issues of patient care and safety, including home visits and use of assistive devices
- Facilitating use of community resources, including barrier-free opportunities and support groups

Considering the Family Context

Try to answer the following questions when assessing a patient's family context.

- Where is the patient in the life cycle, and what have been the patient's roles and responsibilities?
- How have the roles, responsibilities, and expectations of family members been altered?
- Is there lost income and/or added expense?
- What family problems may be exacerbated by this crisis?
- How has the family coped with crises in the past?
- How will the likely course of the disability affect the family?
- How is the family making sense of the experience? Do they have a specific cultural perspective or religious belief?
- To what communities do they belong that may be a source of help or strength?
- Do they need referral for family counseling?

If the patient is to be discharged home, the occupational therapist typically accompanies the patient on a predischarge visit to check for safety and to organize installation of assistive devices. This is a good time to facilitate social participation by helping the patient and family become aware of community resources and barrier-free opportunities. The therapist also connects the patient and family with specific support or advocacy groups through which they may share problem solving, feel a sense of camaraderie, and be empowered if they choose to work to improve the system for themselves and others.

Some patients are discharged to separate quarters or to institutional settings. Community connection is espe-

cially important to the adaptation of those living independently as they test their social self following a new disability. Discharge of a family member to a long-term care facility involves wrenching decisions and can feel like abandonment, especially to families whose traditional values include loyalty and strong bonds among members (Turner & Alston, 1994). This is true even when it seems clear to the clinical community that taking the patient home would seriously overtake the resources of the family. The occupational therapist acknowledges these feelings and helps organize ways to maintain family relationships even though the disabled member will not be living at home.

In certain cases family stress may be extreme, communication difficult, and reactions overwhelming. Social workers or psychologists specifically trained for treating couples and families may serve a critical role in marshaling resources, modeling expression and compassion, and guiding acceptance of change. The occupational therapist is alert to the possible necessity for a specialized couples or family referral (Box 35-3).

Partnership and Sexuality

The unique role of occupational therapists in addressing both activity and meaning places them in an ideal position to include sexual well-being among treatment goals. Sexual well-being correlates with adjustment and satisfaction in other areas of life and is an important component of the partnership bond (Woods, 1984). As one of the activities of daily living, sexual activity merits an accepting, problem-solving focus.

To acknowledge and accept the sexual identity of their patients, occupational therapists become aware of their own beliefs and values and suspend judgment when these values differ from their patients'. Even when the primary sexual counseling is done by another team member, such as a nurse, occupational therapists are prepared to recognize intimate needs within different stages of the life cycle and alternative lifestyles. They are prepared to initiate discussion of sexual activity, including safe practices, without being seductive or eroding clinically appropriate boundaries. Embarrassment or a sense of undesirability may prevent patients from raising sexual concerns themselves. The occupational therapist acquires sufficient medical and psychological background related to disabilities and sexuality to anticipate patients' needs and questions and to organize appropriate referrals.

Because desire, sexual responsiveness, sensory channels, and mobility may be altered by disability (Basson, 1998; Hulter & Lundberg, 1995), the occupational therapist explicitly helps the disabled person by encouraging him or her to reconceptualize sexuality and

Case Example

MR. D.: ADAPTATION PROCESS AFTER STROKE

I felt a Cleaving in my Mind—
As if my Brain had split—
I tried to match it—Seam by Seam—
But could not make them fit—

The thought behind, I strove to join
Unto the thought before—
But Sequence ravelled out of Sound—
Like Balls—upon a Floor—

Emily Dickinson (1830–1886)

This case study follows the structure introduced in the chapter for incorporating psychosocial components in treatment planning. The patient described, Mr. D., was in active inpatient rehabilitation for 3 months followed by periodic home visits. Medical complications contributed to his unusually long length of stay. During the years following his stroke and after a second stroke until his death, he continued to correspond with me, his occupational therapist. He expressed the wish that his experiences be used to help others. He often quoted this Emily Dickinson poem; the accompanying series of drawings that show growing awareness are his (Fig. 35-2).

Patient Information

Mr. D. was a 53-year-old right-handed white man with severe right thalamic hemorrhage that had rapid severe onset and steady improvement. His presenting problems included left hemiparesis; left homonymous hemianopsia; left neglect and anosognosia; disorientation to time and place; deficits in perception, attention, memory, and visuospatial processing; and complete dependence in activities of daily living. Mr. D. had superior verbal ability, advanced education, good family support, and adequate health insurance. In midlife he was a husband, father, former college dean and public administrator, and the family's primary breadwinner.

Facilitating Adaptation

- ► Practice model: integrated.
- ► Practice structure: individual, daily, inpatient treatment.

Initial Treatment Goals

During his initial inpatient rehabilitation, treatment goals addressed Mr. D.'s anticipated improvements in physical functioning and the therapist's plans to aid in adaptation. Mr. D. will do the following:

- ► Improve his orientation to time and place
- ► Demonstrate competence in basic self-care skills
- ► Improve awareness and positioning of and range of motion in left upper extremity

- ► Compensate for left visual field deficits during self-care tasks with cues from therapist
- ► Maneuver the wheelchair for short distances

The therapist will do the following:

- ► Begin therapeutic alliance
- ► Identify motivating factors and past occupational roles
- ► Encourage continuity through drawings and narrative
- ► Open lines of communication with family

Revised Goals

As Mr. D.'s physical function improved and as he continued to adapt, his revised goals and the therapist's intentions reflected these changes. Mr. D. will do the following:

- ► Compensate for neglect and visual field deficits in the context of reading and writing tasks
- ► Initiate social interaction through improved telephone management skills
- ► Walk short distances with an assistive device
- ► Participate in a home visit for assessment of safety and equipment
- ► Carry out exercises to maintain left arm range of motion

The therapist will do the following:

- ► Encourage partnership in setting priorities for goals
- ► Address existential questions
- ► Continue drawings and narrative
- ► Help Mr. D. explore vocational requirements and expectations
- ► Meet with family to share information, process feelings, discuss reintegration and home care, and provide information about community resources

Factors in the Adaptation Process

- ► Personality: Initially wary, disoriented to time and place, confabulatory. Later cooperative, refined, responsive. Increasing depression as denial lifted. Closely identified with vocational role.
- ► Ways of coping: Formed strong therapeutic alliance. Motivated, tried to override fatigue. Sought and offered information, shared concerns. Insisted on control in priorities for goals: reading and writing rather than activities of daily living. Offered feedback; complained if sufficient time was not allowed for enjoyment of his successes. Maintained significant denial during hospitalization about severity of losses and limited vocational prospects. Made phone contact with colleagues and friends. Started stroke support group but felt "little in common with the members other than disability."

▶ Existential questions: Continued to see himself as "whole" in his dreams. Troubled by lost mobility but more significantly by altered emotions. Described no longer "feeling as deeply" as he remembered. Wondered how much he was "still himself." Longed to return to his former life.

▶ Attributions: "No one is really invulnerable; you just never imagine it will be you." Attributions about the stroke were unrelated to lifestyle (stress, smoking) or religious issues.

▶ Metaphors: Identified with artists and poets, "Seeing in a different way, seeing what others cannot see." Used letters, poetry and self-portraits to express his experience. (See series of drawings.)

The Healing Context

The role of the family: Mrs. D. saw lifestyle issues as in part responsible for the stroke, especially cigarettes. She actively supported her husband's recovery and sought and offered information. She validated Mr. D.'s identity issues, confirming the importance of favoring intellectual goals related to work and leisure over independence in activities of daily living. She became increasingly realistic about the severity of Mr. D.'s work limitations and the likelihood that she would have to work outside the home. She orchestrated adaptation of their home and hired a home health aide for his personal care.

▶ Substance abuse: Though he did not have access to cigarettes while hospitalized, he had not made an active choice to quit, so this remained a concern.

▶ Pain: Mr. D. had a subluxated left shoulder; sling and wheelchair tray offered some relief.

▶ Depression: Depression reportedly increased after discharge as denial lifted and the possible extent of lasting disabilities became clearer. Mr. D. continued outpatient rehabilitation and with the support of wife and teenage children entered psychotherapy.

Discussion

The process of psychological reorganization and the associated adaptation to disability may be seriously disrupted by lasting alteration and instability in attention, perception, information processing, abstract thought, and memory following damage to the brain. The patient's internal experiences may be of chaos, terror, loss of control, inability to communicate, even a sense of dismemberment. The sense of discontinuity following brain damage is sometimes extreme (Grosswater & Stern, 1998).

In this case, the period of severe disorientation lifted, but the right hemisphere lesion left significant alterations in perception of self and environment. Initial treatment goals addressed the discontinuity in the patient's experience, helping to make connections in the world and sense of self before and after the brain damage, reducing anxiety and diminishing isolation.

The occupational therapist provided a sympathetic, consistent, relaxed, supportive, protective environment with well-defined boundaries and limited frustrations. Selected activities were intrinsically motivating and provided opportunities for skill acquisition, expression, and success within a carefully paced program of engagement and reinforcement.

During the later stages of recovery, as denial decreased and capacities for introspection grew, the overarching goal became giving up the view of the old self as flawless or ideal and recognizing and embracing the present self as valuable in its own right. Mrs. D. supported his social reintegration and led the family efforts at adaptation and problem solving.

CLINICAL REASONING
in OT Practice

Effect of Stroke-Related Deficits on the Adaptation Process

Mr. D.'s cognitive-behavioral deficits associated with right hemisphere brain damage initially appeared to limit his ability to appreciate his circumstances and adjust to his condition. He retained the ability, however, to verbalize his concerns and comprehend verbal input from others. How might the therapist's plans and goals specific to adaptation have changed if Mr. D. had impairments typically associated with left hemisphere lesions (e.g., communication deficits)?

---

sexual activity more broadly and to explore new possibilities for sexual expression. When the disabled individual has a consistent sexual partner, the therapist offers the opportunity to include him or her in teaching or treatment sessions. A satisfying sexual relationship is learned; it is based on more than simple instinct or appetite and does not have to be unplanned or spontaneous to be fulfilling (Woods, 1984). The disabled person and his or her sexual partner may learn to adapt to periods of fatigue, continence timing, or requirements for special positioning.

Fears may contribute to the disabled person's hesitancy about sexual activity. Fear of rejection may be based on altered appearance or related to patients' misconceptions about others' perceptions of the needs and desires of disabled people. These fears can discourage efforts to establish or maintain relationships. In some cases, especially when this coincides with depression or

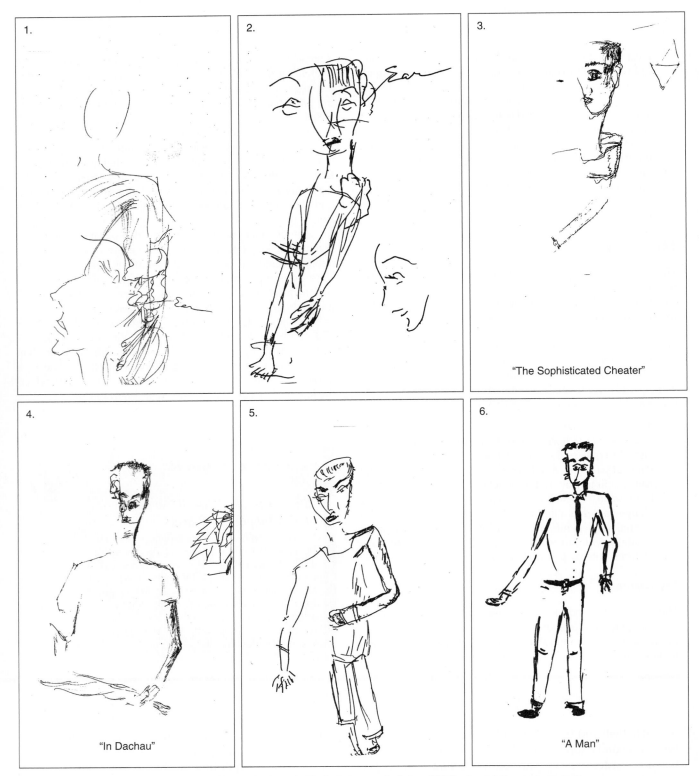

1.

2.

3.

"The Sophisticated Cheater"

4.

5.

6.

"In Dachau"

"A Man"

Figure 35-2 Six serial self-portraits drawn by Mr. D. during months 3, 4, and 5 following right hemisphere stroke.

social isolation, referral for psychotherapy is important. Patients with certain diagnoses may have been warned about the danger of overexertion and may harbor fears about heart attacks or strokes. Some patients fear being injured by sexual activity or anticipate increases in their pain. Here a physician knowledgeable in sexual medicine can be a critical resource. Informed and sensitive medical management, sometimes including medications, can help disabled individuals successfully address problems and reclaim their sexual selves.

In some settings, disabled individuals are vulnerable to sexual exploitation or abuse, especially when cognitive or verbal limitations prevent them from reporting their experiences or serving as reliable witnesses in a court of law. A significant fear of parents of disabled young adults relates to their children's vulnerability in this regard (Hallum & Krumholtz, 1993). Occupational therapists who work with such patients are aware and alert to these possibilities and meet legal and ethical requirements for reporting concerns.

Complicating Factors

Substance abuse, pain, depression, and posttraumatic stress disorder are common complications of illness and injury that hinder adaptation and mandate specific treatments.

Substance Abuse

Illicit drug use in our society is highest among those who are marginalized and culturally or economically disenfranchised (Li & Ford, 1998; Moore & Li, 1998), among them many disabled individuals. Social isolation, losses producing painful feeling states, and traumatic experiences related to injury confer special vulnerability and suggest reasons disabled individuals are at higher than normal risk for substance abuse. Consistent with this observation, disabled vocational rehabilitation clients were shown to have higher use of illicit drugs in all categories, including crack cocaine and heroin, than the general public (Moore & Li, 1994).

Alcohol and drug use have been implicated not just as reactions to but also as causative agents in disability, most notably in relation to auto accidents. Research evidence points to alcohol as having a role in a significant number of spinal cord injuries (Heinemann et al., 1990). Beyond health complications such as malnutrition and liver disease, which may affect all abusers, disabled abusers may be at increased risk for adverse drug interactions, falls due to balance or mobility impairments, and sores and gastrointestinal bleeding that may go undetected because of sensory losses (Heinemann, 1993; Yarkony, 1993).

In studying users' history of drug choice, Khantzian (1990), who posited a self-medication theory of substance abuse, found that many had experimented with various classes of drugs and settled on any that offered a particular type of relief. For example, individuals used stimulants to relieve depression and hyperactivity, opioids to mute psychologically disorganizing feelings such as rage and aggression, and alcohol to break emotional constriction and allow for release or connection. Primary motivations for substance abuse, he concluded, are difficulties in managing feelings, low self-esteem, lack of supporting relationships, and poor self-care, which are particularly common among individuals with abusive or traumatic histories or severely deprived circumstances.

Meyer (Meyer, R. [1999, June 16]. Our models of addiction: Their promise and their problems: unpublished documents. *Psychiatry Grand Rounds*, Cambridge Health Alliance, Cambridge, MA.) studied not only the neurobiology of addiction but its sociology as well. He concluded that for some individuals, drug use becomes a "career." Drug seeking grows into a main source of activity and occupation, especially when no compelling or achievable alternative can be perceived. The addict's lifestyle then becomes a further barrier to other avenues of fulfillment.

As members of the treatment team, occupational therapists are alert to the possibility of substance abuse, prepared to make appropriate referrals, and able to participate in humane, respectful care (Box 35-4). Well-designed substance abuse treatment addresses appropriate stages of recovery; is sensitive to ethnic, cultural, and linguistic differences; and is responsive to patients' particular needs (Health Alliance, Cambridge Hospital [1995]. "Mental Health and Addictions Team." Unpublished document). Treatment addresses the factors that

---

BOX 35-4
PROCEDURES FOR PRACTICE

Addressing Substance Abuse

Considering Substance Abuse

- ▶ Take an occupational history. Was the patient functioning in work or school? Was the patient maintaining relationships?
- ▶ Are any family members likely to be helpful in understanding the patient's history?
- ▶ Is there any evidence that substance abuse was a primary cause of the condition?
- ▶ Might the condition have provoked substance abuse?
- ▶ Are there predisposing factors such as depression, trauma, family history of substance abuse, or membership in a marginalized group?
- ▶ Does evidence support need for referral?

Treatment Goals for Substance Abuse

- ▶ Improve health habits and self-care
- ▶ Develop skills in self-regulation and impulse control
- ▶ Experience group participation; learn to communicate needs; learn to give and receive support
- ▶ Prepare for constructive vocational role
- ▶ Value a clean and sober identity
- ▶ Connect with community resources to maintain change

may have predisposed the individual to substance abuse, not just the behavior itself. Suggested treatment goals for substance abuse are listed in Box 35-4.

Pain

While pain is not a diagnosis in itself, it accompanies many illnesses, injuries, and disabilities. More than a simple sensation, pain is a perception that emerges at the intersection of body, mind, and culture. Pain is an ineffable private experience that each individual must learn to interpret, but it is also a universal phenomenon with broad influence on society at large. A major contributor to health care use and a significant reason for lost workdays and disability benefits, pain also adds significantly to family and marital discord (Grunebaum, J. [1996]. "The importance for effective treatment of understanding the interpersonal context in which pain occurs," unpublished manuscript). An estimated 50 million Americans are partially or fully disabled by pain, with arthritis, headaches, and back pain among the largest contributors (Mayday Fund, 1998).

The Personal Experience of Pain

The daily reality of the individual in pain often includes sleeping difficulties, problems concentrating, and decreased mobility, which limit work, recreation, and sexual expression. Altered moods, especially agitation or lethargy with depression, are common among those who have had pain over an extended period, multiple assessments without diagnosis, or multiple treatments without relief. Grief over lost mastery and diminished life roles and feelings of rage, helplessness, victimization, and defectiveness can result, leading to social withdrawal. Prompt and preemptive treatment of pain is a treatment priority, ideally before roles, relationships, and even identity become irretrievably eroded (Bridle, 1999; Carr & Goudas, 1999).

Pain Treatment

A full pain treatment program includes pharmacological, educational, physical, and psychological components and is administered through a team of clinicians including an occupational therapist. Group and individual treatments are often combined. Education presents a mind–body pain model that both gives recognition to the stress and distress that accompany pain and supports the efficacy of several avenues of treatment (Solet, 1995). Recognition and validation are necessary elements because pain patients sometimes feel that no one understands or cares about the extent of their suffering (Main & Spanswick, 1991).

The mind–body model encourages patients to view their pain not as a simple response to tissue damage but

as a complex experience that can be affected by many factors, such as positioning for activities, ways of thinking, and emotional reactions (Fields, 1997). Diary keeping (self-monitoring) provides information about which specific factors affect an individual's pain experience; this is vital for collaboration in treatment planning. Diary keeping also documents evidence of improvement, which bolsters patients' motivation and supports treatment compliance (see Clinical Reasoning Box below).

CLINICAL REASONING
in OT Practice

Cognitions Associated With Pain

Chronic pain is commonly associated with certain elements of self-narrative. As part of effective pain treatment, the individual must learn to become aware of and change thoughts or cognitions that are undermining function and self-esteem (Gallagher, 1997; NIH, 1997). The statements that follow might be uncovered through monitoring or in dialogue. Using the first two as examples, write positive alternative statements for the other examples of Rumination and Retribution, Punishment in the spaces provided below.

Helplessness

▶ The pain prevents me from doing all the things I want to do.
▶ The pain makes me bad at everything I used to be good at.
▶ There is no point in trying.

Alternatives

▶ When I pace myself, I get things accomplished.
▶ It is harder to do some things, but I can still do many things well.

Dependency

▶ Everyone should take over for me because of the pain.
▶ I can't be expected to do anything when I feel like this.

Alternative

▶ Some things are harder to accomplish, but I can still do them. I will ask for help when I truly need it.

Rumination

▶ I have to attend to the pain every minute to be sure it is not getting worse.

Alternative

▶

Retribution, Punishment

▶ I must have done something to deserve this.

Alternative

▶

The physical components of a pain treatment program can include instruction in body mechanics, and stretching, strengthening, aerobic exercise, pacing, massage and acupuncture. The psychological components can include the relaxation response, biofeedback, cognitive therapy (modification of thought patterns), affect management (control of emotional reactions), and training in assertive communication (Caudill, 1995; Gallagher, 1997). Each of these treatment components may contribute a degree of relief and help patients in managing their pain, even when complete relief is out of reach.

Depression

Theoretical debate over the origins of depression continues, with some focusing on traumatic or psychologically damaging losses and others favoring biological and genetic predispositions. The frontal lobes, which mediate executive functions such as goal-directed activity, have been implicated in the neurobiological processes associated with depression (Powell & Miklowitz, 1994). Clinicians sometimes mistakenly believe that depression is simply a stage or normal reaction to a disabling illness or injury, and that it therefore can be left untreated. In some cases, depression is part of a larger picture that includes swings in energy level and emotions called bipolar disorder, or manic depressive psychosis. But depression, whatever the cause, undermines all areas of functioning and, when severe, is life threatening. As many as 15% of those who suffer from depression or bipolar disorder commit suicide each year; suicide is the ninth leading cause of death in the United States (Nemeroff, 1998).

Diagnosis and Treatment of Depression

Patients whose motivation to participate in treatment is sapped by significant or unrelenting depression not only lose a critical opportunity to reorganize life skills and identity in a protected hospital setting but also fare poorly if depression remains untreated after discharge. Evidence supporting this relationship of mood to physical health is becoming clearer. Research demonstrates that depression is a risk factor for future heart disease (Denollet, 1998) and that depression increases the risk of dying after a heart attack or stroke (Nemeroff, 1998).

Making a diagnosis of depression in cases of ill, injured, or disabled patients can be complicated; symptoms customarily associated with depression, such as sleep or appetite change, can be directly related to the primary conditions for which some disabled patients are seeking care. In addition, actual brain damage may alter neurobiology.

Because occupational therapists often have a close

BOX 35-5
SAFETY BOX

Indications for Psychiatric Referral

- Inability or unwillingness to comply with treatment
- Substance abuse
- Uncontrolled pain
- Traumatic flashbacks or dissociation
- Depression with suicidal tendency
- Mania
- Hostility, agitation
- Paranoia, unwarranted fears
- Hearing voices, delusions
- Social isolation or withdrawal
- Extended denial
- Unresolved religious or existential crisis
- Overwhelming guilt
- Family upheaval

and continuous relationship with their patients, their observations of behaviors, feelings, and ways of thinking contribute important information to diagnosis. The occupational therapist looks not only for somatic or bodily symptoms but also for cognitive and emotional signs of depression. These include indecisiveness, inability to concentrate, diminished interest or loss of pleasure in formerly enjoyable activities, feeling of worthlessness or excessive guilt, and recurrent thoughts of death or suicide (Nemeroff, 1998).

Patients with bipolar disorder commonly receive diagnostic attention during a depressive phase, and the full scope of their psychiatric illness is not always clear. Because the implications for treatment are different, especially in terms of medications, it is important when considering depression also to look for any personal or family history of mania symptoms, which include very high energy, sleeplessness, pressured speech, grandiose thinking, unbridled spending, and even delusions (Ghaemi & Sachs, 1999). Patients' lack of insight into and inability to report their own psychological state during manic periods is the rule.

The occupational therapist documents concerns about depression or mania in the medical record, including supporting observations, and brings this information to the attention of the treating physician or team so as to organize referral for psychiatric evaluation (Box 35-5). Assessment for antidepressant and mood stabilizing medications and psychotherapy is a high priority. Occupational therapy goals for depression treatment include restoring self-care and appetites, improving feelings of mastery through meaningful goal-directed activities, and encouraging social integration.

Posttraumatic Stress Disorder

Individuals injured or disabled through a war, natural disaster, accident, abuse, or violent crime are at risk for the psychological symptom complex called **posttraumatic stress disorder (PTSD)**. Even those who have witnessed terror or extreme helplessness but are not themselves physically injured may develop PTSD. Symptoms may include hyperarousal (vigilance), nervousness, fearfulness, nightmares, flashbacks, ruminations, and mental absence or dissociation (Herman, 1992).

Individuals with symptoms of PTSD require immediate referral to be evaluated for specialized psychotherapy and medication. Coordination between caregivers is critical to a positive outcome for these patients. They need a safe, predictable environment in which they can reflect on, describe, and try to make sense of their experiences. Because listening to these experiences can be disturbing, strong team support and supervision are important for all involved caregivers, including occupational therapists.

Summary Review Questions

1. Write a letter from the rehabilitation hospital to a close friend or family member describing your feelings and efforts to cope following a disabling accident.
2. Explain why it might be useful to have command of more than one model of practice.
3. Using the components of adaptation, ways of making meaning, and the complications described in the chapter, generate five short hypotheses through which to understand why a patient might seem unmotivated in treatment.
4. Present briefly the four stages from injury to rehabilitation as described by Morse and O'Brien. In what ways are stage theories helpful? What wrong assumptions can they produce?
5. What stresses might disabled patients' families or partners experience? What are three ways occupational therapists ease those stresses?
6. Respond to this patient's question: "Why go on living with a severe disability?"
7. Describe four indications that would cause you to seek psychiatric consultation or referral for your patient. What feelings or reactions in yourself would lead you to seek extra support or supervision?
8. What components would you expect treatment for pain and depression to have in common and why?
9. Why use group treatment? What might be offered that is different from individual treatment?

Acknowledgments

I thank the patients who have who have been my teachers for 26 years as an occupational therapist; Cambridge Health Alliance medical librarian Jenny Lee, for her generous help in the literature search; my writing group colleagues; Harvard seniors Matt Stratton and Jonathan Patton for proofreading; sons David and Paul and husband Mike Solet, for draft reading and extended patience; and editors Mary Radomski and Cathy Trombly, for their confidence in offering me the opportunity to contribute.

References

Ader, R. (1981). *Psychoneuroimmunology.* Orlando, FL: Academic.

Alonso, A., & Swiller, H. (1993). *Group Therapy in Clinical Practice.* Washington: American Psychiatric Association.

AOTA (1995a). Position paper: Occupational performance: Occupational therapy's definition of function. *American Journal of Occupational Therapy, 49* (10), 1019–1020.

AOTA (1995b). Position paper: The psychosocial core of occupational therapy. *American Journal of Occupational Therapy, 49* (10), 1021–1022.

Basco, M. R. (1993, Summer). The cognitive behavior therapist's role in diabetes management. *Behavior Therapist,* 180–182.

Barasch, I. B. (1993). *The Healing Path: A Soul Approach to Illness.* New York: Putnam.

Basson, R. (1998). Sexual health of women with disabilities. *Canadian Medical Association Journal, 159* (4), 359–362.

Bauby, J. (1997). *The Diving Bell and the Butterfly.* New York: Random House.

Benson, H. (1995). Commentary: Religion, belief and healing. *Mind/Body Medicine, 1* (3), 158.

Betz, C. L. (1998). Adolescent transitions: A nursing concern. *Pediatric Nursing, 24* (1), 23–30.

Bridle, M. J. (1999). Are doing and being dimensions of holism? *American Journal of Occupational Therapy, 53* (6), 636–639.

Broyard, A. (1992). *Intoxicated by My Illness.* New York: Fawcett Columbine.

Buning, M. E. (1999). Fitness for persons with disabilities: A call to action. *OT Practice, 8,* 27–32.

Burns, D. (1990). *The Feeling Good Handbook.* New York: Plume.

Carr, D. B., & Goudas, L. C. (1999). Acute pain. *Lancet, 353,* 2051–2058.

Caudill, M. A. (1995). *Managing Pain Before It Manages You.* New York: Guilford.

Dangoor, N., & Florian, V. (1994). Women with chronic physical disabilities: Correlates of their long-term psychosocial adaptation. *International Journal of Rehabilitation Research, 17,* 159–168.

Davidhizer, R. (1997). Disability does not have to be the grief that never ends: Helping patients adjust. *Rehabilitation Nursing, 22* (1), 32–35.

Denollet, J. (1998). Personality and coronary heart disease: The type-D scale-16. *Annals of Behavioral Medicine, 20* (3), 209–226.

Dickinson, E. (Franklin, R. W., Ed.) (1999). *The Poems of Emily Dickinson.* Cambridge, MA: Belknap.

Edinger, J. D., & Erwin, C. W. (1992, November–December). Common sleep disorders: Overview of diagnosis and treatment. *Clinical Reviews,* 60–88.

Fields, H. L. (1997). Brain systems for sensory modulation: Understanding the neurobiology of the therapeutic process. *Mind/Body Medicine, 2* (4), 201–206.

Frank, G. (1996). Life histories in occupational therapy clinical practice. *American Journal of Occupational Therapy, 50,* 251–264.

Franz, C. E., & White, K. M. (1985). Individuation and attachment in personality development: Extending Erikson's theory. *Journal of Personality, 53* (2), 224–256.

Gal, B. (1999, Summer). Veterinary update: Pets keep people healthy. *Veterinary Economics,* 3–4.

Gallagher, R. M. (1997). Behavioral and biobehavioral treatment in chronic pain: Perspectives on effectiveness. *Mind/Body Medicine, 2* (4), 176–186.

Gardner, D. (1999, April/May) The protective barrier in brain injury. *TBI Challenge,* 8–12.

Ghaemi, S. N., & Sachs, G. (1999, April 10). Practical psychiatric update: Improving assessment and treatment of the bipolar spectrum. *American Occupational Therapy Association Conference Proceedings,* Boston.

Grosswater, Z., & Stern, M. J. (1998). A psycho-dynamic model of behavior after central nervous system damage. *Journal of Head Trauma Rehabilitation, 13* (1), 69–79.

Groves, J. E. (1978). Taking care of the hateful patient. *New England Journal of Medicine, 298,* 883–887.

Hallum, A., & Krumholtz, J. D. (1993). Parents caring for young adults with severe physical disabilities: Psychological issues. *Developmental Medicine and Child Neurology, 35,* 24–32.

Hasselkus, B. R. (1991). Ethical dilemmas in family caregiving for the elderly: Implications for occupational therapy. *American Journal of Occupational Therapy, 45,* 206–212.

Hasselkus, B. R. (1994). Working with family caregivers: A therapeutic alliance. In B. R. Bonder & M. B. Wagner (Eds.), *Functional Performance in Older Adults* (pp. 339–351). Philadelphia: Davis.

Hawkins, A. H. (1993). *Reconstructing Illness: Studies in Pathography.* West Lafayette, IN: Purdue University.

Heinemann, A., Mamott, B., & Schnoll, S. (1990). Substance abuse by persons with recent spinal cord injuries. *Rehabilitation Psychology, 35,* 217–228.

Heinemann, A. W. (1993). *Substance Abuse and Physical Disability* (pp. 93–106). New York: Hawor.

Helfrich, C., Kielhofner, G., & Mattingly, C. (1994). Volition as narrative: Understanding motivation in chronic illness. *American Journal of Occupational Therapy, 48,* 311–317.

Herman, J. L. (1992). *Trauma and Recovery.* New York: Basic.

Hull, J. (1990). *Touching the Rock: An Experience of Blindness.* New York: Pantheon.

Hulter, B. M., & Lundberg, P. O. (1995). Sexual function in women with advanced multiple sclerosis. *Journal of Neurology, Neurosurgery, and Psychiatry, 59* (1), 83–86.

Humphrey, R., Gonzalez, S., & Taylor, E. (1992). Family involvement in practice: Issues and attitudes. *American Journal of Occupational Therapy, 47,* 587–593.

Johnson, J. (1986). Wellness and occupational therapy. *American Journal of Occupational Therapy, 40,* 753–758.

Jonsson, A. T., Moller, A., & Grimby, G. (1998). Managing occupations in everyday life to achieve adaptation. *American Journal of Occupational Therapy, 53,* 353–362.

Kabat-Zinn, J. (1991). The power of breathing: Your unsuspected ally in the healing process. In *Full Catastrophe Living: The Wisdom of Your Body and Mind to Face Stress, Pain, and Illness* (pp. 47–58). New York: Delacorte.

Kahana, J. R., & Bibring, G. (1964). Personality types in medical management. In N. Zinberg (Ed.), *Psychiatry and Medical Practice in a General Hospital* (pp. 108–123). New York: International Universities.

Kautzman, L. N. (1992). Linking patient and family stories to caregivers' use of clinical reasoning. *American Journal of Occupational Therapy, 47,* 169–173.

Kemp, J. K. (1993). Psychological care of the older rehabilitation patient. *Geriatric Rehabilitation, 9,* 841–857.

Khantzian, E. J. (1990). Self-regulation and self-medication factors in alcoholism and the addictions. In M. Galanter (Ed.), *Recent Developments in Alcoholism* (vol. 8, pp. 255–271). New York: Plenum.

Kilborn, P. T. (1999, May 31). Disabled spouses increasingly face a life alone and a loss of income. *The New York Times,* A8.

Kielhofner, G. (1992). *Conceptual Foundations of Occupational Therapy.* Philadelphia: Davis.

King, G. A., Shultz, I. Z., Steel, K., Gilpin, M., & Cathers, T. (1993). Self-evaluation and self-concept of adolescents with physical disabilities. *American Journal of Occupational Therapy, 47,* 132–140.

Kleinman, A. (1988). *The Illness Narratives: Suffering, Healing, and the Human Condition.* New York: Basic.

Kubzansky, L. D., Kawachi, I., Weiss, S. T., & Sparrow, D. (1998). Anxiety and coronary heart disease: A synthesis of epidemiological, psychological, and experimental evidence. *Annals of Behavioral Medicine, 20* (2), 47–58.

Laatsch, L., & Shahani, B. T. (1996). The relationship between age, gender and psychological distress in rehabilitation inpatients. *Disability and Rehabilitation, 18,* 604–608.

Larson, D. B., & Milano, M. A. G. (1995). Are religion and spirituality clinically relevant in health care? *Mind/Body Medicine, 1* (3), 147–158.

Lazarus, R. S., & Folkman, S. (1984). *Stress, Appraisal, and Coping.* New York: Springer.

Levine, C. (1999). The loneliness of the long-term care giver. *New England Journal of Medicine, 340,* 1587–1590.

Levine, S. (1987). The changing terrains in medical sociology: Emergent concerns with the quality of life. *Journal of Health and Social Behavior, 28,* 1–6.

Li, L., & Ford, J. A. (1998). Illicit drug use by women with disabilities. *American Journal of Drug and Alcohol Abuse, 24,* 405–418.

Lynch, J. W., Kaplan, G. A., & Shema, S. J. (1997). Cumulative impact of sustained economic hardship on the physical, cognitive, psychological and social functioning. *New England Journal of Medicine, 337,* 1889–1895.

Main, C. J., & Spanswick, C. C. (1991). Pain: Psychological and psychiatric factors. *British Medical Bulletin, 47,* 732–742.

Main, T. F. (1957). The ailment. *British Journal of Medical Psychology, 30* (3), 129–217.

Mairs, N. (1996). *Waist High in the World.* Boston: Beacon.

Mayday Fund (1998). Facts and figures about pain in America. *Pain Link Resources.*

Mazor for Rosh Hashanah and Yom Kippur: A Prayer Book for the Days of Awe (1972). New York: Rabbinical Assembly.

Miner, L. (1999, March 25). The psychosocial impact of limb or digit amputation. *OT Week,* 10–11.

Moore, D., & Li, L. (1994). Substance abuse among applicants for vocational rehabilitation services. *Journal of Rehabilitation, 60,* 48–53.

Moore, D., & Li, L. (1998). Prevalence and risk factors of illicit drug use by people with disabilities. *American Journal on Addictions, 7* (2), 93–102.

Morse, J. M., & O'Brien, B. (1995). Preserving self: From victim, to patient, to disabled person. *Journal of Advanced Nursing, 21,* 886–896.

Nemeroff, C. B. (1998, June). The neurobiology of depression. *Scientific American,* 42–49.

Pasciewicz, P. V. (1987). *The Experience of a Traumatic Closed Head-Injury: A Phenomenological Study.* Unpublished doctoral dissertation; The Union Institute (formerly Union for Experimenting Colleges and Universities), Cincinnati, OH.

Pennebaker, J. W. (1995). *Emotion, Disclosure, and Health*. Washington: American Psychological Association.

Powell, K. B., & Miklowitz, D. J. (1994). Frontal lobe dysfunction in the affective disorders. *Clinical Psychology Review, 14*, 525–546.

Quigly, M. C. (1995). Impact of spinal cord injury on the life roles of women. *American Journal of Occupational Therapy, 49*, 780–786.

Rankin, W. (1985, November). A theologian's perspective on illness and the human spirit. *Linacre Quarterly*, 329–334.

Rena, F., Moshe, S., & Abraham, O. (1996). Couples' adjustment to one partner's disability: The relationship between sense of coherence and adjustment. *Social Science Medicine, 43* (2), 163–71.

Rolland, J. S. (1993). Mastering family challenges in serious illness and disability? In F. Walsh (Ed.), *Normal Family Processes* (2nd ed., pp. 444–473). New York: Guilford.

Rowe, C. E., & MacIsaac, D. S. (1991). *Empathic Attunement: The Technique of Psychoanalytic Self Psychology*. Northvale, NJ: Jason Aronson.

Saetersdal, B. (1997). Forbidden suffering: The Pollyanna syndrome of the disabled and their families. *Family Process, 36*, 431–435.

Simkins, C. N. (1999, April/May). Pediatric brain injury may last a lifetime. *TBI Challenge*, 4–5.

Solet, J. M. (1991). *Coping and injury attribution in head-injured adults*. Unpublished doctoral dissertation, Boston University, Boston, Massachusetts.

Solet, J. M. (1995, Aug. 17). Educating patients about pain. *Occupational Therapy Week*, 3–4.

Sontag, S. (1988). *Illness as Metaphor and AIDS and Its Metaphors*. New York: Anchor.

Spencer, J., Young, M. E., Rintala, D., & Bates, S. (1995). Socialization to the culture of a rehabilitation hospital: An ethnographic study. *American Journal of Occupational Therapy, 49*, 53–62.

Stone, A. A., & Porter, M. A. (1995). Psychological coping: Its importance for treating medical problems. *Mind/Body Medicine, 1* (1), 46–54.

Thoren, P., Floras, J. S., Hoffman, P., & Seals, D. R. (1990). Endorphins and exercise: Physiological mechanisms and clinical implications. *Medicine and Science in Sports and Exercise, 22*, 417–428.

Turner, W. T., & Alston, R. J. (1994). The role of the family in psychosocial adaptation to physical disabilities for African Americans. *Journal of the National Medical Association, 86*, 915–921.

Walker, L. G. (1999). Psychological intervention, host defenses, and survival. *Advances in Mind-Body Medicine, 15* (4), 273–281.

Wiltshire, S. F. (1994). *Seasons of Grief and Grace: A Sister's Story of AIDS*. Nashville: Vanderbilt University.

Woods, F. W. (1984). *Human Sexuality in Health and Illness*. St. Louis: Mosby.

Yarkony, G. M. (1993). *Medical Complications in Rehabilitation*. New York: Hawor.

Zegans, L. (1991). The embodied self: Integration in health and illness. *Advances: Journal of the Institute for the Advancement of Health, 7* (3), 29–45.

Suggested Reading

Barasch, I. B. (1993). *The Healing Path: A Soul Approach to Illness*. New York: Putnam.

Bauby, J. (1997). *The Diving Bell and the Butterfly*. New York: Random House.

Broyard, A. (1992). *Intoxicated By My Illness*. New York: Fawcett Columbine.

Hull, J. (1990). *Touching the Rock: An Experience of Blindness*. New York: Pantheon.

Jamison, K. R. (1996). *An Unquiet Mind*. New York: Random House.

Luria, A. R. (1972). *The Man With a Shattered World*. Cambridge: Harvard University.

Luria, A. R. (1968). *The Mind of a Mnemonist*. Cambridge: Harvard University.

Mairs, N. (1996). *Waist High in the World*. Boston: Beacon.

Rogers, A. G. (1995). *A Shining Affliction*. New York: Viking.

Sacks, O. (1970–1985). *The Man Who Mistook His Wife for a Hat*. New York: Simon & Schuster.

Weber, R. J. (2000). *The Created Self: Reinventing Body, Persona, and Spirit*. New York: Norton.

Wiltshire, S. F. (1994). *Seasons of Grief and Grace: A Sister's Story of AIDS*. Nashville: Vanderbilt University.

36

Optimizing Access to Home, Community, and Work Environments

Shoshana Shamberg

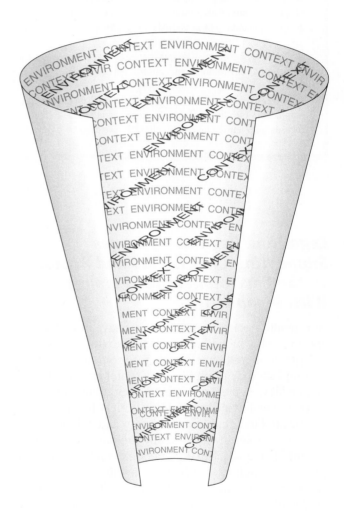

LEARNING OBJECTIVES

After studying this chapter, the reader will be able to do the following:

1. Understand the legal and regulatory issues related to accessible design guidelines and civil rights for people with disabilities in order to assist clients, caregivers, and professionals in promoting independent living and access to the environment.
2. Describe the contributions of occupational therapy practitioners in the implementation of independent living services and access to home, job site, and community.
3. Define and analyze barriers in the environment that may affect the independence and quality of life for a person with functional limitations.
4. Outline strategies and solutions for removing environmental barriers and maximizing safety, independence, and accessibility.
5. Apply principles of universal design to construction and modification of accessible environments.

*T*his chapter introduces the principles and interventions to promote independence, safety, and access to the environment for persons with functional limitations. Because occupational therapists often must advise clients or consumers about their rights and available resources in this realm, legal and regulatory issues related to accessibility are reviewed. Next, the contributions and competency requirements for two primary roles for therapists in the area of accessibility are discussed. The chapter concludes with a review of strategies and specific solutions that maximize accessibility to home, community, and work for persons with disabilities.

Legal and Regulatory Issues Supporting Civil Rights and Access to the Environment for Persons With Disabilities

Historically, occupational therapists have provided training to assist individuals with disabilities to live as independently as possible in the community. This is accomplished by promoting environments and attitudes that facilitate a person's right to decide how and where he or she will live. Two major historical initiatives have contributed to occupational therapy practitioners' influence and role in successfully helping clients work toward that goal: The Independent Living Movement (ILM) and federal legislation specifically addressing accessibility and discrimination issues. This culmination of decades of regulation to eliminate discriminatory practices is typified by the Americans with Disabilities Act (ADA) of 1990. Occupational therapy practitioners who are knowledgeable about these laws provide valuable consultation and information to help integrate people with disabilities into the mainstream of society with greatest independence and quality of life. This **client-centered approach** to service delivery empowers the client to advocate for his or her own needs with knowledge and a wide array of resources.

Independent Living Movement

The ILM differs from the medical model in that it is consumer oriented and directed (American Occupational Therapy Association, 1993). Independent living is defined as control over one's life based on the choice of acceptable options that minimize physical and psychological reliance on others in making decisions and performing everyday activities (Frieden & Cole, 1985). Services to increase quality of life for people with disabilities were established in accordance with the Comprehensive Rehabilitation Services Amendment of the Rehabilitation Act of 1973. This initiated the ILM, which models itself on the civil rights movement. The goal is accomplished through ILM centers, which provide referral and direct services in housing, attendant care, transportation, recreation, housing, and social and vocational counseling. These centers are important because they provide a support system to consumers, often educating the family support network or compensating for the lack of one. Centers for independent living are unique community-based nonprofit nonresidential programs that are substantially controlled by consumers with disabilities (Johnson, 1986).

With this client-centered method of service delivery, the client and caregivers define what they want and need, and the occupational therapists help them meet their goals. The role of the occupational therapy practitioner varies with the work setting and/or the needs of the consumer. The practitioner may act as consultant, advocate, case manager, and often as a provider of both nonmedical and traditional occupational therapy services in the home or community.

Legislation and Governmental Regulation of Accessibility

Over the past 50 years, a number of key legislative initiatives paved the way for fully ensuring that all citizens, including people with disabilities, have access to community, job, and residential environments. Federal legislation addressing accessibility issues began in 1954 with the Hill Burton Act (PL 83-565) to correct construction and design problems in federally funded hospitals. The Architectural Barriers Act of 1968 (PL 90-480) created the U. S. Architectural and Transportation Barriers Compliance Board (ATBCB), which was authorized to study architectural design and develop standards for the construction of accessible buildings. Their findings are reported in the Minimum Guidelines for Accessible Design (MGRAD) (Box 36-1). The Rehabilitation Act of 1973 (PL 93-112) expanded the powers of the ATBCB, which was now authorized to enforce federal accessibility requirements in federally funded buildings, federally funded programs, subsidized and public housing, and transportation facilities. These standards are based on MGRAD and guidelines of the American National Standards Institute (ANSI), a private organization (Reed, 1992).

The Fair Housing Amendments Act (FHAA) of 1988 established the Fair Housing Act Accessibility Guidelines (FHAAG) for multifamily housing of four units or more and civil rights housing protection for persons with disabilities. The FHAA mandates accessibility compliance and civil rights protection in private housing. People with disabilities are provided equal access to housing and a mechanism for filing complaints when their civil rights are violated. According to this law, the resident cannot be denied the opportunity to modify the rented home to meet individual needs for accessibility. However, the cost of the modification is the responsibility of the renter. The landlord may require that the work be done by an approved professional, and an escrow account may be established in which the tenant must place funds in the amount of the cost of returning the residence to its original state. Modifications that may be easily used by other tenants and do not change the nature of the residence are not required to be returned to the original state. Such modifications include widened doorways, levered handles, grab bar solid blocking, and the like. A ramp may have to be removed, cabinets under counters reinstalled, and tub returned to the bathroom from which it was removed to create an accessible shower stall (U.S. Department of Housing and Urban Development, 1989).

In 1990, with congressional approval of the ADA, 43 million Americans with disabilities were awarded civil rights protection by extension of equal rights protection established by the Civil Rights Act of 1964. The ADA is an attempt to correct the many loopholes of earlier legislation aimed at providing services and rights for peoples with disabilities and a method of enforcing specialized regulations through the courts. ADA stipulates that state and local accessibility regulations must be considered in the design or modification of both public and private spaces, including businesses, schools, parks and other recreational facilities, state and local government buildings, and public transportation. The ATBCB used both the Uniform Federal Accessibility Standards (UFAS) and FHAAG standards to create the Americans with Disabilities Act Accessibility Guidelines (ADAAG).

Federal, state, and local governments have established **accessible design guidelines**. These regulate the type, location, design, and layout of public and in some cases private spaces. These guidelines were created to achieve greater accessibility for persons with disabilities to participate as fully as possible in society. Most building design is based on the functional abilities and physical stature of an average person. The application of universal design principles to the construction of homes and public spaces can make those environments

---

BOX 36-1
Abbreviations of Terms Frequently Used by Accessibility Consultants

ANSI
American National Standards Institute

MGRAD
Minimum Guidelines for Accessible Design

504
Section 504 of The Rehabilitation Act (1973)

ATBCB
Architectural and Transportation Barriers Compliance Board

UFAS
Uniform Federal Accessibility Standards

FHAA
Fair Housing Amendments Act (1988)

FHAAG
The Fair Housing Act Accessibility Guidelines

ADA
American with Disabilities Act (1990)

ADAAG
American with Disabilities Act Accessibility Guidelines

safer, more comfortable and usable for all persons and can compensate for changes in function due to aging or disability—an environment that is adaptable to the changing needs of an individual, eliminates barriers, and minimizes the need for costly structural changes later on (Shamberg & Shamberg, 1996a).

Occupational Therapy Roles in Optimizing Accessibility

Occupational therapists are uniquely qualified to help people with disabilities to target problems that may affect their access to the environment. Within the context of optimizing access to the environment, occupational therapy practitioners may choose to assume one of two roles: (1) generalist on a rehabilitation team, who facilitates minimal or short-term adaptations that allow discharge from hospital to home and/or work or (2) accessibility specialist, who consults with contractors, agencies, and consumers to build accessible structures or directs permanent modifications to existing home, work, and community environments. The special-

ist must obtain training and information not traditionally provided by occupational therapy continuing education (see Resources). This practitioner often networks with other professionals for cross-training, including architecture, interior design, landscape architecture, rehabilitation engineering, industrial design, assistive technology, community housing agencies, government regulatory agencies, disability organizations, and building construction. Many government and private agencies and organizations provide this specialized information via training, audiovisual materials, Internet resources, and publications (see Resources).

Expectations and Competency Requirements of the Generalist

Occupational therapy education emphasizes the importance of the dynamic interplay between the individual and the environment and its influence on functional performance, independence, and safety. The occupational therapy practitioner is competent to serve as an accessibility generalist with skills to evaluate the special

---

BOX 36-2
PROCEDURES FOR PRACTICE

Therapeutic Intervention to Promote Safety and Independence: Principles of Work Simplification

► Use both hands to work with symmetrical motions when possible.
► Lay out work areas within normal reach. Work where the areas of both hands overlap and arrange supplies in a semicircle within easy reach. Plan storage within normal reaching ranges in the working area. Arrange storage at first point of use; have extras of the things you need at more than one work center, for example, measuring cups, spoons, knives, and so on. Create fixed workstations where there is a designated location for each job so that supplies and equipment can always be kept there ready for immediate use.
► Slide heavy objects rather than lifting and carrying. For example, slide pots from sink to range. Use a wheeled cart if counters are not contiguous.
► Avoid holding and grasping; instead, use utensils that rest firmly or suction cups or clamps, so both hands are free to work.
► Let gravity work for you by using a laundry chute, refuse chute, gravity-fed flour and sugar bins, or a pan below the level of a cutting board.
► Store small tools so that they are in the proper position to grasp and start working immediately. Store the egg beater so its handle can be grasped in the left hand without shifting. Create efficient storage by using a pegboard on the wall with hooks for hanging, magnetic racks for knives and utensil storage, step shelves to maximize tight spaces with less reaching, and vertical storage racks.

► Have machine controls and switches within easy reach. Change the location and position of switches by using extension cords and minimize unplugging and plugging by using a multiplug outlet or extension cord with a single on–off switch.
► Whenever possible, sit to work in a comfortable chair and adjust the work surface or chair height for upright posture and forearm support. When you are seated, place feet flat on the floor or use a footrest. Use a chair with back support, especially in the lower back. Use a support cushion where needed and slope the seat slightly to the back so that you don't slide forward. Ensure enough knee room to allow you to face the job to be done.
► Use the height appropriate for you, the worker, as well as the job. Jobs requiring hand activity need a higher work surface than those requiring arm motion or pressure. Since body proportions differ, use individualized measurements when possible. The arms and shoulders of a seated or standing person should be relaxed without raising hands above the level of elbows. A work surface a few inches lower than the elbows allows a person to work without hunching the shoulders and enables proper leverage for the work to be done.
► Create pleasant working conditions with a minimum of stress and strain. Natural lighting, halogen lighting, adequate ventilation, comfortable clothing, pleasing colors and music, windows looking onto natural settings, and organization of the environment facilitate this goal.

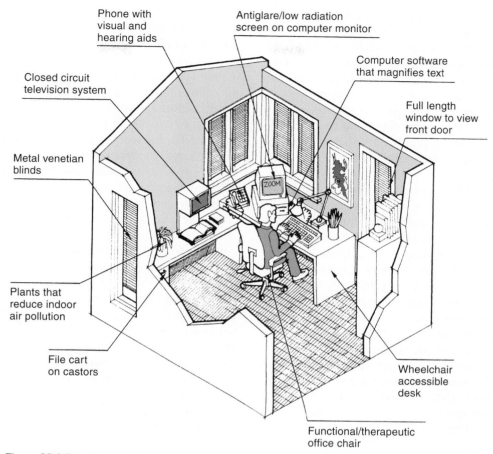

Phone with visual and hearing aids

Antiglare/low radiation screen on computer monitor

Computer software that magnifies text

Closed circuit television system

Full length window to view front door

Metal venetian blinds

ZOOM

Plants that reduce indoor air pollution

File cart on castors

Wheelchair accessible desk

Functional/therapeutic office chair

Figure 36-1 Example of universal-design office. (Reprinted with permission from Canadian Mortgage and Housing Corporation Open House Design Team. 1992. *Open House Guidebook* [p. 6]. Ottawa: CMHC Innovation Division.)

needs of the individual by observing and assessing the ability to perform daily activities, simultaneously considering the demands of the environment, assistance needed, and requirements for modification and adaptation. Generalists advise consumers about relatively simple adaptations to the home or job site; provide off-the-shelf adaptive equipment, such as reachers, grab bars, and tub benches; instruct in work simplification strategies (Box 36-2 and Fig. 36-1); and refer consumers to specialists who help them find more detailed information and technical assistance. Often the rehabilitation team works closely with the specialist before the client's discharge so that information about the client and caregivers can be coordinated and organized for a smooth transition from hospital to the community and home (Shamberg & Shamberg, 1996b).

Expectations and Competency Requirements of the Specialist

Specially trained occupational therapy practitioners may provide consultation and guidance to facilitate compli-

ance with government regulations by consulting architects, engineers, contractors, business owners, private and public agency personnel, disability advocates and service providers, case managers, caregivers, and consumers. These clinicians typically make recommendations about design, adaptive equipment, auxiliary aids, policy changes, **reasonable accommodations** (alternative methods of providing equivalent services), and environmental adaptations to remove barriers (Shamberg, 1993). This specially trained practitioner is known as an **accessibility consultant**.

An accessibility consultant may be trained in one or more specialty areas, such as occupational therapy, physical therapy, architecture, interior design, landscape architecture, industrial design, or rehabilitation engineering. Usually consultants have some familiarity with the technical assistance each professional is trained to provide. A team approach to accessibility services ensures that the many facets of assessing, designing, constructing, or modifying an environment are coordinated and consistent with the consumer's needs, financial resources, and priorities. The accessibility consultant's general knowledge of government regulations, universal and adaptable design concepts, architectural products, building construction, specific disabilities, functional performance, **assistive technology**, and adaptations is necessary to understand the issues of implementation (Hiatt, 1993). Often the role of the occupational therapy specialist is to analyze the physical environment as it relates to human performance, determine specific functional and environmental problems, and formulate appropriate solutions in collaboration with the client and family support network.

Specialists may also be employed in work-hardening programs, in which they play a significant role in assisting employees, employers, and human resource personnel in determining reasonable accommodations. A reasonable accommodation is "any modification or adjustment to an environment that will enable a qualified applicant or employee with a disability to perform essential job functions" (Equal Employment Opportunity Commission & Department of Justice, 1991, p. 3). An occupational therapy practitioner trained in accessibility issues has knowledge of architectural barriers, design, construction, equipment, and installation, as well as knowledge of accessibility guidelines required by government regulations. This knowledge enables the practitioner to make the most appropriate recommendations (Kornblau et al., 2000).

Collaboration Between Generalist and Specialist

Under optimal circumstances, the occupational therapy accessibility generalists and specialists collaborate with patient and family to promote long-term accessibility to home, work, and community (see Case Example).

Generalist

Beginning at admission, hospital-based generalists provide evaluation and treatment that address the access needs and issues with patient, family, and rehabilitation team. Preparation for discharge may include home visits, community outings, and use of homelike or simulated community spaces during rehabilitation. Simulated community spaces demand that patients combine newly learned functional skills to handle real-world challenges that require memory and problem solving as well as mobility. Designed by Patricia Moore, an industrial designer and gerontologist, and David Guynes, an architect, Easy Street and Independence Square are examples of this type of environment (Shamberg et al., 1996). The independent living trial apartment, typically a part of the rehabilitation center, is also an environment designed to simulate a patient's home. The patient's family

or other social supporters stay in this simulated home prior to discharge home and receive comprehensive training. Problem solving and intervention to promote generalization of skills during all of these accessibility experiments facilitate adaptation to the environment and allow patient and therapist to identify new foci for rehabilitation intervention (Shamberg et al., 1996).

The occupational therapy generalist assists the patient, family, and team to select the most appropriate site of discharge. Accessible housing options may be integrated into existing housing stock or multifamily settings, with group living arrangements or a unit adapted for a specific tenant. Housing geared to specialized populations, such as seniors, people with developmental disabilities, or the hearing impaired, provide maximum accessibility and varied levels of care and assistance. Life care communities provide a continuum of care from independent single family home or townhouse to assisted living and nursing home care. Assisted-living centers are increasingly popular, especially in urban and suburban communities, for seniors who want to maintain the maximum independence but may require such assistance as transportation, medication management, meals, laundry, bathing, and dressing. The occupational therapy practitioner often acts as a consultant to match the client's needs and abilities to available services and options.

After a home assessment (see Chapter 10) and prior to discharge, the generalist helps patient and family select necessary adaptive equipment and facilitates its assembly, delivery, and/or installation. He or she trains the patient and family to use this equipment and communicates with home health providers about anticipated needs after discharge. Occupational therapists teach clients to use proper body mechanics while transferring and using equipment and to organize the environment using the principles of work simplification to help clients perform daily activities with minimal assistance and stress. As a general rule, the hospital-based therapist assists the patient and family as they make low-cost or short-duration adaptations to the home, adaptations that the patient may be expected to outgrow as he or she continues to recover. These modifications at a minimum ensure safe and direct access to at least one exterior entrance, a bathroom, and the bedroom. Finally, if permanent and substantive modifications will be needed, the generalist calls in a specialist.

Specialist

The accessibility consultant provides a detailed environmental assessment and specialized product information, carefully researched using information from the design, building, and rehabilitation industries. A thorough functional assessment is conducted, ideally while the person is functioning at home. Information is coordinated with the client's rehabilitation team for effective and efficient problem solving and carryover of the functional skills gained during hospitalization. This can also minimize the stress of community reintegration. However, if assessment with the client on site is not possible, videotaping of the home while the person is an inpatient can provide a means of targeting environmental barriers. Major areas of concern are safety, means of mobility, balance, manipulation, grasp, sitting and/or standing reaching range, sensory skills, cognitive skills, endurance, and the ability to use equipment in the home for daily activities. Medical history, precautions, prognosis, progression of the condition, life changes, social and occupational roles, leisure activities, and support system are also considered (Letts et al., 1994).

The evaluator walks throughout the exterior and interior of the home with the client, beginning where the client gets out of the car or public transportation, and continues along an accessible route to all areas of the home used by the client. Access and use of the following environmental elements are carefully considered (Shamberg et al., 1996):

- ▶ Parking; driveway; exterior walkways, steps, and handrails
- ▶ Outdoor lighting and doorways
- ▶ Lawn maintenance
- ▶ Doorbells, mailbox, or mail chute
- ▶ Interior hallways
- ▶ Space planning in each room, furniture, floor surfaces
- ▶ Environmental controls, such as lights, electrical plugs, thermostat, stove and oven, fan
- ▶ Environmental control units (ECU) for interior lighting, telephones, stereo, television
- ▶ Interior stairs, handrails
- ▶ Bathroom fixtures, water controls, environmental supports
- ▶ Kitchen appliances, storage, closets, laundry facilities
- ▶ Basement access, location of breaker and fuse boxes
- ▶ Personal emergency response systems, fire extinguishers, smoke alarms, intercom system, security system, and emergency escape routes

The occupational therapy accessibility specialist collaborates with contractors and designers knowledgeable in accessibility issues to determine the design, structural feasibility of the suggestions, and the costs of the recommended modifications, equipment, and installation. The client, in collaboration with the team, sets priorities for the suggestions in terms of immediate

requirements to maximize functional goals, safety, and use of the environment for daily activities within an allotted budget. The modifications are generally made in phases: once the client is able to move and function in the bedroom, bathroom, and entrance environments, renovations can be phased in until full access to all areas used by the patient is achieved. In addition to training patient and family to use environmental adaptations and equipment, the social needs of the family and person can be addressed as problems arise. Role changes may result from a disability that prevents the client from returning to a previous job or duties in the home. Transitions to this new status can be less stressful if adequate preparation is provided (Shamberg et al., 1996).

Strategies and Solutions to Optimize Home, Work, and Community Accessibility

This section discusses strategies and solutions from the broad to the specific. First, it reviews principles for designing accessible spaces for all citizens (knowledge necessary for occupational therapy accessibility specialists who collaborate with design and construction professionals). Second, it outlines solutions for specific environmental barriers (knowledge necessary for both generalist and specialist).

Types of Accessible Design

When providing consultation to designers, contractors, families, and patients, occupational therapists appreciate the breadth of access and functional performance strategies and aids that may be available to consumers. The following terms help to clarify the various ways that accessible environments can be created and labeled. This assists in communication with other professionals on the implementation team, especially the designers and building contractors.

- ▶ Environments created using the elements of **universal design** are accessible, adaptable, aesthetically pleasing (nonmedical appearance), and often cost-effective. Universal design eliminates barriers and need for major structural modifications and provides features that can be used by people with a wide range of abilities and needs across the life span. This design minimizes the need for major costly structural modifications to accommodate a functional impairment or age-related decline (American Association for Retired Persons, 1996). Universal design is used in the construction of both public and private spaces and is incorporated in the various

Case Example

COLLABORATION BETWEEN GENERALIST AND SPECIALIST TO OPTIMIZE ACCESSIBILITY

Client Background

Mr. Q. is a 39-year-old man with T2 paraplegia as a result of a skiing accident. He and his wife of 15 years co-own a landscaping company, including a greenhouse and tree nursery, and have 3 young children. About 2 years ago, they purchased their dream house, a 75-year-old two-story farmhouse on 10 acres. Mr. Q. is actively participating in occupational therapy as part of his acute rehabilitation following the injury, with an anticipated length of stay of approximately 8 weeks. Mr. Q., family, and the rehabilitation team plan an overnight visit home approximately 3 weeks before his discharge home.

Recommendations for Temporary Accessibility

Based on the results of a home assessment, the occupational therapist makes recommendations for temporary adaptations to the home that will facilitate both the overnight pass and subsequent visits home as he prepares for discharge. These recommendations focus on maximizing Mr. Q.'s ability to bathe, toilet, and get in and out of the house:

▶ Temporarily convert the first-floor dining room to Mr. Q.'s bedroom and bathroom, as his previous bed and bath are on the second floor and inaccessible.
▶ Rent a commode and portable shower for use in makeshift bathroom.
▶ Rent or construct a temporary portable or modular ramp to allow Mr. Q. to get in and out of the front door of the house.
▶ Contact an accessibility specialist to begin plans for achieving permanent access to home and business.
▶ Provide ongoing support and training for the family to assist in Mr. Q.'s care. Target extended family, friends, and community support networks to assist the family financially, physically, and emotionally during this transition time and beyond as needed.

Recommendations for Permanent Accessibility

During this transition, the occupational therapy accessibility specialist conducts a thorough environmental assessment of the house. The assessment identifies a number of barriers and potential problems: parking, driveway, walkways, entrances, type of lighting, door hardware, hallways, floor surfaces, space planning in each room, type of furniture, kitchen and bathroom layout and use of appliances and fixtures, stairs, bedrooms, basement, safety, utilities, security, environmental controls, adaptive equipment, home and lawn maintenance, and leisure space. The accessibility specialist also collaborates with an architect and building contractor knowledgeable in accessible design and remodeling to obtain price estimates for modifications. The specialist then meets with Mr. and Mrs. Q. and the team to establish priorities and plans. The following short-term goals focus on access to key areas of the house and grounds by the time of his discharge from the rehabilitation center:

▶ Independence in entering and leaving the house
▶ Independent access to a bathroom to enable independence in toileting, grooming, bathing
▶ Independent access to his bedroom, including bed and closet
▶ Independent access to kitchen to enable independence in meal preparation

These long-term goals focus on resumption of self-enhancement and self-advancement roles and were projected for completion within 6 weeks of discharge:

▶ Independent access to the work environment
▶ Independent access to all living spaces in the house, including recreational space, living room, laundry room, and garage

The accessibility consultant also provides Mr. and Mrs. Q. with information about a variety of funding resources to pay for any modifications and equipment not covered by Mr. Q.'s medical insurance. These include grants, special loans, and creative home equity financing. Within a couple of days Mr. Q.'s social worker obtains the documentation necessary to submit applications for funding. Processing takes 2 to 6 weeks.

Short- and Long-Term Accessibility Solutions

Accessibility goals are met through a number of strategies, some of which are detailed below.

Accessibility to the Home Environment
▶ Creation of one no-step entrance into the home along a continuous route from the driveway and construction of a wraparound ramp to the front porch.
▶ Creation of unobstructed spaces in each room with adequate turning radius for the wheelchair (5 feet square). Low-profile furniture, such as the coffee table, moved near the wall. Lamps and cords placed near a wall, out of the way of the wheelchair.
▶ Installation of a stair glide for access to the second floor.

▶ Creation of a master bedroom and bathroom on the first floor with wheel-in shower and a retractable shower bench, grab bar support, barrier-free shower doors, hand-held shower head on an adjustable height track, open-bottom sink with counter space, retractable cabinet doors, and angled mirror over the sink.

▶ Installation of home automation system that controls heating, air conditioning, lights, television, stereo, and security system from a central location.

▶ Installation of adjustable-height counters in the kitchen with easy-glide pull-out bottom cabinets for storage, open-bottom stove top with side-mounted controls, staggered burners, and angled mirror.

Accessibility of the Work Environment

▶ Designation of two accessible parking spaces near entrance

▶ Installation of a ramp to the entrance along with an automatic door opener

▶ Removal of Mr. Q.'s top desk drawer to provide adequate access for his wheelchair

▶ Installation of an intercom that allowed Mr. Q. to communicate with his employees while avoiding unnecessary travel in his wheelchair

▶ Adaptation of all controls such that lights, intercom, telephone and other necessary equipment are within easy reaching range for Mr. Q. from his wheelchair

▶ Modifications to the bathroom that is accessible from his office

---

CLINICAL REASONING
in Occupational Therapy

Temporary Versus Permanent Accessibility Solutions

Consider the effect of the temporary accessibility solutions versus the permanent solutions on Mr. Q.'s psychosocial adjustment to his disability as well as his resumption of roles. Describe a hypothetical day for Mr. Q. a year post injury if only the temporary solutions were implemented. Describe a hypothetical day for Mr. Q. a year post injury after the permanent solutions were implemented.

---

federal guidelines (Abledata, 1995). It addresses the general needs of people with a wide range of functional abilities and limitations.

▶ An *accessible environment* may be used, approached, and entered easily, especially by persons with disabilities. It is not necessarily designed to address a specific functional limitation.

▶ An *adaptable environment* is one that is built or modified so that adaptation for individual and changing needs can be accomplished without major structural changes. Universal design features address the natural effects of aging, which may result in physical, sensory, and/or cognitive decline (Abledata, 1995).

▶ *Lifespan design* incorporates accessible and adaptable features for use as occupants grow older to accommodate changes in functional ability (Shamberg, 1993).

▶ A *barrier-free environment* is built or altered to remove obstacles and maximize accessibility. It is usually designed to address the specific needs of individuals with functional limitations. An example of barrier-free design is a wide, flat entryway to accommodate wheelchairs. By modifying physical space, equipment, tasks, and behavior, a person can compensate for age-related changes or disability

and maximize comfort, safety, and independence. Often the environment produces greater barriers to a person's functional performance than the actual disabling condition (Center for Universal Design, 1997).

Interventions to Access Public Spaces in the Community

UFAS, the guideline designated in Section 504 of the Rehabilitation Act, regulates the design of federally funded buildings and services. This includes recreational facilities, schools, hospitals, libraries, museums, government buildings and programs, and subsidized housing. ADAAG, the guideline designated by the ADA, regulates the design of spaces used by the public, including privately owned, state, and local buildings. These include schools, post offices, transportation facilities, stores, theaters, doctor offices, amusement parks, and so on. Accessibility means that all people, including those with disabilities, must be able to approach, enter, and use all points of contact. The occupational therapy practitioner assesses the functional and environmental issues affecting a client's ability to use these environments or services and consults with designers and building contractors to create the ability for persons with disabilities to participate in activities in the environment. (Shamberg, 1993).

Legally mandated design guidelines provide a basis from which to formulate solutions to eliminate barriers. In public spaces, specified measurements and parameters are designated. In private homes, FHAAG provides guidelines for multifamily and rental housing. If there are offices, businesses, or a day care center on the premises, these must comply with accessible design guidelines under UFAS or ADAAG. Local building code guidelines, if stricter, take priority for compliance. In public housing, individual accessibility needs must be considered and accommodated if not an "undue hardship" or structurally unfeasible. All guidelines provide recommendations for design of architectural features, installation of equipment, and space planning, including height, width, type, and configuration of elements and fixtures. Examples of these include doorways, ramps, steps, grab bars, handrails, and handles (Box 36-3).

Community spaces must also include accessible parking and accessible routes to approach and enter buildings and recreational sites, such as parks. Curb cuts and sidewalks with a continuous and unobstructed pathway wide enough for wheelchairs provide access

---

BOX 36-3
PROCEDURES FOR PRACTICE

Accessible Design of Architectural Elements of Public Spaces and Multifamily Homes

The occupational therapy practitioner considers the following major elements of the environment when consulting about public spaces and multifamily homes as specified in FHAAG and ADAAG:

Accessible route—An accessible site must have a continuous unobstructed path connecting all elements and spaces of a building or facility, such as route from parking space to the entrance.

Signage—ADAAG specifies the proportion, size, location, symbol usage, and level of contrast for character signage. Letters must contrast with background and must be raised and have Braille markings. Raised letters or numbers used to mark buildings, rooms or offices must be placed on the right or left of the door 54 to 66 inches off ground or floor level.

Parking spaces—Accessible parking spaces are required in every parking lot that services employees or visitors. The parking spaces must be convenient and marked for use for people with disabilities. Accessible spaces must have a minimum width of 12 feet, 5 feet of which serves as a drop-off zone and must be connected by an accessible route to an accessible entrance.

Approaches—Paths must be a minimum of 36 inches wide. Pathways should be constructed of firm, smooth, nonslip continuous surfaces. Ramps must have handrails, curb guards, and nonslip surfaces. Landings must be provided at the base and top of each ramp. These landings must be no more than 30 feet apart.

Doors and doorways—A doorway must have a clear opening of 36 inches (32 inches with door open) and must be operable by a single effort. Doorway entrances must be level at grade (0.5 inch or lower threshold). Fire doors are exempt from accessibility guidelines. Turnstile or revolving entrances are not accessible to those who use wheelchairs, and an alternative must be provided.

Stairs—Stairs must be designed to have consistent tread and riser dimensions, be equipped with handrails, drain properly, and have adequate lighting and nonslip surfaces.

Elevators—Elevators should be automatically operated and should have a cab door at least 32 inches wide, protective door and reopening devices, door and signal timing for hall calls, a door delay for cab calls, and an area large enough for wheelchair accessibility.

Controls—Switches and controls for light, heat, ventilation, windows, curtains, fire alarms, and all similar controls must be placed within reach of people in wheelchairs, preferably approximately 42 inches off the floor.

Warning signals—Warning signals must be both visual and audible in nature and located at appropriate accessible heights as designated by ADAAG. Fire or exit signage must be at least 7 feet from the floor.

Lighting—Adequate nonglare lighting should be provided, and electrical outlets and rocker-style or pressure-sensitive switches must be located at accessible heights.

Public telephones and water fountains—A public telephone must be placed so that the coin slot, dial, and headset are reachable from a wheelchair. Phones for people with hearing impairments should be labeled as such, with clear visual operating instructions. Coin slots should not be more than 54 inches off the floor. Similarly, water fountains should be fully accessible. The fountain should not be recessed. Its controls should be on the front of the unit. A wall-mounted unit should not be more than 36 inches off the floor. An accessible cup dispenser and a telephone amplification device are examples of reasonable accommodations.

Bathrooms—Toilet stalls should have grab bars. Toilet partitions should be rearranged and widened to increase maneuverability. Clearance under sinks and counters is necessary. Insulation on hot water pipes under sinks is important. Lowering paper dispensers, raising toilet seats, providing an accessible flushing lever, and lower mirrors or full-length mirrors are appropriate.

Automated teller machines—ATMs must be usable for people with disabilities. Accommodations may be as simple as the installation of an angled mirror to enable a person in a wheelchair to see the screen or may run to major redesign and retrofitting. Tactile cues, Braille, and/or voice prompts must be provided for people with visual impairments.

throughout the community. Auditory signals on elevators and traffic intersections, varying textures on ground and floor surfaces, contrasting the color of surfaces and edges for cueing, increased lighting, large print and Braille or raised-letter signage, and scrolled handrails for directional cues provide access for the persons with visual impairments. Visual and vibrating signals on alarms and electronic devices, Telecommunications Devices for the Deaf (TDDs), amplification devices, closed captioning, and sign language interpreters provide access for persons with hearing impairments. Ramps, lifts, elevators, seating along a route, and handrails provide safe access for persons with mobility or endurance impairment. Unobstructed aisles to allow for wheelchair access in stores and placement of items on shelves within reach are also necessary. A designated salesperson can also be provided if assistance is needed. A firm pathway along a continuous route that is wide enough for a wheelchair enables access to a park, playground, beach, golf course, or other recreational site.

All of these accommodations enable persons with disabilities to participate fully in society. The occupational therapist assists the client, employer, and facility manager to target barriers in the environment and provide the most appropriate equipment and modifications to facilitate compliance with ADA and independent living in the community. Occupational therapy practitioners providing accessibility consultation can also provide inservice and training programs to sensitize people to the needs of those with disabilities to minimize discriminatory attitudes and policies.

Interventions for Access in the Work Environment

Title I of the ADA ensures that workers with disabilities are given the accommodations that enable them to perform the tasks required for their job (see Chapter 33). No qualified person with a disability can be denied access to the job site because of a functional limitation. Examples of accommodations are computer adaptations, such as voice input and output software, large-print screens, adapted keyboards, accessible workstations and bathroom, adapted telephones, TDDs, Braille and large print materials, sign language interpreter, and adapted controls on equipment (Fig. 36-1). Accessible parking spaces must be designated and a continuous and unobstructed route must allow entry to the building via a no-step entrance or ramp. Wheelchair equipment must also be accessible to the worker if required on the job. Doors must open with 5 pounds or less of pressure or with electronic controls. An intercom system to a person designated to open the door may be an accommodation

if security is an issue. A continuous and unobstructed route must also be provided for the person's workstation and office. Access to water fountains or an accessible cup dispenser is also required. Telephones, copy machines, and other office equipment must be located at an accessible height and within an approachable area.

Interventions for Access to the Home Environment

Some persons with disabilities achieve access to home environments by purchasing or renting an existing space in which principles of universal design were employed. Occupational therapy accessibility specialists may have contributed to their design and construction by providing suggestions for the removal of barriers. Access to home may also be achieved by modifying an existing space, employing the expertise of specialists or generalists.

Designing New Accessible Homes
The occupational therapy practitioner uses universal design as a guide to understanding the issues involved in creating an accessible home. The concept of **visitability**, created by Eleanor Smith of Concrete Change in Atlanta, GA, suggests that all environments be designed so that people can visit one another. The features of a visitable environment facilitate inclusion in the community for people with mobility impairments. Where this concept has been used in the design of housing developments and other residential projects, a person using a wheelchair can visit the neighbors and take a baby carriage, bike, or heavy packages into the home without lifting and climbing up stairs. Visitability suggests basic standards for access, including at least one no-step entrance, access to the main floor of the home, and access to a bathroom with an accessible toilet, sink, and light switch. Private homes are not required to be accessible; however, it is often recommended that basic features of access be incorporated into the design in case of future need. This eliminates the need for major and often costly modifications needed later on (Concrete Change, 2001).

Modifying Existing Homes to Achieve Accessibility
The FHAAG, the guideline of the FHAA, regulates the design of private multifamily housing. As previously discussed, rental property must be altered to make accommodations for individual needs if **structurally feasible**, and the tenant must pay for the modifications. The landlord is not required to provide an accessible environment but cannot deny a person permission to renovate the environment to fit his or her specific needs.

Specific Solutions for Designing Accessible Homes or Modifying Existing Homes

Instructions for achieving accessibility in a variety of home environments are reviewed. These ideas are applicable to the design of new spaces or modification of existing homes. Box 36-4 has suggested modifications for various functional limitations. The following specifications are from Leibrock (1995) and Steinfeld (1996).

Parking, Entrances, Ramps, Stairs, and Handrails

Provide a continuous and unobstructed route from the parking area to the dwelling, elevators, and apartment or house entrances. Eliminate any obstructions or protruding surfaces along this route. Provide accessible parking in direct and close access to the accessible entrance. Install motion-sensitive, photosensitive, or automatically timed lighting along this route for security and visual cueing for safety and direction. Construct walkways and hallways at least 48 inches wide with smooth, even,

continuous surfaces. Ensure that there is access to at least one entrance either with no steps or with a ramp or porch lift.

Build ramps according to the functional needs of the client and caregivers, considering configuration and slope (1 foot of length for every 12 to 20 inches of height). Construct a level platform at the top and bottom of the ramp with adequate maneuvering space and clearance on the latch side of the door (Fig. 36-2). Indoor and outdoor ramp specifications include the type and location of floor surface, grading, width, handrails, landings, and edgings.

Install adequate handrails and environmental supports along both sides of walkways, stairs, ramps, and hallways and extend these beyond the top and bottom stairs for maximum stability. Construct stairs with adequate riser heights and widths, nonslip surfaces like stair treads and textures, and low-pile carpets glued to the floor. Use of a contrasting color or reflective tape along

---

BOX 36-4
PROCEDURES FOR PRACTICE

Examples of Suggested Modifications for Specific Functional Limitations

The following are examples of environmental modifications for persons with visual impairments:

▸ Bright lighting, either with high wattage bulbs or multiple bulbs. Use nonglare lighting with sconces or shades. Halogen lighting is recommended for close work and task lighting in work areas for extra lighting when needed. Use switches that can provide adjustable light intensity for different tasks.

▸ Window treatments that allow for light filtering and adjustment and awnings on the outside of windows when direct sunlight is the most intense.

▸ Contrasting colors of surfaces to define objects and spaces, especially background and foreground, such as light switch covers contrasting with walls, chair seat contrasting with floor, wall contrasting with floor, countertops contrasting with sink, dark food on light-colored cutting board and the reverse, step edges contrasting with step surface.

▸ Tactile indicators, raised letters, or voice output on controls and signage. Use of large print with high contrast from the background. Varying textures to provide cues for directionality and dangerous situations.

▸ Elimination of busy and confusing patterns on such surfaces as rugs, upholstery, and wallpaper.

▸ Elimination of clutter and obstacles from access routes throughout the environment and removal of low-profile furniture or moving it against walls out of access routes.

▸ Visual aides such as closed-circuit television, magnifiers, large prints computer screens with high contrast, talking devices.

▸ Illuminated switches for appliances and lights. Large knobs and handles that contrast in color and have a nonslip surface.

▸ Bathroom grab bar system that contrasts with the wall and that has a 1.5-inch diameter and a nonslip surface. Colored tape may be wrapped around the bar to create a pattern.

The following are common environmental modifications to address the needs of persons with hearing impairments:

▸ Use of TDDs for telephone communication. Use of fax machine and telephone relay system.

▸ Handy access to paper and writing implement for communication.

▸ Vibrating or visual signal devices, such as alarm clocks, smoke alarms, telephone, doorbell, baby monitor to place under pillow or bed when sleeping.

▸ Closed caption features on television and videos. Use of closed-loop or amplification devices for use in group settings or large spaces.

▸ Access to oral and sign language interpreters when needed.

▸ Amplification devices to eliminate background noises and increase volume of desired noise.

▸ Arrange furniture so people sit facing each other and ensure that there is adequate lighting so the person can use visual cues when speaking.

(continued)

BOX 36-4
PROCEDURES FOR PRACTICE

Examples of Suggested Modifications for Specific Functional Limitations (Continued)

The following suggestions address the needs of persons with mobility impairments:

- Ranch-style houses with at least one no-step entrance. The house should be on a flat lot with continuous sidewalks and street access from house to house and block to block. The house should be in an area with accessible public spaces like banks, shopping centers, library, post office, medical offices, parks, and recreation centers.
- Open, unobstructed spaces in each room with adequate turning radius for the wheelchair.
- Bathroom off the master bedroom with a wheel-in shower, transfer space on at least one side of the toilet, pull-down grab bars to use when needed.
- Open-bottom sink with counter space and a GFI outlet within easy reach.
- Either a built-in transfer bench or portable one in the shower. Barrier-free shower doors or a shower curtain. Hand-held shower head on an adjustable height track.
- Wheelchair stair lift providing access to the finished basement.
- Patio or deck off the back door and master bedroom with access to a garden area.
- Environmental control system (ECU) to regulate the thermostat, lighting, television, stereo, and so on from one portable control unit.
- Wheelchair-accessible home office with computer station.
- Adjustable-height countertops, cabinets, and sinks.
- Wall oven and microwave at accessible heights.
- Stovetop with staggered burners and front or side controls.
- Angled mirror over the stove to show contents of pots for a seated person.
- Accessible switches for exhaust ventilation and fire extinguisher.

- Low-maintenance lawn covering and landscaping. Raised, vertical, or container beds for gardening from a wheelchair.
- Garbage can on wheels.
- Wheelchair-accessible table tennis, pool table, swimming pool with a lift.

The following recommendations address the needs of persons with mild dementia living in their own homes:

- Environment cues and assistive devices to address safety and memory deficits and communication deficits.
- Personal emergency response system with medication management. Training in use of devices and monitoring of ability to learn.
- Automatic medication management system that is set up weekly by a home care nurse.
- Burglar alarm and posted fire escape plan. Client instructed in emergency response and escape, with periodic reinforcement to ensure carryover of learning. Smoke alarms that are hot-wired with battery backup.
- Emergency lighting in case of power failure.
- Daily call to monitor self-care ability.
- Meals on Wheels and use of microwave with electric hot water pot. Electric range or microwave oven rather than gas stove. Step by step instructions for each appliance and any safety precautions on or next to the device. Ongoing monitoring for safety awareness and proper use.
- Preprogrammed telephone numbers used most for one-button speed calling.
- Well-organized environment to compensate for any problem solving or memory deficits. Labeled cabinets or doors removed in the kitchen for viewing their contents.

each stair edge makes it easy to see the edge of each stair, especially the top and bottom ones (Steinfeld, 1996).

Doorways

Eliminate door thresholds or construct them 0.5 inch high or less, with beveled edges on both sides. Provide kick plates along the bottom of each door to prevent scratches and gouging from wheelchairs and walkers. Install lower peepholes or provide windows along the side of the entrance doors so the client can view visitors from a seated position. Construct doorways at least 36 inches wide with at least a 32-inch clearance when the door is open. Installation of swing-clear hinges provides a low-cost alternative by providing an additional 2

inches of clearance when the door is open. Ensure that door pressure is 5 pounds or less or install automatic door openers and keyless locks to eliminate the need for grasping and manipulating doorknobs and keys. Install levered door handles or doorknob adapters to minimize grasping and turning motions.

Kitchens and Bathrooms

Ensure that each room has enough area for a wheelchair to turn and maneuver, usually a minimum of 60 inches of diameter, or 5 feet square. In tight spaces, such as in a kitchen and bathroom, open cupboards under countertops and sinks and open shower stalls can be used for this turning area (Figs. 36-3 and 36-4). Multilevel or adjustable sink, cabinet, and countertop heights provide

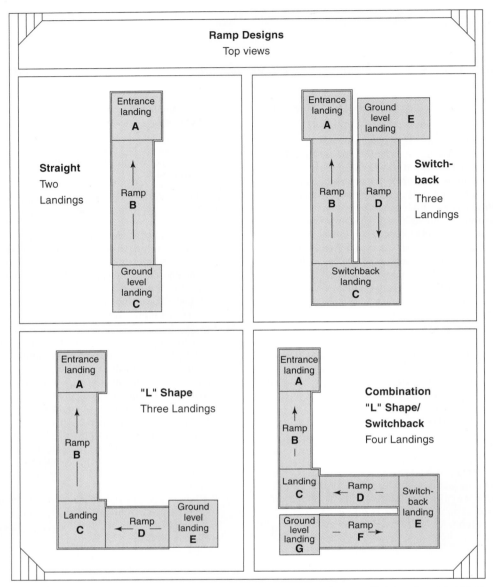

Figure 36-2 Typical ramp specifications. For an outdoor uncovered ramp, the ratio of height to length is 1:20 (for every inch of height, 20 inches of length). For a covered outdoor or indoor ramp, the ratio is typically 1:12. Landings are needed wherever the ramp changes direction and at 30-foot intervals on long ramps. The landing at the top of the ramp should be 5 × 5 feet for adequate maneuvering. The bottom of the ramp must have at least 5 feet of level area at the termination point. Recommended widths of ramps range from 36 to 48 inches with handrail grasping surface 30 to 34 inches high. (Reprinted from Henson J. 1988. *Building a Ramp* [p. 7]. Little Rock, AR: Arkansas Department of Human Services, Division of Rehabilitation Services.)

accessibility from standing and seated positions. Install sink pipes against the back wall and insulate hot water pipes to prevent burns. Use single-lever faucet handles and/or automatic faucets, hand dryers, and soap and shampoo dispensers for a person with limited hand function and upper body strength. An angled mirror on the wall in front of the bathroom sink is helpful for seeing from a seated position. A side-mounted medicine cabi-

net enables easy reaching into and seeing the contents. Install nonglare lighting with accessible controls for lights, ventilation fan, and auxiliary heating. A ground fault intercept (GFI) outlet prevents electrocution during use of electrical appliances near a sink or other source of water.

Use a toilet seat adapter or install a toilet 17 to 19 inches high for level wheelchair transfers and minimal bending when getting up and down. (For a child or person with a small stature, heights should be appropriately determined.)

An accessible shower stall or a shower room provides easy and safe access to the bathing area for a person with mobility problems (Fig. 36-3). Install a grab bar system throughout the bathroom, especially around the toilet and tub or shower to ensure adequate and appropriate grasping surfaces, locations, and heights to ensure stability in this space. Use of a hand-held shower head on an adjustable height track enables a person to bathe from either a seated or standing position. Provide recommendations for the most appropriate shower chair or transfer bench for maximum stability and safety within the constraints of the space. Tub lifts, which lower or raise a person, provide access and safe transfer for someone with poor stability. Use of a rubberized mat and tub strips provide a nonslip floor surface. Contrasting color of surfaces, such as the toilet and floor or grab bar and wall, define surfaces for people with visual or cognitive impairments. Installation of an emergency call system or telephone mounted within

reach from the floor enable someone living alone to call for help.

A U- or L-shaped configuration in the kitchen design can provide efficiency of movement and work (Fig. 36-4). In the kitchen, install cabinets with toe space at the bottom to clear the wheelchair footrests. Use a side-by-side shallow refrigerator with adjustable shelves and drawers. To minimize reaching and bending, place plastic boxes, lazy Susans, and pull-out shelving in the back of the refrigerator and kitchen cabinets. Install a wall oven at an accessible height along with a pull-out shelf underneath that provides a stable surface for transferring hot items from the oven and a work surface to use from a seated position. A side mounted oven door minimizes reach into the hot oven. Ensure that appliances and sinks have counter space on both sides so heavy items can be slid from one place to another without excessive lifting. Install nonglare task lighting over work areas for extra lighting when needed. Install a shallow sink with an open bottom, single-lever faucet controls, and retractable water hose for maximum use and access. Ensure that a fire extinguisher is

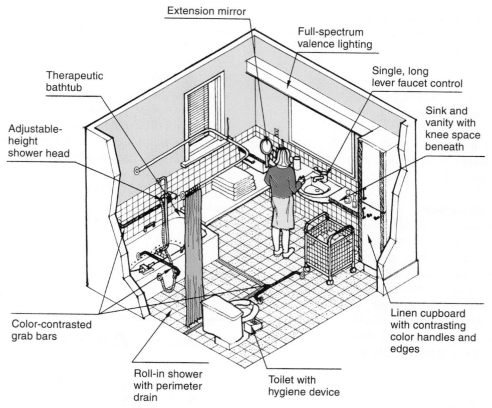

Figure 36-3 Example of universal-design bathroom. (Reprinted with permission from Canadian Mortgage and Housing Corporation Open House Design Team. 1992. *Open House Guidebook* [p. 10]. Ottawa: CMHC Innovation Division.)

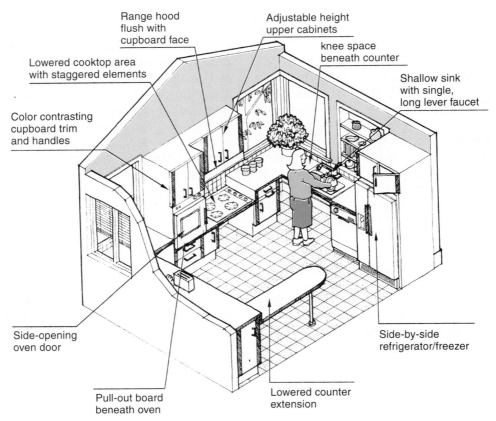

Range hood
flush with
cupboard face

Adjustable height
upper cabinets

knee space
beneath counter

Lowered cooktop area
with staggered elements

Shallow sink
with single,
long lever faucet

Color contrasting
cupboard trim
and handles

Side-opening
oven door

Side-by-side
refrigerator/freezer

Pull-out board
beneath oven

Lowered counter
extension

Figure 36-4 Example of universal-design kitchen. (Reprinted with permission from Canadian Mortgage and Housing Corporation Open House Design Team. 1992. *Open House Guidebook* [p. 14]. Ottawa: CMHC Innovation Division.)

mounted at an accessible height and location. A message board or tape recorder can be used for notes and directions on the use of small appliances. Use large knobs or buttons on stove, dishwasher, and microwave controls for ease in turning. Install a strip plug outlet with a single on–off switch at the front of a counter for ease in using small appliances.

Furniture and Floor Surfaces

Ensure that furniture seating is firm and high enough for smooth transfers and movements from sit to stand. Sturdy armrests with a good grasping surface provide stability for good body mechanics while getting up and down. An electronically controlled lounge chair or a spring-loaded seat lifter increases independence and safety. Provide dense short-loop carpet, preferably glued down, or install with a dense, firm thin pad. Finish wood floors with a matte or natural finish. Install linoleum with a nonslip finish.

Environmental Controls

Elevator controls must be accessible from a wheelchair and should have tactile and auditory indicators for each floor. Light switches should be at least 36 inches from the floor, and telephone jacks and electrical plug outlets should be 18 to 24 inches from the floor. Illuminated switches are easy to find in the dark and in the daytime indicate whether a light is off or on, especially useful for stairways and basements. Photosensitive night lights along hallways and rooms that one may use in the middle of the night, such as the bathroom, provide low nonglaring light. ECUs can enable a person to regulate thermostats, lighting, stereo, and television from a single location or portable control unit (see Chapter 17). Intercoms to entrances and other rooms and remote-controlled door openers can decrease the need to move quickly and unnecessarily.

Summary Review Questions

1. What federal legislation related to civil rights for persons with disabilities led to the development of the ADA and the accessibility guidelines used to guide architectural design? Why is knowledge of these important to the occupational therapy practitioner who consults on accessibility?

2. What is the role of and knowledge needed by the occupational therapy practitioner to provide services with a client-centered approach? What are some of the roles of the generalist and the specialist? Who are the members of the accessibility team and what are their roles in helping the client and caregivers achieve independence and safety while performing activities of daily living?

3. What are some of the functional limitations and environmental barriers that affect the safety and independence of a person at home, at the job site, in the community?

4. What are some of the design and product solutions that help to create a barrier-free environment in the each area of the home? What are some interventions that can assist a person and family in the transition from the rehabilitation setting to the community?

5. How can the concepts of universal design be applied to the design of communities, homes, and job sites to create independence and safety in the most integrated setting?

Resources

Training Programs and Accreditations in Housing Accessibility and Modification

PRIME (Professional Resources In Management Education, Inc.) · 1820 S. W. 100th Ave., Miramar, FL 33025. 954-436-6300. Fax 954-436-0161.

Lifease, Inc. · Margaret Christenson, MPH, OTR, FAOTA, 800-961-3273.

RESNA Assistive Technology Practitioner (ATP) and Assistive Technology Supplier (ATS) Credentialing Program · RESNA, 1700 N. Moore St., Suite 1540, Arlington, VA 22209-1903. 703-524-6686 (V). 703-524-6639 (TTY). 703-524-6630 (TTY).
http://www.resna.org

National Resource Center on Supportive Housing and Home Modification · University of Southern California, Andrus Gerontology Center, 3715 McClintock Ave., Los Angeles, CA 90089-0191. 213-740-1364. Fax 213-740-7069.
http://www.homemods.org

Technical Assistance and Organizations

AbleData · 800-346-2742.
www.abledata.com

Abilities O.T. Services Inc. · 3309 W. Strathmore Ave., Baltimore, MD 21215-3718. 410-358-7269. Fax 410-358-6454.
shoshamberg@yahoo.com

Access Board (ATBCB) · 800-872-2253.

Adaptive Environments Center, Inc. (AEC) · 347 Congress St., Suite 301, Boston, MA 02210. 617-695-1225. Fax 617-482-8099.
http://www.adaptenv.org

Accessible Space, Inc. (ASI) · 2550 University Ave., Suite 330 N., St. Paul, MN 55114. 800-466-7722. Fax 651-645-0541.
http://www.accessiblespace.org

American Association of Homes and Services for the Aging (AAHSA) · 901 E St. NW, Suite 500, Washington, DC 20004-2011. 202-783-2242. Fax 202-783-2255.
http://www.aahsa.org

American Association of Retired Persons (AARP) · 601 E St. NW, Washington, DC 20049. 202-434-6120.
http://www.aarp.org

American National Standards Institute (ANSI) · 212-868-1220.

American Occupational Therapy Association (AOTA) · 4720 Montgomery Ave., PO Box 31220, Bethesda, MD 20814-1220. 301-652-2682.
http://www.aota.org

Association for Safe & Accessible Products (ASAP) · 50 Washington St., Norwalk, CT 06854. 203-857-0200.

Center for Universal Design · North Carolina State University, School of Design, Box 8613, Raleigh, NC 27695-8613. 800-647-6777.
www.ncsu.edu/ncsu/design/cud

Christmas in April—Rebuilding Together · 1536 Sixteenth St. NW, Washington, DC 20036-1402. 800-4-REHAB-9. Fax 202-483-9081.
http://www.rebuildingtogether.org

Concrete Change · 600 Dancing Fox Rd., Decatur, GA 30032. 404-378-7455.
http://concretechange.home.mindspring.com/

Consortium for Citizens with Disabilities (CCD) Housing Task Force
http://www.c-c-d.org/tf-housing.htm

Disability Rights Education Defense fund · 202-986-0375.

Easter Seals · 230 West Monroe St., Suite 1800, Chicago, IL 60606. 800-221-6827. 312-726-6200. 312-726-4258 (TTY).
http://www.easter-seals.org/resources/easy.asp

Fannie Mae · 3900 Wisconsin Ave. NW, Washington, DC 20016-2892. 202-752-7000.
http://www.fanniemae.com

Future Home Foundation Inc. · Att: Dave Ward, curator, 12900 Jarrettsville Pike, Phoenix, MD 21131. 410-666-0086.
cdavidward@aol.com

Habitat for Humanity International (HFHI) · 1 Habitat St., Americus, GA 31709-3498. 800-422-4828 (800-HABITAT). 912-924-6935.
http://www.habitat.org

U. S. Department of Housing and Urban Development (HUD). 800-827-5005.
www.hud.gov/fhe/fheo.html.

Independent Living Centers · for a listing of local centers call the national office at 314-531-3055.

IDEA—Center for Inclusive Design & Environmental Access · School of Architecture & Planning, State University of New York at Buffalo, Buffalo, NY 14214-3087. 716-829-3485. Fax 716-829-3256.
http://www.ap.buffalo.edu/~idea

Industrial Design Society Of America, IDSA-UD Special Interest Section · 1141 Walker Rd., Great Falls, VA 22066. 703-759-0100. Fax 703-759-7679.
http://www.idsa.org

National Association of Home Builders Research Center · 400 Prince George's Center Blvd., Upper Marlboro, MD 20774-8731. 301-249-4000. Fax 301-249-0305.
http://www.nahb.org

National Association of the Remodeling Industry (NARI) · 4900 Seminary Rd., Suite 320, Alexandria, VA 22311. 800-966-7601. 703-575-1100. Fax 703-575-1121.
http://www.nari.org

National Home Modification Action Coalition (NHMAC)
http://www.homemods.org

National Kitchen & Bath Association (NKBA) · 687 Willow Grove St., Hackettstown, NJ 07840. 800-367-6522. 800-843-6522. Fax 908-852-1695.
http://www.nkba.org

National Resource Center on Supportive Housing & Home Modification · University of Southern California, Andrus Gerontology Center, 3715 McClintock Ave., Los Angeles, CA 90089-0191. 213-740-1364. Fax 213-740-7069.
http://www.homemods.org

Paralyzed Veterans of America (PVA) · 801-18th St. NW, Washington, DC 20008. 800-424-8200 (V). 800-795-4327 (TTY). Fax 202-785-4452.
http://www.pva.org

Remodeling Online
http://www.remodeling.hw.net

RESNA · 202-857-1199.
http://www.resna.org

Technical Assistance Collaborative, Inc. · One Center Plaza, Suite 310, Boston, MA 02108. 617-742-5657. Fax 617-742-0509.
www.tacinc.org

TRACE Research and Development Center · University of Wisconsin at Madison, 5901 Research Park Blvd., Madison, WI 53719-1252. 608-262-6966.
www.trace.wisc.edu

Universal Designers & Consultants, Inc. (UDC) · 6 Grant Ave., Takoma Park, MD 20912. 301-270-2470 (V-TTY). Fax 301-270-8199.
http://www.UniversalDesign.com\

Volunteers for Medical Engineering · Baltimore, MD. 410-455-6395.

References

Abledata (1995, January). Informed Consumer Guide to Accessible Housing, *Macro International*, 1–11.

American Association of Retired Persons (1996, Summer/Fall). *Housing Report*, 4–7.

American Health Consultants (1996). Improve patient lives: Evaluation can lead to independence. *Case Management Advisor*, 7, 101–113.

American Occupational Therapy Association. (1993). Statement: The role of OT in the independent living movement. *American Journal of Occupational Therapy*, 47, 11–12.

Architectural Transportation Barriers Compliance Board or Access Board. (1991). *UFAS Retrofit Manual*. Washington: US Access Board.

Canadian Mortgage Housing Corporation. (1992). *Maintaining Seniors' Independence: A Guide to Home Adaptations*. Ottawa: Project Open House.

Concrete Change. (2001). Accessed June 6, 2001 at http://concretechange.home.mindspring.com.

Center for Universal Design. (1997). The principles of universal design. *UD Newsline*, 1, 4–6.

Frieden, L., & Cole, J. A. (1985). Independence: The ultimate goal of rehabilitation for spinal cord-injured persons. *American Journal of Occupational Therapy*, 39, 734–739.

Hiatt, L. G. (1993). *Design for Aging: Strategies for Collaboration Between Architects and Occupational Therapists, Aging Design Research Program*, Rockville, MD: American Institute of Architects.

Johnson, J. (1986). Centers for independent living: A new concept in promoting independence. *AOTA Physical Disabilities Special Interest Newsletter*, 9 (3), 4–5.

Kornblau, B., Shamberg, S., & Klein, R. (2000). Americans with Disabilities Act Position Paper: Occupational Therapy and the Americans with Disabilities Act, adopted by AOTA Representative Assembly 2000.

Leibrock, C. (1985). *Easy Home Access Checklist*. Fort Collins: Colorado State University.

Letts, L., Law, M., Rigby, P., Cooper, B., Stewart, D., & Strong, S. (1994). Person-environment assessments in occupational therapy. *American Journal of Occupational Therapy*, 48, 616–617.

Reed, K. (1992). History of federal legislation for persons with disabilities. *American Journal of Occupational Therapy*, 46, 401–407.

Shamberg, A., & Shamberg, S. (1996a). Blueprints for Independence. *OT Practice*, 1, 22–29.

Shamberg, A., & Shamberg, S. (1996b, July/August). Building functional foundations. *Home Health Care Dealer*, 141–143.

Shamberg, S. (1993). The accessibility consultant: A new role for occupational therapist under the ADA. *Occupational Therapy Practice*, 4, 14–23.

Shamberg, S., Steins, S., & Shamberg, A. (1996). *Personal Enablement Through Environmental Modifications: Physical Medicine & Rehabilitation Secrets*. Philadelphia: Hanley & Belfus.

Steinfeld, E. (1996). *A Primer on Accessible Design*. Buffalo: Center for Inclusive and Environmental Access.

U.S. Department of Housing and Urban Development. (1989). *Federal Register*, 54:13, 3247.

37

Preventing Occupational Dysfunction Secondary to Aging

Bette R. Bonder and Glenn Goodman

LEARNING OBJECTIVES

After studying this chapter, the reader will be able to do the following:

1. Describe normal age-related changes in the cognitive–neuromuscular substrate, first-level capacities, developed capacities, abilities and skills, activities and habits, tasks and life roles, and competency and self-esteem.
2. Discuss activity patterns of older adults as related to self-care, work, and leisure.
3. Describe considerations in assessing the function of older adults.
4. Discuss interventions through which occupational therapists can facilitate function in older adults.
5. Describe the factors that make intervention following illness or injury for older adults different from that for younger adults.

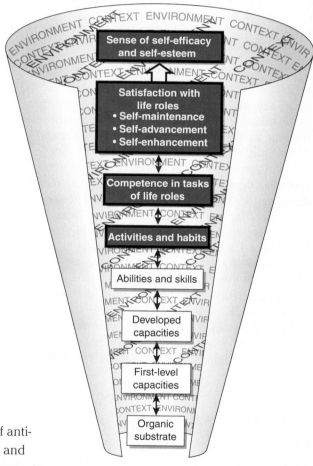

*L*ife expectancy has increased markedly with the advent of antibiotics, vaccinations for disease, improvement in trauma care, and other medical technology. In 1990, 12% of U. S. citizens were over age 65. By 2020, the proportion will increase to 21% (Treas, 1995). The most rapid growth is and will continue to be among the **oldest old**, those over age 85. Most older adults reside in the community. Only 5% of American citizens over age 65 are in institutions such as nursing homes (Rowe & Kahn, 1998). However, all older adults undergo some physiological changes that affect performance. In addition, older individuals have an average of two or three chronic diseases (Rowe & Kahn).

These figures have considerable import for health care providers, particularly occupational therapists, who are concerned with assisting individuals to maintain or regain ability to perform valued

---

---

daily activities. Enhancing functional performance of older adults can have economic, social, and personal benefits for these individuals, their families, and society as a whole.

The emphasis in this chapter is on the normal aging process. Older adults are of course subject to all of the illnesses and injuries that affect younger persons, as well as some that are far more likely to occur in older individuals, such as cerebrovascular accidents, dementing illnesses, and cancer. Other chapters in this volume address mechanisms by which therapists can provide effective intervention for these conditions. When illness or injury occurs, however, the therapist must put the consequences in the context of the individual's life stage, which makes understanding normal aging essential. There are some special considerations in intervening with older adults, and those are also discussed in this chapter.

Normal Aging

Changes that accompany normal aging occur in every sphere, both internal to the individual, including the cognitive–neuromuscular substrate, first-level capacities, and developed capacities, and external to the individual, as in social situations and responses to the physical environment. It is essential to remember, however, the wide range of variation among individuals. All of us know individuals who at age 55 have stooped shoulders, shuffling gait, and poor vision and hearing and whose favorite activity is napping. We also know some who at age 80 have a vigorous stride and engage in activities that would exhaust many a younger person. The existence of

a physical change does not necessarily lead to a commensurate decrement in function. This section considers typical cognitive–neuromuscular, first-level, and developmental changes that accompany normal aging. These changes occur to varying degrees among older adults, with varying effects on performance.

Cognitive–Neuromuscular Substrate

There is no question that genetic factors influence the aging process (Finch, 1990). Perhaps most important from the perspective of aging is the contribution of genetics to predisposition to illness and disability, including type II diabetes, some cancers, and high blood pressure (Finch). The interaction of genetic predisposition with personal behaviors and environmental circumstances leads to expression of genetic tendencies. Thus it may be possible to reduce risk of most genetic disorders by half or more through modification of behaviors (Rowe & Kahn, 1998). For example, exercise can reduce risk of high blood pressure and heart disease even in individuals with a strong genetic risk (Blair et al, 1996).

First-Level Capacities

This section summarizes age-related changes in the following systems and capacities that allow for reflex-based responses: sensory, neuromuscular, cardiovascular, and cognitive.

Sensory Changes

Some sensory changes normally occur with aging; others result from disease processes common among older adults (Aiken, 1995; Hooper, 2001). One role of the occupational therapist is to evaluate the level of dysfunction caused by sensory changes and to determine strategies to compensate for problems that interfere with abilities, activities, tasks, and life roles.

Changes typically occur in all sensory spheres, including vision, hearing, gustation, olfaction, touch, and vestibular sensation. Changes in multiple sensory channels require careful intervention to optimize function. Furthermore, decrements may occur at the level of reception or of interpretation or integration (Ayres, A. J. [1985]. *Developmental dyspraxia and adult-onset apraxia.* Unpublished paper presented at Sensory Integration International, Torrance, CA.), that is, either peripherally or centrally in the nervous system.

Vision

In 1995, 18% of noninstitutionalized persons 70 years of age and older were visually impaired, defined as full or partial blindness or other trouble seeing. The prevalence of visual impairment increases with age, from 13% of persons 70 to 74 years of age to 31% of those 85 years of age and over. Cataracts, glaucoma, and macular degeneration are primary causes of visual impairment among the older population (U. S. Department of Health and Human Services, 1999).

Deterioration of near vision, called **presbyopia**, begins to affect most people when they are about age 40. The lens loses its elasticity and becomes less able to focus because of weakness in the ciliary body (Lewis, 1990). Presbyopia is easily accommodated through the use of a well-known assistive device: eyeglasses.

Another common change is development of degenerative opacities (cataracts) of the lenses, which lead to decreased sensitivity to colors, increased sensitivity to glare, and diminished acuity (Hooper, 2001).

Several diseases, including diabetic retinopathy and retinitis pigmentosa, can affect the retina at any age. The effects of these diseases, both of which may lead to total blindness, are most pronounced in the elderly population, because both are progressive degenerative diseases (Hooper). Macular degeneration, a disorder causing loss of central vision as the macula deteriorates, is most common among older individuals. Most older individuals with macular degeneration retain sufficient peripheral vision to assist in mobility but not enough for activities such as reading or watching television (Hooper).

Musculature that controls eye movement tends to lose strength and tone (Sullivan, 1984). There may be a reduction in tear secretion (Furukawa & Polse, 1978) and degenerative changes in the sclera, pupil, and iris (Kasper, 1978). Results of such changes include excessive dryness, loss of light–dark accommodation, and poor night vision. Finally, decreased color vision and

changes in the vitreous body that affect retinal function (Lewis & Bottomly, 1994) occur with aging.

Hearing

As many as 50% of older adults have severe hearing loss, especially for high frequencies (Aiken, 1995). Conductive hearing loss may be the result of problems in the external or middle ear, such as wax buildup, eustachian tube blockage, or stiffness of the ossicles and membranes (Medina, 1996). Age-related sensorineural hearing loss, known as **presbycusis**, results from dysfunction of the sensory hair cells of the cochlea, neural connections from the cochlea to the cerebral cortex and brainstem, or vascular changes in the auditory system (Lewis, 1990). Functional consequences of these changes include difficulty hearing high-frequency sounds, distinguishing consonants during conversation, and filtering background noise during conversation.

Taste and Smell

Thresholds for taste and smell increase with age (Aiken, 1995; Kiernat, 1991). This has several functional implications. First, the ability to appreciate food flavor is closely related to olfaction (Medina, 1996). Inability to detect aromas may cause food to seem tasteless, possibly resulting in secondary nutritional disorders. Safety may become a concern, as individuals may not be able to detect harmful odors such as natural gas, spoiled food, or smoke (Davis & Kirkland, 1988). Smoking or environmental exposures may exacerbate age-related changes in taste and olfaction.

Tactile Changes

Studies of tactile changes related to aging are sparse and inconclusive (Kiernat, 1991). The existing data seem to indicate that older adults are particularly susceptible to hypothermia and hyperthermia (Aiken, 1995). Losses in vibratory and touch sensitivity are minimal to moderate and occur in less than 50% of subjects over age 50 (Kenshalo, 1977). Loss of position sense is most common in the lower extremities (Davis & Kirkland, 1988). Some sources report a reduction of sensory receptors and a decrease in ability to feel pain with aging (Aiken; Medina, 1996).

Vestibular Function

Vestibular changes are particularly significant because of the importance of falls as a health risk for older adults. Approximately 33% of older adults fall each year (Perry, 1982), and 15% of these individuals are subjected to serious health consequences, such as broken hips (Tinetti et al., 1988). In fact, falls are the leading cause of accidental death in persons over age 65 (Baker et al., 1984).

Older adults have more postural sway than younger adults (Kalish, 1975), a condition that is exacerbated when vision is impaired. Vestibular righting response diminishes with age (Cape, 1978), which can lead to problems in maintaining balance. Age-related changes in static balance (Potvin, 1980), dynamic balance (Newman, 1995), and gait (Winter et al., 1990) appear to increase the probability of falls.

Neuromuscular Changes

The central nervous system, peripheral nervous system, and musculoskeletal system all appear to alter with age.

Central Nervous System

With age the cerebrum atrophies (Lewis & Bottomly, 1994; Medina, 1996) and cerebrospinal fluid space increases. There is a loss and atrophy of neurons, particularly in the precentral gyrus, postcentral gyrus, superior temporal gyrus, and Purkinje cells of the cerebellum (Lewis & Bottomly, 1994). The number of synapses falls, and neurotransmitter systems change. In addition, plaques, fibrillary tangles (Dayan, 1970) and other cellular abnormalities have been found in the brains of functionally normal older adults. Responses to stimuli as measured by electroencephalogram also slow down (Keller et al., 1985).

Peripheral Nervous System

Two major age-related changes in the peripheral nervous system have been identified. Conduction velocity decreases with advancing age (Lewis & Bottomly, 1994), and motor nerve fibers reduce in number (O'Sullivan & Swallow, 1968). However, some sources indicate that the manifestations of nervous system deterioration (reduced sensibility, coordination, cognitive abilities, reaction time) observed with aging do not correspond to the relatively small physical changes seen at the cellular level (Lewis & Bottomly; Medina, 1996). Also, variation between individuals makes functional and structural generalizations problematic (Medina).

Musculoskeletal System

Age-related changes in muscles, joints, and bones are reviewed next.

Muscles. The number and size of muscle fibers decrease with age (Lewis & Bottomly, 1994; Medina, 1996). Other studies report an increase in fatty and connective tissue (Swallow, 1966); decreased strength (Fiatarone et al., 1990); and loss of type II fast-twitch anaerobic muscle fibers that are responsible for phasic movement (Lewis & Bottomly). Decreases in muscle flexibility and endurance have also been reported to occur with aging (Newman, 1995).

Joints. There is a steady decline in joint function after age 20. Ligaments and tendons become less resilient and more prone to injury (Lewis & Bottomly, 1994; Medina, 1996). The quantity and viscosity of synovial fluid decreases with aging (Aiken, 1995; Medina). Cartilage becomes opaque, with an increase in cracks and fraying (Medina). However, the effects of weight bearing and stress on joints and the effects of diseases such as the various kinds of arthritis make the rate and nature of cartilage deterioration highly variable. Once cartilage is destroyed or damaged, it does not regenerate. This has special significance to the elderly, who must rely on prevention or corrective surgery to manage the potentially disabling effects of loss of cartilage (Lewis & Bottomly).

Bones. The progressive loss of bone mineral content with aging results in loss of bone mass and density. The rate of these changes is affected by diet, exercise, and gender (Aiken, 1995; Lewis & Bottomly, 1994; Medina, 1996). Osteoporosis has been studied extensively. Women after age 39 have a rate of bone loss double that of men. Postmenopausal women are affected most. The rate of degeneration slows by age 70 (Medina).

Effect of Disease on the Musculoskeletal System. Arthritis, osteoporosis, connective tissue diseases, orthopaedic injuries from falls and trauma, and repetitive motion disorders are most prevalent in elderly individuals (Aiken, 1995; Tideiksaar, 2001). About 64% of women and 49% of men over age 70 report having some chronic form of arthritis. In 1996, hip fractures alone were responsible for more than 300,000 hospitalizations among persons 65 years of age and older, of whom 80% were women. Among persons 85 years of age and older, 90% of women and 54% of men had measurably reduced hip bone density.

Cardiovascular Changes

The cardiovascular system loses efficiency with age, the result of changes in the frequency and regularity of the conduction system (Dean, 2001), a reduction in pacemaker cells (Lewis & Bottomly, 1994), alterations in blood pressure (Newman, 1995), changes in the elasticity, length, and thickness of the arteries (Lewis & Bottomly; Medina, 1996), a decrease in heart rate and stroke volume (Dean; Medina), and a general thickening of specific heart tissues, such as the atria and valves (Lewis & Bottomly).

Aging affects every component of the cardiopulmonary system (Dean, 2001). There is a decrease in elastic tissues and an increase in fibrous tissue. This especially affects the medium and small airways constructed of smooth muscle. The joints of the chest wall stiffen, the muscles of the diaphragm flatten, and the chest wall becomes more barrel shaped and less compliant (Dean).

New research suggests that the effects of aging on the cardiovascular system once thought to be irreversible and consistent are highly variable among individuals (Chodzko-Zajko, 2001) and cultures (Keith, et al. 1994) and reversible with exercise and dietary changes (Chodzko-Zajko).

Cognitive Changes

Because it is difficult to differentiate between first-level and developed capacities in cognition, the following discussion combines these two aspects of age-related changes. Age-related changes occur in intelligence, problem solving, abstract reasoning, memory, memory processing, and attention. In all of these functions, changes are most noticeable after age 70, although they have been documented in younger subjects (Ivnik et al., 1995; Lindenberger et al., 1993).

As measured by the *Weschler Adult Intelligence Scale*, intelligence quotient decreases with advancing age, largely the result of decreases in the performance rather than verbal subscales (Riley, 2001). Performance subscales may depend on **fluid intelligence** (the ability to use new information), whereas verbal subscales may use **crystallized intelligence** (recall of stored memories) (Rockey, 1997). In particular, flexibility in reasoning tasks seems to decline (Riley), although older adults show wide individual variation in these cognitive tasks. Problem-solving skills also seem to become less efficient (Albert & Heaton, 1988).

To remember, one must attend to the matter to be recalled and be able to receive information through sensory channels. The information must be processed (interpreted) and stored. Initial storage may be relatively short term. Overall, well older adults do not have memory loss in processing and short-term storage of information, although some have difficulty encoding large amounts of information at once (Arenberg, 1982).

However, there are noticeable decrements in long-term memory and encoding (Cattell, 1963). Older adults have more trouble recalling information than do younger ones (Rabbitt, 1982), although retrieval difficulty is not as noticeable for recognition. For example, on seeing a name, an older person may remember the face and personality of an acquaintance but on seeing the person, have difficulty retrieving the name. This difficulty is much less pronounced when the information has practical significance. Remote or very long-term memory appears not to decline. However, this finding is more anecdotal than data based and must be accepted with caution (Riley, 2001).

Another common phenomenon is increased difficulty with word finding, accompanied by subtle deficits in short-term memory, such as difficulty remembering names or where one put an object. Dubbed age-associated memory impairment, this irritating but not disabling condition seems to begin in late middle age. (Helkala et al., 1997). In most instances, the individual remembers the information later. For some individuals, memory training has helped minimize associated functional decrements (Riley, 2001).

A Special Note About Dementia

Dementing illnesses are extremely common among older adults. **Dementia**, characterized by forgetfulness, difficulty finding words, and other cognitive loss, is not a normal condition of aging. Rather, it is the result of any of several disease processes (Corcoran, 2001). Some, such as depression, sensory deprivation syndrome, malnutrition, and drug toxicity, are reversible. Other dementias are not reversible. Alzheimer's disease, the most common form of dementia, is a progressive disorder that eventually leads to total disability and death.

It is beyond the scope of this chapter to deal with the methods for intervening with individuals with dementing disorders. However, health care professionals should be familiar with the early symptoms of cognitive disorder, such as difficulty finding words, forgetfulness about everyday events and procedures, and lack of recollection of familiar individuals. When noted, these symptoms should be carefully evaluated by a **geriatrician**, a physician trained to work with older individuals. Reversible causes may be treated relatively easily. If the individual has an irreversible dementing illness, a variety of management strategies can help informal and formal caregivers to cope with resulting problems. This enhances quality of life for both the ill person and the caregivers. One excellent source of information about management is *The 36-Hour Day* (Mace, Rabins, & McHugh, 1999).

Developed Capacities: Changes in Voluntary Responses

Changes in organic substrates and first-level capacities may impair such voluntary responses as rising from a chair and gait speed (Fiatarone et al., 1990). Weakness in ankle dorsiflexion and knee extension have been correlated with falls in older individuals (Tideiksaar, 2001).

Loss of dexterity and coordination with aging is well documented. Scores on the *Jebsen Hand Function Test* (Jebsen et al., 1969), the *Nine-Hole Peg Test* (Mathiowetz, Weber et al., 1985), and the *Box and Block Test of Manual Dexterity* (Mathiowetz, Volland et al., 1985) all decline with age. These appear to interfere with

Case Example

MRS. P.: OCCUPATIONAL THERAPY TO PREVENT PERFORMANCE LOSS

Client Information

Mrs. P. is a 73-year-old woman who lives alone in a ranch-style house in a small town. Her grown daughter visits about four times a year, her son once a year. Mrs. P. was divorced 12 years ago and never remarried. Mrs. P. worked as a nurse for more than 20 years at a large university hospital. Now she works 2 days a week at a nursing home three blocks from her house, where she reviews charts for quality assurance. Mrs. P. has always enjoyed work and feels that the staff are close friends. Other than her income from the job, Mrs. P.'s only source of funds is Social Security.

Throughout her adult life Mrs. P. has been in a sorority consisting of about a dozen women who have been friends since they were young women. They live nearby. For many years she was a member of a women's group that raised funds for the ballet in the nearby city. When she is at home, Mrs. P. enjoys working on a dollhouse that she built.

Mrs. P. has a long history of health problems. She survived breast cancer when she was in her 40s, and 3 years ago she had surgery to remove a cancerous tumor from her colon. She has high blood pressure, controlled with medication. She also has a significant hearing loss that is gradually worsening.

Reason for Referral to Occupational Therapy

Recently Mrs. P.'s sorority sisters noted changes in her social behavior (missing meetings, not answering her phone, refusing social invitations) and contacted her son with their concerns. He urged his mother to make an appointment with her family physician, her primary care provider for the past 30 years. During the visit, the physician discovered that her high blood pressure has worsened, as has her hearing. She also reported being very tired and having difficulty managing around the house. The physician ordered a series of medical tests and asked a home health agency to send an occupational therapist to evaluate the home and Mrs. P.'s function. He assured her that her son agreed to pay for this evaluation.

Occupational Therapy Assessment

Mrs. P. agreed to a home visit by the occupational therapist. The therapist decided to evaluate Mrs. P.'s home and her performance of basic self-care and instrumental activities of daily living. The therapist used the *Check It Out Check-List* (Pynoos & Cohen, 1990), the *Interest Checklist*, and the *Self Assessment of Occupational Functioning*. She also asked Mrs. P.

to give her a tour of the house and to describe problems encountered in daily tasks.

Problem List and Solutions

The therapist and Mrs. P. discussed these concerns and worked jointly toward identifying potential solutions. Since the therapist was asked to do an evaluation, not to provide long-term intervention, she must provide Mrs. P. with sufficient information to address her concerns.

1. Home safety—Mrs. P. acknowledged that the house was cluttered with old papers, knickknacks, and clothes. She was reluctant to throw anything away but agreed to have her daughter store some of the items for her. Mrs. P. also indicated that she had no funds to replace the worn carpet, although both agree that worn spots and loose edges contribute to falls. She and the therapist identified several possible sources of funds and discussed the possibility of taking the carpet up entirely.
2. Physical deconditioning—Mrs. P. indicated that she had much less energy than she used to, quickly becoming short of breath when walking around the house. She agreed to begin a gradual plan of physical activity, starting with a stroll around the block each day.
3. Social isolation—Mrs. P.'s hearing loss was quite noticeable. The therapist encouraged her to see an audiologist to have her hearing evaluated. Mrs. P. expressed concern about paying for a hearing aid but agreed to ask her son for help.

Mrs. P. indicated that her friends were all in poor health and "no fun" anymore. She also said she was worried about falling at work. She was unwilling to discuss any alternatives for maintaining ties with her friends but agreed that she could discuss her concerns about work with her supervisor.

Treatment Plan and Outcome

Mrs. P. and her occupational therapist developed a time line for Mrs. P. to call her doctor, her daughter, her son, and her boss, and Mrs. P. and her therapist agree that the therapist will make a follow-up call to check on her progress in 2 weeks. On follow-up, the therapist learned that Mrs. P. had accomplished a great deal. Mrs. P.'s physician determined that she had pernicious anemia and instituted monthly injections of B_{12}. Mrs. P. reported that she already felt more energetic.

Mrs. P. was now walking around her yard twice a day. Her daughter came to visit and helped her organize the house. Her son sent a check for a new hearing aid. Mrs. P. had not yet talked with her boss and was worried about doing it. She and the therapist practiced the conversation to provide Mrs. P. with a strategy. A week later, Mrs. P. called the therapist to tell her she was back at work.

Analysis of Reasoning

In this case, the occupational therapist provided an assessment and recommendations but left implementation of the plan to this capable client and family.

CLINICAL REASONING
in OT Practice

Intervention to Prevent Performance Decrements

The occupational therapist focused on screening and prevention in this consultative intervention. How might the therapist's assessment and intervention approaches have been different if Mrs. P.'s function had deteriorated to the extent that she was placed in a long-term care facility?

---

some self-care activities, such as placing a plug in a wall socket and cutting with a knife (Potvin, 1980).

Abilities and Skills: Physical Capacity

The following changes in physical capacity typify skills and abilities that are affected by normal aging: postural alignment, sway, and instability with postural changes (Tideiksaar, 2001); gross motor coordination (Lewis & Bottomly, 1994); fine motor coordination and dexterity (Mathiowetz, Weber et al., 1985); strength and endurance (Aiken, 1995; Lewis & Bottomly; Medina, 1996); walking speed, step length, and step height (Lewis & Bottomly; Tideiksaar); and reaction time (Lewis & Bottomly).

Activities and Habits

As with physiological change, activity patterns are highly individual (Bonder, B. R., & Martin, L. [1998]. *Meaning of activity for older women.* Unpublished paper presented at the American Occupational Therapy Association Annual Conference, Indianapolis; Bonder & Martin, 2000). In fact, older adults have great freedom of choice in our culture. Some older adults engage in many activities; others focus on one or two. For example, some older adults report activities that are related primarily to family, while others may be active in volunteer work, several hobbies, social relationships, and care of their personal needs.

Self-Care

A significant issue for older adults has to do with level of independence in self-care, that is, "everyday competence" (Willis, 1991). If personal ability is compromised, the issue is availability and acceptance of assistance. Most older adults have difficulty with at least one

or two self-care activities (Bonder & Fisher 1990; Treas, 1995), especially cutting toenails, a problem solved with pedicures or visits to a podiatrist. Heavy housework, such as mopping floors and washing windows, is difficult for many individuals and may be hired out or done by family members. In addition, most elders spend more time on self-care activities than they did when younger (Christiansen & Hammecker, 2001). Issues of time can be significant when self-care consumes such a significant proportion of the day that other desired activities cannot be pursued.

Ability to bathe and urinary and bowel incontinence are issues that can influence life-altering decisions for elders. Those who are unable to bathe or who are incontinent are most likely to be placed in institutional settings, an event that most elders wish to avoid.

The importance of habits must be emphasized. There is evidence that when a familiar task is undertaken in a familiar environment, the effect of aging on performance is reduced (Rogers et al., 1997). Where such habits can be followed closely, task performance is improved.

Most older adults accommodate to age-related changes well by modifying routines or finding and accepting assistance. This is true especially when the activity is one for which it is socially acceptable to receive help. Help with driving, cooking, or managing finances is often acceptable. Some older adults are determined to do for themselves, while others are accepting, even relieved, when they can rely on others to take care of them.

Substantial disability in self-care is most likely to be perceived when there is a sudden change due to illness or change in social circumstances rather than the gradual ones that affect most well elders. If the change is loss related, emotional reactions that typically accompany loss must be addressed. However, changes perceived as positive, such as a move to a long-desired

Case Example

OCCUPATIONAL THERAPY INTERVENTION TO OPTIMIZE PERFORMANCE IN SPITE OF AGE-RELATED DETERIORATION

Patient Information

Mrs. S., an 80-year-old nursing home resident, has five children. Four of them live within 50 miles. Mrs. S. worked as the personal secretary for the provost of a small college for 20 years. She had a variety of interests, including reading, cooking, and baking; participating in church and local theater; and gardening.

Mrs. S. faced a number of challenges in her life, including the early death of her father, the Great Depression, her husband's absence for 3 years of service in World War II, raising a child with schizophrenia, the early and sudden death of her husband (she was 51 when he died), and adjusting to a move from her home to an apartment and now to a nursing home.

Mrs. S.'s medical history is fairly typical for a person her age. She developed osteoarthritis in both knees, resulting in several microscopic surgeries and two total knee replacements. She was hospitalized for a brief bout of depression secondary to menopause. She has presbyopia with resulting losses of both near and far vision that are well corrected with eyeglasses. She has severe hearing loss in both ears that is partially corrected with hearing aides.

She also had a series of strokes that began when she was 70. The strokes left her with mild spasticity, about 50% of proximal upper extremity active range of motion, and only a mass grasp in her left hand. She had full use of lower extremities except for a loss of about 15° of right active knee flexion and mild spasticity and weakness in the left lower extremity. She lost approximately 25% of the visual field on the left side to hemianopsia but can accommodate for this by turning her head. Mrs. S. also had mild dysarthria and dysphagia. She dribbled urine because of changes in bladder function and weak sphincter musculature. She wore a small protective pad and took medication to control this. She was hospitalized a year ago for an attempted suicide and major depression as a result of the breaking of her knee replacement and difficulty adjusting to the idea of another major surgery. She received psychiatric services and a long rehabilitation stay after she agreed to have the knee replacement. Her recovery from the knee replacement was very good except for her complaint of chronic pain in the knee that has not responded to medication.

Prior to the failure of her first knee replacement she was totally independent in all basic activities of daily living. After her knee replacement and rehabilitation stay, a trial in her assisted living facility became problematic because of her declining ability to walk, transfer to the bathroom, and inability to do her own personal care. She and her family decided that Mrs. S. should be admitted to a nursing home, where she would receive closer supervision and assistance for her personal care.

Reason for Referral to Occupational Therapy

Nursing home staff was concerned about Mrs. S.'s safety and social withdrawal. Mrs. S. was still using a wheeled walker but found placing her left hand on the walker handle difficult. She was able to move from her bed to the bathroom independently but had several recent falls. She dressed independently if her clothes were placed on a chair beside her bed. However, she displayed poor judgment in activities such as bending too far over the edge of the bed and dangerously reaching for things she dropped on the floor. She also tripped over things while walking. She used a wheelchair on outings with her family and with the activities program at the nursing home. Mrs. S. rarely smiles, and nursing staff reports difficulty getting her to participate in group activities or outings, even though she was physically able to do so. Her family was supportive. Her oldest daughter had power of attorney and durable medical power of attorney. Mrs. S. paid privately for nursing home care and had funds remaining to cover about two more months of care. She was willing to pay privately for brief occupational therapy intervention.

Assessment

After reviewing the medical records, the occupational therapist evaluated Mrs. S.'s life roles, tasks, activities, skills, abilities and developed capacities. Mrs. S. was interviewed along with her oldest daughter and primary nurse. Some of the critical questions raised during the interviews:

▶ What safety issues are you most concerned about?
▶ What is your level of satisfaction with life right now? What do you think could be done to improve it?
▶ What things do you like to do right now? What things irritate you?
▶ If you could change five things around here to make things better for yourself, what would you change?
▶ What worries you most? What makes you happiest?
▶ Do you have any goals to improve yourself, your environment, or your living situation?

Problem List

The interviews and evaluation revealed the following problems:

▶ Mrs. S. tends to get upset and take things into her own hands when she has to wait for assistance. This results in unsafe or dangerous behavior and activities.
▶ Mrs. S. gets depressed and does not feel like socializing with others, especially residents with problems similar to hers or worse.

► Mrs. S. needs some meaningful activities to replace the wide variety of activities that formerly gave her pleasure.

► Mrs. S. needs some modifications to her environment to increase safety and orientation to reality and current events.

► Mrs. S. is easily embarrassed and has difficulty asking for personal assistance, especially with urination and personal hygiene.

► Mrs. S. would like more interaction and visits from her family.

Occupational Therapy Goals

The following goals were agreed upon by Mrs. S, her family, and the nursing staff:

► Mrs. S. will request and wait for assistance or supervision for trips to the bathroom or will use a female urinal at bedside.

► Mrs. S. will call for assistance should she drop any item on the floor that is not within easy reach of her long-handled reacher. Otherwise she will continue to dress herself independently with setup at bed or chair level.

► Mrs. S. will attend at least two outings per week with family or with the nursing home activities program. She will provide constructive criticism to the staff as to how the activity could be improved.

► Mrs. S. will learn to propel her wheelchair so that she can safely navigate throughout the building without falling. She will be supervised for walks to the bathroom or in the hall.

► Mrs. S. will choose and successfully complete three leisure activities within a month using adaptive equipment or techniques recommended by the occupational therapist.

► Mrs. S. will complete a list of things that she is unhappy with as well as a list of things she is grateful for and review them with her daughter at least once a week to encourage her to express her feelings appropriately.

Treatment Plan

The occupational therapist decided to see Mrs. S. once or twice a week for a month to achieve these goals. Mrs. S. agreed to pay for the therapy as she did not qualify for skilled services under Medicare regulations. Direct intervention:

► Instruction in safety for mobility within her room

► Adjustment of call signal button and chairs and removal of throw rugs and other barriers to safe mobility in the room

► Provision of long-handled reachers and instruction in use of them

► A session to assess safety issues during dressing and hygiene activities

► Suggestions for adaptive equipment for playing cards, reading, and plant care

► A daily calendar and structured time to read the paper or watch the news on television for current events

► A meeting with Mrs. S. and her family at the end of the month to review progress on goals and to make decisions about continuance of therapy or discharge.

The occupational therapist suggested referrals to physical therapy for a program to maintain or enhance mobility and physical conditioning, speech pathology to review issues related to dysphagia and dysarthria, and social work to help Mrs. S. and her family apply for Medicaid or other support, as financial concerns were becoming an issue. The therapist consulted the nursing and activities staff and provided written copies of suggestions for the staff to facilitate accomplishment of the therapy goals. Suggestions were also made to Mrs. S. and her family to explore a visit to a chronic pain specialist for the knee pain and to a urologist for follow-up on bladder control issues.

Analysis of Reasoning

The occupational therapist, aware that Mrs. S.'s occupational dysfunction stemmed from multiple factors, created a treatment plan that included referrals to other rehabilitation disciplines. The clinician gathered information about Mrs. S.'s background, goals, and status to project therapy outcomes and time frame. Long-term success of this intervention depended on collaboration with patient, family, and nursing home staff.

CLINICAL REASONING
in OT Practice

Intervention in Spite of Age-Related Deterioration

What strategies did the therapist use to collaborate with patient, family, and nursing home staff? What else could be done to ensure that stakeholders maintain their contribution to Mrs. S.'s function long after the occupational therapy intervention is complete?

---

retirement location, can also cause unanticipated emotional difficulties.

Work

Emerging patterns in work and retirement reflect increasing diversity in the older population (Sterns et al., 2001).

For example, some older adults are creating a trend to earlier retirement followed by a second career in a different area, a return to part-time work, or a move to volunteer work.

Physiological changes seen in normal aging do not typically interfere with work abilities (Sterns et al., 2001).

Elders require somewhat different kinds of in-service training to maintain or expand competency, requiring slightly more time than younger adults to learn new skills. They respond best to learning that is based on practical examples. If these special needs are accommodated, however, they are as capable of maintaining their skills as younger persons.

There is substantial evidence that voluntary retirement is not viewed as a negative event (Richardson, 1993). However, when retirement is involuntary, either as a result of a personal situation such as failing health or external events such as layoffs, individuals are likely to be dissatisfied with retirement.

Retirement often does not mean the cessation of productive activity (Herzog & House, 1991). Herzog and House note that individuals who engage in volunteer work, child care, other service for family members, or other forms of unpaid service report that these have value both to them and to others.

Leisure

Leisure is extremely important to older adults (Bundy, 2001). It provides a sense of identity for individuals who are no longer working. It appears to delay onset of some disabling conditions, and it is linked to life satisfaction. Furthermore, it offers opportunities for expression of important personal meanings (Bonder & Martin, 2000). For older adults, the line between leisure and work may be indistinct, with activities providing both a sense of usefulness to others and satisfaction of personal need for engagement and challenge.

There is a general belief, consistent with activity theory, that maintaining a high level of activity is positive (Rosenfeld, 1997). However, this theory has been challenged by some who believe that an important component of later life is reflection and life review (Ekerdt, 1986; Rowles, 1991).

Tasks and Life Roles

Elders also have greater personal choice in determining their tasks and life roles than do younger individuals. While some individuals must continue to work to support themselves, most have the option of retiring from paid employment. Those who have children typically have finished rearing them. Since living in certain school districts is no longer an issue, some elders opt to sell their home and move to an apartment or to new community.

Satisfaction of Emerging Personal Needs and Meanings

In recent years researchers have made increasing attempts to understand the occupations of older adults (Bonder, B. R., & Martin, L. [1998]. *Meaning of activity for older women.* Unpublished paper presented at the American Occupational Therapy Association Annual Conference, Indianapolis; Bonder & Martin, 2000; Rudman et al., 1997). In particular, researchers are interested in knowing what is important to elders and how their occupations contribute to life satisfaction, defined as a positive evaluation of one's life (Rapkin & Fischer, 1992), both present and past.

Occupational therapists theorize that individuals are most satisfied with their lives when they engage in a variety of occupations that balance self-care, work, and leisure (Kielhofner, 1995). Research suggests that this is true for older adults as well as younger individuals (Bonder, B. R., & Fisher, A. G. [1990]. *Roles and activities of older adults.* Unpublished paper presented at the Gerontological Society of America, San Francisco, CA; Elliott & Barris, 1987; Ogilvie, 1987). Ogilvie found that individuals who were able to express their identities through occupation were more satisfied with their lives than those who had limitations.

Elimination or Alteration of Roles

Clearly, while elders often make choices about self-enhancement roles, far less choice is involved in elimination of tasks associated with changes in social roles. Death of a spouse, siblings, and friends dramatically shift occupational tasks. Many elders find that they must modify their roles to accommodate them. As an example, one woman who had made her living as a weaver found that she could no longer sit at a large floor loom. She chose to weave at a small table loom or use finger looms (Bonder, in press). The salient issue seems to be the ability to find outlets for expression of personal meaning (Bonder & Martin).

Additional Roles

Elders not only lose or choose to end previous roles; they also add roles. An elder who stops paid employment becomes a retiree and may become a volunteer. A parent whose children are grown may become a grandparent. A notable rite of passage in the United States is the receipt of the letter at age 50 that indicates one is eligible for membership in the American Association of Retired Persons; individuals electing to join add this role, too.

New chosen roles can enhance life satisfaction. In some instances, even roles that are not chosen may be satisfying. For example, some elders become not only grandparents but surrogate parents for their grandchildren. As many as 10% of elders are custodial grandparents (Fuller-Thompson et al., 1997). While this may be perceived as a burden, many grandparents express great satisfaction with this role.

Competence and Self-Esteem: Psychosocial Changes

Psychosocial status may well be a more significant predictor of occupational function than any other factor. Highly motivated, enthusiastic individuals tend to fare well, often in spite of what appear to be substantial physical limitations. Practitioners must attend to situations in which the individual, following an injury or illness, becomes depressed, loses motivation, and becomes increasingly disabled.

Changes in psychosocial status must be separated into those that are psychological and those that are social. For a well older adult, the former relate to developmental tasks of later life. The latter relate to external factors, including major life changes such as retirement and the loss of social contacts through moves, retirement, or death of peers.

A number of theorists have attempted to identify the normal psychological processes that accompany aging. Among the theories are disengagement, activity, continuity, and life span models. The principal characteristics of these theories are noted in Table 37-1. Although each theory has appeal, each also has limitations in explaining the psychological functioning of older individuals, and all remain to be carefully tested.

Social changes are also less than clear. It is well established that older individuals have significant losses of social contacts (Bye, Llewellyn & Christi, 2001). However, it is less clear how or whether individuals compensate for those losses. For example, loss of a spouse is devastating for most older individuals (Bye). Some individuals compensate for the loss within a year or so, while others never recover.

Impediments to Occupational Function

We review two categories of barriers to occupational function: disease and environmental factors.

Impact of Disease

Almost all older adults eventually fall ill or have an injury that may call for secondary or tertiary preventive interventions, that is, minimizing consequences early in treatment or enhancing rehabilitation once severe disability has occurred. Some special characteristics of older adults must be considered in planning intervention:

► **Differential severity of condition**—Some conditions that are relatively innocuous in younger individuals can have severe consequences for older individuals (Rowe & Kahn, 1998). One example is

TABLE 37-1
Summary of Theories of Psychological Processes of Older Adults

Theorists	Constructs
Disengagement Theory. Cummings and Henry (1961)	1. Elderly withdraw from activity. 2. Elderly disengage emotionally from people and events.
Activity Theory. Havighurst (1963) Longino & Kart (1982)	1. Elderly strive to maintain activity. 2. High levels of activity correlate with well-being.
Continuity Theory. Atchley (1989)	1. Elderly attempt to continue activities that were always important to them. 2. Elderly perceive activities as continuous. 3. Elderly adapt activity to compensate for change. 4. Successful aging is characterized by degree of continuity achieved.
Lifespan Theories. Neugarten (1975) Levinson et al. (1986) Erikson (1963)	1. Old age is continuation of the developmental process, representing a new development stage. 2. Tasks specific to the stage can be identified. 3. Successful aging results from accomplishing tasks.
Model of Human Occupation. Kielhofner (1995)	1. Individual is an open system. 2. Subsystems are volition, habituation, performance. 3. Effectiveness of development of each subsystem reflects successful performance.

Reprinted with permission from Bonder, B. R. (1994). The psychosocial meaning of occupation. In B.R. Bonder & M. Wagner (Eds.), *Functional Performance in Older Adults*, p. 31. Philadelphia: Davis.

influenza, which is unpleasant for younger adults but may be lethal for older ones. On the other hand, cancers that may be terminal in younger adults are often quite slow growing in older individuals, leading to much less severe outcomes.

► **Multiple health problems**—Otherwise well older adults are likely to have two or three chronic health problems (Treas, 1995), each of which may require a different intervention. A common example is a client who has both rheumatoid arthritis and osteoporosis. Although moderately strenuous weight-bearing exercise may be the treatment of choice to prevent bone loss, such activity may exacerbate the arthritis.

► **Duration of recuperation**—Older adults generally recuperate more slowly than younger ones. Even if the eventual outcome is every bit as good, it is likely to take the older individual longer to arrive at that point. Treatment often ends too soon for older individuals.

▶ **Attitudes of care providers**—Some health care professionals tend to be less aggressive in rehabilitation of older adults than younger individuals (Barta-Kvitek et al., 1986). This may be appropriate in some circumstances, but professionals must exercise considerable caution in assuming bad outcomes.

▶ **Consequences of dysfunction**—Most elders prefer to live independently, or "age in place" (Rowe & Kahn, 1998). It is their wish to remain in the living situation to which they have grown accustomed. However, illness and dysfunction can lead to a decision to institutionalize. Functional abilities are central to such decisions. In particular, bathing and toileting abilities influence family decisions. For this reason, occupational therapists often find that elders want to emphasize these abilities in treatment.

Environmental Factors

As with all clients, environmental factors, both physical and social, can have a profound influence on function. Issues described in Chapters 9 and 10 should be carefully considered during interaction with elderly clients, since changes to the personal, social, cultural, and environmental context can greatly facilitate personal abilities.

Facilitators of Occupational Function

Clinicians consider each patient's age as they plan assessment and treatment to optimize occupational function.

Assessment

Careful assessment is vital to successful intervention focused on supporting functional performance of older adults. Perhaps most attention has been given to assessment of self-care (Wilkins et al., 2001). However, it is important in assessing older adults to be cognizant of the goals of that individual (Rapkin & Fischer, 1992). Assessment should begin with identification of the individual's goals and proceed to determination of factors that support or impede those goals.

Several instruments may be helpful in determining those goals. The *Canadian Occupational Performance Measure* (Pollack, 1993) involves interview of the client and joint identification of goals for therapy. These goals then become the measures of outcome (see Chapter 3). Other instruments that may be helpful include the *Role Change Assessment* (Jackoway et al., 1987) and *Interest Checklist* (Matsutsuyu, 1963).

Legislation, particularly the Omnibus Budget Reconciliation Act (OBRA) (Glantz & Richman, 1991), requires that persons in nursing homes have an environmental assessment, but such assessment should be done in community settings as well. A number of good environmental assessment instruments are available (Mann, 2001; Tiedeksaar, 2001) (see Chapter 10). It is important to evaluate both the physical and the social environment to understand fully the individual's situation.

Therapists must be aware that some assessment is mandated by third-party payers. For example, the U. S. government has implemented a minimum data set (MDS) (Health Care Financing Administration, 1999) for residents of nursing homes, and the Outcomes Assessment Information (OASIS) for home health. Furthermore, accreditation bodies such as the Joint Commission on Accreditation for Healthcare Organizations (1999) require that a patient's age be considered in both assessment and treatment planning.

Intervention

An important role for occupational therapists working with older adults is prevention of functional disability. Intervention may include prevention, screening, environmental modifications, modification or substitution of activities, educational interventions, and acceptance of individual needs and wishes by health care providers.

Prevention

The wellness movement (Gallup, 1999) is based on the principle of maximizing both health and performance. Activities such as stress management, exercise to increase physical fitness, maintenance of adequate nutrition, safe driving habits, avoidance of alcohol and drugs, cessation of smoking, and activities to increase safety are associated with this model (Bonder, 2001). In prevention programs, occupational therapists work with other health care providers to maximize the individual's physical and functional well-being. The occupational therapist may emphasize activities that encourage socialization and physical fitness, modification of the environment to reduce the possibility of accidents, and identification of roles and activities that are satisfying to the individual. Such interventions have demonstrated benefit (Clark et al., 1997).

Screening

During the course of prevention activities, occupational therapists should be alert to potential problems (Wilkins et al., 2001). If individuals who are nutritionally compromised or who have recently had a life-changing loss receive early intervention, disability may be minimized or avoided. For example, if a client becomes unable to drive because of increasing visual impairment, the

BOX 37-1
PROCEDURES FOR PRACTICE

Environmental Modifications for Elderly Individuals

Cognitive Problems
- Reduce clutter.
- Label drawers and cabinets by their contents; for individuals who have dementia or other serious cognitive deficits, pictures may be easier to understand than words.
- Use color, texture, and lighting changes to provide location cues, such as changes from carpet to tile signaling the move from dining area to hallway.
- Use timers as reminders for specific functions.
- Put safety off-switches on stoves and furnaces.

Visual Problems
- Use high tone colors and low gloss finishes to improve visual acuity and depth perception (Tideiksaar, 2001).
- Incorporate devices to increase magnification or enlarge print, contrasting colors, and dependence on other sensory systems such as touch.
- Maintain a consistent environment to allow the visually impaired individual to function more effectively.
- Write with felt-tipped pens and in bold print to help improve visibility (Mann, 2001).
- Access optometrists, ophthalmologists, and staff at sight centers or the Society for the Blind for helpful input.
- Provide high-intensity, low-glare light; avoid fluorescent lights; and put glare-reducing screens over televisions and windows (Tideiksaar, 2001).
- Teach compensatory techniques to individuals who have reduced peripheral vision or who have only peripheral vision (Kasper, 1978).

Hearing and Communication Problems
- Refer for a thorough evaluation from a speech pathologist, audiologist, or otolaryngologist.
- Speak slowly and clearly and use a deep voice with someone who has high-frequency loss; do not shout.

- Make sure the individual can see you when you speak (Hooper, 2001).
- Write messages if necessary.
- Select activities for which verbal interaction may not be essential, such as bowling, swimming, checkers, and walks.
- Check that hearing aids are fitted and used properly and that batteries are fresh; remember that these aids do not restore normal hearing and may not help everyone with hearing impairment.
- Use visual cues, such as flashing lights, to get the client's attention.

Neuromuscular, Motor, or Mobility Problems
- Make sure the environment is free of hazards such as slippery floors, poorly marked stairs, and architectural barriers.
- Adjust the height of chairs, beds, dressers, clothes, and toilet seats, and provide a bath chair if needed; ensure that grab bars are within easy reach.
- Provide task-oriented treatment in the individual's environment; numerous repetitions enhance learning, and simulated activities may not be easily transferred to real situations.
- In institutional settings, keep in mind OBRA regulations that mandate reduced use of restraints. Careful evaluation of seating can eliminate the need for restraints; for example, a chair that is higher in front than in back can make it more difficult to rise, and well-fitted chairs can enhance balance.

Self-Care: Toileting and Continence Problems
- Make sure that the bathroom is physically accessible. Add grab bars, nonskid mats.
- Mark the bathroom clearly. Use large, clear words, pictures, and color code if necessary.
- Reduce liquid intake prior to bedtime.
- Institute regular reminders to use the bathroom.
- Use behavior modification techniques to assist elders to notice full bladders.

---

therapist may acquaint him or her with community transit services or help make contact with friends and relatives who can provide occasional transportation. Such an intervention helps reduce the likelihood of social isolation, which can lead to depression and perhaps to significant disability.

Environmental Modifications
If it is not feasible to increase the individual's performance ability, another highly effective intervention is to reduce some demands through alteration of the environment (Box 37-1).

Technological Aids to Function
Numerous technological assists can maximize function (Box 37-2). Some are simple, such as an alarm on the

doorknob to warn family members that a person is wandering away or automatic off-switches on stoves to reduce fire hazard. Others, such as the computer-operated Smart House, are highly sophisticated and expensive.

There are limits to the application of technology with older clients. Some clients may resist learning to use the new technologies. Devices can break down and may be expensive to repair. Acquiring the devices may be expensive and not covered by insurance. It is difficult to keep up with advances, and sometimes a new and better device appears on the market as soon as a client has purchased an expensive piece of equipment. However, many older adults enjoy technological devices, quickly learn to use them, and with them gain considerable independence.

BOX 37-2
PROCEDURES FOR PRACTICE

Assistive Technology for Problems Associated With Aging

- Telephones with amplifiers, large-print numbers, one-touch dialing and memory features; cordless, cellular, or digital phones; external speakers
- Screen magnification, print enhancements, and voice synthesizers for computer screen reading
- Assistive listening devices, telecommunication devices (TDDs), and closed captioning for television; devices to convert auditory output to flashing lights for smoke detectors, telephones, and doorbells

- Life call systems that provide a link with emergency services
- Advances in cataract and other optical surgery, including lens implants or laser surgery
- Advances in technology for mobility, such as wheelchair seating systems, power carts that are easy to disassemble, lightweight wheelchairs, wheeled walkers with brakes and built-in seating systems, and adaptive controls for cars

BOX 37-3
PROCEDURES FOR PRACTICE

Promoting Activity Choice for Intervention With Elders

- Link older adults with activities that express important personal meanings, especially connectedness with others, spirituality, service to others, and self-expression (Bonder & Martin, 2000).
- Recognize the vast individual variability in selection of activities that express personal meanings. One individual may choose to express spirituality through attendance at church, another through meditation.
- Find out what specific self-care activities are perceived as vital to elders who are concerned about remaining in their homes.

- Remember that older adults persist for longer periods with activities that are purposeful (Nelson, 1988).
- Employ reminiscence as a means to establish and maintain connections with others.
- Use activity inventories to stimulate an older client to think about what he or she values.
- Adapt the activity or help the client identify an activity that meets similar needs when preferred activities become too difficult for a client. To do so, ascertain what component of the activity is meaningful. For example, if he or she likes to cook because it is a way to socialize, substituting an activity that is not social will not be satisfying.

Modification and Substitution of Activity

Activity analysis, a cornerstone of occupational therapy, can be particularly helpful in assisting older clients. The process involves matching present skills, interests, and motivation with activities that are stimulating, challenging, enjoyable, goal directed, and purposeful. Some specific suggestions are presented in Box 37-3.

In conclusion, intervention with older adults requires understanding of the normal developmental processes that affect performance as well as the special life circumstances of older adults. To be most effective, intervention must address all spheres of function. The special factors that alter intervention with older adults must be taken into account. With older adults, the goal of good quality of life as measured by satisfying activities is in reach in many situations. Thoughtful intervention by occupational therapists can ensure it.

Summary Review Questions

1. In a well elderly individual, what are the most typical changes in sensation? How can they affect function?
2. How do normal neuromuscular changes that accompany aging affect mobility? How can these changes ultimately affect occupational function?
3. What are some key differences in the cognitive complaints of adults with age-associated memory impairment versus Alzheimer's disease? Describe ways the therapeutic response to these complaints may differ.
4. In general, what effect does retirement have on an older individual who has planned for the event?

5. What is the first step an occupational therapist should take in assessing the status of an older individual?

6. What factors are important in selecting substitute activities for an older adult?

7. In deciding about technological interventions, what factors must be considered to ensure acceptance of the device?

8. What factors complicate intervention with an older adult who falls ill or is injured?

References

Aiken, L. (1995). *Aging: An Introduction to Gerontology.* Thousand Oaks, CA: Sage.

Albert, M. S., & Heaton, R. K. (1988). Intelligence testing. In M. S. Albert & M. B. Moss (Eds.), *Geriatric Neuropsychology* (pp. 13–32). New York: Guilford.

Arenberg, D. (1982). Changes with age in problem solving. In F. I. Craik & S. Trehub (Eds.), *Aging and Cognitive Processes* (pp. 221–235). New York: Plenum.

Atchley, R. C. (1989). Continuity theory of normal aging. *Gerontologist, 29,* 183–190.

Baker, S., O'Neil, B., & Kark, R. (1984). *The Injury Fact Book.* Lexington, MA: Lexington.

Barta-Kvitek, S. D., Shaver, B., Blood, H., & Shephard, K. (1986). Age bias: Physical therapists and older patients. *Journal of Gerontology, 41,* 706–709.

Blair, S. N., Kampert, J. B., Kohl, H. W. 3rd, Barlow, C. E., Macera, C. A., Paffenbarger, R. S. Jr., & Gibbons, L. W. (1996). Influences of cardiorespiratory fitness and other precursors on cardiovascular disease and all-cause mortality in men and women. *Journal of the American Medical Association, 276,* 205–210.

Bonder, B. R. (in press). Culture and occupation: A comparison of weaving in two traditions. *Canadian Journal of Occupational Therapy.*

Bonder, B. R. (2001). The psychosocial meaning of activity. In B. R. Bonder & M. B. Wagner (Eds.), *Functional Performance in Older Adults* (2nd ed.). Philadelphia: Davis.

Bonder, B. R., & Martin, L. (2000). Personal meanings of occupation for women in later life. *Women and Aging, 12,* 177–193.

Bye, R. A., Llewellyn, G. M., & Christi, K. E. (2001). The end of life. In B. R. Bonder & M. B. Wagner (Eds.), *Functional Performance in Older Adults* (2nd ed. pp. 500–519). Philadelphia: Davis.

Bundy, A. (2001). Leisure. In B. R. Bonder & M. B. Wagner (Eds.) *Functional Performance in Older Adults* (2nd ed.). Philadelphia: Davis.

Cape, R. (1978). *Aging: Its Complex Management.* New York: Harper & Row.

Cattell, R. B. (1963). The theory of fluid and crystalline intelligence. *Journal of Educational Psychology, 54,* 1–22.

Chodzko-Zajko, W. (2001). Biological theories of aging: Implications for functional performance. In B. Bonder and M. Wagner (Eds.) *Functional Performance in Older Adults* (2nd ed., pp. 28–41). Philadelphia: Davis.

Christiansen, C., & Hammecker, C. (2001). Activities of older adults: Self-care. In B. R. Bonder & M. B. Wagner (Eds.). *Functional Performance in Older Adults* (2nd ed., pp. 155–178). Philadelphia: Davis.

Clark, F., Azen, S. P., Zemke, R., Jackson, J., Carlson, M., Mandel, D., Hay, J., Josephson, K., Cherry, B., Hessel, C., Palmer, J., &

Lipson, L. (1997). Occupational therapy for independent-living older adults: A randomized controlled trial. *Journal of the American Medical Association, 278,* 1321–1326.

Corcoran, M. A. (2001). Dementia. In B. R. Bonder & M. B. Wagner (Eds.), *Functional Performance in Older Adults* (2nd ed., pp. 287–304). Philadelphia: Davis.

Cummings, E. M. & Henry, W. E. (1961). *Growing Old: The Process of Disengagement.* New York: Basic.

Davis, L., & Kirkland M. (Eds). (1988). *The Role of Occupational Therapy With the Elderly.* Rockville, MD: American Occupational Therapy Association.

Dayan, A. (1970). Quantitative histological studies on the aged human brain: I. Senile plaques and neurofibrillary tangles in "normal" patients. *Acta Neuropathologica, 16,* 85–94.

Dean, E. (2001). Cardiopulmonary development. In B. R. Bonder & M. B. Wagner (Eds.) *Functional Performance in Older Adults* (2nd ed., pp. 86–120). Philadelphia: Davis.

Ekerdt, D. J. (1986). The busy ethic: Moral continuity between work and retirement. *Gerontologist, 26,* 239–244.

Elliott, M. S., & Barris, R. (1987). Occupational role performance and life satisfaction in elderly persons. *Occupational Therapy Journal of Research, 7,* 215–224.

Fiatarone, M., Marks, E., Ryan, N., Merideth, C., Lipsitz, L., & Evans, W. (1990). High intensity strength training in nonagenarians. *Journal of the American Medical Association, 263,* 3029–3034.

Finch, C. E. (1990). *Longevity, Senescence and the Genome.* Chicago: University of Chicago.

Fuller-Thompson, E., Minkler, M., & Driver, D. (1997). A profile of grandparents raising grandchildren in the United States. *Gerontologist, 37,* 406–411.

Furukawa, R., & Polse, K. (1978). Changes in tearflow accompanying aging. *American Journal of Optometric Physiology and Optometry, 55,* 69–74.

Gallup, J. W. (1999). *Wellness Centers: A Guide for the Design Professional.* New York: Wiley.

Glantz, C., & Richman, N. (1991). *Occupational Therapy: A Vital Link to Implementation of OBRA.* Rockville, MD: American Occupational Therapy Association.

Havighurst, R. J. (1963). Successful aging. In R. H. Williams, C. Tibbitts, & W. Donahue (Eds.), *Processes of Aging* (vol. 1, pp. 299–320). New York: Atherton.

Health Care Financing Administration (1999). MDS 2.0 Information Site. Retrieved on December 6, 1999 from the World Wide Web. http://www.hcfa.gov/medicare/hsqb/mds20/.

Helkala, E. L., Koivisto, K., Hanninen, T., Vanhanen, M., Kuusisto, J., Mykkanen, L., Laasko, M., & Riekkinen, P. (1997). Stability of age-associated memory impairment during a longitudinal population-based study. *Journal of the American Geriatrics Society, 45,* 120–121.

Herzog, A. R., & House, J. S. (1991, winter). Productive activities and aging well. *Generations,* 49–54.

Hooper, C. R. (2001). Sensory and sensory integrative development. In B. R. Bonder & M. Wagner (Eds.), *Functional Performance in Older Adults* (2nd ed., pp. 121–137). Philadelphia: Davis.

Ivnik, R. J., Smith, G. E., Malec, J. F., Petersen, R. C., & Tangalos, E.G. (1995). Long-term stability and intercorrelations of cognitive abilities in older persons. *Psychological Assessment, 7,* 155–161.

Jackoway, I. S., Rogers, J. C., & Snow, T. L. (1987). The *Role Change Assessment:* An interview tool for evaluating older adults. *Occupational Therapy in Mental Health, 7,* 17–37.

Jebsen, R., Taylor, N., Trieschmann, R., Trotter, M., & Howard, L. (1969). An objective and standardized test of hand function. *Archives of Physical Medicine and Rehabilitation, 50,* 311–319.

Joint Commission on Accreditation of Healthcare Organizations

(1999). *Comprehensive Accreditation Manual for Hospitals.* Oakbrook Terrace, IL: Author.

Kalish, R. (1975). Basic processes. In R. Kalish (Ed.), *Late Adulthood: Perspectives on Human Development* (pp. 156–174). Monterey, CA: Brooks/Cole.

Kasper, R. (1978). Eye problems of the aged. In W. Reichel (Ed.), *Clinical Aspects of Aging* (pp. 393–402). Baltimore: Williams & Wilkins.

Keith, J., Fry, C., Glascock, A., Ikels, C., Dickerson-Putman, J. Harpending, H., & Draper, P. (1994). *The Aging Experience: Diversity and Commonality Across Cultures.* Thousand Oaks, CA: Sage.

Keller, W., Largen, J., Burch, N., & Maulsby, R. (1985). Physiology of the aging brain: Normal and abnormal states. In H. Johnson (Ed.), *Relations Between Normal Aging and Disease* (pp. 165–190). New York: Raven.

Kenshalo, D. (1977). Age changes in touch, vibration, temperature, kinesthesis, and pain sensitivity. In J. Birren & K. Schaie (Eds.), *Handbook of the Psychology of Aging* (pp. 562–579). New York: Van Nostrand, Reinhold.

Kielhofner, G. (1995). *A Model of Human Occupation: Theory and Application.* Baltimore: Williams & Wilkins.

Kiernat, J. (1991). *Occupational Therapy and the Older Adult.* Rockville, MD: Aspen.

Lewis, C. (1990). *Aging: The Health Care Challenge.* Philadelphia: Davis.

Lewis, C., & Bottomly, J. (1994). *Geriatric Physical Therapy: A Clinical Approach.* East Norwalk, CT: Appleton & Lange.

Lindenberger, U., Mayr, U., & Kleigl, R. (1993). Speed and intelligence in old age. *Psychology and Aging, 8,* 207–220.

Longino, C. F., & Kart, C. S. (1982). Explicating activity theory: A formal replication. *Journal of Gerontology, 37,* 713–722.

Mace, N. L., Rabins, P. V., & McHugh, P. R. (1999). *The 36-Hour Day: A Family Guide to Caring for Persons with Alzheimer Disease, Related Dementing Illnesses, and Memory Loss in Later Life* (3rd. ed.) Baltimore: Johns Hopkins University.

Mann, W. C. (2001). Technology. In B. Bonder & M. Wagner (Eds.), *Functional Performance in Older Adults* (2nd ed., pp. 429–447). Philadelphia: Davis.

Mathiowetz, V., Volland, G., Kashman, N., & Weber K. (1985). Adult norms for the *Box and Block Test* of manual dexterity. *American Journal of Occupational Therapy, 39,* 386–391.

Mathiowetz, V., Weber, K., Kashman, N., & Volland G. (1985). Adult norms for the *Nine Hole Peg Test* of finger dexterity. *Occupational Therapy Journal of Research, 5,* 24–38.

Matsutsuyu, J. (1963). The *Interest Checklist. American Journal of Occupational Therapy, 32,* 628–630.

Medina, J. (1996). *The Clock of Ages: Why We Age-How We Age-Winding Back the Clock.* New York: Cambridge University.

Nelson, D. (1988). Occupation: Form and performance. *American Journal of Occupational Therapy, 42,* 633–638.

Neugarten, B. L. (1975). *Middle Age and Aging.* Chicago: University of Chicago.

Newman, L. (1995). *Maintaining Function in Older Adults.* Newton, MA: Butterworth Heinemann.

Ogilvie, D. M. (1987). Life satisfaction and identity structure in late middle-aged men and women. *Psychology and Aging, 2,* 217–224.

O'Sullivan, D., & Swallow, M. (1968). Fiber size and content of the radial and sural nerves. *Journal of Neurology, Neurosurgery and Psychiatry, 31,* 464–470.

Perry, B. (1982). Falls among the elderly living in high rise apartments. *Journal of Family Practice, 14,* 1069–1073.

Pollack, N. (1993). Client-centered assessment. *American Journal of Occupational Therapy, 47,* 298–301.

Potvin, A. (1980). Human neurologic function and the aging process. *Journal of the American Geriatric Society, 28,* 1–9.

Pynoos, J., & Cohen, E. (1990). *Home Safety Guide for Older People: Check it Out, Fix it Up.* Washington: Serif.

Rabbitt, P. (1982). How do old people know what to do next? In F. I. Craik & S. Trehub (Eds.), *Aging and Cognitive Processes* (pp. 79–97). New York: Plenum.

Rapkin, B. D., & Fischer, K. (1992). Framing the construct of life satisfaction in term of older adults' personal goals. *Psychology and Aging, 7,* 138–149.

Richardson V. E. (1993). *Retirement Counseling.* New York: Springer.

Riley, K. (2001). Cognitive development in later life. In B. R. Bonder & M. Wagner (Eds.), *Functional Performance in Older Adults* (2nd ed., pp. 139–152). Philadelphia: Davis.

Rockey, L. S. (1997). Memory assessment of the older adult. In P. D. Nussbaum (Ed.), *Handbook of Neuropsychology and Aging,* New York: Plenum.

Rogers, J. C., Holm, M., & Stone, R. (1997). Evaluation of daily living tasks: The home care advantage. *American Journal of Occupational Therapy, 51,* 410–422.

Rosenfeld, M. (1997). *Motivational Strategies in Geriatric Rehabilitation.* Bethesda, MD: American Occupational Therapy Foundation.

Rowe, J. W., & Kahn, R. L. (1998). *Successful Aging.* New York: Pantheon.

Rowles, G. D. (1991). Beyond performance: Being in place as a component of occupational therapy. *American Journal of Occupational Therapy, 45,* 265–271.

Rudman, D. L., Cook, J. V., & Polatajko, H. (1997). Understanding the potential of occupation: A qualitative exploration of seniors' perspectives on activity. *American Journal of Occupational Therapy, 51,* 640.

Sterns, H., Laier, M. P., & Dorsett, J. G. (2001). Work and retirement. In B. R. Bonder & M. Wagner (Eds.), *Functional Performance in Older Adults* (2nd ed. pp. 179–195). Philadelphia: Davis.

Sullivan, N. (1984). Vision in the elderly. In E. Stilwell (Ed.), *Handbook of Patient Care for Gerontological Nurses* (pp. 2–9). Thorofare NJ: Slack.

Swallow, M. (1966). Fiber size and content of the anterior tibial nerve of the foot. *Journal of Neurology, Neurosurgery and Psychiatry, 29,* 205–212.

Tideiksaar, R. (2001). Falls. In B. R. Bonder & M. Wagner (Eds.), *Functional Performance of Older Adults* (2nd ed., pp. 267–286). Philadelphia: Davis.

Tinetti, M., Speechley, M., & Ginter, S. (1988). Risk factors for falls among elderly persons living in the community. *New England Journal of Medicine, 319,* 1701–1707.

Treas, J. (1995). *Older Americans in the 1990s and Beyond.* Washington: Population Reference Bureau.

U. S. Department of Health and Human Services. (1999). *Health, United States, 1999.* Retrieved June 6, 2001 from the World Wide Web. http://www.cdc.gov/nchs/data/hus99.pdf.

Wilkins, S., Law, M., & Letts, L (2001). Assessment of functional performance. In B. R. Bonder & M. B. Wagner (Eds.), *Functional Performance in Older Adults* (2nd ed.). Philadelphia: Davis.

Willis, S. L. (1991). Cognition and everyday competence. In K. W. Schaie (Ed.). *Annual Review of Gerontology and Geriatrics, 11,* 80–109. New York: Springer.

Winter, D., Patla, A., Frank J., & Walt, S. (1990). Biomechanical walking pattern changes in the fit and healthy elderly. *Physical Therapy, 70,* 340–347.

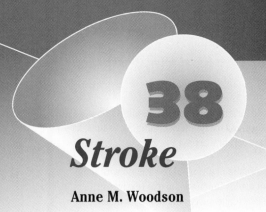

38

Stroke

Anne M. Woodson

LEARNING OBJECTIVES

After studying this chapter, the reader will be able to do the following:

1. Define stroke, or cerebrovascular accident, and briefly describe the causes, incidence, and impairments and disabilities that can result from stroke.
2. Describe the continuum of care for individuals recovering from stroke, including the interdisciplinary team, the various settings for care, and the phases of recovery and intervention.
3. Describe methods for evaluating occupational performance and component abilities and capacities of patients recovering from stroke.
4. Suggest goals and methods for treatment to improve the occupational performance and component abilities and capacities of patients recovering from stroke.
5. Analyze the effectiveness of occupational therapy intervention in improving a patient's quality of life and adjustment to life with stroke.

*S*troke, or cerebrovascular accident (CVA), describes a variety of disorders characterized by the sudden onset of neurological deficits caused by vascular injury to the brain. Vascular damage in the brain disrupts blood flow, limits oxygen supply to surrounding cells, and leads to brain tissue death or infarction. The mechanism, location, and extent of the lesion determine the symptoms and prognosis for the patient. This chapter focuses on patients with stroke, but nonvascular brain trauma or disease, such as gunshot wounds or tumors, may manifest many of the same neurological deficits and may be treated similarly.

GLOSSARY

Aphasia—Language disorder caused by brain damage that affects production and/or comprehension of written or spoken language.

Apraxia—Impairment of organized, controlled movement or motor planning not explained by motor or sensory impairment.

Backward chaining—Process of breaking a task into steps and guiding or assisting learner through all but the last step, which learner performs independently. Preceding steps of task are added until learner can perform entire sequence independently.

Hemiparesis—Weakness or partial paralysis on one side of the body caused by brain damage.

Hemiplegia—Paralysis on one side of the body caused by brain damage.

Hemorrhage—Bleeding resulting from the rupture of a blood vessel.

Homonymous hemianopsia—Visual field deficit caused by brain damage in which patient cannot perceive half of visual field of each eye.

Ischemia—Loss of blood flow through a vessel resulting in an insufficient supply of blood and oxygen to surrounding tissues, as when a blood clot blocks a cerebral artery.

Learned nonuse—Phenomenon observed in patients with hemiparesis in which patient avoids functional use of involved arm after failed attempts to use it and successful attempts to use uninvolved arm.

Postural adaptation—Ability of body to maintain balance automatically and remain upright during alterations in position and challenges to stability.

Shoulder subluxation—Incomplete dislocation of humerus out of glenohumeral joint caused by weakness, stretch, or abnormal tone in the scapulohumeral and/or scapular muscles.

Unilateral neglect—Disturbance in the ability to notice, orient, or respond to stimuli in space on side of body opposite site of brain damage.

Causation

Strokes are usually classified by the mechanism and location of the vascular damage. The two broad causes are **ischemia** and **hemorrhage**. Ischemic strokes result from a blockage of a cerebral vessel and can further be categorized as caused by thrombosis or embolism. Thrombosis is the stenosis or occlusion of a vessel, usually as a result of atherosclerosis. This occlusion is typically a gradual process, often with preceding warning signs, such as transient ischemic attack (TIA). Embolism is dislodged platelets, cholesterol, or other material that travels in the bloodstream and blocks a vessel. Ischemic strokes are the most common type, representing roughly 80% of strokes (Roth & Harvey, 1996).

Hemorrhagic strokes result from a rupture of a cerebral blood vessel. In such strokes, blood is released outside of the vascular space, cutting off pathways and leading to pressure injuries to brain tissue (Caplan & Stein, 1986). Hemorrhages, which are either intracerebral (bleeding into the brain itself) or subarachnoid (bleeding into an area surrounding the brain), may be caused by hypertension, arteriovenous malformation, or aneurysm (Bartels, 1998). CVAs caused by hemorrhage account for only an estimated 20% of strokes, but they can be the most catastrophic (Rolak & Rokey, 1990), accounting for an estimated third of stroke deaths.

Location of Involvement

Most lesions are either anterior circulation strokes, which present signs and symptoms of hemispheric dysfunction, or posterior circulation strokes, which display signs and symptoms of brainstem involvement (Simon et al., 1989). Another distinction related to location of CVA is whether the lesion results from large-vessel or small-vessel disease. Thrombosis occurs most often in the large cerebral blood vessels. Small-vessel, or lacunar, strokes are very small infarctions that occur only where small arterioles branch off the larger vessels in deeper portions of the brain, such as the basal ganglia, internal capsule, thalamus, and pons. Lacunar strokes can produce distinctive syndromes (Bartels, 1998), and they have a good prognosis for almost complete recovery (Rolak & Rokey, 1990).

Incidence

Stroke is the third leading cause of death in the United States and is the most common cause of chronic disability among adults (National Stroke Association, 1994). It is estimated that more than 700,000 persons have first or recurrent CVAs in the United States each year (Broderick et al., 1998) and that two-thirds of patients survive, bringing the number of stroke survivors in the U. S. population at any one time to approximately 3 million (Gresham et al., 1995). Stroke is the single most common diagnosis among patients seen by occupational therapists in the United States (American Occupational Therapy Association, 1996).

The projected aging of the U. S. population is expected to raise the incidence of stroke, as 72% of stroke victims are aged 65 or older. Men have a greater risk of stroke than women in all but the oldest age groups, and the risk for African Americans is double that of other groups (Gresham et al., 1995).

Medical Management

Acute stroke care focuses on determining the cause and site of the stroke, preventing progression of the lesion, preventing secondary medical complications, and treating acute neurological symptoms (Bartels, 1998). Advances in the use of technology and pharmaceuticals have transformed acute stroke care from mainly supportive to possible prevention and intervention. Brain imaging, including computed tomographic (CT) and magnetic resonance (MR) scans, can distinguish ischemic from hemorrhagic lesions and define their location, size, and vascular territory (Caplan, 1998).

In acute ischemic stroke, treatment concerns include restoration of blood flow and limitation of neuronal damage (Bartels, 1998). Antiplatelet and anticoagulation drugs, such as aspirin and heparin, are frequently used to improve flow through occluded vessels and prevent further clotting or thrombosis. Newer pharmacological treatments include thrombolytic drugs, such as tissue plasminogen activator (t-PA), that can open occluded cerebral vessels and immediately restore circulation (Bartels, 1998). Their use is limited, however, by the associated increased risk of hemorrhage and the fact that to be effective they must be administered within 3 to 6 hours after onset (Fisher & Bogousslavsky, 1998). With hemorrhagic stroke, acute treatment includes control of intracranial pressure, prevention of rebleeding, maintenance of cerebral perfusion, and control of vasospasm (Bartels, 1998).

Recovery From Stroke

The degree and time course of recovery from stroke are not easy to predict (Chollet et al., 1991). Gains in function after stroke are attributed to spontaneous recovery in the brain as well as to interventions that influence neural mechanisms and adaptation. It is difficult to distinguish between the two, however, because most patients receive some sort of intervention early post stroke and attempt their own readaptations to their environment (Bach-y-Rita & Balliet, 1987). Langton Hewer (1990) described a model of stroke recovery that includes both intrinsic and adaptive recovery. Intrinsic, or neurological, recovery refers to the remediation of neurological impairments, such as return of movement to a paralyzed limb. Adaptive, or functional, recovery entails regaining the ability to perform meaningful activities, tasks, and roles without full restoration of neurological function, such as using the unaffected hand for dressing or walking with a cane or walker. Most patients gain some degree of both intrinsic and adaptive recovery (Langton Hewer, 1990). Rehabilitation, including occupational therapy, is designed to promote maximum possible functional recovery from stroke.

Neurological Impairments and Recovery

Each survivor of a CVA has a unique combination of deficits determined by the location and severity of the lesion. Table 38-1 lists the most commonly encountered neurological impairments following stroke and describes the possible effect of each on occupational functioning. The most typical manifestation of CVA is **hemiparesis** or **hemiplegia**. Hemiparesis ranges from mild weakness to complete paralysis on the side of the body opposite the site of the CVA.

Certain impairments are associated with lesions in a particular hemisphere. For example, left CVA may cause right hemiparesis, aphasia or other communication deficits, and/or apraxia or motor planning deficits. Right CVA may result in left hemiparesis, visual field deficits or spatial neglect, poor insight and judgment, and/or impulsive behavior (Brodie et al., 1994).

Many patients do not regain full movement or function of the upper extremity. Studies found that 69% of patients admitted to a rehabilitation unit following CVA had mild to severe upper extremity dysfunction (Nakayama et al., 1994), but only 14–16% of stroke survivors with initial upper extremity hemiparesis regained complete or nearly complete motor function (Nakayama et al., 1994; Parker et al., 1986). Historically, motor recovery in the patient with hemiparesis is described as progressing from proximal to distal movement and from mass, patterned, undifferentiated movement to selective, coordinated movement (Brunnstrom, 1970; Fugl-Meyer et al., 1975; Twitchell, 1951). Therapists now rarely see such a distinct progression of motor recovery in patients, perhaps because improved medical treatments limit brain damage or because of arbitrarily shortened time frames for rehabilitation services.

TABLE 38-1
Neurological Impairments Following Stroke

Neurological Deficit	Possible Effect on Occupational Function
Hemiplegia, hemiparesis	Impaired postural adaptation, bilateral integration Impaired mobility Decreased independence in any or all ADL, IADL
Hemianopsia, other visual deficits	Decreased awareness of environment; decreased ability to adapt to environment Impaired ability to read, write, navigate during mobility, recognize people and places, drive. Can affect all ADL
Aphasia	Impaired speech and comprehension of verbal or written language; inability to communicate, read, or comprehend signs or directions. Decreased social, community involvement; isolation
Dysarthria	Slurred speech, difficulty with oral motor functions such as eating, altered facial expressions
Somatosensory deficits	Increased risk of injury to insensitive areas Impairment of coordinated, dexterous movement
Incontinence	Loss of independence in toileting Increased risk of skin breakdown Decreased social, community involvement
Dysphagia	At risk for aspiration Impaired ability to eat or drink by mouth
Apraxia	Decreased independence in any motor activity (ADL, speech, mobility), decreased ability to learn new tasks or skills
Cognitive deficits	Decreased independence in ADL, IADL; decreased ability to learn new techniques; decreased social interactions
Depression	Decreased motivation, participation in activity; decreased social interaction

Studies estimating the frequency of neurological impairments following stroke indicate a much lower rate of impairment with passage of time. For example, the Stroke Data Bank, looking at patients shortly after hospital admission, found an 88% incidence of hemiparesis (Foulkes et al., 1988), while the Framingham Study (Gresham et al., 1979) found only a 48% incidence of hemiparesis in patients 6 or more months post stroke.

Rehabilitation, it is suggested, provides the demands and retraining necessary for central nervous system reorganization leading to decreased impairment (Bach-y-Rita, 1981; Moore, 1986).

Functional Recovery

Much attention is given to the functional outcomes of patients surviving stroke. While residual neurological deficits can lead to permanent impairments, disabilities and handicaps, impairments alone do not predict levels of disability or occupational functioning (Kelly-Hayes et al., 1998).

Important aspects of functional recovery include the amount of assistance required to carry out daily living tasks and whether a stroke survivor can resume function at home. Studies indicate that independence in activities of daily living (ADL) improves with time after an acute stroke. A large retrospective study using *Barthel Index* of ADL scores (Mahoney & Barthel, 1965) found that 6 months post stroke, 47% of 494 stroke survivors were independent in self-care, 9% were dependent, and 44% were partially independent. In other reports, 75–85% of patients surviving stroke were able to return to their homes; 60–78% gained independence in walking; and 22% of patients with first-time thrombotic strokes were living in nursing homes a year after onset (Brown et al., 1999; Gresham et al., 1979; Wade & Langton Hewer, 1987; Wilson et al., 1991).

Few studies have addressed the recovery of instrumental activities of daily living (IADL), such as home management, vocational, leisure, or community skills. Most persons surviving stroke report decreased levels of activity, socialization, and overall quality of life (Gresham et al., 1979; Tangeman et al., 1990).

Factors Influencing Recovery

Research in stroke outcomes has sought to identify characteristics and indicators that predict survival rate, neurological recovery, functional recovery, length of hospitalization, and discharge disposition (Wilson et al., 1991). No simple predictors have been identified from numerous prospective studies. Patients with similar impairments after stroke may achieve wide ranges in outcomes: individuals with mild neurological impairments may end up with serious disabilities or handicaps, while other individuals with severe residual stroke impairments achieve satisfactory functional recovery (Kelly-Hayes et al., 1998).

The type, size, and site of the brain lesion, of course, influence the extent and course of recovery. The presence and severity of coexisting disease, such as diabetes, heart disease, and peripheral vascular disease, can impede optimal functional recovery. One study of recovery of mobility after stroke found that more than 30% of patients who had reduced mobility 2 to 7 years post stroke had causes other than stroke, particularly arthritis and dementia, as the primary deterrents to mobility (Collen & Wade, 1991). Some studies have indicated that advancing age adversely affects recovery after stroke (Andrews et al., 1984; Granger et al., 1992), but age is difficult to isolate as a predictor of outcome because of the increased incidence of coexisting disease and preexisting functional limitations in older stroke survivors (Cifu & Lorish, 1994).

Other factors associated with poor functional outcomes include severe initial motor deficits, dependence in basic ADL, prior stroke, persistent bowel and urinary incontinence, severe visuospatial deficits, severe cognitive impairments, depression, severe aphasia, altered level of consciousness, poor social supports (e.g., lives alone) and poor sitting balance (Cifu & Lorish, 1994; Gresham et al., 1995). Factors that may predict good quality of life after stroke include married status, good family support, independence in basic ADL, access to continued services, and return to work (Cifu & Lorish, 1994).

Time Frame for Recovery

It has traditionally been reported that recovery of function following stroke occurs most rapidly during the first 1 to 3 months but slower improvement can continue up to a year (Wade, 1992). A study that followed persons post stroke for 6 months after discharge from an inpatient rehabilitation unit found continued improvements in neuromuscular function, mobility, and ADL performance (Ferruci et al., 1993). Individual stroke survivors who have successfully resumed life roles or taken on new ones report the process of recovery as continuing years after onset of stroke, with gains reported both in component skills and task performance (Buscherhof, 1998; Newborn, 1998).

Unfortunately, increasing restrictions on health care services at every level have limited long-term studies of individuals recovering from stroke. There is a tendency among policy makers to regard stroke as an acute disorder following a circumscribed recovery course rather than as a chronic, changing condition. Most studies of functional outcomes following stroke have focused on an individual's level of independence in basic self-care and his or her ability to return home. These are outcomes that can realistically be achieved within the duration of inpatient rehabilitation programs. Few studies have tracked the ability of persons surviving stroke to resume previous life roles or to develop meaningful new roles. Although it is estimated that two-thirds of those surviving strokes achieve independence in basic ADL (Jorgensen et al., 1995), most are limited in higher physical and social functioning and are unable to return to work (Duncan et al., 1997).

Spectrum of Care

Because the brain damage resulting from stroke has the potential to affect any aspect of an individual's health and functioning, a wide array of disciplines are involved in caring for survivors of stroke. A patient recovering from stroke may receive care in multiple settings as he or she progresses from onset through a rehabilitation program to a return to the community. Coordination of services and ongoing communication among patients, families, and care providers at each step of rehabilitation is mandatory for optimum outcomes.

Interdisciplinary Team

Ideally, members of the stroke rehabilitation team include the patient, the patient's family, the primary physician (internal medicine, family medicine, or geriatrics), a neurologist or physical medicine specialist (physiatrist), rehabilitation nurse, occupational therapist, physical therapist, social worker, speech–language pathologist, clinical psychologist, therapeutic recreation specialist, and dietitian. Team members vary with the patient's needs and available resources. Frequent communication in the form of clear documentation, team meetings, and individual exchanges among members is vital for effective and efficient teamwork.

Settings for Care

Occupational therapists treat patients recovering from stroke in a variety of settings, including acute-care hospitals, skilled nursing facilities, inpatient rehabilitation centers, outpatient clinics, and home care settings. A study of 1991 Medicare claims for rehabilitation services found that 73% of patients who survived stroke received services in one or more of these settings, with 17% treated in inpatient rehabilitation programs, 23% admitted to nursing facilities, and 40% receiving either home health or outpatient services (Gresham et al., 1995). To facilitate a patient's transition from one setting for care to another, occupational therapists should be familiar with services offered in the patient's area and communicate pertinent information to the next setting, particularly the patient's goals of resuming life roles.

Assessment

A vast array of evaluations exists to identify stroke impairments and disability. To help in the selection and ordering of assessment tools, therapists are guided by models of practice and evidence-based practice guidelines. Because occupational function is the focus of occupational therapy, assessment of a patient post stroke begins with determination of roles, tasks, and activities important to that individual. From this context, the occupational therapist assesses the individual's competence in performing these valued roles, tasks, and activities. Where disabilities are discovered, further evaluation identifies specific impairments in abilities and capacities and residual abilities that can lead to restoration of function.

In response to growing demands for standards of quality health care, the U. S. Department of Health and Human Services' Agency for Health Care Policy and Research (now called Agency for Healthcare Research and Quality) published the *Post-stroke Rehabilitation Clinical Practice Guideline* (Gresham et al., 1995). Concerning assessment, this guideline recommends that practitioners "use well-validated standardized measures" throughout acute care and rehabilitation to achieve consistency of treatment decisions, facilitate team communication, and monitor progress for each survivor (Gresham et al., 1995, p. 7). Often, multiple assessment instruments must be used throughout this process because of the wide variation in individual stroke manifestations and the patient's changing needs over the course of recovery. The guideline recommends specific assessments based on the instrument's validity, reliability, sensitivity to change, and practicality.

Therapists should be familiar with commonly used standardized stroke deficit scales because they are frequently used as an interdisciplinary summary of baseline function and as indicators of recovery or treatment outcomes. The *National Institute of Health Stroke Scale* (Brott et al., 1989) is a brief, well-validated tool that can be administered by physicians, nurses, or therapists. Items scored include consciousness, vision, extraocular movements, facial palsy, limb strength, ataxia, sensation, speech, and language. The *American Heart Association Stroke Outcome Classification* (Kelly-Hayes et al., 1998) was devised to summarize the neurological impairments, disabilities, and handicaps that occur post stroke. This classification formula records the number of neurological domains affected (motor, sensory, visual, language, cognitive, affective), the severity of these impairments, and the functional (ADL) performance rating resulting from these impairments. Such a classification system, it is hoped, can be used to assess recovery, determine response to various treatments, and track long-term effects of stroke on survivors.

Assessment of Occupational Performance

The patient's ability to perform the self-care, recreational, and vocational tasks that he or she hopes to continue are evaluated by observation (Wade & Langton Hewer, 1987) rather than report, because there can be a difference between what a patient can do and actually does. Evaluation to determine a patient's level of occupational functioning is administered early to predict answers to the following questions: (1) Where will the patient live, and what physical adaptations will be necessary? (2) How much and what type of assistance will the patient need? (3) What roles will the patient be able to fulfill, and how will he or she spend his or her time? (Wade, 1992).

A patient's ADL performance in a structured clinical setting may not indicate performance at home. For example, patients who can put on and remove clothes during therapy sessions may not be able to find and retrieve their clothes in a cluttered closet, select clothing appropriate for the weather, or initiate the dressing routine without prompting (Campbell et al., 1991). Conversely, a patient may be unable to master simple meal preparation in the unfamiliar environment of a clinic kitchen but may readapt easily to this task upon return home. A home evaluation can help determine what resources and means a patient has to achieve independence in tasks as well as assessing safety and accessibility (see Chapter 10).

Self-Care

Methods for assessing self-care, or basic ADL, and examples of evaluation tools are discussed in Chapter 3. Measures of disability in ADL recommended by the *Post-Stroke Rehabilitation Clinical Practice Guideline* (Gresham et al., 1995) are the *Barthel Index* (Mahoney & Barthel, 1965) and the *Functional Independence Measure* (Keith et al., 1987). These interdisciplinary measures are well known and widely used in stroke research. Their use can strengthen the team approach to stroke, with occupational therapists typically completing the self-care portions of these assessments and practitioners of other disciplines completing portions pertaining to bowel and bladder control, mobility, communication, cognition, and social interaction. Other useful measurements mentioned in the guideline include the *Katz Index of ADL* (Katz et al., 1963) and the *Kenny Self-Care Evaluation* (Schoening & Iversen, 1968).

Instrumental Activities of Daily Living

A patient's goals and probable discharge situation may direct a therapist to evaluate more complex areas of occupational performance. To have a satisfactory independent life, a stroke patient must competently perform IADL, such as shopping, meal preparation, housekeeping, use of the telephone, financial management, access to transportation, and desired leisure activities. Measures of IADL recommended by the *Post-Stroke Rehabilitation Clinical Practice Guideline* include the *Frenchay Activities Index* (Holbrook & Skilbeck, 1983) and the *Philadelphia Geriatric Center Instrumental Activities of Daily Living*

Scale (Lawton, 1988). The *Frenchay Index* is a self-report tool developed specifically for patients with stroke that looks at how frequently a patient engaged in various activities, such as washing clothes, going on social outings, and gardening, prior to a stroke and frequency of participation in the same activities afterward. The stated purposes of this evaluation are to record changes in patterns of activity after stroke and to reflect quality of life rather than to measure performance in survival skills. The *IADL Scale*, on the other hand, is an observed measure that ranks quality of performance of activities such as using a telephone, managing medications, and handling finances.

When appropriate, potential for driving and return to work may be evaluated by an occupational therapist or other specialist trained in these areas. A patient's ability to resume driving and/or vocational tasks is discussed later in this chapter; see also Chapters 31 and 33.

Assessment of Component Abilities and Capacities

Observation of a patient's ADL performance suggests to the therapist probable deficits in components of independent functioning, which can be measured directly by administration of selected tests. Areas to be evaluated include postural adaptation, specific components of upper extremity function, and motor learning ability.

Postural Adaptation

Postural adaptation, or postural control, refers to the individual's ongoing ability to remain upright against gravity for stability and during changes in body position (Bobath, 1990; Warren, 1990). Because so many daily living tasks depend on this skill (e.g., putting on socks, getting in and out of a bathtub, housework, and participating in sports), the recognition and treatment of deficits in postural adaptation constitute an important aspect of therapy for stroke patients. Evaluation and treatment limited to a patient securely supported in bed or in a wheelchair fail to address most usual daily tasks that require dealing with gravity. A person with hemiplegia typically has decreased trunk control, poor bilateral integration, and impaired automatic postural control. As a result, the patient must devote considerably more effort to remaining upright, with decreased ability to focus on purposeful tasks (Warren, 1991). When engaging in a challenging activity, the hemiplegic patient often resorts to a developmentally lower-level compensatory strategy to help maintain stability, such as using upper extremities to help with standing balance (Warren, 1990).

Postural adaptation capacities such as balance can best be observed during the performance of meaningful functional activities, although the *Berg Balance Scale* (Berg et al., 1989) has been listed as a recommended tool in the *Post-Stroke Rehabilitation Clinical Practice Guideline*. Determining status of a patient's trunk control after stroke is an important starting point for assessing component capacities or skills, because poor trunk control can lead to increased risk of falls, contracture, and deformity and decreased visual feedback, limb movement, tolerance for sitting and standing, and swallowing effectiveness secondary to head and neck malalignment (Gillen, 1998a). A patient's posture and balance, both static and dynamic, can be observed and noted while the patient is seated and standing and during self-care tasks such as dressing, transfers, and bathing. Table 38-2 compares functional seated posture with dysfunctional positioning typically observed in patients recovering from stroke.

Upper Extremity Function

Occupational therapists are the clinicians most often involved with the evaluation and treatment of motor deficits in the hemiplegic or hemiparetic upper extremity. Evaluation of the involved upper extremity should address sensation; the mechanical and physiological deterrents to movement; the presence and degree of active or voluntary movement; the quality of this movement, including strength, endurance, and coordination; and the extent of function resulting from movement.

Somatosensory Assessment

During evaluations of sensory deficits in the stroke patient, it is important to remember that sensation is a component of function and not a focus for treatment except as it relates to the ability to perform usual daily living tasks. Somatosensory disturbances are frequent in patients who have had acute strokes but rarely occur in isolation (Bogousslavsky et al., 1988).

Most tests of sensation require attention, recognition, and response to multiple stimuli; sensory testing is therefore difficult in patients with aphasia, confusion, and other cognitive deficits. It is often necessary to determine the patient's level of comprehension and communication, including yes–no reliability. An expressively aphasic patient can nod, gesture, point to written or pictured cues, or select a stimulus object from an array of objects. When testing with standard procedures is not possible, information may still be gained from observing a patient's reactions to the testing. The presence of gross protective sensation (flinching when pricked with a sharp pin) can be documented even if discriminatory perception cannot be determined.

Patients who have had mild CVAs and who have intact primary sensory awareness may need to be tested for more subtle discriminatory problems using the two-point discrimination test (Callahan, 1990) or the

TABLE 38-2
Common Impairments in Sitting Posture Seen After Stroke

Body Part	Normal Sitting Posture Ready for Function	Abnormal Sitting Posture Typical of Stroke
Head, neck	Neutral	Forward Flexed to weak side Rotated away from weak side
Shoulders	Symmetrical height Aligned over pelvis	Uneven height Involved shoulder retracted
Spine, trunk	Straight from posterior view Appropriate lateral curves Lateral trunk muscle lengths equal bilaterally	Curved from posterior view Thoracic kyphosis Shortened lateral trunk muscles on one side, elongation on opposite side
Arms	Not used to maintain static upright posture Relaxed	Use of stronger arm to maintain upright posture Increased or decreased muscle tone in involved arm
Pelvis	Symmetrical weight bearing through both ischial tuberosities Neutral to slight anterior pelvic tilt Neutral rotation	Asymmetrical weight bearing Posterior pelvic tilt One hip retracted forward
Legs	Hips at 90° flexion Knees aligned with hips; hips in neutral adduction or abduction and internal or external rotation Feet under knees Feet flat on floor, able to bear weight	Hips in more extension Hips adducted so that knees touch or involved hip externally rotated so that knees wide apart Feet in front of knees Feet not flat on floor, unable to bear weight

Moberg Pick-up Test (Dellon, 1981). Such testing is indicated when motor return is good but hand dexterity remains impaired. Chapter 6 provides details of sensory assessment.

Mechanical and Physiological Components

Factors that can interfere with movement and function of the hemiplegic upper extremity include limitations in passive range of motion, joint malalignment, abnormal muscle tone, and pain. Interview and medical records can help determine whether these conditions result from stroke or were present prior to onset. Passive movement restrictions in the joints and soft tissues of the extremity may result from an individual's anatomy and lifestyle or from premorbid conditions such as arthritis or injury. Limitations may result more directly from the stroke, with sudden and prolonged immobilization of joints due to weakness or spasticity in muscles. Persistent stereotyped positioning of joints without counteracting movement results in the shortening and eventual contracture of muscles, tendons, and ligaments. In the shoulder, adhesions, tendinitis, and bursitis are common complications of hemiparesis, and all can result in limited range of motion (Andersen, 1985; Caillet, 1981). Edema secondary to reduced circulation and loss of muscle action can further limit passive joint motion, particularly in the hand. Goniometric measurement of passive range of motion is usually not indicated unless treatment is specifically aimed at increasing passive motion, such as when trying to eliminate an elbow flexion contracture. More useful in assessing patients with stroke is a comparison of the involved extremity to the uninvolved arm to determine probable baseline joint motion.

Shoulder subluxation, or malalignment of the glenohumeral joint, is secondary to weakness or spasticity of the scapulohumeral and/or scapular muscles (Caillet, 1981). In hemiparesis, downward rotation of the scapula and/or lateral flexion of the spine may lead to a downward, backward, and medial orientation of the glenoid fossa. The humerus is thus susceptible to downward (inferior) subluxation from the pull of gravity. In anterior subluxation, the head of the humerus is displaced anteriorly in the glenoid fossa, and the humerus tends toward hyperextension; this pattern is associated with hypertonicity of surrounding muscles (Byrne & Ridgeway, 1998; Ryerson & Levit, 1997). Superior subluxation, also associated with muscle hypertonicity, occurs when the humeral head becomes locked under the coracoid process in a position of elevation, abduction, and internal rotation.

Evaluation of inferior subluxation can be done by palpation: the patient's arm hangs freely with trunk stabilized while the examiner palpates the subacromial space for the separation between the acromion and the head of the humerus. The distance separating the two is measured in finger widths, that is, the number of fingers that can be inserted in the space (Bohannon & Andrews, 1990), or a scale of 0 to 5 can be used, with 1 equaling half a finger width (Hall et al., 1995). The evaluator palpates both shoulders for comparison. There are no known clinical methods to quantify the degree of anterior or superior subluxation, although observation of trunk–shoulder alignment and palpation can detect their presence. Palpation of a space posterior to the head of the humerus suggests anterior subluxation, while superior subluxation is suspected if no space is felt (Hall et al., 1995).

Abnormal muscle tone is a common component of movement deficits in hemiplegia but is also associated with range-of-motion limitations and pain. Definitions of states of increased and decreased muscle tone and methods for evaluating muscle tone are found in Chapter 5. See Chapters 4 and 9 for descriptions of pain evaluation.

Voluntary Movement

Determining the amount and quality of voluntary movement a patient can produce is one of the first steps in assessing movement potential (Warren, 1991). The patterns of motion available are different for each stroke patient . Movement can change dramatically or subtly with time; hence it requires careful reassessment throughout recovery. Factors to consider when evaluating motor control of the involved upper extremity:

▶ Can the patient perform reflexive but not voluntary movement? Examples: Patient demonstrates active elbow extension in the involved arm when balance is disturbed (equilibrium reaction) or flexes the hemiparetic elbow while yawning (associated reaction) but cannot perform these movements on request.
▶ Do proximal segments (neck, trunk, shoulder, hip) stabilize as needed to provide firm support for movement of the distal parts? Example: A patient cannot keep his balance when attempting arm movement and can raise his hemiparetic arm only with pronounced lateral bending of the trunk and excessive elevation of the shoulder girdle.
▶ Can voluntary movement be performed unassisted against gravity, or is assistance required in the form of positioning, support, or facilitation? Example: A patient can bring her hand to her mouth only by flexing her elbow in a horizontal plane with gravity eliminated.
▶ Can voluntary movement be performed in an isolated fashion or only in a synergistic pattern? Example: A patient can reach for an object on a table only with a pattern of shoulder abduction, elbow flexion and trunk flexion, rather than with the more

efficient pattern of shoulder flexion and elbow extension.
▶ Can reciprocal movement (the ability to perform agonist–antagonist motion in succession in an individual joint) (Daniel & Strickland, 1992) be performed with practical speed and precision? Example: A patient cannot produce a smooth pattern of elbow extension-flexion-extension in order to grasp a glass, take a drink, and set it back on the table but can perform both movements separately.

One of the major movement difficulties following stroke is attaining the capacity and ability to isolate and control single muscle actions and combine them in a pattern appropriate for the task at hand. In motor patterns typical in hemiplegia, movement initiated in one joint results in automatic contraction of other muscles linked in synergy with that movement. This results in limited, stereotyped movement patterns rather than adaptive, selective motions. Typical stereotyped patterns are described as flexor or extensor synergy patterns according to the motion at the elbow (Brunnstrom, 1970) (see Chapter 24). There is considerable variation in synergistic patterning, and many abnormal stereotyped patterns may result from compensatory movements, unnecessary movement, muscle tension resulting from exertion or stress, or in response to gravity (e.g., pronation). Abnormal patterns of muscle activation in hemiparetic patients can further be seen in the inability to control activation and deactivation of agonist–antagonist muscle pairs to produce, for example, the rapid alternating movements necessary to brush teeth (Bourbonnais & Vanden Noven, 1989).

Several methods for evaluating voluntary movement post stroke are described in Chapters 5 and 21 to 24. Valid and reliable evaluation tools recommended by the *Post-Stroke Rehabilitation Clinical Practice Guidelines* include the *Fugl-Meyer Assessment of Motor Function* (Fugl-Meyer et al., 1975) (Chapter 24) and the *Motor Assessment Scale* (Carr et al., 1985) (Chapter 22).

Strength and Endurance

Muscle weakness ranging from slightly less than normal strength to total inability to activate muscles has been recognized as a limiting factor in the rehabilitation of patients with hemiplegia (Carr & Shepherd, 1987; Duncan & Badke, 1987; Trombly & Quintana, 1985). Traditionally, manual muscle strength testing has not been recommended for stroke patients except for those who regain isolated muscle control, because the presence of spasticity or synergy patterns was felt to confound accurate assessment of strength. Clinical studies, however, suggest that strengthening of hemiplegic upper extremity musculature is appropriate for many patients

(Bohannon, 1987; Bohannon & Smith, 1987; Trombly, 1992). The motor assessment evaluations described in this chapter and techniques described in Chapter 4 are recommended to establish baseline levels of muscle strength.

Reduced endurance, seen as a decrease in the ability to sustain movement or activity for practical amounts of time, is an important limiting factor in the motor performance of stroke patients because it affects the patient's ability to participate fully in rehabilitation (Warren, 1991) (see Research Note). Decreased endurance can be the result of physical and/or mental fatigue caused by the exertion required to move weakened limbs (Brodal, 1973) or the result of comorbid cardiac or respiratory conditions (see Chapter 4).

Functional Performance

Assessing functional use of a hemiparetic arm post stroke is problematic, because while occupational performance evaluations identify deficits in ADL and IADL, they do not accurately reflect a patient's ability to use the affected arm for tasks. As observed in a population-based study, recovery of function in more than half of patients with significant upper extremity paresis was achieved only with compensatory use of the unaffected arm

(Nakayama et al., 1994). Similarly, physical component skill evaluations may predict a patient's potential for functional use of a hemiparetic arm but are not measures of occupational performance. Many tests are described in the literature as useful for evaluating function of the involved upper extremity. Okkema and Culler (1998) reviewed 13 evaluations that include functional or task-oriented items and concluded that few of these tests are actually functional; that is, few use relevant real-life activities. Most of these tests can be categorized as task-oriented evaluations, with portions or simulations of familiar activities.

One difficulty in measuring function after stroke results from the normal differences in performance ability between dominant and nondominant arms (Bornstein, 1986). Eating with utensils, combing hair, and writing, for example, are normally performed by the dominant arm; testing the ability of a hemiparetic nondominant arm to perform these tasks is not relevant or useful to a patient. Because the arm has a wide range of functions, any single test assesses only a portion of the actual possible functions (Wade, 1989). Therapists must choose tests that seem best suited for the individual patient.

One functional test developed specifically for use with stroke patients is the *Action Research Arm Test* (Lyle,

---

RESEARCH NOTE

Fatigue After Stroke

Ingles, J. L., Eskes, G. A., & Phillips, S. J. (1999). Archives of Physical Medicine and Rehabilitation, 80, 173–178

ABSTRACT

The objective was to determine the frequency and outcome of fatigue, its effect on functioning, and its relationship to depression in patients 3 to 13 months post stroke. Participants included 88 individuals from a pool of consecutive patients previously admitted to an acute stroke service who were willing and able to complete the self-report questionnaires and 56 elderly control subjects living independently in the community. The main outcome measures were the *Fatigue Impact Scale*, a self-report measure of the presence and severity of fatigue and its effect on cognitive, physical, and psychosocial functions, and the *Geriatric Depression Scale*. Results showed that the frequency of self-reported fatigue was greater in the stroke group (68%) than in the control group (36%; $p < .001$) and was not related to time post stroke, stroke severity, or lesion location. Among the stroke group, 40% reported that fatigue was either their worst or one of their worst symptoms. Patients attributed more functional limitations to fatigue than did control subjects with fatigue. Although fatigue was accompanied by depressed mood in a substantial number of subjects in the stroke group (29%), an even greater number (39%) reported fatigue without feelings of depression. The authors concluded that while fatigue was independent of depression, the effect of fatigue on functional abilities was strongly influenced by depression.

IMPLICATIONS FOR PRACTICE

▶ Fatigue is expected to be a problem soon after stroke but is not always considered a deterrent to functional capacity or occupational therapy treatment several months post stroke. Therapists should recognize the long-term effect of fatigue symptoms when planning therapy in community or home programs.

▶ Training in energy conservation and work simplification techniques, including pacing and balancing of rest with activity, are appropriate for patients with stroke.

▶ The use of objective measures of functional and physical performance and standardized measures of fatigue and depression can help patients and families understand the effect of fatigue on function and recommend treatments to lessen that effect.

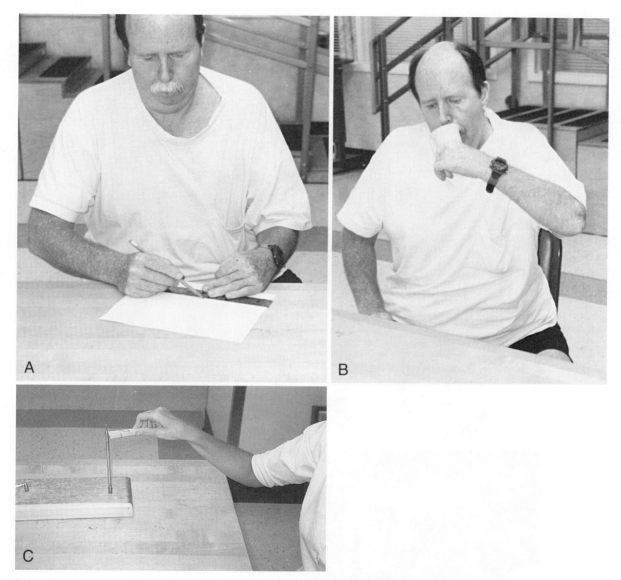

Figure 38-1 *Frenchay Arm Test* tasks. **A.** Stabilizing a ruler while drawing a line. **B.** Drinking from a handleless cup. **C.** Removing and replacing clothespin.

1981). This test is divided into four categories, grasp, grip, pinch, and gross movement, and has 19 items that are graded on a 4-point scale. This test can be quickly administered, was found to have high validity and reliability, and correlates well with the *Fugl-Meyer Assessment of Motor Function* (DeWeerdt & Harrison, 1985). However, the test requires specific handmade and difficult to obtain materials, and items tested are simulations rather than true functional tasks.

The *Frenchay Arm Test* was developed as a battery of functional tasks used to study recovery after stroke (DeSouza et al., 1980). The most recent abbreviated version includes 5 tasks (Heller et al., 1987) requiring use of the affected arm (Fig. 38-1). The test takes little time to

administer and materials are easy to assemble. Validity and reliability were established, but this test has relatively low sensitivity for patients on the low and high ends of the performance scale (Okkema & Culler, 1998).

A standardized test developed by occupational therapists specifically to evaluate patients' ability to use the hemiplegic upper extremity for purposeful tasks is the *Functional Test for the Hemiplegic/Paretic Upper Extremity* (Wilson et al., 1984; Wilson, D. J., Baker, L. L., & Craddock, J. A. [1984]. Protocol: Functional Test for the Hemiplegic/Paretic Upper Extremity. Unpublished manuscript. County Rehabilitation Center, Rancho Los Amigos, Occupational Therapy Department, Downey, CA). This test consists of 17 tasks divided into 7 functional

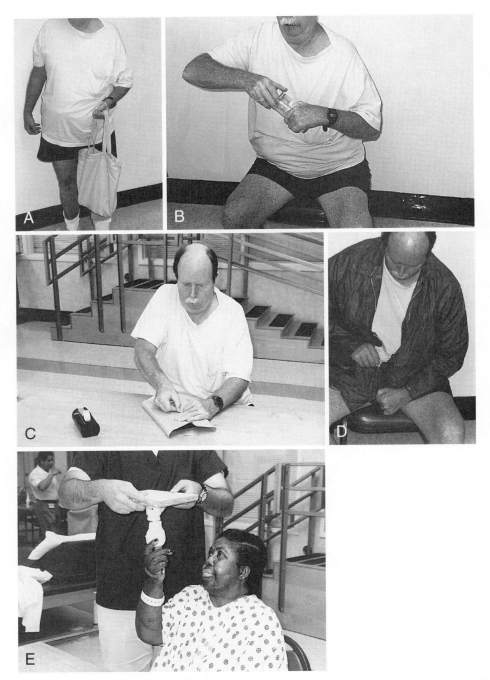

Figure 38-2 *Functional Test for the Hemiplegic/Paretic Upper Extremity*, sample tasks. **A.** Holding a pouch with a 1-pound weight. **B.** Stabilizing a jar while removing lid. **C.** Stabilizing a package while wrapping. **D.** Hooking and zipping a zipper. **E.** Putting in light bulb.

levels that range from absence of voluntary movement to selective and coordinated movement (Figs. 38-2 and 38-3). The tasks follow a pattern of increasing difficulty and complexity and reflect Brunnstrom's hierarchy of motor recovery in hemiplegia. This test was found to have interrater reliability and validity, and scores showed a strong correlation to scores on the *Fugl-Meyer*

Assessment of Motor Function (Filiatrault et al., 1991). The *Functional Test for the Hemiplegic/Paretic Upper Extremity* is dominance neutral in that most items are activities normally performed by either arm or bilaterally. Disadvantages of this test are that it does not provide specific information about why a patient has failed a task (Wilson et al., 1984), and uses pass–fail scoring rather

FUNCTIONAL TEST FOR THE HEMIPLEGIC/PARETIC UPPER EXTREMITY

Patient Name _E.G. (L CVA)_

LEVEL	TASK	DATE: 6-17-99 EXAMINER: AMW		DATE: 7-13-99 EXAMINER: AMW		DATE: 8-12-99 EXAMINER: AMW	
		GRADE	TIME	GRADE	TIME	GRADE	TIME
1	Patient is unable to complete higher level tasks						
2	A. Associated reaction	(NA)		(NA)		(NA)	
	B. Hand into lap	+	2 sec	+	2 sec	+	2 sec
3	C. Arm clearance during shirt tuck	+	5 sec	+	5 sec	+	3 sec
	D. Hold a pouch	+	15 sec	+	15 sec	+	15 sec
	E. Stabilize a pillow	+	25 sec	+	14 sec	+	8 sec
4	F. Stabilize a jar	+	12 sec	+	8 sec	+	5 sec
	G. Stabilize a package	+	75 sec	+	66 sec	+	40 sec
	H. Wringing a rag	+	32 sec	+	15 sec	+	10 sec
5	I. Hold a pan lid	+	20 sec	+	20 sec	+	19 sec
	J. Hook and zip a zipper	+	55 sec	+	22 sec	+	15 sec
	K. Fold a sheet	−	>3 min	+	90 sec	+	50 sec
6	L. Blocks and box	+	35 sec	+	20 sec	+	18 sec
	M. Box on shelf	−	helped w/ L. hand	+	15 sec	+	7 sec
	N. Coin in coin gauge	−	unable to pick up dime	−	dropped dime	+	15 sec
7	O. Cat's cradle			−		+	45 sec
	P. Light bulb			−		+	30 sec (difficult)
	Q. Remove rubber band					+	15 sec

Figure 38-3 *Functional Test for the Hemiplegic/Paretic Upper Extremity.* Copyright 1980 by the Occupational Therapy Department, Rancho Los Amigos Hospital, Downey, California. Reprinted with permission. See Wilson, Baker, and Craddock (1984) and Wilson, D. J., Baker, L. L., & Craddock, J. A. (1984). Protocol: Functional Test for the Hemiplegic/Paretic Upper Extremity. Unpublished manuscript. County Rehabilitation Center, Rancho Los Amigos, Occupational Therapy Department, Downey, CA, for a description of the items.

than an ordinal scale, which makes it difficult to use for documenting partial progress.

Motor Learning Ability

Motor learning ability refers to a patient's ability to learn and organize movement for adaptation to the environment (Warren, 1991). The motor learning model of rehabilitation states that regaining the ability to perform purposeful tasks entails setting a recognizable goal, practicing, and receiving feedback (Carr & Shepherd, 1987). The development of patients' self-monitoring skills and problem-solving abilities should be part of occupational therapy for survivors of stroke (Sabari, 1998a) so that they can learn to apply remaining abilities and what they learn in the clinic to their target environment. In this context, it is essential to assess factors that can affect a patient's ability to learn or relearn, including visual function, speech and language disorders, motor planning ability, cognitive disorders, and psychosocial adjustments. Use of these categories is somewhat artificial, since they operate as parts of an integrated system; it is difficult to discern or separate, for example, cognitive functioning from visual-perceptual or speech/language skills. These classifications are meant to assist the therapist in recognizing the components of learning impairments that follow stroke.

Visual Function

The visual system is a complex of almost all parts of the central and peripheral nervous system; any type or degree of brain damage therefore is expected to have some effect on the function of the visual system (Warren, 1999). Chapter 7 describes assessments of vision and visual perception.

The most common visual disturbance associated with stroke is **homonymous hemianopsia**. Hemianopsia is a visual field defect affecting half of the visual field. Homonymous means the deficit involves both eyes. A patient with left homonymous hemianopsia has decreased or absent vision in the nasal field of the right eye and the temporal field of the left eye. Deficits in visual attention in stroke patients are hemi-inattention, hemineglect or **unilateral neglect**. Unilateral neglect is a failure to notice, orient, or respond to stimuli on one side of visual space (Heilman & Valenstein, 1979). Patients can have hemianopsia without neglect or hemi-inattention without a visual field deficit, but neglect, the most severe form of decreased visual attention, usually indicates a visual field deficit in addition to hemi-inattention (Warren, 1999). Neglect is almost always associated with right hemisphere damage and is most often associated with parietal lobe lesions (Shinsha & Ishigami, 1999). It is highly predictive of poor functional recovery (Halligan et al., 1989).

Because visual deficits are disabling to the degree that they prevent completion of necessary ADL, observation of the patient's functional performance provides the most valuable information concerning the visual system (Warren, 1993, 1999). Patients with significant field deficits or unilateral neglect may display behaviors such as not noticing food on the left side of the tray, shaving only the right side of the face, or bumping into walls or furniture on the left while walking.

Speech and Language

Disturbances in the ability to communicate or to comprehend verbal or written information can significantly affect the ability to resume or relearn usual activities. **Aphasia** is an acquired language disorder that can cause impairment in listening, speaking, reading, writing, arithmetic, or using appropriate gestures (Cherney, 1995). Stroke is the leading cause of aphasia, with damage to the left cerebral hemisphere the usual origin. A simplified clinical classification of aphasia recognizes fluent and nonfluent aphasias, based on the patient's ability to produce speech (Goodglass & Kaplan, 1983). In the fluent aphasias, patients can easily produce spontaneous speech, but auditory comprehension and understanding of language is limited. The most common type of fluent aphasia is Wernicke's aphasia, or receptive aphasia, characterized by the smooth articulation of speech but marked by incorrect word or sound substitutions and the inability to name objects, repeat phrases, or follow commands. Reading and writing impairments are also common to this disorder (Sarno, 1994). Nonfluent aphasia is speech output that is difficult to produce, characterized by slow, awkward articulation with limited vocabulary and grammar usage in the presence of relatively well-preserved auditory comprehension. An example is Broca's aphasia or expressive aphasia, in which the patient can follow commands but cannot name objects, repeat phrases, or convey ideas. Patients with nonfluent aphasia may be able to sing familiar songs or speak in other automatic ways, such as praying (Goodglass & Kaplan, 1983) or swearing. Patients with nonfluent aphasia may also have agraphia, or the inability to express themselves in writing. Global aphasia is a term for a severe aphasia with dysfunction across language production and comprehension; it designates severity rather than a specific type of aphasia (Sarno, 1994).

Dysarthria is a speech disorder characterized by slurred speech, drooling, or decreased facial expression caused by paralysis or incoordination of the speech musculature (Trombly, 1989). Oral apraxia is another communication problem in which the patient has difficulty initiating and sequencing the movements necessary to produce speech. In these disorders, the patient can understand and express symbolic language.

The speech–language pathologist evaluates functions and dysfunctions of speech and speech musculature. The occupational therapist needs to confer with the speech–language pathologist to learn the results of a patient's communication evaluation, support the patient's language goals, and request suggestions for the most effective communication strategies (Sarno, 1994).

Motor Planning

Motor planning deficits, or **apraxia**, are deficits of skilled, organized, purposeful movement sequences that cannot be explained by motor or sensory impairments. These deficits are best identified during performance of daily living tasks. Clinical manifestations of motor planning difficulties include the following (Warren, 1991):

► Failure to orient the head or body correctly to a task, such as a patient attempting a toilet transfer who tries to sit on the toilet before correctly positioning body in front of it.

► Failure to orient the hand properly to objects and/or poor tool use, such as a patient who has to be reminded of the correct way to hold a pen when writing with the uninvolved hand.

► Difficulty initiating or carrying out a sequence of movements, such as a patient with nearly normal motor performance who cannot put on a shirt without step-by-step verbal and physical cueing.

► Movements characterized by hesitations and perseveration, such as a patient who after brushing his teeth, is handed a razor and asked to shave. After a delay the patient brings the razor to his mouth and tries to brush his teeth with it.

► Movements that can be performed only in context or in the presence of a familiar object or situation, such as a patient who does not follow a command to move hand to mouth unless given something to eat or drink.

These deficits are most pronounced during learning sessions, such as when training in wheelchair propulsion or one-handed buttoning, and in activities with multiple steps, such as making a sandwich.

Cognition

Disorders in higher brain functions, including problems with attention, orientation, concentration, memory, reasoning, judgment, or problem solving, are common after stroke (Gresham et al., 1995). Cognitive dysfunction can interfere with learning and the achievement of rehabilitation goals. It is also a source of safety concerns in areas of function such as mobility, meal preparation, and self-medication, which all affect discharge planning (Osmon et al., 1992). Cognitive impairment can be assessed during evaluation and treatment of occupa-

tional performance by focusing on the adaptive abilities of planning, judgment, problem solving, and initiation, which are as important in every functional routine as the physical components (Campbell et al., 1991). Chapter 8 describes specific assessment techniques. Mental status screening tests recommended by the *Post-Stroke Rehabilitation Clinical Practice Guideline* are the *Mini-Mental State Examination* (Folstein et al., 1975) and the *Neurobehavioral Cognitive Status Examination* (Kiernan et al., 1987). Therapists must be careful to differentiate between cognitive deficits and communication difficulties common to stroke (Gresham et al., 1995).

Psychosocial Aspects

Adjustment to disability is a critical component of rehabilitation, although effective measures of adjustment have not been described (Morris, 1998). Patients may appear poorly motivated, express hopelessness, or refuse to participate in therapy (Fraley, 1998), and these conditions restrict their ability to learn ways to return to a quality life.

Most patients have natural emotional reactions to their stroke, including denial, anxiety, anger, and depression (Czyrny et al., 1990). Mood disorder or psychosocial dysfunction is common and does not merely reflect expected grief response to loss of function (Stern & Bachman, 1991), as these disorders have been found to be present in stroke survivors even with good physical recovery (Labi et al., 1980). Depression is the most frequently reported reaction to stroke, with studies projecting that an average of 33–50% of patients develop depression requiring treatment (Remer-Osborn, 1998). Depression tends to develop over time and is more likely to be seen as rehabilitation proceeds than during the acute period post stroke (Gresham et al., 1995). Depression in stroke is both a physiological result of biochemical changes in the brain and a reaction to the personal losses of patients who realize, with time, that they will not fully recover. The boundaries between the organic causes and the reactive changes are not clear-cut (Kaufman & Becker, 1991).

Denial, an adaptive emotional mechanism employed to cope with depression or anxiety, is seen when the survivor of stroke is unable or unwilling to acknowledge the short- and long-term consequences of stroke (Remer-Osborn, 1998). It presents a challenge for the rehabilitation team because the patient may deny the need for treatment, set unreasonable personal goals, and fail to accommodate to the condition in the expectation of complete recovery (Versluys, 1995).

Emotional lability is an emotional response, such as laughing or crying, disproportionate to the emotional stimulus (Remer-Osborn, 1998). A patient may cry whenever seeing a family member or when asked about a valued activity. It is estimated that 18% of patients have emotional lability following first stroke (Morris et al., 1993).

Emotional reactions, compounded by cognitive, perceptual, and language impairments, may lead to behavioral outcomes including frustration, anger, impatience, irritability, overdependence, insensitivity to others, and rigid thinking (Versluys, 1995). These responses can further result in impaired personal interactions, inability to perform social and leisure activities or roles, and eventual isolation. Patients a year or more post stroke have reported decreased socialization and quality of life in spite of improved physical functioning (Ahlsio et al., 1984; Angeleri et al., 1993). Evaluation of the patient's and family's adjustments to the stroke, to rehabilitation, and to the prospect of living with the aftermath of the stroke can be done through interview and observation and by sharing information with other members of the rehabilitation team. The *Post-Stroke Rehabilitation Clinical Practice Guidelin*e suggests two validated measures of quality of life, recognizing that quality of life is difficult to define, much less measure reliably (Gresham et al., 1995). These tools are the *Medical Outcomes Study 36-Item Short-Form Health Survey* (Ware & Sherbourne, 1992) and the *Sickness Impact Profile* (Bergner et al., 1981). Both are meant to monitor progress after return to the community, and neither is specific to stroke. A new *Stroke-Specific Quality of Life Scale* has been found valid, reliable, and responsive in early trials (Williams et al., 1999).

Treatment

A careful interpretation of evaluation results helps determine a patient's assets and deficits in areas of occupational functioning. Possible goals for patients recovering from stroke:

▶ The patient will gain competence in valued and necessary basic ADL and IADL in order to perform at the highest level of independence possible in the desired postdischarge setting.

▶ The patient will improve postural control in order to perform daily living tasks requiring balance and changes in body position.

▶ The patient will gain increased somatosensory perception and/or will employ compensatory strategies in order to perform ADL safely.

▶ The patient and/or caregiver will demonstrate appropriate management techniques for the hemiparetic upper extremity to prevent the development of pain and other secondary mechanical or physiological movement restrictions.

▶ The patient will gain the necessary strength, endurance, and control of movement of the involved

upper extremity in order to use the involved upper extremity spontaneously during the performance of ADL.

▶ The patient will gain visual function or will employ compensatory strategies in order to resume previously performed ADL safely.

▶ The patient will improve motor planning ability in order to relearn old methods or learn new methods of performing ADL.

▶ The patient and/or caregiver will demonstrate appropriate strategies for improving or compensating for cognitive deficits during the performance of ADL.

▶ The patient and/or caregiver will be able to verbalize the reality and impact of emotional reactions to stroke and identify coping strategies or resources to help in the adjustment to living with a stroke.

▶ The caregiver will demonstrate appropriate methods and problem-solving strategies for assisting the patient with ADL and with home activities to improve component skills.

▶ The patient will gain competence in tasks and activities necessary to resume valued roles or to assume new meaningful roles in the community.

Safety of the patient is a concern during and after treatment (Box 38-1). In this chapter description of

BOX 38-1
SAFETY BOX
Precautions With Stroke Patients

▶ In the acute period after stroke, ascertain the patient's medical status and stability daily before treatment. Know the symptoms of progressing or recurrent stroke.

▶ Determine whether cardiac or respiratory precautions apply for a particular patient and monitor accordingly, watching for signs of cardiac distress and blood pressure changes, including dizziness, breathing difficulties, chest pain, excessive fatigue, and altered heart rate or rhythm.

▶ Guard against falls by providing appropriate supervision and assistance during transfers and other transitional movements.

▶ To avoid shoulder injury or pain, never pull or lift a patient by or under the weak arm during transfers or other transitional movements.

▶ Use appropriate precautions in the presence of insensitive skin, particularly if a patient also has visual field deficits and/or unilateral neglect.

▶ Ascertain a patient's ability to swallow and follow recommended management techniques during feeding.

▶ Provide appropriate supervision for patients who demonstrate impulsive behavior and/or poor safety awareness.

▶ Teach the patient, family members and other health care workers about safety concerns for an individual patient.

occupational therapy for stroke patients is divided into three stages: the acute phase, rehabilitation phase, and reentry to the community. For most patients, progression of recovery and provision of services are not this clear-cut. For a variety of reasons, many patients do not have access to the full spectrum of services with smooth continuity of care. Any treatment described, therefore, may apply to any or all other stages for a particular patient and should be viewed as part of a continuum of care adapted to meet changing needs over time (Sabari, 1998b). Specific recommendations from the *Post-Stroke Rehabilitation Clinical Practice Guideline* are included and indicated by colored print. These recommendations are backed by research evidence and/or expert opinion.

Acute Phase

Stroke rehabilitation begins "as soon as the diagnosis of stroke is established and life-threatening problems are under control" (Gresham et al., 1995, p. 53). Length of stay in acute hospital beds is typically just long enough for necessary diagnostic tests, initiation of appropriate medical treatment, and for making decisions and arrangements for the next phase of rehabilitation. Patients soon after stroke may need to be seen bedside because of precautions, monitoring, and varying levels of consciousness. During this phase, the patient must adjust to the sudden, unexpected shift from usual life roles to the role of patient (Fraley, 1998).

Early Mobilization and Return to Self-Care

The patient with acute stroke should be mobilized as soon after admission as is medically feasible. The patient should be encouraged to perform self-care as soon as medically feasible and if necessary should be offered compensatory training to overcome disabilities. The early introduction of basic ADL such as rolling in bed, sitting on the side of the bed, transferring to a wheelchair or commode, self-feeding, grooming, and dressing helps the patient reestablish some control over the environment and begins to improve occupational functioning and component abilities and capacities (Gresham et al., 1995). Even at this early stage, the occupational therapist's assessment of a patient can help determine the most appropriate setting for rehabilitation and discharge. Discharge planning should begin at the time of admission. Goals are to determine the need for rehabilitation, arrange the best possible living environment, and ensure continuity of care after discharge. The occupational therapist in an acute-care setting should take an active role in rehabilitation triage, basing recommendations on the patient's identified deficits and abilities (Radomski, 1995).

Lowering Risk for Secondary Complications

As part of the stroke care team, the occupational therapist should practice methods to prevent or lessen complications resulting from stroke.

Skin Care

It is estimated that 14.5% of patients with stroke develop pressure sores. Those who are comatose, malnourished, obese, or incontinent or who have severe paralysis or muscle spasticity are at greatest risk (Roth, 1991). The occupational therapist helps patients maintain skin integrity by doing the following:

▶ Using proper transfer and mobility techniques to avoid undue skin friction
▶ Recommending appropriate positioning for bed and sitting and participating in scheduled position changes as needed
▶ Assisting with wheelchair and seating selection and adaptation
▶ Teaching patient and caregiver precautions to avoid injury to insensitive skin and involved side of body
▶ Watching for signs of skin pressure or breakdown on a patient (bruising, redness, blisters, abrasions, ulceration), especially over bony areas, and alerting nursing or medical staff as appropriate

Maintaining Soft Tissue Length

Contractures, or shortening of skin, tendons, ligaments, muscles, and/or joint capsule, may result from the immobilization following stroke. Risk factors include muscle spasticity, postural malalignment, and improper positioning, including lack of variation in positioning (Gillen, 1998b). Contractures restrict movement, may be painful, and may limit functional recovery (Gresham et al., 1995). The appropriate management is therefore a preventive program of proper positioning and soft tissue and joint mobilization. Suggested bed positioning for patients with stroke, based on a literature review (Carr & Kenney, 1992), is summarized in Box 38-2. However, bed positioning, like any treatment, must be adapted to meet the individual needs of the patient. Care must be taken to protect the weak upper extremity when the patient is upright because stretching of the shoulder joint capsule is most likely to occur early after stroke when the limb is flaccid (Andersen, 1985). Specific techniques for supporting the hemiparetic shoulder are discussed later in this chapter. Resting hand splints may be worn at night to prevent soft tissue shortening (Milazzo & Gillen, 1998), but their use must be frequently reassessed, as splints prevent sensory input, discourage active movement, and can lead to extensor tendon shortening.

Controlled and frequent movement of body parts is the preferred method to prevent contractures. When a

Case Example

MRS. H.: RIGHT CEREBROVASCULAR ACCIDENT

Patient Information

Mrs. H. is an 82-year-old widow who lived alone independent in ADL and IADL except for community transportation. She was found unresponsive at home by a neighbor and diagnosed with a large right middle cerebral artery infarction.

During her acute hospital stay, an occupational therapist evaluated Mrs. H. and reported inconsistent levels of awareness, no spontaneous movement on the left side, and signs of left hemianopsia and spatial neglect. Treatment consisted of involving the patient in simple self-care tasks and initiating a bed positioning and mobility program in conjunction with nursing and physical therapy to prevent secondary complications. Ten days post stroke, Mrs. H. was able to sit in a wheelchair for 1-hour periods, follow one-step commands consistently, and perform simple grooming and bed mobility tasks with minimal assistance. She was transferred to an inpatient rehabilitation unit for more intensive treatment.

Upon admission to the rehabilitation unit, Mrs. H. was incontinent of bowel and bladder and had a small area of skin breakdown over her coccyx. The speech–language pathologist reported swallowing difficulties and recommended a pureed diet with no thin liquids. Physical therapy described Mrs. H. as requiring maximum (75%) assistance to perform a scooting transfer and unable to sit unsupported or to stand. The therapeutic recreation specialist found that Mrs. H. had led a sedentary life and enjoyed going to church, visiting with neighbors and family, reading her Bible, and watching television. A psychologist reported her verbal comprehension and memory to be good, although Mrs. H. expressed frustration at her continued hospitalization and stated that she expected a full recovery and return home. The social worker reported that Mrs. H.'s family consisted of four adult grandchildren and their families, who were unable to change their work or living situations to care full time for Mrs. H. The family was supportive and hopeful that Mrs. H. could return home with a hired care provider, although they were willing to consider skilled nursing home placement if Mrs. H. did not gain sufficient functioning to return home.

Reasons for Referral to Occupational Therapy

Mrs. H. was referred to occupational therapy to address deficits in self-care, decreased awareness of left visual spatial field, and management of the left arm and to assist in determination of optimum discharge plans.

Occupational Therapy Problem List

► Requires maximum (75%) assistance for lower body dressing, toileting, and bathing because of poor sitting balance and mobility
► Requires minimal (25%) physical assistance with maximum verbal cueing to perform grooming, eating, and upper body dressing because of decreased attention to left visual space and left side of body
► Unable to perform simple IADL tasks or to engage in leisure activities
► At risk for injury or complications in left arm because of lack of voluntary movement, decreased sensation, and visual spatial neglect
► Limited insight into impairments and disabilities resulting from stroke and the predicted course of recovery

Occupational Therapy Goal List

Patient will be able to do the following:

► Perform feeding, grooming, upper body dressing with supervision and minimal cueing.
► Perform lower body dressing, toilet transfers, and bathing on a tub bench with moderate (50%) assistance.
► Maintain sitting balance on the side of bed for at least 2 minutes while engaged in upper body activity.
► Properly position left arm during change of position in bed and while seated in wheelchair.
► Independently operate television by remote control and tape recorder for books on tape.
► Independently perform stretching and range-of-motion activities for left hand, wrist, forearm and elbow. Perform stretching and range of motion activities for shoulder with moderate assistance.

Patient's family will be able to do the following:

► Demonstrate proper techniques for positioning
► Assist with self-care
► Assist with left arm mobility
► Encourage attention to left visual field

Treatment Plan and Discharge Status

The treatment program during Mrs. H.'s 2-week inpatient rehabilitation stay consisted of (1) an activity program emphasizing basic and instrumental ADL training to address sitting balance, transitional movements, management of left upper extremity, and attention to and scanning of the left visual field and (2) patient and family education regarding the consequences and course of recovery of stroke, safety awareness and prevention of secondary impairments, and compensatory techniques and adaptations to promote functional independence.

At discharge, Mrs. H. was able to feed herself, perform simple grooming activities, and use her television and tape recorder with setup and supervision. Status in all other ADL remained unchanged. Sitting balance remained poor, and left spatial neglect remained pronounced. Mrs. H. required maximum assistance with protection and mobilization of left arm. Mrs. H. was transferred to a skilled nursing facility, where she would continue occupational and physical therapy. Mrs. H.'s family attended family training sessions prior to discharge and was provided with written instructions of material covered in training.

Analysis of Reasoning

Mrs. H. had many deficits that predicted poor functional outcome and a long recovery period, so emphasis was placed on (1) improving basic capacities (balance, visual attention),

which would allow her to succeed in simple meaningful activities, rather than focusing on other deficits such as lack of voluntary movement in the left arm; (2) prevention of secondary complications; and (3) education to assist with continuity of care in a new setting and to allow the patient and family to feel they could contribute to the recovery process.

CLINICAL REASONING
in OT Practice

Role of Family and Caregiver in Continuing Therapeutic Goals

One of the problems interfering with Mrs. H.'s progress in inpatient rehabilitation was her left visual field deficit and unilateral neglect. How would this problem affect Mrs. H.'s awareness of and involvement in her new environment at a skilled nursing facility? How would this problem affect her performance of self-care tasks and valued leisure activities? How would the therapist explain this problem to the patient and family? What instruction could the therapist give family members so that they could help Mrs. H. learn to compensate for her visual perceptual deficits? What adaptations could they make in Mrs. H.'s environment?

BOX 38-2
PROCEDURES FOR PRACTICE

Recommended Bed Positioning for Patients With Hemiplegia

Supine Positioning
- Head and neck slightly flexed
- Trunk straight and aligned
- Involved upper extremity supported behind scapula and humerus with a small pillow or towel, shoulder protracted and slightly flexed and abducted with external rotation, elbow extended or slightly flexed, forearm neutral or supinated, wrist neutral with hand open
- Involved lower limb with hip forward on pillow, nothing against soles of feet

Lying on the Unaffected Side
- Head and neck neutral and symmetrical
- Trunk aligned

- Involved upper extremity protracted with arm forward on pillows, elbow extended or slightly flexed, forearm and wrist neutral, and hand open
- Involved lower extremity with hip and knee forward, flexed and supported on pillows

Lying on the Affected Side
- Head and neck neutral and symmetrical
- Trunk aligned
- Involved upper extremity protracted forward and externally rotated with elbow extended or slightly flexed, forearm supinated, wrist neutral, and hand open
- Involved lower extremity with knee flexed
- Uninvolved lower extremity with knee flexed and supported on pillows

Data from Carr & Kenney (1992)

---

patient cannot use the involved side to engage in meaningful activities, therapists should initiate supervised active or active-assistive movement activities. When active movement is not possible, therapists should

see that immobile body parts go through passive range of motion at least once daily. If performing passive range of motion on the involved arm, ensure proper scapulo-humeral rhythm by relaxing and mobilizing the scapula

Case Example

MR. G.: LEFT CEREBROVASCULAR ACCIDENT

Patient Information

Mr. G. is a 38-year-old man with a history of hypertension who had abrupt onset of right-sided weakness and loss of speech. Having been found to have had a left subarachnoid hemorrhage, he spent 9 days in acute care and 2 weeks on an inpatient rehabilitation unit before being discharged home to live with his wife and two children aged 10 and 12. During his hospitalization, Mr. G. made rapid progress and regained most of his speech and movement on the right side. Upon discharge, Mr. G. could perform self-care tasks, simple meal preparation, and household walking using a straight cane with supervision and increased amount of time. He had mild apraxia resulting in delays initiating and sequencing multistep tasks. He had decreased control of his right arm, particularly when he tried to raise it above shoulder level or attempted fine motor activities.

Reason for Referral to Occupational Therapy

Mr. G. was referred to outpatient occupational therapy to continue progress in ADL and IADL independence and to assist with resuming community roles. He also had outpatient physical therapy to work on improving balance and upgrading gait and speech therapy to improve word retrieval and higher-level reading and math skills. Mr. G.'s goals for occupational therapy were to function safely alone at home after his wife returned to work, to improve function of his right dominant arm, and to return to work as soon as possible. Mr. G. worked in the parts department of an automobile dealership. His job included inventory, ordering, stocking, and pickup and delivery of parts. His wife was a teacher who was home for the summer but planned to return to work when school started in 2 months. Initial outpatient assessment included the *Functional Test for the Hemiplegic/Paretic Upper Extremity* (Wilson, Baker, & Craddock, 1984; Wilson, D. J., Baker, L. L., & Craddock, J. A. [1984]. Protocol: Functional Test for the Hemiplegic/Paretic Upper Extremity. Unpublished manuscript. County Rehabilitation Center, Rancho Los Amigos, Occupational Therapy Department, Downey, CA) to determine level of functional use of his right arm (Fig. 38-3).

Occupational Therapy Problem List

▶ Requires supervision and extended time to complete bathing, grooming and dressing because he has dynamic balance concerns, delays in initiation, and poor coordination of right arm.

▶ Unable to perform activities involving right shoulder flexion or abduction above 90° or right-hand fine motor prehension or manipulation.

▶ Requires supervision and/or increased time to perform home IADL tasks (writing checks, preparing meals).

▶ Unable to perform tasks required for job, including using computer, lifting boxes up to 50 pounds, and driving.

▶ Unable to resume leisure activities, including bowling and coaching son's baseball team.

▶ Depressed, anxious over loss of independence and role functioning, financial uncertainties.

Occupational Therapy Goal List

▶ Perform morning self-care independently in 45 minutes or less

▶ Assume partial meal preparation and laundry tasks to help wife

▶ Use right arm to comb hair and to place and retrieve objects on shelf at eye level

▶ Use right hand to tie shoelaces, manipulate coins, sign name, and perform simple computer functions

▶ Participate in gross motor recreational activities with children (swimming, table tennis)

▶ Perform job simulation activities for 2 hours without rest break

▶ Complete predriving evaluation

▶ Be able to use community transportation independently

Treatment Plan

Mr. G. was seen twice a week for 2 months. Treatment consisted of the following: (1) Task-specific training in ADL, IADL, and job activities. Activities were adapted, graded, and added as Mr. G. gained competency. (2) Repetitive task-oriented program to improve motor planning, postural adaptation, and right arm strength and control. This program was designed to be carried over to home. (3) Education concerning safety issues, adaptations to home and activities, social supports, and available community resources.

All goals were achieved. Mr. G. continued to go to the outpatient clinic for monthly follow-up visits after his wife returned to work. He was referred for behind-the-wheel driving assessment and training. He initiated application procedures for his state's vocational rehabilitation financial aid and training services.

Analysis of Reasoning

Mr. G. had problems that seemed to respond best to familiar, meaningful, repetitive treatment activities. Treatment was designed to provide structure to substitute for his loss of employment, to allow him to resume alternative roles at home, and to allow him to explore the feasibility of returning to his previous job. Because Mr. G. showed potential for continued improvements beyond the period of insurance reimbursement, his therapist actively encouraged Mr. G. and his family to monitor and promote his recovery away from the clinical setting.

CLINICAL REASONING
in OT Practice

Use of ADL and IADL to Improve Component Impairments: Occupation-As-Means

Although he showed rapid recovery, Mr. G. was unable to resume occupational roles after returning home because of residual impairments. How would training in meal preparation and laundry activities help to lessen Mr. G.'s particular impairments? How could these activities be graded to increase active shoulder range of motion? Improve hand dexterity?

Upgrade balance requirements? What compensatory strategies could Mr. G. use to improve initiation and sequencing of kitchen and laundry tasks? What safety techniques should he employ? How could his therapist explain to Mr. G. the benefits of practicing job-related activities that were once easily performed but are now difficult?

---

before elevation of the arm and by manually assisting upward rotation of the scapula (Bobath, 1990). The humerus should be externally rotated during abduction to prevent impingement of the supraspinatus between the greater tubercle of the humerus and the acromion process (Caillet, 1981). Whenever possible, a patient should attend closely to passive movement as a first step in relearning motion (Carr & Shepherd, 1987). A study using positron emission tomography (PET) on early poststroke patients who had no active movement showed that passive elbow movements elicited some of the same brain activation patterns as active movement in more recovered patients (Nelles et al., 1999).

Fall Prevention

For patients hospitalized with stroke, falls are the most common cause of injury (Gresham et al., 1995). Factors that increase the risk of falls include advanced age, confusion, impulsive behavior, mobility deficits, poor balance or coordination, visual impairments, and communication deficits that interfere with a patient's ability to request assistance in a timely manner. Treatment that helps to prevent falls includes detecting and removing environmental hazards, optimizing motor control, recommending appropriate adaptive devices, and teaching safety measures to the patient and family.

Patient and Family Education

Early in recovery, support for patients who have had strokes and their families may best be provided in the form of education to promote a realistic understanding of the consequences of stroke and the purposes and methods of various treatments (Gresham et al., 1995). A study of patients hospitalized with acute stroke found that fewer than half knew that stroke was caused by a vascular injury to the brain (Wellwood et al., 1994). All aspects of occupational therapy assessment and treatment for survivors of stroke should be considered opportunities for education: to engage cooperation and participation in the identification of meaningful treatment goals, to highlight residual abilities as well as disabilities, and to promote carryover of treatment gains. Because the period after stroke is stressful, emotional, and tiring for both the patient and family, education sessions provided during the acute phase should be brief, simple, and reinforced as needed with repetition or appropriate learning aids (See Chapter 9).

Rehabilitation Phase

Part of discharge planning during the acute phase of stroke is screening for rehabilitation services. Rehabilitation choices depend on a patient's condition, the social support system, and the resources available in a community. To qualify for further treatment in a rehabilitation program, a patient must be medically stable, have at least one functional disability, have sufficient endurance to sit supported at least an hour, and be able to learn and to participate actively in therapy (Gresham et al., 1995). Patients who do not meet these criteria should continue to receive appropriate medical or support services at home, in a skilled nursing facility, or in a chronic care facility; they may be reassessed later for rehabilitation services. Patients who meet these criteria are referred for inpatient rehabilitation programs, for multidisciplinary rehabilitation services at a skilled nursing facility, or for treatment by one or more disciplines in home care or in an outpatient clinic.

During this phase of recovery, the patient and family are focused on getting better and are usually more concerned with recovering lost function than on adapting to a life of chronic disability (Sabari, 1998b). Successful occupational therapy intervention coordinates a patient's striving for restoration of function with the potential for compensation and alternative occupational roles.

Treatment to Improve Performance of Occupational Tasks

The occupational therapist's primary goal in stroke rehabilitation is to improve independence in daily living tasks, hence the patient's quality of life. **Patients with persistent, nonremediable functional deficits should be taught compensatory methods for performing important tasks and activities, using the affected limb when possible and when not, the unaffected limb.** Many consider that early ADL training focusing on compensatory techniques results in faster success and is therefore more cost-effective and more satisfying to the patient, who again feels competent (Nakayama et al., 1994). Others contend that when ADL training focuses entirely on one-handed techniques, the patient fails to relearn bilateral movements and instead develops unilateral habits (Bobath, 1990; Carr & Shepherd, 1987; Taub et al., 1993). Skilled occupational therapy intervention combines both compensatory and remedial treatment strategies and attempts to reduce both disabilities and impairments by engaging the patient in meaningful activities. Putting on a front-buttoning shirt, for example, besides helping a patient gain independence in the task of dressing, addresses the following component abilities, capacities, and conditions:

► Joint and soft tissue integrity (self-stretching or relaxation techniques for involved arm in preparation for dressing, positioning of arm on a surface to prevent stretching of weak shoulder structures)
► Voluntary movement and function of involved upper extremity (abducting shoulder to put on a sleeve, extending elbow to push the hand through the sleeve, pinching one side of the shirt to stabilize while buttoning)
► Somatosensory perception (the texture of the shirt, the position of the affected arm)
► Postural adaptations (anterior pelvic tilt, trunk rotation, weight shifting)
► Visual–perceptual skills (finding the shirt in the visual field, distinguishing top from bottom, finding the sleeve opening)
► Cognitive skills and emotional reactions (sequencing, attention span, frustration tolerance, motivation)

ADL training with stroke patients begins with simple tasks and gradually increases in difficulty as a patient gains competency (Gresham et al., 1995). Several studies discerned a hierarchy of achievement of self-care skills. Results of one study showed that 31% of stroke survivors needed help with dressing and 49% required assistance with bathing 6 months post stroke (Wade & Langton Hewer, 1987). Aspects of dressing that are particularly difficult for stroke patients are putting a sock and shoe on the affected foot, lacing shoes, and pulling up trousers or pants (Walker & Lincoln, 1990). A study that investigated the relationship between dressing abilities and cognitive, perceptual, and physical deficits found that in general, lower extremity dressing correlates more with motor performance and upper extremity dressing correlates more with cognitive or perceptual performance (Walker & Lincoln, 1991). **Adaptive devices should be used only if other methods of performing the task are not available or cannot be learned. The device should have proven reliability and safety, and the patient and/or caregiver should be thoroughly trained in its proper use.**

As the patient progresses, occupational performance tasks other than basic self-care may have to be addressed. Homemaking and home management skills are practiced with patients who have sufficient motor, cognitive, and perceptual abilities to enable success and safety in these tasks (Trombly, 1989). Avocational interests, including adapted methods of continuing familiar hobbies, is an important area of treatment. Many stroke survivors are faced with increases in leisure time because of inability to go back to work; however, a reduction in social and leisure activities has been found to be a common sequel to stroke (Jongbloed & Morgan, 1991). Chapter 30 discusses specific techniques for regaining independence in ADL for those with loss of the use of one side of the body.

Treatment to Improve Component Abilities and Capacities

Performance component goals are based on the impairments associated with an individual's stroke (Sabari, 1998a) and are directly linked to occupational performance goals. The goals and modalities used to address these component deficits must be purposeful and meaningful from the patient's point of view (Trombly, 1995a). Thus, a floor game may be used to improve sitting balance needed to don socks, or resistive grasp activities may be taught to strengthen muscles needed to squeeze a tube of toothpaste. Treatments for stroke deficits are described individually in the following sections, but most patients in rehabilitation programs have multiple interacting problems necessitating efficient, integrated treatment plans that address several deficit areas at once (Warren, 1991).

Postural Adaptation

The ability to make automatic postural adjustments, including trunk control and the maintenance of balance, is a prerequisite for successful performance of occupational tasks. Part of the occupational therapist's role in training a patient in ADL independence post stroke is in teaching the patient the safest, most effective and efficient "ready" position for engaging in activities (Table 38-2) and strategies for adapting to changes in body position. Various techniques can be used to accomplish these goals as long as the therapist has a clear understanding of each patient's particular strengths and weaknesses regarding stability and mobility. Treatment to improve postural control for the performance of daily living activities is aimed at reestablishing the prerequisites for mature postural adaptation, including these abilities (Warren, 1990):

1. To produce full range of movement in the trunk and extremities
2. To differentiate body parts from one another, such as rotating the shoulders independently of the hips
3. To stop and hold movement at midrange to stabilize against gravity
4. To increase and decrease postural tone in body segments automatically and appropriately to support movement and/or stability
5. To move both sides of the body symmetrically

The incorporation of transitional movement patterns (i.e., strategies to change body positions, such as from supine to side-lying or seated to standing) and the use of strategically placed activities allow patients to practice effective postural adjustment while focusing on the task at hand (Warren, 1990).

Upper Extremity Function

Bilateral use of the upper extremities is crucial to efficient and effective occupational performance. Patients recovering from stroke usually place a high priority on regaining function in the involved arm. The occupational therapist must determine which deficits most affect a patient's upper extremity performance and plan realistic multilevel, task-oriented treatment to restore function or promote adaptation to the loss of function.

Somatosensory Deficits. Treatment for sensory dysfunction of stroke patients has not been systematically developed, although therapists attempt remediation as well as compensation for these deficits (Trombly, 1989). Remedial treatment entails a sequence of presentation of a tactile stimulus, response by the patient, exact feedback, and practice (Weinberg et al., 1979). Compensatory treatment entails substituting intact senses for those lost or dysfunctional. Therapists must determine the appropriateness of either type of treatment for individual patients. For example, sensory retraining is unrealistic for patients with minimal voluntary movement, visual field neglect, or poor cognitive skills.

Yekutiel and Guttman (1993) conducted a controlled trial in which 20 hemiplegic patients 2 or more years post stroke received systematic sensory training for the hemiplegic hand for 6 weeks. Their sensory reeducation program included exploring with each patient the nature and extent of sensory loss, selecting sensory tasks of interest to the patient that promoted learning, and encouraging constant use of vision and the uninvolved hand to teach tactics of perception. At the end of the training period, the treatment group showed significant gains in all sensory tests after training as compared to before, whereas the control group showed no changes.

Treatment to restore tactile awareness and teach compensation for sensory loss is discussed in Chapter 27. Therapists should provide patients with repetitive stimulation of high enough intensity to be appreciated but should avoid aversive stimuli to prevent withdrawal or increased spasticity (Dannenbaum & Dykes, 1988; Eggers, 1984). One method of providing stimulation is to encourage the patient to use the involved hand in ADL as soon as possible. The use of different textures (e.g., foam, terry cloth, Velcro) on weight-bearing surfaces or on the holding surfaces of commonly used utensils such as cups, forks, and pens can increase sensory input to the affected hand.

Mechanical and Physiological Components of Movement. Techniques for maintaining soft tissue length and avoiding pain in the involved upper extremity initiated during the acute phase of stroke recovery should be continued and adapted in response to changes in the patient's movement or muscle tone. As the patient in a rehabilitation program gains in mobility, measures should be taken to protect weak upper extremity structures from stretching or injury due to the effects of gravity and improper movement. Box 38-3 summarizes handling techniques for an affected upper extremity.

Treatment of problems related to the hemiplegic shoulder centers on prevention and management of symptoms and underlying causes. The use of a sling as a

BOX 38-3
PROCEDURES FOR PRACTICE

Proper Handling of the Hemiparetic Upper Extremity

- Teach the patient as early as possible to be responsible for the positioning of the arm during transfers, bed mobility, and other activities involving change of position.
- Use gait belts or draw sheets, rather than the affected arm, to assist the patient in moving his or her body.
- Avoid shoulder range of motion beyond 90° of flexion and abduction unless there is upward rotation of the scapula and external rotation of the humerus (Gresham et al., 1995).
- Avoid overhead pulley exercises, as they appear to increase the frequency of pain in the shoulder because neither scapular nor humeral rotation occurs, and the force may be excessive (Kumar et al., 1990).

prevention or treatment for subluxation of the hemiplegic shoulder is controversial (Andersen, 1985; Gresham et al., 1995) because of questions of effectiveness and the potential for secondary complications. Reasons for using slings are to reduce the subluxation of the glenohumeral joint, provide support for the arm, protect against trauma, and prevent or reduce pain. Carr and Shepherd (1987) found that radiographs of hemiplegic shoulders in slings revealed no significant reduction of subluxation. Gillen (1998b) reports that no available sling can correct malalignment of the scapula on the ribcage, and Bobath (1990) maintained that flexor spasticity in the upper extremity is reinforced with the use of a sling. Pain control is a valid reason for use of a positioning device; however, the relation between subluxation and shoulder pain is unclear. Several studies have found no association between shoulder pain and subluxation after stroke (Arsenault et al., 1991; Bohannon & Andrews, 1990), including one that found a low correlation between shoulder pain after stroke and subluxation, age, or arm motor function but a high correlation between shoulder pain and limited passive shoulder external rotation (Zorowitz et al., 1996). These studies support a general recommendation that shoulder supports not be issued uniformly to all patients with shoulder subluxation. If considering a sling, therapists should address the following questions (Andersen, 1985; Ridgway & Byrne, 1999). A positive response to these questions might indicate a sling:

- Does pain or edema increase when the arm hangs down?
- Is the patient's balance during standing, walking, or transfers improved by the use of a sling?

- Does the patient demonstrate an inability to attend to and protect the arm during movement?
- Will the patient or caretaker be able to independently put on and take off a sling correctly?

A positive response to the following questions might contraindicate a sling:

- Would the sling prevent or hinder active movement or function in the arm?
- Would a sufficiently supportive sling impair circulation or cause excessive pressure on the neck?
- Would the sling put the patient at risk for contracture as a result of immobilization?
- Would a sling decrease sensory input and promote unilateral disregard?

Alternative positioning methods and devices for shoulder support include taping of the shoulder and scapula (Ridgway & Byrne, 1999), wheelchair lapboards and armrest troughs, use of a table while seated or standing, putting the hand in a pocket or under a belt, or using an over-the-shoulder bag while standing (Gillen, 1998b) (Fig. 38-4). Functional electrical stimulation has been used to prevent or improve shoulder subluxation. Studies evaluating the effectiveness of this treatment showed benefits during treatment but reduction of gains after treatment was discontinued (Linn et al., 1999). Any patient with shoulder pain that persists and consistently interferes with function or progress in therapy should be referred to specialists best qualified to diagnose and treat specific shoulder problems.

Along with protection, patients learning to manage their involved arm should know techniques of active, active-assistive, or passive movement designed to maintain range of motion, stretch tight tissues, or relax hypertonicity. The combination of positioning for comfort and muscle imbalances brought on by spasticity and weakness can lead to the development of stereotyped nonfunctional positioning for the hemiplegic upper extremity with shoulder retraction, adduction and internal rotation, elbow flexion, forearm pronation, and wrist and finger flexion. Therapists should emphasize frequent changes of position to prevent contractures and pain.

Even in the absence of motor recovery, normal movement is an important model for movement reeducation (Van Dyck, 1999). The patient needs to concentrate on relearning movement by feeling and thinking about the movement (Trombly, 1989). Methods of teaching self–range-of-motion entail bilateral activities such as having the patient clasp his or her hands while leaning forward to reach for the floor or pushing both hands forward with arms supported on a table (Eggers, 1984). Advantages of these activities are that they can easily be given a functional context, such as picking up objects off the floor or dusting a table, and the patient can monitor his or her own pain threshold and is therefore not apprehensive about movement of the arm (Andersen, 1985). Nelson et al. (1996) found in a study of persons with hemiplegia that using a simple dice game to achieve bilaterally assisted forearm supination brought better results (more range of motion, more repetitions) than use of a rote exercise routine. Self-management of range of motion should be closely supervised and may not be appropriate for patients who have decreased awareness of the involved side, who move too quickly, who do not respect pain, or who lack a mobile scapula.

Hand edema is a frequent complication of hemiplegia. Edema control techniques include elevation of the hand, massage, and use of pressure gloves (Daniel & Strickland, 1992). Patients with minimal voluntary movement should avoid allowing the hand and arm to hang down for long periods. Prolonged hand edema can lead to limited passive movement, pain, and soft tissue contractures. Hand edema and pain combined with trophic changes are early signs of shoulder–hand syndrome and should be addressed vigorously to prevent further loss of functional potential (Trombly, 1989) (see Chapter 42).

Voluntary Movement and Function. Chapters 21 to 26 describe various treatment approaches to promote motor abilities and capacities in the patient recovering from stroke. Therapists usually employ a variety of techniques rather than a single one in response to the complex multiple factors that interfere with upper extremity use in an

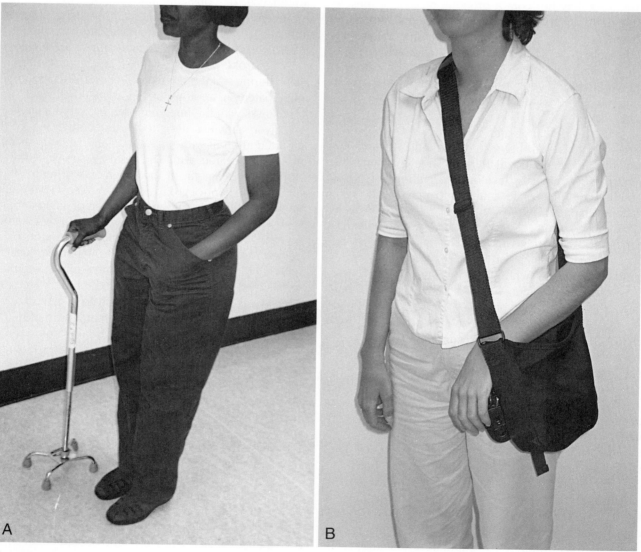

Figure 38-4 Alternative methods for supporting the hemiplegic arm while standing. **A.** Hand in pocket. **B.** Use of shoulder bag.

individual patient. Patients who have functional deficits and at least some voluntary control over movements of the involved arm or leg should be encouraged to use the limb in functional tasks and offered exercise and functional training directed at improving strength and motor control, relearning sensorimotor relationships, and improving functional performance.

Success in restoring voluntary movement in the hemiplegic upper extremity has been limited, perhaps because knowledge about the nature and components of movement deficits after stroke is limited (Basmajian, 1989; Trombly, 1992). Spasticity, for example, has traditionally been described as a major barrier to normal movement and function in the patient with hemiplegia (Bobath, 1990). However, clinical studies (Bourbonnais & Vanden Noven, 1989; Fellows & Thilmann, 1994) suggest that movement deficits in hemiparetic upper extremities may be more a problem of agonist muscle weakness than antagonist muscle spasticity. Voluntary movement deficits in the patient with hemiplegia include problems of muscle force production and control, of abnormal muscle activation and inhibition patterns, and of synergistic organization. In short, the patient finds it difficult or impossible to use available movement in an adaptive way.

In light of the range and complexity of possible motor impairments and the myriad of treatment strategies available, the occupational therapist should design treatment to fit the patient's level and to guide and extend combinations of muscle action into meaningful tasks (Carr & Shepherd, 1987). As Mathiowetz and Haugen (1994, p. 736) wrote, "Recovery from brain damage is a process of discovering what remains to perform tasks." In analyzing reaching performance, Wu et al. (1998) found that persons with stroke produced movements that were less efficient, less direct, less smooth, and slower than movements produced by neurologically intact subjects. This and a subsequent study (Trombly & Wu, 1999) also suggest that providing a meaningful object within a functional context during treatment (e.g., reaching for food on a plate) leads to improved performance over exercise or reaching for a neutral target.

Therapists should review the wide range of possible functions of the upper extremity to select activities patients can succeed in. In normal function, the hand performs as a prehensile tool, and the arm places the hand in a wide variety of different and precise positions (Savinelli et al., 1978). Bard et al. (1964) proposed a classification of function of the upper extremity, including (1) nonmanipulatory activities, (2) prehension and manipulation, and (3) skilled individual finger movements, such as typing. Nonmanipulatory activities, such as weighting down a checkbook while writing, can be incorporated into functional activities by patients who have limited movement or no voluntary hand movement.

It is important to promote functional use of the involved upper extremity early and consistently, because patients tend to have difficulty translating limited upper extremity movement into functional use. They often report that their arm is "dead" or "useless" despite sufficient arm movement for simple activities. Movement may return spontaneously, but it appears that function or purposeful use of the arm is enhanced with therapeutic intervention and practice (Blanton & Wolf, 1999). Based on studies involving both animal and human subjects, Taub et al. (1993) described a phenomenon of **learned nonuse**: the person with hemiparesis notices negative consequences of efforts to use the affected limb, reinforced by successful compensatory use of the unaffected limb (Blanton & Wolf, 1999). The intervention called forced use, or constraint-induced movement therapy, has been described to counteract the effects of learned nonuse. In a comparative clinical study, Taub et al. (1993) restrained the unaffected upper extremities of chronic stroke patients (at least 1 year post onset) in slings during waking hours for 2 weeks. This group also participated in sessions of intensive practice of functional tasks with the impaired arm. A comparison group was given activities designed to encourage use of the impaired arm but without practice and without restraint of the unimpaired arm. The restraint subjects showed greater improvement on measurements of motor function than the control group and showed carryover of this function to life tasks and maintenance of gains during a 2-year follow-up period. A single-subject study (Blanton & Wolf, 1999) looked at the same intervention in an individual who was only 4 months after stroke, using a mitt rather than a sling to constrain the uninvolved hand for the patient's safety. Supervised practice sessions focused on everyday use of the involved hand and return to preferred ADL. After a 2-week treatment period, this patient's motor abilities, including quality and quantity of use, improved in the involved arm. Patients included in these and related studies had to meet minimal voluntary movement requirements including the ability to initiate 20° or more of wrist extension and 10° or more of finger extension. Based on these criteria, it is estimated that approximately 20–25% of patients with chronic stroke may benefit from this treatment (Blanton & Wolf, 1999).

Strength, endurance, and coordination can be graded in functional tasks to increase the motor performance of the involved upper extremity. Carefully selected resistive activities have been shown to improve both manual muscle test scores and occupational performance (Flinn, 1995). More studies are needed to determine the effectiveness of specific clinical strengthening methods in rehabilitating stroke patients. Because decreased physical and mental endurance can limit participation and performance in therapy, treatment should be carefully graded to compensate for and improve reduced endurance. Length of treatment sessions, energy requirements, and need for rest periods should be monitored to meet patients' needs.

Coordinated movement is the product of successful control of the strength, range, speed, direction, and timing of movement. Because almost all purposeful activity requires coordination, encouraging use of the affected extremities in self-care tasks or leisure activities is an appropriate way to improve coordination. Treatment should progress from unilateral activities, in which the patient can concentrate fully on control of the hemiparetic arm, to bilateral simultaneous activities, in which both arms perform the same movement together (such as lifting and carrying a box and catching and throwing a large ball), to bilateral alternating activities, in which the two arms perform different movements at the same time (such as sorting and assembling nuts and bolts). Grading fine motor activities entails progressing from gross to precise manipulation tasks and attempting more difficult patterns of grasp and pinch. Because hand and arm control for patients with hemiplegia becomes more difficult as the arm moves away from the body, the placement of activities should be varied. Writing is a highly coordinated task that is frequently a goal for stroke patients who need at least to be able to sign documents. Training in writing may be necessary if a patient plans to use the hemiparetic hand or the uninvolved nondominant hand.

Motor Learning Ability

Because occupational therapists mainly teach skills, they must address the learning process to help patients improve performance in daily living skills. Learning to dress, for example, entails performing the task effectively and efficiently in a variety of circumstances or contexts (Carr & Shepherd, 1987). In this approach, therapists can best assist patients with stroke by imparting problem-solving techniques and by helping them develop their own effective movement strategies to deal with objects and structures in their environment (Sabari, 1998a).

Visual Dysfunction. Chapter 28 describes treatment for patients with visual deficits. In general, therapists can employ either of two basic approaches for patients with visual problems following stroke, determined by the extent of visual impairment and a patient's intact capabilities (Warren, 1999). With an active approach, the goal of therapy is to improve a patient's visual perceptual processing, either by improving component skills, such as visual scanning ability, or by training in

compensatory skills, such as turning the head to the left. With a passive approach, treatment emphasis is on altering the patient's environment to improve occupational performance, such as positioning all food in the right visual field before a meal.

There is no research to support the effectiveness of visual training procedures used with patients following stroke (Herman, 1992; Neistadt, 1990; Warren, 1993). Results of one study (Weinberg et al., 1977), however, suggest that visual–perceptual deficits following stroke must be confronted and patients taught for treatment to be effective. Sharing results of objective evaluations with the patient and family, giving feedback on the effects of visual deficits on functional performance, and teaching patients to recognize and correct errors in performance have been suggested as techniques for increasing a patient's awareness of his or her deficits (Warren, 1993).

Studies have shown that visual training skills do not necessarily generalize to daily living tasks (Neistadt, 1990; Wagenaar et al., 1992). To ensure transfer of training, Toglia (1991) recommended a multicontext approach of practicing strategies in multiple environments with varied tasks and component demands. Therapists, for example, can provide a stronger learning event by reinforcing a visual searching task (finding all the forks in a dishwasher bin) with touching and moving the targets (picking up the forks and putting them in the correct space in a drawer). Training must be specific to the individual's deficits and goals for occupational functioning. A patient with hemianopsia and unilateral visual neglect who is unsafe with wheelchair propulsion and is not interested in reading or writing as a leisure activity will benefit more from specific environmental scanning activities in a wheelchair (obstacle courses, grocery shopping) than from paper-and-pencil or computer activities.

Speech and Language Disorders. Occupational therapists should work closely with speech–language pathologists to contribute to a patient's improvement in speech and language functioning. Therapists can promote proper posture as an assist to respiration and eye contact important to speech. Therapy sessions also provide a social context supportive of communication (Sarno, 1994). Whenever possible, therapists should incorporate speech and language goals into their treatment sessions, such as requiring verbal responses (counting repetitions of an activity or naming objects used) or addressing functional reading and writing tasks (reading signs and recipes, writing checks). Occupational therapists can assist in selecting and adapting a nonverbal form of communication for a patient, such as writing, drawing, use of a communication board, and gestures. Suggestions for working with patients with aphasia and their families include the following (American Heart Association, 1994; Rubio, 1998):

► Avoid unnecessary noise: turn off television, find a quiet space.

► Do not speak to the patient or request speech when he or she is engaged in a physical activity.

► Allow enough time for the patient to respond; do not rush or force communication; do not switch topics quickly.

► Never assume that the person with aphasia can't understand what's being said; never allow others to ignore the person with aphasia.

► Speak slowly and clearly using simple, concise language; do not speak loudly unless hearing is impaired; do not talk down as if to a child.

► Use demonstration, visual cues, and gestures as needed to help with comprehension.

Motor Planning Deficits. Motor planning deficits are serious learning disorders, among the most difficult to rehabilitate (Duncan & Badke, 1987). Because of the complexity of this impairment, the emphasis of treatment is on teaching compensatory skills rather than on remediation (Warren, 1991), with goals of competent performance of desired habitual or novel activities (Gresham et al., 1995). Suggestions for treatment include manually guided movement, repetitive graded use of objects and contexts to evoke more automatic responses, explaining clearly the components of a task, **backward chaining**, and practicing activities as closely as possible to the patient's usual context or routine (Gresham et al., 1995). Language can facilitate movement planning; it assists in the sequencing of actions required for a task, helps focus concentration and identify mistakes, and reduces perseveration (Warren, 1991). Therapists can have patients verbalize step by step what they have done and are going to do, for example, "I have taken the cap off the toothpaste. Now I will pick up my toothbrush and put toothpaste on it."

Cognitive Deficits. Treatment to optimize cognitive abilities is discussed in Chapter 29. As in other areas of dysfunction, treatment for cognitive problems after stroke can include retraining of specific component skills, teaching compensation techniques or substitution of intact abilities, and/or adaptation of the environment (Gresham et al., 1995). Examples include using prompts or cues to shape desired behavior; providing feedback on performance with suggestions and strategies for improvement; providing visual aids, such as memory logs, checklists, maps, or diagrams for memory; sequencing for organization deficits; simplifying; grading environment and tasks

for patients with attention deficits; and family education and supervision for safety.

Psychosocial Adjustment. Patients and families usually need assistance in making healthy emotional adjustments after stroke. It may be unreasonable to expect compliance to treatment instructions when patients and their families are coping poorly with the losses associated with stroke (Evans et al., 1992). Patients typically employ hope and determination to cope with hospitalization, the hard work of rehabilitation, and changes in body image, but many cling to the belief that they will be "normal" again (Sabari, 1998b). Therapists should reinforce the efforts of the rehabilitation team and encourage patients and families to talk about their reactions to stroke and their comprehension of its progression and prognosis (Daniel & Strickland, 1992). Especially in light of the shortening time frames for rehabilitation, therapists should make sure patients and families understand that recovery from stroke does not end with discharge from a hospital or rehabilitation program. Therapists should also help patients and families to realize that the ultimate goal of rehabilitation is not complete recovery from physical and intellectual impairments but the ability to resume valued life roles.

Therapists should recognize the signs and symptoms of depression and inform appropriate team members if treatment has not been initiated. For the patient with emotional lability, both patient and family need to be reassured that lability is a symptom of the stroke and that control will improve with time (Carr & Shepherd, 1987). The therapist can instruct the patient in techniques such as deep breathing or redirecting attention to help him modify his behavior (Carr & Shepherd, 1987). Group activities, social interactions, and community outings are important methods for allowing a patient to practice roles from before the stroke and realize that the patient role is a temporary transition to getting on with life in spite of residual impairments.

Transition to the Community

"For many stroke survivors and their families, the real work of recovery begins after formal rehabilitation. One of the most important tasks of a rehabilitation program is to help those involved to prepare for this stage of recovery" (Gresham et al., 1995, p. 143).

Discharge Planning

Discharge planning takes place throughout the rehabilitation phase. Successful planning allows the patient and family to feel comfortable with the decisions made for discharge, feel capable of maintaining gains and continuing progress without the intense level of support provided by rehabilitation specialists, and feel able to monitor for changes requiring adjustments or further intervention. Occupational therapists assist in identifying the most appropriate discharge setting; training the patient, family, and caregiver in essential skills; and arranging for continuity of care with community services (Gresham et al., 1995). Factors determining discharge setting include patient's and family's preferences, level of patient's disabilities, level of caregiver's support, and safety and accessibility of the home (Gresham et al., 1995). Often a patient with a fairly high level of physical functioning cannot return home because there is no caregiver or the residence is unsafe or inaccessible, whereas a more disabled patient can return home because a healthy spouse is willing to assume the role of caregiver and the residence is safe and accessible. Therapists perform a major role by participating with patients and families in home visits and safety assessments and recommending necessary home alterations or adaptive equipment.

Patient, Family, and Caregiver Education

Ideally, every treatment session is an opportunity to teach the patient, family, or caregiver techniques and problem-solving strategies for use after rehabilitation. While learning styles vary, patients and their families are best served by a combination of demonstration, experiential sessions, and written instructions. Repetition is important, and caregivers should demonstrate rather than simply verbalize ability to assist the patient safely and independently. At the time of discharge from a rehabilitation program, patients and their families are often overwhelmed with information from several disciplines that they must try to assimilate. After formal therapy sessions have ended, many patients and caregivers report good intentions of following home programs as prescribed but admit that the routine of daily activity leaves little time or energy for carrying out therapeutic recommendations at home. The most effective home programs therefore are those that incorporate treatment for component limitations into self-care and leisure routines (Van Dyck, 1999). An example: "Before bathing or dressing, briefly perform the following stretching movements to get the best posture and arm movement for these tasks." This is more likely to be complied with than "Perform the following exercises, 10 repetitions each, at least twice a day." Home programs should, of course, be individualized and should remind the patient of skills already mastered, of skills the patient can reasonably expect to gain, and of possible problems common to stroke. Patients and families should be well informed of sources for information or assistance as new capabili-

ties or problems evolve. Fall prevention is a necessary component of the home program and should encourage greater independence in mobility while identifying and reducing the risks of falls (Gresham et al., 1995).

Resuming Valued Roles and Tasks

While most individuals who have had stroke improve in basic functional abilities such as walking and self-care, most have limitations in physical and social role functioning (Duncan et al., 1997). Sabari (1998b) refers to the third phase of stroke recovery as that of reestablishing social roles and suggests that this is the critical phase in defining one's quality of life. Occupational therapists should facilitate this adaptive process by helping patients set and achieve reasonable goals for task performance so as to assume adapted or new roles.

Work

For patients who expect to resume working, prevocational or vocational evaluation and appropriate work readiness training should be encouraged (see Chapter 33). Black-Schaffer and Osberg (1990) undertook a study of 79 working-age stroke patients who underwent comprehensive inpatient rehabilitation with an emphasis on prevocational and vocational goals. The researchers found that 49% were able to return to full- or part-time competitive employment, homemaking, or full-time university studies. The study also revealed that a greater percentage of patients with aphasia were unable to return to work and that 58% of patients who returned to work acknowledged that their jobs required modifications. A later study of 200 patients following stroke with a mean age of 44 years found that 30% returned to employment (employment defined as earning at least minimum wage in full- or part-time work), 10% did volunteer work, 1% worked as homemakers, 9% were in sheltered work, and 46% were unemployed, including those in continuing therapy programs, school or training programs, and the retired (McMahon & Crown, 1998). This study found a higher (38%) rate of return to work for patients with aphasia but a lower rate for those with cognitive and perceptual deficits. The factors generally found to predict likelihood of returning to work included independence in self-care, young age, high educational and occupational levels, stable marital status, and high cognitive capacities (McMahon & Crown; Weisbroth et al., 1971).

Leisure and Recreation

Throughout rehabilitation, valued leisure activities should be identified, encouraged, and enabled. Effective therapy incorporates leisure interests into treatment so that the patient recovering from stroke can begin to analyze the effects of impairments on valued activities and anticipate strategies for return to these activities. A study of 40 individuals discharged from rehabilitation programs post stroke found that those with a large variety of interests were more likely to resume at least one leisure activity than those with limited leisure interests (Jongbloed & Morgan, 1991). Other factors influencing leisure participation include family and social support, transportation or financial barriers, attitudes toward altered leisure performance, and amount of free time available (Jongbloed & Morgan, 1991; Whyte & Supon, 1998). Many patients following stroke report decreased time and energy for leisure pursuits because of the increased demands of self-care. Many do not accept performance of a valued activity at a lower standard; for example, a patient with hemiparesis may give up golf rather than play at a reduced level of performance. Many patients, particularly those who were working at the time of their stroke, do not have established leisure roles or do not admit to any leisure interests. Methods to promote leisure and recreation after stroke include adaptations to a valued activity, including ways to overcome physical barriers in the home or community; introduction of new leisure activities suitable for a patient's abilities; and education and advocacy regarding available community resources (Gresham et al., 1995).

Sexuality

Surveys of patients and their spouses show that typical effects of stroke on sexuality include decreased libido, impaired erectile functioning in men, decreased vaginal lubrication in women, and decreased frequency of sexual activity (Korpelaineu et al., 1999). Causes may be physiological (decreased motor, sensory, or cognitive functioning; dependency in ADL; decreased endurance; incontinence; coexisting disease; or side effects of medications), or psychosocial (poor self-image, depression, role changes, impaired communication ability, fear of impotence, fear of recurring stroke) (Farman & Friedman, 1998; Gresham et al., 1995; Korpelaineu et al.).

To assist with sexual expression, all therapists can impart the message that patients are permitted to have concerns and seek information about sexual problems after stroke. Therapists should reassure their clients that these problems are common and that sexual activity after stroke is not contraindicated (Farman & Friedman, 1998; Gresham et al., 1995). Other possible interventions include providing or referring to resources to increase the patient's knowledge, encouraging open communication between partners, suggesting adaptations such as changes in positioning or timing, and referring to a qualified specialist (Farman & Friedman; Gresham et al.).

Driving

Because nearly all adults in the United States drive (Warren, 1999), the ability to resume driving is a high priority for most individuals with brain damage (Jones et al., 1983) and is seen as a way to continue community independence and avoid isolation (Gresham et al., 1995). Because of its complexity and danger, driving after stroke is usually not addressed until a patient has returned home and gained a satisfactory level of independence with self-care and short-distance mobility. It has been reported that only 30% of those who drove before stroke are able to resume driving (Fisk et al., 1997). Although it is not known with certainty which deficits necessitate the use of adaptive driving aids or render a stroke survivor unfit to drive (Lings & Jensen, 1991), perceptual and cognitive deficits are recognized as having a serious effect on driving safety (Korner-Bitensky et al., 1998). Hemiparesis alone does not appear to prevent a return to driving, because vehicles or techniques can be adapted to compensate for most motor deficits seen post stroke (Lings & Jensen). There are no standard evaluation procedures for determining the ability of cerebrally injured patients to return to driving, but consistent practices include (1) a predriving evaluation battery to test for visual scanning, visual attention, higher-level visual–cognitive skills, distractibility, mental slowness, problem solving, and ability to follow directions; (2) a driving simulator evaluation; and (3) a road test, both on a protected course and in traffic (Galski et al., 1997; Korner-Bitensky et al.).

Few studies have substantiated the effectiveness of rehabilitation to improve driving-related deficits (Klavora et al., 1995). Current practices include in-car driver retraining, driving simulator training, and attempts to remediate underlying impairments. Sivak et al. (1984) concluded that visual perceptual training may improve driving-related skills and driving performance. Klavora et al. found significant improvement in behind-the-wheel driving assessments in poststroke subjects who trained with Dynavision, an apparatus "designed to train visual scanning, peripheral visual awareness, visual attention, and visual-motor reaction time across a broad, active visual field" (Klavora et al., p. 535). Therapists must remember that the decision to allow a person who has had a stroke to resume driving rests with the state licensing bureau (Gresham et al., 1995) (see Chapter 31).

Community Support and Resources

Methods to reintegrate the patient into the community (e.g., transportation options, dealing with architectural barriers, assistance from family or friends, access to senior citizen centers) should be addressed throughout rehabilitation, because failure to resume premorbid social activities has been significantly correlated with isolation and depression in stroke patients (Feibel & Springer, 1982). Successful reintegration into the community, according to individuals who have had strokes, can take years rather than months (Buscherhof, 1998), continuing after a patient has regular contact with rehabilitation specialists. Acute-care hospitals and rehabilitation facilities should maintain up-to-date inventories of community resources; provide this information to stroke survivors, their families, and their caregivers; and offer assistance in obtaining needed services. In general, supports for patients and their families include educational, instrumental, and emotional supports (Gresham et al., 1995). Educational resources are available through organizations (see Resources) that offer direct audiotaped, videotaped, printed, and/or online information specific to stroke. Instrumental supports are physical assistance programs such as personal provider services, Meals on Wheels, and volunteer groups who can build wheelchair ramps. Emotional support can come from family, friends, mental health professionals, and other survivors of stroke.

Support for long-term caregivers is especially important, since caregivers appear to be at substantial risk for burnout, depression, isolation, and general health problems (Gresham et al., 1995; Han & Haley, 1999). Therapists can encourage and suggest sources for respite care, support groups, or counseling. Many communities, unfortunately, are limited in resources for the patient and family. Therapists can be advocates and consultants for the development of community programs; this can range from referring patients and families to others in the community living with stroke to organizing a stroke club to identifying opportunities for volunteer jobs for patients.

Post Discharge Monitoring

Because of the varying rates of recovery and adjustment after stroke and the trends toward earlier discharges from acute centers and rehabilitation programs, occupational therapists should facilitate provision of services along a smooth continuum. The stroke survivor's progress should be evaluated within 1 month after return to a community residence and at regular intervals during at least the first year, consistent with the person's condition and the preferences of the stroke survivor and family. The 12 months after stroke is considered a high-risk time crucial to the redevelopment of satisfactory life roles (Gresham et al., 1995; Sardin et al., 1994). Relatively little occupational therapy intervention occurs after the more acute stages of stroke recovery, perhaps because of patterns of reimbursement for services after stroke (Fraley, 1998). Radomski (1995) recommends greater emphasis on outpatient programming to enhance qual-

ity of life and health care effectiveness. Occupational performance and component abilities should be assessed during follow-up visits to determine whether a patient is maintaining the functional level achieved during rehabilitation or is progressing or regressing from this level. A period at home often provides patients the opportunity to experience and acknowledge their strengths and weaknesses and focuses their interest on improving specific skills needed to reintegrate into the home and community. Long-term survivors of stroke report the value of timely interventions over an extended period as they slowly regained confidence in a new self and resumed meaningful life roles (Buscherhof, 1998; Newborn, 1998).

Effectiveness of Treatment

In compiling the *Post-Stroke Rehabilitation Clinical Practice Guideline*, a panel of experts and consultants concluded after an extensive review of the literature that "few well-controlled clinical studies document benefits from rehabilitation" (Gresham et al., 1995, p.11). Difficulties in determining effectiveness of treatment for the stroke population include differentiating benefits of rehabilitation from spontaneous neurological recovery after stroke (Gresham et al.); the heterogeneous nature of the population of stroke survivors with their diverse causes and impairments; and the ethical and practical problems inherent in assigning patients to control groups.

Some studies have reported the effects of rehabilitation in general. Wagenaar and Meijer (1991a, b) suggest in an analysis of 165 studies of the effects of stroke rehabilitation that patients benefit from early intervention, that improvements in impairments did not automatically lead to improvements in ADL, and that there were no significant differences among various types of therapy used to remediate motor impairments. A quantitative review of studies (meta-analysis) on the effectiveness of rehabilitation therapy for stroke patients indicated that the average patient who received focused rehabilitation performed at a higher level than approximately 65.5% of patients in comparison or control conditions (Ottenbacher & Jannell, 1993). Although treatment effects were small, they were significantly practical in that small improvements in independent functioning can make the difference between discharge to home and institutionalization. Improvement in performance appears related to early initiation of rehabilitation treatment. Another meta-analysis looking at the effects of intensity of rehabilitation on disability and impairment (Kwakkel et al., 1997) found small but statistically significant improvements in ADL and neuromuscular outcomes associated with higher intensities of rehabilitation. This analysis reports greater gains in neuromuscular functioning than in ADL, supporting the assumption that neurological and functional recovery are not necessarily linked.

Duncan (1997) reviewed clinical trials and summarized evidence for interventions to improve motor control after stroke. The trials compared various therapeutic approaches, such as traditional biomechanical and rehabilitative therapy versus neurodevelopmental or proprioceptive neuromuscular facilitation treatment. Based on this review of research, remediation programs appear to improve motor control in patients with some initial voluntary movement. There were no statistically significant differences among treatment groups receiving various types of sensorimotor treatment as measured for motor or functional outcomes and no evidence that reduction of motor impairment carries over to functional performance.

Trombly and Ma conducted an evidence-based literature review of the effectiveness of occupational therapy interventions on stroke outcomes (Trombly, C.A., & Ma, H.-I. [1999]. *Evidence Based Literature Review on Occupational Therapy and Stroke*. Unpublished manuscript, American Occupational Therapy Association). They analyzed 25 studies completed between 1980 and 1998 that tested the results of a treatment specific to occupational therapy on patients recovering from stroke. This review of outcomes was organized according to the occupational functioning model (roles, tasks, activities, abilities, and capacities) (Trombly, 1995a). Twice as many studies looked at abilities and capacities as at roles, tasks or activities, although it has not been established that gains in component abilities carry over to functional tasks and activities (Wagenaar & Meijer, 1991a, b). This review summarizes evidence regarding the effectiveness of occupational therapy intervention for stroke patients as follows:

▶ There is insufficient evidence that occupational therapy intervention improves role participation or quality of life.

▶ Task-specific training appears to be effective in improving performance of those tasks.

▶ The use of meaningful objects motivates patients to participate longer in therapeutic activity and organizes and improves movement performance better than movement with simulated objects or no objects (exercise).

▶ Resisted hand exercise engages both agonist and antagonist muscle activity, while unresisted exercise localizes muscle activity to the prime mover only.

▶ The effect of occupational therapy on depression or psychological well-being after stroke is not established.

▶ Carefully planned treatment, including both paper-and-pencil activities and functional tasks appears to improve unilateral neglect and cognitive skills.

From these and other surveys of literature, it is clear that more research is essential to determine which treatments are effective for desired outcomes, which patients will most benefit from these services, and what are the best times and settings for treatment (Trombly, C.A., & Ma, H.-I. [1999]. *Evidence Based Literature Review on Occupational Therapy and Stroke*. Unpublished manuscript, American Occupational Therapy Association). Ideally, therapists will conduct randomized controlled trials to produce the strongest evidence in support of specific interventions. Other suggested methods to provide support for treatment include systematic documentation and accumulation of case reports (Trombly, 1995b; Wagenaar et al., 1992), goal attainment scaling in which successful goal achievement is behaviorally defined and rated along with careful description of treatments used, and recording and analysis of patient variables that could affect outcomes (Trombly, 1995b).

Summary Review Questions

1. Name the two main categories of stroke and the subtypes and causes of each.
2. Name six neurological deficits that can result from stroke and describe how each may interfere with dressing.
3. What is the difference between neurological recovery and functional recovery after stroke? How might occupational therapy facilitate both types of recovery in a patient?
4. Name five settings where occupational therapists work with patients recovering from stroke, and describe characteristics of a patient who might be treated in each setting.
5. Define postural adaptation and name three ways impairments in this area affect occupational performance. Describe treatment methods to improve postural control.
6. What mechanical and physiological components of movement should be evaluated in the hemiplegic upper extremity? What methods can be used to prevent development of a painful shoulder?
7. What variables should be considered during evaluation for voluntary movement in the hemiplegic upper extremity?
8. What factors can affect a stroke patient's ability to learn and organize movement? Describe how deficits in each of these areas affect self-care.

9. Select a treatment activity for a patient recovering from stroke and describe how this activity can both increase ADL independence (reduce disability) and improve component abilities and capacities (reduce impairment).

10. Describe methods to assist a poststroke patient resume self-enhancement and self-advancement roles after discharge from rehabilitation services.

Resources

National Stroke Association · 96 Inverness Drive East Suite 1, Englewood, CO 80112-5112. 303-649-9299. 800-STROKES (800-787-6537). www.stroke.org

American Stroke Association (division of American Heart Association) · 7272 Greenville Avenue, Dallas, TX 75231-4596. 888-4STROKE (888-478-7653).
www.strokeassociation.org
www.americanheart.org

Stroke Support Groups—listings of local stroke clubs from above web sites or organizations.

National Aphasia Association · P. O. Box 1887, Murray Hill Station, New York, NY 10156-0611. 800-922-4622.
www.aphasia.org

References

Ahlsio, B., Britton, M., Murray, V., & Theorell, T. (1984). Disablement and quality of life after stroke. *Stroke, 15,* 886–890.

American Heart Association. (1994). *Caring for the Person with Aphasia.* [Brochure]. Dallas, TX: Author.

American Occupational Therapy Assocoation. (1996). 1995 member survey data. Bethesda, MD: Author.

Andersen, L. T. (1985). Shoulder pain in hemiplegia. *American Journal of Occupational Therapy, 9,* 11–19.

Andrews, K., Brocklehurst, J. C., Richards, B., & Laycock, P. J. (1984). The influence of age on the clinical presentation and outcome of stroke. *International Rehabilitation Medicine, 6,* 49–53.

Angeleri, F., Angeleri, V. A., Foschi, N., Giaquinto, S., & Nolfe, G. (1993). The influence of depression, social activity, and family stress on functional outcome after stroke. *Stroke, 24,* 1478–1483.

Arsenault, A. B., Silodeau, M., Dutil, E., & Riley, E. (1991). Clinical significance of the V-shaped space in the subluxed shoulder of hemiplegics. *Stroke, 22,* 867–871.

Bach-y-Rita, P. (1981). Central nervous system lesions: Sprouting and unmasking in rehabilitation. *Archives of Physical Medicine and Rehabilitation, 62,* 413–417.

Bach-y-Rita, P., & Balliet, R. (1987). Recovery from stroke. In P. W. Duncan & M. B. Badke (Eds.), *Stroke Rehabilitation: The Recovery of Motor Control* (pp. 79–107). Chicago: Year Book.

Bard, G., Hirschberg, G. G., & Tolleson, G. C. B. (1964). Functional testing of the hemiplegic arm. *Journal of the American Physical Therapy Association, 44,* 1081–1086.

Bartels, M. N. (1998). Pathophysiology and medical management of stroke. In G. Gillen & A. Burkhardt (Eds.), *Stroke Rehabilitation: A Function-Based Approach* (pp. 1–30). St. Louis: Mosby.

Basmajian, J. (1989). The winter of our discontent: Breaking intolerable time locks for stroke survivors. *Archives of Physical Medicine and Rehabilitation, 70,* 92–94.

Berg, K., Wood-Dauphinee, S., Williams, J. I., & Gayton, D. (1989). Measuring balance in the elderly: Preliminary development of an instrument. *Physiotherapy Canada, 41,* 304–311.

Bergner, M., Bobbitt, R. A., Carter, W. B., Gilson, B. S. (1981). The sickness impact profile: Development and final revision of a health status measure. *Medical Care, 19,* 787–805.

Black-Schaffer, R. M., & Osberg, J. S. (1990). Return to work after stroke: Development of a predictive model. *Archives of Physical Medicine and Rehabilitation, 71,* 285–290.

Blanton, S., & Wolf, S. L. (1999). An application of upper-extremity constraint-induced movement therapy in a patient with subacute stroke. *Physical Therapy, 79,* 847–853.

Bobath, B. (1990). *Adult hemiplegia: Evaluation and treatment* (3rd ed.). London: Heinemann Medical.

Bogousslavsky, J., Van Melle, G., & Regli, F. (1988). The Lausanne stroke registry: Analysis of 1000 consecutive patients with first stroke. *Stroke, 19,* 1083–1092.

Bohannon, R. W. (1987). Relationship between static strength and various other measures in hemiparetic stroke patients. *International Rehabilitation Medicine, 8,* 125–128.

Bohannon, R. W., & Andrews, A. W. (1990). Shoulder subluxation and pain in stroke patients. *American Journal of Occupational Therapy, 44,* 506–509.

Bohannon, R. W., & Smith, M. B. (1987). Assessment of strength deficits in eight paretic upper extremity muscle groups of stroke patients with hemiplegia. *Physical Therapy, 67,* 522–525.

Bornstein, R. A. (1986). Normative data on intermanual differences on three tests of motor performance. *Journal of Clinical and Experimental Neuropsychology, 8,* 12–20.

Bourbonnais, D., & Vanden Noven, S. (1989). Weakness in patients with hemiparesis. *American Journal of Occupational Therapy, 43,* 313–319.

Brodal, A. (1973). Self-observations and neuroanatomical considerations after stroke. *Brain, 96,* 675–694.

Broderick, J., Brott, T., Kolhari, R., Miller, R., Khoury, J., Pancioli, A., Gebel, J., Mills, D., Minneci, L. & Shukla, R. (1998). The greater Cincinnati/Northern Kentucky stroke study. *Stroke, 29,* 415–421.

Brodie, J., Holm, M. B., & Tomlin, G. S. (1994). Cerebrovascular accident: Relationship of demographic, diagnostic and occupational therapy antecedents to rehabilitation outcomes. *American Journal of Occupational Therapy, 48,* 906–913.

Brott, T., Adams, H. P., Olinger, C. P., Marler, J. R., Barsan, W. G., Biller, J., Spilker, J., Holleran, R., Eberle, R., Hertzberg, V., Rorick, M., Moomaw, C. J., & Walker, M. (1989). Measurements of acute cerebral infarction: A clinical examination scale. *Stroke, 20,* 864–870.

Brown, R. D., Ransom, J., Hass, S., Petty, G. W., O'Fallon, W. M., Whisnant, J. P., Leibson, C. L. (1999). Use of nursing home after stroke and dependence on stroke severity. *Stroke, 30,* 924–929.

Brunnstrom, S. (1970). *Movement Therapy in Hemiplegia.* New York: Harper & Row.

Buscherhof, J. R. (1998). From abled to disabled: A life transition. *Topics in Stroke Rehabilitation, 5*(2), 19–29.

Byrne, D. P., & Ridgeway, E. M. (1998). Considering the whole body in treatment of the hemiplegic upper extremity. *Topics in Stroke Rehabilitation, 4*(4), 14–34.

Caillet, R. (1981). *The Shoulder in Hemiplegia.* Philadelphia: Davis.

Callahan, A. (1990). Sensibility testing: Clinical methods. In J. M. Hunter, L. H. Schneider, E. J. Mackin, & A. D. Callahan (Eds.), *Rehabilitation of the Hand: Surgery and Therapy* (3rd ed., pp. 594–610). St. Louis: Mosby.

Campbell, A., Brown, A., Scheldroth, C., Hastings, A., Ford-Booker, P., Lewis-Jack, O., Adams, C., Gadling, A., Ellis, R., Wood, D., Dennis, G., Adeshoye, A., Weir, R., & Coffey, G. (1991). The relationship between neuropsychological measures and self-care skills in patients with cerebrovascular lesions. *Journal of the National Medical Association, 83,* 321–324.

Caplan, L. R. (1998). Stroke treatment: Promising but still struggling. *Journal of the American Medical Association, 279,* 1304–1306.

Caplan, L. R., & Stein, R. W. (1986). *Stroke: A clinical approach.* Stoneham, MA: Butterworth.

Carr, E. K., & Kenney, F. D. (1992). Positioning of the stroke patient: A review of the literature. *International Journal of Nursing Studies, 29,* 355–369.

Carr, J. H., & Shepherd, R. B. (1987). *A Motor Relearning Programme for Stroke* (2nd ed.). Rockville, MD: Aspen.

Carr, J. H., Shepherd, R. B., Nordholm, L., & Lynne, D. (1985). Investigation of a new motor assessment scale for stroke patients. *Physical Therapy, 65,* 175–180.

Cherney, L. R. (1995). Management approaches for aphasia [Foreword, special issue]. *Topics in Stroke Rehabilitation, 2* (1), vi.

Chollet, M., DiPiero, V., Wise, R. J. S., Brooks, D. J., Dolan, R. J., & Frackowiak, R. S. J. (1991). The functional anatomy of motor recovery after stroke in humans: A study with positron emission tomography. *Annals of Neurology, 29,* 63–71.

Cifu, D. X., & Lorish, T. R. (1994). Stroke rehabilitation. 5. Stroke outcome. *Archives of Physical Medicine and Rehabilitation, 75,* S56–S60.

Collen, F. M., & Wade, D. T. (1991). Residual mobility problems after stroke. *International Disability Studies, 13,* 12–15.

Czyrny, J. J., Hamilton, B. B., & Gresham, G. E. (1990). Rehabilitation of the stroke patient. *Advances in Clinical Rehabilitation, 3,* 64–96.

Daniel, M. S., & Strickland, L. R. (1992). *Occupational Therapy Protocol Management in Adult Physical Dysfunction.* Rockville, MD: Aspen.

Dannenbaum, R. M., & Dykes, R. W. (1988). Sensory loss in the hand after sensory stroke: Therapeutic rationale. *Archives of Physical Medicine and Rehabilitation, 69,* 833–839.

Dellon, A. (1981). *Evaluation of Sensibility and Re-education of Sensation in the Hand.* Baltimore: Williams & Wilkins.

DeSouza, L. H., Langton Hewer, R. L., & Miller S. (1980). Assessment of recovery of arm control in hemiplegic stroke patients. I: Arm function tests. *International Rehabilitation Medicine, 2,* 3–9.

DeWeerdt, W. J. G., & Harrison, M. A. (1985). Measuring recovery of arm-hand function in stroke patients: A comparison of the Brunnstrom-Fugl-Meyer Test and the Action Research Arm Test. *Physiotherapy Canada, 37,* 65–70.

Duncan, P. W. (1997). Synthesis of intervention trials to improve motor recovery following stroke. *Topics in Stroke Rehabilitation, 3* (4), 1–20.

Duncan, P. W., & Badke, M. B. (1987). *Stroke Rehabilitation: The Recovery of Motor Control.* Chicago: Year Book.

Duncan, P. W., Samsa, G. P., Weinberger, M., Goldstein, L. B., Bonito, A., Witter, D. M., Enarson, C., & Matchar, D. (1997). Health status of individuals with mild stroke. *Stroke, 28,* 740–745.

Eggers, O. (1984). *Occupational Therapy in the Treatment of Adult Hemiplegia.* London: Heinemann Medical.

Evans, R. L., Hendricks, R. D., Haselkorn, J. K., Bishop, D. S., & Baldwin, D. (1992). The family's role in stroke rehabilitation. *American Journal of Physical Medicine and Rehabilitation, 71,* 135–139.

Farman, J., & Friedman, J. D. (1998). Sexual function and intimacy. In G. Gillen & A. Burkhardt (Eds.), *Stroke Rehabilitation: A Function-Based Approach* (pp. 423–436). St. Louis: Mosby.

Feibel, J. H., & Springer, C. J. (1982). Depression and failure to resume social activities after stroke. *Archives of Physical Medicine and Rehabilitation, 63,* 276–278.

Fellows, S. J., & Thilmann, A. F. (1994). Voluntary movement at the elbow in spastic hemiparesis. *Annals of Neurology, 36,* 397–407.

Ferrucci, L., Bandinelli, S., Guralnik, J. M., Lamponi, M., Bertini, C., Falchini, M., & Baroni, A. (1993). Recovery of functional status

after stroke: A post-rehabilitation follow-up study. *Stroke, 24,* 200–205.

Filiatrault, J., Arsenault, A. B., Dutil, E., & Bourbonnais, D. (1991). Motor function and activities of daily living assessments: A study of three tests for persons with hemiplegia. *American Journal of Occupational Therapy, 45,* 806–810.

Fisher, M., & Bogousslavsky, J. (1998). Further evolution toward effective therapy for acute ischemic stroke. *Journal of the American Medical Association, 279,* 1298–1303.

Fisk, F. D., Owsley, C., & Pulley, L. V. (1997). Driving after stroke: Driving exposure, advice and evaluations. *Archives of Physical Medicine and Rehabilitation, 78,* 1338–1345.

Flinn, N. (1995). A task-oriented approach to the treatment of a client with hemiplegia. *American Journal of Occupational Therapy, 49,* 560–569.

Folstein, M. F., Folstein, S. E., & McHugh, P. R. (1975). Mini-mental State: A practical method for grading the cognitive state of patients for the clinician. *Journal of Psychiatric Research, 12,* 189–198.

Foulkes, M. A., Wolf, P. A., Price, T. R., Mohr, J. P., & Hier, D. B. (1988). The stroke data bank: Design, methods, and baseline characteristics. *Stroke, 19,* 547–554.

Fraley, C. G. (1998). Psychosocial aspects of stroke rehabilitation. In G. Gillen & A. Burkhardt (Eds.), *Stroke Rehabilitation: A Function-Based Approach* (pp. 47–68). St. Louis: Mosby.

Fugl-Meyer, A. R., Jaasko, L., Leyman, I., Olsson, S., & Steglind, S. (1975). The post-stroke hemiplegic patient: I. A method for evaluation of physical performance. *Scandinavian Journal of Rehabilitation Medicine, 7,* 13–31.

Galski, T., Ehle, H. T., & Williams, J. B. (1997). Off-road driving evaluations for persons with cerebral injury: A factor analytic study of predriver and simulator testing. *American Journal of Occupational Therapy, 46,* 324–332.

Gillen, G. (1998a). Trunk control: A prerequisite for functional independence. In G. Gillen & A. Burkhardt (Eds.), *Stroke Rehabilitation: A Function-Based Approach* (pp. 69–89). St. Louis: Mosby.

Gillen, G. (1998b). Upper extremity function and management. In G. Gillen & A. Burkhardt (Eds.), *Stroke Rehabilitation: A Function-Based Approach* (pp. 109–151). St. Louis: Mosby.

Goodglass, H., & Kaplan, E. (1983). *The Assessment of Aphasia and Related Disorders* (2nd ed.). Philadelphia: Lea & Febiger.

Granger, C. V., Hamilton, B. B., & Fiedler, R. C. (1992). Discharge outcome after stroke rehabilitation. *Stroke, 23,* 978–982.

Gresham, G. E., Duncan, P. E., Stason, W. B., Adams, H. P., Adelman, A. M., Alexander, D. N., Bishop, D. S., Diller, L., Donaldson, N. E., Granger, C. V., Holland, A. L., Kelly-Hayes, M., McDowell, F. H., Myers, L., Phipps, M. A., Roth, E. J., Siebens, H. C., Tarvin, G. A., & Trombly, C. A. (1995). *Post-Stroke Rehabilitation. Clinical Practice Guideline 16.* (AHCPR Publication 95-0662). Rockville, MD: U. S. Agency for Health Care Policy and Research.

Gresham, G. E., Phillips., T. F., Wolf, P. A., McNamara, P. M., Kannel, W. B., & Dawber, T. R. (1979). Epidemiological profile of long-term stroke disability: The Framingham study. *Archives of Physical Medicine and Rehabilitation, 60,* 487–491.

Hall, J., Dudgeon, B., & Guthrie, M. (1995). Validity of clinical measures of shoulder subluxation in adults with poststroke hemiplegia. *American Journal of Occupational Therapy, 49,* 526–533.

Halligan, P. W., Marshall, J. C., & Wade D. T. (1989). Visuospatial neglect: Underlying factors and test sensitivity. *Lancet, 2* (8868), 908–911.

Han, B., & Haley, W. E. (1999). Family caregiving for patients with stroke: Review and analysis. *Stroke, 30,* 1478–1485.

Heilman, K., & Valenstein, E. (1979). Mechanisms underlying hemispatial neglect. *Annals of Neurology, 5,* 166–170.

Heller, A., Wade, D. T., Wood, V. A., Sunderland, A., Langton Hewer, R., & Ward, E. (1987). Arm function after stroke: Measurement and recovery over the first three months. *Journal of Neurology, Neurosurgery and Psychiatry, 50*, 714–719.

Herman, E. W. M. (1992). Spatial neglect: New issues and their implication for occupational therapy practice. *American Journal of Occupational Therapy, 46*, 207–216.

Holbrook, M., & Skilbeck, C. E. (1983). An activities index for use with stroke patients. *Age and Ageing, 12*, 166–170.

Jones, R., Giddens, H., & Croft, D. (1983). Assessment and training of brain-damaged drivers. *American Journal of Occupational Therapy, 37*, 754–760.

Jongbloed, L., & Morgan, D. (1991). An investigation of involvement in leisure activities after a stroke. *American Journal of Occupational Therapy, 45*, 420–427.

Jorgensen, H. S., Nakayama, H., Raaschou, H. O., Vive-Larsen, J., Stoier, M., & Olsen, T. S. (1995). Outcome and time course of recovery in stroke: Part I. Outcome. Copenhagen Stroke Study. *Archives of Physical Medicine and Rehabilitation, 76*, 399–405.

Katz, S., Ford, A. B., Moskowitz, R. W., Jackson, B. A., & Jaffe, M. W. (1963). Studies of illness in the aged. The index of ADL: A standardized measure of biological and psychosocial function. *Journal of the American Medical Association, 21*, 914–919.

Kaufman, S. R., & Becker, G. (1991). Content and boundaries of medicine in long-term care: Physicians talk about stroke. *Gerontologist, 31*, 238–245.

Keith, R. A., Granger, C. V., Hamilton, B. B., & Sherwin, F. S. (1987). The Functional Independence Measure: A new tool for rehabilitation. In M. G. Eisenberg & R. C. Grzesiak (Eds.), *Advances in Clinical Rehabilitation* (vol. 2, pp. 6–18). New York: Springer.

Kelly-Hayes, M., Robertson, J. T., Broderick, J. P., Duncan, P. W., Hershey, L. A., Roth, E. J., Thies, W. H., & Trombly, C. A. (1998). The American Heart Association Stroke Outcome Classification. *Stroke, 29*, 1274–1280.

Kiernan, R. J., Mueller, J., Langston, J. W., & Van Dyke, C. (1987). The Neurobehavioral Cognitive Status Examination: A brief but differentiated approach to cognitive assessment. *Annals of Internal Medicine, 107*, 481–485.

Klavora, P., Gaskovski, P., Martin, K., Forsyth, R. D., Heslegrave, R. J., Young, M., & Quinn, R. P. (1995). The effects of Dynavision rehabilitation on behind-the-wheel driving ability and selected psychomotor abilities of persons after stroke. *American Journal of Occupational Therapy, 49*, 534–542.

Korner-Bitensky, N. A., Safer, S., Gelinas, I., & Mazer, B. L. (1998). Evaluating driving potential in persons with stroke: A survey of occupational therapy practices. *American Journal of Occupational Therapy, 52*, 916–919.

Korpelaineu, J. T., Nieminen, P., & Myllyla, V. V. (1999). Sexual functioning among stroke patients and their spouses. *Stroke, 30*, 715–719.

Kumar, R., Metter, E. J., Mehta, A. J., & Chew, T. (1990). Shoulder pain in hemiplegia: The role of exercise. *American Journal of Physical Medicine and Rehabilitation, 69*, 205–208.

Kwakkel, G., Wagenaar, R. C., Koelmen, T. W., Lankhorst, G. J., & Koetsier, J. C. (1997). Effects of intensity of rehabilitation after stroke: A research synthesis. *Stroke, 28*, 1550–1556.

Labi, M. L., Phillips, C., & Gresham, G. E. (1980). Psychosocial disability in physically restored long-term stroke survivors. *Archives of Physical Medicine and Rehabilitation, 61*, 561–565.

Langton Hewer, R. (1990). Rehabilitation after stroke. *Quarterly Journal of Medicine, 76*, 659–674.

Lawton, M. P. (1988). Instrumental activities of daily living (IADL) scale: Original observer-rated version. *Psychopharmacology Bulletin, 24*, 785–787.

Lings, S., & Jensen, P. B. (1991). Driving after stroke: A controlled laboratory investigation. *International Disability Studies, 13*, 74–82.

Linn, S. L., Granat, M. H., & Lees, K. R. (1999). Prevention of subluxation after stroke with electrical stimulation. *Stroke, 30*, 963–968.

Lyle, R. C. (1981). A performance test for assessment of upper limb function in physical rehabilitation treatment and research. *International Journal of Rehabilitation Research, 4*, 483–492.

Mahoney, F. I., & Barthel, D. W. (1965). Functional evaluation: The Barthel Index. *Maryland State Medical Journal, 14*, 61–65.

McMahon, R., & Crown, D. S. (1998). Return to work factors following a stroke. *Topics in Stroke Rehabilitation, 5* (2), 54–60.

Mathiowetz, V., & Haugen, J. B. (1994). Motor behavior research: Implications for therapeutic approaches to central nervous system dysfunction. *American Journal of Occupational Therapy, 48*, 733–745.

Milazzo, S., & Gillen, G. (1998). Splinting applications. In G. Gillen & A. Burkhardt (Eds.), *Stroke Rehabilitation: A Function-Based Approach* (pp. 161–184). St. Louis: Mosby.

Moore, J. C. (1986). Recovery potentials following CNS lesions: A brief historical perspective in relation to modern research data on neuroplasticity. *American Journal of Occupational Therapy, 40*, 459–463.

Morris, J. (1998). The role of psychology in stroke rehabilitation. *Topics in Stroke Rehabilitation, 5* (2), 1–10.

Morris, P. L., Robinson, R. G., & Raphael, B. (1993). Emotional lability after stroke. *Australia and New Zealand Journal of Psychiatry, 27*, 601–605.

Nakayama, H., Jorgenson, H. S., Raaschou, H. O., & Olsen, T. (1994). Compensation in recovery of upper extremity function after stroke: The Copenhagen study. *Archives of Physical Medicine and Rehabilitation, 75*, 852–857.

National Stroke Association. (1994). *The Brain at Risk: Understanding and Preventing Stroke.* Englewood, CO: Author.

Neistadt, M. E. (1990). A critical analysis of occupational therapy approaches for perceptual deficits in adults with brain injury. *American Journal of Occupational Therapy, 44*, 299–304.

Nelles, G., Spiekermann, G., Jueptner, M., Leonhardt, G., Muller, S., Gerhard, H., & Diener, C. (1999). Reorganization of sensory and motor systems in hemiplegic stroke patients: A positron emission tomography study. *Stroke, 30*, 1510–1516.

Nelson, D. L., Konosky, K., Fleharty, K., Webb, R., Newer, K., Hazboun, V. P., Fontane, C., & Licht, B. C. (1996). The effects of an occupationally embedded exercise on bilaterally assisted supination in persons with hemiplegia. *American Journal of Occupational Therapy, 50*, 639–646.

Newborn, B. (1998). Quality of life for long-term recovery in stroke. *Topics in Stroke Rehabilitation, 5* (2), 61–63.

Okkema, K., & Culler, K. (1998). Functional evaluation of upper extremity use following stroke: A literature review. *Topics in Stroke Rehabilitation, 4* (4), 54–75.

Osmon, D. C., Smet, I. C., Winegarden, B., & Gandhavadi, B. (1992). Neurobehavioral cognitive status examination: Its use with unilateral stroke patients in a rehabilitation setting. *Archives of Physical Medicine and Rehabilitation, 73*, 414–418.

Ottenbacher, K. J., & Jannell, S. (1993). The results of clinical trials in stroke rehabilitation research. *Archives of Neurology, 50*, 37–44.

Parker, V. M., Wade, D. T., & Langton Hewer, R. (1986). Loss of arm function after stroke: Measurement, frequency & recovery. *International Rehabilitation Medicine, 8*, 69–83.

Radomski, M. V. (1995). There is more to life than putting on your pants. *American Journal of Occupational Therapy, 49*, 487–490.

Remer-Osborn, J. (1998). Psychological, behavioral, and environmental influences on post-stroke recovery. *Topics in Stroke Rehabilitation, 5* (2), 45–53.

Ridgway, E. M., & Byrne, D. P. (1999). To sling or not to sling? *OT Practice, 4* (1), 38–42.

Rolak, L. A., & Rokey, R. (1990). *Coronary and Cerebral Vascular Disease: A Practical Guide to Management of Patient With Atherosclerotic Vascular Disease of the Heart and Brain.* Mount Kisco, NY: Futura.

Roth, E. J. (1991). Medical complications encountered in stroke rehabilitation. *Physical Medicine Clinics of North America, 2,* 563–578.

Roth, E. J., & Harvey R. L. (1996). Rehabilitation of stroke syndromes. In R. L. Branddem (Ed.), *Physical Medicine and Rehabilitation* (pp. 1053–1087). Philadelphia: Saunders.

Rubio, K. B. (1998). Treatment of neurobehavioral deficits: A function-based approach. In G. Gillen & A. Burkhardt (Eds.), *Stroke Rehabilitation: A Function-Based Approach* (pp. 334–351). St. Louis: Mosby.

Ryerson, S., & Levit, K. (1997). The shoulder in hemiplegia. In R. Donatelli (Ed.), *Physical Therapy of the Shoulder* (3rd ed., pp. 205–228). New York: Churchill Livingstone.

Sabari, J. S. (1998a). Application of learning and environmental strategies to activity-based treatment. In G. Gillen & A. Burkhardt (Eds.), *Stroke Rehabilitation: A Function-Based Approach* (pp. 31–46). St. Louis: Mosby.

Sabari, J. S. (1998b). Occupational therapy after stroke: Are we providing the right services at the right time? *American Journal of Occupational Therapy, 52,* 299–302.

Sardin, K. J., Cifu, D. X., & Noll, S. F. (1994). Stroke rehabilitation: 4. Psychologic and social implications. *Archives of Physical Medicine and Rehabilitation, 75,* S-52–S-55.

Sarno, M. T. (1994). Neurogenic disorders of speech and language. In S. B. O'Sullivan & T. J. Schmitz (Eds.), *Physical Rehabilitation: Assessment and Treatment* (3rd ed., pp. 633–653). Philadelphia: Davis.

Savinelli, R., Timm, M., Montgomery, J., & Wilson, D. J. (1978). Therapy evaluation and management of patients with hemiplegia. *Clinical Orthopaedics and Related Research, 131,* 15–29.

Schoening, H. A., & Iversen, I. A. (1968). Numerical scoring of self-care status: A study of the Kenny Self-Care Evaluation. *Archives of Physical Medicine and Rehabilitation, 49,* 221–229.

Shinsha, N., & Ishigami, S. (1999). Rehabilitation approach to patients with unilateral spatial neglect. *Topics in Stroke Rehabilitation, 6* (1), 1–14.

Simon, R. P., Aminoff, M. J., & Greenberg, D. A. (1989). *Clinical Neurology.* Norwalk, CT: Appleton & Lange.

Sivak, M., Hill, C. S., Henson, D. L., Butler, M. S., Silber, S. M., & Olson, P. L. (1984). Improved driving performance following perceptual training in persons with brain damage. *Archives of Physical Medicine and Rehabilitation, 65,* 163–167.

Stern, R. A., & Bachman, D. L. (1991). Depressive symptoms following stroke. *American Journal of Psychiatry, 148,* 351–356.

Tangeman, P. T., Banaitis, D. A., & Williams, A. K. (1990). Rehabilitation of chronic stroke patients: Changes in functional performance. *Archives of Physical Medicine and Rehabilitation, 71,* 876–880.

Taub, E., Miller, N. E., Novack, T. A., Cook, E. W. III, Fleming, W. C., Nepomuceno, C. S., Connell, J. S., & Crago, J. E. (1993). Technique to improve chronic motor deficit after stroke. *Archives of Physical Medicine and Rehabilitation, 74,* 347–354.

Toglia, J. P. (1991). Generalization of treatment: A multicontext approach to cognitive perceptual impairment in adults with brain injury. *American Journal of Occupational Therapy, 45,* 505–516.

Trombly, C. A. (1989). Stroke. In C. A. Trombly (Ed.), *Occupational Therapy for Physical Dysfunction* (3rd ed., pp. 454–471). Baltimore: Williams & Wilkins.

Trombly, C. A. (1992). Deficits of reaching in subjects with left

hemiparesis: A pilot study. *American Journal of Occupational Therapy, 46,* 887–897.

Trombly, C. A. (1995a). Occupation: Purposefulness and meaningfulness as therapeutic mechanisms. *American Journal of Occupational Therapy, 49,* 960–972.

Trombly, C. A. (1995b). Clinical practice guidelines for post-stroke rehabilitation and occupational therapy practice. *American Journal of Occupational Therapy, 49,* 711–714.

Trombly, C. A., & Quintana, L. A. (1985). Differences in response to exercise by post-CVA and normal subjects. *Occupational Therapy Journal of Research, 5,* 39–58.

Trombly, C. A., & Wu, C.-Y. (1999). Effect of rehabilitation tasks on organization of movement after stroke. *American Journal of Occupational Therapy, 53,* 333–344.

Twitchell, T. E. (1951). The restoration of motor function following hemiplegia in man. *Brain, 74,* 443–480.

Van Dyck, W. R. (1999). Integrating treatment of the hemiplegic shoulder with self-care. *OT Practice, 4* (1), 32–37.

Versluys, H. P. (1995). Facilitating psychosocial adjustment to disability. In C. A. Trombly (Ed.), *Occupational Therapy for Physical Dysfunction* (4th ed., pp. 377–389). Baltimore: Williams & Wilkins.

Wade, D. T. (1989). Measuring arm impairment and disability after stroke. *International Disability Studies, 11,* 89–92.

Wade, D. T. (1992). Stroke: Rehabilitation and long term care. *Lancet, 339* (8796), 791–793.

Wade, D. T., & Langton Hewer, R. (1987). Functional ability after stroke: Measurement, natural history and prognosis. *Journal of Neurology, Neurosurgery and Psychiatry, 50,* 177–182.

Wagenaar, R. C., & Meijer, O. G. (1991a). Effects of stroke rehabilitation: A critical review of the literature (1). *Journal of Rehabilitation Sciences, 4* (3), 61–73.

Wagenaar, R. C., & Meijer, O. G. (1991b). Effects of stroke rehabilitation: A critical review of the literature (2). *Journal of Rehabilitation Sciences, 4* (4), 97109.

Wagenaar, R. C., VanWieringen, P. C. W., Nelelenbos, J. B., Meijer, O. G., & Kuik, D. J. (1992). The transfer of scanning training effect in visual inattention after stroke: Five single-case studies. *Disability and Rehabilitation, 14,* 51–60.

Walker, M. F., & Lincoln, N. B. (1990). Reacquisition of dressing skills after stroke. *International Disability Studies, 12,* 41–43.

Walker, M. F., & Lincoln, N. B. (1991). Factors influencing dressing performance after stroke. *Journal of Neurology, Neurosurgery and Psychiatry, 54,* 699–701.

Ware, J. E., & Sherbourne, C. E. (1992). The MOS 36-item short form health survey (SF-36): I. Conceptual framework and item selection. *Medical Care, 6,* 473–483.

Warren, M. (1990). A developmental treatment approach for adults with postural dysfunction. *Occupational Therapy Practice, 1,* 53–62.

Warren, M. (1991). Strategies for sensory and neuromotor remediation. In C. Christensen, & C. Baum (Eds.), *Occupational Therapy: Overcoming Human Performance Deficits* (pp. 632–662). Thorofare, NJ: Slack.

Warren, M. (1993). A hierarchical model for evaluation and treatment of visual perceptual dysfunction in adult acquired brain injury: Part 2. *American Journal of Occupational Therapy, 47,* 55–66.

Warren, M. (1999). *Evaluation and Treatment of Visual Perceptual Dysfunction in Adult Brain Injury, Part I* (continuing education handbook). Lenexa, KS: visABILITIES Rehabilitation.

Weinberg, J., Diller, L., Gordon, W. A., Gerstmann, L. J., Leiberman, A., Lakin, P., Hodges, G., & Ezrachi, O. (1977). Visual scanning training effect on reading-related tasks in acquired right brain damage. *Archives of Physical Medicine and Rehabilitation, 58,* 479–486.

Weinberg, J., Diller, L., Gordon, W. A., Gerstmann, L. J., Leiberman, A., Lakin, P., Hodges, G., & Ezrachi, O. (1979). Training sensory awareness and spatial organization in people with right brain damage. *Archives of Physical Medicine and Rehabilitation, 60,* 491–496.

Weisbroth, S., Esibill, N., & Zugar, R. R. (1971). Factors in the vocational success of hemiplegic patients. *Archives of Physical Medicine and Rehabilitation, 52,* 441–446.

Wellwood, I., Dennis, M. S., & Warlow, C. P. (1994). Perceptions and knowledge of stroke among surviving patients with stroke and their caregivers. *Age and Aging, 23,* 293–298.

Whyte, N. C., & Supon, D. A. (1998). Leisure: Methods to improve skills. In G. Gillen & A. Burkhardt (Eds.), *Stroke Rehabilitation: A Function-Based Approach* (pp. 496–507). St. Louis: Mosby.

Williams, L. S., Weinberger, M., Harris, L. E., Clark, D. O., & Biller, J. (1999). Development of a stroke-specific quality of life scale. *Stroke, 30,* 1362–1369.

Wilson, D. B., Houle, D. M., & Keith, R. A. (1991). Stroke rehabilitation: A model predicting return home. *Western Journal of Medicine, 154,* 587–590.

Wilson, D. J., Baker, L. L., & Craddock, J. A. (1984). Functional test for the hemiparetic upper extremity. *American Journal of Occupational Therapy, 38,* 159–164.

Wu, C.-Y., Trombly, C. A., Lin, K., & Tickle-Degnen, L. (1998). Effects of object affordances on reaching performance in persons with and without cerebrovascular accident. *American Journal of Occupational Therapy, 52,* 447–456.

Yekutiel, M., & Guttman, E. A. (1993). A controlled trial of the retraining of the sensory function of the hand in stroke patients. *Journal of Neurology, Neurosurgery and Psychiatry, 56,* 241–244.

Zorowitz, R. D., Hughes, M. B., Idank, D., Ikai, T., & Johnston, M. V. (1996). Shoulder pain and subluxation after stroke: Correlation or coincidence? *American Journal of Occupational Therapy, 50,* 194–201.

39

Traumatic Brain Injury

Mary Vining Radomski

LEARNING OBJECTIVES

After studying this chapter, the reader will be able to do the following:

1. Describe the similarities and differences in the typical course of recovery for persons with severe, moderate, and mild traumatic brain injury.
2. Select appropriate assessment tools and strategies for persons with traumatic brain injury during acute medical management and inpatient and postacute rehabilitation.
3. Apply information from related chapters of this text to the treatment of motor, cognitive, behavioral, and emotional aspects of traumatic brain injury.
4. Analyze how needs of family members change during recovery and adaptation and determine how to meet their needs in occupational therapy.
5. Anticipate possible roles for occupational therapists in addressing long-term needs of survivors of traumatic brain injury.

P ersons who have had a traumatic brain injury (TBI) often undergo changes in their ability to carry out valued roles, tasks, and activities. In fact, moderate to severe brain injury affects virtually every area of life for the survivor and his or her family. Because these individuals are typically young adults at the time of injury, changes in capacities and abilities may affect their occupational functioning for months, years, or decades. The complex interaction of factors associated with impairment and context require a multidisciplinary approach to treatment. Therefore, occupational therapists who work with patients with TBI must appreciate the contributions and expertise of other team members as they offer the patient all that is unique to occupational therapy.

To enable the reader to appreciate the effect of TBI on society, this chapter begins with a discussion of its incidence and causes. Next, mechanisms of injury are explained. A review of the typical

---

GLOSSARY

Agitation—subtype of delirium that is unique to survivors of TBI in altered states of consciousness in which there are excesses in behavior that include some combination of aggression, disinhibition, restlessness, and confusion.

Anterograde amnesia—Inability or impaired ability to remember events beginning with the onset of a condition (Lezak, 1995).

Diffuse axonal injury—Axonal damage (torn axons, shearing of axon clusters, and reactive swelling of strained and damaged axons) resulting from acceleration or deceleration and contracting waveform movements of the brain matter and accompanying fast rotational propulsion of the brain in the skull (Lezak, 1995).

Hematoma—Masses of blood confined to an organ or space that is caused by a broken blood vessel (Scott & Dow, 1995).

Mild brain injury—Trauma-induced physiological disruption of brain function as manifested by at least one of the following: any period of loss of consciousness, any loss of memory for events immediately before or after the accident, any alteration in mental state at the time of the accident, focal neurological deficit that may or may not be transient (ACRM, 1993).

Posttraumatic amnesia—Inability to remember day to day events after brain injury. The time elapsed from injury to recovery of continuous memory is one indicator of severity of brain damage.

Traumatic brain injury (TBI)—Insult to the brain, not degenerative or congenital, that is caused by an external physical force. This insult may produce a diminished or altered state of consciousness and resultant impairment of cognitive, behavioral, emotional, or physical functioning (BIA, 2000).

---

clinical course of recovery from severe TBI emphasizes how occupational therapy contributes to remediation of impairments and adaptation to deficits throughout the continuum of care. The unique needs of persons with mild brain injury are also highlighted, but it is hoped that readers can determine appropriate evaluation and treatment approaches for persons with moderate TBI, based on descriptions of the two extremes of severity of injury. Because brain injury rehabilitation requires an integration of many aspects of occupational therapy evaluation and treatment, the reader will frequently be referred to other chapters of this text.

Incidence, Prevalence, Causation

The Brain Injury Association (BIA) (2000) defines **traumatic brain injury (TBI)** as an insult to the brain, not degenerative or congenital, that is caused by an external physical force. This insult may produce a diminished or altered state of consciousness, hence impairment of cognitive, behavioral, emotional, or physical functioning. Rates of TBI-related hospitalization have declined by approximately 50% since 1980 because of successes in prevention and a shift in treatment of relatively mild cases from inpatient to outpatient settings (Thurman et al., 1999). However, the BIA estimates that 5.3 million Americans are living with disabilities resulting from TBI. Each year approximately 1.5 million people in the United States sustain a TBI, and an estimated 80,000 to 90,000 each year have onset of disabilities resulting from TBI (Thurman et al.). Beyond the sheer numbers of persons with TBI, demographic characteristics of this population have many implications for society and rehabilitation. According to the Traumatic Brain Injury Model Systems National Data Base, persons with TBI are typically young males aged 16 to 35 years at the time of injury (Harrison-Felix et al., 1996). The overall male-to-female ratio is 2–3:1 (Elovic & Antoinette, 1996). The age group that is second most likely to sustain this type of injury is persons over age 75 (Elovic & Antoinette; National Institutes of Health, 1998). Age of onset appears to be related to cause of TBI (Elovic & Antoinette).

Motor vehicle accidents are the most common cause of TBI, with the highest morbidity and mortality among drivers aged 15 to 19 (Elovic & Antoinette). Falls are the second most common causes of injury, approximately 20–30% of TBI, and the leading cause among the elderly (BIA, 2000; Elovic & Antoinette). Interpersonal violence ranks third, although in some urban areas, the percent of TBI caused by violence may exceed that caused by falls or motor vehicle accidents (Elovic & Antoinette; Harrison-Felix et al., 1996). Alcohol use is a contributing factor to accidents resulting in TBI, with estimates that approximately 50% of people who sustain TBI were intoxicated at the time of injury (Agency for Health Care Policy and Research, 1999). Preinjury alcohol use has implications for outcome, treatment, and long-term adjustment to TBI. Patients who were intoxicated when injured reportedly have a longer hospitalization, longer duration of agitation, and lower cognitive status at discharge than those who were not intoxicated (Kelly et al., 1997; Sparadeo & Gill, 1989). Furthermore, a history of TBI increases a person's risk of TBI. The BIA estimates that after one TBI, the risk of a second is three times normal, and after a second TBI, the risk of a third injury is eight times normal.

Finally, it is important to appreciate the incidence of TBI based on severity. TBI is characterized as mild, moderate, or severe (Box 39-1). Statistics regarding the distribution of severity of injury vary (Elovic & Antoinette, 1996). Most people who sustain a TBI (estimates of 60–80%) have a relatively mild injury, although trauma centers appear to have a much higher proportion of patients with severe injuries (Harrison-Felix et al., 1996).

Mechanisms of Injury and Clinical Implications

A TBI is usually caused by a dynamic loading or impact to the head from direct blows or from sudden movements produced by blows to other body parts. This loading can result in any combination of compression, expansion, acceleration, deceleration, and rotation of the brain inside the skull (Bakay & Glasauer, 1980). The type of damage is directly related to the nature and severity of the injury (Katz, 1992).

Diffuse Versus Focal Injuries

Brain injuries may be diffuse, focal, or both. Motor vehicle accidents and falls produce acceleration, deceleration, and rotation of the brain inside the skull. The brainstem is more stable than the cerebrum, which rotates around the brainstem during impact. The rotation places a stretch or shear force on the long axons that transmit information throughout the brain and brainstem (Leech & Shuman, 1982). These injuries, termed **diffuse axonal injuries**, result in coma because of the damage to the axons in the midbrain reticular activating system.

Coma caused by diffuse axonal injuries may quickly reverse if the axonal damage was mild or may continue as a vegetative state if axons were ruptured. Recovery from coma progresses to a period of confusion with impaired attention and **anterograde amnesia**. When confusion clears, any cognitive impairments become more evident. Impairments may include diminished mental processing speed and efficiency and difficulty with divided-attention tasks, which require the patient to respond simultaneously to two sources of information. There is a reduced capacity for higher-level cognitive functions, including abstract reasoning, planning, and problem solving. Typical behavioral outcomes range from impulsivity, irritability, and exaggerated premorbid traits to apathy and poor initiative (Katz, 1992). Diffuse injuries often include damage to the brainstem and cerebellar pathways, resulting in ataxia, diplopia, and dysarthria (Trexler & Zappala, 1988).

Focal lesions include contusions and lacerations of the brain. Although focal lesions can occur anywhere beneath the impact, they are usually seen at the anterior poles and inferior surfaces of the frontal and temporal lobes. They occur when the brain hits the skull and scrapes over the irregular bony structures at these locations (Katz, 1992). The occipital and parietal lobes, which have smooth surfaces, are less likely to incur damage. The folds of the dural membranes, especially the falx cerebri and the tentorium, can also cause damage to the brainstem, the medial aspect of the occipital lobe, and the superior surface of the cerebellum (Bakay & Glasauer, 1980).

Focal lesions to the prefrontal and anterior temporal areas interrupt connections to subcortical limbic structures and affect modulation of memory, emotion, and drive (Katz, 1992). Damage to the orbitofrontal areas results in impulsivity that is greater than with diffuse damage, but there are no motor impairments of the extremities or of speech (Trexler & Zappala, 1988). Damage to the frontolateral cortex results in hemiparesis, impulsivity, and attentional impairments. There is decreased accuracy and decreased mental flexibility, which affects the quality of performance (Trexler & Zappala).

Cranial Nerve Damage Associated With TBI

Cranial nerves can be torn, stretched, or contused. The olfactory nerve (I) is often abraded or torn when the frontal lobes scrape across the orbital surface of the skull (Leech & Shuman, 1982). The optic nerve (II) may be damaged directly, or vision can be compromised by injury to the eye, the optic tracts, or the visual cortex (Brandstater et al., 1991). Cranial nerves III, IV, and VI, which control eye movements, are all vulnerable to injury (Brandstater et al.; Leech & Shuman). The oculo-motor nerve (III) is stretched when edema, bleeding, or a tumor expands the contents of the skull, causing the uncus of the temporal lobe to herniate into the foramen magnum and compress the brainstem (Leech & Shuman). The abducens nerve (VI) is very long and consequently vulnerable to injury. The facial and vestibulocochlear nerves (VII and VIII respectively) may be damaged if the temporal bone is fractured at the base of the skull (Brandstater et al.; Leech & Shuman). Cranial nerves V and IX to XII are rarely damaged (Leech & Shuman).

Fractures Associated With TBI

The skull may fracture from the force of the blow in the area of or at a distance from the actual impact site. The patient with a brain injury from a motor vehicle accident or a fall may have other systemic trauma, such as fractures of the extremities, shoulder girdle, pelvis, or face; cervical fractures with possible spinal cord injury; abdominal trauma; and pneumothorax or other chest cavity trauma.

Secondary Effects of TBI

Secondary effects of the TBI can occur immediately or develop within hours or days (Jennett & Teasdale, 1981). Trauma can abolish or disrupt autoregulation of cerebral blood flow, the blood–brain barrier, and vasomotor functions, resulting in disordered cerebral energy metabolism, intracranial hypotension, cerebral vasospasm, and increases in intracranial pressure (ICP) and cerebral edema (Jennett & Teasdale; Miller, 1985). Other secondary effects of brain trauma include intracranial hemorrhage, ischemic brain damage, uncal herniation resulting in brainstem compression, general systemic reactions to the neural impairment, electrolyte abnormalities, altered respiratory regulation, intracranial infection, and abnormal autonomic nervous system responses (Lillehei & Hoff, 1985; Miller). Usually by the time the patient is stabilized and occupational therapy ordered, the secondary effects of brain trauma are present and influencing the patient's ability to respond to therapy.

Four Phases of Life for the Survivor of TBI

Based on their review of the literature, authors of the Agency for Health Care Policy and Research evidence report on the effectiveness of rehabilitation for persons with TBI described four phases of life for the adult

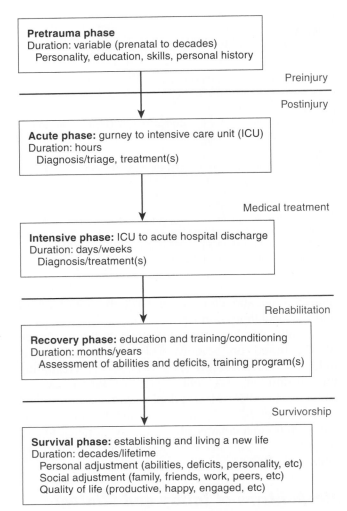

Figure 39-1 Four phases of life of the TBI survivor. (Reprinted with permission from Chestnut, R. M., Carney, N., Maynard, H., Mann, N. C., Patterson, P., & Helfand, M. (1999). Summary report: Evidence for the effectiveness of rehabilitation for persons with traumatic brain injury. *Journal of Head Trauma Rehabilitation*, 14 (2), 176–188.)

survivor of moderate to severe TBI: preinjury, medical treatment, rehabilitation, and survivorship (Fig. 39-1) (Chestnut et al., 1999). While management of TBI is typically a multidisciplinary enterprise, the description of each phase below is based on a typical recovery from severe TBI with emphasis on occupational therapy evaluation and treatment. Note how the role of occupational therapy changes with each phase, increasingly and uniquely focusing on occupational functioning the further the patient progresses in recovery.

Preinjury Phase

"In Chris's first 17 years she became used to being called 'outstanding.' She usually was one of the top students in every honors class . . . . Chris was a fairly good organist and gymnast too. In her first 17 years, outstanding was normal. Outstanding was easy."

(Rain, 2000, p. 6)

Occupational therapists always appreciate the person as distinct from his or her condition, impairment, or disability. People who sustain a TBI bring their personal, social, and cultural backgrounds to recovery (see Chapter 9). Chestnut et al. (1999) suggested that while standard treatments are appropriate for the acute medical treatment phase of TBI, consideration of individual differences becomes increasingly important as patients progress through recovery and adaptation.

Rosenthal and Bond (1990) summarized the importance of understanding premorbid factors that may affect the patient's recovery. They reported that researchers have noted a high frequency of preinjury learning disabilities and behavior disorders in persons with TBI. They suggested finding out about the patient's premorbid cognitive strengths and weaknesses through school records or family interviews and investigating any preexisting neurological conditions, such as previous TBI, epilepsy, dementia, or stroke. Eames et al. (1990) further recommended asking family members how the patient previously reacted to frustration so as to recognize and avoid stress-provoking situations.

Medical Treatment of TBI

"As I gradually regain consciousness in the hospital, I imagine I am having a nightmare .... As I open my eyes and stare around the room at the monitors and plugs and dripping IV bottles, I hope this nightmare will end quickly."

(Rain, 2000, p. 6)

The primary goals of this phase of recovery center on survival, achieving medical stability, and preventing or minimizing the secondary effects of TBI.

Emergency Medical Treatment

Paramedics are typically the first medical specialists to respond to the needs of a person with severe TBI. Once they have ensured an adequate airway and stabilized blood pressure, they usually immobilize the patient on a rigid backboard with the neck in a rigid cervical spine collar (Marion, 1996). Because most secondary brain injury occurs during the first few hours of TBI, vital signs are checked frequently en route to the trauma center, and any deterioration is addressed immediately (Marion, 1996).

Once in the emergency department, the medical team continues to ensure protection of the airway and adequacy of breathing and blood pressure (Marion, 1996). The medical team performs a general assessment of injuries and neurological status, often using the *Glasgow Coma Scale* (*GCS*) (Teasdale & Jennett, 1974). The *GCS* provides an objective assessment of moderate to severe TBI using a 15-point system to test motor, eye-opening, and verbal capabilities (Table 39-1) (Teasdale & Jennett). However, in some cases, alcohol or other drug intoxication or sedation prevents an accurate neurological assessment in the emergency department (Marion).

Computed tomography (CT) of the head is usually obtained within 30 minutes after the patient arrives in the emergency department; it is the most reliable test for determining the presence of intracranial **hematomas** (Marion, 1996). Hematoma, a mass of blood confined to an organ or space and caused by a broken blood vessel (Scott & Dow, 1995) must be evacuated as soon as possible to optimize chances for survival and recovery (Marion).

Intensive Medical Management

After appropriate evaluation and treatment for life-threatening injuries, the patient is taken to the intensive care unit (ICU). Medical treatment aims to optimize cerebral perfusion and brain tissue oxygenation, minimize brain swelling, and maintain all other physiological variables within the normal range (Marion, 1996). The length of stay in the ICU is primarily determined by the ability to manage the patient's brain swelling, which usually subsides within 4 to 5 days (Marion). A physiatrist is typically consulted on the day the patient is admitted to the ICU, and he or she follows the patient

TABLE 39-1
Glasgow Coma Scale

Eye opening (*E*)	Spontaneous	4
	To speech	3
	To pain	2
	Nil	1
Best motor response (*M*)	Obeys	6
	Localizes	5
	Withdraws	4
	Abnormal flexion	3
	Extensor response	2
	Nil	1
Verbal response (*V*)	Oriented	5
	Confused conversation	4
	Inappropriate words	3
	Incomprehensible sounds	2
	Nil	1
Coma score = $(E + M + V) = 3$ to 15		

Reprinted with permission from Jennett, B., & Teasdale, G. (1981). *Management of Head Injuries* (p. 78). Philadelphia: F. A. Davis Company.

throughout the hospital stay and often through reentry to the community. The physiatrist orders rehabilitation services for the coma patient that may begin in the ICU, including occupational therapy. Rehabilitation for patients with alterations in consciousness, as described in this overview, may also occur in medical, rehabilitation, or subacute units or in long-term care facilities.

Patients With Severe Alterations in Consciousness

A person with TBI may exhibit any of a number of states of altered consciousness, depending on the severity of the injury (Scott & Dow, 1995). Various terms are used to describe the continuum from complete consciousness to complete absence of consciousness (Box 39-2). Patients with severe TBI begin in coma, which is a time-limited state (Phipps et al., 1997). Some patients gradually or abruptly recover consciousness directly from coma, while others shift over 2 to 4 weeks into the vegetative state (Phipps et al.). Vegetative patients may still recover consciousness, but they do so gradually, spending long periods in a minimally conscious state in which there is verifiable evidence of conscious processing (Phipps et al.). Giacino and Kalmar (1997) suggested that the distinction between vegetative state and minimally conscious state is important in terms of diagnosis and prognosis. Patients diagnosed with minimally conscious state at admission to rehabilitation attained significantly more favorable outcomes 1 to 12 months post injury than did those in the vegetative state. The ability to sustain visual pursuit eye movement seems to be one of the first signs of the transition out of vegetative state (Giacino & Kalmar) and is an early indicator of possible readiness for rehabilitation (Ansell, 1993).

Assessment

Diagnosis of specific alterations in consciousness and prognostic decisions must be reserved for physicians and other professionals with experience in neurological assessment of patients with impaired consciousness (American Congress of Rehabilitation Medicine, 1995b). However, the rehabilitation team, including occupational therapists, uses a number of objective assessments to monitor changes in function and response to pharmacological, environmental, and behavioral interventions and for early detection of neuromedical complications (O'Dell & Riggs, 1996).

Rancho Los Amigos Levels of Cognitive Functioning Scale. The *Rancho Los Amigos Levels of Cognitive Function Scale* uses behavioral observations to categorize a patient's level of cognitive function (Table 39-2) (Hagen, Malkmus, & Durham, 1979; Hagen, 1998). It helps clinicians to communicate about a patient's level of cognitive function among themselves and with families and to develop appropriate rehabilitation strategies. The first three levels of the *Rancho Los Amigos Levels of Cognitive Functioning Scale* describe the response to stimulation and the environment of patients emerging from coma.

Behavior-Based Assessment Instruments. In addition to the *GCS*, the instruments described in Table 39-3 are all brief assessments that occupational therapists and other rehabilitation team members can use at bedside to evaluate patients with severe alterations in consciousness.

Prognosis and Outcome

In recent years, as the number of patients surviving severe TBI increased, research has focused on finding factors that predict the ultimate outcome of such injuries

---

BOX 39-2
Definitions of Severe Alterations of Consciousness (American Congress of Rehabilitation Medicine, 1995b)

Coma

Denotes unarousability with absence of sleep–wake cycles on electroencephalogram (EEG) and loss of capacity for environmental interaction. Neurobehavioral criteria for this diagnosis:

▶ Patient's eyes do not open either spontaneously or to external stimulation
▶ Patient does not follow commands.
▶ Patient does not mouth or speak recognizable words.
▶ Patient cannot sustain visual pursuits through a 45° arc in any direction when the eyes are held open manually.
▶ These criteria cannot be attributed to use of paralytic agents.

Vegetative State

Indicates complete loss of ability to interact with the environment despite the capacity for spontaneous or stimulus-induced arousal. This state always follows an initial period of coma after TBI and is further characterized by behavioral responses that consist of reflexive reactions only. Sleep–wake cycles may be present on EEG. Neurobehavioral criteria for this diagnosis:

▶ Patient opens his or her eyes spontaneously or after stimulation.
▶ Criteria 2 to 6 under coma are met.

Minimally Responsive State

Describes patients who are no longer comatose or vegetative but are severely disabled. Patients in this state have the capacity for environmental interaction evidenced through observation or testing. Meaningful responses are inconsistent and depend on external stimulation. Patients in this category are sometimes referred to as slow-to-recover (Ansell, 1993). Neurobehavioral criterion for this diagnosis:

▶ Patient demonstrates a meaningful behavioral response after a specific command, question, or environmental prompt.

TABLE 39-2
Rancho Los Amigos Levels of Cognitive Functioning

Level	Description
I	No response: unresponsive to stimuli
II	Generalized response: nonspecific, inconsistent, and nonpurposeful reaction to stimuli
III	Localized response: response directly related to type of stimulus but still inconsistent or delayed
IV	Confused, agitated: response heightened, severely confused, may be aggressive
V	Confused-inappropriate: some response to simple commands, but confusion with more complex commands; high level of distractibility
VI	Confused-appropriate: response more goal directed but cues necessary
VII	Automatic-appropriate: response robotlike, judgment and problem solving lacking
VIII	Purposeful-appropriate *(with standby assistance)*: response adequate *to familiar tasks*, subtle impairments *require standby assistance with acknowledging other people's needs and perspectives, modifying plans*
IX	*Purposeful-appropriate (with standby assistance on request): responds effectively to familiar situations but generally needs cues to anticipate problems and adjust performance; low frustration tolerance possible*
X	*Purposeful and appropriate (modified independent): responds adequately to multiple tasks but may need more time or periodic breaks; independently employs cognitive compensatory strategies and adjusts tasks as needed*

Rancho levels I to VIII are widely used in brain injury rehabilitation. The addition of levels IX and X in 1998 (revisions italicized) describe higher-level cognitive, behavioral, and emotional barriers to optimal functioning.
Adapted with permission from Scott, A. D., & Dow, P. W. (1995). Traumatic Brain Injury. In C.A. Trombly (Ed.), *Occupational Therapy for Physical Dysfunction* (4th ed., p. 710) Baltimore: Williams & Wilkins; Hagen C. (1998). *The Rancho Levels of Cognitive Functioning: The Revised Levels* (3rd ed.) Downey, CA: Rancho Los Amigos Medical Center.

(Scott & Dow, 1995). Early prediction of outcome presumably helps direct expensive medical treatment or rehabilitation to patients who have the best chance for survival with fewer residual impairments and enables the family to make informed, realistic decisions on immediate and long-term care (Davis & Cunningham, 1984; Jennett & Teasdale, 1981). Many researchers have attempted to assess the predictive power of age, clinical observations (such as the *GCS*, pupillary reactions, and eye movements), data from CT, surgical lesion, length of posttraumatic amnesia (i.e., the length of time after the accident before the return of continuous memory), brainstem dysfunction, evoked potentials, increased ICP, or a combination of these factors (Braakman et al., 1980; Bricolo et al., 1980; Karnaze et al., 1985; Salcman et al., 1981). However, even with sophisticated clinical and radiological techniques, during the first days after injury it is not possible to predict outcome with sufficient accuracy to guide early treatment or justify withholding treatment (Marion, 1996). Repeated observations of neurological recovery over weeks or months remain the best means to predict complete or nearly complete recovery (Marion).

As mentioned previously, the *GCS* is often used to predict outcome. An initial score of 8 or below that is maintained for 6 hours post injury predicts mortality 50% or survival with moderate to severe disabilities. Choi et al. (1988) found that a low motor score on the *GCS*, a fixed and dilated pupil, and age greater than 60 years strongly predicted death or severe disability and that the combination of factors had more predictive accuracy than any one of them used independently. The length of posttraumatic amnesia is another frequently used predictor of outcome. Posttraumatic amnesia is a loss of memory of day-to-day events after an injury. Posttraumatic amnesia lasting less than 1 hour indicates mild injury; 1 to 24 hours indicates moderate injury; 1 to 7 days indicates severe injury; and more than 7 days indicates very severe injury (Bond, 1990).

Outcome scales have been developed to allow physicians to correlate "final" recovery levels to early treatment and prognostic indicators. The *Glasgow Outcome Scale (GOS)* is widely used. Its categories are death, vegetative state, severe disability (conscious but dependent), moderate disability (independent but disabled), and good recovery (able to participate in normal social life and return to work), with 90% accurate assessment of prognosis possible 6 months post injury (Jennett & Teasdale, 1981; Satz et al., 1998). The *GOS* does assess some aspects of mental and physical function in assigning outcome categories (Jennett et al.,1981). Some researchers consider that more detailed neuropsychological and/or social factors should be considered in determining outcome (Hall et al., 1985). When these factors are added, more residual disability is identified than by the *GOS*, and improvements in levels of disability are identified more accurately (Hall et al.). Addition of these factors also allows assessment of continued subtle recovery to be made beyond 6 or 12 months post injury (Hall et al.; Najenson et al., 1974).

The therapist is not required to predict but should consider the predictive factors listed herein when deciding on treatment goals or length of rehabilitation efforts. Cognition, personality, and motivation, all of which may

TABLE 39-3
Valid and Reliable Assessment Tools for Altered States of Consciousness

Instrument	Brief Description
Coma/Near Coma Scale[a] (Rappaport et al., 1992)	Measures small clinical changes in patients with severe TBI and nontraumatic brain injuries who function at levels characteristic of near vegetative or vegetative states; consists of 8 parameters, each with a specified number of stimuli and trials. Based on the numerical scoring system, patient falls into 1 of 5 categories: no coma, near coma, moderate coma, marked coma, extreme coma.
Western Neuro Sensory Stimulation Profile[a] (Ansell & Keenan, 1989)	Assesses cognitive function in severely impaired adults (Rancho levels II–IV) and monitors change in noncomatose patients who are slow to recover. Battery consists of 32 items related to arousal, attention, response to stimuli, and expressive communication and results in a profile of 6 subscales that summarize individual patterns of responses.
Coma Recovery Scale (Giacino et al., 1991)	Detects subtle changes in neurobehavioral status; predicts outcome in acute rehabilitation patients with severe alterations in consciousness (Rancho levels 1–IV); consists of 35 items in 6 areas: auditory, visual, motor, oromotor–verbal, communication, arousal. Responses are criterion referenced: specific stimuli administered to elicit specific responses.
Disability Rating Scale[a] (Rappaport et al., 1982)	Single instrument to provide quantitative information on recovery from severe TBI from coma to community; consists of 8 items in 4 categories: arousal and awareness; cognitive ability to handle self-care functions; physical dependence upon others; psychosocial adaptability for work, housework, or school. Scoring takes 30 seconds (if clinician is very familiar with both tool and patient) to 15 minutes (Center for Outcome Measurement in Brain Injury [COMBI], 2000). Thought to be relatively insensitive in detecting problems and progress for persons with mild TBI (COMBI, 2000).
Agitated Behavior Scale[a] (Corrigan, 1989)	Allows objective measurement of agitation, particularly as a serial assessment to evaluate effectiveness of interventions to reduce agitation (COMBI, 2000); consists of 14 items; total score reflects overall agitation, with subscales specific to disinhibition, aggression, and lability.

[a]Available online at http://www.tbms.org/combi.

substantially affect quality of survival (Jennett et al., 1981; Newlon & Greenberg, 1984), are also to be considered in determining treatment goals. Outcome predictions are based on groups of patients, not on individuals, who may have family and character strengths that allow them to recover more completely than anticipated.

Intervention for Patients With Severe Alterations in Consciousness

Rehabilitation for patients with severe alterations in consciousness aims to foster alertness and behavioral responsiveness (Giacino, et al., 1997) and to prevent complications associated with prolonged immobilization (Mysiw et al., 1996). Early intervention is believed to result in shorter rehabilitation stays and higher Rancho levels at discharge (Mackay et al., 1992; Mysiw et al.). However, with little empirical evidence regarding its effectiveness, sensory stimulation remains particularly controversial (Giacino et al., 1997). Giacino et al. (1997) recommended that at a minimum patients with alterations in consciousness receive intervention that includes range of motion exercise, positioning protocols, and tone alteration methods. They suggested that the additional provision of sensory stimulation trials be considered on a case by case basis. Finally, reducing

possible agitation (Eames et al., 1990) and supporting and educating overwhelmed family members are critical aspects of rehabilitation at this phase (Phipps et al., 1997).

For patients with alterations in consciousness, members of the rehabilitation team often have similar roles and responsibilities. For example, both occupational and physical therapists often perform range-of-motion exercises and collaborate to optimize positioning. All team members, including family, follow a consistent sensory stimulation protocol to enhance the reliability and interpretability of observations. For patients at this phase of recovery, intervention typically addresses first-level and developed capacities to lay the foundation for later focus on activities, tasks, and roles (Box 39-3). Because of the medical acuity of many of these patients, occupational therapists attend to the safety precautions summarized in Box 39-4.

Positioning. Occupational therapists collaborate with other members of the rehabilitation team to optimize positioning to normalize muscle tone and ultimately affect motor performance (Rinehart, 1990). Some typical abnormal positions seen in patients with severe traumatic brain injuries include abnormally forward head, protracted and forward-tipped scapulae with or without elevation, posterior pelvic tilt with unilateral retraction and/or elevation, severe trunk tightness with lack of trunk dissociation from neck and head, hip flexor and adductor tightness, and foot plantar flexion and inversion.

The patient's position must be reevaluated frequently. Assistive positioning supports are used intermittently and removed as the patient's neuromuscular status improves. The nursing staff and the patient's family must be made aware of the desired bed and wheelchair positioning and of the wearing schedule for any splints. To reduce abnormal tone and to reduce or prevent contractures, the positioning must continue throughout the day and night.

BOX 39-3
PROCEDURES FOR PRACTICE

Goal Setting for and With Persons With TBI

Occupational therapy treatment goals address changing aspects of occupational functioning as patients with severe TBI progress through recovery and adaptation. Here are some examples based on Chestnut et al. (1999) phases of recovery and adaptation.

▶ Medical treatment phase (treatment focuses on first level and developed capacities)
  ▶ In 3 weeks the patient will make localized responses in less than 15 seconds after the presentation of tactile, olfactory, auditory, or visual stimuli at least 75% of the time to lay the foundation for using a communication board.
  ▶ In 3 weeks the patient will demonstrate improvement in upper extremity range of motion, gaining at least 10% in shoulders and elbows, to facilitate ease and thoroughness with caregiver-provided hygiene activities.
▶ Rehabilitation phase (treatment primarily focuses on abilities and skills, activities and habits, and task competency)
  ▶ In 2 weeks the patient will be able to follow a checklist to carry out personal hygiene tasks with no more than occasional specific cues.
  ▶ In 2 weeks the patient will independently locate and follow a daily schedule in his planner.
  ▶ In 2 weeks the patient will independently follow written and pictorial instructions to carry out his upper extremity range of motion exercises.
▶ Survivor phase (treatment primarily focuses on habits, competency in tasks, and satisfaction with life roles)
  ▶ In 4 weeks the client will use compensatory cognitive strategies to structure his children's afternoon activities.
  ▶ In 4 weeks the client will use an alarm cueing device to improve his completion of time-specific tasks at work.

Bed. Side-lying or semiprone if permitted with good body alignment is preferable to supine if the patient has abnormal posture (Carr & Shepherd, 1980; Farber, 1982). Lying supine triggers an extensor response. In side lying, the head, resting on a small pillow, should be in neutral alignment with the trunk; the bottom upper extremity, in scapular protraction and humeral external rotation; the top upper extremity, in scapular protraction, slight shoulder flexion, and resting on a pillow to avoid horizontal adduction; the bottom elbow flexed; the top elbow extended; wrists in extension; and cones in the hands to decrease spasticity and maintain thumb web spaces. A pillow between the knees decreases hip internal rotation and adduction. The lower leg also may need pillow support to align it with the thigh. The hip and knee are flexed only slightly. Elongation of the lower side of the trunk between the shoulder and pelvis is desirable. A side-lying trunk position may have to be maintained by a pillow or sandbag behind the back and shoulder. Footboards should be avoided, as they elicit extensor thrust. Splints or special shoes (Farber, 1982) that are cut to avoid pressure to the ball of the foot but still maintain ankle flexion to 90° and reduce foot drop are used to avoid stimulating an extensor thrust.

If the patient must be supine, a small pillow under the head is used, with small rolled pillows under that pillow to keep the head in midline if the patient cannot do so. Furthermore, small pillows are placed under the scapulae to protract them, shoulders are positioned in slight abduction and external rotation, elbows are extended, and cones or finger spreaders position the fingers (Charness, 1986). If the pelvis is retracted on one side, a small folded towel is placed behind it, and that leg is positioned in neutral rotation. Some knee flexion should be encouraged by a small towel roll placed under the distal thigh just above the knee.

Wheelchair. Early and correct upright positioning in a wheelchair helps to facilitate arousal by stimulating the visual and vestibular systems, inhibiting abnormal tone, providing normal proprioceptive input, and reducing the likelihood and/or extent of contractures and complications from prolonged bedrest. The pelvis must be positioned correctly before other areas can be addressed. The pelvis should be in a neutral position or have a slight anterior tilt and should be symmetrical, without one side retracted or elevated. Weight bearing equally through both buttocks is essential to improvement of tone. Solid seat and back inserts are necessary, as the typical wheelchair seat and back sag and facilitate posterior pelvic tilt, unequal weight bearing through the hips, and hip internal rotation and adduction. If necessary, a small, flat lumbar roll is placed above the pelvis and below the scapula to facilitate anterior pelvic tilt. If

BOX 39-4
SAFETY BOX

Safety Precautions for Treating Patients in Altered States of Consciousness

The patient with a severe TBI may be referred for occupational therapy before he or she is completely medically stable. Because of systemic injuries, secondary effects of the brain injury itself, disturbance of basic body regulatory systems, and the life support equipment used to treat the patient, precautions may be numerous, and they must be heeded by the therapist. Typical precautions are described here; other precautions may also be necessary and should be ascertained from the nurse, physician, or patient's chart before the evaluation begins.

▸ A major concern with acute brain trauma is control of intracranial pressure (ICP). Sustained increased ICP can be fatal (Jennett & Teasdale, 1981). The patient with an ICP monitor can be readily checked during treatment sessions. The therapist must closely observe patients not on a monitor for pupil changes; decreased neurological responses; abnormal brainstem reflexes; flaccidity; behavioral changes; vomiting; and changes in pulse rate, blood pressure, and respiration rate. Fluids may be restricted, or the patient's head may be positioned in neutral at 30° elevation in an attempt to regulate ICP (Turner, 1985). Turning the patient's head to one side may obstruct the internal jugular vein and result in a sudden increase of ICP (Boortz-Marx, 1985; Parsons, et al., 1985). The neck should be neither flexed nor extended but kept in neutral for maximum venous drainage and decreased ICP. The presence of a family member, gentle touching, quiet talking, and stroking the face have been found to decrease ICP in adults (Mitchell, 1986). Side-lying with the head of the bed elevated is the most desirable position. Side-lying avoids the increased extensor tone promoted in supine. Prone lying is contraindicated with increased ICP and supported sitting at 90° is used as soon as tolerated to help breathing, to provide symmetrical body alignment, and to increase awareness of surroundings (Palmer & Wyness, 1988).

▸ Early posttraumatic epilepsy occurs in 5% of patients with brain injuries, and late-onset epilepsy affects 20% of those with prolonged unconsciousness, depressed skull fracture, or intracranial hematoma (Jennett & Teasdale, 1981; Schaffer, et al., 1985). To reduce the chance of a seizure during treatment, begin tactile stimulation and range of motion slowly to assess the patient's physiological response. Monitor the heart rate, blood pressure, and facial color and any autonomic changes, such as sudden perspiration or increased restlessness. As the therapist becomes more familiar with the patient's responses, he or she gradually increases intensity of stimulation. Use seizure precautions: avoid rapid, repetitive stimuli, such as vibration, flickering lights, and an oscillating fan. If a seizure does occur, ensure that the airway is open, position the patient on his or her side to prevent aspiration of stomach contents, and summon medical assistance (Greenberg, et al., 1993). The patient's limbs should not be restrained during a seizure.

▸ If the patient has had a craniotomy for evacuation of a hematoma, the bone flap may be left off, and the brain may be covered only by scalp to allow the brain to expand. Direct pressure to this site must be avoided.

▸ The patient may have a tear in the dura and cerebrospinal fluid leak. In this case the patient initially is treated with head elevation, antibiotics, and precautions against nose blowing (Jennett & Teasdale, 1981; Schaffer et al., 1985).

▸ If the patient has other systemic trauma, such as fractures or chest cavity trauma, appropriate precautions must be taken when he or she is stimulated or moved. Care must also be taken to avoid disturbing intravenous lines, tracheostomy, nasogastric tube, endotracheal or respirator tubes, and traction for extremity fractures. If the patient has a nasogastric tube, caution must be taken that the patient's head remains above the level of his or her stomach to avoid regurgitation and aspiration (Miller et al., 1990).

---

the pelvis is retracted on one side, wedged back pieces may be helpful for positioning. If unequal weight bearing with habitual elongation of one side of the trunk is occurring, an insert under the habitual weight-bearing buttock may be helpful. The back of the chair may be reclined 10 to 15° to position the trunk and head more appropriately. Hip flexion of 90° can be achieved by a wedge cushion with the high end at the distal thigh. The seat belt should come from the corners of the seat at a 45° angle and fasten over the lower pelvis and hip area to help maintain the anterior pelvic tilt and equal weight bearing through the buttocks. The patient may need firm pads on the outer aspect of the thighs to reduce excessive abduction or a knee abductor to decrease excessive adduction. If the seat belt cannot keep the patient from scooting forward in the chair, a remov-

able padded bar may have to be placed close to the pelvis and femurs.

The trunk, positioned next, should be symmetrical and in midline, with shoulders over pelvis in sagittal, frontal, and horizontal planes. Lateral trunk supports can be used to decrease lateral trunk flexion. Experimentation with the positioning is essential, because trunk control varies among patients. The therapist must not provide too much trunk support, only enough to facilitate the patient's normal movement and control. With a solid seat and back, the patient may not require additional trunk support.

A harness, shoulder straps, or a chest strap may be necessary to prevent forward trunk flexion. These should not fasten directly on top of the shoulders but should extend a little higher before going through the seat back to fasten. An additional seat belt can also be placed horizontally across the anterior superior iliac crests to provide backward pressure (Charness, 1986).

Knees and ankles are flexed to 90°, heels slightly behind the knees in sitting, feet in neutral pronation–supination and inversion–eversion. The footplate should be large enough to support the whole foot. Ankle straps are avoided because they encourage plantar flexion in some patients; a foot wedge, heel loops, an insert behind the foot, special shoes, toe guards, or a combination may be helpful in decreasing abnormal tone and in achieving weight bearing on the heel.

The ideal upper extremity position is neutral scapular elevation or depression with the scapulae in slight protraction, slight shoulder external rotation, and slight flexion and abduction. Elbows are in comfortable flexion and the forearm in pronation. The wrists are in neutral flexion–extension and neutral ulnar–radial deviation; the fingers are relaxed; and the thumb is radially abducted. Excessive scapular retraction may require contouring of the seat back or reclining the seat unit by about 10°. Positioning of shoulder straps, chest straps, and/or lateral trunk supports may help to obtain adequate shoulder position.

A lapboard positioned at the proper height to allow good upper extremity weight bearing is helpful. The lapboard should not be pushed against the patient's abdomen but placed far enough away so the patient can flex forward slightly at the hips. There should be a cutout so that the lapboard fits around the patient, and the lapboard should be large enough to accommodate the whole arm. A V-shaped piece of dense foam can be positioned behind the patient's elbow to decrease elbow flexion and retraction of the arm off the back of the lapboard. The lapboard may also have a contoured surface for the hands. Hand fixation is avoided because it usually causes the patient to pull back against the fixation.

Ideally the head should be in midline, with cervical elongation and the chin tucked in slightly. It is important that positioning eliminate chin jutting and neck hyperextension. The position of the patient's shoulders and upper trunk influences head position. A customized head support may be required (Farber, 1982). Pressure directly to the occipital area elicits increased extensor tone of the head and trunk. Therefore, the pressure to right the head is applied up from the occipital process to each side of midline and around the forehead with a backward and downward pressure. Such a head support has to be fastened to a headrest, which is recessed so that the patient's head cannot push or rest against it. Lateral head supports may be necessary to position the patient's head adequately.

Passive Range of Motion. Passive range of motion (PROM) can be difficult when muscle tone is increased. Inhibitory movements opposite the abnormal tone are performed slowly, holding the stretch until muscles relax (Scott & Dow, 1995). Sudden stretch and inappropriate stimulation and handling should be avoided. Scapular mobility should be addressed before upper extremity PROM to free the scapula and facilitate normal scapular and humeral movement during the rest of PROM (Palmer & Wyness, 1988). PROM within the limits of pain and positioning helps to minimize contractures from heterotopic ossification (Citta-Pietrolungo et al., 1992). See Chapter 20 for a complete discussion of exercise to improve range of motion.

Splinting and Casting. The goals of splinting and casting are to decrease abnormal tone and increase the patient's functional movement. The patient's quality of movement is constantly reassessed to determine continued necessity of the splints or the need for modifications. Splints should be very carefully monitored when used with severely spastic or posturing patients, as they can aggravate abnormal tone and rapidly create pressure areas.

With severe spasticity in elbow, wrist, knee, ankle, or foot, serial casting may be indicated (Malkmus et al., 1980). Serial cylinder casting provides neutral warmth and more even skin pressure and allows for less movement than splints. Casts are usually left on up to 7 days. Dropout casts, which leave a portion of the limb free to relax out of a tightly contracted position; bivalve casts, which are split in two, with moleskin protecting the edges so they can be removed during therapy and nursing procedures; and weight-bearing inhibitory casts, which are fabricated to approximate the ideal weight-bearing posture of the foot or hand, can also be used (Carr & Shepherd, 1980; Malkmus et al.). Hill (1994) found casting more effective than traditional treatment of PROM, stretching, and splinting in reducing contractures in a group of 15 head-injured patients. The effect of casting on spasticity was variable, and Hill recommended further study. Decisions to use serial casting are informed by the patient's cognitive level. If the patient has severe agitation, casts may pose safety problems (Dell et al., 1998). Rinehart (1990) recommended against casting more than one joint if the patient is confused or easily agitated or has short-term memory problems.

Sensory Stimulation. The goals of a sensory stimulation program are to promote arousal, appropriate patterns of movement, and interaction with the environment (Rinehart, 1990). Sensory stimulation programs are individualized to the patient's physical and cognitive functioning, but they always include multiple periods of observation and careful data collection (Mysiw et al., 1996). Clinicians use consistent protocols to standardize the administration of stimuli and data sheets to record observations regarding rate of response and changes in respiration, pulse, blood pressure, head turning, and eye opening (Rader et al., 1989). Responses are measured at the beginning and end of every session and as each sense is stimulated (Rader et al.).

Each stimulus is provided with a desired motor response in mind (Scott & Dow,1995). The response is verbally requested and/or implied through the therapist's handling. Patients at Rancho level II often demonstrate nonspecific responses, such as motor restlessness in response to auditory stimuli. As the patient moves to level III, the responses become more stimulus specific. For example, with oral motor stimulation, one expects a motor response such as lip closure, and certain positional changes aim to facilitate the desired motor response of head righting. As the patient responds more consistently, the therapist attempts to channel those responses into more appropriate interaction with the environment (Scott & Dow).

Tactile, vestibular, olfactory, kinesthetic, proprioceptive, auditory, and visual stimuli are used. Gustatory stimulation may be used if the patient's oral motor status permits. Pleasant and unpleasant and familiar and unfamiliar stimuli are used; stimuli with emotional significance to the patient may be most likely to elicit a response (Scott & Dow, 1995). Trials of organized stimulation periods of 15 to 30 minutes each are scheduled frequently throughout the day. These sessions must be spaced to allow for rest and nursing care. The patient's response to stimulation may be quite slow, because central nervous system processing is slowed or prevented by the damage (Scott & Dow). The therapist should wait for a response to the stimulation and if necessary repeat the stimulus. Box 39-5 describes how to administer various types of stimuli.

Management of Agitation. Once patients begin localizing stimuli, they may become quite agitated and restless

---

BOX 39-5
PROCEDURES FOR PRACTICE

Sensory Stimulation (adapted from Scott & Dow, 1995)

Stimuli are presented in a consistent and meaningful manner, typically one sensory modality at a time. The patient is told what the therapist is doing and often given an instruction specific to a desired response. Minimize competing visual and auditory stimuli by turning off the television, closing the door, or pulling the drape. Give simple, clear verbal feedback on every response elicited such as, "Good. You are turning your head toward my voice." Here are examples of how various types of stimuli are presented.

▸ Tactile stimulation—Rub patient's skin with items of various texture or temperature and use a firm or moving touch on the patient's limbs with verbal cues to orient the patient to his or her body (Farber, 1982). Bathing and dressing are excellent sources of varied input, especially if verbal orientation to body parts being washed or moved is included.

▸ Provide gentle vestibular stimuli by changing body position (from supine to sitting, sitting to side-lying), by head and neck movements, rolling, tilting the bed to sitting, side-to-side or anteroposterior movement of the patient in bed or on a mat, slow spinning, or rocking. Inversion of the head (lying over a large therapy ball or leaning over while seated) helps reduce hypertonicity. **However, this and other forms of vestibular stimulation are contraindicated in a patient with a tracheostomy, elevated ICP, or seizures. The patient's reaction must be closely monitored during and after all vestibular stimulation. Precautions and desired ranges of heart rate, ICP, and blood pressure must be adhered to during stimulation.**

▸ Stimulate the olfactory sense with noxious or pleasant odors, such as spices, almond, vanilla, banana, lemon,

perfume, coffee, or other smells familiar to the patient. This stimulation may be most effective when it is done before the patient is fed. The therapist must offer an effective concentration of the odor. Saturated cotton balls or a sniff bottle are held close to but not touching the patient's nose for 2 to 5 seconds (Farber, 1982). This cranial nerve is sometimes injured in TBI, so olfactory stimulation may not elicit a response (Jennett & Teasdale, 1981). **Avoid odors with fumes, such as ammonia and artificial vanilla, because they irritate cranial nerve V.** A tracheostomy or nasogastric tube eliminates or reduces the air passing through the nostrils, hence reduces the effectiveness of olfactory stimuli.

▸ Auditory stimulation consists of tapes of favorite music or familiar voices, bells, loud alerting noises such as clapping hands, direct conversation to the patient, verbal commands, explanations, and feedback. The therapist uses clear, firm speech, often presenting information to the patient regarding his or her circumstances and whereabouts. During therapy sessions, radios, televisions, and other noises should be eliminated as much as possible so that voice commands for motor responses or the selected auditory stimuli are the most prevalent auditory input.

▸ Provide visual stimulation to elicit attention, focus, and visual tracking with brightly colored objects, a mobile over the bed, mirrors, a flashlight in a darkened room, or pictures of family and friends of the patient. Have the family label the pictures to assist in orienting the patient to them. Environmental changes from the bed to the therapy room or from indoors to outdoors are important sources of visual stimulation.

BOX 39-6
PROCEDURES FOR PRACTICE

Managing Agitation: Rancho Level IV

During this stage of recovery, occupational therapists primarily seek to decrease the patient's agitation by attempting to normalize the environment and employing appropriate physical management methods that allow the patient to move and release energy without jeopardizing safety (Eames et al., 1990). Remember that the patient is not accountable for the agitation, hostility, or aggressiveness (Scott & Dow, 1995). He or she is responding to internal confusion, not specifically to you as a person or professional. At the same time, you must structure your interactions to protect the patient and yourself (Scott & Dow).

Strategies to Normalize the Environment

- Minimize the influence of confusion by asking family members to bring in familiar objects (photographs or belongings) and position them so they are visible to the patient (Eames et al., 1990).
- Work in a quiet environment with minimal distracters that may further alarm or confuse the patient.
- Remove limb restraints during therapy sessions (Scott & Dow, 1995).
- Attempt to maintain a predictable daily structure and routine to reduce confusion (Scott & Dow, 1995).
- Normalize interactions by introducing yourself at each session, telling the patient where he or she is and what you are going to do (Eames et al., 1990). Extend the same courtesies, even to comatose patients, that you would to patients without cognitive impairments (Eames et al.).

Strategies for Physical Management

- Use equipment and devices that maximize freedom of movement along with safety. Mittens without separations for the thumb may keep patients from resisting care or from pulling out tubes (Eames et al., 1990). A floor bed (a mattress on the floor that is surrounded by portable walls lined with therapy mats) allows the patient to move freely in bed without risk of falling (Eames et al.). Extensions to the wheelchair so that it can neither tip over backward nor fit through doorways also allow for safe mobility (Eames et al.).
- Engage the patient in gross motor activities such as face washing, catching a ball, hitting a balloon, putting on simple clothing, if he or she is able (Scott & Dow, 1995). Physical activity, walking, or even being wheeled in the wheelchair may help decrease agitation (Baggerly, 1986).
- Be prepared to change activity at the first sign that the patient is becoming restless or agitated. Consider moving to another environment or offering a drink or snack if the patient has normal oral motor activity (Scott & Dow, 1995). Avoid responding to obscenities or bizarre verbalizations; simply view them as cues to distract the patient with another activity.
- Exude calm, confidence, and acceptance; the patient needs you to provide consistency and predictability that counters his or her confusion.

(Scott & Dow, 1995). Posttraumatic **agitation** is reported to occur in the acute setting in 33–50% of patients with TBI (Sandel et al., 1998) and may last for days or weeks (Malkamus et al., 1980). Agitation is a subtype of delirium unique to survivors of TBI in altered states of consciousness. Agitation causes excesses of behavior that include some combination of aggression, akathisia (motor restlessness or a sense of inner restlessness [Ivanhoe & Bontke, 1996]), disinhibition, and emotional lability (COMBI, 2000; Sandel et al.).

Behavioral disorders associated with TBI have distinct causes and characteristics at various points of recovery (Eames et al., 1990). Eames et al. suggested that efforts to manage behavior be preceded by a contextual assessment in which clinicians attempt to determine what factors are contributing to the problem. Clinicians examine the following variables:

- Personal context—extent and location of brain damage, state of bodily dysfunction, including pain, and premorbid factors such as intellect, personality traits, and coping style

- Social context—persons present during maladaptive behavior; reinforcers
- Physical context—properties of the environment in which problematic behavior occurs

During the period of medical instability, patients may exhibit agitation that stems from posttraumatic confusion and inability to process information (Eames et al., 1990). Patients may demonstrate apparently non–goal directed body movements, such as thrashing; goal-directed behaviors, such as trying to remove life-sustaining tubes or get out of bed; screaming, moaning, or bizarre verbalizations; disinhibited behavior, such as uncontrolled laughter or inappropriate sexual behavior (Eames et al.). The primary aim of behavior management at this phase is to ensure the continuation of medically necessary treatment and to do as little as possible to impede the natural course of recovery (Eames et al.). Box 39-6 has specific suggestions regarding management of agitation during occupational therapy sessions.

Family Support and Education. TBI has almost as many implications for family members as it does for the patient. After a loved one undergoes a severe TBI, family members are typically relieved that the patient has survived but have little experience to help them understand the situation or what lies ahead (Phipps et al., 1997). Television portrayals of people who abruptly "wake" from coma with no apparent deficits may lead families to expect full recovery, and they may have difficulty processing information that is inconsistent with that hope (Phipps et al.). Families of patients with severe TBI, specifically those in coma or a vegetative or minimally responsive state, need support and education from the entire rehabilitation team.

Many families relish the opportunity to contribute to their loved one's recovery. They support the therapist's efforts to position the patient and learn to perform PROM exercises. Family members also make important contributions to the sensory stimulation program by providing information about the patient's preferences, typical manner of responding, and background. They may also receive instruction so they can perform the sensory stimulation protocol and collect data on responses. Families often see a level of responsiveness that is not verifiable by staff, and early in recovery, they tend to interpret unresponsiveness in ways other than as a reflection of cognitive status, such as deafness, lack of interest, or laziness (Phipps et al., 1997). Because the patient's level of responsiveness often drives decisions about what services are appropriate, how long they will be provided, and whether the patient is making progress, tension between the overwhelmed family and rehabilitation team is fairly common (Phipps et al.). By providing the family with clear and concise information that matches their most immediate concerns, therapists can help families begin to understand what has happened in ways that neither inflame expectations nor squelch hope.

Holland and Shigaki (1998) proposed a three-phase model for educating families and caretakers of persons with TBI. They suggested that families benefit from information that is relevant to the patient's stage of recovery and their own stage of adjustment. They recommended that during the first phase (ICU through acute hospitalization), family education should focus on providing basic orientation to help the family decipher what is unfolding and to clarify terms and procedures associated with trauma care and TBI. Family members also need help to understand the disordered and occasionally bizarre behavior associated with agitation and to appreciate it as a natural part of recovery (Eames et al., 1990). Finally, conversations and instructions have to be repeated frequently, as the family is under considerable stress and flux (Livingston, 1990). (See Holland and Shigaki's excellent bibliography of phase-specific materials available for families, some of which are in Spanish.)

Rehabilitation

> "My occupational therapist (OT) has promised to take me to the hospital chapel to play the organ. My mom brought my organ books to the hospital.... Now I can show the therapists that I don't need their exercises ... [and] don't belong here in the hospital."
> (Rain, 2000, p. 6)

Rehabilitation occurs in inpatient, outpatient, and residential settings for weeks, months, or years, though not continuously, until goals are achieved and/or the patient no longer appears to benefit from intervention. In general, the primary goals of inpatient rehabilitation are medical stability, reduction of physical impairments, and acquisition of basic self-care skills. Postacute rehabilitation emphasizes reducing the obstacles of community integration posed by cognitive and behavioral impairments (Malec et al., 2000). However, because of decreases in lengths of stay, often due to expiration of funding, many patients are discharged from inpatient rehabilitation settings without realizing their potential to recover capacities and basic skills (Yody & Strauss, 1999). Postacute rehabilitation therefore increasingly addresses medical needs, fundamental capacities, and basic skill acquisition before or instead of community reentry (Yody & Strauss).

Inpatient Rehabilitation

Patients can fully participate in intensive inpatient rehabilitation when they demonstrate stimulus-specific responses and when posttraumatic confusion and agitation either resolve or do not present a barrier to participation in intensive therapies, such as Rancho levels V and VI. At level V, patients are still disoriented and confused but increasingly goal directed (Heinemann et al., 1990) and capable of teaching–learning interactions (Abreu & Toglia, 1987). They cannot process information at a normal rate or produce an appropriate response to all environmental situations (Scott & Dow, 1995). A patient at this level may require maximum assistance for independent living skills, exhibit significant neuromuscular impairments, need maximum cueing for orientation, display severe memory impairment, possibly show confused verbal and mental processes, and have little carryover of new learning (Scott & Dow). As patients progress to Rancho level VI, they remain inconsistently oriented but begin to be aware of appropriate responses to staff and family and demonstrate carryover for relearned, familiar tasks (Hagen, 1998).

The value and effectiveness of inpatient rehabilitation are generally recognized by providers, consumers, and payers. Najenson et al. (1974) studied the outcome of 169 patients with severe brain injury who underwent a program using postural reflexes, self-care tasks, locomotor tasks, and communication training. The statistics showed that 84% of the patients were independent in daily living skills at discharge. The authors found recovery continuing up to 3 years after injury and stressed the need for continued follow-up of these patients after discharge from a rehabilitation hospital. Gerstenbrand (1972) described a rehabilitation program beginning in the acute stage after trauma that included use of reflexes to influence muscle tone and more active mobilization and socialization techniques later. He briefly stated the results for 170 patients in terms of being back at work and concluded that rehabilitation at full intensity was essential. Cope and Hall (1982) studied two groups of patients with severe brain injuries and compared the time required for rehabilitation and the outcome. The first group were admitted for rehabilitation less than 35 days post injury, and the second were admitted more than 35 days post injury. The researchers concluded that those admitted later required twice as much rehabilitation as those admitted early, despite similar severity of initial injury. Outcome 2 years post injury, however, was not significantly different between groups. Finally, Heinemann et al. (1990) demonstrated that persons with moderate to severe TBI who received inpatient rehabilitation improved in self-care and mobility skills and maintained those gains at follow-up.

Assessment: Inpatient Rehabilitation

Patients with TBI who are in rehabilitation can participate in formal assessment. Occupational therapists often begin by screening vision, visual perception, and cognition. Chapters 7 and 8 detail numerous assessment tools and methods appropriate for persons at this phase of recovery from TBI, such as the *Galveston Orientation and Amnesia Test* (Levin et al., 1979), *Loewenstein Occupational Therapy Cognitive Assessment* (Katz et al., 1989), and the *Patient Competency Rating Scale* (Prigatano et al., 1986). Clinicians must determine the extent to which patients can scan, attend, follow and retain instructions in order to interpret performance on other traditional assessments, including upper extremity strength and function and activities of daily living. A number of tools developed specifically to assess patients with TBI are used in a variety of rehabilitation disciplines, including occupational therapy (Table 39-4). Others are detailed at www.tbims.org/combi.

TABLE 39-4

Valid and Reliable Assessment and Outcomes Tools for TBI Patients in Rehabilitation

Instrument	Brief Description
Supervision Rating Scale (SRS)[a] (Boake, 1996)	Measures level of supervision patient receives from caregivers. Based on interviews with patient and caregiver (such as nurse or family member), clinician rates on 13-point ordinal scale reflecting intensity and duration of supervision needed for safety. Ratings automatically sort patient into one of five levels of supervision: independent, overnight supervision, part-time supervision, full-time indirect supervision, full-time direct supervision.
Functional Assessment Measure[a] (Hall, 1997)	12-item addition to *FIM*; relates to community functioning (i.e., car transfers, employability, adjustment to limitations, swallowing). Makes *FIM* more sensitive to the problems of persons with TBI.
Neurobehavioral Rating Scale (Levin et al., 1987)	27-item clinical rating scale measures common cognitive, behavioral, and emotional disturbances associated with TBI; used to track neurobehavioral recovery, measure behavioral change in response to intervention.
Mayo-Portland Adaptability Inventory[a] (Malec & Thompson, 1994)	Designed for interdisciplinary postacute rehabilitation; covers broad range of observable attributes, such as physical function (including pain and mobility), cognitive capacity, emotional status, social behavior, self-care, work, driving status. Based on team consensus, patient's status on 30 items is rated on a 4-category scale: no impairment; impairment on clinical examination but does not interfere with everyday function; impairment does interfere with everyday function; complete or nearly complete loss of function.
Community Integration Questionnaire[a] (Willer et al., 1994).	15-item instrument to assess home integration, social integration, productivity (employment, volunteer work, school); can be completed by self-report with assistance from family member.

[a]Available online at http://www.tbms.org/combi.
FIM, Functional Independence Measure.

Case Example

MR. R.: OCCUPATIONAL THERAPY DURING ACUTE AND REHABILITATION PHASES OF RECOVERY FROM SEVERE TBI

Patient Information

Mr. R. is a 20-year-old college student who sustained a TBI in a motor vehicle accident. Prior to the accident, Mr. R. was a physics major described by family as dependable and hard-working, with a 3.8 grade point average during his first 2 years of college. In addition to his course work, Mr. R. worked 16 hours a week as a dishwasher in his dormitory. According to his parents and older sister, Mr. R. tends to be quiet and soft-spoken but enjoys the company of a small circle of friends. Leisure interests include golf, cross-country skiing, and playing piano.

Examination in the emergency department revealed a laceration over his forehead and right pneumothorax. His blood alcohol level was 0.226 (more than twice the legal limit). He had an initial *Glasgow Coma Scale* score of 3. Intracranial pressure was elevated. He sustained facial fractures and an undisplaced right suprapubic ramus fracture. Serial CT demonstrated diffuse axonal injury, edema, and right posterior temporoparietal intraparenchymal hemorrhage. Within the first week of the TBI, a tracheostomy and feeding tube were inserted, and shortly thereafter Mr. R. underwent open reduction and internal fixation of the right zygomatic maxillary complex fracture.

Occupational and physical therapy were initiated 2 weeks post injury, with orders for range of motion, positioning, and sensory stimulation 2 days prior to his transfer from ICU to a medical unit. PROM was within normal limits for all extremities; muscle tone was unremarkable. Mr. R. at first did not speak and did not follow commands consistently. Mr. R. was frequently observed to thrash around, primarily moving his left side, and at times his movement appeared purposeful (pulling at tubes, seeming to scratch his right leg with his left foot). He appeared to track objects with his left eye inconsistently. His initial total score on the *Western Neuro Sensory Stimulation Profile* was 23, and he was believed to be functioning at a Rancho level II to III (increasingly responsive to specific stimuli).

Reason for Referral to Occupational Therapy

Mr. R. was transferred to the inpatient brain injury rehabilitation unit and was again referred to occupational therapy and to physical therapy, speech–language pathology, neuropsychology 3 weeks post injury. He was referred to occupational therapy to determine whether an integrated sensory stimulation program would promote recovery and enable him to participate in intensive rehabilitation. Consistent with his acute hospitalization, a family member (typically his mother) was present at most therapy sessions.

Occupational Therapy Problem List

▶ Decreased arousal and attention. During assessment Mr. R. sustained eye contact less than 25% of the time and was awake for approximately 10 minutes of each session.

▶ Decreased and inconsistent visual tracking. During assessment Mr. R. horizontally tracked across midline with both eyes approximately 50% of the time and tracked vertically in one direction somewhat less.

▶ Inability to follow commands consistently. During assessment Mr. R. followed gross motor commands approximately 10% of the time.

▶ Decreased right upper extremity function. Minimal formal assessment of Mr. R.'s right upper extremity function was performed, but he was observed to not use or move it.

▶ Dependence in activities of daily living (ADL). During assessment it was evident that Mr. R. could not contribute to any aspect of ADL.

Initial Occupational Therapy Goal List

Because it was difficult to predict the patient's rate of recovery or response to therapy, the team set goals for 2-week intervals, with the understanding that the patient's length of stay on the rehabilitation unit would be dictated by his apparent ability to profit from intervention. Meanwhile, the patient's family was exploring possible discharge options—to home for continued home-based services or to a subacute rehabilitation facility.

1. Mr. R. will stay awake for two 15-minute sessions per day, demonstrating sensory-specific responses to visual and auditory stimuli 50% of the time.
2. Mr. R. will respond to one-step commands at least 33% of the time, such as during light hygiene activities.
3. Mr. R. will safely sit upright during occupational therapy sessions with proper wheelchair positioning.
4. Mr. R.'s parents will be able to perform systematic sensory stimulation and track responses on data collection form.

Initial Treatment Plan

Mr. R. was seen three times daily, twice in the therapy clinic, with sessions lasting 10 to 30 minutes as tolerated. He participated in daily light hygiene activities in which, for example, he was instructed to turn on the faucet and was handed a wet washcloth and asked to wash his face. Nursing, occupational therapy, and family collaborated to ensure that Mr. R. was fully dressed each morning. As recommended by the therapist, Mr. R.'s parents brought in pictures of friends and family and posted them in the his room. PROM for the right upper extremity was incorporated into his sensory stimulation program, and efforts were made to elicit automatic upper extremity movement by, for example, challenging Mr. R. to catch or hit a balloon. Mr. R. made steady gains in all areas, so that within 3 weeks of his admission to rehabilitation, he followed one-step commands approximately 50% of the time and participated in morning hygiene activities for 15-minute intervals with ongoing verbal and tactile cues. He was able to feed himself with the utensil in his right hand once the therapist scooped food. He started speaking in short phrases approximately 6 weeks after onset and progressed rapidly to whole sentences, indicating, for example, when he had to go to the bathroom. As Mr. R.'s cognitive recovery progressed, the occupational therapist helped him to gain independence in dressing, grooming, and his upper extremity exercise program and to increase his orientation and attention span.

At the time of discharge, Mr. R. needed supervision with grooming and upper extremity dressing and moderate assistance with lower extremity dressing and bathing. Mr. R.'s mother was taught methods to assist him at home. He was able to walk with a quad cane and moderate assistance; he needed contact guard assistance with standing balance. At discharge he was oriented to person, place, and time, scoring in the normal range on the *Galveston Orientation and Amnesia Test*, and demonstrated at least some degree of session-to-session carryover. The therapist recommended 24-hour supervision because of continued impairments in memory, problem solving, and judgment. He was discharged to his parents' home 2 months post TBI with plans to return for daily therapy in the day hospital program (supervised all-day multidisciplinary therapies with return home each evening).

Analysis of Reasoning

At the time of his transfer to the rehabilitation unit and referral to occupational therapy, Mr. R.'s cognitive status posed the primary barrier to his functioning and therefore dictated the focus and structure of his treatment plan. Motor and ADL activities were means by which the therapist promoted arousal, tracking, responsiveness, and Mr. R.'s ability to follow commands. Learning-based intervention could begin in earnest when Mr. R. began to demonstrate session-to-session carryover.

Mr. R. was discharged home before he was fully competent in self-maintenance because his parents were able to provide assistance and supervision and because intensive outpatient services were available. The occupational therapy treatment plan during his 3 weeks in the day hospital focused on use of a memory aid and reestablishing competence in instrumental ADL, including light meal preparation, laundry, checkbook management, and bill paying. His living situation contributed to motivation and improved insight more than the insulated experience of the rehabilitation unit. When he no longer required all-day supervision, he was discharged from the day hospital but continued outpatient occupational therapy three times a week.

CLINICAL REASONING
in OT Practice

Occupational Therapy Intervention in the Survivor Phase of Recovery

Mr. R. had a neuropsychological evaluation a year after he sustained the TBI. Results suggested that despite his considerable neurological and behavioral recovery, Mr. R. demonstrated general cerebral dysfunction that affected his information-processing speed, expressive abilities, abstraction, higher-level reasoning, planning, organization, and memory. Mr. R.'s premorbid attributes, such as above-average intelligence and diligence, appeared to contribute to his recovery, and Mr. R. had plans to reenter college within 2 months of testing. The neuropsychologist advised against this plan, suggesting that Mr. R. allow himself more time to recover and that he further develop compensatory cognitive strategies to optimize the likelihood for successful return to school. The neuropsychologist further recommended that Mr. R. establish connections with a counseling psychologist, anticipating a point when Mr. R.'s expectations to fully resume his career track might clash with his postinjury capabilities. Mr. R. felt that the neuropsychologist was unduly pessimistic, but with encouragement of his parents, he agreed to participate in occupational therapy and at least meet with the counseling psychologist.

Assuming that Mr. R. has not been actively involved in occupational therapy for the past 6 months, what assessment tools and methods would you use to guide your treatment plan? What aspects of occupational functioning do you anticipate having to address in treatment?

Treatment: Inpatient Rehabilitation

Occupational therapy during inpatient rehabilitation is aimed at optimizing motor, visual–perceptual, and cognitive capacities and abilities; restoring competence in fundamental self-maintenance tasks; contributing to the patient's continuing behavioral and emotional adaptation; and supporting the patient's family as they prepare for discharge.

Optimizing Motor Capacities and Abilities. Therapists initially help patients optimize their motor capacities and abilities by engaging them in gross motor activities that they

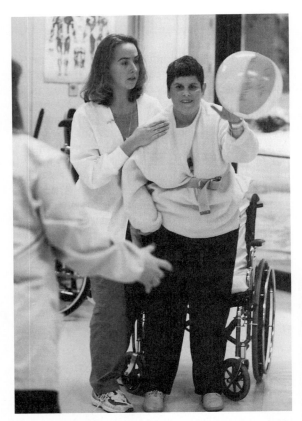

Figure 39-2 Early efforts to optimize motor function focus on eliciting automatic movement. Occupational and physical therapy cotreatment sessions are common.

can perform almost automatically, such as playing catch or hitting a punching bag (Fig. 39-2). Such activities minimize the demands on weakened cognitive capacities, such as attention, concentration, and memory for instructions. Intervention increasingly focuses on refining motor capacities and abilities as the patient's motor and cognitive recovery progress. Occupational therapists use approaches that best match therapy goals and the patient's abilities, many of which are detailed in Chapters 20 to 26.

Optimizing Visual–Perceptual Capacities and Abilities. TBI frequently results in visual–perceptual disturbances that impair occupational function (Bouska & Gallaway, 1991). With TBI, the visual field loss is often in the superior fields; loss of acuity relates to loss of contrast sensitivity; and the oculomotor system is frequently impaired, with poor fixation, deviation of the eyes resulting in diplopia, and difficulty in visual scanning (Scott & Dow, 1995). Limitations in complex visual processing become evident during perceptual evaluation (Warren, 1993). Chapter 7 details specific assessments applicable to patients with TBI. As Quintana

recommends in Chapter 28, intervention for primary visual deficits emphasizes environmental adaptation, compensatory techniques, assistive devices, and patient and family education. It is important to identify possible visual impairments as early as possible so that appropriate patients are referred for ophthalmology assessments and therapists can make an effort to circumvent the influence of visual impairments on performance. The efficacy of perceptual remediation is controversial. Based on her review of research on remedial perceptual retraining, Neistadt was pessimistic about its appropriateness for TBI patients (1994a): "Far and very far transfer from remedial to functional tasks will not occur for clients with diffuse brain injuries and severe cognitive deficits, in either early or late stages of recovery, even with a variety of training tasks and up to 6 weeks of training" (p. 232).

Optimizing Cognitive Capacities and Abilities. Chapter 29 presents four general strategies—remediating the deficit, changing the physical or social context, acquiring behavioral routines, and learning compensatory cognitive strategies—for optimizing cognitive capacities and abilities; all are appropriate for persons with TBI. Inpatients with TBI are typically in a period of relatively rapid improvement, so therapists provide cognitive remediation activities and exercises to challenge and stimulate primary cognitive domains (orientation, attention, memory) in the hope that natural recovery will be enhanced and accelerated. Card or board games, puzzles, and paper-and-pencil tasks, such as word recognition or letter or number cancellation drills, may be used (Scott & Dow, 1995). Computer programs can help retrain the patient's ability to focus attention, increase visual scanning, improve reaction time, improve visual–motor coordination, improve simple problem-solving skills, and increase frustration tolerance. Patients may participate in group treatment, such as an orientation group in which they rehearse and reinforce awareness of date, place, and circumstances.

The effectiveness of cognitive remediation has been questioned (Carney et al., 1999; Salazar et al., 2000), and other methods of optimizing cognitive capacities and abilities should also be employed. For example, occupational therapists often use a dynamic investigative approach (Toglia, 1989) in which cognitive retraining activities become opportunities for assessing performance under a variety of circumstances. Careful activity analysis and logging of observations and environmental variables informs discharge recommendations to families regarding the circumstances in which their loved one is best able to function. Such information is invaluable to families as they assume day-to-day responsibility for structuring the patient's time and activities.

Occupational therapists also use the physical context to optimize patients' cognitive capacities and abilities during this phase of recovery. Specialized brain injury units typically incorporate signage and physical landmarks that enhance orientation and technology, such as monitoring systems, that allow the patient to move even though he or she may be confused and disoriented. Occupational therapists also strategically place familiar pictures and objects, calendars, and clocks in the patient's room to optimize orientation.

Patients in this phase of recovery rarely appreciate the significance and implications of cognitive impairments and therefore are usually not ready to learn to use compensatory cognitive strategies that require initiation and insight. However, occupational therapists often assemble a simple memory log and help patients use it to follow a schedule, reconstruct previous activities and instructions, and remember names of staff.

Restoring Competence in Basic Self-Maintenance Tasks. As previously mentioned, inpatient rehabilitation usually focuses on helping patients reacquire basic self-care skills, such as bathing, dressing, hygiene, and eating. In general, a given self-care task is simplified until the patient is consistently successful in performing it, and then the complexity is gradually increased while the externally provided structure is gradually decreased (Scott & Dow, 1995). Environmental distractions are kept to a minimum. The therapist structures the task, gathers the items to be used, and sequences the task by providing the patient with the appropriate item and instructions, one step at a time. For example, in dressing, the therapist first hands the patient his undershorts and then gives simple verbal instructions and physical assistance as necessary to have the patient put the shorts over his legs and pull them up. The therapist does not present the patient's T-shirt until the shorts are on (Scott & Dow). Initially, the therapist selects solid colors with minimal fastenings to decrease perceptual confusion. The therapist may also choose to limit the task by having the patient do only one or two steps of the entire task (e.g., put on T-shirt only) if the patient has very low endurance, low frustration tolerance, or limited motor skills (Scott & Dow). Selection of the position of the patient (i.e., dressing in bed, sitting in the wheelchair, or sitting on the edge of the bed) and the method of dressing is based on the patient's neuromuscular function (Scott & Dow). Gradually, as the patient becomes more successful in dressing, the therapist decreases verbal and physical cueing, using checklists and/or graded cues (see Chapter 29). Bathing, hygiene training, feeding, and wheelchair transfer training are structured in the same fashion. Occupational therapists can help set the stage for establishing consistent and automatic self-care routines at home by outlining the sequence of steps in which the patient is most successful.

During inpatient rehabilitation, occupational therapists assess the patient's ability to handle other self-maintenance tasks, such as preparing a sandwich, counting and handling money, and using the telephone (Fig. 39-3). Again, a dynamic investigative approach is employed to determine under what circumstances the patient can safely and competently carry out these activities.

Contributing to Behavioral and Emotional Adaptation. Behavioral sequelae may intermittently influence the patient's ability to participate in therapy at this stage. Brain damage itself may cause psychosocial changes, such as irritability, aggressiveness, or apathy (Prigatano, 1992). As the patient becomes more alert, his or her awareness of the situation may increase irritability, uncooperativeness, or mood fluctuations (Scott & Dow, 1995). Patients who lack awareness of deficits may also become frustrated with staff and family who limit their activities. Furthermore, patients who repeatedly fail on a variety of tasks may become depressed or anxious (Prigatano). It is important for occupational therapists to appreciate the state of internal chaos and vulnerability of many patients with TBI at this phase of recovery (Groswasser & Stern, 1998). Without the anchor of intact memory to make connections between experiences, "life is downgraded to a collection of unrelated, disjointed, and sporadic episodes" (Groswasser & Stern, p. 73). Rather than force confrontation of deficits, therapists avoid placing patients in situations that are fraught with frustration and failure and instead structure experiences that reinforce patients' confidence that they still have the potential to accomplish things (Groswasser & Stern). So doing establishes therapeutic trust, the foundation for later phases of

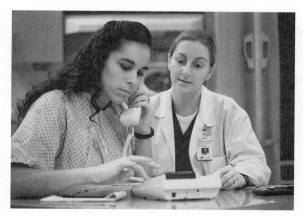

Figure 39-3 Occupational therapists often simulate real-life activities, such as using the telephone book and gathering information over the telephone.

recovery, when patients are better able to compare premorbid and current capabilities. See Chapter 13 for guidelines to establish a therapeutic relationship.

When behavioral sequelae associated with brain injury interfere with progress and the potential for community reintegration, the rehabilitation team establishes an interdisciplinary plan to eliminate socially unacceptable behavior and promote prosocial, adaptive behavior. Eames et al. (1990) pointed out, "Since the primary aim of rehabilitation is a return to the community, simple containment or toleration of disordered behavior within the rehabilitation setting is inadequate because the community at large will not adopt a lenient attitude toward such behavior" (p. 420). These researchers further recommended the following strategies for behavior management during inpatient rehabilitation:

► Manipulate or normalize the environment. For example, if noise and distractions seem to contribute to a patient's irritability and aggressiveness, provide treatment and care in areas that are calm and quiet.
► Identify positive competing behavior, and as a team, consistently and frequently reward all instances of adaptive behavior.
► Withhold all rewards that maintain maladaptive behavior. Use time-outs in a calm, mechanical manner that does not reward the patient with increased social contact.
► Address cognitive impairments that may be contributing to maladaptive behavior.
► Help the patient to learn new skills and to experience success to reduce frustration-induced maladaptive behavior.

Supporting the Patient's Family

Patients' families continue to require information and support to understand the recovery and rehabilitation process and to inform their decision making and discharge planning. Holland and Shigaki (1998) recommended that the rehabilitation team provide the family with information about the following topics: (1) the full spectrum of possible TBI outcomes to enhance realistic expectations; (2) the effects of TBI on family systems and possible alterations in family dynamics post discharge; (3) the benefits, challenges, and responsibilities of caretaking and supervision post discharge; (4) resources available for postacute rehabilitation. Furthermore, by attending occupational therapy treatment sessions, family members encourage their loved one while learning about the patient's strengths and weakness and techniques for helping him or her optimize performance. Participation in inpatient rehabilitation also helps families to frame gains and improvements as continuations of a new start and to minimize expectations of an abrupt

recovery to the "same person" the patient was before the injury (Phipps et al., 1997).

Postacute Rehabilitation

Malec and Basford (1996) described the array of post-acute rehabilitation programs in the literature and possibly available to clients with TBI. (The transition to references to the "client" rather than "patient" signifies the increasingly collaborative therapeutic relationship between therapist and TBI survivor during postacute rehabilitation and survivor phases.) Occupational therapists are typically involved in all of these options, including the following:

► Residential neurobehavioral programs—provide intensive treatment for clients with severe behavioral disturbances
► Residential community reintegration programs—provide integrated cognitive, emotional, behavioral, physical, and vocational rehabilitation to clients who cannot participate in outpatient programs because of severe cognitive and behavioral impairments or lack of availability of outpatient options
► Comprehensive (holistic) day treatment programs—provide integrated, multidisciplinary rehabilitation that emphasizes self-awareness, social skills, and cognitive compensation as precursors to return to work
► Outpatient community reentry programs—provide specific rehabilitation therapies as well as vocational services

Some clients with TBI also receive home-based rehabilitation services.

In their review article comparing outcomes of postacute brain injury rehabilitation with natural recovery after TBI, Malec and Basford (1996) concluded, "Although generally uncontrolled, the studies reviewed document benefits for many individuals with brain injury, including increased independence and a rate of return to independent work or training that exceeds 50% and may reach 60% to 80% for intensive comprehensive (holistic) day treatment programs" (p. 198). Postacute rehabilitation typically is not a continuous sequence of rehabilitation services but more often time-limited, goal-specific series of rehabilitation episodes.

In general, the aim of postacute rehabilitation is to prepare the client to reenter the community, although some programs also offer specialized tracks or pathways that focus on prerequisite physical, behavioral, cognitive, or self-care skills (Abreu et al., 1996). Compensation is emphasized; rarely do these programs focus on deficit remediation. While the occupational therapist's roles and responsibilities vary with the type and even location of the program, this section of the chapter reviews areas that are typically addressed. This section also discusses mild brain injury, as these survivors rarely receive inpatient rehabilitation services.

Occupational Therapy Assessment: Postacute Rehabilitation

Occupational therapists continue to use many of the instruments and methods described earlier in this chapter (Table 39-4) and text. As clients have more real-world experiences and their self-awareness continues to improve, tools like the *Canadian Occupational Performance Measure (COPM)* (Law et al., 1994) become important for identifying treatment goals that are important to the client. Trombly et al. (1998) used the *COPM* to select treatment goals with 16 adults with TBI who were in outpatient occupational therapy and to measure treatment outcome. This instrument, however, is not useful for clients with significant problems with insight and self-awareness, as these individuals are unlikely to view themselves as having problems that can be addressed in therapy (E. S. Davis, personal communication, September 7, 1998). In the aforementioned study, for some clients, progress was marked by self-rated decreases in performance scores at discharge, reflecting improved accuracy of self-appraisal (E. S.

Davis, personal communication, September 7, 1998). See Research Note for further discussion of self-report post brain injury.

Treatment: Postacute Rehabilitation

After discharge from acute rehabilitation, many clients require occupational therapy treatment aimed at teaching them to compensate for residual cognitive and visual–perceptual impairments so that they may resume self-maintenance, self-advancement, and self-enhancement roles.

Optimizing Cognitive Capacities and Abilities. In postacute rehabilitation, clients (usually in Rancho level VII or VIII) may continue to demonstrate specific impairments in short- and long-term memory, reasoning, conceptualization, comprehension, abstract thinking, information processing speed, organization of information, simplification of problems, judgment, and problem solving (Dikmen et al., 1983; Gianutsos, 1980). They may display decreased attention during attempts to store information, inability to determine the salient or relevant details of what they hear or read, decreased ability to structure or associate incoming information appropriately, and decreased cognitive flexibility (Scherzer, 1986). Espe-

---

RESEARCH NOTE

Are Subjective Complaints of Traumatically Brain Injured Patients Reliable?

Sbordone, R. J., Seyranian, G. D., & Ruff, R. M. (1998). Brain Injury, 12, 505–515

ABSTRACT

The complaints of 50 persons with TBI were compared with the report provided by their significant others and then analyzed according to severity of injury and type of complaint (physical, cognitive-behavioral, emotional). Most of the subjects (33 of 50) had severe TBI. Overall, TBI patients complained of significantly fewer problems than their significant others observed. While significant others and persons with TBI tended to agree on the extent of physical problems, persons with TBI rarely complained of cognitive-behavioral or emotional problems. No significant differences were found between the number of subjective complaints reported by patients with mild or moderate TBI and those with severe TBI. Interestingly, however, significant others of patients with severe TBI tended to observe more problems than did significant others of patients with mild or moderate injuries, suggesting even greater underreporting of problems with severe injury. Researchers attribute underreporting of deficits to cerebral trauma and neurologically based lack of self-awareness, as all of the subjects were plaintiffs in personal injury litigation or claimants in a workers' compensation case. In other words, these individuals would stand to gain by overreporting or embellishing their symptoms for financial gain, but in fact they did not appear to do so.

IMPLICATIONS FOR PRACTICE

► During the occupational therapy assessment, the patient's self-report is critical to a holistic client-centered treatment plan. When evaluating patients with TBI, the occupational therapist should consider the possibility they may underreport the cognitive-behavioral and emotional consequences of their injuries.

► Occupational therapists should request input from significant others regarding their observations of TBI patients' cognitive-behavioral and emotional problems and incorporate this information into the assessment.

► Standardized tests can be used to complement patient and significant other reports of cognitive-behavioral problems.

cially if the client also has decreased self-awareness, these impairments will affect his or her ability to make coherent decisions and plan for the future (Scott & Dow, 1995).

Occupational therapists continue to help clients and their families to change the physical and social context to optimize occupational functioning. This may include decreasing stimulus arousal properties and increasing important visual cues at the home and work site to optimize cognitive function. Home and work site visits allow therapists to identify opportunities for these modifications. Also, as clients in postacute rehabilitation have a more stable living situation than they did as inpatients, their occupational therapists can capitalize on consistency of clients' environments and daily activities to help them create routines and habits that minimize the demands of information processing with frequently performed tasks. Occupational therapists also use a variety of activities and exercises, such as computer games, worksheets, crafts and projects, and simulated work tasks, to help clients improve their awareness of strengths and weaknesses. As clients appreciate the significance of residual cognitive impairments and implications for resumption of roles, occupational therapists teach them to use compensatory cognitive strategies, such as day planners, alarm cueing devices, and problem-solving schemata, in the context of personally relevant real world tasks (see Chapter 29).

Optimizing Visual–Perceptual Capacities and Abilities. Similarly, occupational therapists continue to help clients make changes in environment and strategy to circumvent the influence of visual–perceptual impairments. For example, Williams (1995) described occupational therapy intervention for problems with reading and writing of a woman who was more than 12 months post TBI. A comprehensive low vision evaluation performed by an ophthalmologist and occupational therapist revealed adequate central visual acuity, slightly reduced contrast sensitivity, an inferior visual field cut in both eyes, and a dense scotoma bordering the fovea in both eyes. Intervention, which consisted of changes in lighting for reading and writing, oculomotor exercises, and strategy training, ultimately allowed her to resume these valued activities.

Restoring Competence in Self-Maintenance Roles. Clients who have not achieved independence in basic self-care and homemaking tasks continue to work toward those goals in postacute rehabilitation. Giles et al. (1997) used behavioral training to help TBI clients in a transitional living center develop independence in dressing and washing skills in a relatively short period, 11 to 37 days of treatment. Even clients with proficient self-care skills

benefit from treatment that links individual skills to automatic routines (see Chapter 29). Based on performance on the *Rabideau Kitchen Evaluation—Revised* (Neistadt, 1992), Neistadt (1994b) used a meal preparation protocol to help outpatients with TBI learn to prepare a hot beverage and snack. After three 30-minute sessions per week for 6 weeks, participants made gains reflecting improvements in independence and decreased their performance times. Intervention specific to self-care and homemaking always involves input from family and/or caregivers and measures to ensure transfer of newly acquired skills to the client's living environment.

When client and family are satisfied with the client's ability to perform physical daily living skills and homemaking tasks, such as cleaning, meal preparation, and laundry, occupational therapy addresses community and necessary survival skills (Scott & Dow, 1995). Many clients rely on occupational therapy to help them relearn to manage money, write checks, go shopping, use the bank and post office, move in crowds, handle architectural barriers, and use public transportation, the telephone, the newspaper, and the phone book (Scott & Dow). To do so, clinicians again adapt the environment, help clients acquire behavioral routines, and teach clients to use compensatory strategies.

The therapist must carefully assess the amount of supervision and structuring necessary because of impaired judgment and problem-solving ability. The client's ability to bend over and get something from a lower cupboard, climb on an escalator, cross the street safely, organize time adequately, manage finances, and interact with others in a functional manner factor into occupational therapy recommendations regarding the need for continuing assistance or supervision (Scott & Dow, 1995).

Almost as soon as they are discharged from the hospital, many survivors of TBI inquire about their readiness to drive. The client's residual physical, cognitive, perceptual, and visual dysfunction must be thoroughly assessed to determine his or her ability to drive safely. The client's psychosocial status, including self-control, impulse control, and frustration tolerance, must be also carefully considered. A complete history of the medical status, current medications, and driving record is also taken. Simulated driving on a computer is helpful if available. A car can be adapted to compensate for some physical problems (see Chapter 31), and the client can be trained to compensate for visual field neglect (Scott & Dow, 1995). However, no compensation can be made for slowed reaction to emergencies, lack of judgment or problem-solving ability, spatial or directional confusion on the road, impairment in depth perception, or decreased endurance (Jones et al., 1983;

McNeny, 1990). Following evaluation, if the client appears suitable for driving, an on-the-road test covering all driving situations is performed in a dual-control car or the patient's own car, with the assistance of an adaptive driving instructor (Jones et al.). The therapist performing a driving evaluation should be familiar with the department of motor vehicle regulations applicable in that state.

Restoring Competence in Self-Enhancement and Self-Advancement Roles. Occupational therapy plays an important role on the postacute rehabilitation team by helping the client resume previous leisure activities or determine new leisure outlets that are more in line with current abilities. Because lack of initiative and cognitive inflexibility may hinder independence in play and leisure skill, occupational therapists teach clients to use planning and structuring strategies to ensure an optimal balance in their activities.

Many survivors of TBI have to change not only what they do for fun but also with whom they do it. Few friendships withstand the cognitive, behavioral, and emotional upheaval that comes with TBI. Occupational therapy intervention may focus on helping the client initiate new social contacts, participate in support groups, and reestablish the social skills necessary for maintaining and building a social network. Social skills retraining following severe head injury develops skill in social behaviors and facilitates successful social interactions. In general, behavioral learning methods are the most effective for training severely brain-injured individuals to overcome social skill impairments (Giles & Clark-Wilson, 1993). Treatment typically entails instruction and modeling of the social skill, practicing the skill with feedback, and shaping the skill until it is used correctly (Boake, 1991). For example, Yuen (1997) reported how positive talk training (learning to give compliments) in occupational therapy helped a man who was 20 years post TBI to engage in social interactions that were not riddled with what had become his usual style of negative, sarcastic comments. Gutman (1999) described use of a set of guidelines for occupational therapy to help adult men with TBI to achieve greater satisfaction with male social roles.

Once clients reestablish their competence in self-maintenance roles, they are ready to explore return to work. Postacute occupational therapy facilitates that process with prevocational programs that focus on work behaviors and habits, such as punctuality, thoroughness, response to feedback, and ability to take and use notes. Occupational therapists may also link clients with appropriate volunteer jobs where they can employ newly learned compensatory cognitive strategies and build their endurance and work tolerance. Partridge (1997) described occupational therapy within a prevocational program in which therapists assessed clients with TBI in terms of aptitudes and vocational interests and helped them establish realistic vocational goals and action plans.

Contributing to Behavioral and Emotional Adaptation. As clients attempt to resume familiar activities, they cannot escape the awareness that they have changed in some manner (Groswasser & Stern, 1998). Emotional and behavioral difficulties can be attributed to premorbid personality and coping style, cognitive consequences of TBI, and/or grief associated with injury-related losses (Hanks et al., 1999). These emotional and behavioral changes may include social or sexual disinhibition, low tolerance for frustration or stress, reduced insight or judgment, labile affect, irritability, impulsivity, and depression (Jorge et al., 1993; Scott & Dow, 1995). In the extreme, the patient may have paranoia, phobias, confusion, or delusional ideation (Benton, 1979; Brink et al., 1980). Regardless of the specific goals of therapy, occupational therapists support and guide clients with TBI as the clients confront and address impairments and inefficiencies that interfere with performance. Clinicians maintain dual roles as reassuring companion and objective observer by providing sensitive and timely feedback regarding behaviors that could otherwise result in rejection and social isolation in the community. Occupational therapists also respond to indicators that clients may be in need of psychological or psychiatric intervention and make referrals as needed (see Chapters 9 and 35).

Supporting the Client's Family. In most cases, the client's family ultimately provides long-term assistance and support for the survivor, and the family's stresses apparently do not decrease over time as do the stresses related to other traumatic injuries (Muir et al., 1990). As time passes and the client moves through the rehabilitation continuum, the implications of the injury become clearer, and many families feel losses as "partial death" (Muir et al., 1990, p. 436). The person they knew, loved, and depended on to fulfill their expectations is "dead," and long-established roles within the family have changed. Since the course of recovery is unknown (filled with hope, euphoria, and despair), family members undergo mourning that is intense, disorganized, and prolonged (Muir et al.).

Many roles within a marriage change when a spouse has a TBI, including roles as provider and parent. Less discussed are changes in sexual roles because of primary and/or secondary sexual dysfunctions (Griffith et al., 1990). Primary sexual dysfunctions result directly from the brain injury and resultant neural or endocrine disorders influencing sexual interest, activity, responses, and fertility (Griffith et al.). For example, sexual activities may be altered or inhibited by any of a number of motor or sensory disorders, such as hypertonicity or apraxia (Griffith et al.). Secondary sexual dysfunctions—disturbances of psychosocial abilities or sexual responses because of cognitive impairments and psychological reactions—range from hypersexuality syndromes to total apathy and inactivity (Griffith et al.). Partners with TBI may exhibit disinhibited behaviors that are inappropriately provocative or seductive or break unwritten rules regarding personal space and touching (Gronwall et al., 1998). Forgetfulness regarding aspects of personal hygiene further add to the distance and even engender repulsion between previously affectionate partners. Occupational therapists can help clients and their partners resume satisfying sexual roles, first by being willing to discuss matters of intimacy and sexuality. Couples may be referred for medical assessment of primary sexual dysfunctions and counseling for some aspects of secondary sexual dysfunctions. Inappropriate social and sexual behaviors should be addressed in a deliberate and consistent manner by the rehabilitation team.

Finally, occupational therapists continue to support families by providing education. Holland and Shigaki (1998) recommended emphasis on these topics in family education at this phase of recovery and adaptation:

(1) the protracted nature of TBI recovery, (2) the experience of recovery from the patient's perspective, (3) adjustment to and possible management of behavioral and personality changes, (4) sexuality issues, (5) community resources, and (6) home adaptation.

Mild Brain Injury

It is estimated that each year more than a million people in the United States undergo a mild brain injury (Ruff et al., 1996). Mild brain injury has been defined as a traumatically induced physiological disruption of brain function as manifested by at least one of the following: any period of loss of consciousness, any loss of memory of events immediately before or after the accident, any alteration in mental state at the time of the accident, and focal neurological deficits that may or may not be transient (American Congress of Rehabilitation Medicine [ACRM], 1995a). Symptoms of mild brain injury include nausea, dizziness, headache, blurred vision, cognitive deficits, and behavioral changes (ACRM, 1995a). Most people with a mild brain injury return to normal functioning within 1 to 3 months (Ruff et al.). However, approximately 10% of patients continue to have problems a year after injury (Ruff et al.).

Montgomery (1995) described a multifactor explanation for disability after mild TBI. He suggested that personal factors (perfectionism or tendency toward

Case Example

DR. N.: OCCUPATIONAL THERAPY INTERVENTION AFTER MILD TBI

Patient Information

Dr. N. is a 29-year-old single woman who sustained a mild TBI when she fell off her bicycle; she was not wearing a helmet. She reports that she did not lose consciousness and her *Glasgow Coma Scale* score in the emergency department was 13. She was hospitalized for 5 days with a hemorrhagic contusion to the right temporal lobe, a small epidural hematoma over the right occipital region, and significant headaches. Dr. N. returned to work 2 days after her hospital discharge despite continued headaches and balance and memory problems.

Dr. N. has a degree in biochemistry and works as a postdoctoral fellow at a university. Her parents and four siblings reside in another state, and she lives with her significant other of 4 years.

Dr. N. participated in neuropsychological assessment approximately 6 months post injury because cognitive inefficiencies continued to interfere with her function, especially at work. Findings suggested mild impairment for recent verbal

and nonverbal memory and subtle impairment for executive abilities. These cognitive changes contributed to decreased efficiency at work (slowness in problem solving, needing to reread professional literature, frequent note taking). Furthermore, Dr. N. was anxious and depressed. She reported difficulty falling asleep despite overwhelming fatigue. She worried about whether or not she had completed intended tasks, checking and double-checking herself throughout the day. She described herself as easily frustrated, lacking confidence, and overdependent on her significant other. She continued to have headaches approximately 4 days a week. The neuropsychologist expected Dr. N. to maintain her job successfully and pursue premorbid career goals with assistance in adjusting self-expectations and information processing habits.

Reason for Referral to Occupational Therapy

Dr. N. was referred to occupational therapy for assistance in developing compensatory cognitive strategies and behavioral routines that would improve her efficiency at home and work. She was also referred to a psychologist for support and biofeedback to help her manage her headaches.

Occupational Therapy Problem List

► Misattributions and misperceptions regarding personal competence: Dr. N. did not link distracters such as headache and fatigue to episodes of memory failure and absent-mindedness or understand the implications of a limited working memory.
► Inadequate use of external information processing strategies: Dr. N. started writing lots of notes to herself but did not store or refer to them in a systematic manner; she worked off a mental plan each day but could not set priorities among multiple tasks.
► Disruption of personal routines, especially surrounding bedtime: Dr. N. napped for 2 hours after work and spent the evening on household tasks.

Occupational Therapy Goal List

The anticipated length of treatment was four to six sessions.

1. Dr. N. will independently employ compensatory cognitive strategies to increase her effectiveness and efficiency with work and personal tasks.
2. Dr. N. will make changes in her daily routine that contribute to improved balance among work, leisure, and rest.

Treatment Plan

Dr. N. participated in five treatment sessions over 3 months, attending weekly sessions for 3 weeks and two follow-up sessions over 6 weeks. As cognitive inefficiencies were reframed as partly consequences of a working memory overload related to stress and the distraction of physical symptoms, Dr. N. eagerly explored methods to decrease the demands on internal information processing. She purchased a day planner and with input from the therapist established daily and weekly planning routines. Daily and weekly plans helped her set priorities among tasks and allocate time for leisure. She experimented with establishing routines for certain aspects of her "typical" day, scheduling breaks and allocating tasks with low cognitive demands to periods when her energy tended to be low. Her after-work routine changed as well: she set the timer to take a 20- to 30-minute nap followed by a 30-minute walk. She also established a bedtime wind-down routine that ultimately decreased the amount of time she needed to fall asleep.

Analysis of Reasoning

Dr. N. had relatively mild or subtle impairments that changed her cognitive capacity. Similar to many bright individuals, Dr. N. had never thought about her own thinking strategies and did not have a broad repertoire of techniques or habits of mind that she could default to. Furthermore, in her attempts to understand changes resulting from her injury and their implications, Dr. N. failed to appreciate the cumulative effect that subtle impairments, stress, reliance on premorbid cognitive strategies, and distractions associated with pain exerted on her information processing. She was relieved to learn she was not "losing it" and quickly engaged in problem solving with the occupational therapist regarding possible changes in strategies and routines that would buoy her everyday performance. Her relatively brief involvement in treatment shows the benefit of holistic occupational therapy services in dramatically improving an individual's occupational functioning and quality of life.

CLINICAL REASONING
in OT Practice

Implications of Severity of TBI on Treatment Planning

Because Dr. N.'s cognitive impairments were relatively mild, she was aware of cognitive changes and able to learn information-processing principles and independently apply them in novel situations. Explain how the treatment plan would likely change if Dr. N. had sustained a moderate or severe TBI. How might Dr. N.'s cognitive profile be different? What would be the implications in terms of therapist's role, treatment methods, length of treatment, and outcome expectations?

---

negative thinking) interact with transient sequelae of mild brain injury, such as headache and mental inefficiency, that lead to short-term decrements in performance. Premature resumption of normal activities places an undue load on information processing capacities that leads to errors and slowness of performance. Over time, the individual begins to make misattributions of causation, questioning his or her fundamental competence, even sanity (Montgomery). These individuals profit from outpatient rehabilitation services that address residual physical symptoms, provide information and support, and teach them to use cognitive compensatory strategies that decrease the demands on working memory. By normalizing and explaining cognitive inefficiencies, helping reestablish routines, and teaching use of memory backups such as day planners, occupational therapists can play a pivotal role in helping these clients resume premorbid tasks and roles.

Survivorship

"I have been living with multiple effects of a severe TBI for 23 years . . . . Many of these years were spent in lonely isolation, wondering when the nightmare would end . . . . Now, I am focusing my energy on reaching out as well as within to live this life."

(Rain, 2000, p. 6)

The medical treatment and rehabilitation phases of life for the survivor are relatively brief compared to the years, even decades, during which he or she will continue to live with the consequences of TBI. Most survivors ultimately achieve independence in self-care skills and recover motor function (Olver et al., 1996), but cognitive, behavioral, and emotional problems are long-term barriers to good quality of life (Klonoff et al., 1986; Koskinen, 1998). Olver et al. compared outcome after TBI 2 years and 5 years post injury for Australian survivors of moderate to severe injury. Survivors improved in terms of independence in self-maintenance tasks but had more complaints about cognitive, behavioral, and emotional issues at 5 years post injury than at 2 years post injury. More than 60% of their subjects 5 years post injury complained of memory problems, fatigue, and irritability; more than 50% reported that they had lost friends and had become more socially isolated. Koskinen (1998) described a similar pattern in her follow-up study of Finnish survivors of severe TBI 10 years post injury. Subjects indicated that the most unsatisfying aspects of their lives were contacts with friends, sexuality, and leisure activities. Neurobehavioral and emotional consequences of TBI had significant effects on both the quality of life of survivors and level of strain felt by family caregivers.

Olver et al. (1996) reported that fewer survivors were working 5 years post injury than 2 years post (50% of the sample employed at 2 years; 40% at 5 years)—a particular concern, as employment appears to be linked to quality of life after TBI (O'Neill et al., 1998). O'Neill et al. found that being employed part- or full-time contributed to survivors' sense of well being, social integration, and pursuit of meaningful home activities. In fact, individuals who worked part-time had fewer unmet needs, were better integrated socially, and more often engaged in home activities than full-time workers, presumably because of more discretionary time and energy.

These long-term and often unmet needs underscore the importance of intermittent long-term rehabilitation services and community resources for persons with TBI. Unfortunately, most rehabilitation services remain medically oriented, focusing heavily—often exclusively—on intervention for physical impairments. Koskinen (1998) reported that survivors with physical deficits received rehabilitation services over a 10-year period, but physically functioning individuals with cognitive, behavioral, or emotional problems had no possibilities for rehabilitation of any kind.

The contrast between need and service availability is particularly disturbing to occupational therapists who have the education and skills to make a difference in the lives of survivors of TBI. For example, Nelson and Lenhart (1996) described a case in which weekly outpatient occupational therapy sessions over 5 months helped a woman who was 5 years post TBI to improve her ability to handle school, household, and social responsibilities. Trombly et al. (1998) found that adults with TBI met self-identified goals in outpatient occupational therapy; 3 of the 16 participants were more than 2 years post injury.

The survivorship phase of life for persons with TBI presents opportunities for clinicians to employ all that is truly unique to occupational therapy, synthesizing the totality of our education, philosophy, and values to enhance occupational functioning in society. Readers are challenged to consider the following ways to poise themselves for action:

► Recommend that a life care plan be prepared for survivors of moderate to severe TBI (Sherer et al., 2000). Based on expert diagnosis and prognosis, a life care plan delineates the services and items required for the current and long-term care of the survivor as well as the costs of these services (Sherer et al., 2000). The life care plan can be used clinically to plan appropriate long-term care, including intermittent follow-up, and for forensic purposes, such as determination of an appropriate settlement that will provide for the lifetime needs of the injured person (Sherer et al.). In fact, occupational therapists have the background to be credentialed to prepare life care plans for the disabled (K. A. Hobart, personal communication, December 1, 2000).

► Promote to possible referral sources what you as an occupational therapist are able to do to enhance community integration and quality of life for persons with TBI. Join your local brain injury association; connect with your state's vocational rehabilitation division; familiarize yourself with key personnel supporting disabled students at local colleges and universities. Showcase your contribution to clients' occupational function in your documentation. Access resources that will allow you to maintain your expertise (see Resources).

► Establish the kind of therapeutic relationship with clients that will make them want to return to you for help. Respecting the client's readiness for treatment means sometimes not intervening but making sure that he or she knows that your door is open in the future.

► Make sure that the discharge from outpatient occupational therapy incorporates plans for follow-up and clear information regarding possible circumstances in the future when further occupational therapy services may be helpful. Provide information to the survivor and his or her family regarding mechanisms to reinstate services. Remember that the nature of TBI interferes with survivors' ability to advocate for themselves (e.g., lack of initiation, impaired memory), and so you must build in opportunities to discern and respond to their needs.

Summary Review Questions

1. What are some treatment planning implications related to age of onset of TBI? Describe the relevance of the cause of injury, developmental stage, and possible comorbidities.

2. In what ways do occupational therapists use information regarding mechanisms of injury of each patient in the clinical reasoning process? For example, how is the clinical presentation of a diffuse brain injury different from that of a focal brain injury? How can the therapist obtain information about the mechanisms of injury for a given patient?

3. Describe specific ways a patient's preinjury characteristics and background may affect rehabilitation and outcome.

4. Summarize terms used to describe patients in altered states of consciousness and why distinctions between these states are important to the occupational therapist.

5. Analyze the similarities and differences between providing sensory stimulation and managing agitation for a minimally responsive patient.

6. What are some of the frequently cited predictors of prognosis and rehabilitation outcome after TBI? What are the occupational therapy implications of these predictors in planning treatment for patients in terms of goals, length of treatment, and role or needs of the family?

7. Describe the adjustment and adaptation process of the patient with TBI as compared to that of the family. Detail what support and education patients and family members need from occupational therapy during each phase of recovery and adaptation.

8. How might the treatment approach used to optimize cognitive capacities and abilities for an inpatient be different from the treatment approach used in postacute rehabilitation or if the patient returns for services years later?

9. Compare Montgomery's multifactor explanation for disability after mild TBI with your own explanation of disability after severe TBI.

Acknowledgments

The following sections of this chapter were written by Anna Deane Scott and Patricia Weber Dow from *Occupational Therapy for Physical Dysfunction*, 4th edition (1995): mechanisms of injury, prognosis and outcome, bed and wheelchair positioning, passive range of motion, splinting and casting, and driving after TBI. Their material was adapted for use in Boxes 39-4 and 39-5.

Resources

Brain Injury Association (BIA) · Provides information on brain injury, including resources for survivors, families, professionals, and on state BIA associations
http://www.biausa.org

Family Caregiver Alliance · Provides resources for caregivers of individuals with chronic conditions including TBI
http://caregiver.org

Traumatic Brain Injury Model Systems · 17 centers funded by the National Institute on Disability and Rehabilitation Research, National Institute of Health
http://tbims.org

National Institutes of Health Consensus Statement: *Rehabilitation of Persons with Traumatic Brain Injury* · Volume 16, Number 1, October 26-28, 1998. Free copies are available through the NIH Consensus Development Program Information Center, P. O. Box 2577, Kensington, MD 20891
Full bibliography for the NIH Consensus Statement: *Rehabilitation of Persons with TBI*
http://www.nlm.nih.gov/pubs/cbm/tbi.html

Assessment tools used in brain injury rehabilitation available through the Center for Outcomes Measurement in Brain Injury (COMBI)
http://www.tbims.org/combi

Agency for Health Care Policy and Research (AHCPR) Evidence Report/Technology Assessment Number 2, *Traumatic Brain Injury* (AHCPR Publication No. 99-E006). Free copies of this report may be obtained from the AHCPR Clearinghouse by calling 1-800-358-9295 or online at www.ahcpr.gov.

Occupational Therapy Practice Guidelines for Adults with Traumatic Brain Injury (1996) available through the American Occupational Therapy Association (301-652-AOTA)
www.aota.org

References

Abreu, B. C., Seale, G., Podlesack, J., & Hartley, L. (1996). Development of paths of postacute brain injury rehabilitation: Lessons learned. *American Journal of Occupational Therapy, 50,* 417–427.

Abreau, B. C., & Toglia, J. P. (1987). Cognitive rehabilitation: A model for occupational therapy. *American Journal of Occupational Therapy, 41,* 439–448.

Agency for Health Care Policy and Research (1999). *Rehabilitation for Traumatic Brain Injury* (AHCPR publication 99-E006). Rockville, MD: U.S. Public Health Service.

American Congress of Rehabilitation Medicine (1995a). Definition of mild traumatic brain injury. *Journal of Head Trauma Rehabilitation, 8,* 86–87.

American Congress of Rehabilitation Medicine (1995b). Recommendations for use of uniform nomenclature pertinent to patients with severe alterations in consciousness. *Archives of Physical Medicine and Rehabilitation, 76,* 205–209.

Ansell, B. J. (1993). Slow-to-recover patients: Improvement to rehabilitation readiness. *Journal of Head Trauma Rehabilitation, 8*, 88–98.

Ansell, B. J., & Keenan, J. E. (1989). The Western Neuro Sensory Stimulation Profile: A tool for assessing slow to recover head injured patients. *Archives of Physical Medicine and Rehabilitation, 70*, 104–108.

Baggerly, J. (1986). Rehabilitation of the adult with head trauma. *Nursing Clinics of North America, 21*, 577–587.

Bakay, L., & Glasauer, F. E. (1980). *Head injuries*. Boston: Little, Brown.

Benton, A. (1979). Behavioral consequences of closed head injury. In G. L. Odom (Ed.), *Central Nervous System Trauma Research Status Report* (pp. 220–231). Bethesda, MD: National Institute of Neurological and Communicative Disorders and Stroke.

Boake, C. (1991). Social skills training following head injury. In J. S. Kreutzer & P. H. Wehman (Eds.), *Cognitive Rehabilitation for Persons with Traumatic Brain Injury* (pp. 181–189). Baltimore: Paul H. Brookes.

Boake, C. (1996). Supervision rating scale: A measure of functional outcome from brain injury. *Archives of Physical Medicine and Rehabilitation, 77*, 765–772.

Bond, M. R. (1990). Standardized methods of assessing and predicting outcome. In M. Rosenthal, E. R. Griffith, M. R. Bond, & J. D. Miller (Eds.), *Rehabilitation of the Adult and Child With Traumatic Brain Injury* (2nd ed., pp. 59–76). Philadelphia: Davis.

Boortz-Marx, R. (1985). Factors affecting intracranial pressure: A descriptive study. *Journal of Neurosurgical Nursing, 17*, 89–94.

Bouska, M. J., & Gallaway, M. (1991). Primary visual deficits in adults with brain damage: Management in occupational therapy. *Occupational Therapy Practice, 3*, 1–11.

Braakman, R., Gelpke, G. J., Habbema, J. D. F., Maas, A. I. R., & Minderhoud, J. M. (1980). Systematic selection of prognostic features in patients with severe head injury. *Neurosurgery, 6*, 362–370.

Brain Injury Association (2000). *The Costs and Causes of Traumatic Brain Injury*. http://www.biausa.org/costsand.htm.

Brandstater, M. E., Bontke, C. F., Cobble, N. D., & Horn, L. J. (1991). Rehabilitation in brain disorders: 4. Specific disorders. *Archives of Physical Medicine and Rehabilitation, 72*, S332–S340.

Bricolo, A., Turazzi, S., & Feriotti, G. (1980). Prolonged posttraumatic unconsciousness: Therapeutic assets and liabilities. *Journal of Neurosurgery, 52*, 625–634.

Brink, J. D., Imbus, C., & Woo-Sam, J. (1980). Physical recovery after severe closed head trauma in children and adolescents. *Journal of Pediatrics, 97*, 721–727.

Carney, N., Chestnut, R. M., Maynard, H., Mann, N. C., Patterson, P., & Helfand, M. (1999). Effect of cognitive rehabilitation on outcomes for persons with traumatic brain injury: A systematic review. *Journal of Head Trauma Rehabilitation, 14*, 277–307.

Carr, J. H., & Shepherd, R. B. (1980). *Physiotherapy in Disorders of the Brain*. London: Heinemann Medical.

Center for Outcome Measurement in Brain Injury (2000). *List of scales*. http://www.tbims.org/combi/list.html.

Charness, A. L. (1986). *Stroke/Head Injury: A Guide to Functional Outcomes in Physical Therapy Management* (Rehabilitation Institute of Chicago Series). Rockville, MD: Aspen.

Chestnut, R. M., Carney, N., Maynard, H., Mann, N. C., Patterson, P., & Helfand, M. (1999). Summary report: Evidence for the effectiveness of rehabilitation for persons with traumatic brain injury. *Journal of Head Trauma Rehabilitation, 14* (2), 176–188.

Choi, S. C., Narayan, R. K., Anderson, R. L., & Ward, J. D. (1988). Enhanced specificity of prognosis in severe head injury. *Journal of Neurosurgery, 69*, 381–385.

Citta-Pietrolungo, T. J., Alexander, M. A., & Steg, N. L. (1992). Early detection of heterotopic ossification in young patients with traumatic brain injury. *Archives of Physical Medicine and Rehabilitation, 73*, 258–262.

Cope D. N., & Hall, K. (1982). Head injury rehabilitation: Benefit of early intervention. *Archives of Physical Medicine and Rehabilitation, 63*, 433–437.

Corrigan, J. D. (1989). Development of a scale for assessment of agitation following traumatic brain injury. *Journal of Clinical and Experimental Neuropsychology, 11*, 261–277.

Davis, R. A., & Cunningham, P. S. (1984). Prognostic factors in severe head injury. *Surgery, Gynecology and Obstetrics, 159*, 597–604.

Dikmen, S., Reitan, R. M., & Temkin, N. R. (1983). Neuropsychological recovery in head injury. *Archives of Neurology, 40*, 333–338.

Eames, P., Haffey, W. J., & Cope, D. N. (1990). Treatment of behavioral disorders. In M. Rosenthal, E. R. Griffith, M. R. Bond, & J. D. Miller (Eds.), *Rehabilitation of the Adult and Child with Traumatic Brain Injury* (pp. 410–432). Philadelphia: Davis.

Elovic, E., & Antoinette, T. (1996). Epidemiology and primary prevention of traumatic brain injury. In L. J. Horn & N. D. Zasler (Eds.), *Medical Rehabilitation of Traumatic Brain Injury* (pp. 1–28). Philadelphia: Hanley & Belfus.

Farber, S. D. (1982). Neurorehabilitation: A multisensory approach. Philadelphia: Saunders.

Gerstenbrand, F. (1972). The course of restitution of brain injury in the early and late stages and the rehabilitative measures. *Scandinavian Journal of Rehabilitation Medicine, 4*, 85–89.

Giacino, J. T., & Kalmar, K. (1997). The vegetative and minimally conscious states: A comparison of clinical features and functional outcome. *Journal of Head Trauma Rehabilitation, 12*, 36–51.

Giacino, J. T., Kezmarksy, M. A., DeLuca, J., & Cicerone, K. (1991). Monitoring rate of recovery to predict outcome in minimally responsive patients. *Archives of Physical Medicine and Rehabilitation, 72*, 897–901.

Giacino, J. T., Zasler, N. D., Katz, D. I., Kelly, J. P., Rosenberg, J. H., & Filley, C. M. (1997). Development of practice guidelines for assessment and management of the vegetative and minimally conscious states. *Journal of Head Trauma Rehabilitation, 12*, 79–89.

Gianutsos, R. (1980). What is cognitive rehabilitation? *Journal of Rehabilitation, 46*, 36–40.

Giles, G. M., & Clark-Wilson, J. (1993). *Brain Injury Rehabilitation: A Neurofunctional Approach*. San Diego: Singular.

Giles, G. M., Ridley, J. E., Dill, A., & Frye, S. (1997). A consecutive series of adults with brain injury treated with a washing and dressing retraining program. *American Journal of Occupational Therapy, 51*, 256–266.

Greenberg, D. A., Aminoff, M. J., & Simon, R. P. (1993). *Clinical Neurology* (2nd edition). East Norwalk, CT: Appleton & Lange.

Griffith, E. R., Cole, S., & Cole, T. M. (1990). Sexuality and sexual dysfunction. In M. Rosenthal, E. R. Griffith, M. R. Bond, & J. D. Miller (Eds.), *Rehabilitation of the Adult and Child With Traumatic Brain Injury* (pp. 206–224). Philadelphia: Davis.

Gronwall, D., Wrightson, P., & Waddell, P. (1998). *Head Injury: The Facts* (2nd ed.). New York: Oxford University.

Groswasser, Z., & Stern, M. J. (1998). A psychodynamic model of behavior after central nervous system damage. *Journal of Head Trauma Rehabilitation, 13*, 69–79.

Gutman, S. A. (1999). Alleviating gender role strain in adult men with traumatic brain injury: An evaluation of a set of guidelines for occupational therapy. *American Journal of Occupational Therapy, 53*, 101–110.

Hagen, C., Malkmus, D., & Durham, P. (1979). *Levels of Cognitive Functioning, Rehabilitation of the Brain-Injured Adult: Comprehensive Physical Management*. Downey, CA: Professional Staff Association of Rancho Los Amigos Hospital.

Hagen, C. (1998). *Rancho Levels of Cognitive Functioning: The Revised Levels* (3rd ed.) Downey, CA: Rancho Los Amigos Medical Center.

Hall, K. M. (1997). The Functional Assessment Measure. *Journal of Rehabilitation Outcomes Measurement, 1*, 63–65.

Hall, K., Cope, D. N., & Rappaport, M. (1985). Glasgow outcome scale and disability rating scale: Comparative usefulness in following recovery in traumatic head injury. *Archives of Physical Medicine and Rehabilitation, 66,* 35–37.

Hall, K. M., & Johnston, M. V. (1994). Part II: Measurement tools for a nationwide data system. *Archives of Physical Medicine and Rehabilitation, 75,* SC-10–SC-18.

Hanks, R. A., Temkin, N., Machamer, J., & Dikmen, S. S. (1999). Emotional and behavioral adjustment after traumatic brain injury. *Archives of Physical Medicine and Rehabilitation, 80,* 991–997.

Harrison-Felix, C., Newton, C. N., Hall, K. M., & Kreutzer, J. S. (1996). Descriptive findings from the Traumatic Brain Injury Model Systems National Data Base. *Journal of Head Trauma Rehabilitation, 11* (5), 1–14.

Heinemann, A. W., Saghal, V., Cichowski, K., Ginsburg, K., Tuel, S. M., & Betts, H. B. (1990). Functional outcome following traumatic brain injury rehabilitation. *Journal of Neurological Rehabilitation, 4,* 27–37.

Hill, J. (1994). The effects of casting on upper extremity motor disorders after brain injury. *American Journal of Occupational Therapy, 48,* 219–224.

Holland, D., & Shigaki, C. L. (1998). Educating families and caretakers of traumatically brain injured patients in the new health care environment: A three phase model and bibliography. *Brain Injury, 12,* 993–1009.

Ivanhoe, C. B., & Bontke, C. F. (1996). Movement disorders after traumatic brain injury. In L. J. Horn & N. D. Zasler (Eds.), *Medical Rehabilitation of Traumatic Brain Injury* (pp. 395–410). Philadelphia: Hanley & Belfus.

Jennett, B., Snoek, J., Bond, M. R., & Brooks, N. (1981). Disability after severe head injury: Observations on the use of the Glasgow Outcome Scale. *Journal of Neurology, Neurosurgery, and Psychiatry, 44,* 285–293.

Jennett, B., & Teasdale, G. (1981). *Management of Head Injuries.* Philadelphia: Davis.

Jones, R., Giddens, H., & Croft, D. (1983). Assessment and training of brain-damaged drivers. *American Journal of Occupational Therapy, 37,* 754–760.

Jorge, R. E., Robinson, R. G., Arndt, S. V., Starkstein, S. E., Forrester, A. W., & Geisler, F. (1993). Depression following traumatic brain injury: A 1 year longitudinal study. *Journal of Affective Disorders, 27,* 233–243.

Karnaze, D. S., Weiner, J. M., & Marshall, L. F. (1985). Auditory evoked potentials in coma after closed head injury: A clinical-neurophysiological coma scale for predicting outcome. *Neurology, 35,* 1122–1126.

Katz, D. I. (1992). Neuropathology and neurobehavioral recovery from closed head injury. *Journal of Head Trauma Rehabilitation, 1* (2), 1–15.

Katz, N., Itzkovich, M., Averbuch, S., & Elazar, B. (1989). Loewenstein Occupational Therapy Cognitive Assessment (LOTCA) battery for brain-injured patients: Reliability and validity. *American Journal of Occupational Therapy 43,* 184–192.

Kelly, M. P., Johnson, C. T., Knoller, N., Drubach, D. A., & Winslow, M. M. (1997). Substance abuse, traumatic brain injury and neuropsychological outcome. *Brain Injury, 11,* 391–402.

Klonoff, P. S., Snow, W. G., & Costa, L. D. (1986). Quality of life in patients 2 to 4 years after closed head injury. *Neurosurgery, 19,* 735–743.

Koskinen, S. (1998). Quality of life 10 years after a very severe traumatic brain injury (TBI): The perspective of the injured and the closest relative. *Brain Injury, 12,* 631–648.

Law, M., Baptiste, S., McColl, M. A., Carswell, A., Polatajko, H., & Pollock, N. (1994). *Canadian Occupational Performance Measure.* Toronto: Canadian Association of Occupational Therapists.

Leech, R. W., & Shuman, R. M. (1982). *Neuropathology: A Summary for Students.* New York: Harper & Row.

Levin, H. S., High, W. M., Goethe, K. E., Sisson, R. A., Overall, J. E., Rhoades, H. M., Eisenberg, H. M., Kalisky, A., & Gary, H. E. (1987). The Neurobehavioral Rating Scale: Assessment of the behavioral sequelae of head injury by the clinician. *Journal of Neurology, Neurosurgery, and Psychiatry, 50,* 183–193.

Levin, H. S., O'Donnell, V. M., & Grossman, R. G. (1979). *The Galveston Orientation and Amnesia Test. Journal of Nervous and Mental Disease, 167,* 675–684.

Lezak, M. D. (1995). *Neuropsychological Assessment* (3rd ed.). New York: Oxford University.

Lillehei, K. O., & Hoff, J. T. (1985). Advances in the management of closed head injury. *Annals of Emergency Medicine, 14,* 789–795.

Livingston, M. G. (1990). Effect on the family system. In M. Rosenthal, E. R. Griffith, M. R. Bond, J. D. Miller (Eds.), *Rehabilitation of the Adult and Child with Traumatic Brain Injury* (pp. 225–235). Philadelphia: F. A. Davis Company.

Mackay, L. E., Bernstein, B. A., Chapman, P. E., Morgan, A. S., & Milazzo, L. S. (1992). Early intervention in severe head injury: Long term benefits of a formalized program. *Archives of Physical Medicine and Rehabilitation, 73,* 635–641.

Malec, J. F., & Basford, J. S. (1996). Postacute brain injury rehabilitation. *Archives of Physical Medicine and Rehabilitation, 77,* 198–207.

Malec, J. F., Moessner, A. M., Kragness, M., & Lezak, M. D. (2000). Refining a measure of brain injury sequelae to predict postacute rehabilitation outcome: Rating scale analysis of the Mayo-Portland Adaptability Inventory. *Journal of Head Trauma Rehabilitation, 15,* 670–682.

Malec, J. F., & Thompson, J. M. (1994). Relationship of the Mayo-Portland Adaptability Inventory to functional outcome and cognitive performance measures. *Journal of Head Trauma Rehabilitation, 9,* 1–15.

Malkmus, D., Booth, B. J., & Kodimer, C. (1980). *Rehabilitation of the Head Injured Adult: Comprehensive Cognitive Management.* Downey, CA: Professional Staff Association of Rancho Los Amigos Hospital.

Marion, D. W. (1996). Pathophysiology and initial neurosurgical care: Future directions. In L. J. Horn & N. D. Zasler (Eds.), *Medical Rehabilitation of Traumatic Brain Injury* (pp. 29–52). Philadelphia: Hanley & Belfus.

McNeny, R. (1990). Deficits in activities of daily living. In M. Rosenthal, E. R. Griffith, M. R. Bond, & J. D. Miller (Eds.), *Rehabilitation of the Adult and Child With Traumatic Brain Injury* (2nd ed., pp. 193–205). Philadelphia: Davis.

Miller, J. D. (1985). Head injury and brain ischaemia: Implications for therapy. *British Journal of Anaesthesiology, 57,* 120–130.

Miller, J. D., Pentland, B., & Berrol, S. (1990). Early evaluation and management. In M. Rosenthal, E. R. Griffith, M. R. Bond, & J. D. Miller (Eds.), *Rehabilitation of the Adult and Child with Traumatic Brain Injury* (2nd ed., pp. 21–51). Philadelphia: F. A. Davis.

Mitchell, P. H. (1986). Intracranial hypertension: Influence of nursing care activities. *Nursing Clinics of North America, 21,* 563–576.

Montgomery, G. K. (1995). A multi-factor account of disability after brain injury: implications for neuropsychological counselling. *Brain Injury, 9,* 453–469.

Muir, C. A., Rosenthal, M., & Diehl, L. N. (1990). Methods of family intervention. In M. Rosenthal, E. R. Griffith, M. R. Bond, & J. D. Miller (Eds.), *Rehabilitation of the Adult and Child With Traumatic Brain Injury* (pp. 433–448). Philadelphia: Davis.

Mysiw, W. J., Fugate, L. P., & Clinchot, D. M., (1996). Assessment, early rehabilitation intervention, and tertiary prevention. In L. J. Horn and N. D. Zasler (Eds.), *Medical Rehabilitation of Traumatic Brain Injury* (pp. 53–76). Philadelphia: Hanley & Belfus, Inc.

Najenson, T., Mendelson, L., Schechter, I., David, C., Mintz, N., & Grosswasser, Z. (1974). Rehabilitation after severe head injury. *Scandinavian Journal of Rehabilitation Medicine, 6,* 5–14.

National Institutes of Health (1998). *Rehabilitation of Persons with Traumatic Brain Injury. NIH Consensus Statement, 16*(1), 1–41.

Neistadt, M. E. (1992). The Rabideau Kitchen Evaluation—Revised: An assessment of meal preparation skill. *Occupational Therapy Journal of Research, 12,* 242–253.

Neistadt, M. E. (1994a). Perceptual retraining for adults with diffuse brain injury. *American Journal of Occupational Therapy, 48,* 225–233.

Neistadt, M. E. (1994b). A meal preparation treatment protocol for adults with brain injury. *American Journal of Occupational Therapy, 48,* 431–438.

Nelson, D. L., & Lenhart, D. A. (1996). Resumption of outpatient occupational therapy for a young woman five years after traumatic brain injury. *American Journal of Occupational Therapy, 50,* 223–228.

Newlon, P. G., & Greenberg, R. P. (1984). Evoked potentials in severe head injury. *Journal of Trauma, 24,* 61–66.

O'Dell, M. W., Bell, K. R., & Sandel, M. E. (1998). Brain injury rehabilitation. 2. Medical rehabilitation of brain injury. *Archives of Physical Medicine and Rehabilitation, 79,* S-10–S-15.

O'Dell, M. W., & Riggs, R. V. (1996). Management of the minimally responsive patient. In L. J. Horn and N. D. Zasler (Eds.), *Medical Rehabilitation of Traumatic Brain Injury* (pp. 103–131). Philadelphia: Hanley & Belfus.

Olver, J. H., Ponsford, J. L., & Curran, C. A. (1996). Outcome following traumatic brain injury: A comparison between 2 and 5 years after injury. *Brain Injury, 10,* 841–848.

O'Neill, J., Hibbard, M. R., Brown, M., Jaffe, M., Sliwinski, M., Vandergroot, D., & Weiss, M. J. (1998). Quality of life and community integration after traumatic brain injury. *Journal of Head Injury Rehabilitation, 13,* 68–79.

Palmer, M., & Wyness, M. A. (1988). Positioning and handling: Important considerations in the care of the severely head-injured patient. *Journal of Neuroscience Nursing, 20* (1), 42–50.

Partridge, T. (1997). Occupational therapy within a prevocational programme for adults with acquired brain injuries: A case study. *British Journal of Occupational Therapy, 60,* 238–244.

Phipps, E. J., DiPasquale, M., Blitz, C. L., & Whyte, J. (1997). Interpreting responsiveness in persons with severe traumatic brain injury: Beliefs in families and quantitative evaluations. *Journal of Head Trauma Rehabilitation, 12,* 52–69.

Prigatano, G. P. (1992). Personality disturbances associated with traumatic brain injury. *Journal of Consulting and Clinical Psychology, 60,* 360–368.

Prigatano, G. P., Fordyce, D. J., Zeiner, H. K., Rouche, J. R., Pepping, M., & Wood, B. C. (1986). *Neuropsychological Rehabilitation After Brain Injury.* Baltimore, MD: John Hopkins University Press.

Rain (2000). Survivor's voice. *TBI Challenge!, 4,* 6.

Rappaport, M., Dougherty, A. M., Devon, L, & Kelting, B. A. (1992). Evaluation of coma and vegetative states. *Archives of Physical Medicine and Rehabilitation, 73,* 628–634.

Rappaport, M., Hall, K. M., Hopkins, K., Belleza, & Cope, N. A. (1982). Disability Rating Scale for severe head trauma: Coma to Community. *Archives of Physical Medicine and Rehabilitation, 63,* 118–123.

Rinehart, M. A. (1990). Strategies for improving motor performance. In M. Rosenthal, E. R. Griffith, M. R. Bond, & J. D. Miller (Eds.), *Rehabilitation of the Adult and Child with Traumatic Brain Injury,* 2nd edition (pp. 331–350). Philadelphia: F. A. Davis Company.

Rosenthal, M., & Bond, M. R. (1990). Behavioral and psychiatric sequelae. In M. Rosenthal, E. R. Griffith, M. R. Bond, & J. D. Miller (Eds.), *Rehabilitation of the Adult and Child with Traumatic Brain Injury* (pp. 179–192). Philadelphia: F. A. Davis Company.

Ruff, R. M., Camenzuli, L., & Mueller, J. (1996). Miserable minority: Emotional factors that influence the outcome of mild traumatic brain injury. *Brain Injury, 10,* 551–565.

Salazar, A. M., Warden, D. L., Schwab, K., Spector, J., Braverman, S.,

Walter, J., Cole, R., Rosner, M. M., Martin, E. M., Ecklund, J., & Ellenbogen, R. G. (2000). Cognitive rehabilitation for traumatic brain injury: A randomized trial. *Journal of the American Medical Association, 283,* 3075–3081.

Salcman, M., Schepp, R. S., & Ducker, T. B. (1981). Calculated recovery rates in severe head trauma. *Neurosurgery, 8,* 301–308.

Sandel, M. E., Bell, K. R., & Michaud, L. J. (1998). Brain injury rehabilitation. 1. Traumatic brain injury: Prevention, pathophysiology, and outcome prediction. *Archives of Physical Medicine and Rehabilitation, 79,* S-3–S-9.

Satz, P., Zaucha, K., Forney, D. L., McCleary, C., Asarnow, R. F., Light, R., Levin, H., Kelly, D., Bergsneider, M., Hovda, D., Martin, N., Caron, M. J., Namerow, N., & Becker, D. (1998). Neuropsychological, psychosocial and vocational correlates of the *Glasgow Coma Scale* at 6 months post-injury: A study of moderate to severe traumatic brain injury patients. *Brain Injury, 12,* 555–567.

Sbordone, R. J., Seyranian, G.D., & Ruff, R. M. (1998). Are subjective complaints of traumatically brain injured patients reliable? *Brain Injury, 12,* 505–515.

Schaffer, L., Kranzler, L. I., & Siqueira, E. B. (1985). Aspects of evaluation and treatment of head injury. *Neurology Clinics, 3,* 259–273.

Scherzer, B. P. (1986). Rehabilitation following severe head trauma: Results of a three-year program. *Archives of Physical Medicine and Rehabilitation, 67,* 366–374.

Scott, A. D., & Dow, P. W. (1995). Traumatic brain injury. In C.A. Trombly (Ed.), *Occupational Therapy for Physical Dysfunction* (4th ed., pp. 705–733). Baltimore: Williams & Wilkins.

Sherer, M., Madison, C. F., & Hannay, H. J. (2000). A review of outcome after moderate to severe closed head injury with an introduction to life care planning. *Journal of Head Trauma Rehabilitation, 15,* 767–782.

Sparadeo, F. R., & Gill, D. (1989). Focus on clinical research: Effects of prior alcohol use on head injury recovery. *Journal of Head Trauma Rehabilitation, 4* (1), 75–82.

Teasdale, G., & Jennett, B. (1974). Assessment of coma and impaired consciousness: A practical scale. *Lancet, 2,* 81–84.

Thurman, D. J., Alverson, C., Dunn, K. A., Guerrero, J., & Sniezek, J. E. (1999). Traumatic brain injury in the United States: A public health perspective. *Journal of Head Trauma Rehabilitation, 14,* 602–615.

Toglia, J. P. (1989). Approaches to cognitive assessment of the brain-injured adult. *Occupational Therapy Practice, 1,* 36–55.

Trexler, L. E., & Zappala, G. (1988). Neuropathological determinants of acquired attention disorders in traumatic brain injury. *Brain & Cognition, 8,* 291–302.

Trombly, C. A., Radomski, M. V., & Davis, E. S. (1998). Achievement of self-identified goals by adults with traumatic brain injury: Phase I. *American Journal of Occupational Therapy, 52,* 810–818.

Turner, M.S. (1985). Pediatric head injury. *Indiana Medicine, 78,* 194–197.

Warren, M. (1993). A hierarchical model for evaluation and treatment of visual perceptual dysfunction in adult acquired brain injury: Part 1. *American Journal of Occupational Therapy, 47,* 42–54.

Willer, B., Ottenbacher, K. J., & Coud, M. L. (1994). The Community Integration Questionnaire. *American Journal of Physical Medicine and Rehabilitation, 73,* 103–111.

Williams, T. A. (1995). Low vision rehabilitation for a patient with a traumatic brain injury. *American Journal of Occupational Therapy, 49,* 923–926.

Yody, B. B., & Strauss, D. (1999). The effect of decreasing length of stay on long-term TBI patient outcomes. *Journal of Rehabilitation Outcomes Measurement, 3,* 42–50.

Yuen, H. K. (1997). Positive talk training in an adult with traumatic brain injury. *American Journal of Occupational Therapy, 51,* 780–783.

40

Neurodegenerative Diseases

Lois F. Copperman, Susan Jane Forwell, and Lucinda Hugos

LEARNING OBJECTIVES

After studying this chapter, the reader will be able to do the following:

1. Describe four neurodegenerative diseases, including their courses and their symptoms.
2. Describe the occupational therapy approach to addressing neurological complications of human immunodeficiency virus.
3. Select appropriate assessment and evaluation tools for clients with neurodegenerative diseases based on individual clients' characteristics and requirements.
4. Select appropriate interventions for clients with neurodegenerative disease based on individual client's characteristics and requirements.
5. Select appropriate equipment for home, work, and community to help a client with neurodegenerative disease maintain independent function at the highest possible level.

*N*eurodegenerative diseases, such as multiple sclerosis (MS) and Parkinson's disease (PD), amyotrophic lateral sclerosis (ALS), and Guillain Barré syndrome (GBS) are generally chronic and potentially progressive, even fatal. The underlying pathologies of diseases covered in this chapter have mechanisms that attack the peripheral nervous system (PNS) and central nervous system (CNS), resulting in complex and interacting impairments and limitations that affect all aspects of life. Since these diseases commonly affect individuals in the prime of life, interventions may have to address all domains, including employment, community activities and home roles and tasks. Recent research and medical advances have led to new treatments that alter the progressive course of many neurodegenerative diseases and allow people to live longer, more productive lives. However, the underlying diseases are generally not curable, and their causes are only beginning to be understood. Consequently, people with neurodegenerative diseases frequently must cope with both existing impairments and the threat of future losses.

GLOSSARY

Akinesia—Impaired ability to initiate voluntary and spontaneous motor responses, such as the interruption of performance in movement when attention is distracted (e.g., freezing in Parkinson's).

Axon—Process of a neuron that conducts impulses away from the cell body.

Axonal transection—Separation of an axon from its postsynaptic neuron, permanently interrupting action potential propagation.

Bradykinesia—Slowness of body movement.

Cogwheel rigidity—Series of catches in the resistance during passive motion.

Fasciculations—Rapid, flickering twitching movements of a part of a muscle occurring irregularly in time and location.

Muscle atrophy—Reduction in muscle volume and/or size observed as wasting.

Myalgia—Pain in a muscle.

Myelin—Lipid-rich insulating material covering nerve fibers that speeds conduction of impulses.

Neuropathy—Functional disturbance or pathological change in the peripheral nervous system.

Polyneuropathy—Disease involving neuropathies in several nerves.

Rigidity—Hypertonicity of agonist and antagonist muscles that offers a consistent, uniform resistance to passive movement.

This chapter begins with an overview of occupational therapy for persons with neurodegenerative diseases. Broad considerations related to assessment, goal setting, and treatment are reviewed, followed by detailed discussions of MS, PD, ALS, GBS, and also the neurological consequences of human immunodeficiency virus (HIV). The approaches presented for these specific neurodegenerative diseases are applicable to other similar progressive disorders not addressed herein.

Occupational Therapy for Neurodegenerative Diseases

Occupational therapy frequently begins at diagnosis and continues throughout the continuum of comprehensive care. Occupational therapy may take place in inpatient acute care, inpatient rehabilitation, outpatient, in-home, or long-term care settings. Inpatient treatment usually follows a relapse in the disease and/or a crisis. Inpatient acute treatment is generally short and limited to stabilizing symptoms with active medical interventions. Inpatient rehabilitation may last 1 to several weeks, with daily therapy sessions geared to develop new strategies to deal with changed symptoms and to identify and obtain equipment. Outpatient therapy is usually weekly, with 1-hour individual sessions to demonstrate strategies to maximize independence, instruct in home exercise programs, minimize the effects of symptoms on daily activities, and identify and obtain needed equipment.

Occupational therapy in long-term care facilities may be similar to inpatient rehabilitation for people adjusting to changing symptoms or developing palliative care plans for patients whose disease has progressed to the point they cannot be cared for at home.

As neurodegenerative diseases affect most aspects of life, it is imperative for occupational therapy to focus on the activities and occupations that are most relevant, valued, and important to the individual and significant other. Evaluative screens help the therapist to determine which treatable activities are most relevant to the patient and to target these specific areas during assessment. For example, a particular individual may set a high priority on continuing employment and be willing to delegate home and self-care tasks. Assessment and treatment for this person would focus on maximizing independence in activities necessary for work and setting up the support systems needed for home functions. To remain responsive to clients' changing needs and priorities, occupational therapists must also keep an eye on their own coping and objectivity, especially when treating clients whose disease course portends increasing disability or death. Box 40-1 offers suggestions.

Goal Setting

The primary goals of intervention are usually to reduce the effects of disability resulting from disease impairments and to promote maximal independence and quality of life; that is, safe, functional, and comfortable participation in chosen tasks and roles. Because of the unplanned and profound impact of neurodegenerative disease, realistic goal setting is frequently complex, requiring sensitivity, flexibility, and negotiation skills by the therapist. The therapist frequently helps the client modify the behaviors and assumptions of a lifetime while assisting the person to accept realistic new goals. Treatment goals should be flexible and grounded in evidence-based research if possible and acknowledge the probable continuing progression of the disease. Given the progressive nature of many neurodegenerative diseases, regular reassessment, reordering of priorities, and repeated modifications in activities may be necessary.

Treatment

Because of the complexity of the impairments caused by these diseases, intervening in one area may affect several other factors, such as fatigue, pain, and weakness. Interventions are varied and frequently involve significant others, especially as the disease progresses. Here is an overview of ways occupational therapy optimizes performance in key occupational roles for persons with neurodegenerative diseases.

Self-Maintenance Roles

In basic and instrumental activities of daily living, the therapist helps the patient attain safety, maximum independence in priority activities, acceptance and optimal

use of equipment, and energy-conserving participation. Treatment strategies include the following:

▶ Priority setting
▶ Education in areas such as the disease process affecting motor or cognitive changes
▶ Environmental modifications at home and work to promote safety and independence
▶ Exercise such as range of motion to prevent loss of range needed to dress
▶ Behavior modification such as use of energy conservation and time management techniques
▶ Identifying and obtaining equipment to compensate for weakness or other symptoms
▶ Balancing independence with assistance from others

Self-Advancement Roles

The onset of neurodegenerative diseases affects employment in or outside of the home. However, contrary to popular expectations, many individuals can and should continue to work rather than claim disability. Medical treatments affecting disease progression and legislation affecting employment mean that modification of employment is frequently more appropriate than an immediate disability claim. Continued employment has implications for financial independence, health care choices, socialization, and self-esteem. Occupational therapists critically review job expectations and as required, make modifications to the environment, recommend behavioral changes, prescribe equipment, identify resources,

---

BOX 40-1
PROCEDURES FOR PRACTICE

Keys to Avoiding Burnout

Helping persons diagnosed with neurodegenerative diseases is well worthwhile. Occupational therapists can make significant differences in people's lives and help them adjust to difficult circumstances. The following suggestions may help therapists avoid burnout.

▶ Let clients take long-term responsibility for making changes.
▶ Remember that the therapist's role is to give the client tools to manage problems, not cure the disease.
▶ Avoid taking the client's problems home with you, as that will not help the client.
▶ Know the facts about the typical course of neurodegenerative diseases. For example, most people with MS do not end up in a nursing home or even a wheelchair.
▶ Remember that your knowledge of these diseases, medical treatments, and symptom management will make a real

difference to the lives of many people facing difficult problems.
▶ Have realistic expectations of outcomes.
▶ Recognize that neurological research is very promising. Many of these diseases may have a cure in the near future.
▶ Help people stay employed. Work provides financial resources and self-esteem.
▶ Look for short-term gain, not long-term prognosis.
▶ Find or create a team for delivering care to challenging clients.
▶ Get involved in policy making within the department, the profession, or the disease organization.
▶ Vary your schedule with group treatments, a student, a department project, a research project, or teaching a class.

and give recommendations to the individual for the employer. Nonprofit groups such as the National Multiple Sclerosis Society provide resources and are excellent sources of information for both patients and therapists (see Resources).

Self-Enhancement Roles

Maintaining leisure pursuits may be a high priority for individuals with neurodegenerative diseases. Modifications of activities and proper equipment often enable the individual to continue to carry out these important roles.

Specific Neurodegenerative Diseases

The following sections discuss specific neurodegenerative diseases. The first discussion, of MS, is longest and provides the most detailed insights into the clinical reasoning that may be involved in occupational therapy treatment and evaluation for several neurodegenerative disorders. A client with PD who has fatigue, for instance, may benefit from the energy conservation techniques mentioned in the section on MS. However, each neurological disorder has its own underlying pathology, peculiarities, medications, and prognosis. Understanding these issues helps the therapist develop appropriate treatments.

Multiple Sclerosis

MS is the most commonly diagnosed neurological disease that can cause disability in young adults (Stolp-Smith et al., 1997). An estimated 250,000 to 350,000 people in the United States have MS (Kelley, 1996; Anderson et al., 1992). MS causes severe disability in some people, but many continue to lead active and productive lives and are not severely disabled (Stolp-Smith et al.; Rodriguez et al., 1994). Most therapists probably have a skewed perspective, as it is the relatively severely disabled people who typically get referred for therapy. Unfortunately, by the time a person requires wheeled mobility, a tremendous window of opportunity has passed for interventions in ambulation, fatigue management, and employment modifications, among other activities that contribute to quality of life. Therefore, therapists should work to alert physicians to the need for early intervention with persons with MS.

The *multiple* in multiple sclerosis refers to both time and location. The *sclerosis* refers to the hardened, or sclerotic, plaques that are the scar tissue resulting from autoimmune attacks on the white matter (axons and covering myelin). The cause of MS remains unknown. It seems to have an unknown trigger that initiates the autoimmune chain of events in people with genetic susceptibility (Trapp et al., 1998). While this trigger is most likely a virus, none has been positively identified. MS is

considered a neurological disease because of the effects of the damage in the brain and spinal cord. However, it is also an immunological disease because the immune system is activated in response to an initiating trigger.

The CNS **myelin** and **axons** are the targets of the immune response. **Axonal transection** is considered as significant as demyelination in MS damage (Trapp et al., 1998; McGavern et al., 2000). At least temporarily, demyelinated axons may be remyelinated and may still conduct.

Transected axons are permanently destroyed and lose all potential for conduction. At autopsy, Trapp and colleagues (1998) found as many as $11,236 \pm 2775$ transected axons in a cubic millimeter of active lesions in subjects with definite MS compared to 0.7 ± 0.7 in white matter of subjects without brain disease. There is also evidence of continued disease activity even during periods that are clinically quiet (Trapp et al.). The demyelination and axonal damage occur in the presence of inflammation. This may explain the rapid improvement often seen in treatment of relapses with corticosteroid anti-inflammatory agents. Recent pathology research examined actual MS lesions and reported four fundamentally different patterns of demyelination (Lucchinetti et al., 2000). This research suggests that the mechanism and targets of MS may vary between subgroups or stages of MS. There is no cure for MS, but since 1993 drug therapy has slowed its progression (National Multiple Sclerosis Society, 1998).

Diagnosing MS

MS is usually diagnosed when the patient is aged 15 to 50. Peak age of onset is 20 to 30 years. Women are two to three times as likely to get MS as men. Whites of northern European descent have the greatest risk of developing MS (Bourdette, 1997). The incidence of MS increases with distance from the equator, both north and south, similar to the pattern of European settlement (Frankel, 1990; Kurland, 1952). The individual risk is apparently determined by where a person spends the first 15 years of life (Frankel; Alter, 1978) and is about 1:1000 in the United States (Frankel; Hashimoto & Paty, 1986). Having an immediate family member with MS increases the risk to 1:100.

The diagnosis of MS is based on findings of the history, neurological examination, and overall clinical picture. Additional tests, such as analysis of cerebrospinal fluid and magnetic resonance imaging are used only to prove the clinically evident signs and not solely as the basis of the diagnosis. Objective demonstration of two or more white matter lesions in discrete parts of the CNS is necessary to make the diagnosis (Poser et al., 1983). Furthermore, episodes of CNS dysfunction must be reported or demonstrated over time or there must be ongoing progression over 6 months. Finally, there can be no other explanation of these problems. If these criteria are met, the diagnosis of MS is made.

MS can affect any part of the CNS, which results in varied signs and symptoms. The signs and symptoms are a result of inflammation and damage to the myelin covering of neuronal axons and damage to the axons themselves. Impairments include weakness, sensory changes, balance disturbance, visual changes, bowel and bladder disturbance, cognitive changes, dysarthria and dysphagia, dizziness or vertigo, pain, ataxic gait, tremor, sexual dysfunction, depression, spasticity, and fatigue. The most common and pervasive symptom is fatigue (Freal et al., 1984; PVA, 1998). Signs of MS include hyperreflexia, positive Babinski sign, dysmetria, nystagmus, and impaired vibratory or position sensation. The *Expanded Disability Status Scale* (EDSS) (Kurtzke, 1983) is the most commonly used impairment rating instrument utilized by physicians. The presence of several symptoms can readily result in limitations and restrictions such as unemployment and loss of independence.

The Course of MS

The relapsing–remitting course of MS produces clearly defined relapses of acute worsening of neurological function followed by partial or complete improvement and then stable periods of remission between attacks. The term *relapse* is now preferred to *exacerbation*. The most common course of MS at the time of diagnosis, relapsing–remitting MS, often becomes secondary–progressive MS with time (Trapp et al., 1998; Lublin & Reingold, 1996). People with secondary–progressive MS start with a relapsing–remitting course of up to 10 to 15 years following diagnosis. The secondary–progressive diagnosis is typically made when there is continued neurological deterioration. People with primary–progressive MS have continuously declining neurological function from onset (Lublin & Reingold). The fourth main classification of MS is progressive–relapsing (Lublin & Reingold). This differs from relapsing–remitting MS because disease progression continues through the periods between relapses. Two other terms occasionally used to refer to disease classification are benign and malignant (Lublin & Reingold). People with benign MS are fully functional in all their neurological systems 15 years after the disease onset. People with malignant MS have rapid progression leading to significant disability or death in a short period.

Disease-Modifying Medications for MS

Three medications approved for use in the United States have been shown to have positive effects on the disease course: interferon-beta-1a (Avonex); interferon-beta-1b (Betaseron); and glatiramer acetate (Copaxone). They are all approved for treatment of relapsing–remitting disease. Rebif, a fourth medication for relapsing–

remitting MS, is another interferon-beta-1a approved for use in Canada and Europe. These disease-modifying drugs are designed to slow the progression of MS but they are vastly underused (National Multiple Sclerosis Society, 1998). There are many other promising medications for the treatment of MS in human trials. Medications for symptom management, such as Amantadine and Provigil for fatigue and baclofen for spasticity, are typically also necessary.

Clients commonly discuss medications with therapists and ask their opinion on the value of the medications. This is true particularly of MS disease-modifying medications, as they are not designed to improve the patient's condition or reverse disability but rather slow disease progression. Clients often wonder whether it is worth taking the medications when they are not seeing improvement. The therapist's responsibility is to understand and reinforce the importance of continuing to take appropriate medications.

With the increased stability of the disease course that results from these medications, patients may realize greater benefits from rehabilitation intervention, such that they live fuller lives, remain employed, and participate in high-priority activities longer. The costs of these medications may make maintaining employment-related prescription coverage a very desirable outcome of therapy.

Potential Emotional, Social and Economic Consequences

A disease that primarily strikes young adults has substantial economic and employment consequences. Between ages 20 and 40, people typically are entering the labor market, establishing themselves in their careers, and forming families. MS, with its common symptoms of fatigue, weakness, difficulties with prolonged standing or walking, and cognitive problems, can impede productivity both at work and at home. Studies conducted prior to development of disease-modifying medications revealed that more than 70% of individuals with MS were out of the labor force 10 to 15 years after initial diagnosis (Kalb, 1996). However, the influence of disease-modifying drugs, together with employment disability legislation such as the Americans with Disabilities Act, has resulted in opportunities for people to maintain productive paid employment for longer periods. Persons with MS who leave the labor market are likely to have greater social isolation, psychological distress, lower incomes, and more limited access to health insurance than if they had remained employed (Kalb).

The cost of MS to the individual and society is substantial. Although expensive inpatient hospitalizations have been reduced, as most problems are treated in outpatient settings, the total health care costs in the United States averaged $15,122 per person annually in

1994, not including the new disease-modifying medications, which cost approximately $10,000 a year (National Multiple Sclerosis Society, 1998). The average patient's lifetime losses are estimated at $2.2 million in the United States (Kalb, 1996).

Symptoms Typically Addressed in Occupational Therapy

A number of symptoms associated with MS, including fatigue, weakness, cognitive changes, pain, and spasticity, interfere with occupational function.

Fatigue

Fatigue, one of the most common MS symptoms, affects approximately 60–80% of people with MS (PVA, 1998). Fatigue is a main reason people with MS are referred to occupational therapy and a primary contributor to disability. People with MS often report that all of their symptoms tend to worsen when they tire. Fatigue can vary from slight to severe, worsening in the afternoon, and is related to increasing core body temperature. Therapists must be alert to several types of fatigue associated with MS (Box 40-2) (PVA, 1998) and employ multifaceted treatments.

Weakness

Weakness is another common symptom resulting in referral to therapy. Weakness may occur in all parts of the body. One of the most common initial complaints is weakness in the foot dorsiflexors resulting in stumbling or falling, especially on uneven surfaces. Weakness frequently begins in the lower extremities.

Cognition

Approximately 40–60% of people with MS have cognitive problems that vary considerably in severity (Beatty et al., 1995; Rao et al., 1991). Cognitive problems are seen at all

---

BOX 40-2
Types of Fatigue in MS

Primary MS Fatigue
Fatigue directly due to MS disease process. Causation is poorly understood.

Fatigue Due to Poor Sleep
Sleep problems are often related to muscle spasms, depression or urinary problems.

Fatigue Due to Depression

Nerve Fiber or Motor Fatigue
Fatigue probably related to inefficient nerve conduction

Fatigue Due to Impairments, Such as Weakness and Spasticity.

Fatigue Secondary to Medication Side Effects or Infections.

---

stages of the disease and are not directly correlated with motor impairments (Maurelli et al., 1992). Studies have found correlations between cognitive impairments and the extent of brain damage on weighted magnetic resonance brain scans, but the specific locations of lesions do not seem directly related to the type of problem (Rovari et al., 1998; Foong et al., 1997). There is some suggestion that cognitive impairments may be the result of severe widespread damage to the white matter (Rovari et al.). Disease-modifying drugs may slow the progression of cognitive problems (Fischer et al., 2000).

Common cognitive problems of people with MS include word retrieval difficulties; slowed speed of information processing and difficulties learning new material; and problems with attention, concentration, memory, and executive functions, such as diminished judgment, difficulty with abstract reasoning, and reduced verbal fluency organization (National Multiple Sclerosis Society, 1999). Because of the varied locations and severity of MS lesions, people with MS may have other cognitive problems as well. Visual–spatial impairments, for instance, may be reported as a tendency to get lost or a history of motor vehicle accidents.

Cognitive problems are likely to vary somewhat during the day and to increase in the afternoon or when the client is fatigued. The cognitive problems of MS are frequently subtle. Both individuals and their families may be unaware that cognitive problems are related to the disease and are not personality or psychological issues. There is no "MS personality," but executive function problems, such as reduced insight and inflexible thinking, may be mistaken for personality similarities among persons with MS.

Many areas of cognition may remain intact, and screens such as the *Mini-Mental State Exam* are not likely to detect problems (Beatty & Goodkin, 1990). A complete neuropsychological battery of carefully selected relevant tests should be administered by a neuropsychologist skilled in testing people with MS, if possible. Obtaining a baseline of individual cognitive performance on selected tests should be encouraged for documentation of future change and possible future employment disability claim. Identification of cognitive impairments, information about their effects on function, and the development of individualized compensation strategies may reduce the impact of the problems. No medications have been proven effective in treating cognitive problems.

Pain

Pain is estimated to be a problem for 40–60% of people with MS (Moulin et al., 1988). Pain directly due to the neurological lesions is primary; it is usually treated through medications. Pain that is secondary to poor posture, positioning, or spasticity is often relieved by therapy.

Spasticity

Spasticity, often present in MS, is usually greater in the lower extremities than in the upper extremities. Therapists should be familiar with the standard medications for spasticity, such as baclofen and tizanidine, and their side effect of drowsiness, which may increase fatigue (National Multiple Sclerosis Society, 1998). The intrathecal baclofen pump may help to improve function for people with severe spasticity (PVA, 1998).

Adjusting to MS

While only a small percentage of people with MS are severely disabled, the diagnosis is often devastating. The continual need to adjust to changing symptoms and varying impairments and the fear of and uncertainty about the disease process affect self-esteem, relationships, sexuality, physical activities, and recreational interests. From questions about pregnancy to cognitive changes influencing competence or safety, MS subtly or not so subtly affects every role and relationship. The variability of the disease and the hidden nature of many of the symptoms, such as cognitive changes and fatigue, often make it hard to explain to friends, coworkers, and family members.

Initially, people are typically quite preoccupied with their diagnosis, as it represents a major new and unknown threat that has suddenly challenged all their former assumptions about the future. As time passes, particularly if they return to full function, they frequently ignore the diagnosis and pay little attention to MS issues. As long as the inattention does not result in adverse decisions, this may be a fairly healthy attitude. The occupational therapist helps clients process the implications of changes and identifies modifications to minimize their effects. Information about the new symptoms may be all a person needs to make a successful adjustment.

Occupational Therapy Assessment

Assessment of a person with MS has unique features in terms of understanding the individual's history and employing evaluation tools and methods appropriate for this diagnosis.

History

The occupational therapy assessment begins with an interview about the person's goals for therapy and a brief history of symptoms and treatment since diagnosis. This brief history gives the therapist an idea of the course of the disease, previous symptoms, and the person's past coping style. Throughout the history, the therapist actively listens for hints of cognitive difficulties. The therapist should always remember that many people with MS who appear symptom-free have significant hidden impairments. Brief questions regarding dizziness, thinking problems, dropping things, numbness and tin-

gling, manual dexterity, prolonged walking and standing, employment, home physical and social environment, leisure interests, bladder problems, activities of daily living (ADL) and instrumental ADL (IADL), fatigue, sleeping pattern, equipment, muscle cramping, pain, fine motor activities, falling and balance problems, and stiffness can provide clues to what evaluations are likely to be relevant to the person's problems. If possible, particularly if cognitive problems are present, a family member or significant other should be encouraged to sit in on the evaluation if the client consents. The therapist can best probe about symptoms if the client completes selected survey instruments, such as the *Modified Fatigue Impact Scale* (PVA, 1998) and lists all of his or her medications prior to the interview.

Evaluation Tools and Methods

The initial interview and history give the therapist a quick indication of what evaluation tools and methods to use. Upper extremity manual muscle and range of motion tests, manual dexterity, and dynamometer evaluations are routine unless clearly inappropriate. A short evaluation tool being used in MS drug trials is the *Functional Capacity Evaluation* (FCE) from the National Multiple Sclerosis Society which includes a timed 25-ft walk, the *Nine Hole Peg Test*, and the *Paced Auditory Serial Addition Test* (PASAT). Therapists select a variety of other evaluation tools and methods based on the client's history and priorities, including the following:

- ► Fatigue assessment, such as *Modified Fatigue Impact Scale* and qualitative assessment
- ► The *6-Minute Walk Test* to assess endurance and fatigue (Pankoff et al., 2000)
- ► Sleep history or diary
- ► Cognitive screening using standardized evaluations such as the *Rao Cognitive Screen for MS* (Rao et al., 1991)
- ► Vision evaluation
- ► Standardized depression instruments
- ► Gait and/or transfer assessment as appropriate
- ► Bed mobility evaluation
- ► ADL and IADL assessments using standardized instruments if applicable
- ► Dysphagia assessment
- ► Standardized manual dexterity and coordination tests, such as the *9 Hole Peg Test, Box and Blocks*, or *Purdue Pegboard*
- ► Sensory testing, including *Semmes-Weinstein monofilaments* and proprioception
- ► Spasticity assessment using the *Modified Ashworth Scale* or other standardized assessments
- ► Tremor and ataxia assessments
- ► Trigger point evaluation for head, neck, shoulder muscles
- ► Vestibular evaluation

Therapists try to differentiate among various types of fatigue by considering results of some of these assessments. A high score on a depression index, for example, may indicate that depression is contributing to the patient's report of fatigue, while slow times on the *6-minute walk test* may also suggest a nerve fiber or motor fatigue component. Finally, if the person reports repeated falling or safety issues, a home visit may also be appropriate.

Setting Goals

The person with MS, the referral source, and sometimes family or significant others collaborate with the therapist to determine treatment goals. The therapist should not rely exclusively on self-reported goals, since the clients may not understand the nature of their impairments nor treatments available for various symptoms. Frequently, both they and the referring provider mistakenly believe they have to live with problems that in fact are treatable through therapy.

The client's priorities and interests are the cornerstones of goal setting and treatment planning. The therapist's recommendations for intervention will contribute to long-term functional improvement only if the recommendations are in sync with the client's priorities and values during a given episode of care. If the client, for instance, is not interested in obtaining powered mobility equipment, the therapist may discuss its benefits, but obtaining such equipment should not be a goal at that time. Acceptance of equipment, strategies, and treatment options takes time, and the occupational therapist plants the seed for later while pursuing the client's immediate interests.

Interventions

Following the evaluation and a full discussion of the findings, the occupational therapist discusses the various types of interventions that may help the person manage the identified problems. Because of the progressive nature of the disease, occupational therapy is generally compensatory, teaching the client techniques to manage the symptoms and compensate for the impairments rather than reversing them.

Because of the interaction of multiple symptoms, treatment usually addresses a number of symptoms during a given episode of care. Isolated treatment of symptoms is unlikely to be as effective, and concurrent occupational and physical therapy is often indicated. For example, physical therapists may treat fatigue by obtaining gait equipment and promoting aerobic exercises to increase endurance while the occupational therapist instructs the client in energy conservation, identifies adaptive equipment, and helps the client modify home and work tasks. Taken together, these changes may significantly reduce fatigue. Occupational therapy typically addresses one or more of the following: instruction in activity strategies and energy conservation; establishing an appropriate exercise program; addressing pain and spasticity; implementing cognitive compensations; and identifying equipment, environmental, and employment modifications.

Activity Strategies and Energy Conservation

If a client complains of fatigue, the occupational therapist should suspect multiple types of fatigue and direct interventions appropriately. Fatigue treatment begins as the therapist provides written and oral explanations of each relevant underlying type of fatigue in an easily understood fashion. Guidelines for the treatment of fatigue are available (PVA, 1998). At the beginning of intervention, the client typically fills out a detailed activity diary for 5 to 7 consecutive days and makes a list of individual goals and priorities (PVA, 1998). The occupational therapist and client use the diary as a starting point to identify and develop activity modifications to reduce fatigue through a systematic analysis of daily work, home, and leisure activities in all environments relevant to the individual.

Most energy conservation strategies are designed to enable persons with MS to use their limited energy on useful, meaningful activities that are important to them; this approach allows the client to exercise choice and control in everyday occupations. Mathiowetz et al. (2001) demonstrated the effectiveness of instructing a group of people with MS in energy conservation strategies. Essentially, the therapist helps the client analyze activities, understand rest–activity ratios, and identify modifications and equipment to help the individual perform valued tasks and activities. Interventions for fatigue usually entail a combination of energy conservation instruction, behavior modification, and equipment. Recommended changes may include the following:

▶ Decrease prolonged standing and walking by modifying tasks and using powered mobility devices for distances.
▶ Alternate periods of muscle activity with intervals of rest, such as walking, then sitting, then walking.
▶ Teach the client about the relationship between increased body temperature and increased fatigue, a phenomenon probably due to a decrease in the efficiency of nerve conduction in a demyelinated CNS.
▶ Identify modifications to help maintain cooler body temperature, such as layering clothing, purchasing an air conditioner, eliminating hot showers, sitting when showering, using a cooling vest when walking or active, and not using down comforters when sleeping.

▶ Shift important activities to the morning.

▶ Use appropriate equipment, such as a hinged ankle–foot orthosis to reduce the energy required in walking, to compensate for weakness.

▶ Obtain seating systems for trunk support in wheelchairs and properly fit ergonomic chairs with armrests for computer and work activities

Written recommendations and summaries should always be provided at the end of the two to four hour-long sessions usually necessary to treat fatigue. Clients should also be encouraged to return to occupational therapy if changes in their symptoms result in problems in their function; often a follow-up visit in 2 or 3 months is recommended.

Equipment, Behavioral, and Environmental Modifications

Generally, equipment, environmental, and behavioral modifications help patients compensate for weakness, spasticity, tremor, fatigue, ataxia, and cognitive problems. Environmental modifications may help in areas as diverse as providing access to mobility equipment, maintaining independence in ADL, and decreasing the distance to the bathroom. Many standard pieces of adaptive equipment are also helpful in MS. Computers, voice-activated software, and voice-activated memory aids may help decrease limitations due to weakness or tremor. Powered wheeled mobility devices, such as scooters or electric wheelchairs, are frequently effective in limiting fatigue and functional limitations related to weakness and spasticity. Powered mobility devices that are capable of adaptation later, such as adding a tilt feature to an electric wheelchair, allow for changing status. Because of fatigue, self-propelling manual wheelchairs are often not indicated. When appropriate, the therapist identifies needed equipment and helps the client arrange equipment trials. Home and/or work visits may be necessary to identify environmental modifications.

Behavioral changes, such as switching an exercise program from lunch to after work, frequently improve an individual's ability to perform productively. Changing behavior to use the elevator, for instance, might be combined with obtaining a scooter for distance walking and widening the doorways. The combinations of the right equipment, behavior changes, and environmental modifications depend upon the individual's needs and resources. Scheduled rechecks and the development of new modifications as changes occur are recommended; modifications in all three areas are frequently necessary.

Exercise Programs

Occupational therapists help clients achieve the right activity balance by teaching them to monitor the effects of any MS exercise program on both fatigue and their ability to perform high-priority activities. Two common MS symptoms often decrease with regular home exercise. Fatigue may be reduced by a structured aerobic program, and spasticity may be managed with a home stretching program. People with MS who have limited energy must carefully consider the proper time to exercise and the most effective exercises for their particular problems. Exercise often reduces the ability to perform activities immediately afterward for minutes to hours. Since the recovery time varies among individuals, trying different times for exercise is often necessary.

Fatigued clients are often confused by the appearance of a mixed message: the physical therapist or occupational therapist telling them to exercise and occupational therapy recommendations to conserve energy. This confusion is often perpetuated by physicians, MS organizations, and the media. Occupational therapists can help reconcile seemingly conflicting recommendations by helping clients to develop a structured exercise program at a specific time and teaching them to conserve energy in all activities during the rest of the day.

Many clients with MS fatigue unnecessarily because they confuse the energy-consumptive effects of daily activities with the benefits of exercise. For example, a woman with MS may believe she is getting weaker and resolve to take the stairs to strengthen her lower extremities. Unfortunately, the stairs do not provide her with a 25-minute aerobic program, and the resultant fatigue affects her ability to do high-priority activities later in the day. On the other hand, this client may choose to employ energy conservation strategies during her workday to preserve some time and energy for leisure activities with her daughter and 25-minute stationary bike ride in the evening. With the latter approach, this individual invests her limited energy resources in carrying out valued roles and contributes to her long-term health and function.

In general, MS exercise regimens are most likely to be successful if they start slowly and gradually increase time, repetitions, and/or intensity. Keep this principle in mind when making exercise recommendations: a realistic exercise program performed regularly is more desirable than an ideal program that is never followed. Good illustrations and written instructions should accompany every home program.

Aerobic Exercise Programs. An aerobic home program may be recommended as an intervention for fatigue (Petijan et al., 1996; PVA, 1998). The particular type of exercise program depends on the individual and often is developed in physical therapy. However, the occupational therapist may help the client figure out ways to integrate exercise into his or her routine and to identify the best timing of the exercise regimen. For a working person with limited time and slight leg weakness, for instance, a home stationary biking program for 25 minutes three or four times a week may be best. Although water exercise is beneficial because the buoyancy helps reduce the effects of weakness, people with MS should be advised to exercise only in cool pools because of their heat sensitivity.

Other Exercise Programs. Stretching and strengthening home exercise programs may be appropriate for a person with MS, according to evaluation findings about spasticity, range of motion, and pain. The stretching program may be done either independently or by a caregiver, depending on the client's ability. Stretching programs for MS generally emphasize relatively few repetitions and holds of 30 to 60 seconds. Therapists consider a number of factors when determining whether or not a strengthening home program is appropriate for a given client, such as individual history, motivation, fatigue level, and interests. If, for example, a client is significantly fatigued, has never stuck with an exercise program, and is not yet compliant with stretching and aerobic exercise programs, a strengthening program is not indicated. In general, a strengthening program is indicated after a motivated client has successfully maintained a stretching and aerobic exercise program. The neurological weakness in MS cannot be reversed by strengthening, but deconditioning weakness may be reduced. An individualized strengthening program may use Thera-Band, free weights, and/or exercise machines.

Spasticity Interventions

Therapists help clients minimize the impact of MS-related spasticity through a number of approaches. In addition to stretching exercises, adapted dressing techniques may prove helpful, such as using a stool to maintain hip flexion to decrease extensor spasm and/or using dressing sticks to compensate for inability to reach the feet. A standing home program may also be employed, using a standing frame for 30 to 60 minutes per day. Therapists evaluate the appropriateness of a standing home program by first assessing the client's tolerance of the equipment in the clinical setting, having the client stand for 3 to 10 minutes while monitoring vital signs and subjective response to activity. Other interventions include resting splints and posture and positioning techniques, such as bringing the hips into 90° of flexion to decrease extensor tone in the lower extremities. The level of intervention and identification of appropriate equipment depends on the severity of spasticity and the extent to which it interferes with function.

Cognitive Compensation

Occupational therapy for cognitive problems helps clients compensate for deficits and inefficiencies. Careful attention to timing of cognitive problems, fatigue levels, the nature of the problem, and the environment in which they occur helps the therapist develop individualized compensations. For example, treating fatigue with energy conservation techniques and mobility equipment often improves cognitive performance. Performance is also optimized as clients schedule cognitively demanding tasks for periods during the day when they typically feel their best, in minimally distracting environments. For example, tasks requiring higher levels of cognitive function should generally be performed in the morning if possible. Employment responsibilities and requirements should be scheduled to reduce the influence of the problems on job performance.

Education of both the client and his or her significant others regarding the problems is often beneficial. As families and others become aware that these problems are due to disease and not personality, the pressures on the individual can be eased and positive modifications can be undertaken. Caution should be exercised in the disclosure of specific cognitive problems to employers, however, with careful consideration given to individual employment circumstances. Examples of modifications include the following:

- Changing the environment to reduce distractions and interruptions
- Using a memory aid, such as a day planner or palm-top computer
- Structuring the environment to reduce clutter and promote organization
- Providing simple step-by-step written home and/or work directions
- Changing the difficult cognitive tasks to the morning
- Doing one activity at a time
- Increasing the time allotted for an activity
- Delegating difficult tasks to others
- Changing teaching style to require patient to repeat the information to be learned

Pain Treatment

For pain related to weakness, interventions such as posture training programs, ergonomic seating, home stretching exercise programs, and focal heat modalities to relieve pain from muscle trigger points may be effective. An individualized ergonomic workstation assessment should be considered if the client has pain related to spending many hours at a desk.

Employment Modifications

All of the problems described in the preceding sections may affect the performance of individuals at work. Many people with MS apply for disability benefits prematurely because they fear problems that may occur later or do

Case Example

MS. K.: OCCUPATIONAL THERAPY TO MAINTAIN SELF-ADVANCEMENT ROLES FOR A YOUNG WOMAN WITH MS

Client Information

Ms. K., a 37-year-old woman diagnosed with relapsing–remitting MS 2 years prior to her first visit to occupational therapy, had recently submitted her resignation to her employer of 15 years. Upset by having to quit her administrative job, she reported the following problems: (1) severe fatigue, which had increased in the past year and resulted in her inability to do her normal household tasks, perform her ADL, and work without becoming exhausted; (2) a marked increase in lower extremity weakness, with decreased ability to perform tasks requiring prolonged walking or standing; (3) a feeling of heaviness and stiffness in upper and lower extremities; (4) decreased manual dexterity; (5) frequent falling; (6) daily headaches; (7) dizziness; (8) bladder problems; (9) vision problems; (10) disturbed sleep, and (11) increased attention and memory problems. Her equipment at the time of her initial therapy visit included a manual wheelchair and a quad cane. She had quit driving. Her husband was very supportive, but they had recently stopped adoption proceedings because of her MS changes. Medications included a bladder medication and an MS disease–modifying drug.

Assessment

The occupational therapy evaluation reported the following areas of concern: decreased strength bilaterally in the lower extremities and her dominant upper extremity; increased tone bilaterally in the lower extremities; decreased sensation and manual dexterity in the dominant upper extremity; high levels of dizziness with head movement; head, neck, and shoulder muscle trigger points; and a high level of fatigue on the *Modified Fatigue Impact Scale*. Ms. K., determined not to give in to the disease, had made no adaptations to reduce fatigue in daily activities. She was scheduled to have a neuropsychological assessment to identify her current baseline function and problem areas. Her equipment was self-selected and inappropriate for her problems. She was not taking any medications to manage spasticity or fatigue. Her seating at home and work was not supportive. Ms. K. purposefully climbed the stairs in the morning and had a desk distant from the bathroom to get exercise, since she had no exercise program.

Recommendations

The occupational therapist recommended one outpatient treatment session a week for 6 weeks. Ms. K. and the therapist established the following long-term treatment goals and worked closely with the physical therapist on gait and exercise issues: (1) get instruction in and adopt energy conservation techniques at home, at work, and in community; (2) identify and obtain powered mobility equipment; (3) decrease daily headaches with head, neck, and shoulder stretching and focal heat; (4) identify and obtain equipment to decrease energy consumption at home and work; (5) with therapist assistance, identify and obtain ergonomic seating and workstation to decrease pain and energy consumption; (6) increase independence in driving with hand controls; (7) continue full- or part-time employment; (8) instruct in vestibular home exercise; and (9) identify and obtain equipment and modifications to decrease cognitive problems at home and work.

Short-Term Goals

After a month of treatment, Ms. K. will do the following:

- Withdraw resignation notice from employer
- Identify and obtain appropriate powered mobility equipment
- Make changes in work area by obtaining a headset and individualized ergonomic chair and have her desk moved closer to the bathroom
- Submit a request to her employer for power automatic door openers on bathroom
- Apply to vocational rehabilitation
- Work with therapist and vendor to install hand controls on her vehicle
- Incorporate at least six energy-saving changes into her daily schedule
- Demonstrate that she can independently perform head, neck, and shoulder stretching exercises

Results

Following the therapy evaluation, Ms. K. withdrew her resignation at her job and began making modifications in her work equipment and behavior. She learned and applied energy conservation techniques and used cooling strategies, primarily wearing a MicroClimate cooling vest at home and work. She returned to her physician and requested spasticity and fatigue medications, which also improved her sleep. Vocational rehabilitation and her employer provided recommended employment-related equipment, including voice-activated computer software, a headset, an ergonomic chair with arm rests and headrest, door openers, hand controls, earmuffs, cubicle dividers, a walker with a seat, and a scooter lift. Her health insurance purchased a scooter, a light cane, and bilateral ankle–foot orthoses on the recommendation of her physical therapist. She also began a stretching, vestibular, and stationary bike home exercise program. Five years later, Ms. K. was still working full-time and was adopting a child.

CLINICAL REASONING
in OT Practice

Identifying Treatment Interventions in MS

In accordance with the outpatient occupational therapy assessment, Ms. K.'s therapist suggested that Ms. K. withdraw her resignation to her employer until after she tried to manage her MS symptoms. What factors influenced this advice, and why would the therapist make this recommendation?

---

not know about possible modifications. With slowed disease progression, interventions can frequently help individuals continue productive employment for many years. Job modifications may include:

► Changing the times at which tasks are performed
► Limiting prolonged walking and standing by changes such as using conference calls rather than walking to meetings, increasing e-mail consultation, using powered mobility devices, and changing to an office near the bathroom
► Alterations in workstations, such as ergonomic chair with armrests, headsets, and mouse and keyboard trays
► Modifying work hours
► Working all or partly at home
► Using voice-activated software and other technology

Occupational therapists can help clients make choices about employment by providing information on the disease and employment legislation, proactive planning, and recommendations on modifications that help minimize employment problems and anxiety. Equipment or assistance may be obtained from health insurance providers, employers, nonprofit groups, and local agencies, such as the state department of vocational rehabilitation. In general, a person with MS considering disability benefits should first attempt job modifications.

Parkinson's Disease (PD)

PD is a chronic, progressive, unremitting, and highly variable condition. It is most common in later adult years; the mean age of onset is 55 to 60 years, with an incidence of 1%, or 1,000 per 100,000 (Stern, 1993). Parkinson's disease is typically defined by the three

cardinal signs, tremor, **rigidity**, and **bradykinesia**, with a fourth, postural instability, often added (Conley & Kirchner, 1999). Tremor, commonly the first complaint, increases with stress and may present as pill-rolling, a tremor unique to PD (Gelb et al., 1999; Uitti, 1998). Rigidity appears somewhat later in the disease process (Conley & Kirchner; Gelb et al.). Bradykinesia is slowness or poverty of movement causing lack of facial expression, or "mask face," and affects walking, participation in activities, and eye blink (Conley & Kirchner). Postural instability begins with reduced arm swing and shorter strides that progress to a shuffling gait. Lack of postural reflexes often results in increasing falls and **akinesia**, or freezing episodes that reduce or eliminate spontaneous initiation of gait and impede turning and crossing thresholds (Conley & Kirchner; Gelb et al.).

Other symptoms of PD, particularly in the middle to later stages, include vocal and swallowing changes, autonomic deficits, psychiatric complications, and dementia (Conley & Kirchner, 1999; Gelb et al., 1999). The swallowing difficulties, related to delayed swallow reflex, residues of food materials, and abnormal tongue control, often result in mild to moderate nutritional depletion (Fuh et al., 1997). Research has shown that overall disease severity is not related to swallowing dysfunction, as a high percentage of those in early stages of the disease have this problem (Fuh et al.).

Dementia related to PD occurs in 15–20% of cases and tends to occur in patients who were relatively old at the time of diagnosis, have a history of long course of the disease, and have high levels of depression (Aarsland et al., 1996). Motor planning and sequencing are the areas of cognitive function that seem to be most affected (Monza et al., 1998). The pathogenesis of PD is related to the loss of dopaminergic neurons of the substantia nigra that provide input to the corpus striatum, which in part modulates the thalamus and its connections to the motor cortex (Conley & Kirchner, 1999). There is also suggestion that further biochemical anomalies in the basal ganglia are present (Conley & Kirchner).

The cause of PD is not well understood, though both hereditary and environmental factors have been investigated. There is some evidence to show that in 5–10% of cases a hereditary pattern has been linked to a chromosome 4 mutation (Muenter et al., 1998). However, it is not clear whether the role of heredity is direct or merely imparts susceptibility to dopaminergic cell degeneration (Conley & Kirchner, 1999). Environmental factors that are thought to contribute to PD include exposure to the neurotoxin MPTP, living on a farm, drinking well water, and exposure to pesticides (Conley & Kirchner; Marder et al., 1998). The cause of PD is likely multifactorial.

Diagnosing PD

In autopsy studies, PD has been shown to be misdiagnosed in 25% of cases (Calne, 1995). In part, the difficulty in diagnosis is a result of the lack of definitive biological markers and tests or techniques. Clinical imaging techniques such as positron emission tomography remain experimental (Conley & Kirchner, 1999). At present diagnosis is based on clinical evidence, using clinical diagnostic criteria, and it is an art as well as a science.

The Course of PD

PD has been described as having either five stages (Hoehn & Yahr, 1967) or three stages (Bradley, 1996) (Box 40-3). These stages are broadly described by presence of symptoms, functional implications, and response to medications.

Potential Emotional, Social, and Economic Consequences

In the initial stages of PD, the degree of physical disability is minimal. The emotional burden and social consequences, however, can be marked. Resting tremor, the common initial symptom of PD rarely resulting in motor disability, is a frequent source of psychological distress (Uitti, 1998). Many individuals report feeling embarrassed or self-conscious about their tremors. In later stages of PD, Peto et al. (1995) found that tremor and rigidity were highly correlated to distress and reduced quality of life. Another study found the highest predictors of poor quality of life for persons with PD were depression, sleep disorders, and increasing dependence (Karlson et al., 1999). Major depression or depressive symptoms have been found in 45% of those with PD, suggesting that early identification and intervention are crucial (Karlson et al.). Persons with PD report fatigue,

pain, and social isolation contributing to distress and compromised quality of life (Friedman & Friedman, 1993; Karlson et al.).

The economic implications of PD are frequently related to the costs of medications, wheeled mobility, accessibility modifications, self-care and safety equipment, and in-home support. If the individual is employed, increasing limitations may require employment modifications and early application for disability benefits accompanied by loss of income. PD-related dementia may decrease the ability of the person to handle finances. An elderly caregiver is also likely to require caregiver assistance and/or respite care during the final stages of the patient's PD. Placement in a long-term care facility is costly.

The social consequences of PD are striking. The individual's ability to interact with those in his or her environment may be affected in the early stages. For example, handwriting may be somewhat shaky and micrographic, which reduces legibility (Conley & Kirchner, 1999; Uitti, 1998). In the intermediate and later stages, the voice softens and becomes a monotone. Reduced facial expression and minimal hand gesturing

---

BOX 40-3
Stages of Parkinson's Disease

Hoehn and Yahr (1967)

Stage 1:
Unilateral symptoms, no or minimal functional implications, usually a resting tremor

Stage 2:
Midline or bilateral symptom involvement, no balance difficulty, mild problems with trunk mobility and postural reflexes

Stage 3:
Postural instability, mild to moderate functional disability

Stage 4:
Postural instability increasing, though able to walk, functional disability increases interfering with ADL, decreased manipulation and dexterity

Stage 5:
Confined to wheelchair or bed

Bradley (1996)

Early:
Not disabling: monosymptomatic; responds well to medication; may remain at this level for years

Nonfluctuating:
Some disability; Levodopa added to medication regimen; 80% of function is restored

Fluctuating:
Function limited; side effects to Levodopa; difficult-to-control symptoms, postural instability, and gait disturbance become debilitating

also contribute to decreased communication with others (Uitti). The person with PD may have waning interest in social and/or previously enjoyed leisure activities.

Occupational Therapy Assessment

In the early stages of PD, occupational therapy is rarely indicated unless there are functional limitations or psychological issues. Occupational therapy is most often required in the intermediate and later stages of the disease (Hoehn and Yahr [1967] Stages 3 to 5). In the intermediate stages, the occupational therapist screens for occupational functioning problems due to reduced mobility, safety issues, fine motor incoordination and dexterity, slowed movements, **cogwheel rigidity**, depressed affect, and swallowing difficulties. Evaluations should include a brief history with screens for impairments and limitations in activities likely to be affected. Examples of individual impairments and limitations in activities that may be included in screening include but are not limited to these:

- ▶ Mobility issues, such as walking on even and uneven surfaces, stair climbing, and driving
- ▶ Quality of movement, bradykinesia, postural instability and rigidity that limit home, community, leisure, and work activities (specifically ask about stumbling and falling)
- ▶ Limited accomplishment of or changed timing of ADL and IADL because of bradykinesia and rigidity
- ▶ Swallowing or other dysphagia problems prolonging eating and reducing intake
- ▶ Freezing that decreases safety and limits home, community, and work tasks
- ▶ Cognitive problems that affect activities and competence
- ▶ Difficulties with coordination and manipulation in home, community, and work activities
- ▶ Fatigue related to decreased endurance, bradykinesia, rigidity, and postural instability
- ▶ Sexual activity limitations related to bradykinesia, rigidity, fatigue, depression, anxiety, and psychosocial problems
- ▶ Sleep disturbances

Setting Goals

Generally, significant others should be included in the evaluation, goal setting, and intervention. However, because PD-related communication problems are possible, it is important to ensure that the significant other's opinions do not dominate the process. The occupational therapist assists in establishing realistic timelines and breaking down the goals to ensure measures of success. It is important to understand the roles of spouse,

children, and/or significant others in goal setting. Their participation is frequently crucial to the viability and success of interventions.

Occupational Therapy Intervention

Interventions vary with the individual's and significant other's priorities and resources, stage of the disease, occupational difficulties identified through the assessment, and activities in which they participate (Box 40-4).

Amyotrophic Lateral Sclerosis

ALS, popularly known as Lou Gehrig's disease, is a late-onset fatal neurodegenerative disease of upper motor neurons (UMN) and lower motor neurons (LMN). ALS is the most common disorder of the motor neurons, with 5 to 8 cases per 100,000 living with ALS at any given time (Mitsumoto et al., 1998). No special test is available to establish the diagnosis. Initial symptoms vary widely, and diagnosis is a careful, multistep system of exclusion. ALS is considered terminal, but prognosis for individual patients is best left to ALS-expert neurologists. Age at onset and the pattern of symptom development in each person provides information used in determining an individual's prognosis. The cause of the disease is unknown.

The average age at onset is 58, although adults as young as 20 have been diagnosed. Age-specific incidence and mortality rates in sporadic ALS increase until the eighth decade, with a peak between 55 and 75 years of age. Gender probably does not influence prognosis.

There is no known cure or effective treatment for ALS, although a number of drug trials are being conducted. Riluzole (Rilutek), an antiglutamate agent, is the only Food and Drug Administration–approved medication for treatment. Medications can assist in the management of symptoms such as **fasiculations**, spasticity, anxiety, insomnia, and excessive saliva but do not affect the progression of the disease. Tracheotomies, gastrostomies and assisted ventilation are used to ease problems with eating and breathing (Mitsumoto et al., 1998).

In ALS, voluntary muscle control is affected, and early manifestations indicating UMN or LMN disease vary with the site of the initial disease process. UMN damage results in general weakness, spasticity, and hyperreflexia. LMN involvement results in weakness or **muscle atrophy** of the extremities, cervical extensor weakness, fasciculations, muscle cramps, and loss of reflexes. Speech, swallowing, and breathing may be affected by damage to the bulbar nerves. Early bulbar involvement and/or advanced age at time of diagnosis are likely to indicate a quicker course of the disease (Mitsumoto

BOX 40-4
PROCEDURES FOR PRACTICE

Occupational Therapy for PD

Interventions related to increased isolation and communication problems:

- Education about timing important activities to synchronize with medication regimen so that participation can occur when medications are at the height of effectiveness
- Modifications of leisure activities to encourage participation and decrease isolation
- Information on support and advocacy groups and other group activities
- Caregiver training regarding issues such as communication modifications, psychological support, and modifying social activities to promote participation
- Development of emergency communication systems
- Identification of writing modifications, including enlarged felt-tip pen and writing when rested
- Identification of communication aids, including speed dial, large-key telephones, dictating devices, and environmental control systems for lights, television, and other frequently used devices

Interventions related to safety:

- Instruction in sit-to-stand techniques, bed mobility
- Instruction in managing freezing, including avoiding crowds, narrow spaces, doorways, and room corners; good, even lighting, especially in doorways, room corners, and narrow spaces, such as doorways; reducing distractions such as trying to talk while walking or carrying objects; reducing clutter or other distractions in a pathway; doing only one activity at a time; not hurrying to answer the phone or door; focusing when changing directions
- Demonstration of equipment to increase independence and safety, such as a raised toilet seat, toilet grab bars, shower bench, sink chair, soap on a rope
- Identifying and prescribing walking aids and mobility equipment
- Developing environmental modifications, such as good, uniform lighting
- Modifying feeding to include small portions, more frequent, longer meals
- Demonstrating home and group exercises to maintain mobility
- Demonstrating changes to improve swallowing, such as altering food consistency and reducing distractions

Interventions to maintain independence and participation:

- Instruction in using adult absorbent underwear if necessary
- Demonstrating voice and facial exercise programs
- Advising on changing sexual activities to occur after resting and urination
- Demonstration of energy effectiveness strategies in home, leisure and work activities
- Modifications to reduce the need for fine motor control, such as clothing with minimal fasteners, Velcro closures

---

et al., 1998). Generally people with ALS develop both UMN and LMN symptoms as the disease progresses. Cognition may be affected, while sensation and eye, bowel, and bladder control typically are not.

The Course of ALS

Six stages of ALS are recognized and described according to clinical features (see Table 40-1). The median duration of life after diagnosis ranges from 23 to 52 months, but a significant proportion of patients survive 5 years or more (Mitsumoto et al., 1998). Focal weakness of the arm, leg, or bulbar area is a common initial symptom (Mitsumoto et al.). Atrophy may begin in the hands, with wasting of the thenar and hypothenar eminences. Atrophy of the shoulder musculature is also common early in the disease. Because of dorsal and palmar interosseous wasting, finger extension is usually affected earlier than grip strength. Walking and bed mobility are affected, and falling is common with lower extremity weakness. Upper and lower extremity weakness makes transfers and getting up from the floor after a fall increasingly difficult. Speech and swallowing problems may arise early in the disease course.

Potential Emotional, Social, and Economic Consequences

ALS is a devastating disease for both victims and their families. Because of the relatively fast progression, frequently involving early loss of upper extremity function and possibly speech and swallowing, the disease quickly affects quality of life and the abilities of people to perform ADL, IADL, and employment tasks.

People with ALS and their families have little time to make psychological adjustment to the diagnosis and its implications before having to deal with their loved one's increasing inability to function independently at home, at work, and in the community. The acceptance by all family members of the devastating diagnosis may affect the willingness of everyone involved to plan and make the changes necessary to maximize the independence of the person with ALS as the level of impairment increases.

Case Example

MR. B.: OCCUPATIONAL THERAPY TO HELP MAINTAIN SELF-MAINTENANCE ROLES FOR A MAN WITH PD

Client Information

Mr. B., a 76-year-old man diagnosed with PD 8 years ago, has been widowed for 4 years and has no children. He lives alone and is determined to remain living at home. He has a housekeeper 4 hours a week who does his laundry and cleans the house. Mr. B. identified the following problems at his outpatient occupational therapy assessment: (1) a history of falling due to PD; (2) difficulties getting off the floor, toilet, bed, and chairs; (3) increased problems walking around the house and in the community; (4) continuing weight loss; (5) difficulties preparing food and eating; (6) problems managing some aspects of dressing; (7) increased social isolation due to bradykinesia, muscle weakness, rigidity, and postural instability; (8) fluctuating pain; and (9) fatigue. He had not seen his physician in 18 months and was prepared to visit him only if "he doesn't throw me into an institution."

Recommendations

The therapist recommended one treatment session each week for 6 weeks and a home safety assessment. The long term treatment goals: (1) maintain independence at home; (2) obtain grab bars, raised toilet seat, bath transfer bench, and other identified safety equipment; (3) rearrange furniture and modify home lighting to increase safety; (4) obtain remote control for TV, radio, lights, and door locks to decrease falls; (5) increase community participation; (6) obtain additional in-home assistance for bathing and meal preparation; (7) obtain loose clothing with easy fasteners; and (8) change diet and meal timing to decrease swallowing problems and increase nutrition.

Initial Short-Term Goals

As a result of his first month of occupational therapy, Mr. B. will do the following:

- ▶ Maximize mobility and decrease frequency of falls through use of assistive devices in bathroom
- ▶ Improve safety in self-care activities by employing in-home assistance for bathing and meal preparation and obtaining loose clothing with loose fasteners
- ▶ Participate in a swallowing assessment to guide decisions regarding possible changes in diet, timing, and/or portions
- ▶ Learn about the symptoms of PD and benefits of working with his physician

Results

Occupational therapy intervention began by teaching Mr. B. about the importance of having his medications reviewed by his physician to minimize the effects of bradykinesia and rigidity. His home was assessed for safety, which resulted in rearranging furniture to increase space, removing throw carpets, improving the lighting, and providing multiple remote controls to minimize the need for walking when medication effectiveness has declined. He was instructed in sit-to-stand techniques and ways to decrease PD freezing. He began an exercise program in physical therapy. Assistance in the home was increased, and the raised toilet seat, bath bench, and grab bars were prescribed and installed. Clothing was altered to reduce buttons and zippers, and new loose clothing was purchased.

A swallowing assessment revealed a delayed swallow and some difficulty with thin fluids. The home assistant was taught about the kinds of foods that would be easiest and safest for swallowing and to provide four small meals rather than two large ones. Mr. B. was able to manage the small meals with the recommended types of food with little difficulty. As driving was not recommended, a neighbor agreed to take him shopping. This worked well as a social outing and allowed Mr. B. to continue a task he enjoyed.

Mr. B. saw his physician and his medications were altered, which reduced his bradykinesia and rigidity. He was taught about the benefits of timing his activities to coincide with his medication regimen to maximize his performance and satisfaction in his chosen activities. Mr. B.'s long-term goal was to continue to live at home. He was advised to visit his physician annually or as needed.

Discharge Recommendations

- ▶ Reevaluate safe independence in the home with the current level of in-home support, access, and socialization in 6 months.
- ▶ Reevaluate swallowing as indicated.

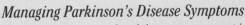

CLINICAL REASONING
in OT Practice

Managing Parkinson's Disease Symptoms

The outpatient occupational therapy assessment indicated to Mr. B.'s therapist that it was important to have a home occupational therapy assessment. Why did the therapist consider it necessary, and how could it be justified to a third-party payer?

People frequently withdraw from employment soon after the diagnosis and may also have to confront economic problems due to loss of income and possibly health insurance. Since men and women in the age group most commonly affected are often still employed and actively involved in family and community activities, the abrupt change in status is often devastating to both the individual and the family.

Occupational Therapy Assessment

The specifics of the occupational therapy assessment depend on the stage of the disease and the individual's needs and priorities. Assessments should be based on clearly defined levels of function and related to the six stages of ALS. Early interventions should be based on the individual's symptoms, and evaluation tools such as the *ALS Functional Rating Scale* (Mitsumoto et al., 1998) and the *Purdue Pegboard* or other timed upper extremity function tests. Standard range of motion and manual muscle testing as well as ADL and IADL assessments should be included in all evaluations. Because of the progression of the disease, reevaluations should be done on repeated visits.

Setting Goals

The progressive nature of the disease necessitates that rehabilitation in ALS be compensatory, focusing on adapting to disability and preventing secondary complications. In general, the treatment goals center on keeping the person as active and independent as possible for as long as possible. Here are some examples of occupational therapy goals for a client with ALS in the early stages:

- ▶ Optimize strength and range of motion through use of home exercise programs
- ▶ Improve level of independence in ADL and IADL through use of assistive or adaptive devices
- ▶ Improve function and decrease pain and fatigue in the head and extremities through use of splints and orthotics
- ▶ Employ joint protection, pain management, energy conservation, and work simplification techniques

As motor function declines, mobility and self-care become increasingly difficult. Home evaluations and/or in-home therapy are important in the later stages of the disease, and treatment goals largely focus on enabling the caregiver to assist the client safely and effectively. The occupational therapist helps the caregiver–client team to do the following:

- ▶ Optimize safety
- ▶ Assess positioning and maintain skin integrity
- ▶ Employ augmentative communication equipment
- ▶ Manage dysphagia
- ▶ Perform safe transfers
- ▶ Identify and obtain appropriate equipment such as hospital bed to allow continued mobility

---

TABLE 40-1

Rehabilitation of Patients With ALS at Various Stages of the Disease

Stage	Characteristic Clinical Features	Activities to Maintain Motor Function	Equipment
I	Ambulatory, no problems with ADL, mild weakness	Normal activities, moderate exercise in unaffected muscles, active ROM exercise	None
II	Ambulatory, moderate weakness in certain muscles	Modification in living; modest exercise; active, assisted ROM exercise	Assistive devices
III	Ambulatory, severe weakness in certain muscles	Active life; active, assisted, passive ROM exercise; joint pain management	Assistive devices, adaptive devices, home equipment
IV	Wheelchair-confined, almost independent, severe weakness in legs	Passive ROM exercise, modest exercise in uninvolved muscles	Assistive devices, adaptive devices, wheelchair, home equipment
V	Wheelchair confined; dependent; pronounced weakness in legs, severe weakness in arms	Passive ROM exercise, pain management, decubitus prevention	Adaptive devices, home equipment, wheelchair
VI	Bedridden, no ADL, maximal assistance required	Passive ROM exercise, pain management, prevention of decubitus ulcers and venous thrombosis, pulmonary toilet	Adaptive devices, home equipment

ADL, activities of daily living;, ROM, range-of-motion exercise.
Data from Sinaki, M. (1980). Rehabilitation. In D. W. Mulder (Ed.), *The Diagnosis and Treatment of Amyotrophic Lateral Sclerosis* (pp. 169–193). Boston: Houghton Mifflin. Reprinted with permission from Mitsumoto, H., Chad, D., & Pioro, E. (1998). *Amyotrophic Lateral Sclerosis. Contemporary Neurology Series*. Philadelphia: Davis.

Throughout the stages of the disease, the therapist remains sensitive to the client's, family's, and caregiver's stress as the demands of caregiving perpetually change. Physical demands, financial concerns, and transformation of the home into a hospital-like setting produce enormous strain on the client and the caregivers (Mitsumoto et al., 1998). Open discussions and close collaboration with clients, caregivers, and the ALS team help to address and plan for the client's changing needs.

Occupational Therapy Interventions

As is true for all recipients of occupational therapy services, client and caregiver goals and priorities drive intervention aims and strategies. When treating clients with ALS, therapists must be particularly sensitive to the client's level of gadget tolerance, financial resources, and social and cultural context and to the overextended caregiver's time. The client's and caregivers' level of psychological distress, depression, and denial should always be included when considering treatment interventions. Psychological counseling and support may be critical to effective rehabilitation. Special considerations for exercise and equipment recommendations with this diagnostic group are briefly reviewed.

Exercise

Active and passive ROM, strengthening, endurance, stretching, and home breathing exercise programs are all appropriate at various stages of the disease. Research indicates they are effective for minimizing secondary complications (Mitsumoto et al., 1998). Attention to overexertion, potential secondary problems, muscle spasms, and careful monitoring of fatigue are important to a successful exercise program. Exercise programs should be modified as the client's status changes. A client may initially be able to perform an independent home stretching program, but as the disease progresses, the program may become too fatiguing or difficult. At that time, the caregiver may have to learn how to perform the program.

Equipment

A variety of assistive and adaptive equipment may help the client achieve the highest possible level of independence. Assistive equipment, such as a neck collar, and adaptive equipment, such as a universal cuff, are frequently helpful. Adaptive equipment should be as simple as possible and must be accepted by the client and caregiver to be effective. Therapists inform clients and caregivers about potentially helpful adaptive equipment at every disease stage.

As the disease progresses, home assessment and client–caregiver consultation inform selection of a wheelchair. Since independent walking becomes diffi-cult in a rapidly progressing disease such as ALS, ordering the wheelchair may need to be expedited. Ideally, a power wheelchair with adaptable controls and the ability to add tilt or recline features enables the client to continue to maximize mobility. Transporting the wheelchair in a vehicle should be considered when making purchase decisions.

Guillain Barré Syndrome

GBS is an inflammatory disease resulting in axonal demyelination of peripheral nerves (Meythaler et al., 1997). Characteristics of GBS include a quickly progressing, symmetrical ascending paralysis starting with the feet; pain, particularly in the legs; absence of deep tendon reflexes; mild sensory loss in glove-and-stocking distributions; cranial nerve dysfunction with possible facial palsy; an autonomic nervous system response of postural hypertension and tachycardia; and respiratory muscle paralysis (Hughes & Rees, 1997; Meythaler et al.). Severity of symptoms varies from so mild that medical attention is unlikely to severe disease that may cause death in approximately 10% of cases (Hughes & Rees).

The cause of GBS is unclear. Its distribution is known to be worldwide, with an incidence of 1.3 to 2 per 100,000 (Hughes & Rees, 1997). Men are slightly more commonly affected than women, and GBS most often occurs in young adults (20–24 years) and the elderly (70–74 years) (Hughes & Rees; Jiang et al., 1997). There is no evidence to support hereditary or familial susceptibility or vaccinations as causal to GBS, though there are reports concerning previous viral infections (Hughes & Rees). Enteritis precedes GBS in 41% of cases, and respiratory tract infections and HIV or AIDS may also precede it (Hughes & Rees; Jiang et al.).

Diagnosing GBS

Diagnosis of GBS entails a detailed history of symptoms and a complete physical and neurological examination that includes nerve conduction velocity tests and possibly a spinal tap (Hughes & Rees, 1997; Muscular Dystrophy Association of Canada, 1997). The medical interventions for GBS attempt to lessen the severity and hasten recovery but do not cure the disease (Muscular Dystrophy Association of Canada). Treatments for GBS include intravenous human immunoglobulin, plasma exchange otherwise known as plasmapheresis, and steroids (Rees et al., 1998). In severe cases ventilation may be required (Muscular Dystrophy Association of Canada; Rees et al.).

The course of GBS

GBS has three phases. In more than 95% of people with GBS, the onset, or acute inflammatory phase, manifests as an acute weakness in at least two limbs that progresses for up to 4 weeks with increasing symptoms (Hughes & Rees, 1997). This is followed by the plateau phase, when the greatest disability is present as are many symptoms described earlier. During this phase, which may last a few days or weeks, there is no significant change. Finally, the progressive period of recovery, when remyelination and axonal regeneration occur, may last up to 2 years, though the average length of this phase is 12 weeks (Jiang et al., 1997; Meythaler et al., 1997). The degree of recovery varies from complete return of function to some residual weakness that may not resolve. The prognosis for 90% of those with GBS is optimistic, as recovery of all or most functions generally occurs (Muscular Dystrophy Association of Canada, 1997).

Potential Emotional, Social, and Economic Consequences

Emotional and psychological reactions often are a response to the rapid onset of symptoms and the degree of disability sometimes associated with GBS. At the height of the acute phase of the disease, should the individual be unable to speak or move, fear of the unknown and frustration are often overwhelming (Muscular Dystrophy Association of Canada, 1997). As recovery progresses and improvement is slow, the psychological adjustment, impatience, and frustration associated with residual disability may be daunting.

Young adults undergo significant educational, employment, and/or economic effects, as they are in their career path, may have debts, and have only small savings. For those who develop GBS in later years, particularly in retirement, the economic effect may be less. Should the recovery phase last several months, the burden on family, colleagues, and/or friends who may be required to absorb the roles previously held by the person with GBS may be profound. This may strain relationships.

Occupational Therapy Approach

The occupational therapist is rarely involved during the acute inflammatory phase of the disease or when the course is relatively mild, producing minimal symptoms, short duration, and few occupational limitations. Referral to occupational therapy is common when the course of GBS is moderate to severe.

Occupational Therapy Assessment

Screening and assessment during the plateau phase typically occurs in intensive care, when the individual is undergoing extensive medical procedures such as plasma exchange or intravenous immunoglobulin. Dur-

ing this period, occupational therapists assess communication, control of the environment as appropriate, comfort, and level of anxiety.

During the recovery phase, occupational therapists assess mobility, self-care, communication, leisure, and reintegration into the workplace as appropriate. As the natural course of GBS is improvement, patients and caregivers tend to be optimistic about recovery. The emotional and psychological consequences are therefore somewhat reduced during the recovery phase.

Setting Goals

The long-term goal is full recovery, so that the individual performs at the same level as prior to the onset of GBS with or without modification.

Occupational Therapy Interventions

Modifications during the plateau phase should be considered temporary. Examples of interventions that may be required:

- ► Developing communication tools, such as sign or picture board
- ► Ensuring access to the nurse call button
- ► Adapting TV and lights to remote control
- ► Modifying the telephone for hands-free use
- ► Modifying positions for lying and sitting to those optimal for function and comfort
- ► Positioning for trunk, head, and upper extremity stability
- ► Teaching about GBS and recommending other support services
- ► Teaching strategies to reduce anxiety

Recovery phase interventions are oriented to the resumption of activities and roles. Examples of interventions that may be required:

- ► Instructing in safe mobility as strength incrementally returns
- ► Demonstrating independent transfers
- ► Training in modified self-care techniques
- ► Providing temporary aids and equipment
- ► Adapting modes of communication according to person's priorities
- ► Encouraging access to the community
- ► Modifying and encouraging routine activities as appropriate
- ► Adapting equipment and modifying behavior in home, leisure, and work activities
- ► Instructing in energy conservation
- ► Providing instruction on and modifying employment roles and tasks

Neurological Complications of Human Immunodeficiency Virus

AIDS is the end result of complications associated with HIV infection (Galantino, 1992; Harvey, 1994). Neurological diseases and dysfunction are manifested throughout the course of HIV disease from early infection to end-stage AIDS. Neurological symptoms in the CNS and PNS are seen in 30–65% of patients, and up to 80–88% are diagnosed at autopsy. In 10% of cases, neurological conditions are the presenting symptoms of HIV or AIDS (Galantino; Koppel, 1998).

HIV is a retrovirus with a long incubation period, often 10 to 15 years. The T helper cells (T4 cells) are the most susceptible to infection. Their depletion deregulates the immune system, setting it up for opportunistic infections and AIDS. A person is designated as having AIDS when the T4 cell count drops below 200 or when the person is diagnosed with an AIDS-defining opportunistic infection.

Significant advances have been made in the treatment of HIV infection in the past 5 years with the introduction of protease inhibitors. Highly active antiretroviral treatment (HAART) is the practice of using three or four medications, usually one protease inhibitor and two or three other antivirals, in combination. Since the introduction of HAART there have been drastic drops in overall incidence of AIDS-related conditions and death. Unfortunately, HAART failure rate has been estimated to be as high as 50%.

The neurological complications of HIV and AIDS can easily be divided into those affecting the PNS and those affecting the CNS. Disorders of the PNS:

▶ Acute demyelinating inflammatory sensorimotor polyneuropathy (GBS)
▶ Chronic inflammatory demyelinating **polyneuropathy**
▶ Mononeuritis multiplex
▶ Distal sensory polyneuropathy, the most common neuropathy of HIV
▶ Progressive inflammatory polyradiculopathy
▶ HIV-associated myopathy

The symptoms of these peripheral neuropathies vary widely and can include pain, weakness, hypersensitivity, loss of vibratory sense, numbness and tingling, fatigue, loss of respiratory muscles, loss of bowel and bladder function, and flaccid paraplegia. Many symptoms can be treated with medications, particularly if they are the result of opportunistic infections. Change in neurological status should immediately be reported to the treating physician.

CNS complications related to HIV and AIDS are generally caused by opportunistic infections, neoplasms, or myelopathies. Clinical manifestations vary, and appropriate imaging, clinical tests, and biopsies are required for the diagnosis. These disorders can produce varying symptoms, including hemiparesis, ataxia, aphasia, seizures, severe headaches, vision problems, paraplegia, loss of bowel and bladder control, depression, and cognitive problems. AIDS dementia complex (ADC) or HIV encephalitis clinically emerges in approximately 66% of patients with HIV symptomatic disease and in 85% of those with AIDS. Cognitive symptoms include apathy, depression, trouble concentrating, memory loss, language impairments, and loss of higher cortical functions. Motor changes include bradykinesia, impaired eye movements, involuntary movements, and ataxia. HAART therapy has been shown to reverse some ADC problems (Price et al., 1999).

Occupational Therapy Approach

Occupational therapists may already be involved with the care of patients with neurological disorders prior to the actual diagnosis of HIV. This underscores the importance of using standard precautions, which are designed to protect the health care worker from being exposed to blood-borne pathogens (Box 40-5).

Occupational Therapy Assessment

Impairments and limitations in activities and participation vary widely depending on the nature of the neurological disorder. The evaluation should include but is not limited to the following areas:

▶ ADL
▶ IADL
▶ Occupational status
▶ Cognitive-perceptual status
▶ Psychosocial status
▶ Vision
▶ Bowel and bladder function
▶ Motor function (strength, range of motion, coordination and balance, muscle tone)
▶ Accessibility of home environment

The therapist should be familiar with the person's history of CNS opportunistic infections and monitor for any relapses of encephalitis. It is important to have a good baseline evaluation of people with HIV, because their status can change quickly with the advent of new opportunistic infections. Changes in status should quickly be referred to the physician for prompt medical invention.

Occupational Therapy Interventions

Therapy interventions for neurological disorders related to HIV vary with the nature of the problem. Significant others should be included, if the person desires, in all goal setting and treatment interventions. Treatment for peripheral neuropathies, such as distal sensory polyneu-

BOX 40-5
SAFETY BOX

Standard Precautions

You must routinely use standard precautions to protect yourself from exposure to blood or body fluids from all patients, regardless of their diagnosis. Standard precautions consist of the use of protective barriers to prevent contamination of the skin, clothing, and mucous membranes (eyes, ears, nose). Hepatitis B virus, Hepatitis C virus and HIV are communicated through blood-borne pathogens. Modes of transmission include sexual contact involving the sharing of body fluid, needlestick, contact with blood through mucous membranes or broken skin, childbirth, receiving blood or blood products, and organ transplantation. Proper use of protective barriers prevents exposure. Protect yourself by always following these recommendations.

► Wear and change gloves.
► Do not wash or decontaminate disposable (single-use) gloves.
► Wear fluid- or moisture-resistant gown, apron, or lab coat when you anticipate contact with bodily fluids.
► Wear surgical cap and/or hood and shoe covers and/or boots when gross contamination is likely.
► Wear mask and eye protection with side shields and face shield when there is potential for splash, spray, or splattering of body fluids to the eyes, nose, or mouth.
► Wash your hands before and after contacting patients.
► Use a pocket mask or other ventilation guard device when doing CPR.

Needlestick or puncture is the most common mechanism for transmission for occupational therapists. To minimize risk use these precautions used by medical personnel:

► Use caution when handling all sharps.
► Do not bend, break, or manipulate items by hand.
► Place disposable sharps in puncture-resistant container immediately after use.
► Do not recap or remove needles from syringe by hand unless no alternative exists.
► Use a device instead of your hand to pick up or remove contaminated needles or other sharp.
► Place reusable sharps in containers that are puncture resistant, leakproof on sides and bottom, and labeled.
► Use a mechanical device to clean up broken glassware.

PROMPTLY report all exposures to your supervisor and health care authorities.

ropathy, include desensitization therapy, compression garments, manual therapy, microcurrent stimulation, balance training, home stretching programs, and splinting (Galantino, 1992; McReynolds, 1995; McReynolds & Galantino, 1996). Therapeutic interventions for inflammatory demyelinating neuropathies are typically similar to those used for GBS (Galantino; Hopp and Rogers,

1989; O'Dell, 1996). Therapy for myelopathies focuses on strengthening (when **myalgias** and elevated creatine phosphokinase have subsided), ADL training, instruction in energy conservation, identification of adaptive equipment, splinting, and the provision of wheeled mobility. In ADC, the occupational therapy depends on evaluation and may include cognitive compensation training, ADL instruction, caregiver training, identification of adaptive equipment, and addressing psychosocial issues (Hopp and Rogers).

Evidence-Based Research on Occupational Therapy for Neurodegenerative Diseases

Although expert consensus (PVA, 1998) may agree that occupational therapy is effective in treating neurodegenerative diseases, unfortunately, little empirical evidence confirms these views. Consequently, typical occupational therapy described here is based on commonly held assumptions about treatment and not on well-designed randomized controlled research trials establishing its effectiveness. Even in the randomized controlled trials that have been published, occupational therapy is frequently not studied alone but is one of several interventions with other rehabilitation therapies (Aisen, 1999; Freeman et al., 1999; Solari et al., 1999), frequently in an inpatient rehabilitation setting (Freeman et al., 1997). Most occupational therapy for persons with these diseases takes place in outpatient, home health, or long-term care facilities, and consequently, the generalizability of these team-based inpatient studies is questionable. The Mathiowetz study of the effectiveness of outpatient group occupational therapy in energy conservation strategies in MS is a notable exception (Mathiowetz et al., 2001). Other problems with existing research are the lack of attention–placebo treatment groups, small numbers of participants receiving multiple interventions, poor internal validity, and failure to select patients carefully and/or control for medications. At a time when evidence-based outcomes are increasingly required for reimbursement, occupational therapists must carry out well-designed research studies of interventions and publish findings in peer-reviewed journals to support the effectiveness of our interventions in achieving positive outcomes.

Summary Review Questions

1. What are the various courses of multiple sclerosis?
2. What primary symptoms of multiple sclerosis may require occupational therapy intervention?

3. What are the main modifications that a therapist might recommend for a woman with severe MS fatigue who is working full-time and has two young children?

4. How can an occupational therapist help a person with neurodegenerative disease stay employed?

5. What factors and symptoms should a therapist consider when ordering wheeled mobility for a patient with neurodegenerative disease?

6. What environmental modifications may be necessary in PD?

7. List the items you would check and primary modifications you might recommend during a home safety visit for a person with a neurodegenerative disease.

8. Why is it important to include the significant others of people with neurodegenerative diseases when developing treatment interventions?

9. What are the standard safety precautions you should use in treating all patients?

10. Plan an outpatient therapy session to treat a person with PD who has akinesia, bradykinesia, and rigidity and who is falling regularly.

Acknowledgment

The section on human immunodeficiency virus was prepared by Margaret A. McReynolds, M.Ed., P. T., Oregon Health Sciences University.

Resources

ALS Association · 21021 Ventura Blvd., Suite 321, Woodland Hills, CA 91364-2206.

Muscular Dystrophy Association, ALS Division · 3300 East Sunrise Drive, Tucson, AZ 85718-3208. 602-529 2000. Publications include *ALS: Maintaining Mobility, Meals* and others

Cleveland Clinic ALS Center · ALS Coordinator, Department of Neurology, 9500 Euclid Ave., Cleveland, OH 44195. Publication: *ALS Care Manual*

National Multiple Sclerosis Society · 733 Third Ave., New York, NY 10017. 800-FIGHT-MS.
www.nmss.org
also local chapters throughout United States and Canada

Paralyzed Veterans of America · 801 Eighteenth St. NW, Washington, DC 20006. 800-424-8200.
www.pva.org

Clearinghouse on Disability Information · U.S. Department of Education, 202-205-8241.
www.ed.gov/offices/oser

Consortium of Multiple Sclerosis Centers · c/o Gimbel MS Center, Holy Name Hospital, 718 Teaneck Rd., Teaneck, NJ 07666. 201-837-0727.

Parkinson's Disease News Letter · 800-947-6658.

Parkinson Foundation of Canada · National Office, 4211 Yonge St., Suite 316, Toronto, Ontario, M2P 2A9, Canada. 800-565-3000.

American Parkinson Disease Association, Inc. · 1250 Hylan Blvd., Suite 4B, Staten Island, NY 10305. 800-223-2732.

National Parkinson Foundation, Inc. · Bob Hope Research Center, 1501 N. W. 9th Ave., Miami, FL 33136-1494. 800-327-4545.

Michael J. Fox Foundation for Parkinson's Research · P. O. Box 2010, Grand Rapids, MN 55745.
www.michaeljfox.org

Cooling Vests

Coolsport (20% discount for people with MS) · 1880 W. Carson St., Torrence, Ca. 40501. 310-618-1590.
www.coolsport.net

MicroClimate Cooling Systems, Inc. · 968 E. Saginaw Rd., Sanford, MI 48657. 800-642-9077.
www.microclimate.com

References

Aarsland, D., Tandberg, E., Larsen, J. P., & Cummings, J. L. (1996). Frequency of dementia in parkinson disease. *Archive of Neurology, 53,* 538–542.

Aisen, M. L. (1999). Justifying neurorehabilitation: A few steps forward. *Neurology, 52,* 8–10.

Alter, M. (1978). Migration and risk of multiple sclerosis. *Neurology, 28,* 1089.

Anderson, D. W., Ellenberg, J. H., Leventhal, C. M., Reingold, S. C., Rodriguez, M., Silberberg, D. H. (1992). Revised estimate of the prevalence of multiple sclerosis in the United States. *Annals of Neurology, 31,* 333–336.

Beatty, W. W., & Goodkin, D. E. (1990). Screening for cognitive impairment in multiple sclerosis: An evaluation of the Mini-Mental State Examination. *Archives Neurology, 47,* 297–301.

Beatty, W. W., Paul, R. H., Wilbanks, S. L., Hames, K. A., Blanco, C. R., & Goodkin, D. E. (1995). Identifying multiple sclerosis patients with mild or global cognitive impairment using the Screening Examination for Cognitive Impairment (SEFCI). *Neurology, 45,* 718–723.

Bourdette, D. (1997). Multiple sclerosis. In R. E. Rakel (Ed.), *Current Therapy* (pp. 937–946). Philadelphia: Saunders.

Bradley, W. E. (1996). *Neurology in Clinical Practice* (2nd ed.). Boston: Butterworth- Heinemann.

Calne, D. B. (1995). Diagnosis and treatment of Parkinson' s disease. *Hospital Practice, 30* (l), 83–86, 89.

Conley, C. C., & Kirchner, J. T. (1999). Parkinson's disease: The shaking palsy. *Post Graduate Medicine, 109* (l), 39–52.

Fischer, J. S., Priore, R. L., Jacobs, L. D., Cookfair, D. L., Rudick, R.A., Herndon, R. M., Richert, J. R., Salazar, A. M., Goodkin, D. E., Granger, C. V., Simon, J. H., Grafrau, J. H., Lezak, M. D., O'Reilly Hovey, K. M., Perkins, K. K., Barilla-Clark, D., Schacter, M., Shucard, D. W., Davidson, A. L., Wende, K. E., Bourdette, D. N., Kooijmans-Coutinho, M. F. (2000). Neuropsychological effects of interferon beta-1a in relapsing remitting multiple sclerosis. Multiple Sclerosis Collaborative Research Group. *Annals of Neurology, 48,* 885–892.

Foong, J., Rozewicz, L., & Quaghebeur, G. (1997). Executive functions in multiple sclerosis: The role of frontal lobe pathology. *Brain, 20,* 15–26.

Frankel, D. I. (1990). Multiple sclerosis. In D. A. Umphred (Ed.), *Neurological Rehabilitation* (2nd ed., pp. 531–549). St. Louis: Mosby.

Freal, J. E., Kraft, G., & Coryell, J. (1984). Symptomatic fatigue in multiple sclerosis. *Archives of Physical Medicine and Rehabilitation, 65,* 135–138.

Freeman, J. A., Langdon, D. W., Hobart, J. S., & Thompson, A.J. (1997). Health-related quality of life in people with multiple sclerosis undergoing inpatient rehabilitation. *Journal of Neurologic Rehabilitation, 10,* 17–20.

Friedman, J., & Friedman, H. (1993). Fatigue in Parkinson's disease. *Neurology, 43,* 2016–2018.

Fuh, J.-L., Lee, R.-C., Wang, S.-J., Lin, C.-H., Wang, P.-N., Chiang, J.-H., & Liu, H.-C. (1997). Swallowing difficulty in Parkinson's disease. *Clinical Neurology and Neurosurgery, 99,* 106–112.

Galantino, M. L. (1992). *Clinical Assessment and Treatment of HIV: Rehabilitation of a Chronic Illness.* Thorofare, NJ: Slack.

Gelb, D. J., Olliver, E., & Gilman, S. (1999). Diagnostic criteria for Parkinson Disease. *Archive of Neurology, 56,* 33–39.

Harvey, C. (1994). HIV Infection and AIDS. In L Oloff (Ed.), *Musculoskeletal Disorders of the Lower Extremity.* Philadelphia: Saunders.

Hashimoto, S. A. & Paty, D. W. (1986). Multiple sclerosis. *Disease-A-Month, 32,* 518.

Hoehn, M. M.. & Yahr, M. D. (1967). Parkinsonism: Onset, progression and mortality. *Neurology, 17,* 427–442.

Hopp, J., & Rogers, E. (1989). *AIDS and Allied Health Professions.* Philadelphia: Davis.

Hughes, R. A. C., & Rees, J. (1997). Clinical and epidemiologic features of Guillain-Barré syndrome. *Journal of Infectious Diseases, 176* (Suppl 2), S92–S98.

Jiang, G. X., Chang, Q., Ehmst, A., Link, H., & de Pedro-Cuesta (1997). Guillain-Barré syndrome in Stockholm County, 1973–1991. *European Journal of Epidemiology, 13* (I), 25–32.

Kalb, R. C. (1996). *Multiple sclerosis: The questions you have—The answers you need.* New York: Demos.

Karlson, K. H., Larsen, J. P., Tandberg, E., & Maeland, J. G. (1999). Influences of clinical and demographic variables in quality of life in patients with Parkinson's disease. *Journal of Neurology, Neuropsychiatry and Psychiatry, 66,* 431–435.

Kelley, C. L (1996). The role of interferons in the treatment of multiple sclerosis. *American Association of Neuroscience Nurses, 28,* 114–120.

Koppel, B. (1998). Neurological complications of AIDS and HIV infection: An overview. In G. Wormser (Ed), *AIDS and Other Manifestations of HIV Infection* (3rd ed., pp. 431–473). Philadelphia: Lippincott-Raven.

Kurland, L. T. (1952). The frequency and geographic distribution of multiple sclerosis as indicated by mortality statistics and morbidity surveys in the United States and Canada. *American Journal Hygiene, 55,* 457.

Kurtzke, J. F. (1983). Rating neurologic impairment in multiple sclerosis: An *Expanded Disability Status Scale* (EDSS). *Neurology, 33,* 1444–1452.

Lublin, F. D., & Reingold, S. C. (1996). Defining the clinical course of multiple sclerosis: Results of an international survey. *Neurology, 46,* 907–911.

Lucchinetti, C., Bruck, W., Parisi, J., Scheithauer, B., Rodriguez, M., & Lassmann, H. (2000). Heterogeneity of multiple sclerosis lesions: implications for pathogenesis of demyelination. *Annals of Neurology, 46,* 907–911.

Marder, K., Logroscino, G., Alfaro, B., Mejia, H., Halim, A., Louis, E., Cote, L., & Mayeux, R. (1998). Environmental risk factors for Parkinson's disease in an urban multiethnic community. *Neurology, 50,* 279–281.

Mathiowetz, V., Matuska, K. M., & Murphy, M. E. (2001). The effects of an energy conservation course for persons with multiple sclerosis. *Archives of Physical Medicine and Rehabilitation, 82,* 449–456.

Maurelli, M., Marchioni, E., Cerretano, R., Basone, D., Bergamaschi, R., Citterio, A., Martelli, A., Sibilla, L., & Savoldi, F. (1992). Neuropsychological assessments in MS: Clinical, neurophysiological and neuroradiological relationships. *Acta Neurologica Scandinavica, 86,* 124–128.

McGavern, D. B., Murray, P. D., Rivera-Quinones, C., Schmelzer, J. D., Low, P. A., Rodrigues, M. (2000). Axonal loss results in spinal cord atrophy, electrophysiological abnormalities and neurological deficits following demyelination in a chronic inflammatory model of multiple sclerosis. *Brain, 123,* 519–531.

McReynolds, M. (1995). Rehabilitation management of the lower extremity in HIV disease. *Journal of American Podiatric Medicine Association, 85,* 394–402.

McReynolds, M., & Galantino, M. L. (1996). HIV patients with distal symmetrical peripheral neuropathy: Effect of microcurrent intervention for reduction of pain and alterations in gait. In M. L. Galantino (Ed.), *Issues in HIV Rehabilitation.* Silver Spring, MD: American Physical Therapy Association.

Meythaler, J. M., DeVivo, M. J., & Braswell, W. C. (1997). Rehabilitation outcomes of patients who have developed Guillain-Barré syndrome. *American Journal of Physical Medicine and Rehabilitation, 76,* 411–419.

Mitsumoto, H., Chad, D., & Pioro, E. (1998). *Amyotrophic Lateral Sclerosis. Contemporary Neurology Series.* Philadelphia: Davis.

Monza, D., Soliveri, P., Radice, D., Fetoni, V., Testa, D., Caffarra, P., Caraceni, T., & Girotti, F. (1998). Cognitive dysfunction and impaired organization of complex motility in degenerative parkinsonian syndromes. *Archive of Neurology, 55,* 372–378.

Moulin, D. E., Foley, K. M., & Ebers, G. C. (1988). Pain syndromes in multiple sclerosis. *Neurology, 38,* 1830–1834.

Muenter, M. D., Forno, L. S., & Hornykiewicz, O. (1998). Hereditary form of parkinsonism: Dementia. *Annals of Neurology, 43,* 6, 768–781.

Muscular Dystrophy Association of Canada (1997). *Guillain-Barré Syndrome.* InfoSMDAC. Toronto: Author.

National Multiple Sclerosis Society (1998). Clinical Bulletin: Disease Management Consensus Statement, New York City. *Neurology, 77,* 231–249.

O'Dell, M. (1996). Physical disability and rehabilitation in HIV infection. In M. L. Galantino (Ed) *Issues in HIV Rehabilitation.* Silver Spring, MD: American Physical Therapy Association.

Pankoff, B., Overend, T., Lucy, D., & White, K. (2000). Validity and responsiveness of the 6 minute walk test for people with fibromyalgia. *Journal of Rheumatology, 27,* 2666–2670.

Paralyzed Veterans of America [PVA]: Multiple Sclerosis Council for Clinical Practice Guidelines (1998). *Fatigue and Multiple Sclerosis.* Clinical Practice Guidelines. Washington: Author.

Petijan, J. H., Gappmaier, E., White, A. T., Spencer, M. K., Mino, L., & Hicks, R. W. (1996). Impact of aerobic training on fitness and quality of life in multiple sclerosis. *Annals of Neurology, 39,* 432–441.

Peto, V., Jenkinson, C., & Fitzpatrick, R. (1995). The development of validation of a short measure of functioning and well being for individuals with Parkinson's disease. *Quality of Life Research, 4,* 241–248.

Poser, C. M., Paty, D., Scheinberg, L., McDonald, W., Davis, F., Ebers, G., Johnson, K., Sibley, W., Silberberg, D., & Tourtellotte, W. (1983). New diagnostic criteria for multiple sclerosis: Guidelines for research protocols. *Annals of Neurology, 13,* 227–231.

Rao, S. M., Leo, G. J., Bernardin, L., & Unverszagt, F. (1991). Cognitive dysfunction in multiple sclerosis. *Neurology, 41,* 685–691.

Rees, J. H., Thompson, R. D., Smeeton, N. C., & Hughes, R. A. (1998). Epidemiological study of Guillain-Barré syndrome in south east England. *Journal of Neurology, Neurosurgery & Psychiatry, 64,* 74–77.

Rodriguez, M., Siva, A., Ward, J., Stolp-Smith, K., O'Brien, P., & Kurland, L. (1994). Impairment, disability, and handicap in multiple sclerosis: A population-based study in Olmsted County, Minnesota. *Neurology, 44,* 28–33.

Rovari, N. M., Filippi, M., Falautano, M., Minicucci, Rocca, V., Marinelli, V., & Comi, G. (1998). Correlation between MR abnormalities and patterns of cognitive impairment in multiple sclerosis, *Neurology, 50,* 1604–1608.

Semchuk, K. M., Love, E. J., & Lee, R.G. (1992). Parkinson's disease and exposure to agricultural work and pesticide chemicals. *Neurology, 42,* 1328–1335.

Solari, A., Filippini, G., Gasco, P., Colla, L., Salmnaggi, A., La Mantia, L., Farinotti, M., Eoli, M., & Mendozzi, L. (1999). Physical rehabilitation has a positive effect on disability in multiple sclerosis patients. *Neurology, 52,* 57–62.

Stern, M. B. (1993). Parkinson's disease: Early diagnosis and management. *Journal of Family Practice, 36,* 439–446.

Stolp-Smith, K. A., Carter, J. L., Rohe, D. E., & Knowland, D. P. (1997). Management of impairment, disability and handicap due to multiple sclerosis. *Mayo Clinic Proceedings, 72,* 1184–1196.

Trapp, B. D., Peterson, J., Ransohoff, R. M., Rudick, R., Mork, S., & Bo, L. (1998). Axonal transection in the lesions of multiple sclerosis. *New England Journal of Medicine, 338,* 278–285.

Uitti, R. J. (1998). Tremor: How to determine if the patient has Parkinson's disease. *Geriatrics, 53,* 30–36.

41
Orthopaedic Conditions

Jane Bear-Lehman

LEARNING OBJECTIVES

After studying this chapter, the reader will be able to do the following:

1. Identify the role of the occupational therapist in assessing and planning treatment for persons with occupational dysfunction secondary to injuries or diseases affecting the musculoskeletal system.
2. Select appropriate assessments and plan treatment according to the stages of recovery following a musculoskeletal injury or disease of the upper extremity.
3. Describe how to accomplish daily life tasks without causing adverse sequelae following fracture or surgery to the hip.
4. State the principles of body mechanics and describe how to apply them to activities and tasks of daily life.

*O*rthopaedic conditions include injuries, diseases, and deformities of bones, joints, and their related structures: muscles, tendons, ligaments, and nerves. These conditions can be caused by traumatic events, such as motor vehicle, recreational, or work-related accidents; by cumulative trauma; or by congenital anomaly. The rising incidence rate of musculoskeletal injuries is attributed to an increase in "individual participation in high-speed travel by land, sea, and air, complex industry, and competitive and recreational sports" (Salter, 1999, p. 417). Furthermore, more individuals are reaching old age, and as they age, the incidence of injuries from falls increases.

The primary complaints of persons treated by orthopaedic surgeons are loss of independent mobility, musculoskeletal deformity, neurological problems that result from disease or injury to the musculoskeletal system, and pain. The primary complaint of persons with musculoskeletal disorders seen in rehabilitation is loss of ability to perform important life activities. Orthopaedic surgery and rehabilitation place equal emphasis on prevention and correction of deformity and disability. The most important aim in orthopaedic rehabilitation is to restore occupational functioning.

This chapter provides an overview of the occupational therapy assessments and treatments used with adult patients who have orthopaedic or musculoskeletal conditions. Specifically, it reviews upper

GLOSSARY

Cervical spine range of motion exercises—Exercises that promote normal movement in the neck: flexion, extension, lateral rotation to the right and left, and lateral bending to the right and left (Hoppenfeld, 1976).

Chronic regional pain syndrome (CRPS)—Painful complications, formerly referred to as reflex sympathetic dystrophy or causalgia, that may occur after an injury and progress over time. The pain exceeds expectations both in magnitude and duration. CRPS may result in significant functional impairment and performance deficits (Mackin, 1997; Stanton-Hicks et al., 1995).

Clinical union—Evidence of bony callus on radiographic examination, although the fracture line is still apparent (Salter, 1999).

Codman's pendulum exercises—Exercises prescribed for most shoulder fractures in early recovery. The standing or sitting patient bends over at the hips so that the trunk is parallel to the floor. The arm assumes a position away from the body and perpendicular to the floor, either with or without a sling. In this gravity-assisted position, the patient moves the arm passively or actively, depending on the surgical protocol, forward into humeral flexion and backward into humeral extension; across and away from the body for shoulder abduction and adduction; and then in a circle for circumduction (Epps & Cotler, 1985; Salter, 1999).

Collar and cuff sling—Sling made from a circle of material placed around the neck; the forearm is placed in the circle and supported only at the wrist. The length of the sling is adjusted to place the radial side of the wrist just below the nipple line (Salter, 1999).

Controlled range of motion—Active or passive movement within a predetermined safe arc. Often the allowed movement begins in the middle of the range and is gradually upgraded toward the full arc as healing occurs. A splint can be used to set the boundaries or block unwanted movement.

Deep pressure tissue massage—Firm manual pressure applied to the skin for about 5 seconds to blanch the underlying scar. This massage is initiated once sutures are removed. On a closed wound, lanolin or Vitamin E can be used. Massage begins at the perimeter and gradually works toward and then over the surgical scar site.

Delayed wound closure—Procedure to allow for further debridement after surgery. The physician elects to close the wound only after there appears to be no risk of infection (Smith, 1995).

Percutaneous pins—Long, slender metal rods used for skeletal traction. They extend from the bone, either proximal or distal to the fracture site, through the skin. One example is a Kirschner wire. They are often used with plaster to fixate a severely comminuted or unstable intra-articular fracture (Frykman & Kropp, 1995).

Secondary intention healing—Wound that the physician has left to heal spontaneously because of host tissue injury, contamination, or presence of a foreign body (Smith, 1995).

Shoulder rolls—Shoulder protraction and retraction performed while the arm is held at the side, to maintain mobility of the scapulothoracic, sternoclavicular, and acromioclavicular joints (Kelley & Clark, 1995).

Skateboard—Cushioned board used to support the forearm and/or hand. It has free-moving ball bearing casters near the four corners on the bottom to allow for unresisted movement on a flat, smooth surface, such as a table.

Trendelenburg gait—Gait pattern that results from a weakened gluteus medius muscle. The patient lurches toward the injured side to place the center of gravity over the hip. It is characterized by dropping of the pelvis on the unaffected side at heel strike of the affected foot.

Volkmann's ischemia—Compartment syndrome that results from increased pressure of progressive edema within the rigid osteofascia of the forearm. The circulation to the enclosed flexor muscles of the forearm and nerves is compromised, and a vicious cycle is established. The tissues outside the compartment are spared (Salter, 1999).

Wall climbing, finger walking, palm gliding—Exercise to develop shoulder flexion. The patient faces the wall, places the injured shoulder's hand on the wall, and either finger walks or glides the palm toward the ceiling and then the floor. For shoulder and scapular abduction, the patient turns parallel to the wall and abducts the shoulder to place the fingers or palm on the wall for finger walking or palm gliding. Commercially available finger climbers can be mounted on the wall or used on a tabletop with set increments for the finger walk; some climbers can be adjusted to different angles to allow for varying degrees of movement.

extremity and hip fractures and their sequelae, hip surgery for trauma and disease, and pain with a focus on low back pain.

Purpose and Role of Occupational Therapy in Orthopaedics

The aim of occupational therapy in orthopaedic rehabilitation is to help the patient achieve maximal function of body and limb to restore occupational functioning. In the acute stage of recovery, the therapist's role is to help relieve pain, maintain joint or limb alignment, and restore function at the injury site. The therapist teaches the patient to achieve safe performance of tasks and activities while protecting the injury site for healing. As healing progresses to **clinical union** and then to consolidation, the occupational therapist retrains the patient in activities of daily living (ADL) and other occupational tasks.

For individuals who have a chronic joint disease, such as osteoarthritis, or cumulative trauma, such as low back pain, the occupational therapist's role depends on the stage of recovery and the directives of the treatment team. The occupational therapist may directly help relieve pain, realign structures, or reduce the stress on soft tissue. Or the occupational therapist may work closely with the physical therapist to relate the functional program to treatment offered in physical therapy to heal the wound. As the acute episode of pain calms, the occupational therapist focuses on an individually tailored education program to help the patient physically and psychologically make the required lifestyle changes to reach and sustain optimal occupational functioning.

Occupational Therapy Evaluation in Orthopaedics

Evaluation is an ongoing process that is carefully coordinated with the stage of recovery. The therapist selects assessments that will provide sufficient information to plan and to direct treatment but will not threaten the injured or inflamed structure during healing. The therapist chooses assessments that correspond to the level of bone healing, the chosen method of reduction and stabilization, and the plan for movement during healing or the acute inflammatory episode. The therapist assesses both participation in life roles and impairments of capacities and abilities.

Participation in Life Roles

Although resumption of life roles may not be possible at the start of the aftercare program, life roles regulate the choices made during treatment planning and serve as

the end point for treatment planning. In addition to noting the activities and tasks the patient can and cannot accomplish, using the assessment tools described in Chapter 3, the therapist observes whether the patient is magnifying the injury and rehabilitation or appears to be adopting a sick role.

Impairments of Abilities and Capacities

Physical impairments are directly measured by various assessment instruments. See Chapter 4 for assessment of pain, edema, range of motion (ROM), strength, and endurance. The surgeon's protocol may stipulate no movement or no force at or near the fracture site, or it may require **controlled range of motion** beginning immediately or within the first 3 to 4 weeks after stabilization (Fig. 41-1). If the surgeon's protocol requires complete rest of the injured bone or joint, ROM measurements are deferred until movement is permissible. If the patient is on a specific program, such as controlled range of motion, the therapist measures the joint, adhering to the precautionary boundaries, and does not allow the patient to exceed the limits of the directive. The adjacent joints are measured, and a treatment program is designed for any adjacent joint that demonstrates less than normal function. Detailed strength testing with applied resistance is deferred until there is bony consolidation or the acute inflammation has calmed. Because of the force required, grip and pinch testing are usually deferred for 2 to 4 weeks following cast removal in forearm fractures. The occupational therapist not only focuses on direct measure of the injured and adjacent anatomical regions but closely observes the patient's total body response in terms of postural changes, pain responses, and psychological reactions.

Occupational Therapy Treatment in Orthopaedics

The most important treatment goal is the restoration of occupational functioning. To achieve this, the patient needs to be directed from the start of recovery to move and to use all joints that are not affected by the injury or the disease. For patients who have an upper limb fracture or a short-term inflammation, the therapist may recommend temporary use of the uninjured hand alone to perform some ADL, assisted by adaptations such as pump bottles for toothpaste and shampoo, a button hook, or a rocker knife. Other ADL may require temporary assistance of another person so as not to disturb the healing region.

When the patient is medically ready, the occupational therapist, through careful activity analysis, ascertains how the patient can safely resume tasks that

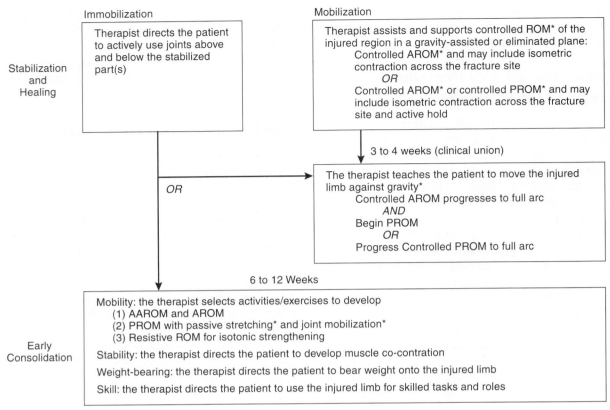

Figure 41-1 Guidelines for therapeutic intervention during fracture healing and consolidation.

correspond with the achieved recovery status to reintegrate the injured or inflamed limb into activity safely. Attention is directed toward redeveloping the function of the injured limb to resume its capacity in mobility, stability, weight bearing, and ultimately for skill (Fig. 41-1). When a condition is chronic, such as hip replacement or low back pain, the therapist recommends alternative methods, adaptive equipment, or environmental modification for safe task completion.

Acute Trauma: Fractures

As long as orthopaedic surgeons have been treating fractures, there has been a controversy between the "movers" and the "resters." The surgeons prescribing rest as a fracture treatment keep their patients immobilized in traction or plaster for long periods after stabilization. However, for many surgeons, the goal in fracture treatment is to mobilize the injured structures as quickly as is compatible with healing and return the patient to work and leisure activities (Salter, 1999).

The goal of fracture treatment is to achieve a precise and effective stabilization for optimal recovery and resolution of function. Closed fractures that are relatively

undisplaced and stable may be managed by protection alone, without reduction or immobilization. Fractures that are undisplaced but unstable do not need reduction but do require positioning and immobilization in a cast or an external splint. Surgical reduction is performed to reduce open fractures and those closed fractures where the bone fragments cannot be approximated accurately by closed manual reduction alone. The bone fragments are brought into a closer anatomical alignment during surgical reduction and are stabilized by insertion of an internal fixation device, such as a nail, pin, screw, rod, compression plate, or an external fixator (Figs. 41-2 and 41-3). Surgical repair also can include prosthetic devices that are implanted to restore joint motion (Apley & Solomon, 1994).

Fracture healing, when the part is immobilized by a cast, splint, or fracture brace (Figs. 41-4 and 41-5), is accomplished through the formation of immature woven bone or external callus. The woven bone then consolidates and remodels so that the fracture is repaired with lamellar bone (Apley & Solomon, 1994). When internal fixation provides complete bone immobilization, external callus does not form, and direct healing occurs. When external callus forms first, more healing time is required. Fracture healing has a general timetable that is confirmed routinely by radiographs to reveal the healing status before advancing the rehabilitation program (Box 41-1). Consolidation or complete fracture repair has occurred when the callus is ossified, the fracture site is no longer tender and painful, and there is no movement when the fractured bone is manipulated (Apley & Solomon).

Rehabilitation begins as soon as the plaster cast dries or within a day or two after reduction. The timing, amount, and kind of activity depend on the place and kind of fracture, the method of fracture reduction selected by the orthopaedic surgeon, and in some instances the age of the patient. Clinical experience has shown that early specific use of the injured limb during healing diminishes or eliminates the need for treatment after immobilization (Salter, 1999). Early movement prevents the unwanted side effects of immobilization: stiff joints, disuse atrophy, and muscle weakness.

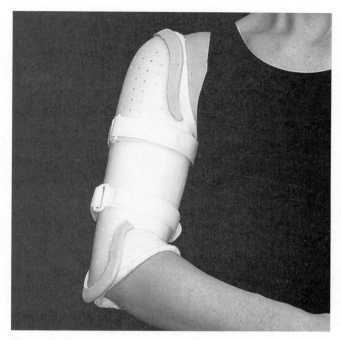

Figure 41-4 Thermoplastic humeral fracture brace to support the length of the humerus during healing. (Courtesy of Smith & Nephew, Inc., Germantown, WI.)

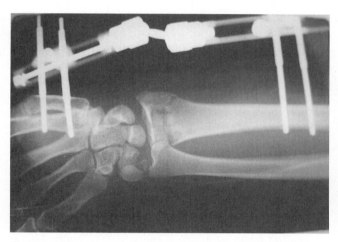

Figure 41-2 An external fixator provides skeletal traction for distal forearm fracture healing as shown in the radiograph. (Courtesy of Robert J. Strauch, MD, New York Presbyterian Hospital, Department of Orthopaedic Surgery, New York, NY.)

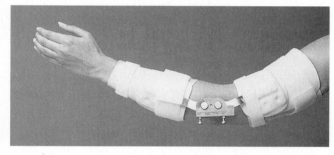

Figure 41-5 Upper extremity fracture brace with adjustable hinge joint designed to position the elbow statically in flexion or extension, block undesirable motion, and allow some free elbow motion. (Courtesy of Smith & Nephew, Inc., Germantown, WI.)

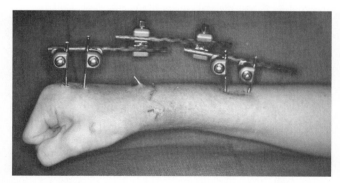

Figure 41-3 External fixator as shown on the forearm. (Courtesy of Robert J. Strauch, MD, New York Presbyterian Hospital, Department of Orthopaedic Surgery, New York, NY.)

Evaluation Process in Aftercare for Fractures

The evaluation is carefully designed and adjusted to the stage of recovery and the kind of fracture. This chapter presents the specialized focus for each fracture by the stage of recovery: immobilization and early mobilization or early consolidation.

Immobilization or Early Mobilization

The therapist identifies the tasks and activities for which the patient needs to learn an adaptation or obtain assistance during the temporary period of restricted movement so that the fracture site remains undisturbed. Measurements of ROM are conducted on adjacent joints. Assessment of active range of motion (AROM) of the

The general estimate of healing time for uncomplicated fractures in tubular bones, according to Apley and Solomon (1994), is as follows:

	Upper Limb	Lower Limb
Callus visible	2–3 weeks	2–3 weeks
Union	4–6 weeks	8–12 weeks
Consolidation	6–8 weeks	12–16 weeks

injured joints depends on the type of protection and stabilization used and the orthopaedic surgeon's protocol for aftercare, as discussed earlier.

Early Consolidation

The therapist determines whether and to what extent the patient can safely reintegrate the injured limb into ADL. The therapist continually assesses the patient's ability to use the injured limb for functional tasks to correspond with clinical progress.

The therapist measures both passive range of motion (PROM) and AROM at joints adjacent to the injury and carefully observes the patient for signs of infection: redness, heat, swelling, pain, loss of function, or changes in circulation. To do so, look at the limb's skin color: purple, dusky, or white coloration indicates alterations in circulation, as does a skin surface that is too warm or too cold to the touch. ***Immediately report abnormal findings to the surgeon.***

Treatment Process in Aftercare for Fractures

Intervention strategies for addressing orthopaedic injuries are based on the stage of recovery and the orthopaedic treatment protocol. The therapist selects and applies intervention strategies that are consistent with the orthopaedic surgeon's immobilization or mobilization plan, the restrictions or precautions, and goals.

Immobilization or Early Mobilization

Early mobilization treatment programs have specific and focused protocols indicating the timing, type, and quantity of desired movement (Fig. 41-1). Advancement of the therapeutic program is determined for each patient on the basis of the fracture configuration, its apparent or tested stability, radiographic signs of fracture healing, and the patient's tolerance (Basti et al., 1994). The cautiously controlled movement usually begins in a gravity-assisted or gravity-eliminated plane. The movement may be active–assistive range of motion (AAROM) or AROM restricted to midrange and gradually upgraded to full ROM. Under careful guidance and manual

handling, isometric contraction of the muscles whose bellies extend across the fracture site is encouraged to facilitate circulation and bone healing. Some protocols require controlled PROM, often followed by an active hold pattern. That is, the therapist passively moves the injured part through the prescribed arc, and then the patient isometrically holds the achieved position briefly.

The therapist may have to fit the patient with a sling, splint, or fracture brace during healing either to add protective support or to begin early controlled movement. To add to a patient's comfort during stabilization in an external fixator, the therapist may recommend and fabricate a supportive static splint. Thermoplastic splinting alone is often used to achieve relative immobilization for fractures of the metacarpals and phalanges (see Chapters 14 and 42). Following the initial treatment of closed reduction of fractures in the shaft of long bones, the surgeon may prescribe a functional fracture brace as shown in Figures 41-4 and 41-5 (Salter, 1999). The lightweight thermoplastic fracture brace allows for motion above and below the fracture site and minimizes detrimental effects of prolonged immobilization. The metal hinge controls the amount of movement available. The patient is closely monitored for circulation, biomechanical alignment, and desired (controlled) movement. The therapist adjusts the shell to facilitate comfort, to respond to changes such as a reduction of limb volume, and to adjust the amount of movement the splint permits.

Patients whose fractures have been stabilized with an external fixator (Figs. 41-2 and 41-3) or externally exposed pins need to learn routine pin maintenance to prevent infection and possible osteomyelitis. The therapist teaches the patient to use alcohol or hydrogen peroxide to clean the pin and cover the pin with gauze, depending upon protocol (Collins, 1993; Smith, 1995). The surgeon's protocol is followed for wound management for open fractures that are healing with **delayed wound closure** or by **secondary intention** (Smith, 1995).

Early Consolidation

Therapy usually begins with focused, active use of the limb. Active therapy consists of activities and tasks to remediate the use of the muscle in the injured region as an agonist, antagonist, and fixator in static cocontraction (Mennell, 1945). The therapist directs the patient in a graduated program to resolve the presenting impairments and to reintegrate the limb into normal and customary use for functional tasks and role performance. If secondary changes are noted in the adjacent body parts or if there is a change in body posture, therapy is also directed to resolving those impairments.

Should edema persist even with elevation and active muscle contraction, additional methods, such as compression gloves or sleeves and retrograde massage, are applied. To ameliorate stiffness and pain, the therapist may introduce modalities such as paraffin, fluidotherapy, or heat packs before or with exercise or activity (see Chapter 18). If stiffness prevails and the fracture is stable, joint mobilization and passive stretching are performed to facilitate the arthrokinetic accessory movements to increase the passive movement potential. Dynamic splinting or the use of continuous passive movement machines may also increase passive mobility over time. Adherent or hypertrophic scar formation after open reduction or soft tissue repair can also limit movement, increase pain, and alter sensation. To prevent this, the therapist teaches the patient **deep pressure tissue massage** and applies continuous pressure to the scar with an agent such as Silastic gel to facilitate scar remodeling (see Chapter 45).

Fractures

The care of fractures challenges both the surgeon and the occupational therapist to help the patient ultimately reincorporate the injured limb into functional performance tasks. To initiate the care of a patient who sustained a fracture, the therapist must understand the anatomy and biomechanics of the extremity and select intervention strategies that are consistent with the physiological process of fracture repair.

Shoulder Fractures

The shoulder complex is the most mobile of all joints in the body. It provides a wide range for hand placement but also provides the important functions of stabilization for hand use, lifting and pushing, elevation of the body, and weight bearing (Skyhar & Simmons, 1992; Smith et al., 1996). The shoulder is considered the most challenging portion of the body to rehabilitate. After traumatic, degenerative, or surgical shoulder lesions, the therapy goals are delicately balanced to relieve pain, restore movement and muscle strength, and allow for callus formation and the approximation of the bony fragments in the injured region (Skyhar & Simmons).

Immobilization of the shoulder results in stiffness and pain; therefore, nonoperative and postoperative therapy programs call for a specific regimen of PROM, AAROM, or AROM within a controlled, guarded range. Shoulder fractures are closely monitored by radiographs as initial controlled PROM and AAROM begin. There is controversy with regard to PROM. Some argue that passive motion is contraindicated, particularly in the elderly (Goldstein, 1999). Others say that passive movement is safe if the provided range corresponds to the surgeon's prescribed limitations (Skyhar & Simmons, 1992). Emphasis is on the patient resuming nonresistive functional activities, such as eating and performing basic hygiene, using the injured limb as soon as movement is allowed.

Since immobilization quickly results in stiffness, active shoulder motion begins as soon as the acute pain diminishes in stable shoulder fractures. Unstable shoulder fractures usually require surgical intervention for fixation. The protocols are based on the classification of fracture, the type of surgical procedure, and age and activity level of the patient, and they often follow the guidelines as originally described by Neer (1990). Some postoperative protocols start isometrics for external rotation and shoulder abduction across the repair site immediately to facilitate stability. Assisted isotonic shoulder motions follow about 3 to 4 weeks later, once the shoulder fragments are approximated as confirmed by radiograph (Jackins & Matsen, 1994; Kelley & Clark, 1995). If shoulder stability is achieved with internal fixation, active, pain-free range of motion exercises may begin as early as 7 to 10 days after surgery (Kelley & Clark).

During the first 6 to 8 weeks, isometric exercises, a stimulant for fracture healing and callus formation, are performed along with **wall climbing**, nonresistive therapeutic activities, and **Codman's pendulum exercises**. Codman's exercises are performed with the patient bending over so that the injured upper limb is perpendicular to the floor. In this gravity-assisted plane, the patient does clockwise and counterclockwise circular movements and flexion–extension, abduction, and adduction. ***Codman's exercises may be contraindicated if the upper extremity is edematous.***

Barring complications, when clinical union is achieved at approximately 6 weeks, progressive shoulder exercises for flexion, extension, abduction, and internal and external rotation are started (Kelley & Clark, 1995). Passive stretching, joint mobilization, and resistive exercises begin once there is established clinical union, the inflammation has decreased, and there is no fear of disrupting the fracture (Kelley & Clark; Skyhar & Simmons, 1992).

Therapy for total prosthetic joint replacement of the shoulder varies with the design of the prosthesis and the surgical procedure. It is accepted that the patient requires dedicated effort to perform PROM and AAROM several times a day beginning within the first 2 to 3 days after surgery. The exercises should not cause any pain. The key to a satisfactory functional result is early achievement of shoulder forward flexion and external rotation in the plane of the scapula. Some protocols require the use of continuous passive motion for forward shoulder flexion immediately following surgery (Rockwood, 1990; Salter, 1999).

Codman's pendulum exercises, AROM exercises done lying supine with the opposite hand assisting the affected limb, and use of an exercise wand and an overhead pulley are introduced during the first 2 to 3 days after surgery (Kelley & Clark, 1995). The patient is instructed to begin each of 4 to 6 daily sessions by performing Codman's exercises and passive flexion and external rotation exercises. Since the subscapularis tendon and the rotator cuff are violated during the surgery, some surgeons introduce external rotation slowly in the first 4 weeks, while others incorporate passive external rotation on the second postoperative day (Rockwood, 1990). The preferred position for passive external rotation exercise is with the humerus adducted. For the first 4 to 5 weeks of rehabilitation, external rotation is often limited to what was obtained at the time of wound closure, or the operative ROM value for external rotation (Kelley & Clark).

The patient is instructed in active exercises of the operated extremity: (1) **shoulder rolls**, (2) **cervical spine ROM exercises**, and (3) nonresistive exercises or activities involving the elbow and hand to reduce stiffness and edema (Kelley & Clark, 1995). The therapist teaches the patient to use the operated extremity safely for nonresistive ADL, namely eating, brushing teeth, and writing (Rockwood, 1990). After suture removal at 2 weeks, wall climbing is added to the program. At 6 weeks, with medical advisement, the program is upgraded to include active resistive exercise and activities to strengthen the rotator cuff muscles and the three parts of the deltoid muscle (Rockwood). Weight bearing on the injured arm is not allowed for at least 6 months (Arntz et al., 1993; Skyhar & Simmons, 1992).

Management of humeral shaft or humeral neck fractures is divided into three phases. Phase I includes positioning, Codman's pendulum exercises, and passive assistive exercises. Phase II includes active and early resistive exercises. Phase III includes advanced stretching and strengthening (Basti et al., 1994). Fractures of the humeral shaft and humeral neck both respond well to early passive movement and positioning. Codman's pendulum exercises and passive assistive movement of the shoulder are performed several times a day to prevent stiffness. The occupational therapist may make a fracture brace conforming to the length of the humerus to provide the initial support after a humeral shaft fracture (Fig. 41-4). The therapist must be careful to flare and roll the edges of the shell to prevent compromise to circulation and nerve impingement while allowing available movement. In the case of humeral shaft fracture, there is a risk of radial nerve damage due to the location of the injury relative to the course of the radial nerve (Salter, 1999). Radial nerve injury is characterized by inability to extend the elbow with gravity eliminated or inability to extend the wrist and/or the digits.

For phase II, the therapist encourages active assisted concentric and eccentric exercise, progressing to lightly resistive exercises. These patterns often begin with the patient supine and progress to seated, in which position the weight of the extremity is first supported by the therapist, a **skateboard**, or an overhead suspension sling.

Phase III addresses both stretching and strengthening. As healing permits, the patient can combine shoulder forward flexion with abduction with or without external rotation (Basti et al., 1994). Functional use of the injured extremity is encouraged.

Elbow Fractures

Elbow motion gives the individual the capacity to position the hand near or far from the body for manipulation of objects (Hotchkiss & Davlia, 1992; Smith et al., 1996). These movements are accomplished by two degrees of freedom: flexion and extension at the ulno-humeral joint and pronation and supination at the proximal radioulnar joint. Supracondylar fractures of the humerus are the most common and the most serious elbow fracture (Salter, 1999). These fractures are associated with a high incidence of malunion and have a risk of **Volkmann's ischemia**, a compartment syndrome of the forearm. Ischemia, considered an urgent medical matter, can be caused by edema within a fascia-surrounded compartment or acute elbow flexion that compresses an artery against bone. ***Signs of ischemia include pale, bluish skin color; absence of forearm radial pulse; and decreased hand sensation accompanied by severe pain. Report these signs immediately.*** Immediate action is important because the peripheral nerves can withstand only 2 to 4 hours of ischemia, though they do have some potential to regenerate. The muscle can withstand up to 6 hours of ischemia, but it cannot regenerate (Salter, 1999). Prolonged occlusion allows for the progression to a contracture as the necrotic muscle becomes dense, shortened, fibrous scar tissue.

The uncomplicated supracondylar fracture may be treated with immobilization in a removable plaster cast or thermoplastic splint following open reduction. The elbow is held in 90 to 100° of flexion, and the arm may be supported in a **collar-and-cuff sling** (Salter, 1999). After the first week, the splint is removed daily for gentle, nonresistive active movement in a gravity-eliminated position. Therapy for elbow fractures emphasizes active—not passive—movement and flexion rather than extension to minimize the risk of ischemia and excessive bone formation (heterotopic ossification) (Salter). Many patients achieve close to full movement after 6 to 12 months without specific treatment; some, however, do not achieve complete elbow extension even with therapy (Apley & Solomon, 1994).

Complex elbow fractures are often treated with open reduction and well-secured fixation. Active motion begins 3 to 5 days after surgery. Similar to the supracondylar fracture, the elbow fracture is splinted in flexion rather than extension, because if a contracture occurs, the hand can be raised to the face for eating and hygiene (Salter, 1999). In the elderly, elbow fractures are often treated with a collar-and-cuff sling alone, and active movement begins early to prevent stiffness and pain. A functional arc of motion for daily activities can be regained, but full ROM is not always achieved.

Radial head fractures seldom require immobilization. Undisplaced fractures without loss of joint congruity require protection in a sling for approximately 2 weeks (Salter, 1999). Active pronation and supination exercises are encouraged early. Full supination is more difficult and painful than pronation; months of therapy may be required to reach the maximum potential (Hotchkiss & Davlia, 1992).

Forearm Fractures

Distal forearm fractures are among the most common upper extremity injuries. Most result from a fall on an outstretched hand (protective extension reaction). The fractures of the distal forearm are named for the orthopaedists who first described them: Colles' fracture, Smith's fracture, Barton's fracture (Frykman & Kropp, 1995). These fractures affect the radius and/or the ulna and their articulations. Fixation with **percutaneous pins** is often required. If there has been extensive injury to the distal radioulnar joint, the arm is immobilized in a long cast, one that extends from the metacarpophalangeal joints to the mid humerus, to control for pronation and supination (Cooney & Schutt, 1992; Frykman & Kropp). If reduction is maintained after 3 weeks of immobilization, a short cast may be applied for another 2 to 4 weeks. The short cast allows for elbow flexion and extension to the limits of the cast and for full proximal and distal interphalangeal flexion and extension. The cast covers the distal palmar crease, limiting metacarpophalangeal flexion. Lateral prehension between the thumb and index finger is feasible. Some patients require a static splint to protect or support the forearm for another 2 to 4 weeks after cast removal (Cooney & Schutt).

If the patient demonstrates incomplete movement at the joints above and below the cast or if movement is limited when the cast comes off, therapy is required. Therapy begins with active movement to restore pain-free wrist and forearm ROM and functional use of the forearm, wrist, and hand. Passive stretching and joint mobilization are indicated for a stable fracture with limited movement. The patient is encouraged to resume activities as tolerated. Overhead positioning of a macramé project or use of an inclined board on which a game is mounted incorporates the whole limb into the activity.

Strengthening begins 2 weeks after the stabilizer is removed. Special emphasis is placed on the development of wrist stability, which is achieved through the use of tools such as screwdrivers or scissors that demand a forceful grasp and sustained wrist stabilization (Laester & Carter, 1996). Weight bearing on the consolidated distal forearm begins with the patient leaning on the injured arm as if it were a pillar while the hand rests on a soft surface, such as bed or carpet; then the patient does activities that gradually increase both the amount of weight the arm bears and the density of the surface.

For the patient who is stabilized in an external fixator (Figs. 41-2 and 41-3), early active motion takes place at the joints immediately and above and below it, depending on the directives of the surgeon. With approval, active exercise is performed in the whirlpool for the benefit of wound cleansing, increased circulation from the surging water, and the opportunity to move in a gravity-eliminated environment. The surgeon may ask the therapist to loosen the fixator to initiate early wrist flexion initially and then in the weeks to follow add wrist extension (Collins, 1993). The arc of movement specifically adheres to the surgeon's guidelines; it is judiciously monitored by both therapist and surgeon. After the external fixator is removed altogether, the protocol parallels that of the patient who was stabilized in plaster. Patients require about 9 months to regain maximum wrist motion (Cooney & Schutt, 1992).

Inflammation, edema, and extent of damage at the time of injury may bring on many complications of distal forearm fractures. Sensory status of the skin supplied by the median and ulnar nerves is monitored because of the risk of damage to these nerves secondary to the distal forearm fracture (Frykman & Kropp, 1995) (see Chapter 6).

The most serious complication of distal forearm fracture is **chronic regional pain syndrome** (Mackin, 1997; Stanton-Hicks et al., 1995), formerly called reflex sympathetic dystrophy. The classic symptoms include extreme pain, stiffness, edema, and vasomotor, sudomotor, and trophic changes (Collins, 1993).

Hip Fractures

Intertrochanteric hip fractures are very common in adults over 60 years of age and are more common in women than in men (Salter, 1999). These fractures occur in bone that is markedly weakened by osteoporosis (Salter). Many of these patients have prior medical complications, including congestive heart failure, coronary artery disease, hypertension, chronic obstructive pulmonary disease, or diabetes, that affect the duration and potential of the rehabilitation program (Lowrey & Coutis, 1992; Tinetti et al., 1994).

Hip fractures are treated with closed reduction and immobilization in plaster or open reduction with internal fixation using pins, nails, screws and plate, or rods (Eftekhar, 1993; Salter, 1999). Partial joint replacement is the treatment for some fractures of the neck and head of the femur. In partial joint replacement, the femoral head and neck are replaced by a prosthesis composed of a metal head and stem. After excision of the femoral head, the stem of the prosthesis is inserted distally into the medullary canal of the femur so that its head articulates with the normal acetabulum. If destructive changes have taken place in both the femur and the acetabulum, a total hip arthroplasty is necessary (Apley & Solomon, 1994; Eftekhar; Salter).

Occupational Therapy Following a Hip Fracture and Surgery

The restrictions for weight bearing and hip movement on the operated leg are directly related to the severity and location of the fracture, the surgical approach, the ability of the fixation device or prosthesis to withstand stress, the integrity of the bone, the weight of the patient, and the patient's cognitive status (Goldstein, 1999). The physical therapist teaches the patient to use a walker or crutches, depending on percentage of body weight allowed on the operated limb (Box 41-2). The occupational therapist teaches the patient to complete ADL safely, corresponding to the medical orders and the

BOX 41-3
PROCEDURES FOR PRACTICE

Adapations for ADL After Hip Replacement Surgery

Problem	Adaptation
Bathe feet	Long-handled bath sponge
Get in and out of tub	Nonskid bath mat; grab bar; bath bench
Don, doff socks	Stocking aide
Don, doff shoes	Extended-handle shoe horn
Don pants	Reacher or dressing stick
Transfer to and from toilet, chair, bed	Raised toilet seat, increased height of chair and bed
Sit in and rise from a chair	Wedge cushion with thick end of the wedge at the back of the chair
Open and close cabinets	Relocate frequently used items to eliminate the need to bend, reach; use a reacher

physical therapy progression for postoperative weight bearing. For some patients, preexisting factors or the risk of dislodging the new hip joint may necessitate the assistance of another person for lower extremity dressing and for bathing.

The rate of progression of weight bearing and mobility is individually tailored for the patient by the rate of fracture healing and the patient's response (Goldstein, 1999). Close communication among the rehabilitation team is imperative to provide the patient with the best quality of care and consistency in learning how to function after surgery. Essential to the planned discharge—following a hospital stay of less than a week for most—is the therapist's evaluation of the patient's ability to perform basic and instrumental ADL safely and independently and the need for adapted equipment and/or assistance of others (Bargar et al., 1998).

It is best to teach the patient who is restricted to non–weight bearing or touchdown weight bearing to sit to perform ADL to conserve energy and increase safety. Once the patient can do partial weight bearing, he or she can safely stand while grooming. For some this may be as early as the first week, and for others it may be as late as the third or fourth week (Goldstein, 1999). For at least 6 weeks, and for some patients longer, movement is restricted. Because these restrictions preclude bending over or bringing the foot closer to the hands, adaptations (Box 41-3) are required to resolve problems in bathing, dressing, functional mobility, and home management.

BOX 41-2
Progression of Weight Bearing After Hip Surgery (Goldstein, 1999)

Weight-Bearing Status	Percentage of Body Weight on Operated Limb	Walking Assist Device
Non–weight bearing	0	Walker or crutches
Touchdown weight bearing	10–15	Walker or crutches
Partial weight bearing	30	Walker or crutches
50% weight bearing	50	Cane
Full weight bearing	75–100	Cane or no device

BOX 41-4
SAFETY BOX

Movement Restrictions After Hip Surgery

- No hip flexion beyond 90°
- No hip rotation
- No crossing the operated leg over the unoperated leg
- No adduction of the operated leg

The patient must be reminded that the operated hip is not to be flexed actively or passively or the leg adducted beyond the midline (Box 41-4). Long-handled dressing and grooming devices are provided, and the therapist teaches the patient to bathe and dress the operated side using these devices to avoid bending over (flexion) or crossing the operated leg (adduction). For bathing, if permitted, some patients shower standing and require a grab assist bar and nonskid bath mat in the tub area for safety. Others prefer to sit to conserve energy or feel secure, and they require a bath bench. The bath bench must be high enough so the hip does not flex more than 80 to 90°. These patients also require a nonskid bath mat and grab assist rail. Box 41-5 has the procedure to get into and out of a bathtub after hip surgery.

To reduce hip flexion during sitting and rising, the patient is instructed to use a raised toilet seat, bed, and chair. Bed and chair heights are raised by putting wooden blocks under the legs. To increase mattress and chair cushion firmness and prevent passive hip flexion, plywood is inserted between the mattress and box spring or between the chair cushion and its frame. The patient is encouraged to sit in a reclined position enhanced by a wedge cushion or a small rolled pillow or towel at the junction of the chair's seat and back, as originally described by McKee (1975).

The patient who must sit in a regular-height chair is taught to stand up without overflexing the operated hip. In a chair with armrests, the patient scoots to the front edge of the seat, keeping the operated hip extended, and uses the armrests to push straight up without bending the trunk forward. In a chair without armrests, the patient moves to the side of the chair so that the operated thigh is over the edge with the foot placed at the midline of the chair. This places the operated hip in extension, puts the foot close to the center of gravity, and enables the person to gain momentum to stand without excessive hip flexion. With this technique, the unoperated hip, knee, and ankle are in position for weight bearing.

By 6 weeks, almost all patients walk with a cane, and some walk unassisted; most can return to driving a car, swimming, and work (Goldstein, 1999). Physical restrictions against bending to put on shoes or socks, sleeping on the operated side, and using a regular-height toilet seat are often lifted 8 to 12 weeks after surgery.

Chronic Conditions

Some orthopaedic conditions are chronic. One is progressive hip pain from degenerative disease. When that pain interferes with activities and tasks of daily life despite medication, rest, reduction in lower extremity loading by the use of a cane, walker, or crutches, and physical therapy, hip surgery is indicated (Salter, 1999). After hip replacement surgery, therapists teach the patient to move the operated leg within the ordered weight-bearing and movement restrictions. Another chronic condition seen by therapists who practice in orthopaedics is low back pain. Low back pain secondary to work injury accounts for the highest incidence of disability and economic loss in the United States (Battie & Videman, 1997). This section discusses occupational therapy both after hip replacement surgery and to relieve low back pain to enable occupational performance.

BOX 41-5
PROCEDURES FOR PRACTICE

Transferring Into and Out of a Bathtub After Hip Surgery

To Get Into the Bathtub
1. Stand with feet parallel to the tub with the operated leg next to the bathtub.
2. Shift body weight to unoperated leg.
3. Hold on to a grab assist rail for support.
4. Position the operated leg into hip extension and knee flexion; then abduct the hip to allow the leg to go over the edge of the bathtub.
5. Extend the knee on the operated side once the leg is over the tub edge.
6. Place the foot on the nonskid bath mat inside the tub.
7. When balance is secure, transfer the body weight to the operated leg.
8. Lift the unoperated leg over the edge of the tub and place the foot on the bath mat.

To Get Out of the Bathtub
1. Position self so feet are parallel to the side of the tub and the operated leg leads (goes out of the tub first).
2. Use the same procedure as for getting into the tub.

Case Example

MRS. B.: OCCUPATIONAL THERAPY IN UPPER AND LOWER EXTREMITY FRACTURE

Patient Information

Mrs. B. is a 72-year-old married woman who slipped on a patch of ice 3 days ago when she walked from her house to her car. She sustained a right intertrochanteric hip fracture and fractured her right distal radius in the fall. She was hospitalized after undergoing a cemented total hip replacement. The radius fracture was reduced and will remain immobilized in plaster for approximately 6 weeks. Mrs. B. anticipates returning home to be with her husband and eventually resuming her family and volunteer roles.

Reason for Referral to Occupational Therapy

Mrs. B. was referred to occupational therapy for the duration of her acute-care postoperative hospital stay, approximately a week, to learn how to move safely while adhering to hip protection precautions, to start upper limb exercises and activities, and to begin to resume personal activities of daily living.

Occupational Therapy Goal List

▶ Mrs. B. will be able to transfer safely to and from a chair, bed, and toilet while adhering to the hip protection precautions and respecting right upper limb status and capacity.

▶ Mrs. B. will be able to use biomechanically safe methods that directly correspond to her recovery stages for *both* fractures to bend and to reach while performing functional tasks in the kitchen, bathroom, and bedroom. These methods will be based on the principles of joint protection, energy conservation, and precautions for hip replacement surgery.

▶ Mrs. B. will demonstrate the ability to complete a self–range of motion program for the right upper limb, targeting the joints above and below the forearm cast.

▶ Mrs. B.'s fear of falling will be assessed.

▶ The plan for discharge will be based on the extent of support and supervision Mrs. B. needs while the postoperative hip precautions are required and the anticipated need for ongoing treatment of the arm fracture after cast removal.

Treatment Plan

Therapy focused on Mrs. B.'s ability to return home safely. The program consisted of the following:

▶ Both the occupational therapist and the physical therapist taught Mrs. B. postures and movements that would be safe

for her operated hip during transfers, sitting, standing, lying in bed, and bending and reaching during ADL and IADL. She was taught to use long-handled assistive devices such as reachers, shoehorns, and sponges. Tasks or components of tasks that she could not complete satisfactorily while adhering to the required postoperative hip precautions were identified.

▶ The therapist taught Mrs. B. exercises for the casted upper limb and its use in ADL. Assistive devices to allow one-handed ADL and IADL were tried. Tasks or components of tasks that she could not complete because of forearm fracture limitations were identified.

▶ The therapist taught Mrs. B. methods to conserve energy during ADL and IADL.

▶ The therapist counseled and trained Mrs. B. concerning fall prevention because her fear of falling was found to be high.

▶ Mrs. B. was given a written and illustrated brochure concerning restrictions related to ADL and a treatment plan to be followed for upper extremity exercise after discharge.

▶ The therapist determined that Mrs. B.'s family, with the assistance of a home health aide, could provide the necessary care for ADL and IADL that she could not manage because of hip precautions and limitations of the cast. Therefore, the recommendation was to discharge her home rather than to a skilled nursing facility.

▶ The therapist further recommended that Mrs. B. attend outpatient occupational therapy for treatment of the arm after cast removal.

Analysis of Reasoning

Treatment was guided by Mrs. B.'s goal to return home and resume prior roles and by the limitations imposed by the hip replacement precautions and the forearm cast. In this acute stage of a condition that would eventually heal, the occupational therapist focused on temporary adaptation, introducing one-handed techniques and assistive devices within the restrictions of the postoperative hip protocol and the capacity of the casted forearm. Because Mrs. B. had multiple fracture sites, there was concern that she would require more direct physical assistance and guidance than for an individual fracture, so careful inventory was made of her capabilities and need for help.

Prevention of falls was considered as well as recommendations for future therapy. To keep the momentum of rehabilitation progressing, therapeutic attention after cast removal is essential for psychological support as well as to improve the strength and range of motion of the upper extremity.

Occupational Therapy After Elective Hip Surgery Resulting From Disease

There are a number of surgical procedures for reduction of hip pain. They include osteotomy; arthrodesis, or hip fusion; and partial or total hip arthroplasty. To select the procedure, the orthopaedic surgeon considers not only the patient's age and physical status but also his or her occupational requirements and lifestyle.

Osteotomy is a procedure to change the alignment of the femur to relieve weight bearing on the hip joint. This may be the surgery of choice in the early stages of the osteoarthritic process or if the patient is 60 years of age or younger (Lowrey & Coutis, 1992). When the osteotomy is done, compression plates stabilize the bone, and the patient can begin early postoperative mobilization with passive movement. Only partial weight bearing on the operated leg using crutches is allowed for 6 months, until the bone is healed (Lowrey & Coutis).

Hip joint arthrodesis fuses the acetabulum with the femoral head at about 25 to 30° of flexion and in neutral abduction and rotation. Arthrodesis is considered for patients under age 60 who are in good physical condition and who have only one painful hip. A candidate is one who is not a candidate for a prosthetic hip implant because of heavy physical demands at work or recreational pursuits that are beyond the tolerances of an implant. This is also considered a salvage procedure for those whose prosthetic hip implant has failed. The patient is mobilized a week after the hip fusion and is allowed gradual weight bearing up to full weight in 2 months. Some patients do use a cane for a long time after surgery. The patient requires long-handled devices to assist with reaching the feet during bathing and dressing because of early postoperative flexion restrictions (Dalseth & Lippincott, 1991). In 6 months, when complete healing is established, the patient may be able to put on a sock and shoe when seated by flexing the knee to the side of the chair and reaching behind, using touch without visual guidance. The arthrodesis does leave the patient with a residual disability, but the hip is strong, stable, and pain free and has adequate endurance for standing at work and participating in active sports, such as walking, hiking, sailing, and horseback riding (Kostuik, 1991).

A total hip arthroplasty (THA) surgically replaces the entire hip joint destroyed by disease or trauma. The main benefit of hip replacement is to resolve arthritic pain. Joint replacement surgery can also restore the length of the limb and its alignment, which has the potential to improve range of motion and function (Brewster & Lewis, 1998). This surgery is performed using a hip joint implant prosthesis that replaces both the acetabular cup and the femoral head with metal or metal and plastic implants. During the procedure the greater trochanter is removed with muscle attachments intact and is reflected back to allow the implantation. After the prosthetic placement, the trochanter is wired back into place (Eftekhar, 1993). The postoperative protocol depends on whether the surgeon elected to use a cemented, cementless, or hybrid prosthesis (Bargar et al., 1998; Salvati et al., 1991). The cemented total replacement usually requires 6 weeks of partial weight bearing, and then the patient begins to walk with a cane. The cementless prosthesis, which depends on ingrowth of porous bone for stability, requires 12 weeks of partial weight bearing before a cane is used (Bargar et al.; Wixson et al., 1991). In the case of the hybrid prosthesis, in which the femoral portion is cemented and the acetabulum is uncemented, 6 weeks of partial weight bearing precedes introduction of a cane (Wixson et al.).

The first 2 months following total hip arthroplasty is critical for protection and function of the new hip joint. The postsurgical program is designed to allow for healing of the trochanter and soft tissues and for development of a capsule around the joint for future stability. ***Until soft tissue is healed, hip flexion beyond 90°, hip adduction, and hip rotation are avoided.*** The extremes of these movements during the first 2 months can dislocate the prosthesis. If dislocation occurs, the hip must be surgically realigned, and the patient may be placed in a hip spica cast for 3 weeks, delaying rehabilitation (Eftekhar, 1993). To protect the prosthesis, the occupational therapist instructs the patient in adaptive procedures and in methods to modify the environment to allow for safe performance of ADL and homemaking (Box 41-3). The techniques used to help the patient following a total hip arthroplasty parallel those described earlier under hip fracture surgery: hip flexion and adduction are discouraged, and weight-bearing guidelines are carefully adhered to. Rehabilitation starting as early as the third day after surgery is tolerated even by patients who are considered to be high risk and yields faster achievement of functional milestones (Munin et al., 1998).

For at least 3 weeks and for some patients up to 8 weeks after surgery, the operated hip is positioned in extension and abduction. A splint or a foam abduction wedge is used with the patient lying down or sitting to encourage hip abduction. Once the patient achieves 55° of hip flexion in physical therapy, the patient can sit reclined on a raised chair using a rolled pillow or wedge cushion between the seat and the back of the chair and a foam abduction wedge between the legs. The patient learns to transfer from supine to standing without flexing the operated hip beyond 90° by keeping the knees apart (hips abducted) and sliding out of a raised bed to take weight on the unoperated leg. Some patients use an overhead trapeze bar to assist this transfer.

The patient with a cemented or hybrid total hip prosthesis usually begins partial weight bearing with a walker or crutches immediately after surgery. In some instances these patients can withstand full weight bearing within the first 3 days; however, many orthopaedic surgeons wait 3 weeks before ordering full weight bearing (Goldstein, 1999). The ADL program, which can be taught with the patient standing, uses the bathing and lower extremity dressing techniques described for fractures (Boxes 41-4 and 41-5). The patient with a cementless total hip arthroplasty is usually touchdown weight bearing for the initial recovery phase and is conservatively progressed to partial weight bearing (Goldstein). This necessitates learning ADL from the seated position. Once 50% weight bearing is ordered, the ADL program is upgraded to allow for standing with a cane. The cane is used until the **Trendelenburg gait** disappears.

Usually, after a total hip arthroplasty, patients do not receive outpatient therapy following inpatient rehabilitation, although many may receive home care occupational and physical therapy for safety assessment and/or treatment. Between the second and third month after surgery, patients usually resume all routine daily activities, with the restrictions listed in Box 41-4 still applicable. For some, this restriction may persist for a long time, even for life. For most patients, strenuous sports, such as tennis, skiing, and jogging, are discouraged.

Low Back Pain

Pain is a personal experience that is real and that the patient expresses with sensory and emotional adjectives (Kirkaldy-Willis, 1999; Waddell, 1992). Acute pain is proportional to the physical findings. Chronic pain, pain that lasts for months or years, results in personality changes; is disassociated from the physical problem; and develops into a separate clinical syndrome (Waddell). The goal is to alleviate the pain early to prevent emotional changes (Andersson, 1992; Wilkinson, 1992).

The most common cause of low back pain is soft tissue strain resulting from sustained static posture, frequent lifting while twisting, or exposure to vibration (Battie & Videman, 1997). Most episodes of low back pain are self-limiting: 90% of patients return to work within 2 months. However, 5% of patients have chronic pain and are out of work for more than 6 months (Nordin, 1992).

The primary goal in medically managed back care is to prevent the patient from developing chronic pain. Continued pain, distress, and illness behavior combine to reduce the patient's overall physical activity level, which leads to disuse syndrome, deconditioning

(Waddell, 1992), and occupational dysfunction. If pain is not alleviated, the objective findings over time may have little or no association to a nociceptive stimulus. Chronic pain and disability become increasingly associated with emotional distress, depression, disease conviction (convince self and others that the disease exists), failure to cope, catastrophizing (feelings of total misfortune), and adaptation to chronic invalidism. This situation becomes self-sustaining and is often resistant to traditional medical management alone (Waddell).

The focus is to prevent the development of chronic pain syndrome by adopting practices used in sports medicine treatment to calm the pain and relax the muscles. Bed rest is replaced with early application of physical therapy, a flexibility program, and active involvement in a graduated ADL program (Mooney, 1992; Weinstein & Herring, 1993). As physical therapy helps the patient develop dynamic control of the lumbar spine through flexibility training, stretching, and ROM exercises, the occupational therapist directs the patient in performance of activities in a neutral lumbosacral position (the midpoint of available range between anterior and posterior pelvic tilt). The occupational therapist teaches the patient to understand, manage, and protect the low back by using proper body mechanics and alternative techniques to perform activities at home and at work (Wilkinson, 1992). As endurance training progresses in physical therapy, the occupational therapist upgrades the type and quantity of ADL and work-related task challenges. When return to usual and customary activities is imminent, the treatment addresses safety and prevention of recurrence.

Teaching patients about their back and body mechanics has been part of rehabilitation for many years. The multidisciplinary team usually consists of a physician, a physical therapist, an occupational therapist, and in some instances a social worker or psychologist. The philosophy is that education in anatomy, spine function, and proper body mechanics for daily living and leisure activities will help patients with low back pain take responsibility for long-term management of their back. Patients are taught to live well in spite of back pain and to prevent recurrence or aggravation of symptoms by working and behaving correctly (Andersson, 1992; Kumar & Konz, 1997).

Evaluation of the Patient With Low Back Pain
In the initial interview the therapist asks about the pain history and pain reaction during activity. Inquiry into occupational function determines the person's extent of accommodation and methods for task completion. Observation of actual or simulated performance of tasks may be indicated to reveal the patient's functional limitations and decision-making process.

Treatment of the Patient With Low Back Pain

The occupational therapist facilitates the patient's active participation in tasks and activities that correspond to the medical stage by teaching body mechanics and how to perform safely. Use of relaxation techniques for stress reduction, biofeedback for muscle control, and group educational sessions may also be included in the occupational therapy program. Body mechanics is taught relative to static and dynamic postures and transition patterns (e.g. sit to stand, stand to stoop). The occupational therapist applies the principles of body mechanics to commonly performed tasks to show the patient how to apply the principles to everyday tasks. Emphasis is on both cognitive and motor learning to develop the patient's understanding and ability to self-regulate motor activity safely. Therapeutic activity, including games, crafts, ADL, and work tasks, are selected for practice. Through feedback, the therapist guides the patient's performance during the activities and encourages development of self-regulation.

Body Mechanics

Good body mechanics entails practices to reduce the load or stresses on the spine in various positions or when moving objects. Compression and twisting of the spine are avoided, as are attempts to exert force in positions that poorly support the spine (Box 41-6). Suggestions for application of principles of body mechanics in various postures:

▶ While standing, for example to cook or wash dishes in the kitchen or to brush teeth at the bathroom sink, the patient places one foot on the shelf under the sink or on a low stool to achieve posterior pelvic tilt. This technique is used whenever prolonged standing is a requirement.

▶ To sit, the patient lowers the body by flexing the knees and hips without bending the spine. To do so, the patient places the hands on the chair's armrest, both to guide the descent and to provide support through the transition. A raised seat is recommended, since it requires less muscle power, which reduces pain and stress on the back. A slightly reclined sitting posture is preferred for prolonged sitting. When seated to work at a table, the patient avoids bending over the work by moving the chair close to the work and raising or inclining the work surface as needed.

▶ For tasks that ordinarily require excessive reaching and bending of the spine, such as sweeping, vacuuming, or raking, the patient is taught to move the body close to the task, that is, to walk with the broom or rake rather than reaching with it.

▶ For lifting objects from the floor, the choice of

BOX 41-6

PROCEDURES FOR PRACTICE

Principles of Body Mechanics

The patient is taught to do the following:

▶ Incorporate a pelvic tilt during static sitting or standing to unload the facet joints, aid in pelvic awareness, and decrease muscular tension in the low back.

▶ Position the body close to and facing the task. This aids in balance by getting the object as close to the center of gravity as possible. Objects held away from the body require increased force of all muscles to lift or hold them. Getting close also helps to avoid twisting or bending the spine.

▶ Avoid twisting. Twisting causes stress on the ligaments and small muscles of the spine. Instead, turn the body by stepping with both legs to face the activity.

▶ Use the hip flexors and extensors to lower and raise the body. These are large muscles with leverage and power to handle heavy loads. The joints and muscles of the spine are much smaller, with less leverage and power.

▶ Avoid prolonged repetitive activity or static positions. Take microbreaks and walk briefly or stretch every hour.

▶ Balance activity with rest to facilitate endurance and safety. Incorporate rest periods into the course of a particular activity or alternate between two work patterns that challenge different muscle groups.

▶ Use a wide base of support. Stability while lifting is increased when the feet are at least hip distance apart, with one foot slightly in front of the other.

▶ Keep the back in proper alignment—ear over shoulder, shoulder over hips, hips over knees and feet—to maintain the natural curves of the back. Practice in front of a mirror.

▶ Test a load before lifting to decide whether the lift should be modified. Decide how to modify the lift: get help, split the load into more than one lift, or put the object on wheels.

▶ Stay physically fit. Strong muscles and flexible joints are the best defense against injury or recurrence of an injury.

position depends on the size and weight of the object. To pick up a lightweight object, such as a newspaper, the patient faces the newspaper and lowers both knees in a semisquat (or a ballet position of plié) toward the floor while keeping the back straight and maintaining posterior pelvic tilt. When lifting a large or heavy object or a small child, the patient adds more central support by lowering one knee to the floor (half-kneeling) so that the body is close to and facing the object. The goal is to bring and keep the weighted mass as close to the body's center of gravity as possible. A small child is encouraged to climb up into the lap. Once the object or child is grasped securely, the knee on the floor helps push the body up, and then both legs extend to lift the weight. The patient should be instructed to lift to an intermediate height, such as a chair, if possible, rest briefly, and then lift to carry.

▶ The patient is taught to carry light, well-balanced loads of laundry, groceries, and parcels close to the body. Infants are best transported in a front or back baby carrier or a stroller. Through practice sessions, the patient learns his or her safe load tolerances over given distances and time. It is important that practice employ common items, such as half a gallon of milk, which weighs 4 pounds, or a gallon of bottled water, which weighs 8 pounds.

Summary Review Questions

1. What are the unwanted side effects of immobilization of any fracture?
2. How would you direct your patient to prevent adverse side effects of prolonged immobilization?
3. What is a major treatment goal for any patient with an upper extremity fracture?
4. Why is passive motion not used in the treatment of fractures of the elbow?
5. What are the guiding principles for advancing a patient in the aftercare therapy program following orthopaedic surgery?
6. What is clinical union, and why is it significant in terms of the therapy program?
7. Why are isometric contractions across the fracture site encouraged?
8. What is the occupational therapist's role for the patient who underwent hip replacement surgery after a fractured hip?
9. After a hip fracture or total hip joint arthroplasty, the therapist directs the patient to perform occupational performance tasks safely. What specific tasks may threaten the integrity of the surgical procedure? Why?
10. List precautions that must be taught to a patient with a total hip arthroplasty.
11. Describe how lower extremity dressing should be taught to a patient with low back pain, using all applicable body mechanic principles. Do the same for the tasks of sweeping the floor and working at a computer.

References

Andersson, G.B.F. (1992). Concept and development of back schools. In M. V. Jayson (Ed.), *The Lumbar Spine and Back Pain* (4th ed., pp. 409–415). New York: Churchill Livingstone.

Apley, A. G., & Solomon, L. (1994). *Concise System of Orthopaedics and Fractures* (2nd ed.). London: Butterworth Heinemann.

Arntz, C. T., Jackins, S., & Matsen, F. A. (1993). Prosthetic replacement of the shoulder for the treatment of defects in the rotator cuff and the surface of the glenohumeral joint. *Journal of Bone and Joint Surgery, 75-A,* 485–491.

Bargar, W. L., Bauer, A., & Borner, M. (1998). Primary and revision total hip replacement using the Robodoc system. *Clinical Orthopaedics and Related Research, 354,* 82–91.

Basti, J. J., Dionysian, E., Sherman, P. W., & Bigliani, L. U. (1994). Management of proximal humeral fractures. *Journal of Hand Therapy, 7,* 111–121.

Battie, M. C., & Videman, K. T. (1997). Epidemiology of the back. In M. Nordin, G. B. J. Andersson, & M. H. Pope (Eds.), *Musculoskeletal Disorders in the Workplace: Principles and Practice* (pp. 253–268). St. Louis: Mosby.

Brewster, N., & Lewis, P. (1998). Joint replacement for arthritis. *Australian Family Physician, 27,* 21–27.

Collins, D. C. (1993). Management and rehabilitation of distal radius fractures. *Orthopedic Clinics of North America, 24,* 365–378.

Cooney, W. P., & Schutt, A. H. (1992). Rehabilitation of the wrist. In V. L. Nickel & M. J. Botte (Eds.), *Orthopedic Rehabilitation* (2nd ed., pp. 711–731). New York: Churchill Livingstone.

Dalseth, T., & Lippincott, C. (1991). Postoperative rehabilitation. In H. C. Amstutz (Ed.), *Hip Athroplasty* (pp. 379–390). New York: Churchill Livingstone.

Eftekhar, N. S. (1993). *Total Hip Arthroplasty.* St. Louis: Mosby.

Epps, C. H., Jr., & Cotler, J. M. (1985). Complications of treatment of fractures of the humeral shaft. In C. H. Epps, Jr. (Ed.), *Complications in Orthopaedic Surgery* (Vol. 1, 2nd ed., pp. 277–300). Philadelphia: Lippincott.

Frykman G. K., & Kropp, W. E. (1995). Fractures and traumatic conditions of the wrist. In J. M. Hunter, E. J. Mackin, & A. D. Callahan (Eds.), *Rehabilitation of the Hand* (4th ed., pp. 315–336). St. Louis: Mosby.

Goldstein, T. S. (1999). *Geriatric Orthopaedics: Rehabilitative Management of Common Problems* (2nd ed.). Gaithersburg, MD: Aspen.

Hoppenfeld, S. (1976). *Physical Examination of the Spine and Extremities.* Norwalk, CT: Appleton-Century-Crofts.

Hotchkiss R. N., & Davila, S. (1992). Rehabilitation of the elbow. In V. L. Nickel & M. J. Botte (Eds.), *Orthopedic Rehabilitation* (2nd ed., pp. 733–746). New York: Churchill Livingstone.

Jackins, S., & Matsen, F. A., III (1994). Management of shoulder instability. *Journal of Hand Therapy, 7,* 99–106.

Kelley, M. J., & Clark, W. A. (1995). *Orthopedic Therapy of the Shoulder.* Philadelphia: Lippincott.

Kelsey, J. L., Mundt, D. F., & Golden, A. L. (1992). Epidemiology of low back pain. In M. V. Jayson (Ed.), *The Lumbar Spine and Back Pain* (4th ed., pp. 537–549). New York: Churchill Livingstone.

Kirkaldy-Willis, W. H., & Bernard, T. N. (1999). *Managing Low Back Pain* (4th ed.). New York: Churchill Livingstone.

Kostuik, J. P. (1991). Arthrodesis of the hip. In H. C. Amstutz (Ed.), *Hip Athroplasty* (pp. 929–940). New York: Churchill Livingstone.

Kumar, S., & Konz, S. (1997). Workplace adaptation for the low back region. In M. Nordin, G. J. Andersson, & M. H. Pope (Eds.), *Musculoskeletal Disorders in the Workplace* (pp. 316–328). St. Louis: Mosby.

Laester, G. G., & Carter, P. R. (1996). Management of distal radius fractures. *Journal of Hand Therapy, 9,* 114–128.

Lowrey, C. E., & Coutis, R. D. (1992). Rehabilitation of the hip. In V. L. Nickel & M. J. Botte (Eds.), *Orthopedic Rehabilitation* (2nd ed., pp. 779–789). New York: Churchill Livingstone.

McKee, J. I. (1975). Foam wedges aid sitting posture of patients with total hip replacement. *Physical Therapy, 55,* 767.

Mackin, G. A. (1997). Medical and pharmacologic management of the upper extremity neuropathic pain syndromes. *Journal of Hand Therapy, 10,* 96–109.

Mennell, J. B. (1945). *Physical Treatment by Movement, Manipulation, and Massage.* Philadelphia: Blakiston.

Mooney, V. (1992). Rehabilitation of the spine. In V. L. Nickel & M. J. Botte (Eds.), *Orthopaedic Rehabilitation* (2nd ed., pp. 765–778). New York: Churchill Livingstone.

Munin, M. C. , Rudy, T. E., Glynn, N. W., Crossett, L. S., & Rubash, H. E. (1998). Early inpatient rehabilitation after elective hip and knee arthroplasty. *Journal of the American Medical Association, 279,* 847–852.

Neer, C. S., II (1990). *Shoulder Reconstruction.* Philadelphia: Saunders.

Nordin, M. (1992). Prevention of back pain in industry. In M. V. Jayson (Ed.), *The Lumbar Spine and Back Pain* (4th ed., pp. 551–563). New York: Churchill Livingstone.

Rockwood, C. A. (1990). The technique of total shoulder arthroplasty. In *Instructional Course Lectures* (Vol. 39, pp. 437–447). Park Ridge, IL: American Academy of Orthopaedic Surgeons.

Salter, R. B. (1999). *Textbook of Disorders and Injuries of the Musculoskeletal System* (3rd ed.). Baltimore: Williams & Wilkins.

Salvati, E. A., Huo, M. H., & Buly, R. L. (1991). Cemented total hip replacement: Long term results and future outlook. In H. S. Tullos (Ed.), *Instructional Course Lectures* (Vol. 40, pp. 121–134). Park Ridge, IL: American Academy of Orthopaedic Surgeons.

Skyhar, M. J., & Simmons, T. C. (1992). Rehabilitation of the shoulder. In V. L. Nickel & M. J. Botte (Eds.), *Orthopedic Rehabilitation* (2nd ed., pp. 747–763). New York: Churchill Livingstone.

Smith, K. L. (1995). Wound care for the hand patient. In. J.M. Hunter, E. J. Mackin, & A. D. Callahan (Eds.), *Rehabilitation of the Hand: Surgery and Therapy* (4th ed., pp. 237–250). St. Louis: Mosby.

Smith, L. K., Weiss, E. L., & Lehmkuhl, L. D., & (1996). *Brunnstrom's Clinical Kinesiology* (5th ed.). Philadelphia: Davis.

Stanton-Hicks, M., Janig, W., Hassenbruch, S., Haddox, J. D., Boas, R., & Wilson, P. (1995). Reflex sympathetic dystrophy: Changing concepts and taxonomy. *Pain, 63,* 127–133.

Tinetti, M. E., Baker, D. J., McAvay, G., Claus, E. B., Garrett, P., Gottschalk, M., Koch, M. L., Trainor, K., & Horowitz, R. I. (1994). A multifactorial intervention to reduce the risk of falling among elderly people living in the community. *New England Journal of Medicine, 331,* 821–827.

Waddell, G. (1992). Understanding the patient with a backache. In M. V. Jayson (Ed.), *The Lumbar Spine and Back Pain* (4th ed., pp. 469–485). New York: Churchill Livingstone.

Weinstein, S. M., & Herring, S. A. (1993). Rehabilitation of the patient with low back pain. In J. A. DeLisa (Ed.), *Rehabilitation Medicine: Principles and Practice* (2nd ed., pp. 996–1017). Philadelphia: Lippincott.

Wilkinson, H. A. (1992). *The Failed Back Syndrome: Etiology and Therapy* (2nd ed.). New York: Springer-Verlag.

Wixson, R. L., Stulberg, D., & Mehlhoff, M. (1991). Total hip replacement with cemented, uncemented, and hybrid prostheses. *Journal of Bone and Joint Surgery, 73-A,* 257–269.

42

Hand Impairments

Cynthia Cooper

LEARNING OBJECTIVES

After studying this chapter, the reader will be able to do the following:

1. State principles and general precautions of hand therapy evaluation and treatment.
2. Select splint positions that minimize, prevent, or correct hand deformity.
3. Describe clinical features of common hand impairments.
4. Recognize and foster favorable tissue responses to hand therapy interventions.
5. Promote pain-free occupational functioning of persons with hand impairment.

*H*and problems, which may be cosmetic or functional or both, are hard to hide. Hands function exquisitely to gesture and express, touch and care, dress and feed (Tubiana et al., 1996). Impairment can be devastating. The purposes of this chapter are to introduce readers to the elements of hand therapy, to highlight the breadth of material that hand therapy encompasses, and to identify resources for further study.

The complex arrangement of the hand, with its intimate anatomy and multiarticulate structures, is unforgiving of stiffness, scar, or edema. Injury at one site can lead to stiffness of other parts of the hand. To test this for yourself, passively hold your ring finger in extension and then try to make a fist. This example, called the quadregia effect, demonstrates the interconnectedness of digits, whereby limited movement of one digit may cause restricted motion in uninjured digits (Burkhalter, 1995). For this and other reasons, hand therapists must look at more than the isolated site of injury and must continually reexamine the patient's function.

Hand therapy originated during World War II. Devastating upper extremity injuries of that era and of subsequent wars prompted a team approach to medical care (Hunter, 1986). Today, members of the rehabilitation team in hand therapy can include physicians and physician assistants, nurses, occupational therapists and occupational therapy assistants, physical therapists and physical therapy assistants, and aides or technicians. Workers compensation representatives

GLOSSARY

Antideformity position, intrinsic-plus position—Position of digital MP flexion and IP extension that maintains the length of the collateral ligaments and volar plate.

Buddy straps—Straps between an injured and an adjacent digit to protect or to promote movement.

Carpal tunnel syndrome—Nerve entrapment involving compression of the median nerve at the wrist causing sensory symptoms typically involving the thumb, index, and long fingers and radial half of the ring finger.

Cervical screening—Proximal screening assessment of neck and shoulder to identify causes of or contributors to distal symptoms.

Claw deformity—Position of MP hyperextension and PIP flexion associated with muscle imbalance in ulnar-innervated structures.

Complex regional pain syndrome (CRPS)—New terminology for reflex sympathetic dystrophy. CRPS is characterized by pain that is disproportionate to the injury, along with swelling, stiffness, and discoloration. Sudomotor (sweating) changes are often seen.

Contracture—Lack of passive motion due to tissue shortening.

Counterforce strap—Support or strap used over flexor or extensor muscle wads to support muscles and prevent maximum muscle contraction, decreasing load on the tendon. Often used to reduce symptoms of lateral or medial epicondylitis.

Cubital tunnel syndrome—Nerve entrapment involving compression of the ulnar nerve at the elbow between the medial epicondyle and olecranon. Sensory symptoms affect the small finger and ulnar half of the ring finger. Motor symptoms affect the FCU, FDP of the ring and small fingers, AP, and interossei.

de Quervain's disease—Tenosynovitis involving the abductor pollicis longus and EPB tendons at the first dorsal compartment.

Extensor lag—Inability to extend a joint actively while passively being able to.

Hard end feel—Unyielding quality of joint motion at end range passively. Indicates an established joint restriction.

Kirschner wires—Fixation devices used alone or in conjunction with other forms of fixation to treat unstable fractures of the hand.

Neuroma—Disorganized mass of nerve fibers that can occur following nerve injury. Significant nerve pain with associated hypersensitivity is elicited by tapping over the neuroma.

Oscillations—Rhythmic movements that may be helpful to reduce guarding and pain.

Place-and-hold fisting—Passive motion used gently to achieve a position, with the patient then actively sustaining or holding that position.

Soft end feel—Spongy quality of joint motion at end range passively. Indicates favorable potential for tissue remodeling.

Tenodermodesis—Adherence of skin to tendon, causing restriction of movement.

Tenolysis—Surgical procedure to release tendon adhesions that restrict movement.

or case managers representing payers may also be involved.

Certified hand therapists are occupational therapists or physical therapists with advanced clinical skills who have passed the examination for certification in hand therapy. A minimum of 5 years of clinical experience and other criteria are prerequisites to taking the examination. It is advisable to establish a strong generalist background in occupational therapy before specializing in hand therapy.

Hand therapy differs from other occupational therapy specializations, such as pediatrics or gerontology, because it merges occupational therapy and physical therapy, and it has its own professional organizations. While most hand therapists are occupational therapists, actual clinical practice may often look more like physical therapy than occupational therapy. Occupational therapy hand therapists should embrace an occupational therapy identity by grounding treatment in core concepts of our profession. To this end, hand therapists should not become so focused on specific anatomical structures that they overlook the person attached to the hand. They should instead treat the hand along with the occupational human whose hand it is.

Psychosocial Factors Affecting Therapeutic Outcomes

Why do some people with minor hand injuries wind up with large disabilities and others with devastating injuries have only small disabilities? Adaptive responses to hand impairment are influenced by body image as well as individual functional needs. The personal or symbolic meaning of the hand, self-esteem, family and friend support systems, and coping strategies all influence outcome (Grunert et al., 1991). Whenever possible, encourage patients to participate in their care. Introduce yourself, maintain eye contact, listen well, use nonmedical terminology and instructional diagrams, and encourage some amiable conversation as appropriate (Moskowitz, 1996). It can be helpful to touch patients' hands supportively and to make positive remarks.

Motivation is the most important variable favorably influencing recovery (Chin et al., 1999). Realistic expectations and appropriate communication that emphasizes education are also important (Bryan & Kohnke, 1997; Moskowitz, 1996). Psychological symptoms related to hand trauma resolve best when intervention occurs early (Grunert et al., 1991).

Hand Therapy Concepts

The following concepts are keys to clinical reasoning for all diagnoses of hand impairment. Intervention should not be determined by diagnosis per se. Rather, hand therapy treatment relies on an understanding of anatomy and physiology, wound healing, biomechanics, tissue tolerances, psychosocial issues, and probable outcomes. Because of the infinite variations among people, no two treatment plans should be the same. Hand therapy treatment should never adopt a cookbook approach (Fess, 1990, 1993). To do so is an injustice to patients and to our profession.

Tissue Healing

Tissue heals in phases as follows: inflammation, fibroplasia, and maturation, or remodeling. The inflammation phase lasts several days. It includes vasoconstriction followed by vasodilation, with white blood cell migration to promote phagocytic removal of foreign bodies and dead tissue. Depending on the diagnosis, immobilization to provide rest is often advised during the inflammation phase (Smith, 1995a; Stewart, 1995).

The fibroplasia phase starts at approximately day 4 and continues for 2 to 6 weeks. In this phase, fibroblasts synthesize scar tissue. The wound's tensile strength increases gradually with the increase in collagen fibers.

At this time, active range of motion (AROM) and splints may be appropriate to protect healing tissues and promote balance in the hand (Fess, 1993; Fess & McCollum, 1998).

The maturation, or remodeling, phase may last for years, but tissue is usually more responsive early rather than late in this period. The remodeling phase reflects the changing architecture and improved organization of collagen fibers and associated increased tensile strength. Gentle resistive activity may be appropriate during maturation, but it may also generate inflammatory responses, which should be avoided. Gentle application of corrective dynamic or static splinting may also be appropriate (Bryan & Kohnke, 1997; Fess, 1993). Tissues' tolerances to controlled stress require monitoring throughout all phases of treatment.

As tissue continues to heal, the wound contracts and the scar shrinks. Collagen continues to remodel, as it is constantly doing in uninjured tissue (Smith, 1995a).

Antideformity Positioning

Upper extremity injury and disuse are associated with predictable deforming hand positions. Edema, which typically accompanies injury, creates tension on extrinsic extensor structures. This leads to a zigzag collapse with a resulting deformity position of flexed wrist, hyperextended metaphalangeals (MPs), flexed proximal interphalangeals (PIPs) and distal interphalangeals (DIPs), and adducted thumb (Stewart, 1995).

Hand joints are anatomically destined to stiffen in predictable positions. Specifically, the MP joint is prone to stiffen in extension. This is because the protruding or cam shape of the metacarpal head causes the collateral ligament to be slack in MP extension and taut in MP flexion. Conversely, the interphalangeal (IP) joints are prone to become stiff in flexion because the volar plate folds on itself (Tubiana et al., 1996).

When prolonged or constant immobilization is necessary and range of motion (ROM) is at risk, it is usually best to splint the patient's hand in the **antideformity position**, also called the intrinsic-plus position (Fig. 42-1). This position places the wrist in neutral or extension, the MPs in flexion, the IPs in extension, and the thumb in abduction and opposition. The antideformity position allows the collateral ligaments at the MP joints and the volar plate at the IP joints to maintain their length, which counteracts the forces that promote zigzag collapse. Certain diagnoses, such as flexor or extensor tendon repair, are not compatible with antideformity positioning. The physician can assist in this determination (Stewart, 1995).

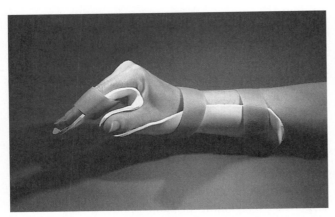

Figure 42-1 Antideformity or intrinsic-plus position: Wrist in neutral or extension; MPs in flexion; IPs in extension; and thumb in abduction and opposition.

The Myth of No Pain, No Gain

Regarding tissue tolerances, the myth of no pain, no gain must be dispelled in hand therapy. A better mindset would be no pain, more gain. Well-intentioned therapists and overzealous family members of patients have too often caused irreversible damage by applying passive range of motion (PROM) forces beyond the tissues' tolerances (Fess, 1993). Pain induced by therapy can also cause **complex regional pain syndrome (CRPS)**, discussed later.

People with upper extremity problems often arrive at therapy prepared for painful treatment. Some patients do not tell the therapist when treatment hurts. It is essential to educate patients about this. In addition, watch the patient's body language and face for signs of pain. Wincing and withdrawing the upper extremity are obvious signals. Proximal guarding is another revealing response. Change the treatment accordingly, and if necessary, try a hands-off approach wherein the therapist coaches and instructs while the patient self-treats.

Passive Range of Motion Can Be Injurious

PROM can be injurious to the delicate tissues of the hand. Specifically, PROM can disturb healing tissues and incite further inflammatory reactions, resulting in increased scar production. PROM can damage articular structures and can even trigger CRPS (Fess, 1993; Tubiana, 1983). Tissue's timeline for remodeling is maximized by noninflaming treatment and is cut short by treatment that is inflaming or provoking. For all of these reasons, if PROM is clinically appropriate, be sure it is done gently and in a pain-free manner. The potential

for harm may be compounded if PROM is performed following external application of heat. Instead, low-load, long-duration splinting is a safer and more effective method for remodeling tissue and increasing PROM (Fess & McCollum, 1998).

Judicious Use of Heat

External application of heat, such as a hot pack, is a popular way to prepare tissues for stretching. Unfortunately, the clinical concerns of externally applied heat have received less attention than they deserve. Heat increases edema, which acts like glue. Heat may degrade collagen and contribute to microscopic tears (Miles et al., 1995). Heat may also incur a rebound effect, with stiffening following its use. ***Do not use heat on patients who have edema or who appear inflamed.*** Overall, it is safer to use aerobic exercise to warm up the tissues of people with hand impairments. If external application of heat is used, elevate the upper extremity, be gentle with exercise, and promote active movement in conjunction with the heat. Continue to monitor for immediate and subsequent signs of inflammation.

Isolated Exercise, Purposeful Activity, and Therapeutic Occupation

Technically, it is necessary to treat hand impairments with a structure-specific approach to isolate and care for the discrete components that are involved. It may seem easiest to accomplish this type of exacting intervention in the form of isolated exercise. Traditional valuing of the appearance of highly technical clinical environments, medical model indoctrination, busy schedules, and financial or material constraints may contribute to the perpetuation of hand therapy identifying itself within an environment that looks like an exercise gymnasium. While some hand therapists do incorporate purposeful activity into treatment, more support is needed for an alternative approach to hand therapy that leads with concepts of therapeutic occupation (Cooper & Evarts, 1998). One way to achieve this is to integrate patient-directed goals and activities of daily living (ADL) into hand therapy. Whenever possible, encourage upper extremity use in ordinary daily activities as appropriate to the diagnosis. Explore the capabilities in the clinic and then teach patients to do so at home. For example, folding socks and underwear can be upgraded to folding heavy towels and jeans, which requires greater strength and endurance.

Purposeful activity elicits adaptive responses that do not occur with exercise alone. Compared to isolated exercise, purposeful activity promotes more coordination and better movement quality (Nelson & Peterson, 1989). An example of isolated hand therapy exercise to increase grip strength is gross grasp with therapy putty or exercise grippers. Examples of purposeful activity to increase strength required for putting away groceries are progressive grasp and release of beans or stacking cups.

Occupation-as-means instills occupational therapy's heritage in what might otherwise be a less function-oriented context (Trombly, 1995). The examples cited above become therapeutic occupation with the use of activity that is meaningful to the particular person to accomplish the therapeutic goal. If the patient enjoys baking, then rolling dough with a rolling pin would be a therapeutic occupation to promote grip function.

Evaluation

History

History taking offers an excellent opportunity to establish therapeutic rapport (Bryan & Kohnke, 1997; Fess; 1995a). Review medical reports, including radiographs, when possible; learn hand dominance, age, occupation, and avocational interests (Aulicino, 1995; Bryan & Kohnke, 1997). Assess occupational performance deficits by asking what the patient cannot do that he or she wants to do, needs to do, or is expected to do. Also discuss the case with the physician.

For trauma, learn date of injury, dates of any surgery, where and how injury occurred, mechanism of injury, posture of the hand when it was injured, and any previous treatment. For nontraumatic problems, learn date of onset, whether the symptoms are worsening, sequence of onset of symptoms, functional effects, and what worsens and/or lessens the symptoms (Aulicino, 1995).

Pain

Pain may be acute or chronic. Acute pain has a sudden and recent onset, usually has a limited course with an identifiable cause, and can last a few minutes to 6 months. Acute pain serves a physiological purpose, signaling the need to protect tissue from further damage. Chronic pain lasts months or years longer than expected and may not serve a physiologic purpose (Maurer & Jezek, 1992). Myofascial pain, which may be chronic or acute, stems from local irritation in fascia, muscle, tendon, or ligament. It has specific reproducible pain patterns and associated autonomic symptoms (Travell & Simons, 1983). Evaluation of pain may include a graphic

representation of pain, in which the patient marks painful areas on a drawing of the human body; analog pain rating scales (see Chapters 4 and 9); joint or muscle palpation to identify areas of local pain or qualitative changes in soft tissue; and trigger point sensitivity (Maurer & Jezek, 1992).

Physical Examination

It is helpful to observe the positioning and use of the patient's upper extremity in the waiting area before the meeting. On examination, look at the entire unclothed upper extremity for posture, guarding and gesturing, atrophy, and edema (Aulicino, 1995). Because distal symptoms are often caused by proximal problems, it is important to perform a **cervical screening**, a proximal screening assessment of neck and shoulder, to identify additional areas requiring intervention. (For more detail on cervical screening, see Cyriax [1982].)

Wounds

Always follow universal precautions. Evaluate wound size in terms of length, width, and depth. Wound drainage (exudate) is bloody (sanguinous), serous (clear or yellow), purulent (pus), or deep or dark red (hematoma). Wound odor is absent or foul (Baldwin et al., 1992).

The three-color concept (red, yellow, or black) dictates wound care. Wounds can be one of or a combination of these three colors. A red wound is healing, uninfected, and composed of revascularization and granulation tissue. A yellow wound has an exudate that requires cleansing and debridement. A black wound is necrotic and also requires debridement. The goal of wound care is to convert yellow and black wounds to red wounds (Evans & McAuliffe, 1995).

Scar Assessment

Observe scar location, length, width, and height. Hypertrophic scars stay confined to the area of the original wound and usually resolve within a year. Keloids proliferate outside the area of the original wound and do not usually become smaller or less pigmented with time. Note any scar tethering or **tenodermodesis**, which is adherence of skin and tendon causing restricted movement. Any wound or scar crossing a joint may form a **contracture**, which restricts passive motion. Immature scar has a red or purplish color imparted by its vascularity. It blanches to touch. Mature scar is flatter and softer. It has neutral color and does not blanch to touch (Baldwin et al., 1992).

Vascular Assessment

Cyanosis, erythema, pallor, gangrene, or grayish color indicates vascular compromise. To test digital capillary refill, apply pressure to the fingernail or distal pad of the involved digit. Color should return within 2 seconds of release of pressure. Compare the refill time to that of uninvolved digits (de Herder, 1992).

Edema

Circumferential measurement is quick to perform and provides a good alternative when it is not possible to use a volumeter (Fess, 1995a). Be consistent with measuring tape placement and tension. Volumetric measurement is contraindicated over open wounds, percutaneous pinning such as Kirschner wires, plaster casts, or vasomotor instability (Fess, 1993). See Chapter 4 for volumetric measurement procedures.

Range of Motion

In hand therapy, ROM is measured as AROM, PROM, or torque range of motion (TROM), a more consistent and objective type of PROM in which the therapist documents the amount of force applied externally to achieve maximal PROM (Breger-Lee et al., 1990). At a minimum, both AROM and PROM should be evaluated and compared to those of the uninjured extremity (Adams et al., 1992) (see Chapter 4). Facilities usually have their own guidelines for measuring ROM. As expected, consistency of retesting is important.

Total active motion or total passive motion measures the sum of composite digital flexion and extension (Box 42-1). This measurement is used in some studies. Normal total active motion and total passive motion are 270° (Fess, 1995a).

Grip and Pinch

When properly calibrated, the Jamar dynamometer is the best instrument to assess grip strength because of its reliability, face validity, and accuracy (See Chapter 4). Hand therapy authorities recommend comparing scores to those of the contralateral extremity rather than using norms (Fess, 1993, 1995a). Goals for grip and pinch strength depend on occupational factors and dominance. There may be approximately 10 to 15% difference in strength between dominant and nondominant hands, with dominant hands usually stronger. Interpretation of maximal effort with grip testing exceeds the scope of this chapter. However, grip testing at all five notch settings of the dynamometer typically reveals a bell-shaped curve when consistent effort is used. (For more on this subject,

BOX 42-1
PROCEDURES FOR PRACTICE

Total Active Motion and Total Passive Motion

▸ Add the measurements for flexion of the MP, PIP, and DIP joints.
▸ Subtract the combined deficits in extension for those joints.

see Smith et al. [1989]). It is routine to measure three pinch patterns, lateral, three-jaw chuck, and tip. As with grip, compare pinch scores to those of the contralateral extremity (Fess, 1992, 1993).

There is no linear relationship between improvement in grip and pinch strength and improvement in function. Rice et al. (1998) noted that even debilitated, deformed hands can be surprisingly functional. These authors found only weak relationships between grip and pinch strength and the forces required to open six containers used commonly in the home. Thus, grip and pinch testing are not substitutes for ADL assessment with contextual relevance (Rice et al., 1998). To promote occupational functioning of people with hand impairments, it is far better to have treatment and goals reflect personally meaningful ADL than grip or pinch strength measures.

Manual Muscle Testing

Manual muscle testing is particularly useful for monitoring progress following peripheral nerve lesions (See Chapter 4). Treatment facilities usually have their preferred method of grading, which may be numerical or descriptive (Shultis-Keirnan, 1992).

Sensibility

Inspect the patient's hand for dryness, moistness, and calluses (See Chapter 6). Blisters may be an alert to injurious hand use due to sensory loss. "Wear marks" illustrate where and how the hand is used and which parts of the hand avoid use, indicating sensory impairment (Callahan, 1995).

Hand therapy does not yet have one tool that evaluates the hand's functional sensibility (Moberg, 1991). The *Semmes-Weinstein Monofilament* and the *Two-Point Discrimination (2PD)* tests are most commonly used in hand therapy. The *Semmes-Weinstein Monofilament Test* assesses pressure threshold, and the *2PD* assesses density of receptors. The *Moberg Pickup Test*

(See Chapter 6) is a functional test appropriate for use on patients with median or median and ulnar nerve lesions.

Dexterity and Hand Function

No one evaluation covers all features of hand function (Jarus & Poremba, 1993). Standard terminology regarding hand function is lacking, and there is limited evidence that the assessment of hand function indicates the patient's actual performance in ADL (Desrosiers et al., 1993; Lynch & Bridle, 1989). Thus, hand function tests should not substitute for ADL assessments but are good measures of improvement.

For dexterity tests to be reliable, therapists must administer them using the standard procedures from the original articles or test manuals, and they must decide whether or not a specific test is valid for the intended use (Mathiowetz & Bass Haugen, 1995; Rider & Linden, 1988). The tests described in this section all require further validation study.

Minnesota Rate of Manipulation Test

The *Minnesota Rate of Manipulation Test* (American Guidance Service, 1969) addresses manual or gross motor dexterity. It assesses the speed and accuracy of repetitive reaching, picking up, manipulating, and placing disks the size of double checkers. It has a 3-foot-long frame with four horizontal rows of openings in which the 60 disks are placed. There are five subtests: placing, turning, displacing, one-hand turning and placing, and two-hand turning and placing. The patient performs the test while standing. Each subtest starts with a practice trial and is tested three to five times. The score is the total time for the subtest trials. This test has been standardized with adaptations for use with patients who are visually impaired (Mathiowetz & Bass Haugen, 1995).

Test–retest reliability ranges from .87 to .95 for two-trial administration. Percentile tables are available, with norms based on young adults (N = 11,000) and on older unemployed adults (N = 3,000.) Box 42-2 presents recommendations for interpretation of a particular patient's score using normative data from a percentile table.

BOX 42-2
PROCEDURES FOR PRACTICE

Interpretation of a Score Using Normative Data

Interpretation of a Score Using Normative Data From a Percentile Table (Mathiowetz & Bass Haugen, 1995)

▸ Administer the test according to standard procedures.
▸ Compare the patient's score with the most appropriate percentile table (e.g., worker category, sex, age).
▸ A patient scoring at the 20th percentile performed better than 20% and worse than 80% of the normative sample.
▸ A score at 2.3 percentile or higher is usually interpreted to be normal or within normal limits.
▸ A score falling between 2.3 and 0.1 percentile is interpreted to be a mild deficit.
▸ A score below 0.1 percentile is interpreted to be a moderate to severe deficit.

Interpretation of a Score Using Normative Data From a Mean and Standard Deviation Table (Mathiowetz, Volland, et al., 1985)

▸ Administer the test according to the standard procedures.
▸ Compare the right-hand score with the right-hand normative data appropriate to the age and sex of the patient. For example, if a 23-year-old man transported 66 blocks within 1 minute with his right hand, his score of 66 would be compared with the mean of 88.2 and the standard deviation (SD) of 8.8 (Table 42-1). Using the formula below, it is found that he scored 2.5 SD below the mean relative to his age group and gender.
▸ Use this formula to determine the SD above or below the mean for a specific patient's score:[a]

   Client's score − mean ÷ SD = SD ± mean
Example:
$$66 − 88.2 = −22.2$$
$$−22.2 ÷ 8.8 = −2.5 \text{ SD}^{a}$$

---

[a]In tests such as the *Box and Block Test*, for which a high score indicates a better performance, a negative score means below the mean. In tests such as the *Nine-Hole Peg Test*, for which a high score indicates a poor performance, a negative score means above the mean (better than average performance). Thus the therapist can document objectively that the patient's right-hand performance on the *Box and Block Test* of manual dexterity was 2.5 SD below the mean. To determine the statistical meaning of the patient's score, the therapist must assume that the *Box and Block Test* scores are normally distributed. In a standard normal distribution table, 97.7% of the sample scores are more than 2 SD below the mean; 2.2% are between 2 and 3 SD below the mean; and 0.1% are more than 3 SD below the mean. By convention, a score that falls 2 SD below the mean or higher is usually interpreted to be normal or within normal limits. A score falling between 2 and 3 SD below the mean is interpreted to show a mild deficit. A score more than 3 SD below the mean is interpreted to show moderate to severe deficit. Thus the example patient would be considered to have a mild deficit in manual dexterity relative to the normative data.

TABLE 42-1

Average Performance of 628 Normal Subjects on the Box and Block Test[a]

Age (Years)	Males		Females	
	Mean	SD	Mean	SD
20–24				
Right-hand	88.2	8.8	88.0	8.3
Left hand	86.4	8.5	83.4	7.9
25-29				
Right hand	85.0	7.5	86.0	7.4
Left hand	84.1	7.1	80.9	6.4
30–34				
Right-hand	81.9	9.0	85.2	7.4
Left hand	81.3	8.1	80.2	5.6
35–39				
Right-hand	81.9	9.5	84.8	6.1
Left hand	79.8	9.7	83.5	6.1
40–44				
Right-hand	83.0	8.1	81.1	8.2
Left hand	80.0	8.8	79.7	8.8
45–49				
Right-hand	76.9	9.2	82.1	7.5
Left hand	75.8	7.8	78.3	7.6
50–54				
Right-hand	79.0	9.7	77.7	10.7
Left hand	77.0	9.2	74.3	9.9
55–59				
Right-hand	75.2	11.9	74.7	8.9
Left hand	73.8	10.5	73.6	7.8
60–64				
Right-hand	71.3	8.8	76.1	6.9
Left hand	70.5	8.1	73.6	6.4
65–69				
Right-hand	68.4	7.1	72.0	6.2
Left hand	67.4	7.8	71.3	7.7
70–74				
Right-hand	66.3	9.2	68.6	7.0
Left hand	64.3	9.8	68.3	7.0
75+				
Right-hand	63.0	7.1	65.0	7.1
Left hand	61.3	8.4	63.6	7.4

[a]Values are number of cubes transferred in 1 minute. Mathiowetz, Volland, et al, 1985.

Box and Block Test

The *Box and Block Test* measures gross manual dexterity. It was developed to test people with severe problems affecting coordination (Fig. 42-2). This test must be constructed according to specific dimensions and published specifications (Mathiowetz, Volland, Kashman, & Weber, 1985). The subject transfers 1-inch blocks from one side of the box to the other. The score is the number of blocks transferred in 1 minute for each hand. Box 42-3 presents procedures for administration of the test. Rec-ommendations for interpretation of a patient's score in terms of normative data from a mean and standard deviation table are shown in Box 42-2 (Mathiowetz, Volland, et al., 1985).

Test–retest reliability of the *Box and Block Test*, established at a 6-month interval, was high (r = .94 for left hands and r = .98 for right hands) (Cromwell, 1976). Interrater reliability reflected strong correlations (r = 1.00 for right hand and r = .999 for left hand) (Mathiowetz, Volland, et al., 1985). Concurrent validity (r = .91) was established with the placing subtest of the *Minnesota Rate of Manipulation Test* (Cromwell, 1976).

The *Box and Block Test* is preferred to the *Minnesota Rate of Manipulation Test* because the normative data for the *Box and Block Test* have a broader range, the patient is allowed to sit while being tested, and it is time limited (Mathiowetz & Bass Haugen, 1995).

Purdue Pegboard Test

The *Purdue Pegboard Test* of finger dexterity (Tiffin, 1968) assesses picking up, manipulating, and placing

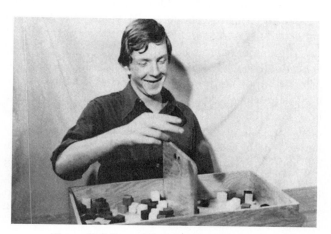

Figure 42-2 *Box and Block Test* of manual dexterity.

little pegs into holes with speed and accuracy. It tests finger or fine motor dexterity (Mathiowetz et al., 1986). It has a wooden board with two rows of tiny holes plus reservoirs for holding pins, collars, and washers. The four subtests are performed with the subject seated. To begin, there is a brief practice. The subtests for preferred, nonpreferred, and both hands require the patient to place the pins in the holes as quickly as possible, with the score being the number of pins placed in 30 seconds. The subtest for assembly requires the patient to insert a pin and then put a washer, collar, and another washer on the pin, with the score being the number of pieces assembled in 1 minute (Mathiowetz & Bass Haugen, 1995). The *Purdue Pegboard Test* manual provides normative data using percentile tables for adults and different categories of jobs and for children 5 to 15 years of age by age and sex.

One-trial administration of the *Purdue Pegboard* produced test–retest reliability of r = .60 to .79. Three-trial administration test–retest reliability ranged from .82 to .91 (Mathiowetz et al., 1986). Administering three trials for the four subtests took more time (20 minutes instead of 10) but provided better reliability. J. M. Gallus ([1999]. *Test–Retest Reliability of the Purdue Pegboard for Individuals With Multiple Sclerosis.* Unpublished master's thesis, University of Minnesota) reported high test–retest reliability (r = .85 to .96) and no practice effects based on individuals with multiple sclerosis. A limitation of the

BOX 42-3
PROCEDURES FOR PRACTICE

Administration Procedures for the Box and Block Test (Mathiowetz, Volland, et al., 1985)

- Place the test box lengthwise along the edge of a standard height table (Fig. 42-2).
- The 150 cubes are in the compartment of the test box to the dominant side of the patient.
- Sit facing the patient to monitor the blocks being transported.
- Give these instructions: *"I want to see how quickly you can pick up one block at a time with your right [left] hand [the therapist points to the dominant hand]. Carry the block to the other side of the box and drop it. Make sure your fingertips cross the partition. Watch me while I show you how."*
- Transport three cubes over the partition in the same direction the patient is to move them.
- After the demonstration, say, *"If you pick up two blocks at a time, they will count as one. If you drop one on the floor or table after you have carried it across, it will still be counted, so do not waste time picking it up. If you toss the blocks without your fingertips crossing the partition, they will not be counted. Before you start you will have a chance to practice for 15 seconds. Do you have any questions? Place your hands on the sides of the box. When it is time to start, I will say 'Ready' and then 'Go.'"*
- Start the stopwatch at the word *go.* After 15 seconds, say "Stop."
- If the patient makes mistakes during the practice period, correct them before beginning the actual testing.
- On completion of the practice period, return the transported cubes to the compartment.
- Mix the cubes to ensure random distribution, and then say, *"This will be the actual test. The instructions are the same. Work as quickly as you can. Ready; go. [After 1 minute:] Stop."*
- Count the blocks transported across the partition. This is the patient's score for the dominant hand.
- If the patient transports two or more blocks at the same time, subtract the number of extra blocks from the total.
- After counting, return the blocks to the original compartment and mix randomly.
- Turn the test around so that the blocks are on the nondominant side.
- Administer the test to the nondominant hand, using the same procedures as for the dominant hand, including the 15-second practice.

Purdue Pegboard Test is that it was developed to select industrial employees. The validity of its use in identifying a need for occupational therapy should be evaluated (Mathiowetz, 1993).

Nine-Hole Peg Test

The *Nine-Hole Peg Test* measures finger dexterity among patients with physical disabilities. This test is sold commercially, or it can be constructed according to published details (Mathiowetz, Weber, Kashman, & Volland, 1985). Test administration is brief, the time it takes to place nine pegs in holes in a 5-inch square board and then remove them. The *Nine-Hole Peg Test* had high interrater reliability (r = .97 for right hand and r = .99 for left hand). Test–retest reliability was moderate: (r = .69 for right hand and r = .43 for left hand) (Mathiowetz, Weber, et al., 1985). There are concerns about the transferability of these norms to data collected with commercial versions of the test that use different materials (Davis, J., Fenlon, P., Proctor, T., & Watson, W. J. [1997]. *The* Nine Hole Peg Test*: A Comparison Study*. Unpublished master's thesis, Kirksville College of Osteopathic Medicine, Kirksville, MO).

The *Purdue Pegboard* is preferred to the *Nine-Hole Peg Test* in the measurement of finger dexterity. Of the two, the *Purdue Pegboard* has better test–retest reliability; it is time limited; it is for both unilateral and bilateral assessment; and its normative data reflect a broader age range (Mathiowetz & Bass Haugen, 1995).

Jebsen Test of Hand Function

The *Jebsen Test of Hand Function* assesses hand function in terms of simulated ADL (Jebsen et al, 1969). It can be administered quickly (Jarus & Poremba, 1993). There are seven timed subtests consisting of writing a sentence, simulated page turning, picking up small common objects, stacking checkers, simulated eating, moving empty cans, and moving heavy cans. Construction specifications and standard procedures are documented (Jebsen et al., 1969). As with all standardized tests, it is important to follow the standard procedures (Jarus & Poremba, 1993). For example, substituting plastic checkers for wooden checkers resulted in significantly lower performance (Rider & Linden, 1988) and thus invalidates the use of norms established for the wooden checkers. Also, reliability statistics do not apply to the adapted test (Fess, 1993).

Test–retest reliability of the *Jebsen Hand Function Test* ranged from .60 to .99, based on 26 patients whose hand impairments had leveled off. No significant practice effect was demonstrated between two sessions with these patients (Jebsen et al., 1969). Although the researchers reported data on reliability of the *Jebsen Hand Function Test*, their data represented patient groups, not

normal subjects (Mathiowetz, Weber, et al., 1985). Stern (1992) confirmed the test–retest reliability with 20 normal subjects, but she also found a significant practice effect for writing and simulated feeding subtests between the first and third sessions.

The *Jebsen Hand Function Test* does discriminate between subjects with and without different physical disabilities (Jebsen et al., 1969; Spaulding et al., 1988). There is a moderate correlation (r = .64) between the Jebsen test and the *Klein–Bell ADL Scale*, suggesting that the Jebsen test may have some usefulness in predicting functional ability, but it would not be an appropriate substitute for an ADL evaluation (Lynch & Bridle, 1989). Norms for adults aged 20 to 94 years (N = 300) are published (Jebsen et al., 1969).

There are several limitations of the *Jebsen Hand Function Test*. One is that it does not really address the proximal upper extremity (Desrosiers et al., 1993). Also, it measures speed, not quality, of hand function (Jarus & Poremba, 1993; Spaulding et al., 1988). In addition, some of its subtests are not representative of ordinary daily activity. Mathiowetz (1993) questioned its content validity when he found that the page turning and feeding subtests do not actually duplicate those tasks in daily life. He also questioned why writing is evaluated as a timed test and why the nondominant hand is tested in handwriting.

TEMPA

TEMPA is an acronym from the French for *Upper Extremity Performance Test for the Elderly* (Desrosiers et al., 1993). It consists of nine tasks, five bilateral and four unilateral, reflecting daily activity. Each task is measured by the three subscores of speed, functional rating, and task analysis. The nine tasks are pick up and move a jar, open a jar and take a spoonful of coffee, pour water from a pitcher into a glass, unlock a lock, take the top off a pillbox, write on an envelope and affix a postage stamp, put a scarf around one's neck, shuffle and deal cards, use coins, and pick up and move small objects. Instructions are in the manual. The test takes about 15 to 20 minutes for an unimpaired elderly subject and about 30 to 40 minutes for an impaired elderly subject (Desrosiers et al., 1993). Advantages of the *TEMPA* are clinical utility, especially with hand patients over 60 years of age; provision of both quantitative and qualitative data; simulation of ADL; test applicability; test availability; and acceptability to patients (Rudman & Hannah, 1998). A possible disadvantage of this test is its cost of approximately $500. Questions have surfaced concerning the quality control in production of the test (Humiston, L. [2000]. *Upper Extremity Performance Test for the Elderly (TEMPA): Normative Data for Ages 20–29*. Unpublished master's thesis, University of Minnesota).

TEMPA norms were established on adults 60 years of age or older (N = 360) by 10-year age groups and by gender. Interrater reliability of the *TEMPA* ranged from .96 to 1.00. Test–retest reliability ranged from .77 to 1.00. Concurrent validity with the *Action Research Arm* test was .90 to .95 and with the *Box and Block Test* was .73 to .78 (Desrosiers et al., 1994, 1995). Some support for construct validity was demonstrated by correlating the *TEMPA* with basic personal care (r = .68) (Desrosiers et al., 1993).

Clinical Reasoning and Treatment

Questions to Ask

Close communication with the patient's physician is always advisable. Choosing which questions to ask depends on the diagnosis and structures involved. General categories of questions may include the physician's expectations for functional recovery; tendon status, such as fraying or vascular compromise; whether the patient is medically cleared for AROM only or active AROM and/or PROM; and whether the patient is medically cleared for low-load, long-duration dynamic splinting.

ADL and Functional Implications

The functional use of the upper extremity and the patient's ability to function occupationally are what really matter. Hand therapists must be careful not to become so focused on the technical aspects of the patient's injury that they overlook the patient's function, personal goals, and life needs. In some circumstances it may actually be better for patients to accept a stiff finger and get on with life using compensatory techniques than to interrupt the flow of their lives for therapy (Merritt, 1998). This may be true if gains are exceedingly slow, if function is not dramatically compromised, or if there are other priorities, such as ill family members, for example.

Goal Setting

Express hand therapy goals in terms that reflect the patient's occupational functioning. Ultimately, the number of degrees achieved in ROM is less important than whether the patient can open a door, get dressed, or return to work. One way to integrate concrete and functional goals is to measure the movement needed to accomplish an appropriate patient-specific functional task and incorporate that measurement into the stated goal. As an example, if a patient wants to be able to splash water on his or her face but lacks forearm supination to do so, have the patient perform the activity with the opposite upper extremity. Measure the supination needed to perform the task. In this instance, the goal could be stated as "sufficient forearm supination (60°) for ability to wash the face" (Skotak, C. personal communication, 1999).

Quality of Movement

Poor quality of movement (called dyscoordinate cocontraction) may result from cocontraction of antagonist muscles. The cause may be habit, fear of pain, guarding, or excessive effort. Poor quality of movement looks awkward and unpleasant. It is important to identify dyscoordinate cocontraction early and to work on retraining a smooth, comfortable, effective quality of motion (Cooper et al., 1999). Pain-free purposeful activity or pain-free therapeutic occupation are the best ways to promote good quality of motion. **Oscillations** are rhythmic movements that may be helpful, but they must be pain-free. Imagery such as pretending to move the extremity through water or gelatin may also help (Cooper et al., 1999). Biofeedback may aid in muscle reeducation as well.

What Structures Are Restricted, and Does PROM Exceed AROM?

Hand therapists strive to be structure specific in identifying and treating upper extremity limitations. It is not adequate to identify a general problem, such as decreased ROM. Rather, it is important to understand and treat the specific structures causing the restriction. Limited PROM may be due to pericapsular structures, such as adhered or shortened ligaments, or actual joint limitations, such as mechanical block or adhesions. PROM that exceeds AROM may be due to disruption of the musculotendinous unit, adhesions restricting excursion of the tendon (Fess, 1993), or weakness. When PROM exceeds AROM, promote active movement and function of the restricted structures with differential tendon gliding exercises, blocking exercises, place-and-hold exercises, and functional splints (discussed later). When PROM equals AROM, discern whether the restriction is joint or musculotendinous or both (See section on joint versus muculotendinous tightness), and promote both passive and active flexibility.

Joint Versus Musculotendinous Tightness

With joint tightness, the PROM of the particular joint *does not change* with repositioning of the joints proximal and/or distal to it. With musculotendinous tightness, the PROM of the particular joint *does vary* with repositioning of joints crossed by that multiarticulate structure.

(Colditz, 1995b). Treat joint tightness with dynamic splinting, static progressive splinting, or serial casting, followed by AROM. Treat musculotendinous tightness the same as extrinsic tightness (discussed later).

Lag Versus Contracture

A lag is a limitation of active motion in a joint that has passive motion available. A joint contracture is a passive limitation of the joint. A patient with a PIP **extensor lag** cannot actively extend the PIP joint even though passive extension is available. A patient with a PIP joint flexion contracture lacks passive extension of that joint.

Treat lags by facilitating motion of the restricted structure with scar management, blocking exercises in mechanically advantageous positions, place-and-hold exercises, static splinting to promote normal length of the involved structure, and functional splints. Treat contractures the same as for joint tightness (discussed later).

An advantageous position to test or treat extensor lag at the PIP level is to maintain MP flexion while trying to extend actively at the PIP. An advantageous position to test or treat extensor lag at the DIP level is to maintain MP and PIP flexion while trying to extend actively at the DIP. This is contraindicated if the diagnosis is acute mallet finger (see section on extensor tendon injury).

Inrinsic Versus Extrinsic Tightness

Compare the PROM of digital PIP and DIP flexion with the MP joint flexed and again with the MP joint extended. With extrinsic tightness, there is less PIP and DIP passive flexion with the MP joint flexed. With intrinsic tightness, there is less PIP and DIP passive flexion with the MP joint extended (Bryan & Kohnke, 1997; Colditz, 1995b).

Treat intrinsic tightness with functional splinting with MPs extended and IPs free. In other words, promote IP flexion with MPs extended. Treat extrinsic extensor tightness with MPs flexed and IPs free, and promote composite digital flexion. Use blocking exercises with an advantageous proximal position (discussed later). Try dynamic or static progressive splinting.

Tightness of Extrinsic Extensors or Extrinsic Flexors

With extrinsic extensor tightness, there is less passive composite digital flexion available with the wrist in flexion than with the wrist in extension. In contrast, with extrinsic flexor tightness, there is less passive composite digital extension available with the wrist in extension than with the wrist in flexion (Colditz, 1995b). Treat extrinsic flexor or extensor tightness with place-and-hold exercises, static splinting comfortably at end range (especially useful at night), dynamic or static progressive splinting during the day, and functional splinting.

Basic Interventions

Edema Control

Elevation, active exercise, contrast baths, and compression have been the mainstays of edema control. Treatment of upper extremity edema has also historically included retrograde massage, string wrapping, compressive garments, and modalities such as an intermittent pressure pump. *Compression garments should not be too tight.*

Exciting new research has challenged hand therapists recently to reexamine the anatomical and physiological bases of our treatment of edema. This inquiry has resulted in a new approach to the treatment of upper extremity edema, called manual edema mobilization (Artzberger, 1997, in press), a technique for stimulating the lymphatic system to remove the excess large plasma proteins that cause sustained edema leading to fibrotic tissue and stiffness. This hands-on technique, which must be learned in workshops that last 2 days or longer, can lead to dramatic and effective results. The approach used in manual edema mobilization is very different from and in some ways opposite to traditional retrograde massage techniques. Furthermore, manual edema mobilization raises questions about whether retrograde massage is sometimes more damaging than helpful. Manual edema mobilization is a wonderful example of the groundbreaking changes in hand therapy, based on scholarly questioning and research, that keep the profession interesting.

Scar Management

Compression (e.g., Isotoner gloves, Tubigrip, or Coban wrap) and desensitization are traditionally used to promote scar softening and maturation. Silicone gel (Baum & Busuito, 1998) helps promote scar maturation, presumably through neutral warmth. Other inserted materials can also be used.

While friction massage has typically been advocated for scar softening, there are recent legitimate questions whether this more aggressive technique may in fact cause inflammation resulting in deposition of even more scar tissue. Manual edema mobilization may be a more effective alternative. Research is needed in this area.

Differential Digital Tendon Gliding Exercises

Tendon gliding exercises maximize total gliding and differential gliding of digital flexor tendons at the wrist. (Fig 42-3) (Rozmaryn et al., 1998; Stewart & van Strien, 1995). Because tendon gliding exercises promote digital and joint motions, they are a mainstay of most home exercise programs.

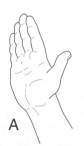 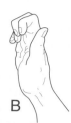 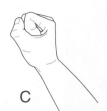 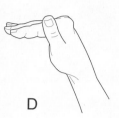 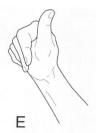

A   B   C   D   E

Figure 42-3 Differential flexor tendon gliding exercises. The five positions: **A.** Straight. **B.** Hook. **C.** Fist. **D.** Table-top. **E.** Straight fist. (Adapted with permission from Rozmaryn, L. M., Dovelle, S., Rothman, E. R., Gorman, K., Olvey, K. M., & Bartko, J. J. [1998]. Nerve and tendon gliding exercises and the conservative management of carpal tunnel syndrome. *Journal of Hand Therapy, 11* (3), 171–179.)

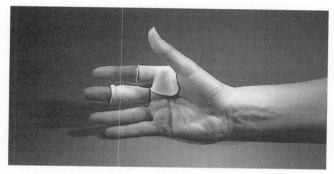

Figure 42-4 Blocking splints. MP splint blocks MP motion, promoting PIP and DIP motion. Digital splint blocks PIP motion, promoting MP and/or DIP motion.

Blocking Exercises

Various blocking tools and splints are available commercially or can be made easily with scraps of splinting materials (Fig. 42-4) (Skirven & Trope, 1994). Digital cylinders blocking the IPs help to isolate and exercise MP flexion and extension. A blocking splint with the MPs extended promotes intrinsic stretch as well as IP flexion. A blocking splint with the MPs flexed promotes extrinsic extensor stretch and recovery of composite fisting. A PIP cylindrical block encourages DIP isolated flexion and flexor digitorum profundus (FDP) excursion at the DIP. A DIP cap facilitates PIP flexion and flexor tendon excursion at the PIP.

Instruct patients who do blocking exercises to exercise comfortably into the end range to remodel the tissue. Teach them to do the exercises frequently and slowly, holding at the comfortable end range for 3 to 5 seconds (Schneider & Berger-Feldscher, 1995).

Place-and-Hold Exercises

Place-and-hold exercises are effective for achieving increased ROM when PROM exceeds AROM. To perform them, use comfortable PROM to position the hand (e.g.,

composite fisting). Then release the assisting hand while the patient tries to sustain the position in a pain-free way (Collins, 1993; Stewart & van Strien, 1995). Place-and-hold exercises can be effective in combination with blocking exercises.

End Feel and Splinting

If there is a **soft end feel** (a favorable spongy quality at end range indicative of potential to remodel), it is reasonable to try low-load, long-duration dynamic splinting for a medically cleared patient. Dynamic splint forces must be prolonged and gentle for tissue to remodel. Forceful splinting is contraindicated because it causes pain and injury, hence inflammation and scar (Brand, 1995; Fess, 1995b). Follow dynamic splint use with activity that challenges and incorporates the limited motion. For a firmer or **hard end feel** (an unyielding quality at end range), try increasing the time in the splint and decreasing the force. If there is a hard end feel, dynamic splinting may not be effective, and serial casting or static progressive splinting may be more useful.

Splints

Functional splints can be used in ordinary daily activity to promote mobility of restricted structures. For example, if the index finger PIP joint lacks flexion and the MP joint moves normally, try a hand-based index finger MP blocking splint, used off and on through the day. When the splint is in use, the patient achieves PIP flexion exercise while performing normal grasping activities.

Buddy straps allow one digit to assist a neighboring digit to achieve greater motion. The offset buddy strap (Fig. 42-5) accommodates different phalangeal lengths of adjacent digits (Jensen & Rayan, 1996). Buddy straps are also useful to retrain keyboard users who habitually maintain the small finger MP in hyperextension or repetitively hyperabduct the small finger when keyboarding.

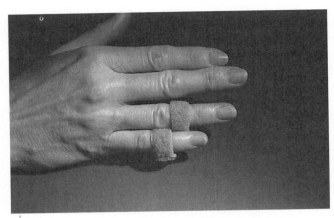

Figure 42-5 Offset buddy straps. Interdigital strap accommodates different phalangeal lengths of adjacent digits. Used to allow one digit to assist the next in achieving motion and for protection.

A dorsal MP flexion blocking splint promotes composite flexion incorporating MP flexion and is particularly helpful when there is extrinsic extensor tightness. If the patient has difficulty incorporating MP flexion into composite fisting and instead extends the MPs while flexing the IPs, a dorsal hood maintaining MP flexion promotes recovery of composite fist incorporating MP flexion. (See Chapters 14 and 15 for further splinting guidelines.)

Common Diagnoses

Hand therapists 15 years ago treated more hand trauma than cumulative trauma, and surgical cases constituted most of the caseload. Nowadays, many hand therapists see a substantially greater number of patients with a soft tissue diagnosis, such as tendinitis or cumulative trauma disorders.

Stiff Hand

Any upper extremity injury can result in the serious and sometimes irreversible problem of a stiff hand. Even an injury in the proximal upper extremity can cause serious stiffening of the digits. The stiff hand is what hand therapists try to prevent. Edema is the main culprit in the series of events leading to a stiff hand. Edema is a natural response to trauma, occurring in the inflammatory phase. The challenge for hand therapy is to strike a balance between rest and movement. Too much rest may increase the edema. Too much movement may increase the inflammation. The right amount of rest in an appropriate position reduces inflammation and promotes healing. Proximal motion plus well-tolerated hand and wrist exercise and functional use, particularly while elevated, help to reduce edema and restore motion.

Encourage the patient to achieve gentle full arcs of available motion with functional use or exercise instead of performing quick or incomplete arcs of motion that are less effective. Make exercises relevant to occupational functioning or at least goal-oriented whenever possible (e.g., grasping and releasing items). *If the patient's hand is painful or more swollen after use or exercise, it is imperative to decrease temporarily the amount of exercise being performed* (Colditz, 1995b).

Avoid aggressive PROM. It is okay to coax tissues to lengthen within their available comfortable range, but always respect the feeling of tissue resistance, and do not exceed it. Gentle passive motion, if indicated, should be accompanied by joint traction to promote gliding of the joint surfaces. Sustained holding of a position is much more effective than fast jerky stretches, which frequently add to the inflammation (Colditz, 1995b).

During the acute inflammatory stage, static splinting is usually most appropriate. After the inflammation has subsided and while the joint displays a soft end feel, dynamic splinting is productive. Inflamed tissue is not as flexible as uninflamed tissue (Brand, 1995). Watch closely for signs of inflammation and return to static splinting as indicated. Later, if there is a hard end feel, serial static or static progressive splinting is most likely to be needed. Many patients with hand impairments complain of morning stiffness. Night splinting, which can be very helpful for this problem, also corrects tissue tightness that limits daytime use of the hand (Colditz, 1995b).

Tendinitis

Since 1989, more than half of occupational illnesses and disorders in the United States have been due to overuse, cumulative trauma disorder, and tendinitis. Terminology and definitions vary. Some authorities use the terms *tendinitis*, *cumulative trauma disorder*, *repetitive strain injury*, and *overuse syndrome* synonymously; others do not. Those who consider *tendinitis* and *overuse syndrome* to be distinct terms define them thus: Tendinitis is inflammation of tendons and of the muscle–tendon attachment. It is often spontaneous in onset, frequently after a single traumatic event. It sometimes occurs with repetitive use. Tendinitis pain tends to be well localized, with swelling of the tendon sheaths. Tenderness and induration, usually local, are present. Weakness is secondary to pain (Verdon, 1996). In contrast, cumulative trauma disorder or overuse syndrome is due to microtrauma that results from the cumulative effect of repetitive stress on tissues (Pitner, 1990). Overuse syndrome is most likely to occur after long hours of repetitive use in unusual positions. The pain of overuse is diffuse and poorly localized. There is swelling in the muscle bellies and at the musculotendinous junction or muscle origin. With overuse, weakness is general and tenderness is subtle and diffuse (Stern, 1992).

There is an ongoing debate over the cause of musculoskeletal problems, and whether they are work related remains controversial (Terrono & Millender, 1996). Tendons are vulnerable because they are relatively avascular. Repetitive microtrauma can lead to cell damage with acute inflammation, which may become chronic (Pitner, 1990). This musculotendinous injury is associated with a vicious cycle consisting of pain, instability, and dysfunction (Kibler et al., 1992). Biomechanical deficits include muscular weakness, inflexibility, and scar tissue. Early treatment of an acute traumatic case typically has a better prognosis than after the injury has become chronic.

Evaluation

An overaggressive evaluation that provokes pain can set the treatment timetable back significantly and undermines the trust of and rapport with the patient. Start the evaluation with a cervical screening to look for proximal causes of distal symptoms. Compare both extremities. Assess for pain that may be local or diffuse, swelling, sensory changes, and loss of function. Tendinitis typically is accompanied by pain with AROM, with resistance, and with passive stretch of the involved structures. Compare subjective and objective findings, but remember that symptoms are often elusive and may occur dynamically or intermittently. Patients who seem angry or hostile may understandably be depressed over their loss of function.

It is essential to identify the activity causing the pain. Occupational therapists possess unique skills for ergonomic-related activity analysis and activity modification. It is best to observe the actual activity. If this is not possible, simulate the activity. Ergonomic risk factors for tendinitis include forceful, rapid, repetitive movements. A movement is considered repetitive if it is performed more than once every 30 seconds or for more than half the total work time (Idler, 1997). Additional risk factors include a history of soft-tissue problems, pressure and shear forces, stress and muscle tension, and hypermobility (Keller et al., 1998).

Treatment

Treat the acute phase with rest, ice, compression, and elevation of the involved structures. Anti-inflammatory physical agent modalities may be useful at this time (See Chapter 18). Splinting is individualized to patient's and physician's preferences (Johnson, 1993). Splinting may be most beneficial and least problematic at night. Although some physicians advocate immobilization for weeks (Idler, 1997), there are also clinical compromises

associated with disuse from immobilization (Bulthaup et al., 1999; Skirven & Trope, 1994). Soft supports may be very helpful. In weighing the advantages and disadvantages of splint use, consult closely with the referring physician, try to avoid pain, and monitor the clinical responses.

After the inflammation subsides, upgrade treatment to restore normal function through gradual mobilization balanced with rest. Most important, pain must be avoided. Instruct in tendon gliding exercises in a pain-free range appropriate to the particular structures involved. Progress from isometric exercises with gentle contractions of involved structures to isotonic exercises (Johnson, 1993). Gradually introduce low-load, high-repetition strengthening in short arcs of motion. Then increase the arc of motion and modify proximal positions to be more challenging if appropriate for work simulation. Instruct in gentle flexibility exercises in a pain-free range. It is often difficult for patients to learn to perform slow and pain-free passive stretch. Aerobic exercises and proximal conditioning are essential (Pitner, 1990).

Prevent reinjury through education (Furth et al., 1994). Simulation and biofeedback (see Chapter 25) can promote biomechanically efficient upper extremity use. Teach the patient to avoid reaching and gripping with an extended elbow or a flexed or deviated wrist. First solve the easily recognizable issues, such as obviously poor posture or trunk twisting with reaching and lifting. Instruct in pacing to avoid fatigue that leads to reinflammation. Unsupported upper extremity use is taxing, as are nonsymmetrical upper extremity use, nonfrontal trunk or upper extremity alignment, and unilateral upper extremity work. Many people with distal symptoms recover well by focusing treatment on posture, conditioning, and proximal strengthening. Using hand-held tools with ergonomic design can be helpful (Johnson, 1993). Even a small ergonomic adjustment, such as learning to lift bilaterally with proper body mechanics or making use of a telephone headset instead of laterally flexing the neck and elevating the shoulder to hold the receiver, can often lead to dramatic improvement.

Lateral Epicondylitis, or Tennis Elbow

Lateral epicondylitis involves the extrinsic extensors at their origin. The extensor carpi radialis brevis is most commonly involved. There is pain at the lateral epicondyle and extensor wad (the proximal portion of the extensor muscles) (Wuori et al., 1998). This diagnosis is differentiated clinically from radial tunnel syndrome, in which tenderness occurs more distally over the radial tuberosity. Test for radial tunnel syndrome with the middle finger test (positive if there is pain secondary to resisting the middle finger proximal phalanx while the patient maintains elbow extension, neutral wrist, and MP extension) or by percussing distally to proximally over the superficial radial nerve. This percussion test is positive if it elicits paresthesias (Skirven & Trope, 1994; Terrono & Millender, 1996).

Exercises should include proximal conditioning and scapular stabilizing. Use built-up handles. If using a splint, support the wrist in extension, especially at night. Splinted wrist position recommendations range from neutral to about 30°. Also try a **counterforce strap**, a strap placed over the extensor wad to prevent full muscle contraction and to reduce the load on the tendon during the day with activity (Skirven & Trope, 1994; Wuori et al, 1998). *Avoid applying the counterforce strap too tightly; this can cause radial tunnel syndrome.*

Medial Epicondylitis, or Golfer's Elbow

Medial epicondylitis involves the extrinsic flexors at their origin (Johnson, 1993). The flexor carpi radialis (FCR) is most commonly involved. There is pain at the medial epicondyle and flexor wad (the proximal portion of the flexor muscles) and pain with resisted wrist flexion and pronation. Exercise should promote proximal conditioning. Avoid end ranges with forceful activity. Provide built-up handles. If using a splint, maintain the wrist in neutral, and try a counterforce strap over the flexor wad.

De Quervain's Disease

De Quervain's disease is tendinitis involving the abductor pollicis longus (APL) and extensor pollicis brevis (EPB) tendons at the first dorsal compartment. It is the most common upper extremity tenosynovitis. There is a positive Finkelstein's test, which is exquisite pain with passive wrist ulnar deviation while flexing the thumb (Fig. 42-6) (Mooney, 1998). This diagnosis occurs frequently among golfers, knitters, racquet sports play-

ers, mail sorters, and filing clerks (Verdon, 1996). Thumb posture in sustained hyperabduction at the computer space bar may also be provoking (Pascarelli & Kella, 1993). Differential diagnosis is for carpometacarpal (CMC) arthritis, scaphoid fracture, intersection syndrome, and FCR tendinitis (Stern, 1992).

Teach patients to avoid wrist deviation, especially in conjunction with pinching. Provide built-up handles. If splinting, use a forearm-based thumb spica, leaving the IP free. Watch for irritation from the radial splint edge along the first dorsal compartment (Skirven & Trope, 1994).

Intersection Syndrome

Intersection syndrome presents as pain, swelling, and crepitus of the APL and EPB muscle bellies approximately 4 cm proximal to the wrist, where they intersect with the wrist extensor tendons (extensor carpi radialis brevis and extensor carpi radialis longus). This diagnosis associated with repetitive wrist motion occurs in weight lifters, rowers, and canoers (Servi, 1997). Differential diagnosis is for de Quervain's disease (Stern, 1992), and both diagnoses can occur concomitantly. Teach patients to avoid painful or resisted wrist extension and forceful grip. Splinting is the same as for de Quervain's disease.

Extensor Pollicis Longus Tendinitis

Also called drummer boy palsy, tendinitis of the extensor pollicis longus (EPL) reveals pain and swelling at Lister's tubercle (a dorsal prominence at the distal radius around which the EPL passes). It is less common than other forms of tendinitis, but if left untreated, it can lead to tendon rupture. EPL tendinitis is associated with activities requiring repetitive use of the thumb and wrist, as seen in drummers. Rupture of the EPL may occur in persons with rheumatoid arthritis or Colles' fracture (Verdon, 1996).

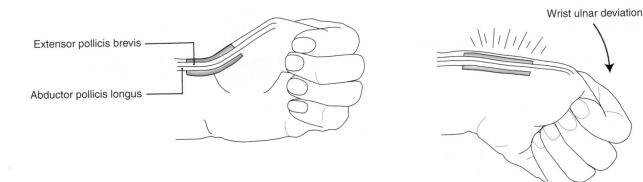

Figure 42-6 Finkelstein's test for de Quervain's disease. (Adapted with permission from American Society for Surgery of the Hand. [1990]. *The Hand: Examination and Diagnosis* (3rd ed.). New York: Churchill Livingstone.)

Help patients to identify and eliminate provocative activities. Enlarge the girth of utensils. The splinting choice is a forearm-based thumb spica that includes the IP.

Extensor Carpi Ulnaris Tendinitis

Tenosynovitis of the extensor carpi ulnaris (ECU) occurs fairly frequently. It causes pain and swelling distal to the ulnar head and is associated with repetitive ulnar deviation motions. Subluxation of the ECU tendon elicits a painful snap with forearm supination and wrist ulnar deviation. Differential diagnosis includes instability of the distal radioulnar joint (Stern, 1992) and ulnocarpal abutment or tears of the triangular fibrocartilage complex.

Teach patients to avoid ulnar deviation with activities. Splinting consists of a forearm-based ulnar gutter or a wrist cock-up splint.

Flexor Carpi Radialis Tendinitis

With tendinitis of the FCR, there is pain over the FCR tendon just proximal to the wrist flexor creases. Differential diagnosis is for a volar ganglion (Stern, 1992) or arthritis of the scaphotrapeziotrapezoid joint. Splinting consists of a wrist cock-up in neutral or a position of comfort.

Flexor Carpi Ulnaris Tendinitis

Flexor carpi ulnaris (FCU) tendinitis is more common than FCR tendinitis. It causes pain along the volar-ulnar side of the wrist. Inflammation occurs where the FCU inserts at the pisiform. Differential diagnosis is pisiform fracture and pisotriquetral arthritis (Verdon, 1996) or triangular fibrocartilage complex injury. Teach patients to avoid wrist flexion with ulnar deviation. Splinting consists of a forearm-based ulnar gutter.

Flexor Tenosynovitis, or Trigger Finger

Trigger finger is also called stenosing tenosynovitis of the digital flexor. The usual cause is stenosis at the A-1 pulley, which is part of the fibro-osseous tunnel that prevents bow-stringing of the digital flexors (Culp & Taras, 1995). There is tenderness over the A-1 pulley of the digital flexor (Fig. 42-7) along with pain with resisted grip and painful catching or locking of the finger in composite flexion (Kirkpatrick & Lisser, 1995).

The origin of this impairment can be inflammatory or not. There is a strong association with diabetes and rheumatoid arthritis (Kirkpatrick & Lisser, 1995). Medical management often consists of a mixture of steroid and local anesthetic injected into the flexor sheath. The injection may be repeated a few times. Therapy consists of splinting the MP in neutral to prevent composite

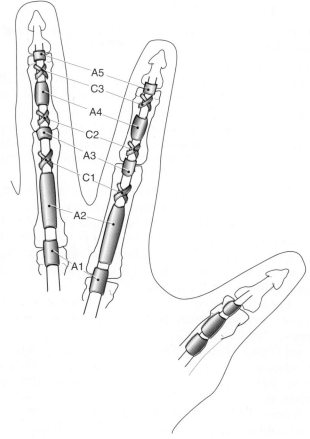

Figure 42-7 Pulley system. (Adapted with permission from Reiner, M. [1991]. *The Illustrated Hand*. St. Paul: Minnesota Hand Rehabilitation.)

digital flexion (preventing triggering) while promoting tendon gliding, and place-and-hold fisting that avoids triggering. Built-up handles, padded gloves, and pacing strategies are helpful. Instruct the patient to avoid triggering, as this reinflames the tissue. See the classic article by Evans et al. (1988). If symptoms persist, the surgeon will surgically release the A-1 pulley.

Nerve Injury

When injury or disease occurs to a neural structure in the upper extremity, there is a high likelihood that multiple areas of neural pathology will develop. This phenomenon is known as the double or multiple crush syndrome (Posner, 1998). Remembering this concept lessens the possibility of missing relevant clinical findings.

The various mechanisms of nerve injury include acute or chronic compression, stretch ischemia, electrical shock, radiation, injection, and laceration (Smith, 1995b). Compression and laceration, impairments that are commonly seen by hand therapists, are described next.

Nerve Compression

Median Nerve Compression at the Wrist, or Carpal Tunnel Syndrome

Carpal tunnel syndrome is the most common upper extremity nerve entrapment (Concannon et al., 1997). It results from compression of the median nerve at the wrist. The carpal bones form the floor of the carpal tunnel. The transverse carpal ligament, also called the flexor retinaculum, forms the roof of the tunnel (Szabo, 1998) and acts as a pulley for the flexor tendons during gripping (Netscher et al., 1998).

Inside the carpal canal there are nine flexor tendons (four FDP, four flexor digitorum superficialis [FDS], and the flexor pollicis longus) and the median nerve, which is most superficial (Fig. 42-8). Swelling or thickening of the tendons can lead to pressure on the nerve, resulting in sensory symptoms in the distribution of the median nerve (Hunter, Davlin, & Fedus, 1995).

Carpal tunnel syndrome occurs with greatest frequency among women 40 to 60 years of age and is frequently bilateral (Lam & Thurston, 1998). Typical complaints include hand numbness, particularly at night or when driving a car, along with pain and paresthesias in the distribution of the median nerve (thumb through radial ring finger pads), and clumsiness or weakness (Mooney, 1998). Associated diagnoses include rheumatoid arthritis, Colles' fracture, diabetes, deconditioning (Mooney, 1998), obesity (Lam & Thurston, 1998), and thyroid disease (Szabo, 1998). Transient carpal tunnel syndrome is fairly common in pregnancy (Stolp-Smith et al., 1998). Carpal tunnel syndrome may be associated with repetitive use (Keir et al., 1998) or flexor tenosynovitis (Donaldson et al., 1998) due to increased friction between the tendons and nerve (Mooney, 1998). For these people, focus treatment on resolving the tendinitis.

Evaluation

Perform a cervical screening, and evaluate posture, ROM, grip and pinch, and manual muscle testing looking for independent excursion of FDP and FDS. Also do Tinel's, Phalen's, *Semmes-Weinstein monofilament*, and two-point discrimination tests (Sailer, 1996). Tapping at the volar wrist elicits Tinel's sign, which is a sensation of tingling or electric shock if the median nerve is compromised. Phalen's test provokes sensory symptoms in the median nerve distribution if positive, created by maintaining the wrist in flexion for 60 seconds (Tubiana et al., 1996). Phalen's test should be done with extended elbows to avoid confusing these findings with a positive elbow flexion test (See section on cubital tunnel syndrome). Advanced cases of carpal tunnel syndrome reveal thenar atrophy of the abductor pollicis brevis, which can be functionally debilitating (Aulicino, 1995; Concannon et al., 1997).

Treatment

Conservative medical management may include steroid injection (Terrono & Millender, 1996). Conservative therapy for carpal tunnel syndrome includes night splinting with the wrist in neutral, because this position minimizes pressure in the carpal tunnel; exercises for median nerve gliding at the wrist (Fig. 42-9); differential flexor tendon gliding exercises (Fig. 42-3); aerobic exercise; proximal conditioning; ergonomic modification; and postural training (Donaldson et al., 1998; Rozmaryn et al., 1998). Teach patients to avoid extremes

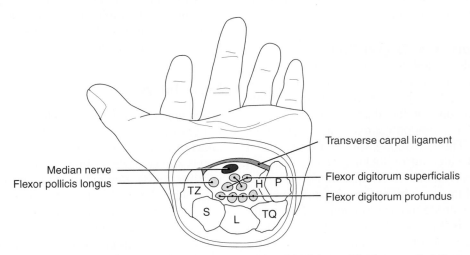

Figure 42-8 Carpal tunnel cross-section. TZ, trapezium; S, scaphoid; L, lunate; TQ, triquetrum; P, pisiform; H, hook of Hamate. (Adapted with permission from Reiner, M. [1991]. *The Illustrated Hand*. St. Paul: Minnesota Hand Rehabilitation.)

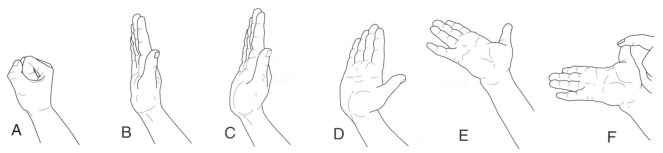

Figure 42-9 Median nerve gliding exercises at the wrist. Positions: **A.** Neutral wrist with finger and thumb flexion. **B.** Fingers and thumb extended. **C.** Wrist and fingers extended with thumb in neutral; **D.** Thumb extended. **E.** Forearm supinated. **F.** Thumb gently stretched into extension. (Adapted with permission from Rozmaryn, L. M., Dovelle, S., Rothman, E. R., Gorman, K., Olvey, K. M., & Bartko, J. J. [1998]. Nerve and tendon gliding exercises and the conservative management of carpal tunnel syndrome. *Journal of Hand Therapy, 11* (3), 171–179.)

of forearm rotation or of wrist motions and to avoid sustained pinch or forceful grip. Provide padded gloves and built-up handles (Sailer, 1996). Thick padded steering wheel covers are helpful.

Surgical intervention consists of decompression of the carpal tunnel by division of the transverse carpal ligament (Hunter, Davlin, & Fedus, 1995). Carpal tunnel release is one of the 10 most frequent surgeries performed in the United States (Rozmaryn et al., 1998). Postoperative therapy, when necessary, consists of edema control, scar management, desensitization as needed, nerve and tendon gliding exercises (Skirven & Trope, 1994), and eventual strengthening. Many therapists postpone strengthening exercises until at least 6 weeks following carpal tunnel release to avoid inflammation. Patients with new and mild symptoms tend to recover best (Aulisa et al., 1998).

Ulnar Nerve Compression at the Elbow or Cubital Tunnel Syndrome

Cubital tunnel syndrome is the second most common upper extremity nerve entrapment and is the most commonly compressed site of the ulnar nerve, at its location between the medial epicondyle and the olecranon (Posner, 1998). Typical complaints include proximal and medial forearm pain that is aching or sharp; decreased sensation of the dorsal and palmar surfaces of the small finger and the ulnar half of the ring finger; and weakness of interossei, adductor pollicis, flexor carpi ulnaris, and flexor digitorum profundus of the ring and small fingers. Clawing may be more evident if the FDP is not involved, because the long flexors are unopposed. Wartenberg's sign, the inability to adduct the small finger, and Froment's sign, in which effort at lateral pinch elicits thumb IP flexion due to weakness of the adductor pollicis, may be seen. Grip and pinch strength are decreased, and patients complain of dropping things (Khoo et al., 1996; Posner, 1998). Symptoms are worse

when the elbow is flexed repeatedly or is kept in flexion because this position dramatically reduces the volume of the cubital tunnel (Bozentka, 1998). Understandably, symptoms may increase at night if the person sleeps with the elbow flexed (Blackmore & Hotchkiss, 1995).

Cubital tunnel syndrome may result from trauma, such as a blow to the elbow or fracture or dislocation of the supracondylar or medial epicondylar area, or it may be due to chronic mild pressure on the elbow. Associated diagnoses include osteoarthritis, rheumatoid arthritis, diabetes, and Hansen's disease (Osterman & Davis, 1996).

Evaluation

Tapping over the cubital tunnel elicits a positive Tinel's sign. However, Tinel's sign may also be positive in 20% of normal people (Khoo et al., 1996). The elbow flexion test is positive if passively flexing the elbow and holding it flexed for 60 seconds produces sensory symptoms (Tetro & Pichora, 1996). Keep the wrist neutral while performing the elbow flexion test so as not to confound the findings with Phalen's test. Look for digital clawing and for muscle atrophy in the first web space, hypothenar eminence, and medial forearm. Perform grip and pinch testing and manual muscle testing as appropriate, and test sensation (Osterman & Davis, 1996).

Treatment

Conservative therapy for cubital tunnel syndrome includes edema control; splinting or padding the elbow; and positioning guidelines to avoid leaning on the elbow, to avoid elbow flexed postures and to avoid elbow-intensive activity (Khoo et al., 1996). Elbow splinting helps prevent sleeping with the elbow flexed. Types of splints include elbow pads or soft splints, pillows, and anterior or posterior thermoplastic splints. The splinted elbow position for sleeping is usually about

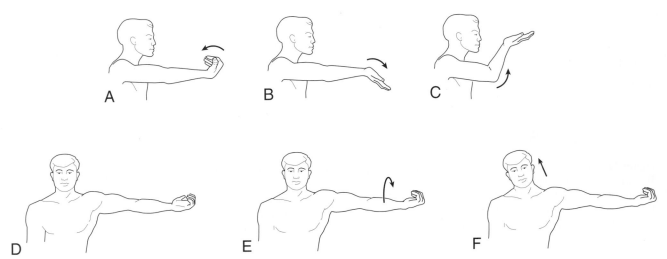

Figure 42-10 Ulnar nerve gliding exercises. **A.** Extend the arm with elbow straight and wrist and fingers flexed. **B.** Extend the wrist and fingers. **C.** Flex the elbow. **D.** Abduct the shoulder with wrist and fingers flexed. **E.** Externally rotate the shoulder. **F.** Laterally flex the neck. (Adapted with permission from Byron, P. M. [1995]. Upper extremity nerve gliding programs used at the Philadelphia Hand Center. In J. M. Hunter, E. J. Mackin, & A. D. Callahan [Eds.], *Rehabilitation of the Hand: Surgery and Therapy* [4th ed., p. 954]. St. Louis: Mosby.)

30° of flexion. Additional therapy includes proximal conditioning, postural and ergonomic training, and ulnar nerve gliding exercises (Fig. 42-10)

Radial Nerve Compression, or Posterior Interosseous Nerve Syndrome

Posterior interosseous nerve syndrome is purely motor. It presents two clinical pictures. In one paralysis affects all muscles innervated by the posterior interosseous nerve, with inability to extend the MP joints of thumb, index, long, ring, or small fingers. Wrist extension occurs only radially because of paralysis of extensor digitorum and ECU. In the other presentation of this syndrome, the person cannot extend the MP joint of one or more digits. Paralysis may spread to other digits if it is not treated on a timely basis (Spinner, 1995).

A common site of entrapment of the posterior interosseous nerve is at the supinator muscle, where it pierces the two heads of this muscle. Other causes include soft tissue tumors, rheumatoid arthritis with synovial proliferation, and radial head fractures or dislocations (Spinner, 1995). Therapy focuses on maintaining PROM and splinting to prevent deformity and promote function.

Nerve Laceration

Nerve lacerations are categorized as complete or partial. Stretching and contusion injuries can occur along with the laceration. Nerve reconstruction is primary if within 48 hours, early secondary if within 6 weeks, and late secondary after 3 months. The advantages associated with primary repair are that nerve stump retraction is limited and electrical stimulation can be used to identify distal fascicles (Smith, 1995b).

A **neuroma**, a disorganized mass of nerve fibers, can follow nerve injury. There is significant nerve pain elicited by tapping over the neuroma, with hypersensitivity limiting functional use of the hand. Desensitization techniques are helpful, along with padding over the painful area to promote functional use (Smith, 1995b).

Following nerve injury, therapy emphasizes promotion of function with ADL training and adaptive equipment and assists in prevention of deformity with splinting and appropriate PROM. Hand therapy provides valuable education to patients about their diagnosis and general recovery sequence and teaches protective guidelines to compensate for sensory loss. Hand therapy monitors changes in sensory and motor function and helps prevent joint contractures and imbalance by reevaluating ROM, sensation, and muscle status. Splint modifications are based on clinical changes over time.

Low Median Nerve Lesion

Median nerve laceration at the wrist results in low median nerve palsy, with denervation of the opponens pollicis (OP) and abductor pollicis brevis of the thumb and of the lumbricals to the index and long fingers. Clawing of the index and long fingers does not usually occur because the interossei remain ulnarly innervated. There is also loss of sensation of the radial side of the hand. With the absence of thumb abduction and opposition, the thumb rests in adduction, where it may become contracted. Fabricate a hand-based thumb abduction splint to maintain balance, to substitute for lost thumb opposition, and to prevent overstretching of denervated muscles (Colditz, 1995a).

Median nerve laceration creates serious functional loss of manipulation and sensibility of the thumb, index, and long fingers. Motor recovery usually occurs before sensory recovery. Be sure to teach compensatory strategies to avoid reinjury while sensibility is impaired (Colditz, 1995a). Instruct the patient to perform PROM to maintain joint mobility. Fabricate splints to sustain thumb abduction and digital MP flexion with IP extension to promote functional hand use and to counteract the deforming forces of the injury.

High Median Nerve Lesion

Injury near or at the elbow is called a high median nerve injury. Along with the motor loss identified earlier, there is denervation of FDP to index and long fingers, FDS to all digits, pronator teres, and pronator quadratus. The median nerve is considered the most important sensory nerve, and its loss severely compromises hand function. In therapy, prepare patients for probable tendon transfers by preventing deformity with splinting and by maintaining PROM of pronation, of digital MPs in flexion, of digital IPs in extension, and of thumb CMC abduction (Colditz, 1995a; Tubiana et al., 1996). Visual cues, adaptive devices, and modified handles may help compensate for the functional loss.

Low Ulnar Nerve Lesion

Laceration of the ulnar nerve at the wrist level is called a low ulnar lesion. This injury results in loss of most of the hand intrinsics. Denervation of the adductor digiti minimi, flexor digiti minimi, and opponens digiti minimi results in flattening of the hand with loss of the ulnar transverse metacarpal arch; denervation of thumb. Adductor pollicis (AP) and deep head of flexor pollicis brevis resulting in loss of thumb adduction and MP support; denervation of dorsal and volar interossei resulting in loss of digital abduction or adduction; and denervation of lumbricals to the ring and small fingers resulting in extrinsic imbalance. The ring and small fingers present a **claw deformity**, a position of MP hyperextension and PIP flexion associated with muscle imbalance in ulnar-innervated structures. Fine manipulation skills are compromised (Colditz, 1995a). Sensory loss involves the ulnar digits.

Splinting for ulnar nerve palsy aims to prevent overstretching of the absent ring and small finger intrinsics. An MP blocking splint that maintains slight MP flexion and prevents MP extension is recommended (Colditz, 1995a) (See Chapter 14). Teach patients to compensate for sensory loss and to maintain passive range of the MPs in flexion and the IPs in extension. Built-up handles in conjunction with the MP blocking splint may be helpful.

High Ulnar Nerve Lesion

A high ulnar nerve lesion is often identified with trauma at or proximal to the elbow. There is involvement of the muscles listed earlier and denervation of FDP of ring and small fingers and of FCU. Ring and small finger clawing is less apparent with the high lesion but becomes noticeable as the FDP are reinnervated and are unopposed by the still-absent intrinsics. Splinting and treatment are the same as for a low ulnar nerve lesion. If the FDP is absent, teach the patient to maintain full PROM of the IPs of the ring and small fingers to prevent contractures (Colditz, 1995a).

Low Radial Nerve Lesion

Low radial nerve injury of the deep motor branch is called posterior interosseous palsy. Presentations vary (see section on radial nerve compression), but brachioradialis and extensor carpi radialis longus function is usually present. Efforts to extend the wrist yield strong radial deviation. MP extension is affected. Sensation on the dorsal radial hand is affected. Therapy is similar to that described for radial nerve compression, with emphasis on maintaining PROM for wrist, thumb, and digital extension and splinting to promote tenodesis for functional pinch, grip, and release.

High Radial Nerve Lesion

A high radial nerve injury is seen commonly with humeral fractures because this nerve spirals around the humerus. Sensory loss occurs on the dorsal–radial hand, which interferes less with function than does sensory loss on the palmar hand. Triceps function remains, but the supinator and all wrist and finger extensors are out. Tenodesis is lost (Colditz, 1995a; Tubiana et al., 1996).

Splinting restores tenodesis and may be useful for many months during the wait for reinnervation, which occurs at approximately 1 inch per month. A variety of static and dynamic splints are available; the dynamic splints are most useful functionally. Many patients make good use of both types of splints. Because of these splints' functional value, compliance tends to be good. It is important to maintain joint suppleness while awaiting reinnervation or reconstructive surgery (Colditz, 1995a).

Fractures

Distal Radius Fracture

Distal radius fractures are among the most common upper extremity fractures (Frykman & Kropp, 1995). Hand therapists frequently treat patients with this diagnosis. Distal radius fractures should not be confused with fractures of the carpal bones. The main complication associated with distal radius fracture is traumatic arthritis due to poor articular congruency (Leibovic, 1999). Decreased wrist ROM, decreased grip strength, alteration of the carpal alignment, and instability may ensue. Other complications include tendon rupture, compression of the median or ulnar nerve, and CRPS (Reiss, 1995).

Therapy During Immobilization

Appropriate early therapy can make a huge difference in the patient's overall functional recovery. If digits are allowed to become swollen and stiff, the long-term functional results can be devastating. These fractures are common among older people with osteoporosis and balance problems. Temporary loss of independence following fracture can trigger an irreversible downward spiral in their occupational functioning.

Typical medical management of Colles' fracture is cast immobilization, usually above-elbow with the elbow in 90° of flexion to prevent forearm rotation during the first 3 weeks. When the patient is put in a short arm cast and the elbow is freed, begin elbow AROM for flexion and extension, but avoid resisted elbow motion so as not to stress the fracture healing (Reiss, 1995). Do not perform elbow PROM without medical clearance, and be very gentle. Biceps tightness commonly follows elbow immobilization.

Certain fractures require an external fixator and/or internal fixation. (See Research Note.) Some physicians delay the referral of patients to therapy, but postponing the initiation of therapy can result in significant problems with edema and decreased ROM. It is a good idea to communicate with referring physicians and encourage routine early therapy referral for this diagnosis.

While the patient is in an external fixator, provide pin site care as the physician prescribes using sterile technique and universal precautions (Bryan & Kohnke, 1997). Teach the patient digital ROM and tendon gliding exercises, and instruct in precautions related to cast wearing. It is critical to monitor for cast tightness, for this can cause CRPS. Call the physician if the cast is too tight. Discourage the use of slings, for they promote unnecessary proximal stiffness and disuse (Collins, 1993).

Insidious onset of shoulder restrictions is problematic and best avoided. Physicians most assuredly appreciate therapists' input regarding early signs of this problem. To prevent a frozen shoulder, proximal ROM is a high treatment priority (Skirven & Trope, 1994). Instruct in shoulder flexion, abduction, internal rotation, and external rotation (Collins, 1993). Perform as thorough a physical assessment as tolerated and as cast constraints permit. This may have to be done in phases. Early identification of guarding, excessive pain, or autonomic signs can alert the team to the possibility of CRPS (Reiss, 1995).

Following distal radius fracture, the recovery of function depends on restoration of motion and strength and on maximizing the length–tension relationship of the digital flexors and extensors (Collins, 1993). Edema

---

RESEARCH NOTE

Load Relaxation and Forces with Activity in Hoffman External Fixators: A Clinical Study in Patients With Colles' Fractures

Winemaker, M. J., Chinchalkar, S., Richards, R. S., Johnson, J. A., Chess, D. G., & King, G. J. W. (1998). Journal of Hand Surgery, 23A, 926–932

ABSTRACT

Small-frame Hoffman external fixation bars with strain gauges to quantify bending and torsional forces were applied to four patients with displaced metaphyseal fractures of the distal radius. Measurements were taken during surgery and 1, 3, and 6 weeks after surgery during ADL and hand therapy mobilization. Radiographs were taken before and after reduction and at each subsequent visit. Significant changes in external fixator forces were measured during ADL and hand therapy mobilization, but these returned to baseline after the activities were performed. The most provocative activities studied were twisting a doorknob and lifting heavy objects.

IMPLICATIONS FOR PRACTICE

▶ Twisting a doorknob and lifting heavy objects were the most provocative activities of those studied.
▶ The findings from this study suggest that patients with unstable distal radius fractures should be cautioned not to use the involved extremity to twist a doorknob or to lift heavy objects.
▶ A limitation of the study was that external fixator bar forces were surmised to be proportional to the forces transmitted to the fracture site, but these measurements may be affected by factors such as muscle action, pin loosening, and ancillary fixation. Further study and larger sample size are needed.

can contribute to decreased ROM at uncasted areas (Tubiana, 1983). Patients are often surprised that uninjured and uncasted areas can stiffen.

The goals of early therapy during immobilization are to normalize edema and to achieve as nearly normal AROM of uncasted areas as possible (Collins, 1993). During this period, intrinsic tightness, extrinsic tightness, and digital joint tightness may occur (Skirven & Trope, 1994). The chance of tendon adherence is increased following open reduction and its accompanying incisional scar (Tubiana, 1983). Various blocking splints may be used with functional activity and exercise to resolve joint or musculotendinous tightness (Fig. 42-4). Differential tendon gliding exercises are extremely important. Frequent exercise throughout the day is better than a few long sessions. It is generally advised to perform exercises every hour or two, perhaps 5 to 10 repetitions each, maintaining the end position comfortably for 3 to 5 seconds. Incorporate exercises into purposeful activity and ADL as much as possible (Bryan & Kohnke, 1997).

If extrinsic musculotendinous tightness persists, it may be appropriate to add night static progressive splinting or low-load, long-duration dynamic splinting in conjunction with exercise to normalize extrinsic length (Collins, 1993). Consult the physician before making this determination.

Therapy After Cast or Fixator is Removed

When fracture immobilization is discontinued, physicians often recommend a custom-fabricated volar wrist splint. This is protective and can be corrective to help restore functional wrist motion (usually extension). This temporary support is particularly helpful if the patient maintains habitual wrist flexion, for this doggy paw posture leads to development of the undesirable deformity position of MP extension, PIP flexion, thumb adduction and extension discussed earlier (Skirven & Trope, 1994).

Following removal of the cast or external fixator, there is usually measurable limitation in ROM, with patients reporting awkwardness and decreased function (Byl et al., 1999). Consult the physician for medical clearance and guidelines for forearm and wrist ROM. ***Do not initiate PROM of the wrist without medical clearance, as this may be injurious.*** Teach the patient to wean off the protective splint according to the physician's guidelines, which are individualized. Edema control continues to be the highest priority until it is resolved. AROM and ADL can help correct the edema.

At any time, but especially in this early stage, overzealous therapy is harmful. Patients and families who think they should be aggressive in their home programs need education and reinforcement to avoid overdoing it. Use written material and illustrations to teach them how to observe tissue responses and monitor inflammation (Colditz, 1995b). Temperature elevation over the joints of digits may indicate that treatment is eliciting an inflammatory reaction and should be adjusted accordingly (Fess, 1993).

It is extremely important to retrain the wrist extensors to function independently of the extensor digitorum (Laseter & Carter, 1996). Have the patient practice wrist extension with available composite digital flexion, being especially sure the MPs are flexed. Then have the patient flex the wrist with digits relaxed but extended, to isolate the wrist flexors. Because substitution patterns are hard to overcome, early training of biomechanically efficient movement is best. Progressive grasp-and-release activities reinforce this tenodesis training. It is also important to retrain the extensor digitorum to function independently of the intrinsics. Have the patient extend the MPs with the IPs slightly flexed to isolate the extensor digitorum.

Gradually upgrade therapy with increasingly challenging motions, combined motions, and activities aiming to restore joint suppleness and musculotendinous lengths. Dexterity activities, such as cat's cradle, and games such as pick-up sticks promote spontaneous functional movements. Sorting drawers and folding small items of clothing are good home activities. Initiate graded functional strengthening with medical clearance, usually after good motion has been achieved. Again, it is easy to be too aggressive with these patients. Upgrade carefully, monitor patient and tissue responses, and adjust the treatment accordingly.

Scaphoid Fracture

Some 60% of carpal fractures affect the scaphoid (also called the navicular) bone. The mechanism of injury is usually a fall on the outstretched hand (called FOOSH). There may also be associated ligamentous injury. Tenderness in the anatomical snuffbox, a depression at the base of the thumb between the EPL and EPB tendons, where snuff used to be placed, is a classic finding. Scaphoid fracture may be difficult to confirm radiographically initially and may not become apparent until 3 weeks following injury due to resorption at the fracture site. Once fracture is confirmed, the thumb is usually included in the cast, with the IP joint free.

Because of the pattern of vascular supply, proximal scaphoid fractures may be at risk for developing avascular necrosis. Casting time may be long for this reason. Hand therapy principles are the same as for distal radius fracture (Frykman & Kropp, 1995).

Case Example

MS. P.: HAND THERAPY FOR DISTAL RADIAL FRACTURE

Patient Information

Ms. P. is a 49 year-old athletic computer software manager with dominant right hand. She is single and lives alone. Ms. P. fell on an outstretched hand while on vacation out of state, sustaining a comminuted displaced right distal radius fracture. She was initially treated with closed reduction and a long-arm cast. Ten days later, after returning home, she underwent open reduction internal fixation of the right distal radius with percutaneous pins, synthetic bone graft material, and application of an external fixator. Family members came to stay with her to assist with self-care and ADL needs. At the time of her injury, she was looking forward to a kayaking vacation.

Ms. P. was referred to outpatient hand therapy the day after surgery. She had significant pain, edema, and increased autonomic signs. Her digital ROM was significantly limited actively and passively. She had visceral responses (nausea) when trying to look at her hand or at the fixator.

Reason for Referral to Hand Therapy

Ms. P. was referred to hand therapy to maximize functional abilities while her hand was immobilized and to promote wound and fracture healing, edema control, and mobility of non-immobilized structures.

Hand Therapy Problem List

▶ Disruption of independent living and job performance; interruption of frequent job-related travel
▶ Inability to sleep or to perform self-care or home activities due to pain, significant edema of the upper extremity including the digits, and decreased ROM of upper extremity, including the digits
▶ Risk of CRPS with degradation of functional and clinical status as evidenced by increased autonomic signs

Hand Therapy Goal List

▶ Normalize autonomic signs and ameliorate pain interfering with function and sleep
▶ Promote spontaneous pain-free use of the right upper extremity in daily activity
▶ Achieve independent self-care and assisted homemaking and resume job-related travel and engagement in athletic activity

Treatment Plan

Ms. P. began a home program of education about the expected clinical course and recovery; pin site care; edema control; and shoulder, elbow, and digital ROM in pain-free ranges. Emphasis was on shoulder active exercise and upper extremity elevation. A week after surgery, Ms. P.'s autonomic signs were resolving. Her digits remained edematous, and AROM was still limited throughout the upper extremity except for her shoulder, which was functional.

At 2 weeks after surgery, digital AROM and PROM were slowly improving but still limited (Fig. 42-11, *A* and *B*). Ms. P.'s home program was upgraded to include edema control, functional grip and release activities, blocking exercises with thermoplastic supports, place-and-hold exercises, night composite digital extension static splinting, and day dynamic digital composite extension splinting. Differential digital flexor tendon gliding was restricted by adherence at the volar distal forearm incisional site, which was still healing. She had extrinsic extensor tightness, extrinsic flexor tightness, and intrinsic tightness. Fortunately, Ms. P. was not developing PIP flexion contractures. She had been relying on her nondominant left hand for handwriting and all self-care. She returned to work soon after surgery and was once again traveling frequently on business.

At 3 weeks after surgery, when incisional sites were healed, manual edema mobilization began, and all functional activities, splints, and exercises were upgraded in a pain-free fashion. Silicone gel was applied to incision sites at night for scar management. Ms. P. continued to make slow but measurable progress. Her physician reported good radiographic alignment.

At 6 weeks after surgery, Ms. P.'s fixator was removed. Her physician reported good reduction and stability of the distal radioulnar joint. She was severely limited in forearm pronation and supination and in wrist AROM and PROM. She was instructed in pain-free forearm and wrist AROM. A thermoplastic volar wrist splint was fabricated for support and to correct limited wrist extension. Ms. P. began to resume use of her right upper extremity for handwriting intermittently and for home activities as tolerated. Although she was very compliant with her home program, her progress was slow. She had improved but was still limited in all ROM of the elbow, forearm, wrist, and hand and was still compromised functionally by musculotendinous tightness. She had become quite adept at using her left hand for dexterity tasks.

At 10 weeks after surgery, Ms. P. began to demonstrate dramatic gains in suppleness (Fig. 42-20, *C* and *D*). She was significantly improved in digital edema and in all ROM. Elbow extension was normal. Forearm supination and pronation were better, with AROM being equal to PROM. Isolated wrist extension was improved. Digital composite fisting and FDP and FDS differential tendon gliding were nearly normal, and tightness of the extrinsic flexors was almost fully resolved. Ms. P. was using her right hand for all handwriting and grooming and for driving her sports car. She was eager to begin simulating kayaking, as she had kept her plans for a kayaking vacation. Ms. P. said that her dynamic splints and night static composite extension splints were helpful to her, so these were modified and upgraded. Strengthening exercises were gradually and cautiously upgraded as well.

Analysis of Reasoning

Ms. P.'s progress was slower than average. Her tissue formed more scar than usual with that injury. While a therapist following textbook timelines might have been inclined to upgrade her program earlier, this would have set her progress back because of the residual edema and stiffness. She had maintained a soft end feel throughout her therapy, and this critical detail permitted a slow but steady, tolerable approach to remodel her tissues. She was dependable and actively engaged in her program. Her functional outcome was excellent eventually, and she was able to enjoy her kayaking vacation.

CLINICAL REASONING
in Hand Therapy Practice

Effects of CRPS on Functional Use of the Involved Extremity

Initially, Ms. P. demonstrated a guarded upper extremity position associated with autonomic signs. How might upper extremity posturing influence pain, edema, and ROM? What should the home program emphasize to promote autonomic normalization?

Effects of Edema on Upper Extremity Pain, ROM, and Function

Persistent edema of Ms. P.'s hand worsened her pain, stiffness, and function. What treatment techniques are helpful in resolving upper extremity edema?

Effects of Substitution Patterns on Wrist and Hand Function

Ms. P. could not isolate her wrist extensors from her extensor digitorum function. This interfered with recovery of normal grasp and release patterns. What clinical problems contribute to the inability to isolate wrist extensors? What functional exercises would help retrain isolated wrist extension with simultaneous grip (i.e., normal tenodesis patterns)? What choice of splint or splints might help recover these motions?

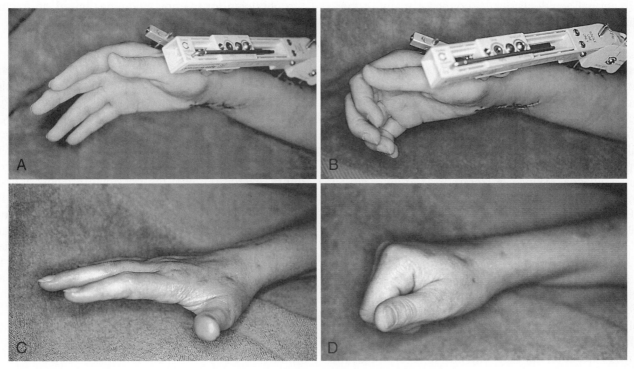

Figure 42-11 At 2 weeks post surgery, Ms. P.'s active digital extension (**A**) and flexion (**B**); at 10 weeks post surgery, Ms. P.'s active digital extension (**C**) and flexion (**D**).

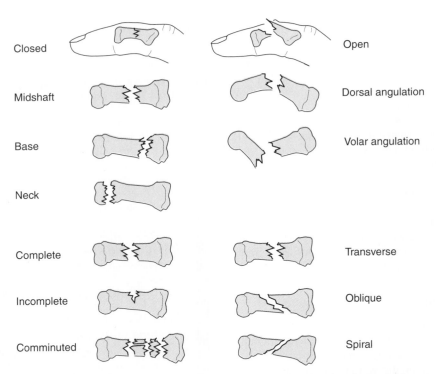

Figure 42-12 Fracture terminology. (Adapted with permission from American Society for Surgery of the Hand. [1990]. *The Hand: Examination and Diagnosis* (3rd ed.). New York: Churchill Livingstone.)

Nonarticular Hand Fracture

Fracture occurs more often in the hand than any other area, and more than 50% of hand fractures occur at work. Motor vehicle accidents, household injuries, and recreational accidents also account for many of these injuries (Meyer & Wilson, 1995). (Fig. 42-12).

Distal Phalanx Fracture

Distal phalanx digital fractures typically result from a crushing injury and occur most often in the thumb and middle finger. Tuft fractures occur at the distal tip. They are extremely painful, in part because there is often a subungual (i.e., beneath the nail) hematoma (Meyer & Wilson, 1995). Following a distal phalanx fracture, hypersensitivity, pain, and decreased ROM of the DIP joint may occur (Skirven & Trope, 1994). Monitor closely for signs of DIP extensor lag, or the inability to extend the DIP joint actively despite passive extension (Meyer & Wilson, 1995).

Middle Phalanx Fracture

At the middle phalanx, fractures angulate according to their relation to the FDS insertion. Medical management and early positioning guidelines vary among caregivers. Following middle phalanx fractures, decreased PIP and DIP ROM are common problems. Fractures at this site may require long immobilization time for healing, with resulting stiffness. When the patient is medically cleared

for therapy, isolated FDS exercises are very important. Here, too, PIP joint flexion contractures are serious complications that can occur in as little as 2 weeks of immobilization in flexion (Tubiana, 1983). Consult with the physician for therapy guidelines based on fracture stability and healing (Russell, 1999).

Proximal Phalanx Fracture

At the proximal phalanx, fractures tend to angulate with a palmar apex. This deforming force is due to the action of the intrinsic muscles on the proximal fragment (Meyer & Wilson, 1995). With proximal phalanx fractures, a hand-based splint in intrinsic-plus (antideformity) position is useful at night. A digit-based extension splint provides support and protection in the day except during exercise. Again, the physician provides therapy guidelines based on fracture stability and healing. PIP joint flexion contractures are the most likely and difficult complication (Tubiana, 1983). Watch for these and catch them early. Better yet: avoid them with appropriate splinting and structure-specific exercise. PIP extensor lag and flexor tendon adherence at the fracture site are other serious problems (Meyer & Wilson, 1995; Vahey et al., 1998).

Metacarpal Fracture

Unless there is associated trauma, metacarpal fractures at the base are frequently stable. Metacarpal fractures at the shaft may be transverse, oblique, or spiral. Metacarpal fractures at the neck are common, occurring most often in the small finger. They may result in muscle imbalance between the intrinsics and extrinsics (Meyer & Wilson, 1995).

With metacarpal fractures, dorsal hand edema is a frequent complication that can contribute to MP joint dorsal capsular tightness. If there is associated soft tissue injury, intrinsic contracture or extensor digitorum adherence may occur (Skirven & Trope, 1994). Appropriate early therapy and preventive edema control are important (Meyer & Wilson, 1995).

Unstable fractures require fixation to achieve stability and allow early ROM. **Kirschner wires**, a common form of fixation used for hand fractures, may be used alone or in conjunction with additional fixation. Other forms of internal fixation include tension band wires, lag screws, plates, and mini external fixators (Leibovic, 1999). Functional recovery relates to anatomical restoration. To maximize functional outcomes, the ideal situation allows for early motion. Preventing stiffness of uninvolved digits is a high priority that can itself be challenging. Prolonged immobilization is associated with edema and pain. Persistent edema results in joint and tendon scar and adhesions; atrophy occurs, as well as osteoporosis (Meyer & Wilson, 1995).

Collateral Ligament Injury

PIP Joint Sprain

PIP joint sprains often result from sports involving balls. Their severity, which may be underappreciated (Dawson, 1994), is described as grade I through grade III. In grade I, the ligament remains intact but there is diffuse individual fiber disruption. In grade II, there is complete disruption of one of the joint capsule's major retaining ligaments. In grade III, there is complete disruption of one collateral ligament in addition to injury to dorsal and/or volar capsular structures (Wilson & Hazen, 1995). Pain, decreased ROM, and risk of flexion contracture are the most common problems associated with grade I and II injuries. Joint instability may occur with grade III injuries (Benson & Bailie, 1996).

Therapy focuses on edema control, joint protection, and ROM. Buddy straps are helpful to protect or to promote movement. They may be offset to improve fit (Fig. 42-5) (Jensen & Rayan, 1996). Splinting is both protective and corrective. A dorsal extension blocking splint is often ordered early on for volar plate injuries associated with dorsal PIP joint dislocation (Fig. 42-13) (Lairmore & Engber, 1998). Persistent thickening about the joint commonly occurs, interfering with recovery of ROM (Benson & Bailie, 1996).

Skier's Thumb

Disruption of the ulnar collateral ligament of the thumb MP joint occurs with acute radial deviation. This diagnosis, which may entail avulsion of bone fragment at the ligamentous insertion, is often seen among people who fall while skiing (Lairmore & Engber, 1998). Injury to the radial collateral ligament of the thumb MP occurs only one-tenth as often (Wilson & Hazen, 1995). Following surgical repair, the wrist and thumb are casted. When therapy begins, IP ROM is the priority, as full MP flexion may not be achieved, especially among older patients. Avoid resistive exercise until medically cleared. Then begin with lateral pinch but avoid tip pinch until further medical clearance, which may not be for 12 weeks, as tip pinch is strenuous on the injured structures (Wilson & Hazen, 1995). Use a hand-based spica splint for protection. Scar hypersensitivity due to the underlying radial sensory nerve is common.

Flexor Tendon Injury

Surgical repair of flexor tendon injury is a complex undertaking performed by specialists in the field. Like the surgery, hand therapy for these patients is a complicated and specialized area. Therapy can be time-consuming, and it entails substantial education of the patient, with subtle but significant changes in splinting and exercise at every session to promote function while protecting fragile repaired structures. Multiple structures are often involved, and there are many precautions and contraindications that vary according to the details of the patient's surgery and the surgeon's specifications and preferences. It is essential to maintain close communication with the patient's surgeon. A therapist experienced in the treatment of these patients should closely supervise their care.

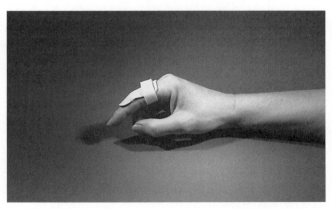

Figure 42-13 Dorsal PIP extension–blocking splint. Protective digit-based splint maintains slight PIP flexion. Used to prevent full extension to protect volar plate injury.

Five anatomical zones describe flexor tendon injury to the index, long, ring, and small digits (Fig. 42-14). Zone I is from the insertion of the FDS to the insertion of the FDP. Zone II is the area where the FDS and FDP both lie within the flexor sheath, from the A-1 pulley to the FDS insertion. This region has memorably been dubbed "no man's land" to reflect the technical challenge and historically poor prognosis for repair in this area (Wang & Gupta, 1996). Zone III describes the area from the distal edge of the carpal tunnel to the A-1 pulley of the flexor sheath, including the lumbrical muscles. Zone IV is where the flexor tendons lie under the transverse carpal ligament in the carpal tunnel. Injuries in this zone may include the median and ulnar nerves. Zone V is the area from the forearm flexor musculotendinous junction to the border of the transverse carpal ligament (Culp & Taras, 1995).

Physicians usually indicate specific postoperative positioning guidelines to protect repaired structures

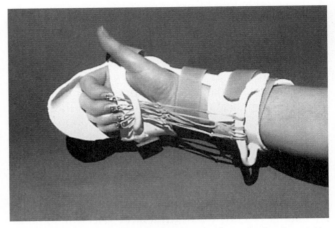

Figure 42-15 Modified Kleinert splint. Dorsal splint maintains the wrist in 30° of flexion, MPs in 70° of flexion, and IPs in extension. Rubber band attachments provide passive digital flexion.

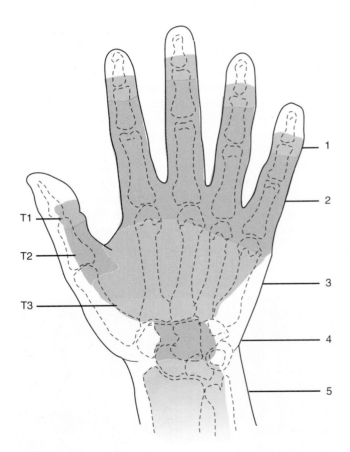

Figure 42-14 Flexor tendon zones. (Adapted with permission from Kleinert, H. H., Schepel, S., & Gill, T. [1981]. Flexor tendon injuries. *Surgical Clinics of North America, 61*, 267–286; Stewart, K. M., & van Strien, G. [1995]. Postoperative management of flexor tendon injuries. In J. M. Hunter, E. J. Mackin, & A. D. Callahan [Eds.], *Rehabilitation of the Hand: Surgery and Therapy* [4th ed., pp. 433–462]. St. Louis: Mosby.)

following flexor tendon repair. The goals are twofold and contradictory: to minimize adhesion formation (Skirven & Trope, 1994) and to prevent gap or attenuation of the repaired tendon (Silva et al., 1998). These dual goals highlight the complexity of therapy associated with this diagnosis. Various protocols exist for controlled mobilization, using a dorsal splint with the wrist in about 30° flexion, MP joints in about 70° flexion, and IP joints ideally in extension (Wang & Gupta, 1996). The involved IP joints may have to be in some flexion if a digital nerve has been repaired. The Duran protocol entails passive digital flexion and extension within the protective splint, to achieve 3 to 5 mm of differential digital tendon excursion. With this protocol, gentle active motion begins with medical clearance about 4 or 5 weeks after surgery (Culp & Taras, 1995).

The passive flexion–active extension protocol, also called the Kleinert protocol, uses rubber band attachments to the fingernails to provide passive digital flexion within the protective dorsal splint (Fig. 42-15). The patient performs gentle active digital extension and the rubber band provides passive digital flexion within the confines of the protective splint. Exercises are gradually increased to 10 repetitions comfortably every waking hour. At night, the digits may be strapped carefully and comfortably to the dorsal hood of the splint to counteract the tendency to develop PIP or DIP flexion contractures (Wang & Gupta, 1996).

The Chow protocol uses a combination of the Duran and Kleinert techniques. With advances in suture techniques, some caregivers are advocating early active motion protocols (Cannon, 1993; Winters et al., 1998).

When the physician gives medical clearance to discontinue the dorsal protective splint, begin a graded program to promote functional movement. Edema control and scar management remain high clinical priorities. Assess closely and determine tissue-specific limitations that guide the therapy program. Tendon gliding exercises and place-and-hold exercises are typical early techniques. Corrective splinting is useful, along with ADL, graded activity, and upgraded exercise as appropriate.

Staged Flexor Tendon Reconstruction

Staged flexor tendon reconstruction is a complex two-part procedure. It is highly advisable to have an experienced hand therapist supervise the treatment. Staged flexor tendon surgery is chosen when there is significant scarring of the tendon yet potential for eventual function. It may be used in cases of flexor tendon rupture or when primary repair was not possible, such as a complex injury involving bone and multiple tissues. In the first stage, a tendon implant replaces the scarred tendon; capsular contractures are released; and pulleys are reconstructed. The implant, which may be active or passive, stimulates formation of a new biological sheath. In the second stage, after about 3 months, a tendon graft replaces the implant (Hunter, Taras, Mackin, Maser, & Culp, 1995).

Extensor Tendon Injury

Therapy of extensor tendon injuries is complicated and requires supervision by experienced hand therapists. There are various protocols for immobilization, controlled passive motion, or active short arc of motion following extensor tendon repair (Evans, 1995; Thomes & Thomes, 1995).

Seven zones describe the digital extensors for the index, long, ring, and small fingers, and five zones describe the thumb extensors (Fig. 42-16). Injury in zones I and II leads to a mallet deformity (Evans, 1995), which follows disruption of the terminal extensor tendon and manifests itself as DIP extensor lag (Fig. 42-17) (Brzezienski & Schneider, 1995). Depending on the nature of the problem, in nonoperative cases, therapy may include continuous splinting of the DIP in extension for 6 to 8 weeks as determined by the physician while the tendon heals. It is essential to maintain normal PIP ROM during immobilization at the DIP. When initiating ROM of the DIP after the terminal tendon has healed, watch closely for recurrence of DIP extensor lag and resume splinting as needed to recover DIP extension (Evans, 1995). Some physicians recommend continuation of night splinting when DIP AROM is begun (Brzezienski & Schneider, 1995; Crosby & Wehbe, 1996).

Extensor injuries in zones III and IV lead to a boutonniere deformity, an imbalanced digital position of PIP flexion and DIP hyperextension (Fig. 42-18). The deformity is due to volar displacement of the lateral bands secondary to involvement of the central slip (Coons & Green, 1995; Rosenthal, 1995). In nonoperative cases, splint the PIP in full extension for 6 weeks and promote DIP active and passive flexion to prevent stiffness of the oblique retinacular ligament (Coons & Green, 1995). In operative cases, follow the physician's guidelines, which may vary in timing and technique of mobilization and splinting. When the patient is medically cleared to begin PIP active exercises, watch closely for PIP extensor lag and modify therapy and splinting accordingly (Crosby & Wehbe, 1996).

Injury in zones V and VI may be treated by immobilization or by controlled early motion (Evans, 1995). Specific positioning and motion guidelines vary from surgeon to surgeon and are modified according to each patient's tissue responses. Multiple complex splints may be needed to achieve a program that balances rest and motion appropriately.

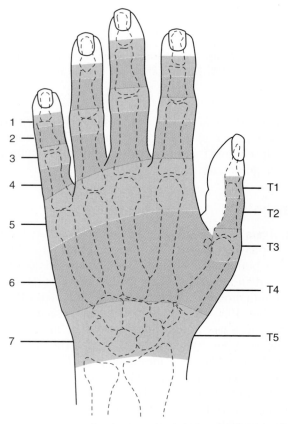

Figure 42-16 Extensor tendon zones. (Adapted with permission from Kleinert, H. H., Schepel, S., & Gill, T. [1981]. Flexor tendon injuries. *Surgical Clinics of North America, 61,* 267–286; Evans, R. B. [1995]. An update on extensor tendon management. In J. M. Hunter, E. J. Mackin, & A. D. Callahan [Eds.], *Rehabilitation of the Hand: Surgery and Therapy* [4th ed., pp. 565–606]. St. Louis: Mosby.)

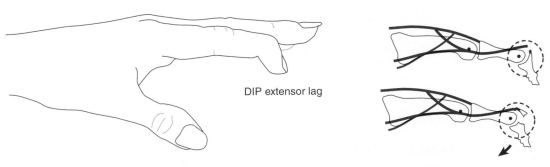

Figure 42-17 Mallet deformity. (Adapted with permission from American Society for Surgery of the Hand. [1990]. *The Hand: Examination and Diagnosis* (3rd ed.). New York: Churchill Livingstone.)

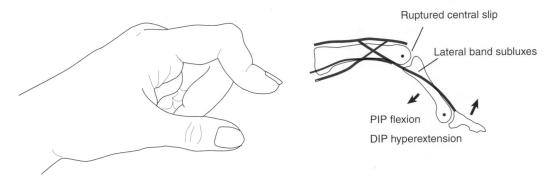

Figure 42-18 Boutonniere deformity. (Adapted with permission from American Society for Surgery of the Hand. [1990]. *The Hand: Examination and Diagnosis* (3rd ed.). New York: Churchill Livingstone.)

Injury in zone VII is likely to result in restrictions due to development of adhesions (Evans, 1995). Communicate closely with the surgeon for specific positioning and motion guidelines.

Tenolysis

Tenolysis is a surgical procedure to release tendon adhesions that restrict movement. Physicians do not usually perform this procedure until injured tissues have matured and PROM is maximized, as demonstrated by a plateau in progress during therapy. (Schneider & Berger-Feldscher, 1995). Therapy following tenolysis may begin as early as a few hours after surgery. The first few days following surgery are considered crucial. The physician's referral should include information on the integrity of the tendon and expected ROM goals based on intraoperative findings (Schneider & Berger-Feldscher, 1995). First priorities are edema control and ROM; observe and respect these fragile tissues' tolerances.

Complex Regional Pain Syndrome

Any upper extremity injury, whether as minor as a paper cut or as major as a complex crush injury, has the potential to result in devastating reflex sympathetic dystrophy (RSD), recently renamed complex regional pain syndrome (CRPS) by the International Association for the Study of Pain (IASP). The IASP has suggested transitional use of RSD in parentheses after the new terminology because it would be unrealistic to expect immediate abandonment of this familiar term (Stanton-Hicks et al., 1995). In this chapter, CRPS is understood to be synonymous with RSD.

CRPS type I follows a noxious event. Pain that is not limited to the territory of a single peripheral nerve occurs spontaneously, and it is disproportionate to the inciting noxious event. There is edema, with abnormality of skin color or abnormal sudomotor activity in the painful area since the onset. The diagnosis of CRPS is excluded by other existing conditions that may cause the pain and dysfunction (Stanton-Hicks et al., 1995).

CRPS type II is the same as type I except that it develops after a nerve injury, whereas type I does not involve a nerve injury. CRPS type III refers to a group not otherwise specified, for patients who do not fulfill the criteria for types I or II (Stanton-Hicks et al., 1995).

Pain that is disproportionate to the injury is the hallmark of CRPS (Wong & Wilson, 1997). Constant attention to the patient's pain level and autonomic responses can lead to early medical management, if not prevention, of this challenging problem. The earlier this problem is diagnosed, the more successfully it may resolve (Bryan & Kohnke, 1997; Walsh, 1995).

Over the years many terms have been used to describe CRPS, including causalgia, Sudeck's atrophy, and shoulder–hand syndrome (Fealy & Ladd, 1996). Although clinical presentation is variable, traditional hand therapy literature identifies five clinical types as minor causalgia, minor traumatic dystrophy, shoulder–hand syndrome, major traumatic dystrophy, and major causalgia (Lankford, 1995).

Historically, the four cardinal symptoms and signs of CRPS have been identified as pain, swelling, stiffness, and discoloration. Secondary symptoms and signs include osseous demineralization, sudomotor changes (sweating), temperature changes, trophic changes, vasomotor instability, palmar fasciitis (thickening of palmar fascia), and pilomotor activity (goose pimples or hair standing on end) (Lankford, 1995, p. 782).

Literature refers to people with CRPS as hypersympathetic reactors, who experience cold hands and feet, fainting, sweaty palms, heart palpitations, hyperventilation, and vasoconstriction. Authorities have unfairly labeled these people as hysterical personality types. There is no good evidence supporting a predispositional personality profile for this diagnosis. There is, however, a lot of methodologically bad evidence, unfortunately stigmatizing those with the diagnosis and biasing caregivers (Lynch, 1992).

Elegant animal studies have shown that self-protection through immobilization, intended to avoid pain, is itself a risk factor for the diagnosis of CRPS. People with CRPS must learn to use the extremity in ways that are pain free and biomechanically efficient. Normalizing sensory input also helps interrupt the vicious cycle of pain and stiffness (Byl & Melnick, 1997).

Therapy for CRPS

The most important therapy guideline is no PROM or painful treatment. The first thing is to control the pain. This includes management through medications, sympathetic blocks such as stellate ganglion blocks, and modalities such as transcutaneous electrical nerve stimulation (TENS) as appropriate. Close communication with medical experts specializing in pain management is ideal.

Provide vasomotor challenge through stress loading (described later), temperature biofeedback, and posture changes during activity. Hardy and Hardy (1997) recommend resetting the sensory thresholds through contrast, vibration, and desensitization (See Chapter 27). Water aerobics and functional activities are excellent ways to provide active movement incorporating reciprocal mo-

tion. Use stress loading routinely with patients who are at risk for CRPS. Stress loading is proposed to change sympathetic efferent activity. While the physiological mechanisms of stress loading are not known (Carlson & Watson, 1988), it is popular among hand therapists for treating active CRPS, not the sequelae.

The two components of stress loading are "scrubbing the floor" (performed literally on all fours if possible), in brief sessions, 3 times per day initially, and carrying a weighted briefcase, done with the extremity in extension. The weight should be light and tolerable. Be sure it is not too heavy. Scrubbing and carrying achieve compressive loading and distraction of the upper extremity (Walsh, 1995). If actual scrubbing cannot be tolerated, substitute comfortable weight-bearing exercises.

The frequency and duration of scrub and carry are upgraded as tolerated. If wrist ROM limitations or injury precautions do not allow the patient to assume the scrub position, positions may be adapted to accomplish comfortable weight bearing (See Chapter 23).

Avoid PROM or other therapy until the pain and swelling begin to subside, and then monitor responses closely. Incorporate traditional hand therapy, including splinting and other nonaggravating modalities with edema control, joint ROM, differential tendon gliding, restoration of musculotendinous lengths, strengthening, desensitization, physical agents including transcutaneous electrical nerve stimulation and ultrasound as appropriate, and functional activity within tolerance. Manual edema mobilization is effective with this diagnosis.

Perhaps with CRPS more than other diagnoses, patient-directed therapy is essential. It is better to perform gentle, pain-free active exercises frequently for short periods than fewer and longer sessions. Light massage and active exercise help to interrupt the pain cycle. Make the exercise program bilateral and include reciprocal upper extremity motions (Byl & Melnick, 1997). Allow the progress to be as slow as necessary to prevent worsening of symptoms. This diagnosis can be overwhelming and discouraging. Provide the patient with appropriate encouragement and reassurances that progress can be made over time.

CRPS typifies the difficult clinical problems that hand therapists are trying to avert or avoid. Treatment programs that are progressing well can be suddenly and unexpectedly derailed by this disorder. For this reason, it is advisable to approach all hand therapy patients supportively and with a very careful eye, regardless of their diagnosis.

Osteoarthritis

Idiopathic osteoarthritis (OA) is the most common type of OA. In the upper extremity, it often affects the DIP and

PIP joints. Osteophytes at the DIP are called Heberden's nodes, and osteophytes at the PIP are called Bouchard's nodes. For painful DIP nodes, small cylindrical splints or light Coban wrap may promote function while decreasing pain (Melvin, 1989).

Hand therapy for osteoarthritis focuses on alleviating symptoms through education in principles of joint protection, protective and supportive splinting, and provision of adaptive devices for ADL. For osteoarthritis of the thumb CMC, a hand-based thumb spica splint (Fig. 42-19) is often extremely helpful (Swigart et al., 1999). Some therapists prefer to use a forearm-based spica splint, particularly when there is pantrapezial involvement rather than just CMC joint involvement (Melvin, 1989).

Thumb CMC arthroplasty is a common postoperative diagnosis seen by hand therapists. Surgical techniques and timelines for therapy vary among physicians. Patients are often sent to therapy a few weeks after surgery for fabrication of a static forearm-based thumb spica splint with the IP free. The physician indicates appropriate guidelines for AROM according to the particular surgical procedures performed. Postoperative therapy goals are to promote pain-free stability and function. ADL modification and joint protection remain a priority.

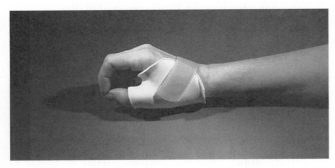

Figure 42-19 Hand-based thumb spica splint. Used to provide pain relief and promote functional pinch.

Rheumatoid Arthritis

Unlike osteoarthritis, rheumatoid arthritis (RA) is a systemic disease that primarily affects the synovium. Its debilitation and crippling can be severely disabling. Rheumatoid arthritis presents as inflammation of synovial membranes of joints and of tendon sheaths, with redness, swelling, pain, and heat in the areas of involvement (Melvin, 1989; Swanson, 1995a).

Digital involvement at the DIP is less common than at the PIP. If DIP involvement does occur, a mallet finger may result. Involvement at the PIP may result in swan-neck or boutonniere deformities. (See section on extensor tendons for clinical management of mallet and boutonniere deformities.) A swan-neck deformity presents as MP flexion, PIP hyperextension, and DIP flexion (Fig. 42-20). Fabricate a digital dorsal splint in slight PIP flexion to minimize deforming forces and enhance FDS function. At the level of the MP joints, deformity usually manifests as MP ulnar drift and palmar subluxation (Melvin, 1989). Thumb deformities include boutonniere (primary thumb MP involvement) and swan-neck (primary CMC involvement) deformities. The thumb may also demonstrate stiff, unstable, and painful joints at the levels of the IP, MP, or CMC (Swanson, 1995b). Rheumatoid arthritis often affects the wrist. This is significant because the wrist is anatomically critical to proper hand function. Wrist involvement is compounded by concomitant hand deformity. Synovitis at the wrist can lead to flexor or extensor tendon ruptures (Melvin, 1989).

In evaluating patients with rheumatoid arthritis, observe deformities and abnormal posture, any atrophy, and skin condition. Identify crepitus of joint or tendon, palpable nodules, tendon integrity, and joint stability. Ask about morning stiffness, fatigue, and pain. The appearance of the deformity (cosmesis) is also relevant (Philips, 1995).

The goals of upper extremity splinting for rheumatoid arthritis include reducing inflammation, supporting

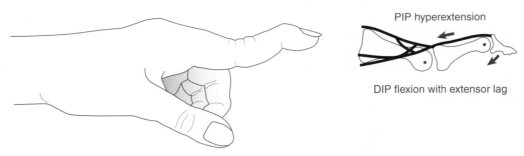

PIP hyperextension

DIP flexion with extensor lag

Figure 42-20 Swan-neck deformity. (Adapted with permission from American Society for Surgery of the Hand. [1990]. *The Hand: Examination and Diagnosis* (3rd ed.). New York: Churchill Livingstone.)

weak tissues, and minimizing deforming forces. Splinting also provides functional assistance. Splinting is used especially in the acute stage, when inflamed structures are at risk for further damage. Forearm-based resting splints may support the wrist and entire hand, the wrist and MPs, or only the wrist.

Determine splint design according to the pathomechanics of the disease. Involved MP joints are at risk for volar subluxation. Therefore, splint the wrist in neutral or slight extension, the MP joints in available extension, and the PIP joints in slight flexion (Philips, 1995). Radial deviation of the wrist encourages ulnar drift of the digits at the MP joints because of the zigzag deformity. A splint to correct MP ulnar drift often improves the biomechanics of hand use. Talk with the patient to identify individual preferences and needs in terms of ADL and joint protection. Adapt the straps and practice with patients to be sure they can open and close them. For some people who require bilateral splints, it may be easier to use one at a time on alternate nights (Philips, 1995).

Conclusion

Wilson (1998) states, "The hand is not merely a metaphor or an icon for humanness, but often the real-life focal point—the lever or the launching pad—of a successful and genuinely fulfilling life" (p. 14). Occupational therapy can be the launching pad for people with hand impairments to reestablish fulfilling lives.

Summary Review Questions

1. Why should painful treatment be avoided? What signs are indicative of overaggressive treatment?
2. Name the phases of tissue healing and approximate timelines.
3. Define joint versus musculotendinous tightness, intrinsic versus extrinsic tightness, and tightness of extrinsic extensors versus extrinsic flexors.
4. Describe the antideformity position of the wrist and hand and explain why it is used.
5. What function is lost with a low radial nerve injury? What kind of splinting is appropriate, and why?
6. What distribution of sensation is usually impaired with carpal tunnel syndrome? What musculature might be atrophied in an advanced case? What night splint position is best for carpal tunnel syndrome, and why?
7. Describe complex regional pain syndrome and discuss treatment priorities for this diagnosis.
8. What symptoms are associated with a trigger finger?
9. Name four self-care or home activities that are safe and therapeutic for a person in a short arm cast with a healing distal radius fracture.

Acknowledgments

Heartfelt thanks to John L. Evarts, BS, for the photography and his valuable ideas, contribution to content, and ongoing support; to Cecelia M. Skotak, OTR, CHT, for her detailed review and excellent suggestions; to Virgil Mathiowetz, PhD, OTR, for substantial help with the section on dexterity and hand function; and to Michelle Pressman, MS, OTR, and Kevin Renfree, MD, for their input.

Resources

Brochures

American Society for Surgery of the Hand · 303-771-9236. www.arthritis.org
> *Arthritis of the Basilar Joint of the Thumb*
> *Carpal Tunnel Syndrome*
> *Dupuytren's Disease*
> *Trigger Finger/Trigger Thumb*

Arthritis Foundation · 800-283-7800.
> *Osteoarthritis*
> *Carpal Tunnel Syndrome*
> *Using Your Joints Wisely.*

Consumer Guides and Books

American Occupational Therapy Association · 301-652-2682. http://www.aota.org
> Dellon, A. L. (1997) · *Somatosensory Testing and Rehabilitation.* Bethesda, MD: AOTA.
> Lee, K., & Marcus, S. (1990) · *Home Rehabilitation Exercises: Hand.* Rockville, MD: AOTA.
> Melvin, J. L. (1995) · *Rheumatoid Arthritis: Caring for Your Hands.* Bethesda, MD: AOTA.

Minnesota Hand Rehabilitation, Inc. · 612-646-4263.
> Reiner, M. (1991) · *The Illustrated Hand.* St. Paul: Minnesota Hand Rehabilitation.

CD ROM

Primal Pictures Ltd. · +44-171-494-4300
> McGroutier, D. A., & Colditz, J. (1998) · *Interactive Hand Therapy.* London, UK: Primal Pictures.

Video

American Occupational Therapy Association · 301-652-2682. http://www.aota.org
> Apfel, E. (1995) · *Carpal Tunnel Syndrome: Causes and Treatments.* Bethesda, MD: AOTA.
> Apfel, E. (1995) · *Trigger Finger: Surgical and Conservative Treatment Approaches.* Bethesda, MD: AOTA.

Tests

Physiopro · 805 rue Longpre, Sherbrooke, Quebec, Canada J1G 5B8. *TEMPA.*

References

Adams, L. S., Topoozian, E., & Greene, L. W. (1992). Range of motion. In J. S. Casanova (Ed.), *Clinical Assessment Recommendations* (2nd ed., pp. 55–70). Chicago: American Society of Hand Therapists.

American Guidance Service (1969). *The Minnesota Rate of Manipulation Tests: Examiner's Manual.* Circle Pines, Minnesota: Author.

Artzberger, S. (in press). Manual edema mobilization: Treatment for edema in the subacute hand. In E. J. Mackin, A. D. Callahan, A. L. Osterman, & T. M. Skirven (Eds.), *Rehabilitation of the Hand and Upper Extremity* (5th ed.). St. Louis: Mosby.

Artzberger, S. M. (1997). Edema control: New perspectives. *American Occupational Therapy Association Physical Disabilities Special Interest Section Quarterly, 20* (1), 1–3.

Aulicino, P. L. (1995). Clinical examination of the hand. In J. M. Hunter, E. J. Mackin, & A. D. Callahan (Eds.), *Rehabilitation of the Hand: Surgery and Therapy* (4th ed., pp. 53–75). St. Louis: Mosby.

Aulisa, L., Tamburrelli, F., Padua, R., Romanini, E., Lo Monaco, M., & Padua, L. (1998). Carpal tunnel syndrome: Indication for surgical treatment based on electrophysiologic study. *Journal of Hand Surgery, 23A* (4), 687–691.

Baldwin, J. E., Weber, L. J., & Simon, C. L. (1992). Wound/scar assessment. In J. S. Casanova (Ed.), *Clinical Assessment Recommendations* (2nd ed., pp. 21–28). Chicago: American Society of Hand Therapists.

Baum, T. M., & Busuito, M. J. (1998). Use of a glycerin-based gel sheeting in scar management. *Advances in Wound Care, 11*, 40–43.

Benson, L. S., & Bailie, D. S. (1996). Proximal interphalangeal joint injuries of the hand. *American Journal of Orthopedics, 25* (8), 527–530.

Blackmore, S. M., & Hotchkiss, R. N. (1995). Therapist's management of ulnar neuropathy at the elbow. In J. M. Hunter, E. J. Mackin, & A. D. Callahan (Eds.), *Rehabilitation of the Hand: Surgery and Therapy* (4th ed., pp. 665–677). St. Louis: Mosby.

Bozentka, D. J. (1998). Cubital tunnel syndrome pathophysiology. *Clinical Orthopaedics and Related Research, 351*, 90–99.

Brand, P. W. (1995). The forces of dynamic splinting: Ten questions before applying a dynamic splint to the hand. In J. M. Hunter, E. J. Mackin, & A. D. Callahan (Eds.), *Rehabilitation of the Hand: Surgery and Therapy* (4th ed., pp. 1581–1587). St. Louis: Mosby.

Breger-Lee, D., Bell-Krotoski, J., & Brandsma, J. W. (1990). Torque range of motion in the hand clinic. *Journal of Hand Therapy, 3* (1), 7–13.

Bryan, B. K., & Kohnke, E. N. (1997). Therapy after skeletal fixation in the hand and wrist. *Hand Clinics, 13* (4), 761–776.

Brzezienski, M. A., & Schneider, L. H. (1995). Extensor tendon injuries at the distal interphalangeal joint. *Hand Clinics, 11* (3), 373–386.

Bulthaup, S., Cipriani, D. J., & Thomas, J. J. (1999). An electromyography study of wrist extension orthoses and upper-extremity function. *American Journal of Occupational Therapy, 53* (5), 434–440.

Burkhalter, W. E. (1995). Mutilating injuries of the hand. In J. M. Hunter, E. J. Mackin, & A. D. Callahan (Eds.), *Rehabilitation of the Hand: Surgery and Therapy* (4th ed., pp. 1037–1056). St. Louis: Mosby.

Byl, N. N., Kohlhase, W., & Engel, G. (1999). Functional limitation immediately after cast immobilization and closed reduction of distal radius fractures: Preliminary report. *Journal of Hand Therapy, 12* (3), 201–211.

Byl, N. N., & Melnick, M. (1997). The neural consequences of repetition: Clinical implications of a learning hypothesis. *Journal of Hand Therapy, 10* (2), 160–174.

Callahan, A. D. (1995). Sensibility assessment: Prerequisites and techniques for nerve lesions in continuity and nerve lacerations. In J. M. Hunter, E. J. Mackin, & A. D. Callahan (Eds.), *Rehabilitation of the Hand: Surgery and Therapy* (4th ed., pp. 129–152). St. Louis: Mosby.

Cannon, N. (1993). Post flexor tendon repair motion protocol. *Indiana Hand Center Newsletter, 1*, 13.

Carlson, L. K., & Watson, H. K. (1988). Treatment of reflex sympathetic dystrophy using the stress-loading program. *Journal of Hand Therapy, 1* (4), 149–154.

Chin, K. R., Lonner, J. H., Jupiter, B. S., & Jupiter, J. B. (1999). The surgeon as a hand patient: The clinical and psychological impact of hand and wrist fractures. *Journal of Hand Surgery, 24A* (1), 59–63.

Colditz, J. C. (1995a). Splinting the hand with a peripheral nerve injury. In J. M. Hunter, E. J. Mackin, & A. D. Callahan (Eds.), *Rehabilitation of the Hand: Surgery and Therapy* (4th ed., pp. 679–692). St. Louis: Mosby.

Colditz, J. C. (1995b). Therapist's management of the stiff hand. In J. M. Hunter, E. J. Mackin, & A. D. Callahan (Eds.), *Rehabilitation of the Hand: Surgery and Therapy* (4th ed., pp. 1141–1159). St. Louis: Mosby.

Collins, D. C. (1993). Management and rehabilitation of distal radius fractures. *Orthopedic Clinics of North America, 24* (2), 365–378.

Concannon, M. J., Gainor, B., Petroski, G. F., & Puckett, C. L. (1997). The predictive value of electrodiagnostic studies in carpal tunnel syndrome. *Plastic and Reconstructive Surgery, 100* (6), 1452–1458.

Coons, M. S., & Green, S. M. (1995). Boutonniere deformity. *Hand Clinics, 11* (3), 387–402.

Cooper, C., & Evarts, J. L. (1998). Beyond the routine: Placing therapeutic occupation at the center of upper-extremity rehabilitation. *OT Practice, 3* (6), 18–22.

Cooper, C., Liskin, J., & Moorhead, J. F. (1999). Dyscoordinate contraction: Impaired quality of movement in patients with hand disorders. *OT Practice, 4* (3), 40–45.

Cromwell, F. S. (1976). *Occupational Therapist's Manual for Basic Skill Assessment: Primary Prevocational Evaluation.* Altadena, CA: Fair Oaks.

Crosby, C. A., & Wehbe, M. A. (1996). Early motion after extensor tendon surgery. *Hand Clinics, 12* (1), 57–64.

Culp, R. W., & Taras, J. S. (1995). Primary care of flexor tendon injuries. In J. M. Hunter, E. J. Mackin, & A. D. Callahan (Eds.), *Rehabilitation of the Hand: Surgery and Therapy* (4th ed., pp. 417–431). St. Louis: Mosby.

Cyriax, J. (1982). *Textbook of Orthopaedic Medicine.* (8th ed., Vol. 1) London: Bailliere Tindall.

Dawson, W. J. (1994). The spectrum of sports-related interphalangeal joint injuries. *Hand Clinics, 10* (2), 315–326.

de Herder, E. F. (1992). Vascular assessment. In J. S. Casanova (Ed.), *Clinical Assessment Recommendations* (2nd ed., pp. 29–39). Chicago: American Society of Hand Therapists.

Desrosiers, J., Hebert, R., Bravo, G., & Dutil, E. (1995). Upper extremity performance test for the elderly (TEMPA): Normative data and correlates with sensorimotor parameters. *Archives of Physical Medicine and Rehabilitation, 76*, 1125–1129.

Desrosiers, J., Hebert, R., Dutil, E., & Bravo, G. (1993). Development and reliability of an upper extremity function test for the elderly: The TEMPA. *Canadian Journal of Occupational Therapy, 60* (1), 9–16.

Desrosiers, J., Hebert, R., Dutil, E., Bravo, G., & Mercier, L. (1994). Validity of the TEMPA: A measurement instrument for upper extremity performance. *Occupational Therapy Journal of Research, 14* (4), 267–281.

Donaldson, C. C., Nelson, D. V., Skubick, D. L., & Clasby, R. G. (1998). Potential contributions of neck muscle dysfunctions to initiation and maintenance of carpal tunnel syndrome. *Applied Psychophysiology and Biofeedback, 23* (1), 59–72.

Evans, R. B. (1995). An update on extensor tendon management. In J. M. Hunter, E. J. Mackin, & A. D. Callahan (Eds.), *Rehabilitation of the Hand: Surgery and Therapy* (4th ed., pp. 565–606). St. Louis: Mosby.

Evans, R. B., Hunter, J. M., & Burkhalter, W. E. (1988). Conservative management of the trigger finger: A new approach. *Journal of Hand Therapy, 1* (2), 59–68.

Evans, R. B., & McAuliffe, J. A. (1995). Wound classification and management. In J. M. Hunter, E. J. Mackin, & A. D. Callahan (Eds.), *Rehabilitation of the Hand: Surgery and Therapy* (4th ed., pp. 217–235). St. Louis: Mosby.

Fealy, M. J., & Ladd, A. L. (1996). Reflex sympathetic dystrophy: Early diagnosis and active treatment. *Journal of Musculoskeletal Medicine, 13* (3), 29–36.

Fess, E. E. (1990). Hands, changes, quality, and survival. *Journal of Hand Therapy, 3* (1), 1–6.

Fess, E. E. (1992). Grip strength. In J. S. Casanova (Ed.), *Clinical Assessment Recommendations* (2nd ed., pp. 41–45). Chicago: American Society of Hand Therapists.

Fess, E. E. (1993). Hand rehabilitation. In H. L. Hopkins & H. D. Smith (Eds.), *Willard and Spackman's Occupational Therapy* (8th ed., pp. 674–690). Philadelphia: Lippincott.

Fess, E. E. (1995a). Documentation: Essential elements of an upper extremity assessment battery. In J. M. Hunter, E. J. Mackin, & A. D. Callahan (Eds.), *Rehabilitation of the Hand: Surgery and Therapy* (4th ed., pp. 185–214). St. Louis: Mosby.

Fess, E. E. (1995b). Principles and methods of splinting for mobilization of joints. In J. M. Hunter, E. J. Mackin, & A. D. Callahan (Eds.), *Rehabilitation of the Hand: Surgery and Therapy* (4th ed., pp. 1589–1608). St. Louis: Mosby.

Fess, E. E., & McCollum, M. (1998). The influence of splinting on healing tissues. *Journal of Hand Therapy, 11* (2), 157–161.

Frykman, G. K., & Kropp, W. E. (1995). Fractures and traumatic conditions of the wrist. In J. M. Hunter, E. J. Mackin, & A. D. Callahan (Eds.), *Rehabilitation of the Hand: Surgery and Therapy* (4th ed., pp. 315–336). St. Louis: Mosby.

Furth, H. J., Holm, M. B., & James, A. (1994). Reinjury prevention follow-through for clients with cumulative trauma disorders. *American Journal of Occupational Therapy, 48* (10), 890–898.

Grunert, B. K., Matloub, H. S., Sanger, J. R., Yousif, N. J., & Hettermann, S. (1991). Effects of litigation on maintenance of psychological symptoms after severe hand injury. *Journal of Hand Surgery, 16A,* 1031–1034.

Hardy, M. A., & Hardy, S. G. P. (1997). Reflex sympathetic dystrophy: The clinician's perspective. *Journal of Hand Therapy, 10* (2), 137–150.

Hunter, J. M. (1986). Philosophy of hand rehabilitation. *Hand Clinics, 2* (1), 5–24.

Hunter, J. M., Davlin, L. B., & Fedus, L. M. (1995). Major neuropathies of the upper extremity: The median nerve. In J. M. Hunter, E. J. Mackin, & A. D. Callahan (Eds.), *Rehabilitation of the Hand: Surgery and Therapy* (4th ed., pp. 905–916). St. Louis: Mosby.

Hunter, J. M., Taras, J. S., Mackin, E. J., Maser, S. A., & Culp, R. W. (1995). Staged flexor tendon reconstruction using passive and active tendon implants. In J. M. Hunter, E. J. Mackin, & A. D. Callahan (Eds.), *Rehabilitation of the Hand: Surgery and Therapy* (4th ed., pp. 477–514). St. Louis: Mosby.

Idler, R. S. (1997). Helping the patient who has wrist or hand tenosynovitis. *Journal of Musculoskeletal Medicine, 14* (1), 21–35.

Jarus, T., & Poremba, R. (1993). Hand function evaluation: A factor analysis study. *American Journal of Occupational Therapy, 47* (5), 439–443.

Jebsen, R. H., Taylor, N., Trieschmann, R. B., Trotter, M. J., & Howard, L. A. (1969). An objective and standardized test of hand function. *Archives of Physical Medicine and Rehabilitation, 50,* 311–319.

Jensen, C., & Rayan, G. (1996). Buddy strapping of mismatched fingers: The offset buddy strap. *Journal of Hand Surgery, 21* (2), 317–318.

Johnson, S. L. (1993). Therapy of the occupationally injured hand and upper extremity. *Hand Clinics, 9* (2), 2889–2898.

Keir, P. J., Bach, J. M., & Rempel, D. M. (1998). Fingertip loading and carpal tunnel pressure: Differences between a pinching and a pressing task. *Journal of Orthopedic Research, 16* (1), 112–115.

Keller, K., Corbett, J., & Nichols, D. (1998). Repetitive strain injury in computer keyboard users: Pathomechanics and treatment principles in individual and group intervention. *Journal of Hand Therapy, 11* (1), 9–26.

Khoo, D., Carmichael, S. W., & Spinner, R. J. (1996). Ulnar nerve anatomy and compression. *Orthopedic Clinics of North America, 27* (2), 317–337.

Kibler, W. B., Chandler, T. J., & Pace, B. K. (1992). Principles of rehabilitation after chronic tendon injuries. *Clinics in Sports Medicine, 11* (3), 661–671.

Kirkpatrick, W. H., & Lisser, S. (1995). Soft-tissue conditions: Trigger fingers and de Quervain's disease. In J. M. Hunter, E. J. Mackin, & A. D. Callahan (Eds.), *Rehabilitation of the Hand: Surgery and Therapy* (4th ed., pp. 1007–1016). St. Louis: Mosby.

Lairmore, J. R., & Engber, W. D. (1998). Serious, often subtle, finger injuries: Avoiding diagnosis and treatment pitfalls. *Physician and Sportsmedicine, 26* (6), 57–69.

Lam, N., & Thurston, A. (1998). Association of obesity, gender, age and occupation with carpal tunnel syndrome. *Australian and New Zealand Journal of Surgery, 68* (3), 190–193.

Lankford, L. L. (1995). Reflex sympathetic dystrophy. In J. M. Hunter, E. J. Mackin, & A. D. Callahan (Eds.), *Rehabilitation of the Hand: Surgery and Therapy* (4th ed., pp. 779–815). St. Louis: Mosby.

Laseter, G. F., & Carter, P. R. (1996). Management of distal radius fractures. *Journal of Hand Therapy, 9* (2), 114–128.

Leibovic, S. J. (1999). Bone and joint injury in the hand: Surgeon's perspective. *Journal of Hand Therapy, 12* (2), 111–120.

Lynch, K. B., & Bridle, M. J. (1989). Validity of the Jebsen-Taylor hand function test in predicting activities of daily living. *Occupational Therapy Journal of Research, 9* (5), 316–318.

Lynch, M. E. (1992). Psychological aspects of reflex sympathetic dystrophy: A review of the adult and paediatric literature. *Pain, 49,* 337–347.

Mathiowetz, V. (1993). Role of physical performance component evaluations in occupational therapy functional assessment. *American Journal of Occupational Therapy, 47* (3), 225–230.

Mathiowetz, V., & Bass Haugen, J. B. (1995). Evaluation of motor behavior: Traditional and contemporary views. In C. A. Trombly (Ed.), *Occupational Therapy for Physical Dysfunction* (4th ed., pp. 157–185). Baltimore: Williams & Wilkins.

Mathiowetz, V., Rogers, S. L., Dowe-Keval, M., Donahoe, L., & Rennells, C. (1986). The *Purdue Pegboard:* Norms for 14- to 19-year-olds. *American Journal of Occupational Therapy, 40* (3), 174–179.

Mathiowetz, V., Volland, G., Kashman, N., & Weber, K. (1985). Adult norms for the *Box and Block Test* of manual dexterity. *American Journal of Occupational Therapy, 39* (6), 386–391.

Mathiowetz, V., Weber, K., Kashman, N., & Volland, G. (1985). Adult norms for the Nine Hole Peg Test of finger dexterity. *Occupational Therapy Journal of Research, 5* (1), 24–38.

Maurer, G. L., & Jezek, S. M. (1992). Pain assessment. In J. S. Casanova

(Ed.), *Clinical Assessment Recommendations* (2nd ed., pp. 95–108). Chicago: American Society of Hand Therapists.

Melvin, J. L. (1989). *Rheumatic Disease in the Adult and Child: Occupational Therapy and Rehabilitation* (3rd ed.) Philadelphia: Davis.

Merritt, W. H. (1998). Written on behalf of the stiff finger. *Journal of Hand Therapy, 11* (2), 74–79.

Meyer, F. N., & Wilson, R. L. (1995). Management of nonarticular fractures of the hand. In J. M. Hunter, E. J. Mackin, & A. D. Callahan (Eds.), *Rehabilitation of the Hand: Surgery and Therapy* (4th ed., pp. 377–394). St. Louis: Mosby.

Miles, C. A., Burjanadze, T. V., & Bailey, A. J. (1995). The kinetics of the thermal denaturation of collagen in unrestrained rat tail tendon determined by differential scanning calorimetry. *Journal of Molecular Biology, 245*, 437–446.

Moberg, E. (1991). The unsolved problem: How to test the functional value of hand sensibility. *Journal of Hand Therapy, 4* (3), 105–110.

Mooney, V. (1998). Overuse syndromes of the upper extremity: Rational and effective treatment. *Journal of Musculoskeletal Medicine, 15* (8), 11–18.

Moskowitz, L. (1996). Psychological management of postsurgical pain and patient adherence. *Hand Clinics, 12* (1), 129–137.

Nelson, D. L., & Peterson, C. (1989). Enhancing therapeutic exercise through purposeful activity: A theoretical analysis. *Topics in Geriatric Rehabilitation, 4* (4), 12–22.

Netscher, D., Steadman, A. K., Thornby, J., & Cohen, B. J. (1998). Temporal changes in grip and pinch strength after open carpal tunnel release and the effect of ligament reconstruction. *Journal of Hand Surgery, 23A* (1), 48–54.

Osterman, A. L., & Davis, C. A. (1996). Subcutaneous transposition of the ulnar nerve for treatment of cubital tunnel syndrome. *Hand Clinics, 12* (2), 421–433.

Pascarelli, E. F., & Kella, J. J. (1993). Soft-tissue injuries related to use of the computer keyboard. *Journal of Occupational Medicine, 35* (5), 522–532.

Philips, C. A. (1995). Therapist's management of patients with rheumatoid arthritis. In J. M. Hunter, E. J. Mackin, & A. D. Callahan (Eds.), *Rehabilitation of the Hand: Surgery and Therapy* (4th ed., pp. 1345–1350). St. Louis: Mosby.

Pitner, M. A. (1990). Pathophysiology of overuse injuries in the hand and wrist. *Hand Clinics, 6* (3), 355–364.

Posner, M. A. (1998). Compressive ulnar neuropathies at the elbow: 2. Treatment. *Journal of the American Academy of Orthopedic Surgeons, 6* (5), 289–297.

Reiss, B. (1995). Therapist's management of distal radial fractures. In J. M. Hunter, E. J. Mackin, & A. D. Callahan (Eds.), *Rehabilitation of the Hand: Surgery and Therapy* (4th ed., pp. 337–351). St. Louis: Mosby.

Rice, M. S., Leonard, C., & Carter, M. (1998). Grip strengths and required forces in accessing everyday containers in a normal population. *American Journal of Occupational Therapy, 52* (8), 621–626.

Rider, B., & Linden, C. (1988). Comparison of standardized and non-standardized administration of the *Jebsen Hand Function Test*. *Journal of Hand Therapy, 1* (3), 121–123.

Rosenthal, E. A. (1995). The extensor tendons: Anatomy and management. In J. M. Hunter, E. J. Mackin, & A. D. Callahan (Eds.), *Rehabilitation of the Hand: Surgery and Therapy* (4th ed., pp. 519–564). St. Louis: Mosby.

Rozmaryn, L. M., Dovelle, S., Rothman, E. R., Gorman, K., Olvey, K. M., & Bartko, J. J. (1998). Nerve and tendon gliding exercises and the conservative management of carpal tunnel syndrome. *Journal of Hand Therapy, 11* (3), 171–179.

Rudman, D., & Hannah, S. (1998). An instrument evaluation framework: Description and application to assessments of hand function. *Journal of Hand Therapy, 11*, 266–277.

Russell, C. R. (1999). Bone and joint injury in the hand: Therapist's commentary. *Journal of Hand Therapy, 12* (2), 121–122.

Sailer, S. M. (1996). The role of splinting and rehabilitation in the treatment of carpal and cubital tunnel syndromes. *Hand Clinics, 12* (2), 223–241.

Schneider, L. H., & Berger-Feldscher, S. (1995). Tenolysis: Dynamic approach to surgery and therapy. In J. M. Hunter, E. J. Mackin, & A. D. Callahan (Eds.), *Rehabilitation of the Hand: Surgery and Therapy* (4th ed., pp. 463–475). St. Louis: Mosby.

Servi, J. T. (1997). Wrist pain from overuse. *Physician and Sportsmedicine, 25*, 41–44.

Shultis-Kiernan, L. (1992). Manual muscle testing. In J. S. Casanova (Ed.), *Clinical Assessment Recommendations* (2nd ed., pp. 47–53). Chicago: American Society of Hand Therapists.

Silva, M. J., Hollstien, S. B., Fayazi, A. H., Adler, P., Gelberman, R. H., & Boyer, M. I. (1998). The effects of multiple-strand suture techniques on the tensile properties of repair of the flexor digitorum profundus tendon to bone. *Journal of Bone and Joint Surgery, 80A* (10), 1507–1514.

Skirven, T., & Trope, J. (1994). Complications of immobilization. *Hand Clinics, 10* (1), 53–61.

Smith, G. A., Nelson, R. C., Sadoff, S. J., & Sadoff, A. M. (1989). Assessing sincerity of effort in maximal grip strength tests. *Archives of Physical Medicine and Rehabilitation, 68*, 73–80.

Smith, K. L. (1995a). Wound care for the hand patient. In J. M. Hunter, E. J. Mackin, & A. D. Callahan (Eds.), *Rehabilitation of the Hand: Surgery and Therapy* (4th ed., pp. 237–250). St. Louis: Mosby.

Smith, K. L. (1995b). Nerve response to injury and repair. In J.M. Hunter, E. J. Mackin, & A. D. Callahan (Eds.), *Rehabilitation of the Hand: Surgery and Therapy* (4 ed., pp. 609–626). St. Louis: Mosby.

Spaulding, S. J., McPherson, J. J., Strachota, E., Kuphal, M., & Ramponi, M. (1988). *Jebsen Hand Function Test*: Performance of the uninvolved hand in hemiplegia and of right-handed, right and left hemiplegic persons. *Archives of Physical Medicine and Rehabilitation, 69*, 419–422.

Spinner, M. (1995). Nerve lesions in continuity. In J. M. Hunter, E. J. Mackin, & A. D. Callahan (Eds.), *Rehabilitation of the Hand: Surgery and Therapy* (4 ed., pp. 627–634). St. Louis: Mosby.

Stanton-Hicks, M., Janig, W., Hassenbusch, S., Haddox, J. D., Boas, R., & Wilson, P. (1995). Reflex sympathetic dystrophy: Changing concepts and taxonomy. *Pain, 63*, 127–133.

Stern, E. B. (1992). Stability of the Jebsen-Taylor Hand Function Test across three test sessions. *American Journal of Occupational Therapy, 46* (7), 647–649.

Stewart, K. M. (1995). Therapist's management of the complex injury. In J. M. Hunter, E. J. Mackin, & A. D. Callahan (Eds.), *Rehabilitation of the Hand: Surgery and Therapy* (4th ed., pp. 1057–1073). St. Louis: Mosby.

Stewart, K. M., & van Strien, G. (1995). Postoperative management of flexor tendon injuries. In J. M. Hunter, E. J. Mackin, & A. D. Callahan (Eds.), *Rehabilitation of the Hand: Surgery and Therapy* (4th ed., pp. 433–462). St. Louis: Mosby.

Stolp-Smith, K. A., Pascoe, M. K., & Ogburn, P. L. (1998). Carpal tunnel syndrome in pregnancy: Frequency, severity, and prognosis. *Archives of Physical Medicine and Rehabilitation, 79* (10), 1285–1287.

Swanson, A. B. (1995a). Pathomechanics of deformities in hand and wrist. In J. M. Hunter, E. J. Mackin, & A. D. Callahan (Eds.), *Rehabilitation of the Hand: Surgery and Therapy* (4th ed., pp. 1315–1327). St. Louis: Mosby.

Swanson, A. B. (1995b). Pathogenesis of arthritic lesions. In J. M. Hunter, E. J. Mackin, & A. D. Callahan (Eds.), *Rehabilitation of the Hand: Surgery and Therapy* (4th ed., pp. 1307–1313). St. Louis: Mosby.

Swigart, C. R., Eaton, R. G., Glickel, S. Z., & Johnson, C. (1999). Splinting in the treatment of arthritis of the first carpometacarpal joint. *Journal of Hand Surgery, 24A* (1), 86–91.

Szabo, R. M. (1998). Acute carpal tunnel syndrome. *Hand Clinics, 14* (3), 419–429.

Terrono, A. L., & Millender, L. H. (1996). Management of work-related upper-extremity nerve entrapments. *Orthopedic Clinics of North America, 27* (4), 783–793.

Tetro, A. M., & Pichora, D. R. (1996). Cubital tunnel syndrome and the painful upper extremity. *Hand Clinics, 12* (4), 665–677.

Thomes, L. J., & Thomes, B. J. (1995). Early mobilization method for surgically repaired zone III extensor tendons. *Journal of Hand Therapy, 8* (3), 195–198.

Tiffin, J. (1968). *Purdue Pegboard: Examiner Manual.* Chicago: Science Research Associates.

Travell, J. G., & Simons, D. (1983). *Myofascial Pain and Dysfunction: The Trigger Point Manual.* Baltimore: Williams & Wilkins.

Trombly, C. A. (1995). Occupation: Purposefulness and meaningfulness as therapeutic mechanisms. 1995 Eleanor Clarke Slagle Lecture. *American Journal of Occupational Therapy, 49* (10), 960–972.

Tubiana, R. (1983). Early mobilization of fractures of the metacarpals and phalanges. *Annals de Chirurgie de la Main, 2* (4), 293–297.

Tubiana, R., Thomine, J.-M., & Mackin, E. J. (1996). *Examination of the Hand and Wrist* (2 ed.). London: Martin Dunitz.

Vahey, J. W., Wegner, D. A., & Hastings, H. (1998). Effect of proximal phalangeal fracture deformity on extensor tendon function. *Journal of Hand Surgery, 23A* (4), 673–681.

Verdon, M. E. (1996). Overuse syndromes of the hand and wrist. *Primary Care, 23* (2), 305–319.

Walsh, M. T. (1995). Therapist's management of reflex sympathetic dystrophy. In J. M. Hunter, E. J. Mackin, & A. D. Callahan (Eds.), *Rehabilitation of the Hand: Surgery and Therapy* (4th ed., pp. 817–833). St. Louis: Mosby.

Wang, A. W., & Gupta, A. (1996). Early motion after flexor tendon surgery. *Hand Clinics, 12* (1), 43–55.

Wilson, F. R. (1998). *The Hand: How Its Use Shapes the Brain, Language, and Human Culture.* New York: Pantheon.

Wilson, R. L., & Hazen, J. (1995). Management of joint injuries and intra-articular fractures of the hand. In J. M. Hunter, E. J. Mackin, & A. D. Callahan (Eds.), *Rehabilitation of the Hand: Surgery and Therapy* (4 ed., pp. 377–394). St. Louis: Mosby.

Winters, S. C., Gelberman, R. H., Woo, S. L. Y., Chan, S. S., Grewal, R., & Seiler, J. G. (1998). The effects of multiple-strand suture methods on the strength and excursion of repaired intrasynovial flexor tendons: A biomechanical study in dogs. *Journal of Hand Surgery, 23A* (1), 97–104.

Wong, G. Y., & Wilson, P. R. (1997). Classification of complex regional pain syndromes: New concepts. *Hand Clinics, 13* (3), 319–325.

Wuori, J., Overend, T. J., Kramer, J. F., & MacDermid, J. (1998). Strength and pain measures associated with lateral epicondylitis bracing. *Archives of Physical Medicine and Rehabilitation, 79,* 832–837.

43

Spinal Cord Injury

Michal S. Atkins

LEARNING OBJECTIVES

After studying this chapter, the reader will be able to do the following:

1. Define key terms and concepts central to spinal cord injury and its care.
2. Value the physical, psychosocial, and occupational challenges associated with spinal cord injury.
3. Describe the tests and procedures appropriate for occupational therapy assessment.
4. List the roles and priorities of the occupational therapist in each of the treatment phases.
5. Recognize functional expectations of patients with various levels of injury.

A spinal cord injury (SCI) is a devastating event that disrupts every facet of life. Diminished physical capacities, inability to get around and carry out daily routines, and feelings of confusion and despair are coupled with loss of gainful employment and questions about the ability to return home. The occupational therapist may share this burden. With such devastating losses, where does the therapist begin? How do we help patients rebuild a sense of efficacy and self-esteem? How do we set priorities for our treatment interventions?

This chapter provides beginning answers to these questions. It outlines occupational therapy evaluations, goal setting, and treatments used with persons with SCI and introduces epidemiological data, definitions, and classifications of injuries. Next, it discusses the course after injury, followed by occupational therapy evaluations and interventions. Case studies of people who were recently injured are presented. Research data, resources, and suggested readings are listed to assist the therapist in exploring SCI beyond the material outlined in this chapter.

GLOSSARY

Dermatome—"The area of the skin innervated by the sensory axons within each segmental nerve (root)" (ASIA, 2000, pg. 5).

Complete injury—"Absence of sensory and motor function in the lowest sacral segment" (ASIA, 2000 pg. 7).

Incomplete injury—"Partial preservation of sensory and/or motor function below the neurological level and including the lowest sacral segment" (ASIA, 2000 pg. 7).

Long opponens splint—Static resting, wrist-hand orthosis. The hand and wrist are maintained in functional position; the thumb is positioned in abduction; and the fingers are free to flex with gravity.

Myotome—"The collection of muscle fibers innervated by the motor axons within each segmental nerve (root)" (ASIA, 2000, pg. 6).

Paraplegia—Loss or impairment in motor and/or sensory function in the thoracic, lumbar, or sacral segments of the cord resulting in impairment in the trunk, legs, and pelvic organs and sparing of the arms (ASIA, 2000).

Tenodesis grasp—Passive opening of the fingers when the wrist is flexed and closing of the fingers when the wrist is extended (Wilson et al., 1984).

Tetraplegia—Loss or impairment in motor and/or sensory function in the cervical segments of the spinal cord resulting in functional impairment in the arms, trunk, legs, and pelvic organs (ASIA, 2000).

Epidemiology

Spinal cord injury is relatively rare, afflicting approximately 10,000 people a year in the United States. The numbers of people with SCI alive today in the United States is estimated to be in the range of 183,000 to 203,000 (Stover et al., 1995). Most SCI occur to young males. A ratio of four injured males per female persists over the past decades (National Spinal Cord Injury Statistical Center, 2000). The average age of injury is 31.8 years, with 50% of those injured aged 16 to 30 (National Spinal Cord Injury Statistical Center).

The National Spinal Cord Injury Statistical Center (NSCISC), a federally funded organization established in 1973, collects SCI epidemiological data in the United States. The causes of SCI as tracked by NSCISC from 1973 to 1997 are as follows: approximately 43%, motor vehicle accidents; 22%, falls or hit by object; 19%, violence; and 11%, sports injuries. Other causes, such as nontraumatic SCI, account for the remaining 5% (Becker & DeLisa, 1999). Nontraumatic SCI is caused by spinal stenosis, tumors, ischemia, infection, and myelitis (McKinley et al., 1999). In large metropolitan areas in the United States, violence and more specifically, gunshot wounds are on the rise and are the leading cause of SCIs (Nobunaga et al., 1999). In other countries violence accounts for only a small fraction of injuries.

In the United States, ethnic distribution of injured persons includes 59.1% Whites, 27.6% African Americans, 7.7% Hispanics, 2.1% Asians, 0.4% Native American, 0.5% unknown and 2.5% unclassified (NSCISC, 2000). This distribution shows greater representation of minority groups than the ethnic distribution of the U. S. population. NSCISC also notes a trend in the rise of injuries to minority groups (Nobunaga et al., 1999).

Most persons with SCI (59.3%) have completed high school, and 59.6% were employed at onset. Generally, the level of education of injured individuals is somewhat lower and the unemployment rate higher than in the general population. Considering the young age of onset, it is not surprising that most persons are single when the injury occurred (Stover et al., 1995).

The clinical implications of the SCI epidemiological data have great relevance to the work of occupational therapists. Therapists must appreciate that the patients' ethnic, gender, socioeconomic, and educational backgrounds may differ from their own (see Chapter 9). Additionally, sexual, bowel, and bladder management issues must be addressed with great sensitivity, and therapists must become comfortable with their role in these matters (Trieschmann, 1988).

Course After Spinal Cord Injury

Spinal cord injury causes a disruption in the motor and sensory pathways at the site of the lesion (Fig. 43-1). Because the nerve roots are segmental, a thorough evaluation of motor and sensory function can identify the level of lesion (Fig. 43-2). For example, if the spinal cord is completely severed at the level of the sixth cervical nerve root, motor and sensory information below that level no longer can travel to and from the brain. This results in paralysis of muscular activity and absence of sensation below the level of injury (Hollar, 1995).

Immediately after the injury there is a period of spinal shock characterized by areflexia at and below the level of injury. Spinal shock may last hours to days or weeks. As soon as spinal shock subsides, reflexes below the level of injury return and become hyperactive. At the level of injury, areflexia may remain as the reflex arc is interrupted.

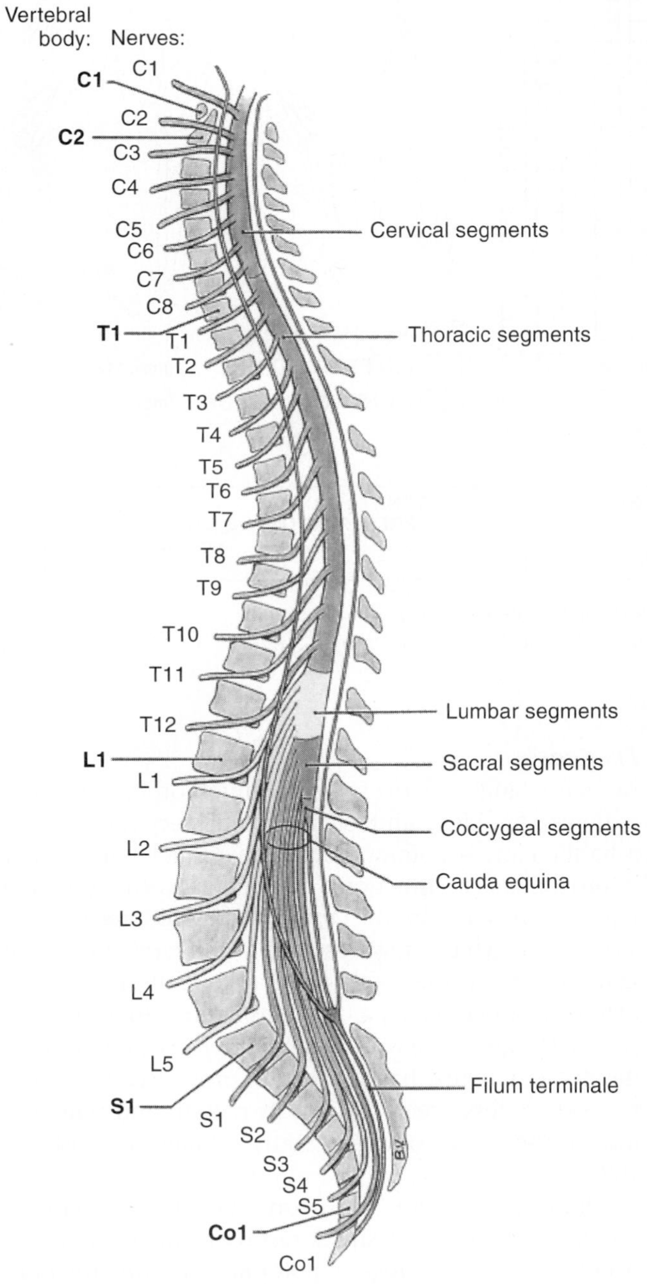

Neurological Classification of SCI

To understand the typical course of recovery from SCI, occupational therapists must be familiar with commonly used terms that describe SCI impairment and know how levels of impairment relate to prognosis.

Definitions

Tetraplegia results in functional impairment in the arms, trunk, legs, and pelvic organs. The term *tetraplegia*, which has replaced *quadriplegia*, is defined as an impairment in motor and/or sensory function in the cervical segments of the spinal cord (ASIA, 2000). It is caused by damage to neural elements within the vertebral canal and the term is not used to describe injuries to peripheral nerves. **Paraplegia** refers to motor and sensory impairment at the thoracic, lumbar, or sacral segments of the cord. Likewise, it refers only to damage to the neural elements inside the vertebral canal. Paraplegia results in sparing of arm function and, depending on the level of the lesion, impairment in the trunk, legs, and pelvic organs. The terms paraparesis and quadriparesis, which were used in the past to describe incomplete injuries, should no longer be used (ASIA, 2000).

The neurological level is diagnosed by the physician according to the motor and sensory level. The motor level is determined by testing 10 key muscles on each side of the body and the sensory level, by testing sensation of 28 key points on each side of the body (Fig. 43-2). The neurological level is the lowest level at which key muscles grade 3 out of 5 or above on manual muscle testing (MMT) and sensation is intact for this level's **dermatome**. Also, the level above must have normal strength and sensation. For example, a person is diagnosed as having C6 tetraplegia when radial wrist extensors test 3 out of 5 and sensation is intact for the C6 dermatome. Furthermore, all motor and sensory status above the C6 level is intact. Skeletal level refers to the level of greatest vertebral damage (ASIA, 2000).

A functional level, a term used by occupational and physical therapists, refers to the lowest segment at which strength of key muscles is graded 3+ of 5 or above on MMT and pain sensation is intact. Key muscles are those that significantly change functional outcomes (Occupational Therapy Department [1990]. Functional goals for patients with quadriplegia, Unpublished form. Rancho Los Amigos National Rehabilitation Center, Downey, CA). The ASIA muscle list for the physician's motor examination (Fig. 43-2) includes only some of the

Figure 43-1 Spinal cord and spinal nerves in relation to the vertebrae. (Reprinted with permission from Agur A. M. R. [1991]. Grant's Atlas of Anatomy (9th ed.). Baltimore: Williams & Wilkins.)

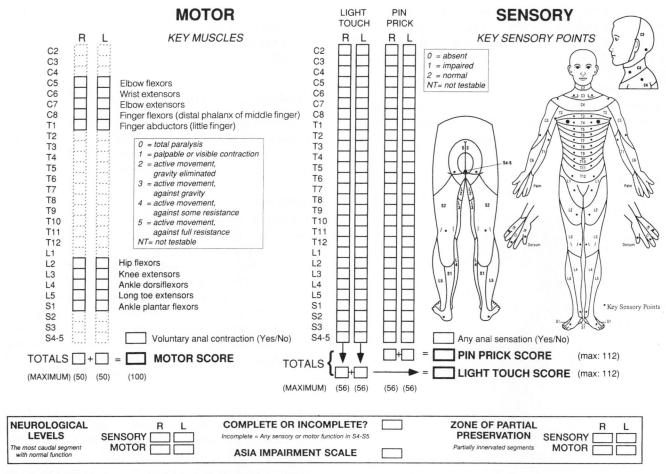

Figure 43-2 Standard Neurological Classification of SCI. (Courtesy of the American Spinal Injury Association [ASIA, 2000]. This form may be copied freely but should not be altered without permission from the American Spinal Injury Association.)

muscles considered important to determine a functional level.

Two other terms commonly used with spinal cord–injured patients are **complete** and **incomplete** injuries (Box 43-1). Complete injury consists of absence of sensory or motor function in the lowest sacral segments (S4-S5) (ASIA, 2000). The term *incomplete injury* should be used only when there is partial preservation of sensory and/or motor function below the neurological level and including the sacral segment (ASIA, 2000). The physician tests innervation at the lowest sacral segment, including anal sensation and sphincter contraction.

The term *zone of partial preservation* is used for patients with complete injuries who have partial innervation in dermatomes below the neurological level (ASIA, 2000). A patient may have a C5 neurological level complete injury although radial wrist extensors innervated by C6 are functional (zone of partial preservation). Finally, some specific cord lesions cause a common pattern of clinical findings (Box 43-1).

Prognosis

Not surprisingly, recovery is very much on the minds of patients, families, and staff. Neural recovery during rehabilitation is common and can result in significant improvement in function. In patients with complete injuries, muscles in the zone of partial preservation strengthen, which may result in significant functional change. This is true especially if a key muscle, such as extensor carpi radialis, strengthens enough to enable the person to extend the wrist and hold objects. Patients with incomplete injury have a better prognosis and their recovery is less predictable in its pattern and outcome than those with complete injury (Waters & Yoshida, 1996).

Immediately after the injury, all reflexes cease to function. When spinal shock resolves, patients have an excellent chance to regain motor and sensory function. However, as time after injury increases, the recovery rate declines. Most motor and sensory return in both complete and incomplete injuries occurs in the first 6 months post onset, and the rate of recovery is minimal after a year (Waters & Yoshida, 1996; Waters et al., 1995).

As patients and significant others hope for complete recovery, it is important for the therapist to maintain hope while planning a realistic course of treatment. Research data can assist the clinician in predicting recovery and outcomes. One such source is the booklet *Recovery Following Spinal Cord Injury: A Clinician's Handbook* (Waters et al., 1995). However, be cautious about sharing this information with patients when they are most vulnerable.

Long-term survival of people with SCI has improved dramatically over the past 50 years. For people who survive the first year after injury—the year with the highest mortality rates—life expectancy is only slightly less than for the able-bodied population (DeVivo & Stover, 1995).

Impairments and Their Therapeutic Implications

Paralysis is the most common result of SCI. This injury is accompanied by a variety of frequent complications. The therapist must be aware of these impairments to provide a safe therapeutic environment and educate patients in understanding how to live a safe and healthy life.

Respiration

Many patients with SCI have compromised breathing. This is true especially for individuals with cervical injuries. Respiratory complications, specifically pneumonia, have been identified as the leading cause of death in the first year of life after SCI (DeVivo & Stover, 1995). In lesions above C4, damage to the phrenic nerve results in partial or complete paralysis of the diaphragm. These patients require ventilatory support (Fig. 43-3). Lower cervical and thoracic spine injuries can result in paralysis of other breathing muscles, such as the intercostals, abdominals, or latissimus dorsi (Kendall et al., 1993). Patients with such injuries do therefore have impaired respiration.

Use of proper techniques and infection control standards are important for respiratory care. Under the direction of the physician, the physical and respiratory therapists and the health care team work to achieve adequate bronchial hygiene and to facilitate good breathing at rest and during activities. Good communication with the team allows the occupational therapist to support breathing goals.

BOX 43-1
Definitions Box
ASIA Impairment Scale

The following scale is used in grading the degree of impairment:

A = Complete
No sensory or motor function is preserved in the sacral segments S4-S5.

B = Incomplete
Sensory but not motor function is preserved below the neurological level and includes the sacral segments S4-S5.

C = Incomplete
Motor function is preserved below the neurological level, and more than half of key muscles below the neurological level have a muscle grade less than 3.

D = Incomplete
Motor function is preserved below the neurological level, and at least half of key muscles below the neurological level have a muscle grade greater than or equal to 3.

E = Normal
Motor and sensory function are normal.

Clinical Syndromes

Central Cord Syndrome
Incomplete injury most common to the cervical region in which the center part of the cord is damaged. This lesion results in greater weakness in the upper limbs than in the lower limbs, with sacral sparing (ASIA, 2000).

Brown-Sequard Syndrome
Half of the cord is damaged, causing ipsilateral proprioceptive and motor loss and contralateral loss of pain and temperature sensation (ASIA, 2000).

Anterior Cord Syndrome
Lesion with variable motor and sensory loss and preservation of proprioception (ASIA, 2000).

Conus Medullaris Syndrome
Lesions to the sacral cord and lumbar nerve roots within the spinal canal; commonly results in areflexic bladder, bowel, and lower limbs (ASIA, 2000).

Cauda Equina Syndrome
Lower motor neuron injury to the lumbosacral nerve roots within the spinal canal; results in areflexic bladder, bowel, and lower limbs (ASIA, 2000).

To receive a grade of C or D, a person must have sensory or motor function in the sacral segments S4-S5. In addition, the individual must have either (1) voluntary anal sphincter contraction or (2) sparing of motor function more than three levels below the motor level.
ASIA Impairment scale reprinted with permission from the American Spinal Injury Association (2000). *International Standards for Neurological Classification of Spinal Cord Injury.* Chicago: Author.

Autonomic Dysreflexia

Autonomic dysreflexia, a sudden dangerous increase in blood pressure, is a possibly life-threatening complication associated with lesions at the T6 level or above (Box 43-2). It is brought on by an unopposed sympathetic response to noxious stimuli. Some of the more common causes of autonomic dysreflexia are distended bladder,

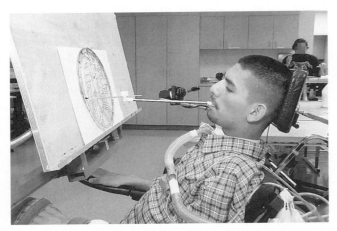

Figure 43-3 A person with C2 complete tetraplegia, ventilator dependent, using a mouthstick.

urinary tract or other infection, bladder or kidney stones, fecal impaction, pressure sores, ingrown toenails, invasive procedures such as urinary catheterization or enema, and pain. The main symptoms are hypertension and a pounding headache (Consortium for Spinal Cord Medicine, 1997).

Orthostatic Hypotension, or Postural Hypotension

Orthostatic hypotension is a sudden drop in blood pressure occurring when a person assumes an upright position (Box 43-2). Most common in patients with lesions at the T6 level and above, it is caused by impaired autonomic regulation. There is a decrease in the returning blood supply to the heart, commonly because of blood pooling in the lower extremities. Orthostatic hypotension is aggravated by a prolonged stay in bed. When the patient attempts to sit up, the blood rushes down to the legs. The patient may complain of light-headedness or dizziness and may faint on moving from reclined to upright. The therapist must use caution when sitting the patient up by having the patient move slowly and in stages and letting the blood pressure adjust to the change. Elevating the head of the bed, using a tilt table, or using a reclining wheelchair can accomplish this. To control this problem further, patients

---

BOX 43-2
SAFETY BOX

Autonomic Dysreflexia, or Sympathetic Hyperreflexia

Individuals with injuries at the T6 level or above may develop dangerously high blood pressure in response to a noxious stimulus. This condition is brought about by unopposed hyperactivity of the autonomic nervous system. If not promptly treated, autonomic dysreflexia may result in a stroke or sudden death. An increase of 20 mm Hg or more in systolic blood pressure is a sign that must be attended to. A pounding headache is the most common symptom. Other signs and symptoms include heavy sweating, flushed skin, goose bumps, blurry vision, a stuffy nose, anxiety, difficulty breathing, and chest tightness (Consortium for Spinal Cord Medicine, 1997a).

Take the following steps:

1. Ask the person to stop any ongoing activity, as it may further increase blood pressure.
2. Check blood pressure. If high:
3. Have the person sit up with head elevated to avoid excessive blood pressure to the brain.
4. Loosen clothing, abdominal binder, and any other constrictive devices.
5. Check the urinary catheter for kinks or folds and straighten any.
6. Continue to monitor blood pressure and seek medical assistance, which may include bladder irrigation, manual fecal evacuation, and medications.

Orthostatic, or Postural, Hypotension

In contrast to autonomic dysreflexia, in orthostatic hypotension, blood pressure drops to dangerously low levels in response to assuming an upright position. If it is not treated immediately, the person may lose consciousness. Symptoms of orthostatic hypotension include light-headedness, pallor, and visual changes. To resolve the problem:

1. Check blood pressure.
2. If the person is in bed, lower the head of the bed.
3. If the person is in a wheelchair, lift his or her legs and observe for signs of relief. If symptoms persist, recline the wheelchair to place the head at or below the level of the heart.
4. If symptoms persist, put the patient to bed.
5. Continue to monitor blood pressure and seek medical assistance. Do not leave the patient unattended until a nurse or a physician is present.

Principles for treatment of autonomic dysreflexia are derived from Consortium for Spinal Cord Medicine (1997a) and Zejdlik (1991).

Principles for treatment of postural hypotension are derived from Zejdlik (1991).

benefit from wearing abdominal binders and elastic stockings (Zejdlik, 1991).

Pressure Ulcers and Pressure Relief

Pressure ulcers are a common problem for people with SCI. Most patients do not have the sensory feedback that periodically cues them to shift position in their bed or wheelchair. The constant pressure caused by maintaining a static position without shifting weight can lead to skin breakdown. All patients must be placed on a weight-shifting pressure-relief schedule.

Although most pressure relief efforts are aimed at the buttocks, many other parts of the body are vulnerable in patients with higher lesions. All insensate areas must be inspected daily. For high tetraplegic patients these areas may also include the spine of the scapula and the back of the head.

The pressure relief program is successful only if patients with SCI incorporate this practice in their daily routines following hospitalization. They must become responsible for carrying out pressure relief procedures themselves or for asking assistance in doing so. In bed, patients must change their position every 2 hours and in a wheelchair, they must relieve pressure on their buttocks every hour for 1 minute (Hill, 1986).

Bowel Function and Management

Persons with complete SCI lose the ability to defecate voluntarily. Patients with injuries above the sacral segments achieve this function reflexively. Bowel function can be facilitated with oral and suppository medications or digital stimulation—anal insertion and manipulation of a finger or a special tool called a dill stick to facilitate reflex defecation. Patients with incomplete injuries may have mixed bowel function. Examples of this are persons who have only partial voluntary control of their sphincter, making waiting to get to a bathroom impossible. A thorough evaluation of the bowel by the physician and clear communication to all team members are vital for a well-managed program. The occupational therapist must participate in bowel programs of patients with tetraplegia who have the desire and potential either to become independent or to assist in managing their bowel. Precautions must be carefully followed, as an independent bowel program carries some risks. The person has impaired and/or absent sensation in the hand and anal area, which requires full visual compensation. A history of hemorrhoids or other bowel problems must be reviewed prior to goal setting. When bowel evacuation practices become regulated, they may pose no complications. Most individuals, after discharge, opt to carry out their bowel program in the morning every other day and can complete the procedure within 45 minutes (Kirshblaum et al., 1998).

Bladder Management

Like bowel function, bladder function is controlled in the S2-5 spinal segments. Therefore, all persons with complete lesions at and above the S2-5 levels lose their ability to void voluntarily. To avoid complications these patients must empty their bladder routinely. An indwelling catheter is commonly inserted soon after the person is admitted to the acute care hospital. Although some patients choose the indwelling catheter, an effort is made to find other ways to empty the bladder (Yarkony & Chen, 1996). The rehabilitation team must be aggressive in offering voiding alternatives to prevent urinary tract infections, another leading cause of complications in the SCI population. Intermittent catheterization is the manual insertion of a catheter into the bladder at fixed intervals of approximately 6 hours. It is the preferred method of bladder care (Zejdlik, 1991). With intermittent catheterization most men can stay dry, whereas women often need to wear a diaper, as their shorter urethra is more prone to leakage.

Sexual Function

The need for emotional and physical intimacy does not diminish after SCI, and questions about intimacy, sexuality, fertility, and reproduction must be answered by a team of sensitive and knowledgeable professionals (Adler, 1996). SCI affects both sexual intercourse and reproduction. Usually, male patients with complete injuries are unable to have psychogenic (voluntary) erections and ejaculations. They can, however, have reflex erections that may be controlled by stimulation, such as pulling the pubic hairs (Ducharme & Gill, 1997). Patients with complete injuries at S2-5 lose bowel, bladder, and genital reflexes and have a complete loss of erection. As with physical performance, male fertility is decreased after SCI. However, advances in technology provide ways for male patients to sustain an erection and improve the chances of fathering children (Ducharme & Gill).

Although sexual and reproductive functioning is less affected in women, sex, fertility, and menopause are still issues of concern. Some consequences related to these issues are dysreflexia and bladder incontinence during intercourse and complications of pregnancy and delivery (Jackson & Wadley, 1999).

For both males and females, other psychological, social, and physical issues add to the difficulty in resuming satisfying sexual roles. Problems with mobility, dependency, and societal role expectations are some of the issues the person with SCI must face. Knowledgeable members of the team must address sexual issues with patients. Individual counseling, often by a psychologist, takes place after a thorough evaluation by a physician. These four areas are typically addressed: sexual satisfaction, sexual function, fertility, and desirability. Patients learn that despite their injury, they can continue to be desirable and have an active sex life (Ducharme & Gill, 1997).

Temperature Regulation

Many people with SCI cannot regulate body temperature, which can lead to hypothermia or heat stroke (Zejdlik, 1991). Because of decreased sensation, patients may become severely sunburned or frostbitten. Education in the importance of neutral temperatures and the prevention of skin exposure to sun and severe temperatures is an important part of the occupational therapy program (Hill, 1986).

Pain

Acute and chronic pain (duration of more than half a year) is common after SCI. Considering the violent nature of most injuries, it is not surprising that most patients have pain at onset and that pain persists for a long time (Fairholm, 1991). Although many types of pain are present, they are most commonly classified thus:

- ► Mechanical pain—Local soft tissue pain associated with the injury. Mechanical pain, common in the shoulder of the tetraplegic patient, may be caused by direct trauma, muscle imbalance, and overuse of weak muscles (Fairholm).
- ► Radicular pain (also called segmental root pain)— Pain that often follows the segmental distribution of the nerve.
- ► Central pain (also called deafferentation or neurogenic pain)—Pain that originates in the spinal cord and is thought to be the result of misdirected neural sprouting after the injury.

Most of the SCI population has some chronic pain (Fairholm, 1991). For many the pain contributes to disability and depression. The occupational therapist's contribution to pain management includes a thorough evaluation (see Chapter 9). Although treatment goals are often directed toward reducing impairments, our main contribution is in changing habits and roles and facilitating engagement in meaningful activities despite pain.

Fatigue

Physiological, psychological, and environmental factors all contribute to patients' fatigue. Persistent pain, antispasmodic medications, and prolonged bed rest are physical factors that can make the patient feel tired or sleepy. This is often compounded by restless nights interrupted by hospital routines, such as repositioning patients in bed and waking them for checking vital signs and administering medications. Occupational therapists must be aware of these constraints and observe and listen to the patient. They must find the optimal waking hours for activities and report nighttime sleep disturbances, any changes of behavior that medication may affect, and other factors.

Spasticity and Spasms

An injury to the spinal cord often results in an increase in transmission within the synaptic stretch reflex. This results in spasticity. Spasticity develops into clonic or tonic spasms triggered by sensory stimuli such as sudden touch, infection, or other irritation (Trombly, 1989). Management of spasticity is important in maximizing a patient's functional independence. Severe spasticity may hinder function; for example, the hypertonicity of the hip and knee adductors can make donning pants difficult. The most common way to decrease spasticity is to use a muscle relaxant, such as Baclofen. An intrathecal pump, motor point, or nerve blocks may be used in severe cases. Spasticity can lead to contractures, so routine positioning in bed (Fig. 43-4) and in the wheel-

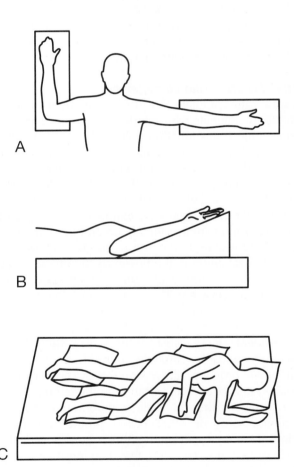

Figure 43-4 Positioning in bed. **A.** Alternate the arm in shoulder abduction and external rotation. **B.** Side view of A, showing placement of foam wedge. **C.** During side lying keep the upper back flat on the bed to protect the weighted shoulder.

BOX 43-3
RESEARCH NOTE

Access to the Environment and Life Satisfaction After Spinal Cord Injury
Richards, J. S., Bombardier, C. H., Tate, D., Dijkers, M., Gordon, W., Shewchuk, R., & DeVivo, M. J. (1999). *Archives of Physical Medicine and Rehabilitation, 80, 1501–1506*

ABSTRACT

Researchers evaluated 650 adults with traumatic SCI either 1 or 2 years post injury to determine any relation between satisfaction with life after SCI and accessibility of the environment. The *Craig Handicap Assessment and Reporting Technique* subscale was used to measure access to the environment. Sample questions: "Can you enter and exit your home without assistance from someone?" "Can you use your transportation independently?" The *Satisfaction With Life Scale* was also administered. Results showed that patients who had greater access to the environment reported greater satisfaction with life 1 and 2 years post injury. Positive correlation was also noted between accessible environments and self-perceived health. The authors suggest that feeling healthy and living productive, busy lives inside and outside the home are positively associated with satisfaction with life.

IMPLICATIONS FOR PRACTICE

▶ Occupational therapy evaluation of individuals with SCI must include an early detailed examination of the discharge context.
▶ The occupational therapist must work with the patient, family, and SCI team to remove environmental barriers, such as access to transportation.
▶ Occupational therapy must contribute to research and educate legislators in our professional beliefs and values regarding the right of people with SCIs to full participation in all of life's roles.

---

chair and range of motion are essential; patient and family must participate in these measures for continuity of care (see Chapter 5).

Deep Vein Thrombosis

Deep vein thrombosis is the formation of a blood clot, most often in a lower extremity or the abdomen or pelvic area. A clot may develop further and dislodge from the venous wall, forming an embolus. This condition poses a threat to the patient, as the embolus may travel and occlude pulmonary circulation (Consortium for Spinal Cord Medicine, 1997b; Zejdlik, 1991). The therapist helps prevent this condition by observing any asymmetry in the lower extremities in color, size, and/ or temperature. When deep vein thrombosis is identified, the patient must have complete bed rest and anticoagulants to prevent embolus (Consortium for Spinal Cord Medicine, 1997b; Zejdlik, 1991). This is a good time to inform the patient and family about the symptoms, prevention, and care of deep vein thrombosis.

Heterotopic Ossification

Heterotopic ossification, pathological bone formation in joints, has been recorded in 15 to 20% of SCI cases (Zejdlik, 1991). It is a condition in which connective tissue calcifies around the joint. Heterotopic ossification usually appears 1 to 4 months after injury. The symptoms are a warm, swollen extremity, fever, and/or range of motion limitations. Most often seen in the hip and shoulder joints, it can result in joint contractures. Posi-

tioning in bed and in the wheelchair and daily range of motion prevent or control heterotopic ossification. As the first indication of heterotopic ossification most typically is range of motion limitation, the occupational therapist must use each range of motion session to monitor joint ranges, especially those with spastic muscles (Garland, 1991).

Psychosocial Adaptation

As mentioned before, SCI dramatically disrupts life (Box 43-3) (see Chapters 9 and 35). What coping mechanisms are enlisted to enable the individual to adjust to these dramatic life challenges? Despite inconclusive and conflicting research, many authors agree that reactions to SCI may include periods of shock, anxiety, denial, depression, internalized and externalized anger, adjustment, and acknowledgment. These coping behaviors may be enlisted in a different order, and some may be skipped (Livneh & Antonak, 1997).

Depression

Although it is not universal, many patients have varying degrees of depression, sadness, or grief (Consortium for Spinal Cord Medicine, 1998a). Logically, we associate depression with the grieving time right after the injury; however, depression may persist long after the injury. Fuhrer et al. (1993) estimated that after SCI, up to 25% of men and 47% of women have symptoms of depression. Depressive symptoms are also associated with lack of social and occupational involvement. Injured individuals who show more symptoms of depression participate less in worker, volunteer, and student roles. Interestingly, level of injury does not appear to be associated with depressive symptoms. Individuals with a high cervical lesion are not necessarily more commonly or intensely depressed than individuals with paraplegia (Fuhrer et al., 1993).

To understand the complexity of the psychosocial adjustment to SCI, we must also examine the reactions of the patient's family and significant others. The family and significant others may also go through these psychological reactions. Concurrently, they may have to reassess their future commitment to the injured person. A mother, for example, may grieve and be sad while having to decide whether to take her fully dependent son home after a turbulent adolescence.

Occupational therapists and other health care professionals must also examine their emotional reactions and the influence of these emotions on the patient and therapeutic process. For example, sometimes upon interviewing a newly injured person, I become especially sad as I strongly identify with something in the patient's life narrative (e.g., the struggles of a mother with two young children). I am reminded of my projection, as the patient may be perfectly accepting and cheerful. Furthermore, studies show that health care professionals may overestimate the degree of patients' distress and depression. Patients' description of their own depression is often milder than perceived by the health care professional (Cushman, 1990).

As occupational therapists, we contribute to psychosocial adaptation after SCI as we incorporate the following considerations into evaluation and treatment.

▶ Set aside all preconceived biases about who the patient is and how he or she should feel or behave. Instead, concentrate on learning to know patients, their unique life contexts, and their individual reactions to their trauma.
▶ Provide psychological support. At times when the patient is overwhelmed with sadness, it is okay just to be present and available to the person. It is okay to stop an activity, find a quiet environment, possibly outside, and listen, affirm, and educate.
▶ Select activities with a just-right challenge. After weeks of being dependent, patients find hope by being able to feed themselves or turn on a CD player independently.
▶ Accept patients' emotional state without judging them (Hammell, 1995). If patients are not showing signs of depression or anger, it does not necessarily mean that they are not coping with their injury. They may be using ways of coping that are not the textbook ones. Remember that there is no require-

ment to mourn to learn to accept and live with the injury (Cushman, 1990, p. 195).
▶ Create opportunities for peer education and support. Peers with SCI are often very effective in reaching patients and in making them feel less isolated and more optimistic. Individuals with similar levels of injury can truly understand the pain that comes with SCI and may help the therapeutic process.

Assessment: Getting to Know the Person

Prior to the assessment, the occupational therapist checks the medical chart for medical clearance to begin the evaluation. The patient often has other trauma, such as lacerations of internal organs, closed head injury, and fractures. Special care is taken to review records and communicate with the physician to ensure the safety of the patient. The initial evaluation is often difficult, as the newly injured patient may be sedated, in pain, and/or confused. Furthermore, this assessment may be interrupted by numerous medical procedures and may be restricted by medical and spinal precautions. Therefore, the occupational therapist must be flexible in choosing appropriate evaluation time, in gathering bits of information in interrupted sessions, and in choosing the right tool for the moment when the patient is available. In essence, the evaluation process should not be limited to set scheduled intervals, and the therapist must view each encounter with the patient as part of an ongoing assessment. Information should be also collected from significant others and other team members. Thus, at the end of the assessment period, the therapist assembles all fragments of information into a full, initial evaluation. Treatment begins while the evaluation is in progress. This prevents further complications, such as range of motion limitations and edema. The therapist may also address patients' immediate needs, for example making them more comfortable in bed, which further establishes rapport and trust.

Often various members of the interdisciplinary team repeat parts of the evaluation. A positive trend toward an interdisciplinary team evaluation in which a few members of the team evaluate the patient together brings organized information gathering to the process that is not redundant. Assessment in occupational therapy after SCI includes an occupational history, physical and functional evaluations.

Occupational History

The goals of the initial evaluation include beginning to establish rapport and trust, teaching patients about their potential, and learning about who they are and what is important to them. From the first encounter the therapist also begins to educate the patient and to plan discharge. This is true especially today, when hospital stays have been cut to a bare minimum. In the acute phase and shortly after the injury, patients may be quite limited in their knowledge of the nature of their injury, prognosis for recovery, and potential for function. It is important not to overwhelm the patient with more than can be absorbed at that moment. The therapist must always leave room for hope without deceiving the patient.

To gather deeper understanding of patients' roles, activities, and the meaning behind the activities, use open-ended questions. Charting a typical day's schedule prior to injury allows for creative questioning and enables the therapist to sketch a person's habits, routines, and other activities.

The *Canadian Occupational Performance Measure (COPM)* is an excellent tool for working with the SCI population. It focuses on finding out patients' occupational goals and their priorities (see Chapter 3). If patients are not psychologically ready to formulate goals that are important to discharge, first goals may be directed toward their attaining more control over their immediate environment.

Physical Evaluation

Spinal stability must be established prior to any physical contact with the patient. The occupational therapist must clarify with the primary physician how much movement and load are allowed without jeopardizing spinal integrity.

The physical assessment includes upper extremity range of motion, strength, muscle tone, and sensation (see Chapters 4–6). The therapist also observes the patient's endurance, trunk balance, fatigability, and pain. The appearance of the upper extremities can reveal signs of reflex sympathetic dystrophy, an upper limb disease marked by severe pain and swelling. Such findings are vital for prevention of further deformity by immediately initiating an aggressive treatment regimen.

Functional Evaluation

Selection of appropriate functional evaluations is dictated by level of injury and stage of recovery. Occupational therapists rely on both observation and standardized assessments to evaluate hand function, basic and instrumental activities of daily living (ADL), leisure, school, vocational interests, and aptitudes.

Hand and Wrist of the Patient With Tetraplegia

Evaluation of the hands and wrists is both physical and functional. Most therapists observe hand use while the person is performing activities such as picking up pieces of a game or eating. Some hand tests, such as the *Sullerman Hand Function Test*, also prove useful for assessing the tetraplegic hand (Curtin, 1999). Pinch and grip strength are measured when wrist and hand muscles are functioning.

Activities of Daily Living and Instrumental Activities of Daily Living

Often full ADL evaluation is postponed because of medical and spinal restrictions and predictions regarding length of stay and functional outcomes are rendered without complete data. The *Functional Independence Measure (FIM)* is widely used to assess function; however, some instruments are designed specifically for the patient with SCI, such as the *Quadriplegia Index of Function* (Gersham et al., 1986) and the *Modified Barthel Index* (Yarkony et al., 1987).

Leisure

Persons with SCI have high unemployment rates and much free time (Yerxa & Baum, 1990). Therefore, finding past relevant and meaningful leisure activities is of special importance (see Chapters 3 and 34).

School and Vocation

A full vocational evaluation is rarely performed during acute rehabilitation because patients are focused on more immediate challenges. Many have lost the physical ability to engage in prior occupations. Vocational exploration begins with defining patients' abilities and interests. Observation of factors such as hand function and work habits contribute information for the prevocational team and department of vocational rehabilitation.

Home and Community

The home visit is an invaluable assessment tool for the person with SCI, and the earlier it is performed, the better. This visit allows the therapist to assess home accessibility and safety and to evaluate the capacity of patients and their families to problem solve (Atkins, M. S. [1989]. A descriptive study: The occupational therapy predischarge home visit program for spinal cord injured adults. Unpublished Master's thesis. University of Southern California, Los Angeles.).

Setting Goals: Ordering Priorities for Meaningful and Relevant Activities

Setting treatment goals in the acute phase may seem overwhelmingly difficult for both patient and therapist. Complications seem to hinder progress, and patients are often confused, fearful, and uncertain about their impairments and abilities. Answers to the following questions help patient and therapist set priorities, establish short-term goals, and start treatment while evaluation is still in progress:

▶ What must be done to prevent further deformities and complications?
▶ What activity is important to the patient to engage in right now?

The development of short-term goals stems from the therapist's ability to perform an activity analysis. Short-term goals may address functional performance areas and tasks, underlying problems, or the component skills necessary to perform an ADL. For example, a C4 tetraplegic who wants to use a mouthstick for word processing on the computer must first tolerate sitting upright in the wheelchair for significant periods. Increasing tolerance for sitting upright is an appropriate short-term goal for achieving the independence of mouthstick computer use.

Functional Expectations

Expected functional outcome charts predict the degree of functional independence for a particular level of injury. One such chart was published in a 1999 document, *Outcomes Following Traumatic Spinal Cord Injury: Clinical Practice Guidelines for Health Care Professionals* (Consortium for Spinal Cord Medicine, 1999). The consortium is administered and financed by the Paralyzed Veterans of America. This document, free to the public, is presented here in part. It includes an evidence-based expected functional outcome chart (Box 43-4 and Appendix 43-1).

Age-Specific Considerations

While every patient has unique considerations in treatment planning, this chapter highlights the unique needs of adolescents and older adults.

Adolescence and Young Adulthood

The adolescent with SCI must deal with complicating normal developmental factors coupled with new impairments and disabilities (Smith et al., 1996). Psychological adaptation to the injury may be especially difficult for adolescents, as the injury comes in the midst of development of adult self-image, identity, and independence. The therapist is challenged to maintain a delicate balance between the needs to support patients and families and to encourage the young person to be self-reliant. Warning the family about avoiding overindulgence can lead to more engaged and assertive participation by the patient (Smith et al., 1996). At times, when the adolescent exhibits brooding or defiant behaviors that are harmful to progress, a strict behavioral program

becomes necessary to draw the adolescent into positive participation (Massagli & Jaffe, 1990). Along with establishing independence, primary goals for the adolescent must include the following:

▶ Reentering the student role—Goals may include meeting with school personnel and visiting the school with the patient (Massagli & Jaffe).
▶ Sexual roles—Adolescents must be assured that individuals with SCI can remain sexually active (Massagli & Jaffe, 1990).
▶ Driver role—Initial evaluation and referral may be carried out in the acute rehabilitation phase and may be continued in the transition and adaptation phases. Driving, if possible, may provide the adolescent with a valuable sense of empowerment, independence, and increased motivation.

At times it is hard to remember that adolescents, though on an adult unit, are minors and that all fundamental decisions must be made with parental participation and consent. The parents must be supported and must be part of the team, helping the patient make appropriate choices. Parents must also participate in educational sessions to ensure consistency in treatment, for example with pressure relief.

The Older Adult

Having SCI and being elderly may be considered a dual diagnosis. The physiological process of aging can make rehabilitation from SCI particularly difficult (Teasell & Allatt, 1991). Most geriatric SCIs are attributed to falls that result in lesions at the cervical level (DeVivo & Stover, 1995). The central cord syndrome is common among the elderly SCI population.

The geriatric patient may require downgrading of expected functional outcomes, given physical and/or cognitive limitations (Teasell & Allatt, 1991). Some important factors are decreases in muscle strength, endurance, and physical fitness; joint degeneration; bone decalcification; skin integrity; cognition; vision; and emotional changes (Teasell & Allatt) (see Chapters 9 and 37).

Aging With Spinal Cord Injury

Long-term survival rates of SCI patients have improved dramatically in the past few decades, and many people with SCI live for decades after injury (Devivo et al., 1999). Along with normal aging issues, some unique problems arise in this population. Using the upper limbs for mobility (pushing a wheelchair, transferring), overuse of weak muscles, and muscle imbalance may cause chronic shoulder pain and less often, elbow and wrist pain (Curtis et al., 1999). Other body changes may include skin changes with increasing susceptibility to pressure ulcers, decreased bone density, susceptibility to

BOX 43-4
PROCEDURES FOR PRACTICE

Using Expected Functional Outcomes Charts

Outcome-based practice guidelines can provide estimates of the effect of rehabilitation on functional status or activity restrictions. In Appendix 43-1, the Consortium for Spinal Cord Medicine has put forth its best description, based on outcome studies and expert consensus, of outcomes of people with motor complete SCI 1 year after injury. These outcome guidelines are presented with the full recognition that outcomes are not fully under the influence or control of health care providers. Differences in patient characteristics, the course of medical events, psychological, social, and environmental supports, and cognitive abilities have strong influences on outcomes.

These outcome-based guidelines can be used to establish goals, provide information for quality improvement, and compare performance across facilities with similar populations. When used appropriately, outcome-based practice guidelines provide a benchmark for comparing programs and services while improving both the processes and outcomes of care that have an enduring impact on long-term functioning in the community. Disability outcome measures are generally focused on the degree to which a person can independently complete an important function or activity of daily living (ADL). This definition of disability is consistent with the World Health Organization (WHO) model of disablement in which disability is measured at the level of the person interacting with the environment during daily routines. In the completion of daily tasks, adaptive equipment becomes a crucial adjunct to the independence of the person with SCI.

Appendix 43-1 presents expectations of functional performance of SCI at 1 year post injury for each of 8 levels of injury (C1-3, C4, C5, C6, C7-8, T1-9, T10-L1 and L2-S5). The outcomes reflect a level of independence that can be expected of a person with motor complete SCI, given optimal circumstances.

The categories presented reflect expected functional outcomes in the areas of mobility, activities of daily living, instrumental activities of daily living, and communication skills. The guidelines are based on consensus of clinical experts, available literature on functional outcomes, and data compiled from the Uniform Data System (UDS) and the National Spinal Cord Injury Statistical Center (NSCISC).

Within the functional outcomes for people with SCI listed in Appendix 43-1, the panel has identified a series of essential daily functions and activities, expected levels of functioning, and the equipment and attendant care likely to be needed to support the predicted level of independence at 1 year post injury. These outcome areas include:

▸ **Respiratory, bowel, and bladder function**. The neurological effects of spinal injury may result in deficits in the ability of the individual to perform basic bodily functions. Respiratory function includes ability to breathe with or without mechanical assistance and to adequately clear secretions. Bowel and bladder function includes the ability to manage elimination, maintain perineal hygiene, and adjust clothing before and after elimination. Adapted or facilitated methods of managing these bodily functions may be required to attain expected functional outcomes.

▸ **Bed mobility, bed/wheelchair transfers, wheelchair propulsion, and positioning/pressure relief.** The neurological effects of SCI may result in deficits in the ability of the individual to perform the activities required for mobility, locomotion, and safety. Adapted or facilitated methods of managing these activities may be required to attain expected functional outcomes.

▸ **Standing and ambulation.** Spinal cord injury may result in deficits in the ability to stand for exercise or psychological benefit or to ambulate for functional activities. Adapted or facilitated methods of management may be required to attain expected functional outcomes in standing and ambulation.

▸ **Eating, grooming, dressing, and bathing.** The neurological effects of SCI may result in deficits in the ability of the individual to perform these activities of daily living. Adapted or facilitated methods of managing these activities of daily living may be required to attain expected functional outcomes.

▸ **Communication (keyboard use, handwriting, and telephone use).** The neurological effects of SCI may result in deficits in the ability of the individual to communicate. Adapted or facilitated methods of communication may be required to attain expected functional outcomes.

▸ **Transportation (driving, attendant-operated vehicle, and public transportation).** Transportation activities are critical for individuals with SCI to become maximally independent in the community. Adaptations may be required to facilitate the individual in meeting the expected functional outcomes.

▸ **Homemaking (meal planning and preparation and home management).** Adapted or facilitated methods of managing homemaking skills may be required to attain expected functional outcomes. Individuals with complete SCI at any level will require some level of assistance with homemaking activities. The hours of assistance with homemaking activities are presented in Appendix 43-1.

▸ **Assistance required.** Appendix 43-1 presents the number of hours that may be required from a caregiver to assist with personal care and homemaking activities in the house. Personal care includes hands-on delivery of all aspects of self-care and mobility, as well as safety interventions. Homemaking assistance is also included in the recommendation for hours of assistance and includes activities previously presented. The number of hours presented in both the panel recommendations and the self-reported *Craig Handicap Assessment and Reporting Technique* (CHART) [Whiteneck et al., 1992] data is representative of skilled and unskilled and paid and unpaid hours of assistance. The 24-hour-a-day requirement noted for the C1-3 and C4 levels includes the expected need for unpaid attendant care to provide safety monitoring.

(continued)

BOX 43-4
PROCEDURES FOR PRACTICE

Using Expected Functional Outcomes Charts (Continued)

Adequate assistance is required to ensure that the individual with SCI can achieve the outcomes set forth in Appendix 43-1. The hours of assistance recommended by the panel do not reflect changes in assistance required over time as reported by long-term survivors of SCI (Gerhart et al., 1993), nor do they take into account the wide range of individual variables mentioned throughout this document that may affect the number of hours assistance is required. The *Functional Independence Measure* (FIM) estimates are widely variable in several categories. One does not know whether the representative individuals with SCI in the individual categories attained the expected functional outcomes for their specific level of injury nor whether there were mitigating circumstances such as age, obesity, or concomitant injuries, that would account for variability in assistance reported. An individualized assessment of needs is required in all cases.

▸ **Equipment requirements.** Minimum recommendations for durable medical equipment and adaptive devices are identified in each of the functional categories. Most commonly used equipment is listed, with the understanding that variations exist among SCI rehabilitation programs, and that use of such equipment may be necessary to achieve the identified functional outcomes. Additional equipment and devices that are not critical for the majority of individuals at a specific level of injury may be required for some individuals. The equipment descriptions are generic to provide for variances in program philosophy and financial resources. Rapid changes and advances in equipment and technology will be made and therefore must be considered.

Health care professionals should keep in mind that the recommendations set forth in Appendix 43-1 are not intended to be prescriptive, but rather to serve as a guideline. The importance of individual functional assessment of people with SCI prior to making equipment recommendations cannot be over emphasized. All durable medical equipment and adaptive devices must be thoroughly assessed and tested to determine medical necessity to prevent medical complications (e.g., postural deviations, skin breakdown, or pain), and to foster optimal functional performance. Environmental control units and telephone modifications may be needed for safety and maximal independence, and each person must be individually evaluated for the need for this equipment. Disposable medical product recommendations are not included in this document.

▸ **FIM.** Evidence for the specific levels of independence provided in Appendix 43-1 relies both on expert consensus and data from the FIM in large-scale, prospective, and longitudinal research conducted by NSCISC. FIM is the most widely used disability measure in rehabilitation medicine, although it may not incorporate all of the characteristics of disability in individuals recovering from SCI, it captures many basic disability areas. FIM consists of 13 motor and 5 cognitive items that are individually scored from 1 to 7. A score of 1 indicates complete dependence and a score of 7 indicates complete independence. The sum of the 13 FIM motor score items can range from 13, indicating complete dependence for all items, to 91, indicating complete independence for all items. FIM is a measure usually completed by health care professionals. Different observers, including the patient, family members, and caregivers, can contribute information to the ratings. Each of these reporters may represent a different type of potential bias. It should also be noted that although the sample sizes of FIM data for certain neurological level groups are quite small, the consistency of the data adds confidence to the interpretation. Other pertinent data regarding functional independence must be factored into outcome analyses, including medical information, patient factors, social participation, quality of life, and environmental factors and supports. In Appendix 43-1, FIM data, when available, are reported in three areas. First, the expected FIM outcomes are documented based on expert clinical consensus. The second number reported is the median FIM score, as compiled by NSCISC. The interquartile range for NSCISC FIM data is the third set of numbers. In total, the FIM data represent 1-year postinjury FIM assessment of 405 survivors with complete SCI. Sample size for FIM and Assistance Data is provided for each level of injury. Different outcome expectations should clearly apply to different patient subgroups and populations. Some populations are likely to be significantly older than the referenced one. Functional abilities may be limited by advancing age (Penrod et al., 1990; Yarkony et al., 1988).

▸ **Home modifications.** To provide the best opportunity for individuals with SCI to achieve the identified functional outcomes, a safe and architecturally accessible environment is necessary. An accessible environment must take into consideration, but not be limited to, entrance and egress, mobility in the home, and adequate setup to perform personal care and homemaking tasks.

Reprinted with permission from the Paralyzed Veterans of America (PVA). Consortium for Spinal Cord Medicine. (1999). *Outcome Following Traumatic Spinal Cord Injury: Clinical Practice Guidelines for Health Care Professionals.* Washington DC: Paralyzed Veterans of America.

fractures, impaired cardiovascular fitness, and renal complications. Additional problems may include depression, an increase in functional dependence, and decreased mobility (Whiteneck et al., 1993).

The occupational therapist, using knowledge of energy conservation, joint protection, and activity analysis must communicate with and educate the patient in restructuring activities to accommodate the new condition. An aging patient, once independent in all self-maintenance skills, may need help in the morning to conserve energy for work. A grandmother who wants to interact with her toddler grandson may have to train him to climb onto her lap rather than picking him up.

Treatment

The occupational therapist treats trauma patients in various settings and at various times. Throughout this treatment continuum of acute care, acute rehabilitation, transition, and adaptation, most treatment principles remain the same. However, the focus of care changes as the patient's internal processes and external environment change.

Acute Recovery: Focus on Support and Prevention

Immediately after injury, most patients are admitted into an intensive care unit, where the focus is on preservation of life, stabilizing fluids, electrolytes, and cardiopulmonary and other vital functions. The patient is immobilized in traction, waiting to hear whether surgery is required to stabilize the spine. For prevention of pressure ulcers, the patient is put in a rotating bed (Yarkoni & Chen, 1996). In the intensive care unit medical and surgical procedures take precedence over therapy. The therapist must be flexible, often seeing the patient for brief periods throughout the day. One or two 15-minute sessions per day are often helpful to the patient, who may be in pain, fatigue easily, and become confused or overwhelmed by this fast-paced environment of electronic devices and medical procedures. The occupational therapist's initial contact should be within 24 hours of admission. Treatment begins as the initial evaluation is in progress, allowing the therapist to begin to gain a full picture of the patient (Hammell, 1995). In addition to ongoing patient and family support and education, the goals of therapy in the acute recovery phase:

1. Provide some environmental controls to help the patient get some control.
2. Maintain normal upper limb joint range of motion and prevent deformities (Yarkoni & Chen, 1996; Adler, 1996).

Movement in joints particularly susceptible to contractures are monitored daily. These are scapular rotation, shoulder scaption (the functional motion between abduction and flexion), shoulder external rotation, elbow extension, and forearm pronation. Hands are fitted with resting hand splints. Upper limbs are placed in either abduction or fencing position (Fig. 43-4). Alternating arms between these positions puts all vulnerable joints in stretch.

Range of motion to the hand of the tetraplegic patient is performed in a special way to facilitate **tenodesis grasp**: passive opening of the fingers when the wrist is flexed and closing of the fingers when the wrist is extended (Fig. 43-5) (Wilson et al., 1984). The patient, family, and others are taught how to perform range of motion exercises to facilitate tenodesis. Again, range of motion exercises must be augmented with proper positioning.

Acute Rehabilitation: Focus on Support, Education, and Meaningful Activities

In the 1970s the mean length of stay in acute SCI rehabilitation was 144.8 days. By the late 1990s mean length of stay had decreased to 44 days (NSCISC, 2000). To make matters worse, at present insufficient health care money is being allocated to services for outpatient services, and patients' needs are being only partially met (Trieschman, 1988; Zigler et al., 1998). Consequently, therapists are often frustrated, trying to accomplish too much in too little time. It helps to conceptualize rehabilitation as a lifelong endeavor, with acute rehabilitation being only the beginning phase. Shortened hospital stays serve as a catalyst for making tough decisions about what is most important to accomplish during inpatient stay.

During acute rehabilitation, occupational therapy continues to focus on providing education and support to patients and helping them begin to explore meaningful activities that restore a sense of efficacy and self-esteem. Treatments must always be structured with these overriding goals in mind. This chapter offers basic information. For specific detailed interventions, consult the reference list.

Educating Patients and Family

Each encounter with patients and families must be viewed as an educational opportunity. The style, quantity, and direction of each session must be carefully considered (Hammell, 1995). While patients are learning to put on a shoe, for example, the therapist may ask if they have checked skin integrity and by so doing draw attention to the importance of skin inspection. This discussion may also inform the patient about preferable shoe styles and sizes, pedal edema, and deep vein thrombosis. Nurses, the only team members who see the patient throughout the day, are pivotal in enforcing a daily routine. The therapist must communicate with them daily to ensure a coherent and consistent program.

Case Example

MR. A.: OCCUPATIONAL THERAPY FOR A PERSON WITH TETRAPLEGIA

Patient Information

Mr. A. is a 19 year old man with C6 complete tetraplegia resulting from an ocean diving accident 3 months ago. Mr. A. is a sophomore at a community college. He came to the United States from Samoa to attend college on a football scholarship. Mr. A. is single and lives with fellow students in a rented house near campus. He has a large and supportive family in Samoa. After his injury, Mr. A.'s mother, aunt, and two of his sisters came to be with him for a month. Mr. A. is fluent in English.

Following his injury, Mr. A. was sent to a trauma center, where he underwent posterior fusion surgery to stabilize C4 to C7 vertebrae and was placed in a Philadelphia collar, a rigid collar that limits neck motion. Following surgery Mr. A. was prescribed spine restrictions that allowed only minimal (3+/5) upper limb bilateral resistive activities. This restriction allowed him to perform only light unilateral activities and light to moderate bilateral activities and exercises. During the postoperative hospital stay, Mr. A. was on a rotating bed to prevent pressure sores. The occupational therapist performed daily upper limb range of motion exercise. She established a shoulder positioning program and fitted Mr. A. with prefabricated resting hand splints. In conversations with the patient and his family, the therapist began to explain rehabilitation. The occupational therapist documented that the family was engaged and supportive and that the patient appeared passive and quiet. Mr. A. was transferred to a rehabilitation center 3 weeks post injury.

Reason for Referral to Occupational Therapy

Mr. A. was referred to occupational therapy to address limitations in self-maintenance, self-advancement, and self-enhancement roles and to overcome adverse emotional reactions. Mr. A. was hoping to stay in California and resume his studies. He did not have a discharge destination.

Occupational Therapy Problem List

▶ Moderate depression, lack of engagement with the rehabilitation team, excessive dependency on family
▶ Decreased upper limb strength (*Manual Muscle Test*) and endurance. Summary of findings: Right hand dominant.
  Symmetry in strength with right upper extremity slightly stronger than left
  Scapulas and shoulders: strength 4/5 throughout
  Elbows: 4/5 flexion; 0/5 extension
  Forearms: 4/5 supination; 2–/5 pronation
  Wrist: Extensor carpi radialis longus and brevis: right 3+/5; left 3/5; 0/5 ulnar wrist extension and wrist flexion.
  Fingers and thumb: 0/5

▶ Sensory level: C6 dermatome intact; impaired C7 dermatome and absent below (Fig. 43-2)
▶ Hand use: Drags objects to edge of table; picks up objects with right hand; holds object with 2 hands
▶ Unable to feed, brush teeth, groom, dress, write, phone, use a computer (priorities identified by *COPM*).

Occupational Therapy Goal List

▶ Independently use phone
▶ Independently feed, brush teeth, and groom (*FIM-6*)
▶ Independently write and use the computer
▶ Learn routine SCI precautions for skin care, pressure relief, and bowel and bladder care
▶ Learn to direct own care
▶ Increase upper limb strength and improve hand function (tenodesis hand)
▶ Become independent in upper body dressing
▶ Assist in lower body dressing
▶ Resume student role
▶ Have hope and feelings of independence and competence

Treatment Program

To meet these goals, the 8-week treatment program consisted of the following:

▶ ADL training that included upper body dressing and feeding, brushing teeth, and grooming using a universal cuff
▶ Evaluation for the use of right wrist-driven wrist–hand orthosis with clinic trial equipment. Ordering, checking fit, and training in orthosis use.
▶ Practice tabletop activities: writing, computer skills, telephone use, and other student role activities, such as using a tape recorder and handling books and papers.
▶ Strengthening program with emphasis on wrists. When spinal precautions were lifted, Mr. A. was referred to a progressive resistive exercise physical therapy group.
▶ Education: Individual and group. Group experiential training in topics such as taking public transportation, assertiveness training, and directing care.

Analysis of Reasoning

Treatment priorities were established based on patient-identified goals (*COPM*) and the therapist's knowledge of the capacities and skills necessary to meet those goals (such as developing abilities in hand use through exercise, promoting tenodesis, hand use trial, and selecting appropriate equipment, such as the wrist-driven wrist–hand orthosis). The therapist also anticipated the importance of optimized functional independence and Mr. A.'s ability to maintain health and direct care to discharge planning.

During the sixth week of hospitalization, the initial discharge plan fell through because the person who offered Mr. A. a house and care changed his mind. The team recommended an interim discharge to an independent living center to assist the transition from hospital to independent living, given the absence of family in the United States. This would enable the patient to acquire more skills and more confidence in his abilities prior to returning to school and independent living. As Mr. A. began to emerge from his depression, he became more involved in the program and started socializing with other patients. With a renewed sense of hope, the patient identified a new set of goals prior to discharge. These included visiting a transitional living center, visiting his college, and becoming independent in self-catheterization.

CLINICAL REASONING
in OT Practice: Patient With Tetraplegia

Effects of Depression and Lack of Involvement on Rehabilitation

In interviews and observations in acute care and acute rehabilitation, Mr. A.'s therapists noted that the patient appeared depressed and uninvolved in his care. What could the therapist do to facilitate greater involvement and participation by the patient? What bodily and environmental factors might exaggerate these problems? What bodily and environmental factors might improve these problems?

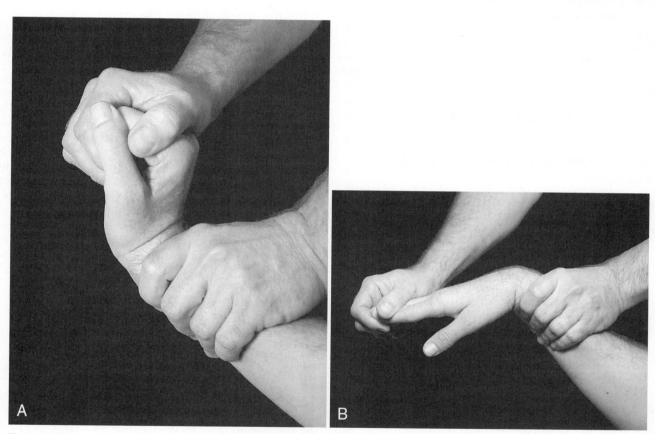

Figure 43-5 Ranging to facilitate tenodesis grasp. **A.** When the wrist is extended, the fingers are flexed. **B.** When the wrist is flexed, the fingers are extended.

Education is often enhanced by learning and problem solving with a peer or in a group (Hammell, 1995; Trieschmann, 1988). Group learning is widely used in SCI centers, to inform and invite group dialogue on topics such as home modifications, accessibility rights, attendant management, assertiveness, travel, and driving. Experiential group activities, such as going to a restaurant, are recommended for building emotional and

Case Example

MR. J.: OCCUPATIONAL THERAPY FOR A PERSON WITH PARAPLEGIA

Patient Information

Mr. J. is a 21-year-old man who was shot once in a drive-by shooting near his home. The injury resulted in T10 complete paraplegia. Mr. J. lives with his working mother and two younger sisters in a rented house. Since dropping out of high school in the 11th grade, Mr. J. has held several unskilled jobs lasting approximately 4 months at each. His jobs have included stacking boxes at a packing company and working as a driver, delivering merchandise.

Following his injury, Mr. J. was in a medical trauma center for 5 days. When medical and spinal stability were established, he was transferred to acute rehabilitation, where he participated in rehabilitation for 5 weeks. At the time of discharge, Mr. J. was independent in self-care skills, transfers, and wheelchair skills. His discharge evaluations stated that he demonstrated an adequate knowledge of spinal injury precautions, such as avoidance of pressure ulcers and use of intermittent catheterization. The occupational therapist noted that although Mr. J. was initially interested in passing his high school equivalency examination (GED) with the goal of entering a community college, he showed no interest in pursuing this goal at discharge.

Reasons for Referral to Outpatient Occupational Therapy

Mr. J. was referred to occupational therapy 6 months after discharge to address bilateral shoulder pain and deficits in self-advancement and self-enhancement roles.

Occupational Therapy Problem List

- Bilateral shoulder pain interfering with function (pain history, *range of motion* and *manual muscle testing*)
- Bathing transfers too strenuous on shoulders (*FIM*)
- Feelings of worthlessness, isolation, and boredom (*COPM* satisfaction with activities 1-3 range)
- Lack of meaningful activities and roles (*Typical Day Form*)
- Lack of transportation (*COPM*)

Occupational Therapy Goal List

The patient will do the following:

- Remain independent in ADL while learning to minimize strain on shoulders.
- List factors that affect shoulder pain.
- Prepare to begin student role (In *COPM* remained a desired goal)

- Develop beginning satisfaction with ability to perform meaningful activities (*COPM*)
- Learn to use public transportation

Treatment Program

The outpatient program, which ran 2 hours twice a week for 6 weeks, included (1) education on shoulder pain, with the need to rest the shoulders and be selective in activities that put extra strain on shoulders; (2) analyzing bathing needs and testing solutions for these needs; (3) participation in an outpatient return to school or work support group with peers; (4) taking the bus and finding routes to and from home; (5) referral to a physical therapy class for shoulder strengthening; (6) visit to a community college and meeting with a disabled student counselor to learn about GED preparatory class.

Analysis of Reasoning

The treatment plan emphasized decreasing shoulder pain by finding an adequate way for the patient to bathe without having to transfer multiple times in compromised positions. To minimize the long-term consequences of overuse, therapy also emphasized adequate upper extremity rest and compliance with medication regimen. When shoulder pain decreased, a physical therapy referral was made to help him initiate strengthening exercise protocol designed to decrease shoulder pain for manual wheelchair users (Curtis et al., 1999). Finally, to decrease the sense of isolation and begin engagement in meaningful activities, the patient entered a peer group, discussing topics necessary to return to school, such as filling in applications, transportation, and organizing daily routines to allow for greater participation.

CLINICAL REASONING
in OT Practice: Patient With Paraplegia

Effects of Overuse on Shoulder Impairment

The outpatient occupational therapy assessment revealed to Mr. J.'s therapist that inappropriate bathing transfers from wheelchair to a chair to the bottom of tub and back contributed to shoulder pain. How can Mr. J. bathe, putting less strain on the shoulders? Keep in mind that Mr. J.'s home is rented. What educational methods and tools would you employ to teach Mr. J. about overuse of shoulders? The therapist determined that Mr. J. needs to come for follow-up appointments. List goals and treatment plan for the follow-up appointments.

social alliances with peers while learning from each other's successes and failures. Educational materials and videos are available through groups such as the Paralyzed Veterans of America and the Spinal Cord Injury Association (see Resources). Participation in self-initiated learning, such as surfing the Internet, empowers the patient. Family education must result in competence in range of motion, positioning, pressure relief, assistance in ADL, and use of equipment. Home and weekend passes provide an excellent opportunity to develop and refine skills.

Encouraging Problem Solving

Our challenge as therapists is to recruit, educate, and empower our patients to be problem solvers. By so doing we encourage active participation, generalization of information, and the transfer of learning to the discharge environment (Radomski, 1998). When planning an outing, ask the group to prepare a list of items to be checked to ensure a safe, successful outing. Upon return to the hospital, encourage discussion of the outing to reflect on ways future outings can be improved. Practical issues like restaurant accessibility to wheelchairs and self-catheterization in public bathrooms may arise.

Focusing on the Discharge Context: Objects, Locations, Activities, and People Central to the Patient

An early home visit can save many hours of therapy as the therapist obtains a visual image of the patient's discharge environment (Atkins, M. S. [1989]. A descriptive study: The occupational therapy predischarge home visit program for spinal cord injured adults. Unpublished Master's thesis. University of Southern California, Los Angeles). Engaging the patient in visualizing postdischarge activities at home helps make treatment relevant. For a bath evaluation, for example, the therapist must look for a setting that resembles the patient's home as closely as possible.

Balancing Self-Maintenance Skills and Meaningful Activities

In acute rehabilitation most patients are relearning skills that they mastered in childhood, such as eating and dressing independently. This training is an important part of our job. For many patients, however, this training is frustrating, time consuming, tiring, and a constant reminder of their impairments and disabilities. The therapist has the difficult task of helping the patient see when relearning skills is valuable and when the skill should be accomplished by an attendant, either for now or permanently. The ultimate goal of rehabilitation is no longer viewed as the attainment of maximal functional independence. Rather, it is the attainment of optimal

desired functional independence. Functional expectations charts (Appendix 43-1) help us understand the range of expectations for a given level of injury considering only the motor and sensory status of the patient. These charts do not answer such questions as these: Why should the patient dress for half an hour when his wife can dress him in 5 minutes? Will it still take that long after adequate training? What will the patient do when his wife is away? Such discussions encourage patients and families to explore the range and consequences of their choices. The novice therapist will find books such as *Spinal Cord Injury: A Guide to Functional Outcomes in Occupational Therapy* (Hill, 1986) and *Physical Management for the Quadriplegic Patient* (Ford & Duckworth, 1987) especially valuable, as they contain photographs that demonstrate various skills, their sequencing, and the use of assistive devices.

Choosing Equipment

Initially, when pain, spinal precautions, and orthoses may stand in the way of accomplishing goals, assistive devices may be handy facilitators. When obstacles diminish, some equipment, such as a dressing stick, can be eliminated. Only essential equipment should be sent home with the patient, since much of it is costly and it may further complicate the person's life. Also, a universal device should be favored over multiple assistive devices (Clark et al., 1997).

Patients and families should be involved in the purchase of any major equipment, including the wheelchair and bathroom equipment. When prescribing a wheelchair or commode, the therapist must consider mobility and positioning. Other factors, such as compatibility to the patient's home and transportation, must be also considered (Hollar, 1995) (see Chapter 16).

Special Treatment Considerations Based on Level of Injury

The level of injury dictates the degree of motor, sensory, and autonomic nervous system impairments. Consequently, treatment considerations and outcomes vary greatly with each level. Most evidence-based data, as in the following discussion of the levels of SCI, describe individuals with complete injuries, as the clinical picture is similar from person to person. Outcome of incomplete injuries cannot be easily predicted or generalized, as impairment varies greatly between individuals.

The Patient With High Tetraplegia: C1 to C4

Patients with complete C1-C3 require an external breathing device, as their diaphragm is either paralyzed or only partially innervated (C3). Most persons with C4 tetraplegia require assistance with ventilation during acute care, but as the diaphragm strengthens, they are able to breath independently. The most common device for assisted breathing is the ventilator, a pneumatic electric machine that forces room air into the lungs. Expiration is passive. This device is attached via plastic tubes directly to a hole in the trachea (Fig. 43-3).

People with complete high tetraplegia are paralyzed from the neck down. These patients require a highly specialized team to stabilize them medically and to prevent further complications, such as respiratory infections and pressure sores. The occupational therapist who works with this population must be comfortable with nursing procedures. These tasks include suctioning (removing secretions from the trachea), manually ventilating the patient with a manual resuscitator (Ambu-bag) and proficiently managing a ventilator (Nead & Hughes, 1997). The rehabilitation team must also be well coordinated, providing the patient and family with care while preparing them for discharge. Patients with high lesions have a myriad of issues to deal with in many domains of their life. It may be surprising to realize that despite seemingly insurmountable obstacles to success, many patients with such lesions live healthy and meaningful lives (Whiteneck et al., 1989).

Some additional roles the therapist may have in treating persons with high cervical injury include teaching them to direct their own care, helping them select specialized and sophisticated equipment for life support, mobility, and ADL, and training them in the use of mouth sticks, rigid long rods held in the mouth that allow the patient to perform activities such as turning pages, drawing, typing, painting, and playing board games (Fig. 43-3) (Hammell, 1995; Adler, 1989).

The Patient With Lower Cervical Injuries: C5-C8

As in the acute recovery phase, physical intervention includes positioning in bed and in the wheelchair (Fig. 43-4), splinting the upper extremities (see Chapter 15), daily upper extremity range of motion, and strengthening. Strengthening, an important goal in this phase, can be performed by using weights, pulley systems, skateboards, suspension slings, mobile arm supports (discussed later), and modalities such as biofeedback and neuromuscular electrical stimulation (Trombly, 1989) (Chapters 18, 20, and 25).

Patients With C5 Tetraplegia

Initially, the deltoids and biceps, key muscles for this level of injury, are weak, so upper limbs require support to function. The mobile arm support, also called a ball bearing feeder, is a mechanical device attached to the wheelchair. This shoulder–elbow support carries the weight of the arm and reduces friction

in motion (Clark et al., 1997; Wilson et al., 1984). The mobile arm support can assist the patient in driving the wheelchair, feeding, hygiene and grooming, and carrying out tabletop activities, such as writing and cooking (Clark et al.; Zigler et al., 1998). If and when the strength of the deltoids and biceps is 3+/5 or greater and endurance is good, patients can engage in activities without mobile arm supports (Zigler et. al.) (see Chapter 14).

Patients with C5 complete tetraplegia need a way to grasp and hold objects, since their wrists and hands are paralyzed. First, the wrist must be stabilized with a splint or orthosis. Next, a device is attached to the hand to enable the person to perform activities. The universal cuff is a simple, inexpensive utensil holder that rests around the palm (Fig. 43-6). Other U- or C-shaped clamps can be attached to objects such a telephone receiver or a shaver. Some splints, devices, and orthoses accommodate the wrist and the hand as a unit. One is the Ratchet wrist–hand orthosis, made of metal and manually controlled. To maximize functional gain with this orthosis, the patient must be carefully trained.

Most patients with C5 tetraplegia can master tabletop activities. However, they lack trunk control and muscles below the shoulder, so they are mostly dependent in dressing and bathing (Appendix 43-1) (Clark et al., 1997; Zigler et al., 1998). With adequate emotional and financial resources persons with C5 tetraplegia engage in meaningful, productive activities. Case in

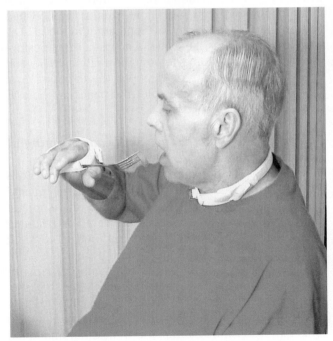

Figure 43-6 A person with C5 complete tetraplegia using a universal cuff.

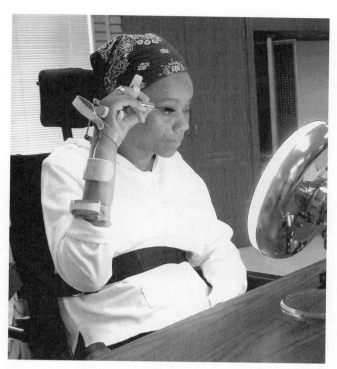

Figure 43-7 A person with C6 complete tetraplegia using the wrist-driven wrist–hand orthosis.

point: Mr. L. is a financial consultant who lives on his own and has part-time attendants. He lives a busy life full of business trips and leisure activities with friends. He attributes his success to much planning and good organizational skills.

Patients With C6 and C7 Tetraplegia

Patients with C6 and C7 tetraplegia may attain significantly higher levels of independence than the C5 patient. The addition of radial wrist extensors allows patients to close their fingers with a tenodesis grasp. This is a critical functional enhancement, as with it light objects may be picked up, held, and manipulated. The wrist-driven wrist–hand orthosis, or the flexor hinge splint and tenodesis splint, is a metal device that transfers power from the extended wrist to the radial fingers, allowing a stronger pinch (Fig. 43-7) (Clark et al., 1997) (see Chapter 14).

More fully innervated proximal scapular and shoulder muscles, such as the rotator cuff, deltoids, and biceps allow for an increase in upper limb strength and endurance. Patients can also roll in bed, and their arms can cross the midline more forcefully, with the addition of the clavicular pectoralis muscle. The ability to use the triceps, the key muscle for C7 tetraplegia, allows the patient to reach for objects above head level, such as items on a store shelf; transfer with greater ease; and push a manual wheelchair.

Patients With C8 Tetraplegia

Hand function is significantly improved with the addition of extrinsic finger muscles and thumb flexors. Hand dexterity and strength are limited by the absence of intrinsic finger and thumb muscles. A person with complete C8 tetraplegia grasps objects with the metacarpophalangeal joints in extension and the proximal interphalangeal and distal interphalangeal joints in flexion. This is called a claw hand or intrinsic minus (Formal & Smith, 1996).

Surgical Options for the Upper Extremities

Restoring hand function is the top priority of many individuals with tetraplegia (Moberg, 1978). To improve hand function, persons with C5, C6, or C7 injuries may have surgical options. These options do not provide for a normal hand but aim to restore pinch and grasp. Tendon transfer surgeries are recommended only after full spontaneous motor and sensory recovery has occurred and no earlier than a year after injury, as some of these procedures permanently alter the musculoskeletal structures (Waters et al., 1996).

Reconstructive surgeries, although not performed as frequently as in the 1970s and 1980s, in part because of the cost, are available for increasing motion and function of the upper extremities. Upper limb reconstructive surgeries may shorten or change the direction of pull of tendons of passive (paralyzed) muscles to provide a mechanical advantage to the thumb or fingers. Other common procedures may entail tendon transfers of functioning muscles. Typically, a proximal functional muscle with strength of 4/5 or above is attached to a tendon of a distal paralyzed muscle. Following the surgery, the patient learns to contract a proximal muscle to move a distal joint (Waters et al., 1996). An example of a hand tendon transfer surgery is the brachioradialis to flexor pollicis longus. This surgery restores lateral pinch by attaching the tendon of a strong (4/5 muscle or above) brachioradialis to a paralyzed flexor pollicis longus. To pinch an object, the patient flexes the elbow while the forearm is in pronation. To improve the stability of the thumb the interphalangeal joint is fused.

The preoperative and postoperative evaluation, education, wound care, and muscle reeducation must be carried out by an experienced therapist. Additionally, consistent communication with the operating physician is vital for favorable outcomes.

A select number of centers worldwide offer a relatively new and complex procedure for achieving hand function. A hand grasp neuroprosthesis, a permanently implanted electrical stimulation system, allows the person with C5-C6 injury to open and close the hand by moving the opposite shoulder. This electrical device is composed of eight electrodes implanted into various muscles; electrode leads; transmitter; and a shoulder sensor. An external controller box on the wheelchair controls the device remotely with no connecting wires. Often the neuroprosthesis surgery is either combined with or follows other hand surgeries that allow for optimal use of the device (Kilgore et al., 1997).

The Patient With Paraplegia

Most people with complete or incomplete paraplegia are independent in self-maintenance, self-enhancement, and self-advancement roles, though they require assistance with heavy housekeeping and physically demanding vocational pursuits (Consortium for Spinal Cord Medicine, 1999). Paraplegics with injuries at T10 and below may attain skills more easily and rapidly than patients with higher injuries. Good trunk control enables a person with low paraplegia to bend down and from side to side without fear of falling forward. Skills performed while upright (e.g., bowel management, lower body dressing, undressing, and bathing) require the patient with a higher injury to secure the trunk by supporting the body with one arm while performing the activity with the other, to prevent falls (Zigler et al., 1998).

Typically, patients with paraplegia have fewer medical complications than those with tetraplegia, and

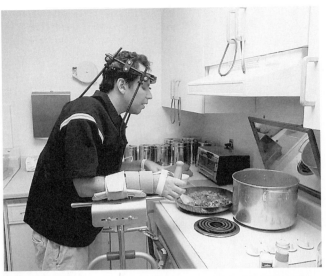

Figure 43-9 A person with ASIA D incomplete tetraplegia cooking while using an arm trough walker. The 8- to 10-pound Halo vest interferes with balance and limits vision.

self-maintenance skills are learned quickly. Thus, the therapist and patient may shift the focus to self-enhancement and self-advancement roles. Community outings are encouraged as soon as possible to facilitate early integration and participation (Zigler et al., 1998; Figure 43-8).

The Ambulatory Patient: Incomplete Paraplegia and Tetraplegia

Typically when we think of spinal cord injuries, we picture a person using a wheelchair. Yet many individuals with incomplete SCI are able to walk (Fig. 43-9). Data shows that there has been an increase in incomplete injuries in the United States in recent decades (Stover et al., 1995). This positive trend brings with it some unique challenges to the patient and occupational therapist.

For expedient and relevant treatment planning, the occupational therapist must clearly understand ambulation goals soon after admission. Early discussion with the physical therapist helps clarify goals and enables the occupational therapist to outline a treatment course that takes walking into consideration. Answers to the following questions guide treatment planning:

1. Will upper extremity aids be needed to assist in walking (e.g., a forearm trough walker)? If so, how will the patient carry objects if both hands are occupied?
2. What lower extremity braces are needed? Will the patient require assistance in donning and doffing the braces?

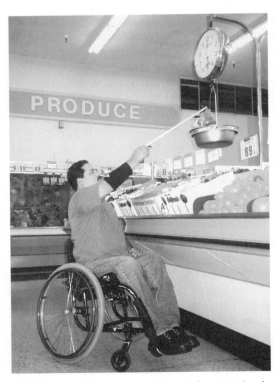

Figure 43-8 A person with paraplegia using a reacher to retrieve hard-to-reach items on a shopping outing.

3. Is the goal walking short distances only? Will the patient need a wheelchair for mobility in the community?

Not surprisingly, ambulatory patients with tetraplegia pose the greatest challenge with their often weak upper extremities. In the wheelchair, equipment such as lapboards, armrests, and mobile arm supports support weak arms and allow for function. When upper limb proximal muscles are weak, hand function becomes difficult or impossible, since the patient lacks a mechanism for bringing the hand to the mouth or face. Various solutions depend on the pattern of upper extremity muscle strength (e.g., a table or a chair mounted mobile arm support). Frequently, however, these solutions are less than optimal.

Concomitant Brain Injury and Cognitive Deficits

Much attention is given to the visible paralysis of the injured patient, while less visible traumatic brain injury may be overlooked and unattended to (Zejdlik, 1991). However, if we think about the velocity of the body at the time of impact in injuries such as motor vehicle accidents and falls, it becomes apparent that head injuries are common. The percentage of patients who suffer concomitant injuries to the brain and spinal cord may be as high as 40 to 50% (Davidoff et al., 1992). These injuries may be diffuse or focal and mild or severe (Zejdlik, 1991). As Chapter 39 is solely devoted to traumatic brain injury, the discussion here is limited to elements that are unique to the dual diagnosis.

The occupational therapist must be vigilant for clues of brain injury in the first encounters with the patient. A period of unconsciousness and posttraumatic amnesia raises a red flag. Therapists should ask patients directly whether they have trouble remembering events or sense any changes in their thinking. However, patients may lack insight. The family often is an excellent source of information, as they usually know the premorbid cognitive status of the patient. The evaluation of the patient is made more challenging with factors such as fatigue, medication side effects, pain, depression, sleep deprivation, and sensory deprivation (Davidoff et al., 1992). A formal screening can determine whether consultation with a communication specialist is indicated. It is common in many hospitals to request such consultations automatically if the patient had any period of unconsciousness or posttraumatic amnesia.

Cognitive deficits in the SCI population may not be limited to those incurred as a result of the injury. Factors such as previous head injuries, learning disabilities, and a history of alcohol and drug abuse are often present,

and they affect the patient's cognitive functioning (Davidoff et al., 1992). The effects of a mild brain injury associated with SCI may diminish over time; however, the prognosis for recovering from a preexisting cognitive deficit is poor (Davidoff et al.).

Transitions: Restoring Roles at Home and in the Community

The dramatic decrease in length of stay has had some negative consequences. More people now require rehospitalizations, and more are being discharged to skilled nursing facilities (Eastwood et al., 1999). To ease the transition from the hospital to the community, the occupational therapist assumes two primary roles: advocate and service provider.

Advocacy

The therapist must be prepared to articulate and document the need for longer hospitalization when the length of stay is inappropriately short and may jeopardize the safety of the patient. The therapist may also be called upon to find resources that allow the patient to continue to receive care and engage in occupations following discharge. Often the patient is referred to an outpatient clinic to continue treatment. With the help of the social worker, liaison nurse or case manager, the therapist can minimize barriers to receiving therapy after discharge. A frequent barrier is lack of transportation. If patients cannot leave home, an agency such as the Visiting Nurses Association may provide occupational therapy services at home for a limited time. Other transitional services, such as support groups and transitional living centers, must be identified. Transitional living centers provide an excellent opportunity to restore competence in desired roles. Unfortunately, such facilities are few and are not adequately funded, despite their documented savings in costs (Hammell, 1995; Trieschmann, 1988).

Service Provision

Most patients continue to gain strength during the first year after their injury and long after their discharge from the acute rehabilitation facility (Waters & Yoshida, 1996). This increase in strength may allow the patient to become more independent. Outpatient programs teach patients to use new movement and offer intensive ADL training. As patients gain strength and endurance and improve their balance, they should be encouraged to reassess and reorder their goals. For example, a patient who once could not carry out a bowel program but who later exhibits normal strength in manual muscle testing of the triceps and latissimus dorsi can begin bowel training.

Customized orthoses, such as the wrist-driven wrist–hand orthosis, are commonly given to the patient soon before discharge because production and adjustment of orthoses require much time. Therefore, orthotic training often begins during the last days of hospitalization and continues during outpatient visits to ensure good fit and use. Outpatient evaluation and training in the use of other equipment is beneficial because the patient and family can use these devices at home immediately.

The outpatient occupational therapist should begin and/or continue working on goals and skills that move the patient toward greater community integration (e.g., driving and vocational evaluation and training). The outpatient education of family members and attendants must continue to assure continuity and progress.

Adaptation: Focus on Facilitation Toward Full Participation

The path from being a dependent patient to becoming a person with a sense of efficacy and self-esteem is long and individual. The occupational therapist must encourage persons with SCI to develop competencies and satisfaction in life roles (Trombly, 1995). While some laws (e.g., Americans with Disabilities Act) aim to encourage individuals with SCI to participate fully in all societal roles, many barriers continue to hinder full participation. The unemployment rate of individuals with SCI is significantly higher than in the general population, and income is lower (Krause et al., 1999).

Yerxa and Baum (1990) studied the pattern of engagement in daily occupations and quality of life among people with SCI. They found that people with SCI had much more free time than their undisabled counterparts. Other studies show that life satisfaction was not related to the level of injury but to social integration, access to the environment, and occupation (Richards et al., 1999). These studies heighten the importance of looking beyond treating impairments and analyzing the daily activities of each individual, revealing meanings of these activities and promoting them.

Occupational therapy literature emphasizes the role of the occupational therapist in helping individuals with SCI analyze their daily life, find solutions to simplify daily routines, and engage in experiential creative problem solving in the community (Hammell, 1995). This occupational therapy role is yet to be fully practiced, since models for independent living are few and only a few of those employ occupational therapists. To fill this role, we must seek work in group homes and governmental agencies and rely less on traditional hospital-based employment. We must also engage in shaping public policy (Baum, 2000).

Summary Review Questions

1. List three key epidemiological factors of the SCI population and describe how these factors influence evaluation and treatment.
2. List three precautions the therapist must consider in planning for an outing with a patient with C5 injury.
3. What is a tenodesis grasp? Why is it important, and how can the occupational therapist facilitate it?
4. List five parts of the initial occupational therapy evaluation of a patient with SCI.
5. Describe a typical feeding setup for a C5 tetraplegic patient.
6. What are the functional expectations for the patient with a C7 injury?
7. You read in the medical chart that a patient lost consciousness at the time of injury. How do you modify your evaluation? Describe how concomitant brain injury may alter your treatment goals and interventions.
8. What are the roles of the occupational therapist in the transition phase?

Acknowledgments

I thank my husband, Richard Atkins, for his assistance in editing this chapter and for countless hours of meaningfully occupying the kids. I also thank the patients and staff at Rancho Los Amigos National Rehabilitation Center, who have inspired and taught me so much over the years. Last, I thank the photographer, Paul Weinreich.

Resources

Information for Patients, Families, and Clinicians Available From Paralyzed Veterans of America (PVA)

Paralyzed Veterans of America · 801 Eighteenth St., NW, Washington, DC 2006. 800-424-8200. 202-872-1300.
www.pva.org

Hammond, M. C., Umlauf, R. L., Matteson, B., Perduta-Fulginiti, S., (1989) · *Yes, You Can! A guide to self-care for persons with spinal cord injury* (2nd ed.) available form Paralyzed Veterans of America (PVA).

Monthly magazines · *Paraplegia News* and *Sports 'n Spokes*

Consortium for Spinal Cord Medicine publications of clinical practice guidelines available to clinicians and consumers · Free guides for people with SCI. Booklets cover topics such as depression, autonomic dysreflexia, and bowel management.

Other Spinal Cord Injury Organizations

American Paralysis Association · 500 Morris Ave., Springfield, NJ 07081. 800-225-0292. 201-379-2690. Hotline 800-526-3456.
www.apacure.com

National Spinal Cord Injury Association · 8701 Georgia Ave., Suite 500, Silver Spring, MD 20910. 800-962-9629. 301-588-6959. www.spinalcord.org

Spinal Cord Injury Network International · 3911 Princeton Dr., Santa Rosa, CA 95405-7013. 800-548-2673. 707-577-8796. Fax 707-577-0605. www.sonic.net/~spinal/

Christopher Reeve Paralysis Foundation · 500 Morris Ave., Springfield, NJ 07081.

Other Sources

Accent on Living · P. O. Box 700, Bloomington, IL 61702. 800-787-8444. *How to Live with a Spinal Cord Injury*

Spinal Network · S. Maddox, Boulder, CO. *Spinal Network: The Total Resource for the Wheelchair Community* (1991).

Louis Calder Memorial Library and University of Miami School of Medicine · WWW Internet Manual. PionTIS. http:/calder.med.miami.edu/pointis

Statistical Data

National Spinal Cord Injury Statistical Center · 1717 6th Ave. South, Room 544, Birmingham, AL 35233-7330. 205-934-3320. Fax 205-934-2709. www.NSCISC@sun.rehabm.uab.edu

Facts and Figures at a Glance www.spinalcord.uab.edu

Publications

New Mobility www.newmobility.com

Paralinks paralinks.net/contents.html

Videos

Rancho Los Amigos Research and Education Institute · *Starting Over* (Parts 1–3). Downey, CA: Author.

Rehabilitation Institute of Chicago. (1990) · *Challenged life: Spinal Cord Injury*. Chicago: Author.

For more complete information on resources:

National Rehabilitation Information Center. (1996) · Spinal Cord Injury: A NARIC Resource Guide for People with SCI and Their Families. *Occupational Therapy in Health Care, 10* (1), 69–83.

References

Adler, C. (1996). Spinal Cord Injury. In Pedretti, L. W. (ed.), *Occupational Therapy: Practice Skills for Physical Dysfunction* (pp. 765–784). St. Louis: Mosby.

Adler, C. (1989). Equipment considerations. In G. Whiteneck, D. P. Lammertse, M. Scott, & R. Mentor (Eds.), *The Management of High Quadriplegia* (pp. 207–231). New York: Demos.

American Spinal Injury Association [ASIA]. (2000). *International Standards For Neurological Classification of Spinal Injury Patients*. Chicago: Author.

Baum, C. (2000). Occupation-based practice: Reinventing ourselves for the new millennium. *OT Practice, 1* (3), 12–15.

Becker, B. E., & DeLisa, J. A. (1999). Model Spinal Cord Injury System trends, and implications for the future. *Archives of Physical Medicine and Rehabilitation, 80*, 1514–1521.

Clark, D. R., Waters, R. L., & Baumgarten, J. M. (1997). Upper limb orthoses for the spinal cord injured patients. In B. Goldberg & J. D. Hsu (Eds.), *Atlas of Orthoses and Assistive Devices* (3rd ed., pp. 291–303). St. Louis: Mosby.

Consortium for Spinal Cord Medicine (1997a). *Acute Management of Autonomic Dysreflexia: Adults With Spinal Cord Injury Presenting to Health care Facilities*. Washington: Paralyzed Veterans of America.

Consortium for Spinal Cord Medicine (1997b). *Prevention of Thromboembolism in Spinal Cord injury: Clinical Practice Guidelines*. Washington: Paralyzed Veterans of America.

Consortium for Spinal Cord Medicine (1998a). *Depression Following Spinal Cord Injury: A Clinical Practice Guideline*. Washington: Paralyzed Veterans of America.

Consortium for Spinal Cord Medicine (1998b). *Neurogenic Bowel Management in Adults With Spinal Cord Injury: Clinical Practice Guidelines*. Washington: Paralyzed Veterans of America.

Consortium for Spinal Cord Medicine (1999). *Outcome Following Traumatic Spinal Cord Injury: Clinical Practice Guidelines for Health care Professionals*. Washington: Paralyzed Veterans of America.

Curtin, M. (1999). An analysis of tetraplegic hand grips. *British Journal of Occupational Therapy, 62* (10), 444–450.

Curtis, K. A., Tyner, T. M., Zachary, L., Lentell, G., Brink, D., Didyk, T., Gean, K., Hall, J., Hooper, M., Klos, J., Lesina, S., & Pacillas, B. (1999). Effect of a standard exercise protocol on shoulder pain in long-term wheelchair users. *Spinal Cord, 37*, 421–429.

Cushman, L .A., & Dijkers, M. (1990). Depressed mood in spinal cord injured patients: Staff perceptions and patient realities. *Archives of Physical Medicine and Rehabilitation, 71*, 191–196.

Davidoff, G. N., Roth, E. J., & Richards, J. S. (1992). Cognitive deficits in spinal cord injury: Epidemiology and outcome. *Archives of Physical Medicine and Rehabilitation, 73*, 275–284.

DeVivo, M. J., Krause, J. S., Lammertse, D. P. (1999). Recent trends in mortality and causes of death among persons with spinal cord injury. *Archives of Physical Medicine and Rehabilitation. 80*, 1411–1419.

DeVivo, M. J., & Stover, S. L. (1995). Long-term survival and causes of death. In S. L. Stover, J. A. Dehisha, & G. Whiteneck (Eds.), *Spinal Cord Injury: Clinical Outcomes From the Model Systems* (pp. 289–316). Gaithersburg, MD: Aspen.

Ducharme, S. H., & Gill, K. M. (1997). *Sexuality After Spinal Cord Injury*. Baltimore: Paul H. Brookes.

Eastwood, E. A., Hagglund, K. J., Ragnarsson, K. T., Gordon, W. A., & Marino, R. J. (1999). Medical rehabilitation length of stay and outcomes for persons with traumatic spinal cord injury—1990-1997. *Archives of Physical Medicine and Rehabilitation, 80*, 1457–1463.

Fairholm, D. (1991). Managing pain. In C. P. Zejdlik (Ed.), *Management of Spinal Cord Injury* (2nd ed., pp. 593–601). Boston: Jones & Bartlett.

Ford, J. R., & Duckworth, B. (1987). *Physical Management for the Quadriplegic Patient* (2nd ed.). Philadelphia: Davis.

Formal, C., & Smith, J. (1996). Upper extremity function in spinal cord injury. *Topics in Spinal Cord Injury Rehabilitation, 1* (4), 1–13.

Fuhrer, M. R., Rintala, D. H., Hart, K. A., Clearman, R., & Young, M. E. (1993). Depressive symptomatology in persons with spinal cord injury who reside in a community. *Archives of Physical Medicine and Rehabilitation, 74*, 255–260.

Garland, D. E. (1991). A clinical perspective on common forms of acquired heterotopic ossification. *Clinical Orthopaedics and Related Research, 242*, 169–176.

Gerhart, K. A., Bergstrom, E., Charlifue, S. W., Menter, R. R., & Whiteneck, G. G. (1993). Long-term spinal cord injury: Functional changes over time. *Archives of Physical Medicine and Rehabilitation, 74*, 1030–1034.

Gersham, G. E., Labi, M. I., Dittmar, S. S., Hicks, J. T., Joyce, S. Z., & Phillips Stehlik, M. A. (1986). The Quadriplegia Index of Function (QIF): Sensitivity and reliability demonstrated in a study of thirty quadriplegic patients. *Paraplegia, 24*, 38–44.

Hammell, K. W. (1995). *Spinal Cord Injury Rehabilitation.* Suffolk, UK: Chapman & Hall.

Hill, J. (1986). Spinal cord injury: A guide to functional outcomes in occupational therapy. Rockville, MD: Aspen.

Hollar, L. D. (1995). Spinal cord injury. In C. A. Trombly (Ed.), Occupational Therapy for Physical Dysfunction (4th ed., pp. 795–813). Baltimore: Williams & Wilkins.

Jackson, A. B., & Wadley, V. (1999). A multicenter study of women's self-reported reproductive health after spinal cord injury. *Archives of Physical Medicine and Rehabilitation, 80*, 1420–1428.

Kendall, F. P., MeCreary, E. K., & Provance, P. G. (1993). *Muscles: Testing and Function* (4th ed.) Baltimore: Williams & Wilkins.

Kilgore, K. L., Peckham, P. H., Keith, M. W., Thrope, G. B., Woulle, K. S., Bryden, A. M., & Hart, R. L. (1997). An implanted upper-extremity neuroprosthesis. *Journal of Bone and Joint Surgery, 79-A*, 533–541.

Kirshblaum, S. C., Gulati, M., O'Conner, K. C., & Voorman, S. J. (1998). Bowel care practices in chronic spinal cord injury patients. *Archives of Physical Medicine and Rehabilitation, 79*, 20–23.

Krause, J. S., Kenman, D., DeVivo, M. J., Maynard, F., Coker, J., Roach, M. J., Ducharme, S. (1999). Employment after spinal cord injury: An analysis of cases from the Model Spinal Cord Injury Systems. *Archives of Physical Medicine and Rehabilitation, 80*, 1492–1500.

Livneh, H., & Antonak, R. F. (1997). Psychosocial adaptation to chronic illness and disability. Gaithersburg, MD: Aspen.

Massagli, T. L., & Jaffe, K. M. (1990). Pediatric spinal cord injury: Treatment and outcome. *Pediatrician, 17*, 244-254.

McKinley, W. O., Seel, R. T., & Hardman, J. T. (1999). Nontraumatic spinal cord injury: Incidence, epidemiology, and functional outcome. *Archives of Physical Medicine and Rehabilitation, 80*, 619–623.

Moberg, E. (1978). *The Upper Limb in Tetraplegia.* Stuttgart: Thieme.

National Spinal Cord Injury Statistical Center (2000). *Spinal cord injury: Facts and figures at a Glance.* Birmingham: University of Alabama. www.spinalcord.uab.edu.

Nead, C., & Hughes, M. B. (1997). Patients with spinal cord injuries who are ventilator dependent: The practitioner's role. *Physical Disabilities: Special Interest Section Quarterly, 20*, 4. Bethesda, MD: American Occupational Therapy Association.

Nobunaga, A. I., Go, B. K., & Karunas, R. B. (1999). Recent demographic and injury trends in people served by the Model Spinal Cord Injury Systems. *Archives of Physical Medicine and Rehabilitation, 80*, 1372–1382.

Penrod, L. E., Hegde, S. K., & Ditunno, J. F. (1990). Jr. age effect on prognosis for functional recovery in acute traumatic central cord syndrome (CCS). *Archives of Physical Medicine and Rehabilitation, 71*, 963–968.

Radomski, M. V. (1998). Problem-solving deficits: Using a multidimensional definition to select a treatment approach. *Physical Disabilities: Special Interest Section Quarterly, 21*, 1. Bethesda, MD: American Occupational Therapy Association.

Richards, J. S., Bombardier, C. H., Take, D., Dijkers, M., Gordon, W., Shewchuk, R., & DeVivi, M. J. (1999). Access to the environment and life satisfaction after spinal cord injury. *Archives of Physical Medicine and Rehabilitation, 80*, 1501–1506.

Stover, S. L., Whiteneck, G. G., & DeLisa, J. A. (eds.) (1995). *Spinal Cord Injury: Clinical Outcome from the Model Systems.* Gaithersburg, MD: Aspen.

Smith, Q. W., Frieden, L., Nelson, M. R., & Tilbor, A. G., (1996). Transition to adulthood for young people with spinal cord injury. In R. R. Benz & M. J. Mulcahey (Eds.), *The Child With a Spinal Cord Injury* (pp. 601–612). Rosemont, IL: American Academy of Orthopedic Surgeons.

Teasell, R., & Allatt, D. (1991). Managing the growing number of spinal cord-injured elderly. *Geriatrics, 46* (6), 78–89.

Trieschmann, R. B. (Ed.) (1988). *Spinal Cord Injuries: Psychological, Social and Vocational Rehabilitation* (2nd ed.) New York: Demos.

Trombly, C. A. (Ed.) (1989). Occupational Therapy for Physical Dysfunction (3rd ed.). Baltimore: Williams & Wilkins.

Trombly, C. A. (1995). Theoretical foundations for practice. In C.A. Trombly (ed.), *Occupational Therapy for Physical Dysfunction* (4th ed., pp. 15–20). Baltimore: Williams & Wilkins.

Waters, R. L., Adkins, R. H., Yakura, J. S., & Sie, I. (1995). Recovery following spinal cord injury: A clinician's handbook. Downey, CA: Los Amigos Research and Educational Institute.

Waters, R. L., Sie, I. H., Gellman, H., & Tognella, M. (1996). Functional hand surgery following tetraplegia. *Archives of Physical Medicine and Rehabilitation, 77*, 86–94.

Waters, R. L., & Yoshida, G. M. (1996). Prognosis of spinal cord injuries. In A. M. Levine (Ed.), *Orthopedic Knowledge Update: Trauma* (pp. 303–310). Rosemont, IL: American Academy of Orthopedic Surgeons.

Whiteneck, G. G., Charlifue, S. W., Gerhart, K. A., Lammertse, D. P., Manely, S., Menter, R. R., & Seedroff, K. R. (eds.) (1993). *Aging With Spinal Cord Injury.* New York: Demos.

Whiteneck, G. G., Charlifue, S. W., Gerhart, K. A., Overholser, J. D., & Richardson, G. N. (1992). Quantifying handicap: A new measure of long-term rehabilitation outcomes. *Archives of Physical Medicine and Rehabilitation, 73*, 519–526.

Whiteneck, G. G., Lammertse, D. P., Manley, S., & Mentor, R. (eds.) (1989). The management of high quadriplegia. New York: Demos.

Wilson, D. J., McKenzie, M. W., Barber, L. M., & Watson, K. L. (1984). *Spinal Cord Injury: A Treatment Guide for Occupational Therapists* (2nd ed.). Thorofare, NJ: Slack.

Yarkony, G. M., Roth, E. J., Heinemann, A. W., & Lovell, L. L. (1988). Spinal cord injury rehabilitation outcomes: The impact of age. *Journal of Clinical Epidemiology, 41*, 173–177.

Yarkony, G. M., Roth, E. J., Heinemann, A. W., Wu, Y. C., Katz, R. T., & Lovell, L. (1987). Benefits of rehabilitation for traumatic spinal cord injury: Multivariate analysis in 711 patients. *Archives of Neurology, 44*, 93–96.

Yarkony, G. M., & Chen, D. (1996). Rehabilitation of patients with spinal cord injuries. In R. L. Braddom (Ed.), *Physical Medicine and Rehabilitation*. Philadelphia: Saunders.

Yerxa, E. J., & Baum Locker, S. (1990). Quality of time use by adults with spinal cord injuries. *American Journal of Occupational Therapy, 44*, 318–326.

Zejdlik, C. P. (1991). Management of spinal cord injury (2nd ed.). Boston: Jones & Bartlett.

Zigler, J. E., Atkins, M. S., Resnik, C. D., & Thompson, L. (1998). Rehabilitation. In A. Levine, F. Eismont, S. Garfin, & J. E. Zigler (Eds.), *Spine Trauma* (pp. 585–606). New York: Saunders.

Suggested Reading

American Spinal Injury Association (2000). International Standards for Neurological Classification of Spinal Injury Patients. Chicago: Author.

Consortium for Spinal Cord Medicine (1999). *Outcome Following Traumatic Spinal Cord Injury: Clinical Practice Guidelines for Health care Professionals.* Washington: Paralyzed Veterans of America.

Ford, J. R., & Duckworth, B. (1987). *Physical Management for the Quadriplegic Patient* (2nd ed.). Philadelphia: Davis.

Hammell, K. W. (1995). Spinal cord injury rehabilitation. London: Chapman & Hall.

Hill, J. (1986). *Spinal Cord Injury: A Guide to Functional Outcomes in Occupational Therapy.* Rockville, MD: Aspen.

Maynard, F. M., Bracken, M. B., Creasey, G., Ditunno, J. F., Donovan, W. H., Ducker, T. B., Graber, S. L., Marino, R. J., Stover, S. L., Tator, C. H., Waters, R. L., Wilberger, J. E., & Young, W. (1997). International standards for neurological and functional classification of spinal cord injury. *Spinal Cord, 35,* 266–274.

Reeve, C. (1998). *Still Me.* New York: Ballantine.

Trieshmann, R. B. (Ed.) (1988). *Spinal Cord Injuries: Psychological, Social and Vocational Rehabilitation* (2nd ed.). New York: Demos.

Zejdlik, C. P. (1991). *Management of Spinal Cord Injury* (2nd ed.). Boston: Jones & Bartlett.

Appendix 43-1: Expected Functional Outcomes

Level C1-3

Functionally relevant muscles innervated: Sternocleidomastoid; cervical paraspinal; neck accessories
Movement possible: Neck flexion, extension, rotation
Patterns of weakness: Total paralysis of trunk, upper extremities, lower extremities; dependent on ventilator

FIM/Assistance Data: Exp = Expected FIM Score / **Med** = NSCISC Median / **IR** = NSCISC Interquartile Range
NSCISC Sample Size: FIM=15 / Assist=12

	Expected Functional Outcomes	Equipment	FIM/Assistance Data Exp	Med	IR
Respiratory	• Ventilator dependent • Inability to clear secretions	• 2 ventilators (bedside, portable) • Suction equipment or other suction management device • Generator or battery backup			
Bowel	Total assist	Padded reclining shower–commode chair (if roll-in shower available)	1	1	1
Bladder	Total assist		1	1	1
Bed mobility	Total assist	Full electric hospital bed with Trendelenburg feature and side rails			
Bed, wheelchair transfers	Total assist	• Transfer board • Power or mechanical lift with sling	1	1	1
Pressure relief, positioning	Total assist; may be independent with equipment	• Power recline and/or tilt wheelchair • Wheelchair pressure relief cushion • Postural support and head control devices as indicated • Hand splints may be indicated • Specialty bed or pressure relief mattress may be indicated			
Eating	Total assist		1	1	1
Dressing	Total assist		1	1	1
Grooming	Total assist		1	1	1
Bathing	Total assist	• Hand-held shower • Shampoo tray • Padded reclining shower–commode chair (if roll-in shower available)	1	1	1
Wheelchair propulsion	Manual: Total assist Power: Independent with equipment	• Power recline and/or tilt wheelchair with head, chin, or breath control and manual recliner • Vent tray	6	1	1–6
Standing, ambulation	Standing: Total assist; Ambulation: Not indicated				
Communication	Total assist to independent, depending on workstation setup and equipment availability	• Mouth stick, high-tech computer access, environmental control unit • Adaptive devices everywhere as indicated			
Transportation	Total assist	Attendant-operated van (e.g., lift, tie-downs) or accessible public transportation			
Homemaking	Total assist				
Assist required	• 24-hour attendant care to include homemaking • Able to instruct in all aspects of care		24*	24*	12–24*

*Hours per day

Expected Functional Outcomes (continued)

Level C4

Functionally relevant muscles innervated: Upper trapezius; diaphragm; cervical paraspinal muscles
Movement possible: Neck flexion, extension, rotation; scapular elevation; inspiration
Patterns of weakness: Paralysis of trunk, upper extremities, lower extremities; inability to cough, endurance and respiratory reserve low secondary to paralysis of intercostals

FIM/Assistance Data: Exp = Expected FIM Score / **Med** = NSCISC Median / **IR** = NSCISC Interquartile Range
NSCISC Sample Size: FIM=28 / Assist=12

	Expected Functional Outcomes	Equipment	FIM/Assistance Data Exp	Med	IR
Respiratory	May be able to breathe without a ventilator	If not ventilator free, see C1–3 for equipment requirements			
Bowel	Total assist	Reclining shower–commode chair (if roll-in shower available)	1	1	1
Bladder	Total assist		1	1	1
Bed mobility	Total assist	Full electric hospital bed with Trendelenburg feature and side rails			
Bed, wheelchair transfers	Total assist	• Transfer board • Power or mechanical lift with sling	1	1	1
Pressure relief, positioning	Total assist; may be independent with equipment	• Power recline and/or tilt wheelchair • Wheelchair pressure relief cushion • Postural support and head control devices as indicated • Hand splints may be indicated • Specialty bed or pressure relief mattress may be indicated			
Eating	Total assist		1	1	1
Dressing	Total assist		1	1	1
Grooming	Total assist		1	1	1
Bathing	Total assist	• Shampoo tray • Hand-held shower • Padded reclining shower–commode chair (if roll-in shower available)	1	1	1
Wheelchair propulsion	Power: Independent Manual: Total assist	• Power recline and/or tilt wheelchair with head, chin, or breath control and manual recliner • Vent tray	6	1	1–6
Standing, ambulation	Standing: Total assist Ambulation: Not usually indicated	• Tilt table • Hydraulic standing table			
Communication	Total assist to independent, depending on workstation setup and equipment availability	Mouth stick, high-tech computer access, environmental control unit			
Transportation	Total assist	Attendant-operated van (e.g., lift, tie-downs) or accessible public transportation			
Homemaking	Total assist				
Assist required	• 24-hour care to include homemaking • Able to instruct in all aspects of care		24*	24*	16–24*

*Hours per day.

Expected Functional Outcomes (continued)

Level C5

Functionally relevant muscles innervated: Deltoid, biceps, brachialis, brachioradialis, rhomboids, serratus anterior (partially innervated)
Movement possible: Shoulder flexion, abduction, and extension; elbow flexion and supination; scapular adduction and abduction
Patterns of weakness: Absence of elbow extension, pronation, all wrist and hand movement; total paralysis of trunk and lower extremities

FIM/Assistance Data: Exp = Expected FIM Score / **Med** = NSCISC Median / **IR** = NSCISC Interquartile Range
NSCISC Sample Size: FIM=41 / Assist=35

	Expected Functional Outcomes	Equipment	FIM/Assistance Data Exp	Med	IR
Respiratory	Low endurance and vital capacity secondary to paralysis of intercostals; may require assist to clear secretions				
Bowel	Total assist	Padded shower, commode chair or padded transfer tub bench with commode cutout	1	1	1
Bladder	Total assist	Adaptive devices may be indicated (electric leg bag emptier)	1	1	1
Bed mobility	Some assist	• Full electric hospital bed with Trendelenburg feature with patient's control • Side rails			
Bed, wheelchair transfers	Total assist	• Transfer board • Power or mechanical lift	1	1	1
Pressure relief, positioning	Independent with equipment	• Power recline and/or tilt wheelchair • Wheelchair pressure relief cushion • Hand splints • Specialty bed or pressure relief mattress may be indicated • Postural support devices			
Eating	Total assist for setup, then independent eating with equipment	• Long opponens splint • Adaptive devices as indicated	5	5	2.5–5.5
Dressing	Lower extremity: Total assist Upper extremity: Some assist	• Long opponens splint • Adaptive devices as indicated	1	1	1–4
Grooming	Some to total assist	• Long opponens splints • Adaptive devices as indicated	1–3	1	1–5
Bathing	Total assist	• Padded tub transfer bench or shower–commode chair • Hand-held shower	1	1	1–3
Wheelchair propulsion	Power: Independent Manual: Independent to some assist indoors on uncarpeted, level surface; some to total assist outdoors	Power: Power recline and/or tilt with arm drive control Manual: Lightweight rigid or folding frame with hand rim modifications	6	6	5–6
Standing, ambulation	Total assist	Hydraulic standing frame			
Communication	Independent to some assist after setup with equipment	• Long opponens splint • Adaptive devices as needed for page turning, writing, button pushing			
Transportation	Independent with highly specialized equipment; some assist with accessible public transportation; total assist for attendant-operated vehicle	Highly specialized modified van with lift			
Homemaking	Total assist				
Assist required	• Personal care: 10 hours/day • Home care: 6 hours/day • Able to instruct in all aspects of care		16*	23*	10–24*

*Hours per day.

Expected Functional Outcomes (continued)

Level C6

Functionally relevant muscles innervated: Clavicular pectoralis; supinator; extensor carpi radialis longus and brevis; serratus anterior; latissimus dorsi
Movement possible: Scapular protractor; some horizontal adduction, forearm supination, radial wrist extension
Patterns of weakness: Absence of wrist flexion, elbow extension, hand movement; total paralysis of trunk and lower extremities

FIM/Assistance Data: Exp = Expected FIM Score / **Med** = NSCISC Median / **IR** = NSCISC Interquartile Range
NSCISC Sample Size: FIM=43 / Assist=35

	Expected Functional Outcomes	Equipment	FIM/Assistance Data Exp	Med	IR
Respiratory	Low endurance and vital capacity secondary to paralysis of intercostals; may require assist to clear secretions				
Bowel	Some to total assist	• Padded tub bench with commode cutout or padded shower–commode chair • Other adaptive devices as indicated	1–2	1	1
Bladder	Some to total assist with equipment; may be independent with leg bag emptying	Adaptive devices as indicated	1–2	1	1
Bed mobility	Some assist	• Full electric hospital bed • Side rails • Full to king standard bed may be indicated			
Bed, wheelchair transfers	Level: Some assist to independent Uneven: Some to total assist	• Transfer board • Mechanical lift	3	1	1–3
Pressure relief, positioning	Independent with equipment and/or adapted techniques	• Power recline wheelchair • Wheelchair pressure relief cushion • Postural support devices • Pressure relief mattress or overlay may be indicated			
Eating	Independent with or without equipment except cutting, which is total assist	Adaptive devices as indicated (e.g., U-cuff, tenodesis splint, adapted utensils, plate guard)	5–6	5	4–6
Dressing	Independent upper extremity; some to total assist for lower extremities	Adaptive devices as indicated (e.g., button; hook; loops on zippers, pants; socks, Velcro on shoes)	1–3	2	1–5
Grooming	Some assist to independent with equipment	Adaptive devices as indicated (e.g., U-cuff, adapted handles)	3–6	4	2–6
Bathing	Upper body: Independent Lower body: Some to total assist	• Padded tub transfer bench or shower–commode chair • Adaptive devices as needed • Hand-held shower	1–3	1	1–3
Wheelchair propulsion	Power: Independent with standard arm drive on all surfaces Manual: Independent indoors; some to total assist outdoors	Manual: Lightweight rigid or folding frame with modified rims Power: May require power recline or standard upright power wheelchair	6	6	4–6
Standing, ambulation	Standing: Total assist Ambulation: Not indicated	Hydraulic standing frame			
Communication	Independent with or without equipment	Adaptive devices as indicated (e.g., tendenosis splint; writing splint for keyboard use, button pushing, page turning, object manipulation)			
Transportation	Independent driving from wheelchair	• Modified van with lift • Sensitized hand controls • Tie-downs			
Homemaking	Some assist with light meal preparation; total assist for all other homemaking	Adaptive devices as indicated			
Assist required	• Personal care: 6 hours/day • Home care: 4 hours/day		10*	17*	8–24*

*Hours per day.

Expected Functional Outcomes (continued)

Level C7-8

Functionally relevant muscles innervated: Latissimus dorsi; sternal pectoralis; triceps; pronator quadratus; extensor carpi ulnaris; flexor carpi radialis; flexor digitorum profundus and superficialis; extensor communis; pronator/flexor/extensor/ abductor pollicis; lumbricals [partially innervated]
Movement possible: Elbow extension; ulnar/wrist extension; wrist flexion; finger flexions and extensions; thumb flexion/extension/abduction
Patterns of weakness: Paralysis of trunk and lower extremities; limited grasp release and dexterity secondary to partial intrinsic muscles of the hand

FIM/Assistance Data: Exp = Expected FIM Score / **Med** = NSCISC Median / **IR** = NSCISC Interquartile Range
NSCISC Sample Size: FIM=43 / Assist=35

	Expected Functional Outcomes	Equipment	FIM/Assistance Data Exp	Med	IR
Respiratory	Low endurance and vital capacity secondary to paralysis of intercostals; may require assist to clear secretions				
Bowel	Some to total assist	• Padded tub bench with commode cutout or shower–commode chair • Adaptive devices as needed	1–4	1	1–4
Bladder	Independent to some assist	Adaptive devices as indicated	2–6	3	1–6
Bed mobility	Independent to some assist	Full electric hospital bed or full to king standard bed			
Bed, wheelchair transfers	Level: Independent. Uneven: Independent to some assist	With or without transfer board	3–7	4	2–6
Pressure relief, positioning	Independent	• Wheelchair pressure relief cushion • Postural support devices as indicated • Pressure relief mattress or overlay may be indicated			
Eating	Independent	Adaptive devices as indicated	6–7	6	5–7
Dressing	Independent upper extremities; independent to some assist lower extremities	Adaptive devices as indicated	4–7	6	4–7
Grooming	Independent	Adaptive devices as indicated	6–7	6	4–7
Bathing	Upper body: Independent Lower extremity: Some assist to independent	• Padded transfer tub bench or shower–commode chair • Hand-held shower • Adaptive devices as needed	3–6	4	2–6
Wheelchair propulsion	Manual: Independent all indoor surfaces and level outdoor terrain; some assist with uneven terrain	Manual: Rigid or folding lightweight or folding wheelchair with modified rims	6	6	6
Standing, ambulation	Standing: Independent to some assist Ambulation: Not indicated	Hydraulic or standard standing frame			
Communication	Independent	Adaptive devices as indicated			
Transportation	Independent car if independent with transfer, wheelchair loading and unloading; independent driving modified van from captain's seat	• Modified vehicle • Transfer board			
Homemaking	Independent light meal preparation and homemaking; some to total assist for complex meal prep and heavy housecleaning	Adaptive devices as indicated			
Assist required	• Personal care: 6 hours/day • Home care: 2 hours/day		8*	12*	2–24*

*Hours per day.

Expected Functional Outcomes (continued)   **Level T1–9**

Functionally relevant muscles innervated: Intrinsics of the hand including thumbs; internal and external intercostals; erector spinae; lumbricals; flexor/extensor/abductor pollicis
Movement possible: Upper extremities fully intact; limited upper trunk stability. Endurance increased secondary innervation of intercostals
Patterns of weakness: Lower trunk paralysis. Total paralysis lower extremities

FIM/Assistance Data: Exp = Expected FIM Score / **Med** = NSCISC Median / **IR** = NSCISC Interquartile Range
NSCISC Sample Size: FIM=144 / Assist=122

	Expected Functional Outcomes	Equipment	FIM/Assistance Data Exp	Med	IR
Respiratory	Compromised vital capacity and endurance				
Bowel	Independent	Elevated padded toilet seat or padded tub bench with commode cutout	6–7	6	4–6
Bladder	Independent		6	6	5–6
Bed mobility	Independent	Full to king standard bed			
Bed, wheelchair transfers	Independent	May or may not require transfer board	6–7	6	6–7
Pressure relief, positioning	Independent	• Wheelchair pressure relief cushion • Postural support devices as indicated • Pressure relief mattress or overlay may be indicated			
Eating	Independent		7	7	7
Dressing	Independent		7	7	7
Grooming	Independent		7	7	7
Bathing	Independent	• Padded tub transfer bench or shower–commode chair • Hand-held shower	6–7	6	5–7
Wheelchair propulsion	Independent	Manual rigid or folding lightweight wheelchair	6	6	6
Standing, ambulation	Standing: Independent Ambulation: Typically not functional	Standing frame			
Communication	Independent				
Transportation	Independent in car, including loading and unloading wheelchair	Hand controls			
Homemaking	Independent with complex meal prep and light housecleaning; total to some assist with heavy housekeeping				
Assist required	Homemaking: 3 hours/day		2*	3*	0–15*

*Hours per day.

Expected Functional Outcomes (continued)

Level T10–L1

Functionally relevant muscles innervated: Fully intact intercostals; external obliques; rectus abdominis
Movement possible: Good trunk stability
Patterns of weakness: Paralysis of lower extremities

FIM/Assistance Data: Exp = Expected FIM Score / **Med** = NSCISC Median / **IR** = NSCISC Interquartile Range
NSCISC Sample Size: FIM=71 / Assist=57

	Expected Functional Outcomes	Equipment	FIM/Assistance Data Exp	Med	IR
Respiratory	Intact respiratory function				
Bowel	Independent	Padded standard or raised padded toilet seat	6–7	6	6
Bladder	Independent		6	6	6
Bed mobility	Independent	Full to king standard bed			
Bed, wheelchair transfers	Independent		7	7	6–7
Pressure relief, positioning	Independent	• Wheelchair pressure relief cushion • Postural support devices as indicated • Pressure relief mattress or overlay may be indicated			
Eating	Independent		7	7	7
Dressing	Independent		7	7	7
Grooming	Independent		7	7	7
Bathing	Independent	• Padded transfer tub bench • Hand-held shower	6–7	6	6–7
Wheelchair propulsion	Independent all indoor and outdoor surfaces	Manual rigid or folding lightweight wheelchair	6	6	6
Standing, ambulation	Standing: Independent Ambulation: Functional, some assist to independent	• Standing frame • Forearm crutches or walker • Knee, ankle, foot orthesis			
Communication	Independent				
Transportation	Independent in car, including loading and unloading wheelchair	Hand controls			
Homemaking	Independent with complex meal prep and light housecleaning; some assist with heavy housekeeping				
Assist required	Homemaking: 2 hours/day		2*	2*	0–8*

*Hours per day.

Expected Functional Outcomes (continued)   **Level L2–S5**

Functionally relevant muscles innervated: Fully intact abdominals and all other trunk muscles; depending on level, some degree of hip flexors, extensors, abductors, adductors; knee flexors, extensors; ankle dorsi-flexors, plantar flexors.
Movement possible: Good trunk stability. Partial to full control lower extremities.
Patterns of weakness: Partial paralysis lower extremities, hips, knees, ankle, foot

FIM/Assistance Data: Exp = Expected FIM Score / **Med** = NSCISC Median / **IR** = NSCISC Interquartile Range
NSCISC Sample Size: FIM=20 / Assist=16

	Expected Functional Outcomes	Equipment	FIM/Assistance Data Exp	Med	IR
Respiratory	Intact function				
Bowel	Independent	Padded toilet seat	6–7	6	6–7
Bladder	Independent		6	6	6–7
Bed Mobility	Independent				
Bed/Wheelchair Transfers	Independent	Full to king standard bed	7	7	7
Pressure Relief/ Positioning	Independent	• Wheelchair pressure-relief cushion • Postural support device as indicated			
Eating	Independent		7	7	7
Dressing	Independent		7	7	7
Grooming	Independent		7	7	7
Bathing	Independent	• Padded tub bench • Handheld shower	7	7	6–7
Wheelchair Propulsion	Independent on all indoor and outdoor surfaces	Manual rigid or folding lightweight wheelchair	6	6	6
Standing/ Ambulation	Standing: Independent Ambulation: Functional, independent to some assist	• Standing frame • Knee-ankle-foot orthosis or ankle-foot orthosis • Forearm crutches or cane as indicated			
Communication	Independent				
Transportation	Independent in car, including loading and unloading wheelchair	Hand controls			
Homemaking	Independent complex cooking and light housekeeping; some assist with heavy housekeeping				
Assist Required	Homemaking: 0–1 hour/day		0–1*	0*	0–2*

*Hours per day.

44

Rheumatoid Arthritis and Osteoarthritis

Y. Lynn Yasuda

After studying this chapter, the reader will be able to do the following:

1. Describe the differences between rheumatoid arthritis and osteoarthritis.
2. Identify joint problems and other clinical sequelae that interfere with meeting occupational functioning goals.
3. Select assessments to optimize occupational functioning for patients with RA and OA.
4. Describe interventions to enable patients to meet their occupational functioning goals.
5. Identify preventive interventions to enable prolonged continuance of desired occupational goals.

*A*lthough there are more than 100 rheumatic diseases, this chapter focuses on only rheumatoid arthritis (RA) and osteoarthritis (OA) because they are the most common rheumatic diseases encountered in an occupational therapy clinic. Both can be disabling and both require intervention to allow optimal occupational functioning. Other rheumatic diseases may have some symptoms similar to RA or OA, and the principles used to manage these two diseases can also be used when encountering others. However, because each rheumatic disease has unique manifestations, occupational therapists must address the unique symptoms as well.

GLOSSARY

Crepitus—Grating, crunching, or cracking sound or sensation during joint or tendon motion.

Energy conservation—Process of saving energy and improving distribution of energy over the time needed to use it (Gerber, 1985)

Joint tenderness—Degree of a patient's discomfort when pressure is applied directly on the joint line.

Joint protection methods—Methods to reduce external stress applied to impaired joints.

Lag—Difference of active ROM subtracted from passive ROM, measured in degrees.

Morning stiffness—Subjective complaint of local or general lack of easy mobility of the joints upon arising. This is a non-specific indication of inflammation in RA; duration is directly proportional to the severity of the inflammatory process. Complaints vary from none to many hours. Patients with OA may also complain of morning stiffness, but it tends to be milder and brief.

Rheumatoid nodules—Firm, usually painless lumps of variable size found in patients with RA. They can be found over areas that are subject to mechanical trauma (e.g. elbows, heels, and hand) and on finger flexor and extensor tendons.

Rheumatoid Arthritis (RA)

RA is a systemic disease that affects joints and sometimes the major organs of the body. Early symptoms include symmetrical polyarticular joint pain and inflammation that persists more than 60 days, **morning stiffness** that may last for several hours after arising, malaise, and fatigue. Primary changes associated with inflammation are **joint tenderness** and swelling. Most patients note swelling and tenderness in at least three joints, including at least one hand joint. Early radiographs show minimal changes. Over long periods, joint tenderness and swelling may improve while progressive deformity and disability develop. Disease progression results in joint space narrowing as a result of cartilage destruction and erosion. Further progression may result in radiographic evidence of joint malalignment. More than half of patients with RA develop radiographic abnormalities within 2 years of onset (Anderson, 1993; Arnett et al., 1988; Pincus, 1996; Wilder, 1993). Muscle weakness and neurological abnormalities may also occur.

The cause of RA remains unknown. Extensive efforts to identify an exogenous infectious agent, such as a bacterium, mycobacterium, mycoplasma, fungus, or virus, have been unsuccessful (Pincus, 1996). Any joint may be affected, but those most commonly involved are the second and third metacarpophalangeal (MCP) joints of the hand, second and third proximal interphalangeal (PIP) joints of the hand, metatarsophalangeal joints, wrists, knees, elbows, and less commonly, shoulder, hip, and distal interphalangeal (DIP) joints (Pincus).

Classification criteria for RA suggest that there are at least three types of disease. Type I exhibits a self-limited inflammatory polyarthritis, which often resolves. Type II is characterized by persistent disease that does not lead to significant long-term consequences. Type III is a progressive disease with radiographic changes and decline in function and reported work disability.

Timing for occupational therapy intervention depends on the severity of the disability and whether the patient can meet his or her occupational functioning goals. The American College of Rheumatology (ACR) has developed a classification system for severity of functional disability in RA. This classification, developed to place patients in clinical trials, also reflects the effects of various therapies on function (Hochberg et al., 1992). Because this classification describes function according to levels, it may be useful as a model for treatment planning (Box 44-1).

This classification does not address specific issues or causes of limitations in usual activities of daily living (ADL). However, it provides a general framework to define advancing disability in RA, in which many complex medical, psychosocial, and environmental issues can affect function. The limits of this classification for an occupational therapist include the possibility that patients may overlap in the levels; for example, a person may be working but need assistance in self-care or may be able to continue with avocational skills although advanced disease has limited function in all other areas. Therefore, each person is assessed according to his or her own goals in the context of his or her environment (Yasuda, 2000). For the purposes of this chapter, the classification is used to identify only major issues that require occupational therapy intervention with advancing disability.

Evaluation

In response to a request for services, the occupational therapist reviews the chart, observes and interviews the patient concerning occupational functioning, and may use screening tests to determine whether referral for occupational therapy is indicated. A patient who risks decline in occupational functioning because of pain; fatigue; loss of strength, endurance, or joint range of motion (ROM); change in environment, including social support; or loss of coping skills or whose function may be improved can benefit from occupational therapy (Backman, 1998; Feinberg & Trombly, 1995).

Assessment begins with a semistructured interview, such as an occupational history and/or the *Canadian Occupational Performance Measure (COPM)* to determine areas of occupational functioning that are important to the person and that are at risk or are compromised (Backman, 1998; Law et al., 1994). As initial patient-identified goals are recognized, all subsequent aspects of evaluation are related to finding out whether more detailed occupational functioning deficits or impairment issues exist. Occupational functioning and performance context assessments may include specific ADL evaluations and environmental analyses, including social support and architectural issues, to determine the influence of the environment on the patient's ability to function (Backman, 1998). Common assessments of impairments of abilities and capacities may include but are not limited to ROM evaluation, strength testing, and evaluation of hand deformities, pain, fatigue, and psy-

chosocial status. Sensory evaluation should be done if systemic involvement has led the patient to make complaints that indicate polyneuropathies or nerve compression (Anderson, 1993).

Occupational History

An occupational history provides information in several areas. It can give information about the balance of rest and activity, the meaning and importance of various occupations, the environmental and social supports and/or barriers to performance, the effect of physical limitations on performance, adjustment to disability, and a sense of self-efficacy. This open-ended interview allows the therapist to learn the patient's perspective on occupational functioning in relation to the severity of the physical impairment.

A common method to learn about an individual's occupational history is to ask the patient about his or her typical day. This open-ended description allows the occupational therapist a beginning opportunity to find out about important occupations that the patient may wish to achieve and beginning information about impairment and context issues that affect the performance of these occupations.

Stage of Adjustment to Disability

To identify the patient's goals, the therapist must recognize the patient's response to the impairment issues that the disease has imposed. This helps establish the treatment plan. For example, a person who recognizes that the diagnosis is accurate and who understands and accepts the consequences of the disease process may design goals that can be met immediately, such as finding appropriate adapted equipment to continue working. Another person may not accept the diagnosis and therefore deny that there are any issues, believe that normalcy will soon return, and feel that dependency on others is appropriate. Many authors have defined stages of adjustment to disability. At least 40 theorists have described this phenomenon (Livneh, 1986a, b). Although the models have not been accepted by all psychologists, they have pragmatic value in approaching treatment planning.

The initial stage of adjustment has been called shock. For the person who has been diagnosed with RA, shock may accompany the diagnosis. Since the time between initial symptoms and diagnosis can be weeks, a period of shock in which there is disorganization, disbelief, and inability to attend to incoming information can occur. Treatment planning includes providing support and hope. Intensive education of the patient may not be effective. In the next stage, which some authors call defensive retreat, the patient may ignore symptoms and diagnosis to maintain psychological stability. During

---

BOX 44-1
American College of Rheumatology (ACR) Revised Criteria for Classification of Functional Status in Rheumatoid Arthritis (Hochberg et al., 1992)

Class I
Completely able to perform usual activities of daily living (self-care, vocational, and avocational)[a].

Class II
Able to perform usual self-care and vocational activities but limited in avocational activities.

Class III
Able to perform usual self-care activities but limited in vocational and avocational activities.

Class IV
Limited ability to perform usual self-care, vocational, and avocational activities.

[a]Usual self-care activities include dressing, feeding, bathing, grooming, and toileting. Avocational (self-enhancement roles) and vocational (self-advancement roles) activities are identified by the patient and are age and sex specific.

this period, a patient may reject splints or **joint protection techniques**, since the hope is that the condition will disappear. These types of interventions must be introduced cautiously. During the next stage of adjustment, sometimes known as acknowledgment, patients may be situationally depressed or angry at having the condition. The therapist may be entreated to try harder to reduce the impairment, or the patient may look for questionable alternative interventions. Clear and attainable objectives established with the patient at this time may be significant in helping the patient to continue to engage in meaningful occupations. Meeting treatment objectives successfully, even in small increments, is important during this period. The ideal stage of adjustment is adaptation. An example of a patient in this stage is the person who wishes to be able to perform a task and requests special assistance in finding a way to achieve this through assistive equipment, environmental adaptations, or other compensatory methods (Livneh, 1986a, b).

Personal Care and Instrumental ADL

Survival skills to live independently in the community include personal care skills and instrumental activities of daily living (IADL) skills. Patients may not always identify these skills as their most important occupational performance goals because they presume that there will be someone to do these tasks for them. However, it is not always possible to obtain assistance; it may in fact be inconvenient to find help. Therefore, many patients can be helped to choose to be able to accomplish these tasks as part of their goals. Backman (1998) described ADL and IADL instruments for occupational therapists working with patients who have rheumatic disease. Observation of skills is important to assess how the person accomplishes tasks. Are joint protection methods used? Is the person aggravating impaired joints while doing these tasks? Are **energy conservation techniques** used? Is adapted equipment used? It is important to ask the person how often these tasks are performed and when assistance is sought. Although during an interview the patient may answer questions about personal care in an idealized manner, it is up to the therapist to aim for accuracy in obtaining the information through interview. For example, consider the following scenario:

"Do you dress yourself?"
"Yes."
"Did you dress yourself this morning before arriving to the clinic?"
"No, because we were in a hurry to get here."
"Did you dress yourself yesterday?"
"No, because it was late and we had to get to church on time."
"Did you dress yourself in the past week?"

"Yes."
"How many days of last week did you dress yourself?"
"Possibly only once or twice, because I had a lot of morning stiffness and it was painful. Besides, my daughter was home to help me."

The reader can see how pursuit of the question is important to identify problems that may need further attention.

With patients who are admitted to the hospital, all morning personal care may be observed. However, the therapist may first encounter a patient with RA as an outpatient. In this case, observation of all personal care activities may not be practical. One study of 45 RA patients found that they appeared more willing to admit difficulties with self-care in a self-administered questionnaire than in a personal interview (Spiegel et al., 1985). The use of a self-administered questionnaire saves time in a comprehensive evaluation. The self-administered *Evaluation of Daily Activity Questionnaire* (Nordenskiold et al., 1998; Nordenskiold et al., 1996) has been tested with women with RA in Sweden. This 102 item checklist asks the respondent to indicate degree of difficulty of various tasks. The therapist can use a scoring procedure to note changes as function improves with the use of assistive devices.

For patients who work, a number of interviews and observational tools exist that are not specific to RA (Backman, 1998). These instruments can be used, but the evaluator must pay special attention to joint and systemic problems unique to this disease as this assessment is done. The person may be able to do tasks, but repetition and effort during a test may not pose the problems that are seen when translated to an 8-hour work day. Another method to look at IADL skills when evaluation time is limited is to simulate key areas that may be problematic. For example, if patients say they cannot reach and place items in cupboards above the counters in the kitchen, having the person lift an item of similar weight to a cupboard in the occupational therapy clinic may provide clues as to whether the problem lies in grip strength, shoulder ROM, pain, or weakness.

An area of ADL that is sometimes overlooked is sexual expression. This area can be problematic for the person with RA because of pain, discomfort, fatigue, limited ROM, and other physical limiting factors. It can be awkward for patients to bring up this topic as part of ADL. The therapist must be sensitive to patients' cultural background in pursuing this aspect of ADL, but this topic should be brought up to allow the patient to discuss problems in this area (Majerovitz & Revenson, 1994). If the sexual expression problems are related to psychological areas unrelated to the disease, a referral to a psychologist may be indicated. In interviewing patients for problems in sexual expression, the approach is similar to that for other aspects of ADL: ask whether the problem is inability to perform activities, impairment of an ability area, or due to contextual or environmental factors. Depending on which factors are problems, provide intervention appropriately.

Range of Motion

Observation and measurement of upper extremity active ROM from an upright position gives the examiner useful information about functional ROM that the patient has for use in occupational functioning (See Chapter 4). Pain is often a reason for limited active ROM against gravity in RA, especially noted in the shoulders, but limited ROM also can be from weakness, contractures, or joint derangement. Radiographs that show osteophytes, erosions, joint narrowing, and other skeletal problems rule out strengthening for the purpose of increasing active ROM. It is important to limit measurement to those areas of concern.

Strength

Testing of muscle groups or motion with the patient in an upright posture provides information about function (See Chapter 4). For example, the patient who actively flexes the shoulder to 60° and takes moderate resistance without pain is likely to be able to lift a light plate to place it on a low shelf above the counter. Testing resistance to joint motions also enables the examiner to record whether pain limits the amount of resistance taken by the joint. It is important to use principles of joint protection in applying resistance to joints at the end of active ROM, to observe the patient's face for an indication of pain, and to stop immediately. Otherwise, the patient may have more pain than usual after leaving the testing session.

Strength in the hand can be measured with grasp meters and pinch meters (See Chapter 42). The Jamar dynamometer is a common instrument that is used to measure grasp. Although the metal of the dynamometer is bothersome to some patients because of deformities and pain, it is still useful, as most objects used in everyday life are inflexible. If, however, a patient has grasp strength less than 5 pounds, the Jamar dynamometer does not provide accurate measures of differences in strength as a result of intervention. In this case, other tools, such as an adapted sphygmomanometer (Melvin, 1989) or the *Grippit* (Nordenskiold & Grimby, 1993) show small increments of change brought about by intervention. Standard pinch meters can be used with patients with RA. However, the standard method of measurement, advocated by Mathiowetz et al. (1985) cannot always be used because of thumb and finger deformities and therefore the norms would not apply. Although the

norms cannot be used for comparison, it can be useful to describe how the pinch was achieved, for example, "the thumb pad is pressed against the index finger proximal phalanx, secondary to limited thumb abduction." Although this may be accompanied by ulnar deviation by the second MCP, this is useful for actively holding a small object. These compensatory mechanisms used by patients with severe deformity must be thoroughly evaluated, especially when surgery to improve hand function is considered. Some patients with severe RA have pinch strength greater than the available gross grasp strength.

Hand Assessment

Among the various hand assessments, Backman and Mackie (1995) have developed one specifically for this population. Others that were not designed for this population can be useful for some purposes (Backman, 1998). Standardized hand assessments are useful as a baseline measure if an intervention is intended to show change in hand function or to assist in decision making for elective hand surgeries. Carroll (1965) developed an instrument to assess the entire upper extremity (*Upper Extremity Function Test*) in the performance of gross and fine motor functional activities.

Endurance

In RA, the ability to sustain functional motion can be limited by fatigue, weakness, or pain. Self-assessment measures of ability to sustain functional performance are useful for determining how fatigue interferes with meaningful occupations. If the patient has to rest all day because the previous day's activity caused fatigue or increased pain, activities of a prolonged, sustained nature must be curtailed to enable participation in occupations of highest choice. This is discussed further under fatigue management.

Pain

Pain can be evaluated during joint examination and/or during performance of occupations. However, sometimes specific knowledge of pain location, severity, and time of day is useful, especially if intervention is to alter any of the parameters of pain. The *Visual Analogue Scale* for pain has been found to be a simple and reliable tool to measure pain (Huskisson, 1974) (See Chapters 4 and 9).

Hand and Wrist Deformities

It is useful to record hand and wrist deformities to determine the best course of action for intervention to allow occupational performance. For each joint of the wrist and hand, the following should be palpated and recorded: (1) swelling, heat, and/or redness (cardinal signs of inflammation); (2) pain; (3) subluxation or dislocation; (4) **crepitus;** (5) tendon rupture; (6) **rheumatoid nodules**.

The following description of common deformities and how they develop will enable the therapist to apply appropriate interventions, such as hand splints, joint protection techniques, and/or patient education programs that dispel myths and increase the patient's understanding of causation of deformity.

Deformities of the Wrist

It is estimated that 95% of persons with persistent RA develop bilateral wrist joint involvement (Wilson, 1986). Three pathological processes alter the carpus directly and produce deformity. These are cartilage degradation, synovial expansion with erosion, and ligamentous laxity. Cartilage degradation is often seen early in RA. Synovial expansion may cause bony erosion and may lead to ruptured tendons, especially the extensor tendons of the ulnar fingers or the flexor pollicis longus (Shapiro, 1996). Even without erosion, synovial expansion can lead to volar subluxation of the proximal carpal row that has been noted in 80% of RA wrists. The new positioning of all of the carpals can elicit pain. If pressure among the carpal links increases during gripping motions, pain increases as intercarpal pressure increases, which leads to a desire to reduce grip strength to reduce pain (Shapiro). Both cartilage loss and synovial expansion can lead to lax ligaments and thence to wrist instability and further carpal derangement, which in turn can lead to a radial shift of the carpus on the radius (Taliesnik, 1989). Even if the synovial destruction stops prior to significant deformity, fibrous ankylosis of some wrist joint surfaces may occur. Synovial erosion that proliferates and causes massive joint destruction, including any combination of tendon ruptures and variants in joint derangement, can produce a floppy wrist (Shapiro).

Deformities of the Metacarpophalangeal Joints

Ulnar drift of the MCP joints is uncommon in the early stages of RA. However, Wilson (1986) reports 45% of patients whose disease has persisted longer than 5 years demonstrate this deformity. Ulnar drift is a combination of deviation of the phalanx from the metacarpal head and a lateral shift of the phalanx upon the metacarpal (Wilson) (Fig. 44-1). The following are contributors to this deformity (Wilson):

1. Synovitis within the MCP joint alters the supporting structures. The radial collateral ligaments, which are weaker than their ulnar counterparts, stretch.

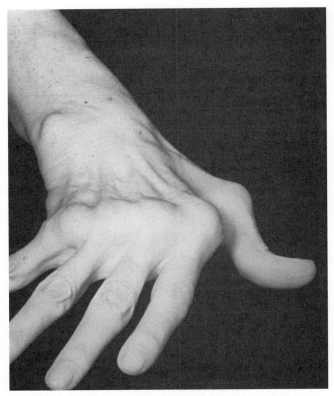

Figure 44-1 MCP ulnar deviation and subluxation. (Reprinted from the ARHP Arthritis Teaching Slide Collection. Used with permission of the American College of Rheumatology.)

2. With resolution of the synovitis, the extensor tendons migrate toward the ulnar side, eventually ending up in the valleys between the metacarpal heads.
3. As the fingers flex, the flexors pull the digit ulnarly unopposed by the weakened radial collateral ligament.
4. Contractures of the intrinsic muscles caused by a reflex protective muscle spasm secondary to the synovitis contribute an MCP volar displacing force. This disrupts the balance of the volar plate, sagittal bands, transverse metacarpal ligament, and collateral ligament.
5. When wrist synovitis causes radial deviation of the wrist, the dynamics of the finger flexor tendons change as they cross the MCP, providing an ulnar force.
6. MCP joint cartilage loss and bony erosion lead to volar subluxation, again allowing the finger flexors to pull ulnarly during flexion.
7. Flexor tenosynovitis can also lead to volar subluxation of the MCP joint.

Because the MCP collateral ligaments normally tighten on MCP flexion, abnormal laxity of the radial collateral ligament at the MCP joint can be evaluated by placing each of the patient's MCP joints in full passive flexion. Each digit is then pushed toward the ulna. In a normal hand the digit has little or no movement laterally. If the radial collateral ligament is stretched, the finger can be easily displaced ulnarly.

When and if the MCP joints become fixed in flexion because of disease, the midpalmar crease may become moist and macerated from lack of exposure to air. This can be accompanied by a foul odor as it becomes difficult for the person to clean the hand; therefore patient, therapist, and physician must be attentive in preventing this deformity.

Deformities of the Interphalangeal Joints

Swan-neck and boutonniere deformities are the most common finger deformities (Rizio & Belsky, 1996) (Figs. 44-2 and 44-3). Synovitis of the PIP joint produces a painful, swollen joint. If synovitis continues, it spreads proximally under the central extensor slip, which becomes attenuated, and between the extensor and intrinsic tendons. When the central slip and lateral bands stretch, they migrate volarly and a boutonniere deformity is produced (Rizio & Belsky; Wilson 1986). Nalebuff (1984) has described three stages of the boutonniere deformity. Stage I exhibits only a slight extensor **lag**, and a slight loss of DIP flexion occurs. A 40° PIP flexion deformity is considered stage II. In stage III, the PIP joint has a fixed flexion deformity.

If the initiating PIP synovitis is anterolateral, it can stretch the transverse retinacular ligament, allowing the lateral band to migrate dorsally, resulting in a PIP joint hyperextension, or swan-neck deformity. Lateral bands in this position prevent the normal volar and lateral shift

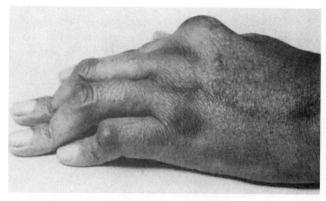

Figure 44-3 Boutonniere deformity: PIP flexion with DIP hyperextension. (Reprinted with permission from Feinberg, J. R. (1992). Effect of the arthritis health professional on compliance with use of resting hand splints by patients with rheumatoid arthritis. *Arthritis Care and Research, 5,* 17–23.)

that allows PIP flexion. With progression of the synovitis, joint erosion and finally destruction occur with fibrous articular adhesions or bony ankylosis (Wilson, 1986). The swan-neck deformity can also be caused by the destructive effect of the synovitis beginning at any one of the three digital joints (Rizio & Belsky, 1996). The disturbance in function in patients with a swan-neck deformity is directly caused by the loss of flexibility of the PIP joint (Rizio & Belsky). Four types of swan-neck deformities have been described (Wilson). Type I deformity is characterized by full flexibility of the PIP joint. Patients complain of transient locking and trouble initiating PIP flexion. Type II deformity exhibits a flexible PIP when the MCP is flexed, but when the MCP is extended, there is limited PIP flexion. When there is significant loss of PIP motion, the deformity is designated type III. In type IV, there is intra-articular destruction and limited motion.

Deformities of the Thumb

Nalebuff's (1984) description of four types of common thumb deformities provides a shorthand for complex problems. Type I, or boutonniere deformity, is the most common and is characterized by MCP joint flexion and IP joint hyperextension (Fig 44-4). This usually occurs when synovitis of the MCP joint stretches the extensor mechanism, including the dorsal capsule, extensor pollicis brevis tendon, and extensor hood. This results in MP flexion; volar subluxation of that joint may occur also. The stretching of the extensor pollicis brevis tendon allows it to displace ulnarly and volarly. Type II begins at the carpometacarpal (CMC) joint and results in MCP flexion and adduction and IP hyperextension. This type is not common. Type III, or swan-neck deformity, is common; it is characterized by MCP joint hyperexten-

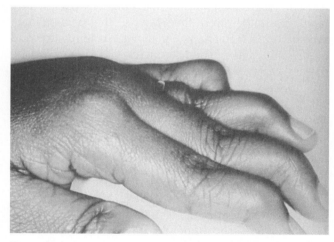

Figure 44-2 Swan-neck deformity: PIP hyperextension with DIP flexion. (Reprinted from the ARHP Arthritis Teaching Slide Collection. Used with permission of the American College of Rheumatology.)

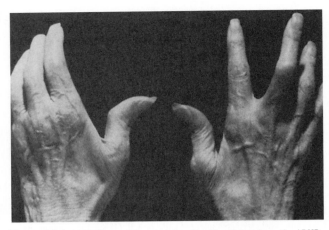

Figure 44-4 Nalebuff type I thumb deformity. (Reprinted from the ARHP Arthritis Teaching Slide Collection. Used with permission of the American College of Rheumatology.)

sion and adduction and IP joint flexion. The origin of this deformity is synovitis at the CMC joint (Stein & Terrono, 1996).

Three other types of thumb deformity have been recognized and classified (Stein & Terrono, 1996). The most common of these is type IV, gamekeeper's deformity. This is characterized by MCP adduction and lateral instability of the MCP joint and is the result of attenuation of the ulnar collateral ligament. As the proximal phalanx deviates radially at the MCP joint, the first MCP assumes an adducted position, and the web space contracts. Type V consists of MCP hyperextension and IP flexion. The first metacarpal is not always adducted, and the CMC joint is usually not involved. Initiating cause is instability or attenuation of the volar plate at the MCP joint. Type VI consists of marked skeletal collapse and loss of bone substance called arthritis mutilans; the thumb becomes quite short and typically is unstable, with skin that appears to be redundant in relation to the underlying skeleton. It is ordinarily associated with similar deformities in the other digits.

Intervention

Intervention addresses the problems identified by evaluation and is guided by the manifestation of the disease, the patient's adjustment to disease progression, and the patient-identified limitations in occupational functioning. The understanding of the altered biomechanical forces on joints, the systemic aspects and progression of the disease, and patients' level of engagement in meaningful occupation drive the occupational therapy intervention. Intervention varies with ACR functional class (Box 44-1) and as the disease progresses from acute (characterized by synovial inflammation and proliferation and systemic symptoms such as fever, and pain) to the subacute, noninflammatory phase and then to the

chronic stage, in which the disease is burned out but deformities are created or remain. ***In all stages, fatigue and exacerbation of pain are avoided.*** The occupational functioning goals identified by patients may be impaired by any of the following:

- ► Limited knowledge of the disease and its progression
- ► Limited knowledge and skill to modify activities at home or in the community to protect joints and conserve energy
- ► Limited ability to manage a full day, balancing between rest and activity
- ► Joint limitations and deformities
- ► Limited strength
- ► Limited knowledge of use of splints
- ► Limited knowledge on how to adapt or modify the environment
- ► Limited sense of self-efficacy to redesign lifestyle

Patient and Family Education

All intervention requires teaching the patient and family about the disease, its symptoms, and how prolonged synovitis can lead to irreversible joint destruction. Physicians and nurses explain how medications work. Occupational therapists must reinforce the importance of following medication guidelines and the reasons for it. Patients must understand that joint deformities cannot be prevented if the disease progresses unchecked without anti-inflammatory or disease-modifying medications. Although not all cases can be controlled easily or well with medications, the large number of choices allows the opportunity to try a variety until the appropriate compound and dosage are discovered. Those who do not respond early to the medication can be discouraged. The occupational therapist teaches adaptation to the disease progression. Besides helping the patient and family to understand the disease, the occupational therapist must instill hope that the use of adaptation and modifications as needed throughout the course of the disease can permit continued meaningful occupational functioning.

Joint Protection

The occupational therapist uses joint protection techniques to reduce pain and deformity. The goals of joint protection are to reduce loading through vulnerable joints, develop strategies to help preserve the present integrity of joint structures, relieve joint pain during activities, and reduce local inflammation (Cordery & Rocchi, 1998). The principles of joint protection described by Cordery and recently revised by Cordery and Rocchi (Box 44-2) require the therapist to apply teaching–learning techniques that will lead to these behavioral changes.

Respect Pain. The pain-sensitive structures in the joint are the fibrous capsule, ligaments, fat pads, and periosteum. Pain during the inflammatory process is common. Pain can also be elicited when attenuated ligaments and deranged joint spaces are aggravated through use that lengthens the ligaments further or resistive motion that compresses the joint spaces (Shapiro, 1996). When pain is present at rest during the inflammatory process, reducing activity level to prevent increasing pain and to promote reduction of inflammation is indicated. In the chronic phase, the aggravating postures or precipitating activities are avoided or adaptations devised.

Maintain Muscle Strength and Joint ROM. Balanced strength around unstable joints can reduce further injury to the capsule, ligaments, and cartilage. Joint protection during therapeutic exercise includes ensuring that muscle pull does not accentuate deformity. Joint position and ROM are critical for optimum functioning of muscles. Limited range at one joint, such as the shoulder, requires exaggerated motions at distal joints to accomplish a task.

In the presence of acute joint inflammation, when range can become limited, joint protection includes use of gentle, pain-free ROM exercise. Attempts to go beyond this range can raise intra-articular pressure and aggravate existing pain.

Use Each Joint in Its Most Stable Anatomical and/or Functional Plane. The most stable anatomical and/or functional plane is one in which muscle, not ligament, provides resistance

to the motion (Cordery & Rocchi, 1998). For example, in a type I thumb deformity with flexible hyperextension of the IP joint, pinch with IP flexion against the pad of the thumb provides increased stability.

Avoid Positions of Deformity and Forces in Their Direction. Avoid external loads and internal forces that facilitate deformity when the degree of disease puts them at risk (Cordery & Rocchi, 1998). Turning resistive round doorknobs when the finger MCP joints are subluxated volarly and ulnarly is an example of force to be avoided by use of a lever door opener.

Use the Strongest Joints Available for the Job. Use of stronger, larger joints that can handle greater forces is a useful principle. Examples of this principle include lifting objects by using the hips and knees instead of bending at the spine; pushing or pulling objects rather than carrying them; and using a belted waist pack rather than holding the purse with hook grasp (Fig. 44-5).

Ensure Correct Patterns of Movement. Incorrect patterns may be the result of pain, tenosynovitis, deformity, muscle imbalance, or habit (Cordery & Rocchi, 1998). For example, to raise the arm, the shoulder hikes (scapular elevation and upward rotation) as substitution for glenohumeral flexion. Using the glenohumeral joint within pain limits keeps this joint mobile. Another example is to push up when arising from a chair by using the flat surface of the palm rather than the dorsum of the fingers to prevent deforming forces toward MCP flexion.

Avoid Staying in One Position for Long Periods. This advice has been recommended for workers in general, as prolonged static postures can lead to muscle fatigue. When fatigued muscles cannot provide stability around a joint, the load transfers to the underlying joint capsule and ligaments that may already be stretched out secondary to disease (Cordery & Rocchi, 1998). Change of position or taking breaks and performing active ROM during activities that are normally prolonged, such as use of the computer, is recommended to prevent muscle fatigue and soreness and subsequent poor patterns of use. This principle is difficult to follow, as patients, like everyone else, want to complete tasks.

Avoid Starting an Activity That Cannot Be Stopped Immediately If It Proves to be Beyond the Person's Ability. This principle requires planning and is not always easy, especially for an unfamiliar task. Fatigued muscles surrounding affected joints can lead to poor patterns of use and increased pain when timely rest is impossible. This principle has been well applied in newer designs of compact walkers that have seats and trays to make them convenient to use

---

BOX 44-2
PROCEDURES FOR PRACTICE

Principles of Joint Protection

- ► Respect pain as a signal to stop the activity.
- ► Maintain muscle strength and joint ROM.
- ► Use each joint in its most stable anatomical and functional plane.
- ► Avoid positions of deformity and forces in their direction.
- ► Use the largest, strongest joints available for the job.
- ► Ensure correct patterns of movement.
- ► Avoid staying in one position for long periods.
- ► Avoid starting an activity that cannot be stopped immediately if it proves to be beyond capability.
- ► Balance rest and activity.
- ► Reduce the force.

From: Cordery, J., & Rocchi, M. (1998). Joint protection and fatigue management. In J. Melvin & G. Jensen (Eds.), Rheumatologic Rehabilitation Series, Vol. 1: Assessment and Management (pp. 279–321). Bethesda, MD: American Occupational Therapy Association, Inc. Reprinted with permission.

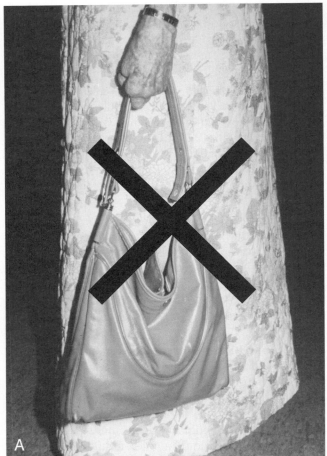

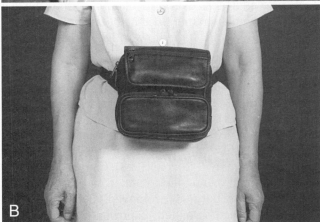

Figure 44-5 How to distribute a load over a larger area and use largest joint available for a task. **A.** Problem: patient carries her handbag using the small joints of the hand. **B.** Solution: Patient uses a belted waist pack. (Courtesy of the Collection of Rancho Los Amigos National Rehabilitation Center, Downey, CA.)

shopping, in the community or in the kitchen. These walkers have enabled many who engage in community activities to sit when desired, rather than searching for and perhaps not finding a sitting surface. Another example of application of this principle is having

patients identify midway locations, such as a chair on the porch which is located between the car and the kitchen. The patient can sit on this chair, if unable to ambulate the complete distance to the target location.

Balance Rest and Activity. People with RA generally need more rest than others. Individuals must plan the balance between activity and rest to accomplish priority activities for the day and week (Gerber, 1985). One method to self-assess priorities is through the use of the workbook *Rehabilitation Through Learning: Energy Conservation and Joint Protection* (Gerber, 1985; see also Furst et al., 1987; Gerber & Furst, 1992).

Reduce the Force. Strong effort or resistive motions can be problematic for involved joints, leading to further destruction and/or pain. In the hand, this can be avoided by building up handles to avoid tight grasp, which can put excessive stress on problematic finger joints and increase compressive forces at the wrist (Shapiro, 1996). Other ways to reduce resistive motions are the use of assistive devices, such as jar openers that use the power of the upper arm rather than involved hand and wrist joints, and lightweight cooking utensils.

Work simplification methods also reduce stress on joints. Rather than carrying objects back and forth in the kitchen repeatedly, placing them all on a rolling cart to push them across the room at one time reduces the force on small hand joints. Stabilizing joints with splints avoids use of internal forces to stabilize them. Resistive activities that push unstable MCP joints toward the ulna should be

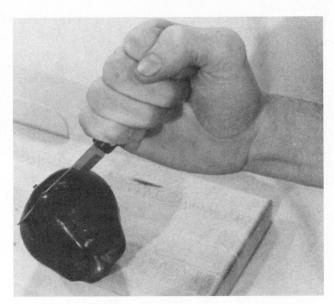

Figure 44-6 Avoidance of ulnar deviation forces. Cutting an apple using a dagger grip on the knife to push the fingers radially.

avoided (Fig. 44-6). However, if a patient's favored leisure activity has been a hobby such as knitting and if satisfactory substitute activities cannot be found, the therapist must assess how the patient can knit without use of undue force. Suggestions include building up the needles and using large doweling for needles, taking frequent rest breaks, searching for loose-weave patterns, and other solutions that patients may suggest. Preventing continuous resistance to stretched radial collateral ligaments may reduce rupture or further attenuation of the radial collateral ligaments.

Fatigue Management

Fatigue has been described as the enduring subjective sensation of generalized tiredness or exhaustion (Belza, 1995). The general fatigue called exhaustion is multidimensional, may originate in the central nervous system, and consists of emotional, behavioral, and cognitive components (Belza). Fatigue severity is associated with joint pain, poor overall mood, depression, fragmented sleep, and reduced functional ability (Belza). To control the effects of fatigue on everyday activities, the therapist teaches the patient to analyze daily activities to determine activities that increase pain and fatigue (Cordery & Rocchi, 1998). Furst et al. (1987) found that rest breaks during the day can support a full day of activity. This was shown in a study of a 6-week course of energy conservation and joint protection training for patients with RA in which participants were taught to take periodic short rest periods during prolonged activities. As a result, 50% of these persons increased the amount of time they were active, compared with 11% of the control subjects (Furst et al., 1985). In the 6-week course the patients used worksheets to determine what may and may not be changed in their daily schedules to self-assess realistic changes. Additional activities provided in the workbook for the course continued this self-analysis to enable patients to plan their fatigue management.

Managing Your Fatigue, a useful brochure published by the Arthritis Foundation, can accompany patient education programs on this topic. It is one of a large series of patient education brochures for people with rheumatic diseases (see Resources).

Maintain Joint Mobility

Patients with RA commonly have limited ROM because of inflammation, joint destruction, weakness, reflex inhibition from pain, or limited use. The cause of the limitation directs the intervention.

During acute joint inflammation, joint motion should be maintained with at least one complete ROM exercise daily. The brochure *Exercise and Your Arthritis* by the Arthritis Foundation (See Resources) is an example of information that patients can follow. It is important not to overstretch inflamed tissues, as tensile strength can be reduced by as much as 50%, leading to tears (Minor, 1996). Active and active–assistive ROM are commonly used during this period. If the patient's effort against gravity leads to discomfort or there is lag in the joint (most notable in the shoulder), passive ROM may be used to ensure that contractures do not occur during this period. It is imperative to pay attention to the patient's response if outside assistance is given, because stoicism and the desire to not lose range may prevent the patient from reacting to pain overtly. Gentle active ROM in the evening can reduce morning stiffness (Minor). However, some have found that the best time for performing this activity is in the morning after they take anti-inflammatory medication.

When joint inflammation has subsided, increasing ROM with gentle, controlled stretching can regain all or some of the loss that occurred during the inflammatory stage. General guidelines for ROM exercises for patients with RA include the following (Coppard et al., 1998; Minor, 1996):

▶ Exercise daily when stiffness and pain are the least.
▶ Take a warm shower or apply heat and/or cold before or after exercise.
▶ Perform gentle ROM exercise in the evening to reduce morning stiffness and in the morning to limber up prior to arising.
▶ Modify exercise (decrease frequency or adapt movement) to avoid increasing joint pain either during or after the exercise. ***Pain following exercise is a guide to reduce the number of repetitions.***
▶ Use self-assistive techniques, such as wand exercises, to perform gentle stretching.
▶ Reduce number of repetitions when the joint is actively inflamed.

Strengthening

Patients with chronic RA are at risk for the ill effects of inactivity, including muscle atrophy and decreased exercise capacity, endurance, and cardiovascular fitness, resulting in a deconditioned state (Komatireddy et al., 1997). Research by Komatireddy et al. suggests that exercise may not be as detrimental as previously believed (Box 44-3).

Isometric exercise is often used prior to or in conjunction with dynamic resistive and aerobic exercise programs. Initially, isometric exercise may be indicated to improve muscle tone, static endurance, and strength and to prepare joints for more vigorous activity (Minor, 1996). Isometric contractions performed at 70% of the maximal voluntary contraction, held for 6 seconds and repeated 5 to 10 times daily, can increase strength

BOX 44-3
RESEARCH NOTE

Efficacy of Low Load Resistive Muscle Training in Patients With Rheumatoid Arthritis Functional Class II and III

Komatireddy, G. R., Leitch, R. W., Cella, K., Browning, G., & Minor, M. (1997). *Journal of Rheumatology, 24,* 1531–1539

ABSTRACT

Researchers randomly assigned 49 patients, classified as RA functional class II and III, with a mean age of 60.5 years and mean time since onset of 10.5 years, to exercise and control (nonexercise) groups for a 12-week resistive muscle training program. A circuit weight training program using 12 to 15 repetitions of a series of 7 exercises using weights and elastic bands was used with the treatment group. Resistance was increased according to the ability and comfort of the patient. A videotape demonstrating the exercises was given to all exercising participants to enable them to continue the program at home at least 3 times per week with a biweekly self-report evaluation.

Efficacy of the exercise program was assessed by evaluation of changes in (1) muscle strength, (2) cardiopulmonary function, (3) functional ability, (4) self-reported health status, and (5) disease activity status. At 12 weeks, a significant improvement was noted in the exercise group for self-report joint count (any peripheral joints that have swelling, tenderness, or pain on motion), *Stanford Health Assessment Questionnaire (HAQ)* score (a self-administered reliable, valid, and sensitive indicator of functional ability in persons with RA), number of painful joints, sit-to-stand time, grip strength, isokinetic knee extension testing at 60°, *Arthritis Impact Measurement Scale* (a valid indicator of both the physical and psychological dimensions of health for persons with arthritis) dexterity score, and time to anaerobic threshold. The control group did not show any measurable improvement. In conclusion, low-load resistive muscle training increased functional capacity as reported by patients. It is a safe form of exercise for those in functional class II and III. Furthermore, the exercise group reported increased confidence and less fear that exercise would increase joint pain and disease activity.

IMPLICATIONS FOR PRACTICE

▶ Occupational therapists should consider the use of strength training in designing programs for patients with RA in functional class II and III.
▶ Low-load resistive muscle work through use of occupations using lightweight objects can be considered for patients in functional class II or III. For example, use of a lightweight vacuum cleaner is a low-load resistive activity.

---

significantly (Minor). Instructions for isometric exercise should include the following cautions: maintain the contraction for no more than 6 seconds; avoid maximal effort, as it is neither necessary nor desirable; exhale during the contraction and inhale during a similar period of relaxation; and avoid contracting more than two muscle groups at a time (Minor).

Dynamic exercise is the form most frequently used to increase strength. It can improve both strength and endurance. Resistance can be supplied by weight of the body part or external resistance in the form of tools, common objects, or a variety of resistive exercise equipment (Minor, 1996). A cautious approach to resistance training is recommended to protect unstable or inflamed joints from damage. The exercise should be performed within the pain-free range. Exercise of 8 to 10 antigravity repetitions should be well tolerated before additional resistance is added (Minor). ***Intensity, frequency, or ROM should be reduced if joint swelling or pain occurs*** (Minor).

Splinting

Hand splints have been used in the treatment of RA for a variety of purposes (Falconer, 1990). The effectiveness of splints for all of these purposes has not been extensively documented, although some studies have addressed pain reduction, grip strength, and comfort of a variety of commercially available orthoses (Kjeken et al., 1995; Nordenskiold, 1990; Stern et al., 1996, 1997; Tijhuis, 1998). The following are some reasons splinting has been found useful with people with RA.

Reduce Inflammation

During the inflammatory process, joint rest by means of immobilization has been found to reduce joint inflammation, as was shown when the ring size was significantly reduced in a small sample of persons with RA who were treated by immobilization versus those not immobilized (Partridge & Duthie, 1963). It is very common for resting hand splints to be prescribed during the inflammatory period. Some patients state that when they awaken in the morning, the hand is more comfortable, having rested in a comfortable position during the night. The joints that are covered by a splint should be determined by the location of the inflammation. For example, if only the wrist is involved, a wrist splint is indicated. If the whole hand and wrist are involved, the orthosis should include all joints. The occupations of the patient may require fitting two orthoses for the inflamed hand. A night resting splint that covers all joints may be alternated with a shorter orthosis that allows the fingers to be free to perform pain-free nonresistive activities during the day.

Provide Support and Reduce Pain to Unstable Joints During Function

During the postinflammatory stage, if unstable or subluxated joints or other joint deformities occur, the external support of an orthosis can enhance stability or prevent joint motion. Stability is provided only to joints posing problems. Feinberg and Brandt (1981) found that when splinting relieved pain, adherence to splint wearing was good. Feinberg (1992) also found that patient education enhanced patient adherence to wearing of splints.

Prevent Undesirable Motion During Occupational Performance

A key example of this is to prevent hyperextension of the finger PIP joints (swan-neck deformity) through the use of a three-point splint that allows flexion but prevents hyperextension. Another example is to use an orthosis in the early stage of the Nalebuff type I deformity of the thumb, hyperextension of the IP joint. Although patients can be taught to remember to flex the IP joint when using a pinch motion, an orthosis that limits hyperextension can be a passive reminder to prevent further hyperextension and stretch to collateral ligaments. Another example that is somewhat controversial is immobilizing the finger PIP joint into extension when an early Boutonniere deformity is seen. Some positive results have been seen in controlling the deformity for a limited time (Palchik et al., 1990).

Increase ROM or Prevent Deformity

Dynamic splinting, using an orthosis with finger extension outriggers, has been commonly used after finger MCP Silastic implant arthroplasty. This use of dynamic orthoses has been proposed for other purposes, such as to reduce contractures secondary to the disease, but there is little evidence to support this outcome or the use of dynamic splinting to prevent deformity.

Position Joints for Occupational Performance

An example of positioning joints for occupational performance is the use of the MCP ulnar deviation orthosis (Fig. 44-7) to permit continued use of the IP joints of the hand, when, if unsplinted, pain would be induced at the MCP joint with activity. Information regarding types of splints and use of custom versus prefabricated orthoses is discussed in Chapters 14 and 15.

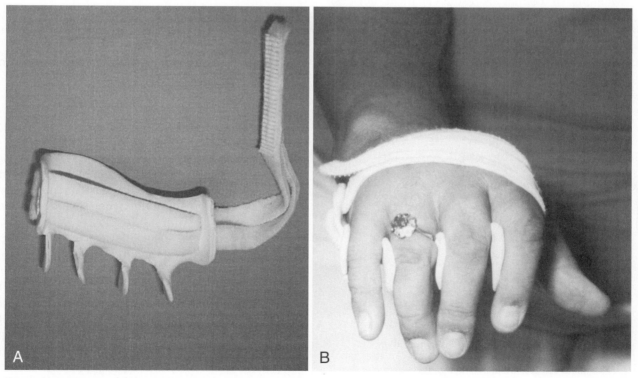

Figure 44-7 Splint to control ulnar deviation of the MCP joints during hand use. **A.** Ulnar deviation correction splint. **B.** Splint in place on the patient's hand. (Courtesy of the Collection of Rancho Los Amigos National Rehabilitation Center, Downey, CA.)

Modify Environment

Ways to modify the environment to maintain the ability to participate in occupations of choice include changing the physical environment, recommending use of assistive devices, and assisting the patient to recognize and choose work or leisure environments that accommodate the disability. Examples of each of these are given for a variety of problems. The reader should be able to recognize readily what joint problems these modifications accommodate. The adaptations generally can be done with equipment from a local hardware store.

Change the Physical Environment

The patient and therapist must think about modifying all environments important to the patient's occupational functioning, especially home and work.

Home

- ▶ Remove doors of cabinets or attach loops to door handles.
- ▶ Lower above-counter cupboards.
- ▶ Replace shelves in low cupboards with swivel or pull-out shelves.
- ▶ Replace standard oven with a microwave oven on a surface that accommodates available reach.
- ▶ Replace doorknobs with lever handles.
- ▶ Replace faucet handles with long lever handles.
- ▶ Use remote control devices to automate on–off switching of commonly used electrical devices, such as light switches.
- ▶ Lower closet rods if reach is limited.
- ▶ Use a rolling cart to move items from room to room (Axtell & Yasuda, 1993).

Work

- ▶ Organize workstation so that shelves are within reach and the table and chairs are at ergonomically correct heights.

BOX 44-4
PROCEDURES FOR PRACTICE

Criteria to Consider When Choosing Assistive Devices

- ▶ Lightweight, durable, compact, attractive in appearance
- ▶ Multipurpose use to prevent need to search for multiple devices
- ▶ Simplicity of operation
- ▶ Reduce stress to all multilinked joints involved in operating the device
- ▶ Suitable for the individual patient's gadget tolerance
- ▶ In accord with the self-image of the user

BOX 44-5
PROCEDURES FOR PRACTICE

Commercially Available Common Assistive Devices

- ▶ **Self-care**—Buttonhook; dressing stick (various lengths can be used for dressing as well as reach for distant items); sock cone; reacher; long-handled sponge; extended handle for managing toilet paper, long-handled comb, electric toothbrush, pump toothpaste dispensers
- ▶ **Meal preparation**—Rolling cart, knob turner for stove, built-up handles on cooking utensils, knives with right-angled handles (Fig. 44-8), electric can opener, jar opener, spring-lever scissors, cutting board with spikes to stabilize food, electric chopper, high kitchen stool, high stool on roller such as EZ Stand Mobile Stool (Fig. 44-9)
- ▶ **Home maintenance**—Long-handled dustpan, bucket on rollers, reachers to pull items out of areas and from floor
- ▶ **Work and school**—Luggage cart, rolling cart, backpack, fanny pack, computer forearm–wrist rest, adapted key holder, built-up handle for writing implements, telephone headset, adapted hand tools, electric stapler and pencil sharpener, car door opener (Fig. 44-10A)
- ▶ **Leisure**—Adapted gardening tools, rolling stool for gardening, card holder, reading rack, embroidery hoop holder, rolling golf cart, knob turner (Fig. 44-10B)

- ▶ Attach forearm and wrist supports to computer areas.
- ▶ Use a rolling cart or luggage roller to transport items from room to room.

Recommend Assistive Devices

Many assistive devices are available to the general public. These devices can assist the person with RA to limit stresses to joints. It is useful to teach patients joint protection principles so they can search independently for the products that produce the least amount of stress to joints. Criteria to consider when helping patients choose devices are found in Box 44-4. There are excellent resources for special devices made for people with joint problems when common everyday products do not accommodate the problems (Box 44-5 and Resources). Generally, selection of these products requires professional advice and an opportunity to try the device to ensure that it will serve the purpose desired by the patient. Therefore, it is important for the occupational therapy clinic to have an array of devices for trial use (Mann, 1998). Keeping current equipment catalogs and using the World Wide Web to assist patients in finding appropriate items helps people with RA to maintain their ability to perform meaningful occupations. A useful database found on the World Wide Web is Abledata; it offers more than 20,000 assistive devices (see Resources). When none of the products available in the general or specialty market solves the problems, the occupational therapist can customize tools in the clinic. Common methods of customizing tools are building up or lengthening handles with materials such as foam tubing, low temperature thermoplastics, plastic tubing, or wooden dowels. Creativity on the part of the therapist is needed to meet the patient's requirements.

Assist the Patient to Recognize and Choose Work or Leisure Environments that Accommodate the Disability

To change previously comfortable daily life routines to accommodate disability requires significant effort. A recent study of lifestyle redesign was implemented with the well elderly. The methods used in this study to enable individuals to implement lifestyle redesign can apply to individuals with RA. Lifestyle redesign suggests that people can achieve greater meaning in their lives by examining the occupations that are most meaningful to them and identifying what prevents them from performing these occupations (Clark et. al., 1997). In lifestyle redesign the individual, through a process facilitated by the occupational therapist, determines what is needed to

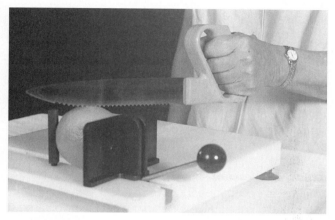

Figure 44-8 Cutting with an angled knife on a cutting board with vegetable spike. (Courtesy of Paul Weinreich, Rancho Los Amigos National Rehabilitation Center, Downey, CA.)

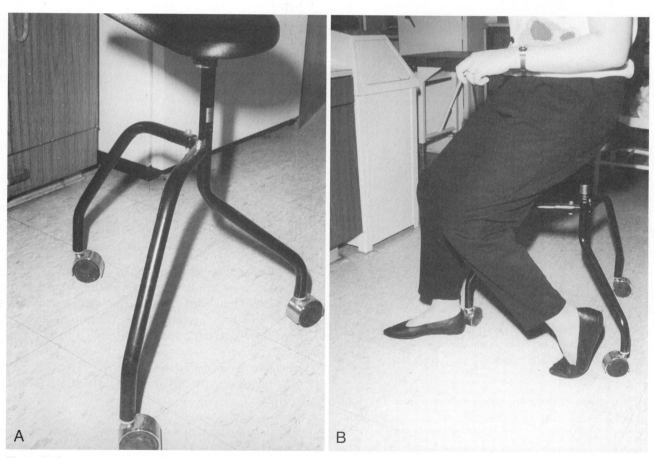

Figure 44-9 EZ Stand Mobile Stool. (Courtesy of the Collection of Rancho Los Amigos National Rehabilitation Center, Downey, CA.)

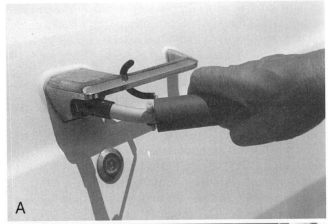

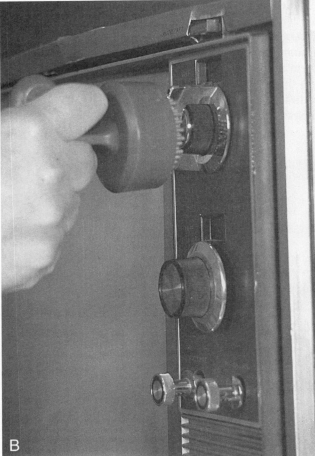

Figure 44-10 Car door opener (**A**) and multipurpose knob turner (**B**). (Courtesy of Rancho Los Amigos National Rehabilitation Center, Downey, CA. Paul Weinreich, photographer.)

perform these important occupations and develops solutions to overcome these barriers to occupational functioning. Although this was intuitively known by occupational therapists, Clark et al. demonstrated that as a result of this lifestyle redesign intervention, people were healthier as demonstrated by scores on tools such as the *SF-36*, a quality of life measure, in contrast to those who did not have this intervention. The intervention included exposure to a number of tasks and activities in small groups. At the same time each individual approached the task determining what had to be done to meet his or her own needs to perform the task again, independent of the group (Jackson et al., 1998).

In those with RA, this lifestyle redesign may have to be done periodically or on an ongoing basis as the disease progresses or as exacerbations and remissions occur. Teaching people to manage lifestyle redesign by emphasizing occupational self-analysis and achievement of individual goals eliminates the need for professional intervention except when a major crisis in the life of the individual occurs.

Sexual Expression

An area of occupational performance that is sometimes overlooked is sexual expression. The focus of assessment is identifying hindrances to sexual expression related to performance area, component, or context. Majerovitz and Revenson (1994) found among 113 couples, of whom 79.6% included one spouse with RA, that there was an association between greater disability and greater dissatisfaction. They suggested that health providers be sensitive to patients' questions and concerns regarding sexuality and openly discuss these issues with both patient and partner. Intervention in the area of sexual expression may include education, development of communication skills, planning for more comfortable sex, and finding more comfortable positions.

Patient Education

Topics included in education address the following issues: Pain and stiffness in joints can lead to avoidance or limited sex. Partners may also fear causing pain. Fatigue, which may be part of the disease process, can reduce desire for sex. Some medications cause fatigue or reduce sexual desire.

Development of Communication Skills

Discussion of sex with a partner is difficult for some. Discussion of needs for intimacy and how a partner feels can lead to more extensive discussion of effects of disease on sexual performance.

Planning for More Comfortable Sex

The following suggestions are from the Arthritis Foundation (1993):

► Plan for sex at a time of day when you generally feel best.
► Time your dose of pain relief medication so that its effect will occur during sexual relations.

▶ Pace your activities during the day to help avoid extreme fatigue.

▶ Practice ROM exercises to relax your joints.

▶ Warm the bed ahead of time with an electric blanket.

▶ Take a warm bath or shower before sex to relax.

Finding More Comfortable Positions

The Arthritis Foundation brochure *Guide to Intimacy and Arthritis* describes positions for sex that reduce stress to commonly involved lower extremity joints (see Resources). Individuals may use the brochure to identify which postures are the least stressful for them. Communicating with a partner is important for trying new postures, letting the partner know what feels good, and finding alternative ways to enjoy sex.

Clinical Outcomes

The described interventions require that the recipient of services redesign his or her life in a variety of ways: from wearing a hand splint to use of assistive devices or changing the routine patterns of daily living. Change of typical routine is not easy, and it has been estimated that at least 50% of patients with RA are noncompliant with therapy irrespective of the nature of the intervention (Belcon et al., 1984; Feinberg & Trombly, 1995). In a study designed to examine the effect of interaction between the patient and the occupational therapist on subsequent splint use, splint use was greater in a group of patients who were treated by a therapist using compliance-enhancing behaviors that included the suggestions in Box 44-6.

Osteoarthritis (OA)

Osteoarthritis is a heterogeneous condition in which biomaterial properties of articular cartilage or bone are abnormal or there is excessive biomechanical loading, such as may occur after trauma to a joint or to normal cartilage or bone, or both. Repetitive impact loading leads to joint failure, which accounts for the high prevalence of OA in specific joints related to vocational or avocational overload. Although articular cartilage is an excellent shock absorber, it is not the only shock absorber that protects the joint from large loads, such as in normal walking. Adaptive protective mechanisms are provided by subchondral bone, which also has shock-absorbing qualities, and periarticular muscles, which not only move a joint but can act as a large "rubber band" that can absorb large amounts of energy to decelerate the body. Muscle weakness, which may occur in association with OA, reduces the effectiveness of this shock-absorbing mechanism (Brandt & Slemenda, 1993).

Joints most commonly involved are the knees, hips, interphalangeal joints, the first CMC joint, and the spine, although other joints can be involved. Common symptoms are joint tenderness, sometimes accompanied by crepitus, pain after use that is relieved by rest, and progression of pain at rest and at night. Morning stiffness in the involved joint generally lasts less than 30 minutes.

BOX 44-6
PROCEDURES FOR PRACTICE

Clinical Suggestions for Enhancing Compliance (Feinberg & Trombly, 1995)

Apply Learning Principles to Patient Education
▶ Patients best remember instructions presented first.
▶ Emphasized instructions are recalled better.
▶ The fewer the instructions, the greater the proportion remembered.
▶ Pace the amount of information to avoid overload.
▶ Use simple, understandable language without medical jargon.
▶ Individualize teaching methods to the patient.
▶ Reinforce essential points by review, discussion, or summary.
▶ Ask the patient to repeat essential elements of the message.
▶ Provide written instructions for home reference.
▶ Devise mechanisms for helping patients to remember advice.

Assess the Patient's Expectations and Experience Concerning the Following
▶ The clinical encounter
▶ His or her beliefs and misconceptions about the cause, severity, and symptoms of the illness and susceptibility to complications or exacerbations
▶ Goals of treatment
▶ Perceptions about the costs and risks versus the benefits of treatment
▶ Existing health-related knowledge, skills, and practices
▶ Degree of adaptation to the disease
▶ Sense of self-efficacy or lack of control and hopelessness
▶ Learning limitations
▶ Extent of family involvement and influence

Encourage the Patient to Assume Responsibility for Disease Management
▶ Use behavioral contracts if necessary
▶ Use other motivational techniques
▶ Encourage the patient that he can be successful with self-management

Use a Facilitating Affective Tone
▶ Listen to the patient
▶ Be approachable
▶ Appear knowledgeable
▶ Inspire trust and confidence
▶ Be enthusiastic and expect positive results

Case Example

MS. B.: RHEUMATOID ARTHRITIS

Patient Information

Ms. B. is 45 years old and has a 3-year history of RA. She has been followed by a rheumatologist for the entire period, with ongoing use of anti-inflammatory medication. Her current major complaint is bilateral wrist pain. The finger MCPs show very mild inflammation, and she does not report pain in them. There are no other notable pain complaints in other joints. Grasp strength is 20 pounds bilaterally. She is a full-time fourth grade school teacher and lives alone in a one-bedroom apartment on the first floor.

Interview with the patient shows that Ms. B. has increased pain after working a full day. Her daily teaching schedule includes an approximate total time of 2 hours writing on the blackboard. She also opens and closes heavy institutional doors at least twice a day. She drives her car to and from work. She carries a full briefcase to and from work. She buys her lunch at the cafeteria daily. The pain subsides over the weekend, when she engages in very few active tasks, such as housecleaning or cooking. She has been having friends cook for her and has let her housecleaning go. Her wrist pain is totally eliminated over 2-week vacations and the summers, when she is not teaching.

Reason for Referral to Occupational Therapy

Ms. B. was referred to occupational therapy to address her complaint of bilateral wrist pain, which is beginning to interfere with her teaching, although she has not had to take time off work. Ms. B. desires to continue to teach full time.

Occupational Therapy Problem List

▶ Wrist pain exacerbated in the course of her work day, especially when she writes on the blackboard
▶ Inability to perform home maintenance
▶ Inability to prepare meals

Occupational Therapy Goal List

1. Explore use of bilateral wrist orthoses for use during function.
2. Explore alternative means to writing on blackboard.
3. Reexamine joint protection measures to prevent wrist pain during home maintenance and meal preparation tasks and activities.

Treatment Plan

The therapist recommended this six-session outpatient program over 6 weeks:

1. Determine and fit appropriate bilateral wrist orthoses to use during function.

2. Explore alternatives for writing on blackboard, such as use of overhead projector and transparency pens or chalk holders to diminish prolonged tight pinch with its secondary potential effect on intercarpal pressures.
3. Explore use of adapted equipment for carrying heavy loads, such as a briefcase. This may include use of a luggage roller, special shoulder straps for carrying the briefcase, or a canvas pack on wheels.
4. Review meal preparation activities and adapted aids to decrease use of prolonged grasp and stress to wrists. This may include use of special jar openers, can openers, and knives that use arms instead of the wrists for power.
5. Review use of tools that can decrease stress to wrists, such as a rolling cart in the kitchen.
6. Identify which activities are the most important to Ms. B. to accomplish each day at work, home, and in the community. Reexamine whether priorities should be set and whether stress to wrist joints is exacerbated with any of these activities.
7. Provide ongoing education on joint protection techniques that emphasizes self-analysis of each activity and examination of alternative methods to accomplish important tasks without undue stress to wrist joints.
8. Explain wearing time of splints and purpose of splints. Train in appropriate donning, doffing and general care of splints.

Analysis of Reasoning:

Teaching Ms. B. strategies for joint protection during occupational performance allowed the patient to learn self-analysis with each new activity that she could continue after the end of therapy. Because of the visibility of splinting, which may have negative connotations at work, education was important to assure that Ms. B. was comfortable wearing the splints in the classroom and that she recognized that the splints allowed performance in the classroom without increased pain at the end of the work day. It was important to teach Ms. B. to recognize independently activities that aggravated wrist pain and find alternative ways to perform or use special tools or adapt the environment so that she could assume control over her disease.

CLINICAL REASONING
in OT Practice

Fatigue Management

Ms. B. returns to see the occupational therapist 6 months after completion of the intervention described in the case example. The interventions relieved the pain that had been exacerbated by her daily occupations, especially at work. She now has a new problem: fatigue in the afternoon while she is teaching. What can be done for fatigue management?

The joint may swell, but the enlargement is generally due to overgrowth of bone and cartilage rather than synovial effusion, as in RA, although synovial effusion can occur. Diagnosis is based on the history, physical examination, and radiographic features of joint space narrowing, sclerosis of bone, marginal osteophytes, and bony remodeling (Stein et al., 1996).

Although OA often progresses, it does so at highly variable rates in different patients, and for some it does not progress. Fewer than half of those with radiographically identifiable OA have symptoms. Knee OA is more likely to result in disability than OA of any other joint (Brandt & Slemenda, 1993). It occurs in 10 to 20% of those aged 65 to 74 years, with women twice as likely to be affected as men.

Spurs at the dorsolateral and medial margins of the DIP joints of the fingers, which generally develop slowly, are called Heberden's nodes. Heberden's nodes can cause volar and lateral deviation of the distal phalanx. Heberden's nodes are 10 times as prevalent in women as in men. A similar enlargement at the PIP joints of the fingers is called Bouchard's nodes. When the first CMC joint is involved, there is tenderness and pain at the base of the metacarpal and a squared appearance of the hand (Brandt & Slemenda, 1993). Precision and power pinches are most at risk when the first CMC is significantly involved. In a review of 99 patients with hand OA, more than half of patients had functional loss. Nearly half of the 99 had a concomitant history of OA of the knee (Altman et al., 1990). McFarlane et al. (1990) found, in following 32 patients with hand osteoarthritis from entry to a year later, that osteophytes, particularly when fast growing, produce pain. The slower the change in size, the less likely that the joint was seriously compromised.

Evaluation

With OA limited to particular joints, the initial interview is spent taking an occupational history to provide information about whether joint problems are compromising occupational functioning. Administering the *COPM* following the initial interview determines which occupational performance tasks are important to reinstitute or improve to a more satisfactory performance level. An examination of joints causing occupational functioning problems determines whether the problem is due to limited motion and/or pain. Following this examination, a simulation or actual observation of problematic activities is done to objectify the report of the patient. Sometimes, a patient's perception of which joints are problematic can be in error because of referred pain from another joint or joints. Since OA commonly affects the larger weight-bearing joints, observation of stooping,

kneeling, and bending to pick up objects are important. If the hand is affected, identifying location of pain during function assists with treatment planning.

Intervention

Patient education concerning unloading and protecting involved joints and strengthening the muscles around joints is the key intervention. Other interventions include modification of the environment, prescription of assistive devices, and lifestyle redesign.

Patient Education

The goal of education is to enable the patient to control long-term management of OA. Understanding how OA affects joints and understanding OA-related joint protection principles and their application to daily living are key areas for education.

Joint Protection

Joint protection principles are appropriate to OA, although the rationale varies from that of RA, since OA is limited to joint involvement without systemic effect. Joint protection guidelines for OA include the following: maintain joint ROM and increase muscle strength and fitness, reduce excessive loading on the joint, avoid pain in activities, balance activity and rest, and avoid staying in one position for long periods (Cordery & Rocchi, 1998).

Maintain ROM, Increase Muscle Strength and Fitness. Maintaining as much ROM as possible allows optimal functioning of muscles by providing biomechanical advantage in the use of the joint and prevents joint contractures. Maintaining daily activities within the limitations of the patient's pain prevents disuse atrophy. Strengthening around an unstable joint can increase stability and reduce pain. Past belief was that any joint compression, such as walking, might aggravate hip and knee OA; however, current practice is to encourage aerobic exercise, such as walking or pool exercises, to reduce pain and improve function in patients with hip or knee OA (Cordery & Rocchi, 1998). Bony enlargement around the CMC joint of the thumb can inhibit motion. When this occurs, a bony block can prevent attempts to increase ROM and lead to further pain; therefore, attempts to increase ROM are avoided.

Reduce Excessive Loading on Joints. Compression of the articular cartilage transmits loads to the underlying subchondral bone, both of which act as shock absorbers. However, in OA the cartilage is too thin to protect against repetitive impact loading, which produces the most destructive effects on cartilage. The principal

Case Example

MRS. S.: OSTEOARTHRITIS

Patient Information

Mrs. S. is 55 years old and lives with her husband in their own home. They owned and operated a small café for 15 years until they retired 5 years ago. Mrs. S. has bilateral OA of the knees that has progressed to the degree that she can walk only short distances at home without incurring knee pain that requires sitting or lying down. The strength in her knees and hips is graded 4. She also has pain in the CMC joint of the right thumb, which is noted especially when she is attempting to cook or garden. On a *Visual Analogue Scale* for pain (1–10), her scores of pain at the knees bilaterally and the right thumb CMC joint after use are 8 to 10. Her right palmar and lateral pinch strength ranges between 3 and 5 pounds.

Reason for Referral to Occupational Therapy

Mrs. S. was referred to outpatient occupational therapy because of her complaints about managing self-care, home skills, and gardening.

Occupational Therapy Problem List

Assessment reveals that Mrs. S. cannot transfer into and out of the bathtub without her husband's assistance. She prefers to stay in her night clothes all day because of knee discomfort when donning and doffing her pants to dress and to use the toilet and loss of interest and identified need to wear day clothes. She also has problems grasping and pinching items in her right hand that require any degree of resistance. This includes opening jars, turning doorknobs, managing can openers, using scissors, opening drawers with small knobs, and managing dials that require twisting, such as on her microwave oven. She has trouble opening the car door and turning the ignition key and generally using any keys.

Treatment Plan

Equipment is identified for her problems with the occupations of most interest to her, namely cooking and gardening. The equipment includes EZ Stand Mobile Stool to use while cooking, walker with seat to use in the garden area, Zim jar opener, lever-handle doorknobs, electric can opener, loop scissors, multipurpose knob turner, yarn loops for drawer handles, adapted car door opener with key holder, and reachers to pick up items from the floor and garden, such as a water hose.

Alternative ways to perform activities include use of a rolling cart in the kitchen. Splinting will be considered for the right CMC joint of the thumb. Mrs. S. will be taught how joints work and the effect of OA on them. Why joint protection techniques reduce pain to joints will also be discussed.

After each session in occupational therapy, a home program was provided and was steadily graduated to allow her to return to her important occupations, cooking and gardening. In the early sessions, the home program emphasized the use of the right CMC thumb splint for her important occupation of preparing sandwiches for herself and her husband for lunch. At the midpoint of the sessions a home program was given to prepare a light meal for self and husband, using the EZ Stand Mobile Stool and using specific joint protection for this activity. She was told to assess whether she felt pain following the activity and bring a report to the following session.

Analysis of Reasoning

Mrs. S. has given up many cherished activities because of bilateral knee pain and right CMC joint pain. Assistive devices, adapted methods, and right CMC thumb splint should enable her to return to these activities.

CLINICAL REASONING
in OT Practice

Joint Protection Principles Applied to Leisure Skills

Mrs. S. has returned to cooking for herself and her husband. She also goes out to the garden two or three times a week to water the plants. She has told the therapist that she would like to participate in leisure activities in the community. What kinds of activities would you suggest and for what reasons?

---

protection to healthy joints is through neuromuscular mechanisms and normally functioning proprioceptors. When we prepare to step down to a landing that is 12 inches beyond what we expected, we feel a spine-tingling sensation, as we did not send messages to our neuromuscular mechanisms and proprioceptors to pre-pare for this joint impact. Factors that lead to muscle fatigue and weakness in OA reduce the effectiveness of this shock-absorbing mechanism (Brandt & Slemenda, 1993). Patients' understanding of joint physiology and the role of the proprioceptors can help them to under-stand which daily occupations use excessive impact loading, such as the effect of carrying heavy loads up and down stairs. This understanding lets the patient recognize the need to use alternative methods to accomplish the task. For example, in this case, to have others carry the load down the stairs or carry small amounts of load in a backpack and use the handrail to reduce the impact load to involved knee joints.

Anatomical bony malalignment may place additional biomechanical stress on one side of an involved joint. Pronation of the foot and varus or valgus knee deformities are common and can be countered with appropriate orthotics. The use of a hand splint can be useful to stabilize an unstable first CMC joint in palmar abduction to reduce pain while engaging in activities requiring pinch. This type of static orthosis is worn only during function to allow joint mobility and avoidance of contractures arising from constant immobilization (Cordery & Rocchi, 1998).

Avoid Pain in Activities. Joint pain produced by engagement in activities is a useful symptom that may indicate stress to joints by use that exceeds the limits of comfort to the involved joint. Examples of this include prolonged kneeling and squatting, both of which can aggravate knee symptoms. Kneeling and squatting can usually be avoided by relocating items from low surfaces to higher levels. Equipment that can be used to avoid kneeling and squatting includes such items as long-handled dustpan and reachers. To avoid lifting heavy loads, when the spine and lower extremities are painful, usual equipment can be replaced by lighter versions made of materials such as aluminum, plastic, or nylon canvas. Examples of this are nylon canvas suitcases and briefcases. A rolling cart and luggage roller can be used. Postures that aggravate back symptoms when the spine is involved, such as prolonged leaning over a desk, can be modified by use of an upright reading rack. Leaning over a railing to pick up an infant from a crib can be avoided by adapting the railing to open to mattress level and sitting to transfer the infant to one's lap or an elevated stroller.

Raising the height and firmness of chairs, toilet seats, beds, and other furniture avoids knee or hip pain during arising. Lateral supports or armrests may also be used to assist with rising from the seated position. To avoid pain when the thumb CMC is affected, the person can use jar openers, electric can openers, electric scissors, and lightweight or large-handled utensils to prevent undue stresses to this joint (Cordery & Rocchi, 1998; Stein et al., 1996).

Balance Rest and Activity. Although fatigue that accompanies systemic disease in RA does not exist in OA, continued use of affected joints, along with other joints, can increase the discomfort level in these joints. Self-monitoring by recognizing onset of pain and discomfort with a routine daily schedule should be used to determine when activity should be stopped to rest the joints. Using a method advocated by Furst et al. (1987) for working with patients with RA, patients with OA can record length of time in a task that is followed by moderate to severe pain and/or fatigue. Using this information, patients can reduce the time in the task to determine whether pain and/or fatigue is reduced. Cordery and Rocchi (1998) advocate rest periods shorter than 30 minutes several times a day between tasks.

Avoid Staying in One Position for Long Periods. People with OA are prone to "gelling" or stiffness and discomfort that follow periods of inactivity. If in addition the activity requires static hold of involved joints over a long time, the muscles surrounding that joint tire and are less effective in supporting the joint (Cordery & Rocchi, 1998). Frequent breaks are important when there is a tendency to perform prolonged static postures. Performing active ROM to affected joints every 15 to 20 minutes may minimize stiffness and facilitate muscle function (Brandt & Slemenda, 1993).

Modify the Environment

Not all patients with OA understand that modification of the environment can prevent undue stresses to involved joints and enable continuation of meaningful occupations. For example, it may be difficult for a patient to give up a previously comfortable chair even though it poorly supports the spine and positions hip and knees in excessive flexion. The patient should be taught to sit in a comfortable chair that has armrests, elevated seat if needed, and firm back for support to prevent further stretching of joint and surrounding structures weakened from OA. Other guidelines that should be taught: Keep commonly used items that need to be transported often, such as table settings at home or files at work, on a rolling cart to avoid overuse of damaged joints. Place commonly used items on countertops rather than storing them in low cupboards to prevent the need to squat. Move to a lower-level bedroom, bathroom, and kitchen to avoid the need to climb stairs. Use computer workstations that are ergonomically correct to support good posture. Use handrails while ascending and descending stairs to reduce load to lower extremity joints.

Assistive Devices

People with OA who have significant involvement of only a few joints may not seek out rehabilitation care and may be unaware of and reluctant to use assistive devices that can prevent loss of participation in meaningful occupations. Instead, it is fairly common to hear about continued use of involved joints with pain until there is sudden termination of important occupations, when the use of assistive devices could have prevented aggravation to joints. Elevated toilet seats and tub benches can be used to eliminate the stress on knees and hips of arising from low surfaces. Using a reacher and dressing stick to pick up items from the floor prevents stooping. Other items used by those with RA can be used by people with OA when they protect the specific joints involved (See Resources).

Lifestyle Redesign

As with the person with RA, it is important for the therapist to work with the patient to examine all activities and to determine which are most important to the individual. The patient is encouraged to decide which can be eliminated or performed differently. The skill of the therapist in helping patients recognize the value of assistive devices or alternative ways of performance is often needed to enable lifestyle redesign, as some devices or alternative ways of performance connote a sense of disability that is not congruent with the person's body image. Crutches, canes, and hand splints are prime examples. People, even some health care professionals, find it difficult to use these devices because they denote a negative body image in spite of their advantages—prolonging walking and functional hand use. Alternatives, which may include change of vocation, also may require significant counseling to enable the patient to recognize the advantages to the change. For example, if the patient's job requires much stooping and lifting and there are no alternatives for this at work, vocational counseling to examine other job opportunities that do not stress involved joints may be indicated.

Summary Review Questions

1. List the primary differences between RA and OA.
2. Describe joint problems that can lead to diminished occupational functioning for people with RA.
3. Describe joint problems that can lead to diminished occupational functioning for people with OA.
4. Besides joint problems, what clinical problems can affect occupational functioning for people with RA?
5. Is a patient with only thumb CMC joint involvement and resultant pain on resistive motion more likely to have OA or RA?
6. Describe joint protection techniques used for people with RA to prevent or restore occupational functioning.
7. Describe compliance-enhancing techniques that enable patients to modify behaviors to enhance occupational functioning.
8. Name several resources for patients with RA and OA to find adapted tools to enhance their occupational functioning.
9. How is splinting used for people with RA and OA to enhance occupational functioning?
10. What assessments are used to optimize occupational functioning for people with RA and OA?

Resources

Arthritis Foundation patient education booklets (partial listing)
Arthritis in the Workplace
Diet and Arthritis
Exercise and Your Arthritis
Gardening and Arthritis
Golf and Arthritis
Guide to Intimacy & Arthritis
Managing Your Activities
Managing Your Fatigue
Managing Your Pain
Travel Tips for People with Arthritis
Osteoarthritis
Rheumatoid Arthritis
Walking and Arthritis
Water Exercise: Pools, Spas and Arthritis
For these or other booklets, call your local Arthritis Foundation chapter or contact the Arthritis Foundation Distribution Center · P. O. Box 1616, Alpharetta, GA 30009-1616. 800-207-8633.
www.arthritis.org/AFStore

Sources for Information or Purchase of Assistive Devices

Abledata
http://trace.wisc.edu

Smith & Nephew, Inc. · One Quality Drive, P. O. Box 1005, Germantown, WI 53011-8205. 800-558-8633.
www.smith-nephew.com/US/

Sammons Preston · P. O. Box 5071, Bolingbrook, IL 60440-5071. 800-323-5547.
www.sammonspreston.com/

Maddak, Inc. · 6 Industrial Rd., Pequannock, NJ 07440-1993. 973-628-7600.
www.maddak.com/

North Coast Medical · 18305 Sutter Blvd., Morgan Hill, CA 95037-2845. 877-213-9300.
www.ncmedical.com/

Ergonomics and Occupational Health Catalogue · AliMed, 297 High St., Dedham, MA 02026. 800-225-2610.
www.alimed.com/

References

Altman, R., Alarcon, G., Appelrouth, D., Bloch, D., Borenstein, D., Brandt, L., Brown, C., Cooke, T. D., Daniel, W., Gray, R., Greenwald, R., Hochberg, M., Howell, D., Ike, R., Kapila, P., Kaplan, D., Koopman, W., Longley, S., McShane, D. J., Medsger, T., Michel, B., Murphy, W., Osial, T., Ramsey-Goldman, R., Rothschild, B., Stark, K., & Wolfe, F. (1990). The American College of Rheumatology criteria for the classification and reporting of osteoarthritis of the hand. *Arthritis and Rheumatism, 33* (11), 1601–1610.

Anderson, R. J. (1993). Rheumatoid arthritis. B. Clinical features and laboratory. In R. H. Schumacher, (Ed.), *Primer on the Rheumatic Diseases* (10th ed., pp. 90–95) Atlanta: Arthritis Foundation.

Arnett, F. C., Edworthy, S. M., Bloch, D. A., McShane, D. J., Fries, J. F., Cooper, N. S., Healey, L. A., Kaplan, S. R., Liang, M. H., Harvinder, S., Luthra, S., Medsger, T. A., Jr., Mitchell, D. M., Neustadt, D. H., Pinals, R. S., Schaller, J. G., Sharpt, J. T., Wilder, R. L., & Hunder, G. G. (1988). The American Rheumatism Association 1987 revised criteria for the classification of rheumatoid arthritis. *Arthritis and Rheumatism, 31,* 315–324.

Arthritis Foundation (1993). *Living and Loving.* Atlanta: Author.

Axtell, L. A., & Yasuda, Y. L. (1993). Assistive devices and home modification in geriatric rehabilitation. *Clinical Geriatric Medicine, 9,* 803–821.

Backman, C. (1998). Functional assessment. In J. Melvin & G. Jensen (Eds.), *Rheumatologic Rehabilitation Series* (Vol. 1, pp. 157–194). Bethesda, MD: American Occupational Therapy Association.

Backman, C., & Mackie, H. (1995). Arthritis hand function test: Inter-rater reliability among self-trained raters. *Arthritis Care and Research, 8* (1), 10–15.

Backman, C., & Mackie, H. (1996). The arthritis hand function test. [AOTA] *Physical Disabilities Special Interest Section Newsletter, 19* (4), 1–2.

Belza, B. L. (1995). Comparison of self-reported fatigue in rheumatoid arthritis and controls. *Journal of Rheumatology, 22,* 639–643.

Belza, B. L. (1996). Fatigue. In S. T. Wegener, B. L. Belza, & E. P. Gall, (Eds.), *Clinical Care in the Rheumatic Diseases* (pp. 117–120). Atlanta: American College of Rheumatology.

Belcon, M. C., Haynes, R. B., & Tugwell, P. (1984). A critical review of compliance studies in rheumatoid arthritis. *Arthritis and Rheumatism, 27,* 1227–1233.

Blank, J. E., & Cassidy, C. (1996). The distal radioulnar joint in rheumatoid arthritis. *Hand Clinics, 12* (3), 499–513.

Brandt, K. D., & Slemenda, C. W. (1993). Osteoarthritis: Epidemiology, pathology, and pathogenesis. In H. R. Schumacher, (Ed.), *Primer on the Rheumatic Diseases* (10th ed., pp. 184–187). Atlanta: Arthritis Foundation.

Carroll, D. (1965). A quantitative test of upper extremity function. *Journal of Chronic Disease, 18,* 479–491.

Clark, F., Azen, S. P., Zemke, R., Jackson, J., Carlson, M., Mandel, D., Hay, J., Josephson, K., Cherry, B., Hessel, C., Palmer, J. M., & Lipson, L. (1997). Occupational therapy for independent-living older adults. *Journal of American Medical Association, 278* (16), 1321–1326.

Coppard, B. M., Gale, J. R., & Jensen, G. M. (1998) Therapeutic exercise. In J. Melvin & G. Jensen, (Eds.), *Rheumatology Rehabilitation Series, Vol. 1: Assessment and Management* (pp. 335–350). Bethesda, MD: American Occupational Therapy Association.

Cordery, J., & Rocchi, M. (1998). Joint protection and fatigue management. In J. Melvin & G. Jensen (Eds.), *Rheumatologic Rehabilitation Series, Vol. 1: Assessment and Management* (pp. 279–321). Bethesda, MD:American Occupational Therapy Association.

Falconer, J. (1990). Hand splinting in rheumatoid arthritis. *Arthritis Care and Research, 4* (2), 81–86.

Feinberg, J. (1992). Effect of the arthritis health professional on compliance with use of resting hand splints by patients with rheumatoid arthritis. *Arthritis Care and Research, 5* (1), 17–23.

Feinberg J., & Brandt, K. D. (1981). Use of resting splints by patients with rheumatoid arthritis. *American Journal of Occupational Therapy, 35* (3), 173–178.

Feinberg, J. R. & Trombly, C. A. (1995). Arthritis. In C.A. Trombly (Ed.), *Occupational Therapy for Physical Dysfunction* (4th ed., pp. 815–830). Baltimore: Williams and Wilkins.

Furst, G., Gerber, L. H., & Smith, C. (1985). *Rehabilitation through learning: Energy conservation and joint protection. A workbook for persons with rheumatoid arthritis.* (Publication 85–2743). Rockville, MD: U.S. Department of Health and Human Services, National Institutes of Health.

Furst, G. P., Gerber, L. H., Smith, C. C., Fisher, S., & Shulman, B. (1987).

A program for improving energy conservation behaviors in adults with rheumatoid arthritis. *American Journal of Occupational Therapy, 41,* 102–111.

Gerber, L., & Furst, G. P. (1992). Validation of the NIH activity record: A quantitative measure of life activities. *Arthritis Care and Research, 5,* 81–86.

Gerber, L. H., Furst, G. P., Smith, C., Shulman, B., Liang, M., Cullen, K., Stevens, M. B., & Gilbert, N. (1987). Patient education program to teach energy conservation behaviors to patients with rheumatoid arthritis: A pilot study. *Archives of Physical Medicine and Rehabilitation, 68,* 422–445.

Hochberg, M. C., Chang, R. W., Dwosh, I., Lindsey, S., Pincus, T., & Wolfe, F. (1992). The American College of Rheumatology 1991 revised criteria for the classification of global functional status in rheumatoid arthritis. *Arthritis and Rheumatism, 35* (5), 498–502.

Huskisson, E. C. (1974). Measurement of pain. *Lancet, 2* (7889), 1127–1131.

Jackson, J., Carlson, M., Mandel, D., Zemke, R., & Clark, F. (1998). Occupation in lifestyle redesign: The well elderly study occupational therapy program. *American Journal of Occupational Therapy, 52* (5), 326–335.

Kjeken, I., Moller, G., & Kvien, T. K. (1995). Use of commercially produced elastic wrist orthoses in chronic arthritis: A controlled study. *Arthritis Care and Research, 8,* 108–113.

Komatireddy, G. R., Leitch, R. W., Cella, K., Browning, G., & Minor, M. (1997). Efficacy of low load resistive muscle training in patients with rheumatoid arthritis functional class II and III. *Journal of Rheumatology, 24* (8), 1531–1539.

Law, M., Baptiste, S., Carswell, A., McColl, M. A., Polatajko, H., & Pollock, N. (1994). *Canadian Occupational Performance Measure* (2nd ed.). Toronto: CAOT.

Livneh, H. (1986a). A unified approach to existing models of adaptation to disability: Part 1. A model of adaptation. *Journal of Applied Rehabilitation Counseling, 17* (1), 5–16.

Livneh, H. (1986b). A unified approach to existing models of adaptation to disability. Part 2. Intervention strategies. *Journal of Applied Rehabilitation Counseling, 17* (3), 6–10.

Majerovitz, S. J., & Revenson, T. A. (1994). Sexuality and rheumatic disease. *Arthritis Care and Research, 7* (1), 29–34.

Mann, W. (1998). Assistive technology for persons with arthritis. In J. Melvin & G. Jensen (Eds.), *Rheumatology Rehabilitation Series, Vol. 1: Assessment and Management* (pp. 369–392). Bethesda, MD: American Occupational Therapy Association.

Mathiowetz, V., Kashman, N., Volland, G., Weber K., Dowe, M., & Rogers, S. (1985). Grip and pinch strength, normative data for adults. *Archives of Physical Medicine and Rehabilitation, 66,* 69–74.

McFarlane, D. G., Buckland-Wright, J. C., Emery, P., Fogelman, I., Clark, B., & Lynch, J. (1990). Comparison of clinical, radionuclide, and radiographic features of osteoarthritis of the hands. *Annals of the Rheumatic Diseases, 50* (9), 623–626.

Melvin, J. L. (1989). *Rheumatic Diseases in the Adult and Child: Occupational Therapy and Rehabilitation* (3rd ed.). Philadelphia: Davis.

Minor, M. A. (1996). Rest and exercise. In S. T. Wegener, B. L. Belza, & E. P. Gall, (Eds.), *Clinical Care in the Rheumatic Diseases* (pp. 79–82). Atlanta: American College of Rheumatology.

Nalebuff, E. A. (1984). The rheumatoid thumb. *Clinics in Rheumatic Diseases, 10,* 589–608.

Nordenskiold, U. (1990). Elastic wrist orthoses. Reduction of pain and increase in grip force for women with rheumatoid arthritis. *Arthritis Care and Research, 3* (3), 158–162.

Nordenskiold, U. M., & Grimby, G. (1993). Grip force in patients with rheumatoid arthritis and fibromyalgia and in healthy subjects. A study with the Grippit instrument. *Scandinavian Journal of Rheumatology, 22,* 14–19.

Nordenskiold, U., Grimby, G., & Dahlin-Ivanoff, S. (1998). Questionnaire to evaluate the effects of assistive devices and altered working methods in women with rheumatoid arthritis. *Clinical Rheumatology, 17,* 7–16.

Nordenskiold, U., Grimby, G., Hedberg, M., Wright, B., & Linacre, J. M. (1996). The structure of an instrument for assessing the effect of assistive devices and altered working methods in women with rheumatoid arthritis. *Arthritis Care and Research, 9,* 21–30.

Palchik, N. S., Mitchell, D. M., Gilbert, N. L., Schulz, A. J., Dedrick, R. F., & Palella T. D. (1990). Nonsurgical management of the boutonniere deformity. *Arthritis Care and Research, 3* (4), 227–232.

Partridge, R. E. H., & Duthie, J. J. R. (1963). Controlled trial of the effect of complete immobilization of the joints in rheumatoid arthritis. *Annals of Rheumatic Disease, 22,* 91–96.

Pincus, T. (1996). Rheumatoid arthritis. In S. T. Wegener, (Ed.), *Clinical Care in the Rheumatic Diseases* (pp. 147–156). Atlanta: American College of Rheumatology.

Rizio, L., & Belsky, M. R. (1996). Finger deformities in rheumatoid arthritis. *Hand Clinics, 22* (3), 531–540.

Shapiro, J. S. (1996). The wrist in rheumatoid arthritis. *Hand Clinics, 12* (3), 477–498.

Spiegel, J. S., Hirshfield, M. S., & Spiegel, T. M. (1985). Evaluating self care activities: Comparison of a self-reported questionnaire with an occupational therapist interview. *British Journal of Rheumatology, 24,* 357–361.

Stein, A. B., & Terrono, A. L. (1996). The rheumatoid thumb. *Hand Clinics, 12* (3), 541–550.

Stein, C. M., Griffin, M. R., & Brandt, K. D. (1996). Osteoarthritis. In S. T.

Wegener, B. L. Belza, & E. P. Gall, (Eds.), *Clinical Care in the Rheumatic Diseases* (pp. 177–182). Atlanta: American College of Rheumatology.

Stern, E. B., Ytterberg, S. R., Krug, H. E., Mullin, G. T., & Mahowald, M. L. (1996). Immediate and short-term effects of three commercial wrist extensor orthoses on grip strength and function in patients with rheumatoid arthritis. *Arthritis Care and Research, 9* (1), 42–50.

Stern, E. B., Ytterberg, S. R., Larson, L. M., Portoghese, C. P., Kratz, W. N. R., & Mahowald, M. L. (1997). Commercial wrist extensor orthoses: A descriptive study of use and preference in patients with rheumatoid arthritis. *Arthritis Care and Research, 10* (1), 27–35.

Taliesnik, J. (1989). Rheumatoid arthritis of the wrist. *Hand Clinics, 5* (2), 257–277.

Tijhuis, G. J., Vlieland, T. P. M., Zwinderman, A. H., & Hazes, J. M. W. (1998). A comparison of the Futuro wrist orthosis with a synthetic Thermolyn orthosis: Utility and clinical effectiveness. *Arthritis Care and Research, 11* (3), 217–222.

Wilder, R. L. (1993). Rheumatoid arthritis: Epidemiology, pathology, and pathogenesis. In R. H. Schumacher, (Ed.), *Primer on the Rheumatic Diseases* (10th ed., pp. 86–89). Atlanta: Arthritis Foundation.

Wilson, R. L. (1986). Rheumatoid arthritis of the hand. *Orthopedic Clinics of North America, 17* (2), 313–343.

Wilson, R. L. (1996). Extensor tendon problems in rheumatoid arthritis. *Hand Clinics, 12* (3), 551–559.

Yasuda, Y. L. (2000). *Occupational Therapy Practice Guidelines for Adults With Rheumatoid Arthritis.* Bethesda: American Occupational Therapy Association.

45

Burn Injuries

Monica A. Pessina and Amy C. Orroth

LEARNING OBJECTIVES

After studying this chapter, the reader will be able to do the following:

1. Differentiate between superficial, superficial partial-thickness, deep partial-thickness, and full-thickness burn injuries.
2. Explain the rationale for splinting and positioning programs for patients with burn injuries.
3. Outline occupational therapy treatment techniques for each phase of burn recovery.
4. Describe potential complications and treatment strategies for hand burns.
5. Discuss the effects of a burn injury on a patient's psychosocial functioning.

*A*pproximately 1.25 million burn injuries occur in the United States each year, resulting in 5,500 fire- and burn-related deaths (Brigham & McLoughlin, 1996). Thermal damage to the skin can be caused by fire, contact with a hot object or hot liquid (scald burn), radiation, chemicals, or electricity. Almost 80% of burn injuries occur in and around the home, and hot food and liquid spills are the most common source of burns to children (Brigham & McLoughlin). There are an average of 51,000 acute hospital admissions annually for burn injuries, of which 23,000 admissions are to regional burn centers designated by the American Burn Association (Brigham & McLoughlin). Although many patients with major burns are treated at these specialized burn care facilities, a large percentage of patients with burn injuries are also treated at local or regional hospitals. Therefore, every occupational therapist should understand the principles of care and rehabilitation of patients with burn injuries. Treatment of these injuries requires a comprehensive approach by a qualified burn treatment team, including a skilled occupational therapist. This chapter explores the unique role of occupational therapy in treatment of burn patients, from the initial injury to the patient's return to independent function. Topics include various phases of burn rehabilitation, scar management, psychosocial issues, and reconstructive surgery. We hope to convey the unique and rewarding aspects of working with patients with burn injuries.

GLOSSARY

Antideformity positions—Positions opposite to common patterns of deformity to prevent contractures.

Blanch—Apply sufficient pressure to interrupt blood flow temporarily: an assessment of capillary flow rate.

Deep partial-thickness burn—Thermal injury that destroys cells from the epidermis to the deep dermal layer.

Debride—Remove eschar and loose or necrotic tissue to prevent infection and promote healing.

Dermis—Layer of skin below the epidermis that contains blood vessels, nerve endings, hair follicles, and sweat and oil glands. Supports the regrowth of new epithelial tissue.

Epidermis—Most superficial layer of the skin; acts as a barrier. It is continually sloughed and replaced.

Eschar—Burned tissue.

Full-thickness burn—Thermal injury in which the epidermis and dermal layers are destroyed.

Superficial burn—Thermal injury that involves only cells in the epidermis.

Superficial partial-thickness burn—Thermal injury in which the epidermis and upper portion of the dermal layer are destroyed.

Wound contracture—Part of normal healing in which myofibroblasts in the wound bed contract in an attempt to close the wound.

Z-plasty—Surgical procedure in which a Z-shaped incision is made and tissue is transposed to increase tissue length.

Burn Classification

In the past, burn depth was classified as first, second, or third degree. Today, the preferred classification system more accurately describes the level of cellular injury. The terms in use are **superficial**, **superficial partial-thickness**, **deep partial-thickness**, and **full-thickness** (Fig. 45-1). Burns typically have mixed depths, which necessitates that the burn team carefully assess the appearance and progress of each area of the wound site. Disruption of any portion of the skin has the potential to interfere with its normal functions, which include temperature regulation, excretion, sensation, vitamin D synthesis, and acting as a barrier against infection and dehydration (Falkel, 1994). Occupational therapists may treat patients with all levels of thermal injury. It is important to differentiate among the classifications to plan appropriate intervention.

Superficial Burns

Superficial burns damage cells only in the **epidermis** (Malick & Carr, 1982; Staley et al., 1994). These injuries are painful and red. They heal spontaneously within approximately 7 days and leave no permanent scar (Malick & Carr).

Superficial Partial-Thickness Burns

Superficial partial-thickness burns damage cells in the epidermis and the upper level of the **dermis** (Malick & Carr, 1982; Staley et al., 1994). The most common sign of a superficial partial-thickness burn is intact blisters over the injured area (Staley et al.). These injuries are also painful because of the irritation of the nerve endings in the dermal layer. Superficial partial-thickness burns heal spontaneously within 7 to 21 days and leave minimal or no scarring (Staley et al.).

Deep Partial-Thickness Burns

Deep partial-thickness burns cause cell injury in the epidermis and severe damage to the dermal layer (Malick & Carr, 1982; Staley et al., 1994). These injuries appear blotchy, with areas of whitish color interspersed throughout the wound (Malick & Carr). The injury site is painful. Pressure sensation is intact but light touch is diminished (Staley et al.). Spontaneous healing of deep partial-thickness burns is sluggish (3–5 weeks) because vascularity in the dermal layer is impaired. Therefore, the risk of significant scarring is increased (Staley et al.). For this reason, deep partial-thickness burns are often grafted to expedite healing and minimize scarring.

Full-Thickness Injury

In a full-thickness injury both the epidermis and the dermal layer are destroyed (Malick & Carr, 1982; Staley et al., 1994). These wounds appear white or waxy and are inherently insensate because of the complete destruction of the dermal nerve endings (Malick & Carr). Full-thickness burns require surgical intervention, such as skin grafting (Malick & Carr; Staley et al.), since there are no dermal elements to support the regrowth of epithelial tissue. Some burns, such as electrical burns, may damage structures below the dermis, including subcutaneous fat, muscle, or bone.

Rule of Nines

A commonly used technique to determine burn size is the rule of nines (Fig. 45-2). The percentage of total body surface area (TBSA) that has been burned is used for the following:

▶ Calculating nutritional and fluid requirements
▶ Determining level of acuity to establish the level of medical treatment needed (i.e., admission to an intensive care unit)
▶ Predicting length of acute hospitalization (often expected to be 1 day per percent TBSA burned)

Phases of Burn Management and Rehabilitation

Identifying specific phases of burn management helps to describe the role of occupational therapy for patients with burn injuries. These include the emergent, acute, and rehabilitation phases. Each of the phases, along with accompanying occupational therapy considerations, are described.

Emergent Phase

The emergent phase of a burn injury is considered to be from initial injury to approximately 72 hours post burn (Grigsby deLinde & Miles, 1995).

Medical Management

During the emergent phase, the medical team attempts to stabilize the patient. This may include fluid resuscitation, establishment of adequate tissue perfusion, and achievement of cardiopulmonary stability. Associated

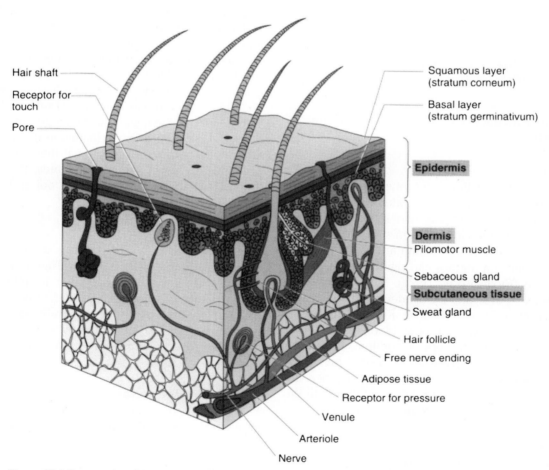

Figure 45-1 Cross-section of the skin. (Reprinted with permission from Willis, M. C. (1996). *Medical Terminology: The Language of Health Care* (p. 90). Baltimore: Williams & Wilkins.)

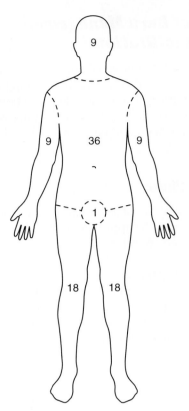

Figure 45-2 Rule of nines. (Reprinted with permission from Malick, M. H., & Carr, J. A. (1982). *Manual on Management of the Burn Patient* (p. 10). Pittsburgh: Harmarville Rehabilitation Center.)

injuries, such as fractures, are evaluated and treated during this time.

Inhalation Injury

An important consideration in the emergent phase is the possibility of an inhalation injury. Damage to the upper airway as a result of inhaling either hot particles or noxious gases results in an inhalation injury. This damages the respiratory epithelium and can impair gas exchange. Inhalation injuries can significantly increase mortality rate (Cioffi & Rue, 1991). Singed eyebrows, soot around the nares, and facial edema are indications of an inhalation injury (Cioffi & Rue). Diagnosis is confirmed by analysis of arterial blood gases, chest radiographs, and bronchoscopy. In addition, edema can quickly develop in the airway and constrict breathing. Therefore, patients with significant burn injuries are usually intubated to maintain an open airway until the risk of airway closure due to edema has diminished.

Escharotomy and Fasciotomy

Circulation can be compromised when burn injuries girdle a body segment. This is due to the inelasticity of the **eschar** (burned tissue) combined with increased

internal pressure within fascial compartments. Local increase in pressure in the extremities compresses blood vessels and reduces blood flow (Sheridan et al., 1995). Symptoms of increased compartmental pressure include paraesthesias, coldness, and decreased or absent pulses in the extremities. In the trunk, inelastic eschar can act as a corset, limiting lung expansion and preventing adequate respiration. In both cases, surgical intervention (escharotomy and/or fasciotomy) is required to relieve the pressure and prevent tissue death. An escharotomy is a surgical incision through the eschar, whereas a fasciotomy is a deeper incision extending through the fascia. Unless exposed tendon is present, the escharotomy region can be mobilized during therapy (Grigsby deLinde & Miles, 1995). However, therapy is contraindicated for an area where a fasciotomy has been performed.

Dressings

After the initial burn assessment, the nursing staff applies dressings. The functions of dressings include protecting the wound against infection, maintaining contact between the topical agent and the wound, superficially **debriding** the wound, and providing comfort for the patient (Grigsby deLinde & Miles, 1995). Debriding is the removal of devitalized tissue from the wound site. Types of topical agents vary widely, although most are widespectrum antimicrobials. Examples include mafenide acetate (Sulfamylon), silver sulfadiazine (Silvadene), and 0.5% silver nitrate solution (Duncan & Driscoll, 1991). As a rule the nursing staff changes dressings twice a day. By periodically participating in dressing removal and application, the occupational therapist makes opportunities to view the healing wounds. This allows the therapist to monitor healing and adjust the therapy program accordingly.

Infection Control

One of the functions of the skin is to act as a barrier against infection (Falkel, 1994). Therefore, a patient with a burn injury is susceptible to infection. It is essential that all staff, family, and visitors adhere to infection control procedures. This includes frequent hand washing, use of gloves when necessary, and avoiding cross-contamination through instruments and equipment (Box 45-1).

Contracture Formation

Patients with burn injuries are at significant risk for contractures. **Wound contracture**, a normal physiological response to an open wound (Greenhalgh & Staley, 1994; Staley et al., 1994), combined with prolonged immobilization, creates an opportunity for permanent soft tissue contracture. Contractures tend to occur in predictable patterns, usually flexed, shortened positions (e.g., elbow flexion, shoulder adduction, knee flexion) and can considerably limit the patient's ability to perform activities of daily living (ADL). For example, decreased elbow extension may limit the patient's ability to dress.

Occupational Therapy Assessment During the Emergent Phase

During the emergent phase, the occupational therapist performs a screen of the patient's needs. A full evaluation is deferred until after the emergent phase, when the patient is more medically stable. During the screen, the therapist notes the distribution of the burn and which joints are involved. This allows the occupational therapist to establish an appropriate splinting and positioning program. It is also during this time that the therapist begins collecting information regarding the patient's functional status before admission, including individual interests and social supports.

Occupational Therapy During the Emergent Phase

Occupational therapy in the emergent phase focuses on the prevention of early contracture formation through the use of splints and positioning programs. It is ideal to initiate occupational therapy intervention as early as

BOX 45-1
PROCEDURES FOR PRACTICE

Hand Washing

Hand washing is the easiest and most effective thing you can do to prevent infections for you and your patients.

When

▶ Before and after all patient contact
▶ After removing gloves used to perform a task involving contact with blood, body fluids, or infectious material
▶ After handling possibly infectious devices or equipment
▶ Before and after preparing and eating food

General Procedure

▶ Dispense paper towel
▶ Push up long sleeves
▶ Wet hands and wrists
▶ Apply antiseptic solution or soap
▶ Use friction to clean between fingers, under nails, and palms and backs of hands; effective scrubbing lasts at least 15 seconds
▶ Rinse hands and towel dry
▶ Turn off faucet using paper towel
▶ Dispose of paper towel in appropriate trash barrel
▶ Waterless hand cleaner can be used until hand washing facilities are available

24 to 48 hours post burn, because collagen synthesis and contracture formation begin during the initial response to thermal injury (Evans & McAuliffe, 1995; Institute for Healthcare Quality [IHQ], 1997).

Splinting

Ideally, splints are fabricated and applied in the initial visit and a positioning program is established and communicated to the team. Table 45-1 describes common contracture patterns, antideformity positions, and appropriate splints. Generally, any joint involved in a superficial partial-thickness injury or worse has the potential for contracture and is usually splinted. Splint wearing times are determined by the patient's ability to use the involved extremity. That is, a decrease in active movement indicates the need for increased splint wearing time. For example, a heavily sedated patient cannot perform active movement, and therefore requires splinting at all times except for therapy and dressing changes. An alert patient who can use his or her affected extremity for functional tasks, such as self-feeding or prescribed exercises, may require the use of splints only at night. Splints are applied over the burn dressing and secured with either gauze wrap or Velcro straps.

Positioning

Antideformity positioning, which is used as an adjunct to splinting for prevention of contractures, can be begun in the first visit. Elevating the upper extremities can also help to minimize upper extremity edema. Elevation can be done with foam wedges, pillows, or specialized arm troughs attached to the bed. A risk of upper extremity elevation is the potential for brachial plexus strain. Symptoms of brachial plexus strain include tingling, numbness, and cold fingers.

Acute Phase

The acute phase begins after the emergent phase and continues until the wound is closed, either by spontaneous healing or skin grafts (Grigsby deLinde & Miles, 1995). The acute phase can last several days to several months, depending on the extent of the burn and the amount of grafting required.

Medical Management

Skin grafting, which occurs primarily in the acute phase, is required when the dermal bed is sufficiently destroyed to prevent or significantly impair spontaneous regrowth of the epithelial tissue (Grigsby deLinde & Miles, 1995). If reepithelialization of the burn site has not occurred within 14 days of the injury or is not expected, grafting would be considered (Kagan & Warden, 1994). Skin grafting is generally performed for all full-thickness

TABLE 45-1
Anticontracture Positioning by Location of Burn

Location of Burn	Contracture Tendency	Anticontracture Positioning and/or Typical Splint
Anterior neck	Neck flexion	Remove pillows; use half-mattress to extend the neck; neck extension splint or collar
Axilla	Adduction	120° abduction with slight external rotation; axilla splint or positioning wedges; watch for signs of brachial plexus strain
Anterior elbow	Flexion	Elbow extension splint in 5–10° flexion
Dorsal wrist	Wrist extension	Wrist support in neutral
Volar wrist	Wrist flexion	Wrist cockup splint in 5–10° flexion
Hand-dorsal	Claw hand deformity	Functional hand splint with MP joints 70–90°, IP joints fully extended, first web open, thumb in opposition (safe position; see Chapter 42)
Hand-volar	Palmar contracture	Palm extension splint
	Cupping of hand	MPs in slight hyperextension
Hip- anterior	Hip flexion	Prone positioning; weights on thigh in supine; knee immobilizers
Knee	Knee flexion	Knee extension positioning and/or splints; prevent external rotation, which may cause peroneal nerve compression
Foot	Foot drop	Ankle at 90° with foot board or splint; watch for signs of heel ulcer

Reprinted with permission from Pessina, M. A., & Ellis, S. M. (1997). Rehabilitation. *Nursing Clinics of North America* (p. 367).

burns and for large, deep partial-thickness burns. Skin grafting entails both excision of necrotic (dead) tissue and the placement of skin or a skin substitute over the wound bed.

Types of Grafts
A variety of grafting procedures are available to the burn team. According to the size of the burn and the medical stability of the patient, the team may opt to use one or more types of grafts described next.

Autografts. Skin harvested from an unburned area of the patient is an autograft. Split-thickness autografts, the most frequently used, are taken at the level of the mid dermis (IHQ, 1997; Staley et al., 1994). Donor sites are ideally selected for the best match of color and texture to the affected area. As donor sites produce mild scarring, their location, when possible, is in an inconspicuous site, such as the upper thigh. The harvested skin can be left as a solid sheet (sheet graft) or perforated to increase surface area (meshed graft) (Staley et al.). Meshing allows the surface area of the harvested skin to cover up to four times the original area. Both sheet and meshed grafts have advantages and disadvantages. A sheet graft has the best cosmetic outcome and is therefore preferred for the face and hands (Duncan & Driscoll, 1991). However, infection and the development of hematoma under a sheet graft can cause complete graft loss and require regrafting. A meshed graft, while less cosmetically appealing (the meshed pattern is retained permanently), covers large areas when the donor site is limited.

In addition, meshed grafts allow drainage of blood and exudate, which prevents hematomas and improves graft adherence (Duncan & Driscoll).

Temporary Grafts. In cases of extensive burn injuries, where there is not sufficient donor skin to cover all of the affected area with autograft, the burn team may opt to use temporary grafts until the donor site has healed sufficiently for reharvesting. These temporary dressings aid in wound management by decreasing infection, stimulating healing and preparing the wound bed for autograft skin, decreasing pain, and protecting exposed tendons, nerves, and blood vessels (Duncan & Driscoll, 1991). Examples include xenografts (medically manipulated bovine skin), allografts (cadaver skin), and biological dressings, such as Biobrane.

Occupational Therapy Assessment During the Acute Phase
During the acute phase, the occupational therapist performs a detailed initial evaluation. This includes a thorough chart review to determine the history of the wound and associated injuries. Previous medical history is also important. Factors such as psychiatric illness, diabetes, or lung disease affect occupational therapy treatment. Areas specifically assessed by the occupational therapist during the initial evaluation:

▶ ADL and instrumental activities of daily living (IADL)
▶ Psychosocial status and support systems

- ▶ Behavior and communication
- ▶ Cognitive-perceptual status
- ▶ Neuromuscular status (range of motion strength, sensation)
- ▶ Activity tolerance

Evaluation is responsive to areas particularly important to patients with burns. It can consist of observation during task performance, interviews with patient and family, and the use of standardized tests such as the *Functional Independence Measure* (Uniform Data System for Medical Rehabilitation, 1997). The potential for permanent scarring and disfigurement may cause significant anxiety and limit the patient's ability to participate in rehabilitation. Thus, early identification of the patient's support systems can improve functional outcomes.

Occupational Therapy During the Acute Phase

Because of the acute medical nature of many burn injuries, treatment in the acute phase focuses on capacities and abilities such as range of motion and strength. These are addressed through continued splinting, positioning, and exercise. Environmental modifications are also initiated. Impaired ability to communicate due to intubation or perioral burns may contribute to anxiety. To address this, the occupational therapist, in collaboration with the burn team, implements alternative communication systems, such as a communication board or eye blink signaling. In the acute phase, the individual's ability to participate in treatment related to self-care, activity tolerance, functional retraining, and scar management is often limited by complex medical issues. These areas are addressed in detail during the rehabilitation phase.

Splinting and Positioning

During the acute phase, the splinting and positioning programs established in the emergent phase are continually monitored and adjusted. Splinting schedules are adjusted to the individual's ability to participate in an exercise and positioning program. For example, if a patient consistently uses an affected elbow for self-feeding and ADL during the day, decreasing the wearing time for the elbow splint to nights and rest periods is appropriate. Conversely, a patient who cannot follow through with an exercise and positioning program because of impaired alertness or poor motivation should wear a splint continuously except for dressing changes and therapeutic exercise. It is imperative to check all splints daily for modifications to ensure proper form and function. In addition, teaching the nursing staff proper fit and application of splints can decrease the potential for complications (Pessina & Ellis, 1997).

Exercise

In the acute phase, splinting and positioning are used in combination with exercise. Exercise is especially important for burned patients to control edema and prevent muscle atrophy, tendon adherence, joint stiffness, and capsular shortening (Harden & Luster, 1991). Exercise programs for burn patients typically follow a continuum with passive exercise at one end and the patient's ability to incorporate specific motions into daily activities at the other. The exercise continuum progresses as follows:

1. Passive range of motion
2. Active assistive range of motion
3. Active range of motion
4. Functional activity

If the patient cannot participate in active exercise because of poor medical status or impaired level of alertness, passive range of motion is indicated. However, active exercise is encouraged whenever possible (Burke Evans et al., 1996; Wright, 1984). Regardless of the entry point on the continuum, the role of the therapist is to guide the patient toward function. Within a single treatment session, a patient may participate in all of these forms of exercise. In fact, functional activities may be used to improve active range of motion. Exercise programs are performed up to five times daily (Wright). Periodic inspection of the wound by the occupational therapist is essential to determine status of wound healing and skin integrity as related to tolerance of the exercise program. Contraindications to exercise include exposed tendons, recent autografts (< 5–10 days), and fractures (Duran-Coleman, 1991; Grigsby deLinde & Miles, 1995; Staley et al., 1994).

Perioperative Care

The 5 to 10 days following a skin graft procedure is the perioperative period. A patient with a large burn injury may make many trips to the operating room for skin grafting. Each surgical procedure begins a new perioperative stage. For example, a patient needing grafting on the trunk, arms, and legs may make three trips to the operating room, with each successive area requiring proper perioperative care. The role of the occupational therapist in the perioperative period is to fabricate custom splints to immobilize the newly grafted areas in antideformity positions. Ideally, splints are fabricated immediately prior to or during surgery and applied at the conclusion of the surgery. These splints usually stay in place, along with the primary dressing, for 5 to 10 days (Duran-Coleman, 1991; Grigsby deLinde & Miles, 1995). During this time, range of motion exercises are contraindicated to allow for graft adherence. After the primary dressing is removed, the burn team assesses the graft adherence and a determination is made regarding the appropriateness of resuming exercise.

Pain Management

The occupational therapist must address pain. Many patients in intensive care cannot verbalize subjective response to manipulation, such as during dressing changes or exercise. In these cases the therapist monitors objective responses to pain, such as blood pressure, heart rate, and respiratory rate and adjusts the treatment accordingly. As a result, the time of the treatment may be changed to allow pain medication to be administered. Decreased repetitions and increased rest breaks during exercise sessions may also be appropriate. Other techniques used to manage pain throughout recovery include distraction techniques, visualization, and having the patient participate in exercises and dressing changes.

Environmental Adaptation

Beginning in the acute phase and throughout recovery, the occupational therapist provides modified call buttons and bed controls, voice-activated telephone systems, modified utensils (Fig. 45-3) and self-care items. These modifications, combined with patient, staff, and family education, can increase a patient's sense of control and independence. The development of environmental modifications is limited only by the patient's motivation and the therapist's creativity.

Patient and Family Teaching

The occupational therapist provides members of the patient's support system with guidance regarding ways to interact with and support the patient during recovery. They may be encouraged to make tape recordings and posters or to bring in favorite music or foods. They may

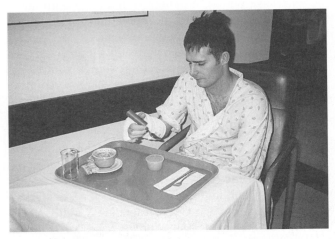

Figure 45-3 Modified utensils can increase independence in the acute phase.

need to learn new ways to touch or comfort their loved one. In addition, the family and friends provide a source of information regarding the patient's vocational and avocational roles and available community resources if the patient cannot communicate this information. An educated family and/or support system can be an important asset for ensuring follow-through of exercise and splinting programs and for encouraging participation in functional activities (Duran-Coleman, 1991).

Discharge Planning

Because hospital stays are generally short, discharge planning begins as soon as possible after admission (Fletchall & Hickerson, 1995; Rivers & Jordan, 1998). Many patients in the acute phase are discharged directly home or leave a burn center for continued care on a rehabilitation unit. Elements to consider during discharge planning are the availability of community resources for outpatient or follow-up care, support systems available to the patient, and physical demands of the home environment. When patients who have sustained major burns cannot return to the hospital where they received acute care, it is important for the inpatient occupational therapist to establish a relationship with a therapist in the patient's community to ensure continuity of care throughout the rehabilitation phase. In accordance with the knowledge and experience of the community therapist, the discharging therapist provides appropriate literature and written, photographic, and/or videotaped descriptions of the rehabilitation program. This establishes a communication channel for the community therapist so questions and concerns can be addressed in a timely manner. Whenever possible, all authorization from third-party payers should be established prior to discharge (Fletchall & Hickerson), to avoid delays in the initiation of outpatient therapy. If a patient can not be discharged directly to home, transfer to an inpatient rehabilitation facility is appropriate, and again early communication with the receiving therapist is necessary to ensure continuity of care. Regardless of the discharge setting, well-briefed patients are best able to advocate for appropriate care.

Team Communication

Communication with all members of the team, including the patient and the patient's family and/or support system throughout hospitalization is essential. During this acute phase, collaboration between the occupational therapist and the burn team is essential for several reasons (Pessina & Ellis, 1997). Teamwork is necessary for these matters:

1. Alerting the team to developing contractures and response to therapeutic intervention

2. Planning for perioperative splinting
3. Clarifying range of motion orders based on graft integrity
4. Teaching the team about environmental modifications or communication systems
5. Advocating on the patient's behalf regarding eventual outpatient needs

Support and Psychosocial Adjustment in the Acute Phase

All patients with burn injuries, regardless of age, exhibit some of the same psychological responses, including withdrawal, denial, fear of death, regression, anxiety, depression, and grief (Wright, 1984). In addition, various factors can influence a burn patient's psychological status. These include emotional trauma arising from the hospital stay, the length of the hospital stay, adjustment to physical changes, adjustment to others' reactions, and location and depth of the burn injury (Baker et al., 1996; LeDoux et al., 1996). Baker et al. refer to two stages of psychosocial recovery: the first alert stage and the predischarge stage. Performance can vary considerably between the two phases. During the first alert stage, the patient initially orients to the burn injury; a severely burned patient may simply be happy to be alive (Baker et al.). It may not be until later, as the patient enters the rehabilitation phase and approaches the predischarge stage, that he or she begins to deal with the limitations in physical function. However, the patient may also exhibit early signs of depression and withdrawal, and early assessment of the patient's psychosocial status is essential. LeDoux et al. state that the burn team can foster healthy coping strategies while working with the burn patient by using these techniques:

1. Identify strengths that each patient can emphasize, reminding him or her of the strength already involved in surviving a painful and frightening experience.
2. Validate sadness and fear.
3. Assist patient to achieve goals; this helps to show hope for the future.
4. Instill a belief that the patient can succeed.

Using these techniques, the occupational therapist can work in conjunction with the burn team to begin to address individual psychological needs (LeDoux et al., 1996).

Rehabilitation Phase

The rehabilitation phase follows the acute phase and continues until scar maturation (Rivers & Jordan, 1998). Scar maturation can take 6 months to 2 years (Rivers & Jordan; Staley et al., 1994). It is considered complete when the scar becomes pale and the rate of collagen synthesis levels off (Grigsby deLinde & Miles, 1995). The level of direct involvement of the occupational therapist during this extended time is varied. It may range from daily inpatient treatment to weekly outpatient treatment to annual clinic visits.

Occupational Therapy Assessment During Rehabilitation Phase

During the rehabilitation phase, the occupational therapist continues to assess capacities and abilities such as range of motion and strength. In addition, functional assessments specific to self-care and homemaking are valuable in guiding treatment planning and preparing for discharge. Standardized tests, such as the *Functional Independence Measure* (Uniform Data System for Medical Rehabilitation, 1997) and the *Valpar Work Samples* (see Resources) are important as they provide objective data.

Occupational Therapy During Rehabilitation Phase

The overall goal of this phase is to facilitate the patient's return to his or her previous level of function. Patients are encouraged to take increasing responsibility for their care, including helping to establish meaningful goals. In addition to range of motion and strength, occupational therapy also focuses on activity tolerance, sensation, coordination, scar management, and self-care and home management skills.

Range of Motion

In addition to the range of motion program established in the acute phase, the patient benefits from daily stretching routines. In the early part of this phase, there is an increased rate of collagen synthesis (Staley et al., 1994), requiring the patient to stretch frequently throughout the day. As the scar matures and the collagen synthesis slows, decreased frequency of stretching is required. At all times, skin integrity must be monitored during stretching to prevent tearing. Massage using a non–water-based cream should precede stretching to help prevent dry skin from rupturing (Rivers & Jordan, 1998). An appropriate stretch consists of bringing the tissue to the point of **blanching**, or becoming pale, and holding it in that position for several seconds. The patient should report tension but not pain. Overzealous stretching can result in tissue tears and edema, which increase joint stiffness. Stretching is initially performed by the occupational therapist. However, with training, the patient and/or caregiver can also complete stretching routines.

Strength

Resistive exercise and graded functional activities can improve strength. For example, a patient may be taught an independent exercise program with resistive rubber ribbon or tubing such as Theraband to increase proximal upper body strength. Patients also gain strength as they perform self-care activities, such as progressing from sitting to standing for hygiene activities.

Activity Tolerance

A key feature of rehabilitation is mobilizing the patient as much as possible. For an inpatient, this includes increased time spent out of bed and trips to the gym and off the nursing unit. For an outpatient, this may mean resuming leisure activities and going on community outings.

Sensation

Newly healed skin and grafted skin may be hypersensitive. Hypersensitivity can be addressed effectively by systematic desensitization. This can be achieved by asking the patient to manipulate objects in the environment with varying textures. Initially, the patient practices holding soft textures, such as cotton balls or lambswool, and then progresses to manipulating objects with rougher textures, such as Velcro or burlap. Sometimes a formal system such as the Downey desensitization program (Barber, 1990) is used (see Chapter 27).

Coordination

Coordination can be impaired by a variety of factors, including limited range of motion, strength, or sensation. Coordination can be improved through the use of selected progressive tasks designed to challenge the patient's skills (Fig. 45-4). For example, a patient may be asked first to take lids off large jars and then smaller containers. The patient may also trace large letters or patterns before attempting to work a crossword puzzle.

Scar Management

Scar tissue formation is a natural response to wound healing (Grisby deLinde & Miles, 1995). It begins in the emergent phase and may take up to 2 years (Poh-Fitzpatrick, 1992). A hypertrophic scar (Fig. 45-5) is a red, raised, and inelastic scar (Abston, 1987). A hypertrophic scar contains an increased number of fibroblasts as compared to normal skin (Abston). Its collagen fibers are arranged in a nodular as opposed to parallel fashion (Abston). There is thought to be a disruption in the balance between collagen synthesis and lysis (Grigsby deLinde & Miles). Any tendency for hypertrophic scarring is unique to each individual. In general, patients with large amounts of pigment in the skin and young patients are most prone to hypertrophic scarring (Staley et al.). Hypertrophic scarring is also inversely related to the depth of the initial burn wound (Staley et al.). In addition to being cosmetically unappealing, hypertrophic scars can limit functional skills by restricting joint range of motion.

Occupational Therapy Assessment of Scars. The *Burn Scar Index* (*Vancouver Scar Scale*) is a standardized assessment tool used to rate the pliability, vascularity, height, and pigmentation of scars (Sullivan et al., 1990). Used periodically, the *Burn Scar Index* can help guide the occupational therapist in determining effective scar management and evaluating the stage of scar maturation.

Occupational Therapy and Scar Management. The occupational therapist attempts to prevent or limit the development of hypertrophic scars. Treatment methods include a combination of techniques, including massage, pressure therapy, and the use of specialized inserts.

Massage. Massage may be useful in reducing scar contracture (Staley et al., 1994). Scar massage is initiated when it is determined that the injured area can withstand slight friction. In addition, scar massage maintains suppleness, as normal sweat and oil gland function is often disrupted. Scar massage also aids in desensitiza-

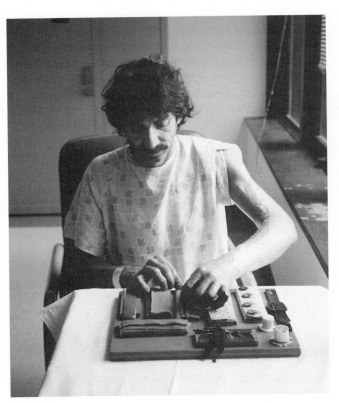

Figure 45-4 Coordination can be addressed with use of simulated or actual functional tasks.

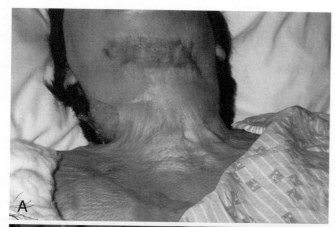

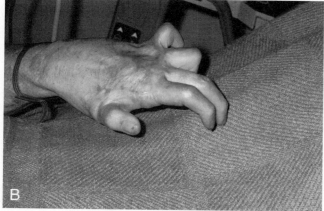

Figure 45-5 Hypertrophic scars on the neck (**A**) and hand (**B**). The hypertrophic scar on the dorsum of the hand causes claw hand deformity.

Wearing time is gradually increased by 2-hour increments until 24-hour wear is tolerated. Tolerance is determined by lack of blisters or open areas. At this point, increased pressure using customized garments such as Jobst or Bioconcepts is indicated (Fig. 45-7). Staley et al. (1994) suggest that the application of 25 mm Hg of pressure is ideal to aid in collagen organization which ultimately helps decrease scar tissue formation. Custom garments cause notable shearing during application and removal and therefore should be used only when the skin is healed sufficiently to withstand these forces. Wearing of custom garments continues until the scar is inactive, or mature, as described earlier. The therapist's role is to initiate the ordering of custom garments and oversee their use. Most providers of custom garments send trained personnel to measure the patient for custom fitting. For facial burns, the patient may use a transparent facial orthosis secured by elastic straps to provide even pressure distribution. These orthoses are usually fabricated by a specially trained orthotist at the request of the therapist.

Inserts are often used in conjunction with pressure garments. They may be constructed from products such as Otoform (Fig. 45-8), Elastomere or closed cell foam. Their purpose is to increase pressure in concave areas, such as the web spaces and the sternoclavicular depression. Silicone inserts have also been demonstrated to be effective in improving some characteristics of hypertrophic scars (Ahn et al., 1989), although the mechanism of action remains to be determined. The design of a scar management program is determined by the available resources, careful clinical observation, and the patient's ability to comply with the program (Evans & McAuliffe, 1995). Periodic outpatient visits to occupational therapy or an established burn clinic throughout the rehabilitation phase allow for monitoring and adjustments of the scar management program.

tion. Scar massage is performed several times daily with deep pressure (enough to blanch the scar temporarily) in either a circular pattern or perpendicular to the long axis of the scar. Lotion is used during massage to reduce friction. Perfume-free lotions are preferred to decrease potential irritation to newly healed skin. Initially, scar massage is the responsibility of the occupational therapist so that skin integrity and tolerance can be monitored. Once an established routine has been developed, the therapist teaches the patient and/or caregivers to assume responsibility for daily scar massage.

Pressure Dressings and Garments. Pressure dressings and garments are another form of scar management that has been advocated in the literature (Chang et al., 1995; Ward, 1991). The flattened, smooth, supple appearance of the scar after application of pressure has been reported clinically, but objective support has been inconclusive (Grigsby deLinde & Miles, 1995; Ward, 1991). The occupational therapist initiates the application of gentle pressure via Tubigrip, elastic bandage wraps, Coban, or Isotoner gloves (Fig. 45-6). Initially pressure dressings are applied for 2-hour intervals.

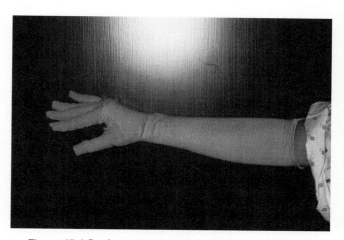

Figure 45-6 Gentle pressure is applied using Coban and Tubigrip.

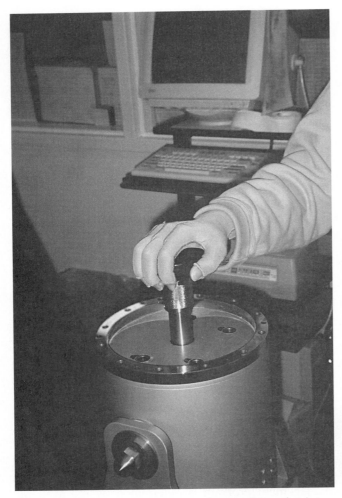

Figure 45-7 Custom pressure garments can be worn while performing simulated functional activity.

Self-Care and Home Management Skills

If neuromuscular limitations impede the patient's performance of functional tasks, the therapist may provide adaptive equipment, such as built-up handles for impaired grasp or long-handled utensils for decreased elbow flexion. Teaching adaptive techniques, such as performing certain activities using two hands for extra support, may also improve function.

Patient and Family Teaching

Patients should understand the rationale for each of the splints and techniques used in their care. They participate in the development of goals, so that they are invested in achieving them. Skin care is an important element in discharge teaching. Patients practice monitoring their skin for breakdown and caring for their skin, including the daily use of a moisturizer. They learn to use a sunscreen with a SPF of at least 15 (reapplied frequently) if they anticipate exposure to the sun (Staley et al., 1991). In addition, patients should have a basic

understanding of wound healing and tissue response to exercise and scar management techniques.

Support and Psychosocial Adjustment During the Rehabilitation Phase

While the patient and family typically focus on survival immediately after injury, many other issues arise during rehabilitation. For example, guilt or embarrassment regarding the injury may lead the patient to withdraw. The patient may also begin questioning his or her ability to return to the role of a parent or provider, which creates anxiety. Patients may fear their ability to maintain relationships and sexual functioning. The increase in activity in the rehabilitation phase not only assists physical rehabilitation but also assists patients to discover how their injury affects their daily lives. Emotional reactions to the realization of loss may produce a wide range of behaviors, such as tears and anger. Patients may also have responses related to posttraumatic stress disorder, such as flashbacks.

One of the most difficult challenges for the burn therapist is caring for patients as they grieve for a functional limitation or loss or alteration in body image

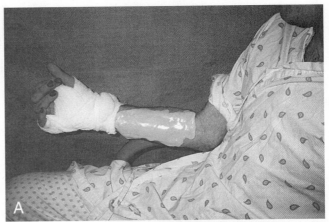

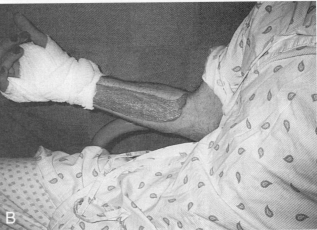

Figure 45-8 A. Use of the Otoform insert. **B.** Without insert.

(Pessina & Ellis, 1997). The occupational therapist supports the patient by encouraging questions and verbalization of feelings about the burn injury (Pessina & Ellis). The occupational therapist also chooses treatment activities to restore confidence and self-esteem. Group activities provide opportunities for socialization and sharing of concerns in a safe environment (Summers, 1991). Because of the extensive contact with the patient throughout all phases of recovery, the occupational therapist is in a unique position to identify and address psychosocial issues, but consultation with other specialists on the burn team (e.g., nursing staff, family members, social workers, and psychologists) is essential.

Potential Complications

In addition to the potential for soft tissue contractures and loss of joint range of motion, other complications may occur in any phase of burn recovery.

Pruritis

Pruritus (persistent itching) is a common complication (IHQ, 1997; Staley et al., 1994), presumably due to nerve regeneration. It usually resolves within 2 years of the initial injury (Poh-Fitzpatrick, 1992). The use of compression garments, skin moisturizers, cold packs, and medications such as antihistamines may alleviate itching (IHQ).

Microstomia

Patients with facial burns in the area of the mouth are at risk for oral commissure contracture (microstomia) (Rivers & Jordan, 1998)—tightening of the musculature around the lip area that limits mouth opening. In extreme cases urgent surgical revision is required. This risk is exaggerated if the patient has undergone prolonged periods without eating or speaking because of intubation or respiratory compromise. In addition to daily scar massage, the therapist can teach the patient facial stretching exercises, such as yawning or grinning widely and pursing lips together. The exercises can be combined with the wearing of a microstomia splint to stretch the oral commissure. The splint may be worn as tolerated, usually starting with 10 minutes and gradually increasing to 60 minutes twice a day. These devices can be purchased or constructed by the occupational therapist. The cognitive level of the patient is an extremely important factor in use of a microstomia device because of the risk of an unexpected airway emergency. For example, a heavily sedated or confused patient may attempt to swallow the device.

Heterotopic Ossification

Heterotopic ossification, or myositis ossificans, is the development of new bone in tissues that normally do not ossify. It occurs in up to 13% of patients with major burns

(Dutcher & Johnson, 1994). The most common location in the burn-injured population is the elbow, though the shoulder, knee, and hip can also be affected (Dutcher & Johnson). Heterotopic ossification causes pain, swelling, and rapid loss of range of motion. The therapist must be aware of the symptoms and alert the team so treatment options, including medications and surgery, can be discussed. Aggressive range of motion is contraindicated.

Heat Intolerance

Heat intolerance is caused by loss of sweating, as split thickness skin grafts do not contain sweat glands (Grigsby deLinde & Miles, 1995; Rivers & Jordan, 1998). To compensate for this, patients may sweat excessively in remaining unburned areas. Patients in extremely hot climates may require additional air conditioners in the home to maintain comfort (Rivers & Jordan). The lack of sweat glands also makes healed grafts susceptible to extreme dryness (Grigsby deLinde & Miles; Staley et al., 1994), and patients are encouraged to use moisturizing cream often throughout the day.

Reconstructive Surgery

An important element in burn recovery is the planning and execution of reconstructive procedures. In spite of diligent efforts by the burn team and patient, contractures may develop. Reconstructive surgery can be useful in correcting these deformities. Surgery is typically performed once the scar tissue is mature; however, it may be necessary to perform reconstructive surgery before scar maturation if a severe functional deficit is present (Robson et al., 1992). For example, an axilla contracture, which limits abduction to 80°, may significantly interfere with dressing and hygiene. A surgical procedure can involve using a **Z-plasty** to elongate soft tissue (Robson et al.; Staley et al., 1994). A skin graft to cover the deficit may be necessary once the contracture is released.

Occupational Therapy Assessment Related to Reconstructive Procedures

When results of functional assessment suggest that the patient's progress toward his or her self-management goals has ceased because of a contracture, the occupational therapist communicates to the burn team the possible need for surgical release of the contracture.

Occupational Therapy Related to Reconstructive Procedures

Postoperatively, the occupational therapist provides a custom splint to immobilize and protect the graft in

Case Example

MS. J.: INPATIENT OCCUPATIONAL THERAPY TREATMENT FOR A WOMAN WITH BURNS

Patient Information

Ms. J. is a 42-year-old woman who sustained a 45% TBSA burn as a result of a house fire. She presented to the emergency department with superficial and superficial partial-thickness burns to her face and neck and deep partial- and full-thickness burns to both upper extremities and hands (dorsal aspect only), chest, and proximal aspect of her bilateral lower extremities. She also sustained an inhalation injury and was intubated and sedated. She was admitted to the Intensive Care Unit. No significant medical history was reported. Occupational therapy was consulted on the first day of admission. In accordance with the initial screen during the emergent phase, the occupational therapist fabricated and applied bilateral elbow extension splints and bilateral hand splints in the position of function. In addition, her upper extremities were positioned in slight elevation using foam wedges. In the acute phase, a full initial evaluation was performed and daily occupational therapy was initiated. Split-thickness skin grafts (STSG) were performed to her chest and upper thighs three days after admission. STSGs were performed to her arms and hands 10 days after admission. After skin grafting was complete, Ms. J. was extubated and moved to a private room. She was on a regular diet and could walk independently. She was noted to be withdrawn and was concerned regarding her ability to care for her daughter.

Reason for Referral to Occupational Therapy

Ms. J. was referred to occupational therapy to prevent contractures that might result in deficits in occupational functioning, to provide patient and family education, and to address psychosocial sequelae related to the burn injury.

Occupational Therapy Problem List

▶ Unable to feed or dress and bathe independently because of impaired strength and range of motion in both upper extremities
▶ Impaired ability to care for her daughter
▶ Withdrawn behavior and feelings of dependency on family
▶ Activity tolerance limited to 5 minutes

Acute Phase

Occupational Therapy Goals

The following short-term goals were established for the acute phase:

▶ Ms. J. will use splinting, positioning, and exercise to prevent loss of range of motion in her upper extremities.
▶ Ms. J. will be able to perform 10 repetitions of active–assistive range of motion of bilateral upper extremities.

Treatment Plan

The occupational therapist recommended treatment 6 days a week for splinting and positioning, exercises and perioperative care. In addition, the occupational therapist implemented a modified call button that Ms. J. could use while her hands were splinted. The therapist encouraged the family to bring in tapes of get-well messages that Ms. J. could listen to with headphones.

Rehabilitation Phase

Occupational Therapy Goals

Short-term goals were revised as follows:

▶ Ms. J. will improve ability to grasp utensils by increasing flexion in her right MP joints from 40 to 75°.
▶ Ms. J. will eat 90% of her meal independently, using adaptive equipment as needed.
▶ Ms. J. will be able to comb her daughter's hair independently.
▶ Ms. J. will be able to type for 5 minutes with minimal errors.
▶ Ms. J. will demonstrate independence in her scar management program.
▶ Ms. J. will cope with anxiety and withdrawal by attainment of goals and through increased knowledge of the burn recovery process.

Treatment Plan

Occupational therapy continued 6 days a week, and Ms. J. was encouraged to participate actively in establishing meaningful goals. A dynamic MP flexion splint was fabricated to address

its new lengthened position. After approximately 10 to 14 days, the therapist initiates an exercise program beginning with gentle active range of motion and progressing to more aggressive exercise as skin integrity

tolerates. Pressure therapy over the newly grafted area minimizes scarring. This includes the use of a pressure garment and an insert fabricated to match the contours of the new graft.

limitations in range of motion. Cylindrical foam was used to build up the handles on her utensils. Ms. J. was taken to the occupational therapy gym as much as possible, and private time with her daughter was added to her daily schedule. She was provided with both verbal and written instruction regarding scar management and skin care. After 35 days in the hospital, Ms. J. was discharged home with outpatient occupational therapy.

Analysis

As discussed throughout the chapter, goals of occupational therapy must address specific needs in each phase of burn recovery. In the acute phase it is imperative to prevent early formation of contractures. Prevention of contractures ensures timely return of functional skills, reduces the need for reconstructive surgery, and minimizes the potential for scarring. The goals in this phase address abilities and capacities, such as range of motion and strength. Abilities and capacities

continue to be addressed as the patient enters the rehabilitation phase, although treatment expands to include valued activities, tasks, and roles. Goals are revised to address individual needs.

CLINICAL REASONING
in OT Practice

Outpatient Occupational Therapy After Burn Injury

As Ms. J. is discharged home, she continues to have limitations that affect her ability to resume tasks and roles of importance. How would you characterize her phase of recovery once she is discharged home? Based on the description of her background, scope of injury, and progress to date, write three possible short-term goals as she begins outpatient treatment.

Return to Work

Returning to work before final scar maturation preserves function and improves the patient's self-concept (Rivers & Jordan, 1998). The physician provides medical clearance for return to work. During the initial evaluation in the acute phase, the occupational therapist gathers information regarding the work history of the patient and specific job demands the patient previously encountered daily. With this information, the occupational therapist can guide treatment activities to prepare for return to the previous level of functioning. For example, if the patient was employed as a mechanic prior to injury, tool use should be incorporated into treatment activities as soon as possible. Patients may need job retraining if the extent of the injury renders the original job demands now unrealistic. In this case, the occupational therapist works with the patient and employer to explore appropriate job modifications.

Return-to-work parameters are ideally based on the percent of body surface area affected, whether the job requires the use of the affected body part, and the depth of the burn (IHQ, 1997). A recent study (Fletchall & Hickerson, 1995) investigated the effectiveness of a daily 6-hour outpatient program beginning immediately after discharge. Patients in this program, with burns to the upper extremity and hands averaging less than 25% TBSA, returned to work in an average of 8 weeks; patients in a similar population who participated in traditional outpatient therapy returned in an average of 19 weeks (Fletchall & Hickerson). In addition, the experimental program was shown to reduce the over-

all costs to the health care payer (Fletchall & Hickerson). Assignment of a case manager early during the inpatient phase also facilitated the progression from rehabilitation to return to work. (Fletchall & Hickerson).

Special Considerations for Hand Burns

Hand burns resulting in significant functional limitations occur quite frequently (Wright-Howell, 1989). The high rate of injury to the hand is because individuals use their hands to protect themselves or to extinguish the fire (Tanigawa et al., 1974). Dorsal hand burns occur more frequently than palmar injuries (Tanigawa et al.). As previously noted, significant edema usually occurs in response to thermal injury. This pulls the hand into a position of deformity (Sheridan et al., 1995) characterized by thumb radial abduction, digital metacarpal hyperextension, interphalangeal joint flexion, and flattening of the palmar arches (Wright-Howell). If this position is maintained, the result is joint contracture and severe functional limitation.

Evaluation of Hand Burns

A comprehensive hand evaluation includes determination of whether range of motion limitations are due to joint stiffness, intrinsic muscle tightness, extrinsic muscle tightness, or inelasticity of skin. Other factors that limit hand flexibility and decrease range of motion include pain, bulky dressings, exposed tendons, and the presence of eschar, which is inelastic. Once the clinician determines the cause of range of motion limitations, an effective treatment plan can be devised.

Treatment of Hand Burns

The occupational therapist must provide appropriate splinting and exercise programs to prevent contracture and expedite functional use of the burned hand. The appropriate splinting position of the hand is described in Table 45-1. In this position, the collateral ligaments of the metacarpophalangeal (MP), proximal interphalangeal (PIP), and distal interphalangeal joints are positioned at length, preventing ligamentous contracture so that maximum digital range of motion is preserved.

Thumb positioning in palmar versus radial abduction is controversial (Sheridan et al., 1995). Radial abduction maintains the first web space at maximum length. However, we prefer palmar abduction, as this is a position of function. Although palmar burns are rarer than dorsal ones, a deep palmar burn can lead to palmar contracture. In this case, a volar hand extension splint is appropriate. However, careful monitoring of MP flexion is critical to prevent shortening of the collateral ligaments. Here is a list of splinting options for the conditions previously discussed (see Chapter 14 for splint illustrations):

- ▶ Dynamic PIP extension splint such as Capaner, LMB, or banana splints for PIP stiffness—start 10 minutes three times a day, increase wearing time as tolerated, not to exceed 60 minutes at a time.
- ▶ Dynamic flexion splint in which the MPs are blocked in full extension while the IPs are passively flexed (for intrinsic muscle tightness)—start 10 minutes three times a day, increase wearing time as tolerated, not to exceed 60 minutes at a time.
- ▶ Forearm-based dynamic flexion splint that offers composite MP–IP flexion (Fig. 45-9) (for extrinsic extensor tightness or inelastic skin that limits composite flexion)—start 10 minutes three times a day, increasing as tolerated but not to exceed 45 minutes.
- ▶ Volar forearm-based static extension splint (for extrinsic flexor tightness)—wear at night.
- ▶ Forearm-based dynamic extension splint (for extrinsic flexor tightness) —wear periodically during the day, starting with 10 minutes three times per day and progressing to 45 minutes as tolerated.

Often individuals do not present with a single limitation; usually a combination of factors limit the individual's ROM. The clinician must determine which factor is the primary source of dysfunction and modify the treatment accordingly. Finally, appropriate splints are always used in conjunction with exercises, func-tional activities, and scar management techniques. Splints should never be used to the extent that they limit or prevent ADL.

Potential Complications of Hand Burns

Normal hand anatomy can be characterized by a balance of levers and pulleys that work harmoniously to achieve motion. Damage to this balanced network results in significant functional limitations.

Extensor Tendon Injury

Extensor tendon injury is often associated with dorsal hand burns, because they lie superficially on the dorsal aspect of the hand. Limitations can be due to direct thermal injury or tendon ischemia (Wright-Howell, 1989). Because of the close proximity of structures, the formation of scar tissue can greatly limit tendon excursion and create imbalance. This can result in contracture development. Boutonniere and swan-neck deformities are the result of extensor tendon damage (Evans & McAuliffe, 1995; Rosenthal, 1995; Wright-Howell).

Web Space Contractures

Web space contractures can be due to overgrafting of the web spaces, muscle shortening (contracture of the adductor pollicis brevis resulting in a first web space contracture), joint stiffness, or skin graft contracture in a normal response to tissue healing. Splints, scar management, and exercise are effective treatment modalities. First web space contractures (between the thumb and index finger) respond well to a web space C-splint (Fig. 45-10) that is lined with Otoform, a silicon gel sheet, or Elastomere. This is usually worn at night for 6 to 8 hours. During the day, the individual performs stretching, massage, and functional activities that encourage full range of motion of the affected area. For example, an

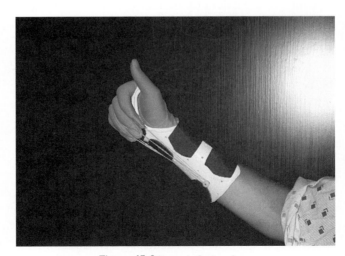

Figure 45-9 Dynamic flexion glove.

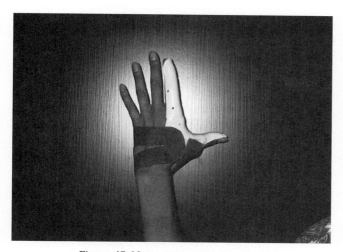

Figure 45-10 C-splint in radial abduction.

individual with a first web space contracture is asked to pick up containers of various sizes, using palmar abduction to promote full abduction of the thumb. A dynamic splint with an insert that exerts pressure over the second, third, and fourth web spaces can be appropriate for digital web space contractures. Another option is the addition of web space inserts under a Jobst or Isotoner glove.

Outcome Studies

The American Burn Association is undertaking research to determine long-term functional outcomes of patients who have sustained major burn injuries. A tool that has been established to address this issue is the *Burn Specific Health Scale* (Blalock et al., 1994). This recently revised scale is a 31-item instrument that includes items in seven categories: simple functional abilities, work, body image, interpersonal relationships, affect, heat sensitivity, and treatment programs. When the scale was administered to 244 patients from 8 burn centers, it was found both reliable and valid (Blalock et al., 1994). Subjects were asked to report their functioning using a 5-point scale, with 1 indicating extremely good function and 5 indicating none at all. The mean values for employed patients in the categories of simple functional abilities, body image, and interpersonal relationships were 4.77, 3.74, and 4.60 respectively (Blalock et al.).

Another study investigated hand function after acute hand burns (Sheridan et al., 1995). The study examined 659 patients with a total of 1,047 hand burns. It was reported that normal function was resumed in 97% of patients with superficial injuries and 81% of patients with deep dermal or full-thickness injuries. Of the patients with severe injuries, which included tendon damage or joint capsule or bone involvement, only 9% had normal function, while 90% were able to compensate for this and independently perform ADL (Sheridan et al.).

Baker et al. (1996) performed an outcome study using the *Burn Specific Health Scale* to identify factors affecting physical functioning and psychological status of 31 adult patients who had sustained burn injuries. The study concluded that minor first-degree burns can significantly affect an individual's physical and psychological functioning (Baker et al.). These results highlight the fact that patients whose burns are not severe may undergo physical and psychological ramifications similar to those of patients with major burn injuries (Baker et al.). Baker et al. also state that the psychosocial influence of a burn injury may in some cases provide a growth experience and actually enhance self-esteem as the patient takes pride in the tremendous accomplishment of recuperation.

Finally, LeDoux et al. (1996) administered to 32 burn survivors two standardized instruments that measured self-perception of competence and adequacy. Many of the patients used denial as a coping mechanism, and this was found to be beneficial to their perception of competence. The study demonstrated that the patients did not accept feelings of being helpless or hopeless but rather seemed to change their value systems to reflect areas they could control. They placed less value on social acceptance, athletic competence, and physical appearance and more value on job competence, romantic appeal, and scholastic appeal—areas they believed they could control and develop (LeDoux et al.). As specialists in the evaluation and treatment of function, occupational therapists have a responsibility to continue to enhance the knowledge base in this area (see Resources).

Summary Review Questions

1. In your own words, what is the primary goal of burn care?
2. How is the role of the occupational therapist unique to the burn team?
3. Describe the differences in treatment approaches for superficial, superficial partial-thickness, deep partial-thickness, and full-thickness burns.
4. What splinting and positioning program would you establish for a patient who is intubated in the ICU with deep partial-thickness burns to the axilla, elbow, and wrist?
5. How would your approach differ with the same patient awake and alert?
6. Describe the correct positioning for a deep dorsal hand burn and explain the anatomical justification behind your answer.

7. What factors would you consider when designing a scar management program for your patient?

8. As the occupational therapist on the burn unit, how would you help to address the psychosocial issues of your patients?

9. List five complications you might encounter as your patient recovers from a significant burn injury.

10. What might you, as an occupational therapist, find difficult about treating a patient with a burn injury? How would you address these issues?

Acknowledgments

We thank the patients, physicians, and staff of the Sumner Redstone Burn Unit at Massachusetts General Hospital and the staff of the occupational therapy and hand therapy departments.

Resources

American Burn Association · National Headquarters Office, 625 North Michigan Ave, Suite 1530, Chicago, IL 60611.
www.ameriburn.org

Journal of Burn Care and Rehabilitation · Sponsored by American Burn Foundation, published by Mosby. 215-629-9200.

National Fire Protection Association. 617-770-3000.
www.nfpa.org

Burn Survivors Online · 28997 Nicholas Rd., Norwalk, WI 54648.
www.alpha-tek.com/burn/

Valpar Work Samples

Valpar International Corporation · P. O. Box 5767, Tucson, AZ 85703-5767.

References

Abston, S. (1987). Scar reaction after thermal injury and prevention of scars and contractures. In J. A. Boswick Jr. (Ed.), *The Art and Science of Burn Care* (pp. 359–371). Rockville, MD: Aspen.

Ahn, S. T., Monafo, W. W., & Mustoe, T. A. (1989). Topical silicone gel: A new treatment for hypertrophic scars. *Surgery, 106*, 781–787.

Baker, R. A., Jones, S., Sanders, C., Sadinski, C., Martin-Duffy, K., Berchin, H., & Valentine, S. (1996). Degree of burn, location of burn, and length of hospital stay as predictors of psychosocial status and physical functioning. *Journal of Burn Care and Rehabilitation, 17* (4), 327–333.

Barber, L. M. (1990). Desensitization of the traumatized hand. In J. M. Hunter, E. J. Mackin, & A. D. Callahan. (Eds), *Rehabilitation of the Hand* (p. 721). St. Louis: Mosby.

Blalock, S. J., Bunker, B. J., DeVellis, R. F. (1994). Measuring health status among survivors of burn injury: Revisions of the Burn Specific Health Scale. *Journal of Trauma, 36*, 508–515.

Burke Evans, E., Alvarado, M. I., Ott, S., McElroy, K., Irwin, C. (1996). Prevention and treatment of deformity in burned patients. In D. N. Herndon (Ed.), *Total Burn Care* (pp. 443–454). Philadelphia: Saunders.

Brigham, P. A., & McLoughlin, E. (1996). Burn incidence and medical care use in the United States: Estimates, trends, and data sources. *Journal of Burn Care and Rehabilitation, 17*, 95–107.

Chang, P., Laubenthal, K. N., Lewis, R. W, Rosenquist, M. D., Lindley-Smith, P., & Kealy, G. P. (1995). Prospective, randomized study of the efficacy of pressure garment therapy in patients with burns. *Journal of Burn Care and Rehabilitation, 16*, 473–475.

Choctaw, W. F., Eisner, M. E., & Wachtel, T. L. (1987). Causes, prevention, pre-hospital care, evaluation, emergency treatment, and prognosis. In B. M. Achauer (Ed.), *Management of the Burned Patient* (pp. 3–19). Los Altos, CA: Appleton & Lange.

Cioffi, W. G., & Rue, L. W. (1991). Diagnosis and treatment of inhalation injuries. *Critical Care Nursing Clinics of North America, 3*, 191–198.

Duncan, D. J., & Driscoll, D. M. (1991). Burn wound management. *Critical Care Nursing Clinics of North America, 3*, 199–220.

Duran-Coleman, L. A. (1991). Rehabilitation of the burn survivor. *Progress Report: A Rehabilitation Journal, 3* (3), 1–8.

Dutcher, K., & Johnson, C. (1994). Neuromuscular and musculoskeletal complication. In R. L. Richard & M. J. Staley (Eds.), *Burn Care and Rehabilitation: Principles and Practice* (pp. 576–602). Philadelphia: Davis.

Evans, R. B., & McAuliffe, J. A. (1995). Wound classification and management. In J. M. Hunter, E. J. Mackin, & A. D. Callahan, (Eds), *Rehabilitation of the Hand: Surgery and Therapy* (pp. 217–235). St. Louis: Mosby–Year Book.

Falkel, J. E. (1994). Anatomy and physiology of the skin. In R. L. Richard & M. J. Staley (Eds), *Burn Care and Rehabilitation: Principles and Practice* (pp. 10–18). Philadelphia: Davis.

Fletchall, S., & Hickerson, W. L. (1995). Quality burn rehabilitation: Cost-effective approach. *Journal of Burn Care and Rehabilitation, 16*, 539–542.

Greenhalgh, D. G., & Staley, M. J. (1994). Burn wound healing. In R. L. Richard & M. J. Staley (Eds). *Burn Care and Rehabilitation: Principles and Practice.* (pp. 70–102). Philadelphia: Davis.

Grigsby deLinde, L., & Miles, W. K. (1995). Remodeling of scar tissue in the burned hand. In J. M. Hunter, E. J. Mackin, & A. D. Callahan, (Eds), *Rehabilitation of the Hand: Surgery and Therapy* (pp. 1265–1303). St. Louis: Mosby–Year Book.

Harden, N. G., & Luster, S. H. (1991). Rehabilitation considerations in the care of the acute burn patient. *Critical Care Nursing Clinics of North America 3*, 245–253.

Institute for Healthcare Quality [IHQ]. (1997). *Quality First Position Paper: Burns.* Minneapolis: Author.

Kagan, R. J., & Warden, G. D. (1994). Management of the burn wound. *Clinical Dermatology, 12* (1), 47–56.

LeDoux, J. M., Meyer, W. J., Blakeney, P., & Herndon, D. (1996). Positive self-regard as a coping mechanism for pediatric burn survivors. *Journal of Burn Care and Rehabilitation, 17*, 472–476.

Malick, M. H., & Carr, J. A. (1982). *Manual on Management of the Burn Patient.* Pittsburgh: Harmarville Rehabilitation Center.

Poh-Fitzpatrick, M. B. (1992). Skin care of the healed burn patient. *Clinical Plastic Surgery, 19*, 745–751.

Pessina, M. A., & Ellis, S.M. (1997). Rehabilitation. *Nursing Clinics of North America, 32*, 365–374.

Rivers, E. A., & Jordan, C. L. (1998). Skin system dysfunction: Burns. In M. J. Neistadt & E. B. Crepeau (Eds.), *Willard and Spackman's Occupational Therapy* (9th ed., pp. 741–755). Philadelphia: Lippincott.

Robson, M. C., Barnett, R. A., Leitch, I. O., & Hayward, P. G. (1992). Prevention and treatment of postburn scars and contracture. *World Journal of Surgery 16* (1), 87–96.

Rosenthal, E. A. (1995). The extensor tendons: Anatomy and management. In J. M. Hunter, E. J. Mackin, & A. D. Callahan (Eds),

Rehabilitation of the Hand: Surgery and Therapy (pp. 519–564). St. Louis: Mosby–Year Book.

Sheridan, R. L., Hurley, J., Smith, M. A., Ryan, C. M., Bondoc, C. C., Quinby, W. C., Tompkins, R. G., & Burke, J. F. (1995). The acutely burned hand: Management and outcome based a ten-year experience with 1047 acute hand burns. *Journal of Trauma, 38,* 406–411.

Staley, M. J., Richard, R. L., & Falkel, J. E. (1994). Burns. In S. B. O'Sullivan, & T. J. Schmitz (Eds), *Physical Rehabilitation: Assessment and Treatment* (pp. 509–532). Philadelphia: Davis.

Summers, T. M. (1991). Psychosocial support of the burned patient. *Critical Care Nursing Clinics of North America, 3,* 237–244.

Sullivan, T., Smith, J., Kermode, J., McIver, E., & Courtemanche, D. J. (1990). Rating the burn scar. *Journal of Burn Care and Rehabilitation 3,* 256–260.

Tanigawa, M. C., O'Donnell, O. K., & Graham, P. L. (1974). The burned hand: A physical therapy protocol. *Physical Therapy, 54,* 953–958.

Uniform Data System for Medical Rehabilitation (1997). *Guide for the Uniform Data Set for Medical Rehabilitation.* Buffalo: University of New York.

Ward, R. S. (1991). Pressure therapy for the control of hypertrophic scar formation after burn injury: A history and review. *Journal of Burn Care and Rehabilitation, 12,* 257–262.

Wright, P. C. (1984). Fundamentals of acute burn care and physical therapy management. *Physical Therapy, 64,* 1217–1231.

Wright-Howell, J. (1989). Management of the acutely burned hand for the non-specialized clinician. *Physical Therapy, 69,* 1077–1089.

46
Amputations and Prosthetics

Felice Gadaleta Celikyol

LEARNING OBJECTIVES

After studying this chapter the reader will be able to do the following:

1. Discuss prosthetic components available and appropriate for upper limb amputation levels.
2. State options for creating prosthetic prescriptions.
3. Plan treatment programs for persons with transradial and transhumeral amputations.
4. Design treatment for pre-prosthetic and prosthetic management of upper and lower limb amputation.
5. Describe the psychosocial implications of amputation for the patient and their impact on therapeutic management.

Amputation can result from several causes:

▶ Traumatic injury that occurs as a result of accidents as in the use of machinery or motor vehicle accidents
▶ Disease such as vascular disease, tumors or infection
▶ Congenital limb deficiencies that present as missing or partially developed limbs

This chapter addresses only adults with **acquired amputation**, that is, amputations that occurred after birth. Discussion of the role of the occupational therapist in providing therapy for adults with lower limb amputation is also included.

GLOSSARY

Acquired amputation—Surgical amputation after birth as a result of trauma or disease.

Body power (BP)—Person's own effort, without an external power source.

External power—Electric or other motor that provides impetus to move the prosthesis or terminal device.

Preprosthetic therapy program—Period from the postsurgical procedure until the permanent prosthesis is received.

Terminal device (TD)—Prosthetic hook, hand, or other prehensile device that is inserted into the wrist unit of the prosthesis.

Transfemoral amputation—Amputation across the axis of the femur; previously called above knee (AK).

Transhumeral amputation—Amputation across the axis of the humerus; previously called above elbow (AE).

Transradial amputation—Amputation across the axis of the radius and ulna; labeled by the larger of two adjacent bones. Previously called below elbow (BE).

Transtibial amputation—Amputation across the axis of the fibula and tibia; labeled according to the larger of two adjacent bones. Previously called below knee (BK).

Voluntary closing (VC) mechanism—TD that remains open until tension is applied to the control cable for grasp.

Voluntary opening (VO) mechanism—TD that remains closed until tension is applied to the control cable to open it.

Incidence, Levels, and Classification of Amputation

There are more than 150,000 persons with amputations in the United States, with a ratio of arm to leg amputations estimated to be 1:3. Some 57% of arm amputations are transradial, that is, below the elbow through the radius and ulna (Esquenazi, 1996; Leonard & Meier, 1998). Trauma rather than disease is the primary cause (close to 75%) of upper limb amputations in adults, with injury occurring primarily to males aged 15 to 45 years in work-related accidents (Leonard & Meier). Amputations of upper limbs can also result from other events, such as gunshot wounds and electrical burns. Disease is the primary reason for lower limb amputations, with peripheral vascular disease and diabetes being the most common causes in people over 60 years of age. Trauma causes 20% of acquired lower extremity amputations, with 5% due to tumors (Leonard & Meier).

When amputation is necessary, the surgeon's aim is to preserve as much limb length as possible and still retain healthy skin, soft tissue, blood supply, sensation, muscles, bones, and joints (Leonard & Meier, 1998). A residual limb that is pain free and functional is the final surgical goal.

Acquired amputations were previously described by such terms as *short above elbow (AE)*, *standard AE*, *very short below elbow (BE)*, and *long BE*. Other terminology has been adopted by the International Standards Organization and endorsed by the American Academy of Orthotists and Prosthetists, the American Academy of Orthopedic Surgeons, and the International Society for Prosthetics and Orthotics (Schuch & Pritham, 1994). The term *trans* is now used to describe an amputation across the axis of a long bone, as with **transhumeral** to replace AE, or the larger of two adjacent bones, as with **transradial** for radius–ulna, or BE. The levels of amputation for the upper extremity are illustrated in Figure 46-1. Often the level of amputation directly affects the use of a prosthesis. The higher the amputation, the more difficult it is to use a prosthesis, because fewer joints and muscles are available for control. Furthermore, the weight of the prosthesis is greater and more complex systems are needed for active control. The level of amputation is only one reason for discarding the prosthesis. There are many reasons a patient may choose not to wear a prosthesis, including the individual's psychological reaction to the amputation.

Psychological Aspects of Limb Loss

"When a man loses his limb, he loses more; he loses his heart."

(Kessler, 1969)

Amputation of an upper limb means losing the ability to hold and manipulate objects, feel these objects, communicate through gestures, and be whole in body. This loss can profoundly influence the person's self-esteem and sense of efficacy. Reactions to amputation are as complex as the unique nature of each human. With each life experience, human personalities evolve and belief systems develop; these beliefs influence how one responds to crisis. Often, an early response to limb amputation is shock and disbelief, and when both upper extremities are amputated, a feeling of helplessness is common. It is also natural for the person to grieve (Dise-Lewis, 1989; Winchell, 1995) and feel a multitude of painful emotions. For example, one may respond with anger, feelings of guilt, denial, hopelessness, bitterness, revulsion, or depression. Sometimes the patient may project negative feelings onto the therapist. The therapist must encourage open discussion and instill a climate of trust and respect. Amputation affects not only physical function but also the patient's life roles in many contexts: maintenance of self, family, and home; self-enhancement, such as engaging in leisure and community activities; and self-advancement as a worker or student (Trombly, 1995). What can the occupational therapist do?

► Give the patient information. Explain the therapy and the expected outcomes; this reduces the patient's fears and anxiety. Often the prosthesis is not up to patients' expectations in that they are anticipating a realistic replacement of their limb. The therapist can prepare the patient during the preprosthetic phase by showing prostheses that are appropriate to the amputation level and by discussing their features while listening to the patient and understanding the patient's life roles. A collaborative relationship between therapist and patient instills a sense of control in the patient.

► Introduce the patient to another person with a similar amputation, and allow them to chat in private. If possible, bring in others with amputations to acquaint the patient with several perspectives. This is probably the single most important action the therapist can take to help the patient adjust. Make referrals to any self-help groups in the area.

► Provide the patient with reference material; topics can include information on coping and adjusting to the amputation, information on prosthetic options, tips on how to manage one's daily life skills independently, and a list of organizations for persons with upper and lower limb amputation (see Resources).

► Communicate with other team members if the patient's behavior appears to be impeding progress. Recommend psychological or spiritual counseling if appropriate.

Rehabilitation: A Team Approach

The core members of the professional team are the physician, prosthetist, and occupational therapist. The social worker, psychologist, and vocational counselor may be called in as needed. Patients are always active, equal members of the team and must be given the opportunity to explain their needs, preferences, and goals. The occupational therapist is critical to the rehabilitation process, since this professional works so closely with the patient and can influence the patient's adjustment. Some aspects of the rehabilitation program may be addressed by other team members, as in the acute postoperative period, when management of the residual limb may be rendered by a physical therapist or a nurse.

Preprosthetic Therapy

The **preprosthetic** therapy program occurs from the postsurgical period until the patient receives the permanent prosthesis. This is a preparatory time for emotional and physical healing.

Postoperative Care

Postoperative care, required immediately after surgery, addresses wound care, maintenance of skin integrity,

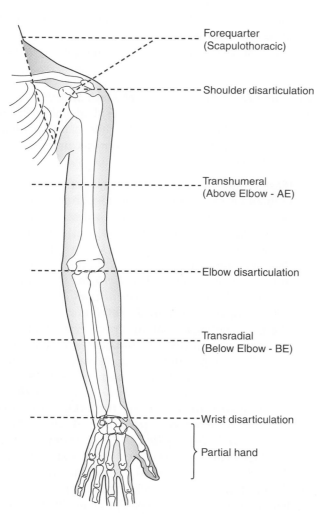

Forequarter
(Scapulothoracic)

Shoulder disarticulation

Transhumeral
(Above Elbow - AE)

Elbow disarticulation

Transradial
(Below Elbow - BE)

Wrist disarticulation

Partial hand

Figure 46-1 Levels of amputations.

joint mobility, reduction of edema, prevention of scarring, and control of pain (Atkins & Meier, 1989a; Malone et al., 1984). This usually occurs in an acute-care setting, with surgeon, nurse, and physical therapist most involved, and continues in an outpatient setting. Outpatient therapy can be provided in a rehabilitation unit, rehabilitation center, or hand clinic. Inpatient admission may be necessary for multiple amputations or other complications, such as extensive burns.

Phantom Limb Sensation

The perception of the presence of the amputated limb is a universal phenomenon that is remarkably real to the patient. The cause of phantom limb sensation is still not clearly understood; research is continuing (Jones & Davidson, 1996; Liaw, 1998). Phantom limb sensation is most common in traumatic amputations. According to Melzack (1989), the "neural system exists within the brain even when the body input is cut off by amputation" (p. 4). These perceptions are strongest with amputations of upper extremities, and the hand and fingers are felt more vividly than the arm.

With time, the distal portions of the phantom limb may move closer to the site of the amputation. Phantom limb sensation often remains, and ordinarily the patient accepts it. The patient may view it as an annoyance during mild burning or tingling sensations or may find it useful, as when learning myoelectric control for externally powered prostheses. Open discussion with the patient regarding this common phenomenon is a must.

Phantom Limb Pain

Phantom limb pain is even less clearly understood, and its causation and management remain controversial; again, research continues (Flor & Elbert, 1995; Geraghty & Jones, 1996). This pain can be felt as extremely intense burning or cramping sensations or shooting pain and is most common in traumatic amputations. Peripheral nerve irritation, abnormal sympathetic function, and psychological factors are thought to be contributory factors.

Often, pain increases with stress. The therapist is advised to avoid emphasizing pain when possible. Treatments for those with severe pain include analgesics and surgery, such as nerve blocks and neurectomies. In the rehabilitation setting, limb percussion, ultrasound, and transcutaneous electrical nerve stimulation (TENS) have been used (Jones & Davidson, 1996). Acupuncture, psychotherapy, hypnotherapy, and relaxation techniques have also been instituted. However, no one approach has proved to be clearly successful.

Preprosthetic Program Guidelines

Occupational therapy during the preprosthetic period includes providing emotional support, ensuring maximal limb shrinkage and shaping, desensitizing the residual limb, maintaining range of motion and strength, and facilitating independence in activities of daily living.

Provide Emotional Support
Establish an ongoing supportive, trusting relationship with the patient and family to facilitate open discussion. Collaborate with the team regarding patient's needs, and refer the patient for counseling if needed. Introduce the patient to others with similar amputations and comparable circumstances, such as similar levels of amputation or vocation.

Instruct in Limb Hygiene and Expedite Wound Healing
► Instruct the patient to wash the limb daily with mild soap and dry it thoroughly.
► Provide wound cleansing, such as debridement or use of a whirlpool; this may be the responsibility of the physical therapist or nurse.
► Use creams to massage at the suture line to loosen crustlike formations.

Maximize Limb Shrinkage with Limb Shaping
The goal is to shrink and shape the residual limb so that it is tapered at the distal end; this allows for optimal prosthetic fit. The following interventions can be used to achieve this goal.

► Elastic bandage. The patient is taught to wrap the limb and is expected to do so independently unless physical or cognitive limitations prevent it. In this case, a family member or friend is instructed. The residual limb must be wrapped in a figure eight diagonal configuration, with most pressure applied at the end of the limb. ***The limb must never be wrapped in a circular manner, as this causes a tourniquet effect and restricts circulation.*** The bandage must conform firmly to the limb and be wrapped in a distal to proximal direction (Fig. 46-2). The wrap should be worn continuously and reapplied immediately if it loosens. ***The patient is advised to remove the bandage two to three times daily to examine the skin for any redness or excessive pressure. A clean bandage should be applied at least every 2 days.*** Bandages can be washed with mild soap and laid flat to dry but not squeezed or machine dried.
► Elastic shrinker. An elasticized sock can be worn in lieu of the bandage if the patient or family members

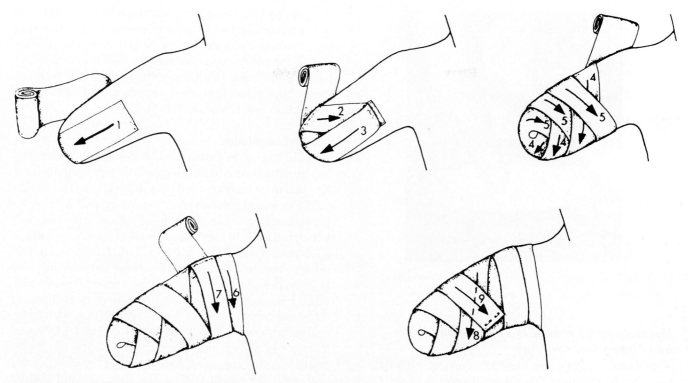

Figure 46-2 Wrapping technique for transhumeral amputation. Repeat diagonal turns as necessary to cover the limb with no constrictions.

do not reliably follow proper wrapping procedures using the elastic bandage. However, the shrinker tends to loosen as the limb shrinks. Although this can be less effective than the bandage, the shrinker is preferable to improper application of the elastic bandage.

▶ Removable rigid dressing. A socket can be fabricated using plaster bandages or fiberglass casting tape. This may be the method of choice for those unable to wrap the limb (Olivett, 1990); however, this cast must be replaced or altered frequently as the limb shrinks, which is time consuming.

▶ Immediate postoperative prosthesis. The immediate postoperative prosthesis is, as the name suggests, applied directly after surgery (Maiorano & Byron, 1990; Malone et al., 1984). This is probably the ideal approach if the rehabilitation team members are available to ensure success.

▶ Early postoperative prosthesis. The early postoperative prosthesis is strongly recommended for bilateral amputations (Lehneis & Dickey, 1992) to reduce dependency for self-care activities. This temporary prosthesis may ensure acceptance and use of the permanent prosthesis. Studies support the premise that early fitting tends to ensure acceptance of

the prosthesis and its use (Kejlaa, 1993; Pinzur & Angelats, 1994).

Desensitize the Residual Limb

The aim is to desensitize the residual limb so that it will accommodate touch and pressure in preparation for encasement in the socket. This goal can be met through the following interventions (see also Chapter 27).

▶ The patient bears weight on the end of the limb against various surfaces. These surfaces are graded from very resilient, such as soft foam, to variously resistant and textured, such as layers of felt, rice, and clay (Fig. 46-3). The patient is to push the limb down into the surface for 5-second intervals and increase the contact time as tolerated.

▶ Massage is useful for desensitizing but is primarily used to prevent or release adhesions and soften scar tissue.

▶ Tapping and rubbing the residual limb and applying a vibrator are also useful.

▶ Residual limb wrapping contributes to desensitizing the limb.

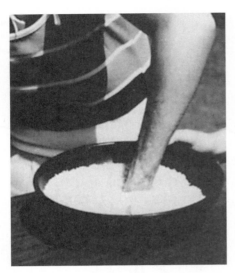

Figure 46-3 Weight bearing into materials of various textures (here, rice) to desensitize limb.

Maintain or Increase Range of motion and Strength of the Limb

A physical conditioning regimen can be instituted to increase or maintain the range of motion of all joints proximal to the amputation. Increasing muscle strength of the residual limb and shoulder area are also goals. Include the contralateral side if limitations are noted. For patients with high-level amputations, a shift of weight and center of gravity can occur, so the therapist provides an exercise program to improve or prevent asymmetry of posture. Mobilization of the limb also increases circulation and reduces edema. This conditioning regimen can be practiced at home, using weight cuffs wrapped around the limb. The BTE Work Simulator can be used in the clinic to strengthen the residual limb in functional patterns. The limb, encased in a cuff, is attached to the Work Simulator, and rotary patterns and pushing and pulling movements are done with increasing measured amounts of resistance. Encourage the patient to include the residual limb in bilateral gross grasp tasks during daily activities.

Facilitate Independence in Daily Living Activities

It is important that the patient develop skills to be proficient without the prosthesis. Ordinarily, the patient with a unilateral amputation receives only one prosthesis; therefore, there may be times when the prosthesis is being repaired and the patient will have to manage without it. Furthermore, the patient may decide not to wear a prosthesis.

Unilateral Amputation

For persons with amputation of the dominant limb, change of dominance activities, such as writing, must receive special attention. Although the patient will instinctively use the remaining extremity, the therapist can introduce a wide variety of activities and provide tips for one-handed techniques for independent activities of daily living (IADL) as needed for home management, communication, desk activities, and community interaction (see Chapters 30–32).

Bilateral Amputation

Establishing some degree of independence is essential for the patient who has undergone bilateral amputations, and this must be addressed promptly (Lehneis & Dickey, 1992) to lessen feelings of dependency and frustration. Immediately provide the patient with a universal cuff, which is useful for holding a utensil or toothbrush; this is a temporary substitute for grasp. Early fitting with a temporary prosthesis on at least one limb is by far the best approach. Adapted devices may be needed (Friedmann, 1989; Heinze, 1988) to assist the patient in performing basic self-care tasks, such as eating, toileting, grooming, and some dressing. Use of the feet should be encouraged if at all possible, and other modifications of performance can be suggested, such as use of the chin, knees, and teeth (Edelstein, 1992). The therapist and patient can analyze tasks and solve problems together. Ordinarily, the longer limb will be chosen as the dominant extremity.

Explore Prosthetic Options

Demonstrate prostheses appropriate to the level of amputation to guide the patient to establish realistic expectations. Arrange a meeting between this patient and a former one, preferably someone with a similar level of amputation, so that they can talk candidly about any issues of concern, which will probably include negative and positive features of prostheses.

Myoelectric Site Testing and Training

Muscle site testing must be instituted for patients choosing a myoelectric prosthesis. The prosthetist and therapist can collaborate to determine whether the patient is a candidate by evaluating electromyographic (EMG) signals. At that time the optimal location for the control site or sites is chosen. The goal is to find a site where the patient can hold a steady contraction for at least 1 to 2 seconds and relax for that time. A myotester or computer program can be used as well as the electronic hand. Ordinarily, the agonist and antagonist are chosen, such as biceps and triceps for transhumeral amputation and typically wrist extensors and flexors are used in transradial amputation. It is possible to use only one muscle to control two functions: a strong contraction controls one function and a weaker contraction controls another; relaxation turns the system off. However, this system is difficult to learn. The skin electrodes are strapped to the limb or encased in a test socket (Fig.46-4) with the electronic controls attached to a motorized hand, computer, or myotester; a biofeedback unit can also be used.

Prescribing the Prosthesis

As a member of the prosthetic team, the occupational therapist contributes to the prescription of the prosthesis. The therapist has come to know the patient in some depth during the preprosthetic program and can contribute information from a social and cultural perspective (Box 46-1).

Prosthetic Components

The components of a prosthesis are frequently categorized in the following sequence, from distal to proximal:

1. **Terminal devices (TD)**
   a. Active prehensors
   b. Passive terminal devices
2. Wrist units
3. Forearm component or sockets
4. Elbow units or hinges
5. Upper arm component or sockets
6. Shoulder units or hinges

Prosthetic Control Choices: Body Powered (Box 46-2)
Terminal Devices

TDs are considered the most important components of the prosthesis. The components for the wrist, elbow, and upper arm are needed to position the arm in space to enable efficient TD use.

TD Prehensors. TD prehensors can be classified as operating by a **voluntary opening (VO) mechanism** or **voluntary closing (VC) mechanism** (Table 46-1). For a VO

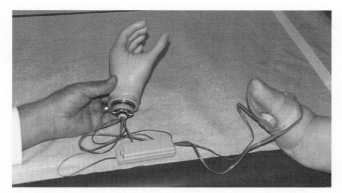

Figure 46-4 Finding the best site for electrode placement for consistent control of electric hand.

BOX 46-1
PROCEDURES FOR PRACTICE
Prescribing the Prosthesis

Consider these factors:

► Residual limb: length, range of motion, skin integrity, strength
► Preference for cosmesis and function
► Activities at work, home, school, community and recreational interests
► Motivation and attitude
► Financial coverage: health care insurance, ability to pay privately
► Cognitive abilities to learn to use prosthetic controls

BOX 46-2
Types of Prostheses

Body Powered (BP) Prosthesis
Body motion is used to apply tension on the control cable to activate the TD and elbow unit.

Externally Powered Prosthesis
Motors for the TD, wrist unit and elbow components are electrically controlled either by a microswitch or by electromyographic (EMG) signals.

Myoelectric Prosthesis
This externally powered prosthesis uses EMG signals to activate electric components. Metal electrodes embedded inside the prosthetic socket are in contact with the patient's skin and pick up EMG signals as the muscle contracts. The signals are amplified and relayed to the electronic TD, wrist unit or/and elbow unit.

Hybrid Prosthesis
Hybrid prostheses combine BP and electrical power control systems.

mechanism, the fingers of the device remain closed by springs for a mechanical hand or by rubber bands for a hook. The force of pinch on the hook can be increased by adding rubber bands, approximately 1 pound for each band, and by adjusting the spring mechanism for the hands. For the Therapeutic Recreational Systems (TRS) VC mechanism, the amount of pinch force can be decreased or increased by the amount of tension pull the patient applies on the cable to close the TD.

Voluntary Opening Hooks. The voluntary opening hook is most widely used, and Hosmer-Dorrance is the primary manufacturer (Fig. 46-5). Hooks of aluminum alloy or stainless steel come in several sizes; some have neoprene rubber–lined fingers. The neoprene lining pro-

TABLE 46-1
Hooks and Hands Compared

Features	Hooks VO (BP)	VC TRS Grip (BP)	Hands Myoelectric	Hands VO (BP)
Cosmesis	Appearance poor	Appearance poor	Cosmetically appealing	Cosmetically appealing
Pinch force	Relies on elastic bands; more bands require more effort to open	Excellent for controlled strong grip >40 lb; relies on force exerted on cable	Strong ~25 lb; proportional control allows fast or slow opening, closing	Pinch force stronger than VO hook but less than myoelectric hand; relies on internal springs
Prehension pattern	Precise, exact pinch	Pinch more precise than hands, less than hooks	Cylindrical grasp, 3-point pinch; configuration same as BP hand	Cylindrical grasp, 3-point pinch; configuration same as myoelectric hand
Weight	Lighter than hands; aluminum to stainless steel; 3–8.7 oz	Aluminum, polymer, stainless steel; 4–16 oz	Heaviest; ~16.2 oz	Heavy; 10.5—14 oz
Durability	Very durable; stainless steel strongest	Very durable and rugged; stainless steel more so	Not durable; delicate internal electronics & glove	Not durable; delicate inner spring mechanism & glove
Reliability	Very good; little servicing needed	Very good; little servicing needed	Good, but cannot be used for rugged activities	Good; cannot be used for rugged activities; needs less servicing than myoelectric
Feedback	Some proprioceptive feedback from tension on harness & limb in socket when operating TD/elbow	Better proprioceptive feedback, as tension on cable must be maintained for sustained grasp	Some feedback through intensity of muscle contraction, particularly for proportional control	Feedback similar to VO hook
Ease of use	Effort increases with more bands on hook	More effort to sustain grasp; lock available	Low effort to activate; lock available	More effort to open; can relax for grasp
Use in various planes	Difficult for high planes	Similar to VO hook	Very good for transradial amputation	Similar to VO hook/ hand because of harness system
Visibility of items grasped	Very good	Good; less than VO	Poor for small items	Poor for small items; similar to myoelectric hand
Cost	Lowest	Higher than hook, less than hands	Highest cost for hand & systems	Higher than hooks; lower than myoelectric

vides a firm grip and prevents slippage. Aluminum hooks are lighter (4 ounces) than stainless steel (8 ounces) and are used for routine activities.

The #7 stainless steel work hook has special features that facilitate holding tools and can withstand the rigors of heavy mechanical activity; however, it weighs 11 ounces. The Hosmer hooks come in right or left and can be differentiated by holding the hook with fingers in pronation; the thumb post closest to the midline indicates its orientation to side; for example, a right hook, when pronated, has the thumb post closest to the body or midline.

Voluntary Closing Terminal Devices. The TRS GRIP voluntary closing terminal device is fast becoming the TD of choice in this category (Fig. 46-6). Strong variable prehension is controlled by the amount of force the

individual can exert. It is conceivable that a grasp of more than 30 pounds can be attained. A locking mechanism can be inserted if requested. These devices are available in aluminum and steel and can be plastic coated. This TD is particularly appealing for people who are active in sports, heavy physical work, or recreational activities. Use of the APRL hook, developed by the Army Prosthetics Research Laboratory, is declining because it contains complex inner mechanisms and tends to require more servicing than most.

Voluntary Opening Mechanical Hands. The Hosmer-Dorrance or Otto Bock mechanical hand is most frequently selected. The VO hands operate similarly to the VO hooks except that in the hand, the thumb and first two fingers open when the cable is pulled. These fingers oppose in a three-point prehension pattern. This is different from the

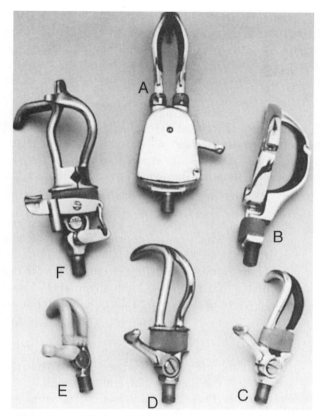

Figure 46-5 Hooks. **A.** APRL VC hook. **B.** Contour hook. **C.** VO 10x hook. **D.** VO #5 stainless steel hook. E. Plastisol-covered VO hook. **F.** Stainless steel #7 VO work hook. *Photo courtesy of Hosmer-Dorrance Corp., Campbell, CA.*

Hosmer hook, in which the cable is attached only to the thumb post so that the finger with the thumb post moves while the other finger remains stationary.

Voluntary Closing Mechanical Hands. The APRL VC hand is available only in men's sizes. The thumb can be manually adjusted and locked in two positions to achieve a 1.5- or 3-inch opening. Otto Bock offers VC hands in several sizes, all of which weigh less than the APRL hand. The VC hands are less popular than the VO hands. TRS also provides VC hands.

Cosmetic Gloves. All prosthetic hands have rubberized coverings (Fryer & Michael, 1992). These gloves are available in a variety of colors and sizes to cover mechanical, passive, and electric hands. A reverse mold of the remaining hand is sent to the manufacturer. The glove is replaced by the prosthetist when damaged. Some of the available choices are described here.

A stock (production) glove is ordered by the prosthetist. The skin color choices are made from a selection of sample swatches. These polyvinyl chloride (PVC) gloves are the least expensive but are susceptible to staining from contact with such items as newsprint,

clothing dyes, and ballpoint ink. The glove can deteriorate with temperature extremes and in sunlight.

A silicone covering is more expensive than PVC. There is a wider range of color choices, and details, such as veins, are painted on the glove to render a more realistic covering. These silicone gloves can withstand extremes of temperature and do not stain as easily as those of PVC.

A custom-sculpted silicone glove, also called an anatomical cover, truly attempts to replicate the individual's remaining hand (Figs. 46-7 and 46-8). The remaining hand is cast in silicone, which duplicates its contours in great detail. It is then reversed. A cosmetic restorationist adds to the realistic appearance of the hand by painting the glove and adding veins and other features. This glove is the most costly.

Passive cosmetic hands and prostheses are chosen when appearance is valued more than function. These prostheses are available to replace any part of a limb, from a single digit to a whole arm.

The Final Choice: Hooks or Hands? Fortunately, the patient can choose from several TDs. It is possible to have several interchangeable hooks and hands. The hook is viewed as most functional for the following reasons:

► Small items can be grasped with precision.
► Visibility is good, an extremely important feature, since tactile sensation is absent.
► It weighs less than the hand.
► It costs less than the hand.
► It is more reliable and requires less maintenance than the hand.
► It can fit in close quarters.

Nonetheless, many people prefer the hand because it is cosmetically more appealing, although heavier, more delicate, and more expensive than hooks.

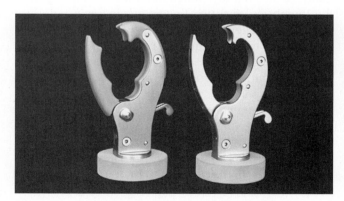

Figure 46-6 Voluntary closing prehensors. **(A)** Grip 3 with polyethylene gripping surface. **(B)** Grip 2S made with titanium, stainless steel, and aluminum materials. *Photo courtesy of TRS, Inc., Boulder, CO.*

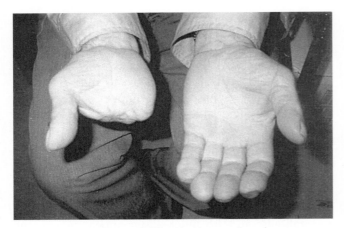

Figure 46-7 Partial hand amputation.

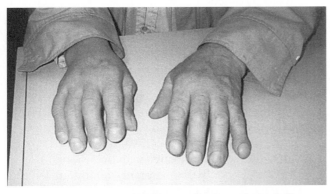

Figure 46-8 Cosmetic anatomical covering for this partial hand. (Courtesy of Michael Curtain, Alternative Prosthetic Services, Southport, CT.)

With the continued development and refinement of externally powered hands, electric hands are being chosen over mechanical hands, particularly by those with transradial amputations, since they offer greater pinch force, can be activated with more ease, and do not require a harness. A mistaken notion is that the electric hand provides more dexterity than the mechanical hand. To the contrary, both hands move identically, with the thumb and first two fingers moving as a unit, in a three-point prehension pattern. They differ in the control system only: the mechanical hand is controlled through cable or **body power (BP)**, and the electric hand is controlled through myoelectric signals or switches, that is, **external power**.

For the individual with bilateral amputations, BP hooks continue to be preferred, because function is of paramount importance. Some individuals choose a different TD for each limb, for example, a BP hook for one side and a myoelectric hand for the other. How can the ideal TDs be chosen? Listen to the patient and consult with the other team members to get varied perspectives. These options are presented to the patient who makes the ultimate choice.

Wrist Units

The wrist unit provides a means to attach the TD to the forearm. It also provides an important function: the terminal device can be rotated to positions of supination, pronation, or midposition before engaging in an activity. This prepositioning is an important substitution movement for reduced or absent active forearm rotation. There are several types of wrist units; the ones described here are the most popular:

▶ Constant friction. This wrist unit contains a nylon threaded insert that surrounds the stud of the TD to hold it in place. An Allen wrench is used to turn a small set screw that applies pressure against the nylon insert, which causes constant pressure against the stud of the TD. Just enough friction must be applied to allow the individual to rotate the TD but not so little that the TD inadvertently rotates while it is being activated by the cable pull. The therapist teaches the patient to use the wrench to make adjustments.

▶ Quick change. These units provide easy disconnection of different TDs. The TD is pressed down into the wrist to eject the TD or to lock it into position.

▶ Wrist flexion. There are two versions of this unit: (1) The Hosmer wrist flexion unit can be manually placed in neutral, 30° of flexion, or 50° of flexion. (2) The dome-shaped Sierra wrist flexion unit can be screwed into a standard wrist unit and can be rotated and flexed to the same angles as the Hosmer unit. Wrist flexion units are indispensable for the person with bilateral amputations because of their usefulness in reaching the midline for toileting, dressing, and eating.

▶ Ball and socket. This unit can be prepositioned around the ball, but it cannot be locked in position.

Transradial (BE) Components

Forearm Socket Designs. The residual limb is encased in the socket of the prothesis with total contact. A standard forearm socket (Fig. 46-9) encases two-thirds of the arm length but can be cut down to allow for more active pronation and supination for a long limb. The supracondylar socket (modified Muenster) is a frequent choice for the short transradial limb; the proximal brim grips the humeral lateral and medial epicondyles and the posterior olecranon (Fig. 46-10). This design is widely used for the myoelectric prostheses. It is self-suspending, with no harnessing necessary.

Elbow Hinges. Elbow hinges connect the socket to the triceps cuff or pad on the upper arm. These can be flexible straps of Dacron or leather or rigid metal hinges. The flexible hinge allows for flexibility around the joint, whereas the rigid hinge offers stability at the elbow joint.

Triceps Cuff. The triceps cuff on the upper arm is connected to the socket by the elbow hinge. It serves as a point of attachment for the cable housing of the control attachment strap.

Harness and Control System. The harness serves two purposes: (1) to suspend, or hold the prosthesis firmly on the residual limb and (2) to allow for force (through body motion) to be transmitted to the control cable that operates the terminal device. Three types of harnesses are most popular for the transradial prosthesis: figure-of-eight, figure-of-nine, and chest strap with a shoulder saddle. The figure-of-eight harness is most often used. Its axilla loop serves as the anchor point (reaction point) from which the other straps are attached; the inverted Y support strap attaches to the anterior support strap of the harness. These two attachments are important because they stabilize the socket to the harness and prevent displacement when heavy loads are carried or lifted. The chest strap with shoulder saddle may be suitable for the patient who cannot tolerate the axilla loop pressure or when stability is needed for heavy work. The shoulder saddle distributes the pressure over a larger area. The figure-of-nine harness is used with the supracondylar socket. Because the socket configuration provides self-

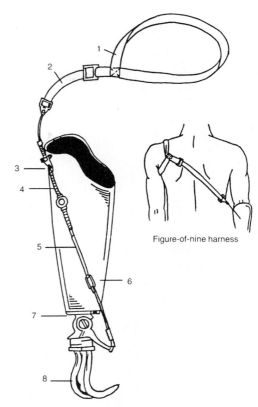

Figure 46-10 Supracondylar prosthesis. 1, Figure-of-nine harness; 2, control attachment strap; 3, lift loop; 4, housing; 5, cable; 6, supracondylar socket; 7, wrist unit; 8, TD. Illustration by Gregory Celikyol.

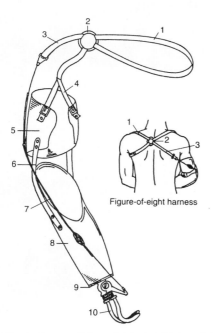

Figure 46-9 Standard transradial prosthesis. 1, Axilla loop; 2, Northwestern University (NU) ring; 3, control-attachment strap; 4, inverted Y strap; 5, triceps cuff; 6, flexible elbow hinge; 7, cable; 8, socket; 9, wrist unit; 10, TD. Illustration by Gregory Celikyol.

suspension, only a control attachment strap is needed to attach the axilla loop to the cable control system.

Transhumeral (AE) Components

Socket Designs. The conventional socket edge is generally just near or above the acromion, depending on limb length. Another design is often selected because it provides more rotational stability, as with the Utah arm. A transhumeral prosthesis with an internal locking elbow is shown in Figure 46-11.

Elbow Units. There are two elbow units for the AE prosthesis: (1) an internal elbow locking unit for a standard or short transhumeral amputation and (2) external elbow locking unit for a long transhumeral or elbow disarticulation amputation.

Friction Units. The friction unit must be manually flexed into place. It is lightweight and is used with passive prosthetic arms. Manual elbow components are also available with a locking mechanism.

External Spring Lift Assist. The external spring lift assist is a clock spring mechanism that is added to the medial side of the elbow. Tightening the mechanism causes in-

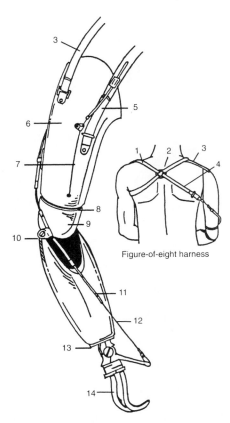

Figure-of-eight harness

Figure 46-11 Standard transhumeral prosthesis. 1, Axilla loop; 2, NU ring; 3. Lateral support strap; 4. Control attachment strap; 5. Elastic anterior support strap; 6. Socket; 7. Elbow lock cable; 8. Turntable; 9. Internal elbow lock unit; 10. Lift loop; 11. Housing; 12. Cable; 13. Wrist unit; 14, TD. Illustration by Gregory Celikyol.

creased tension for elbow flexion and assists in initiating this motion. The patient can adjust it.

Shoulder Hinges. The shoulder hinges can be manually positioned into flexion or extension or abduction or adduction for placement of the arm in space.

Shoulder Disarticulation and Scapulothoracic Components

Most socket designs for shoulder disarticulation and scapulothoracic protheses consist of a plastic laminated shoulder cap or frame socket with carbon fiber reinforcements. Another choice is an endoskeletal passive arm that is lightweight and contains an internal pylon shaft. It is covered with resilient foam contoured to the shape of the arm. A chest strap harness suspends the prosthesis.

Harness and Control Systems. The harness and control systems for a transhumeral amputation are usually of the figure-of-eight or chest strap design. For a shoulder disarticulation prosthesis, the elbow lock can be activated using a chin nudge lever or a manual elbow lock mechanism.

Externally Powered Prosthetic Components

Electric Terminal Devices. Electric-powered hands and hooks can be activated through myoelectric or switch control (Heckathorne, 1992). The electric-powered prehensors are heavier (approximately 1 pound) but provide stronger pinch force (20 to 23 pounds) than the BP types. There are two speed systems: (1) digital control (constant speed), in which muscle contractions cause opening and closing at a given speed; and (2) proportional control (variable speed), in which the speed and pinch force increase in proportion to the intensity of muscle contraction.

Electric Hands. Otto Bock electric hands (Fig. 46-12) are the most popular models. They are available in several sizes. Either a PVC or silicone glove can cover them. The motor in the hand mechanism drives the thumb and first two fingers as a unit to provide palmar (three-point) prehension.

Electric Hooks. The Otto Bock electric Greifer TD is interchangeable with the Otto Bock hand and may be preferred for work that requires prehension force up to 50 pounds. It is bulky, encased in a hard plastic shell with no glove covering, and is less delicate than the hand. It is available in one size. The two fingers move symmetrically in opposition, parallel to one another (Fig. 46-13).

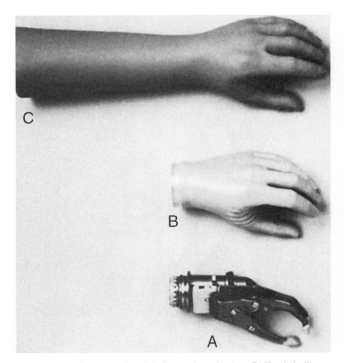

Figure 46-12 Electronic hand. **A.** Internal mechanism. **B.** Hand shell covering. **C.** Glove. Photo courtesy of Otto Bock Orthopedic Industry, Minneapolis, MN.

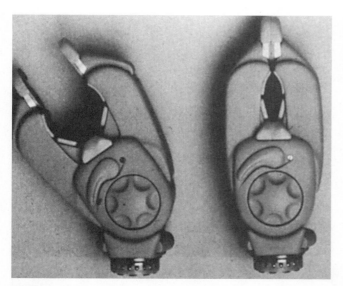

Figure 46-13 Electric Greifer TD in open and closed positions. Photo courtesy of Otto Bock Orthopedic Industry, Minneapolis, MN.

The Hosmer NU-VA Synergetic Prehensor contains motors that drive each of the fingers at different speeds and torque. Therefore, in grasping an object, one finger closes quickly on an object while the other finger applies the force for secure grip.

Electric Wrist Rotation Units. Wrist rotation units, used for pronation and supination, are being prescribed more often. Sears and Shaperman (1998) present a strong case for their use by persons with unilateral and bilateral amputations.

Electric Elbows. These three electric elbow mechanisms are the most popular: the Boston elbow, the NY-Hosmer electric elbow, and the Utah (Motion Control) elbow (Fig. 46-14). These elbows can be controlled by electromechanical switches or by myoelectric control.

The Final Prescription: A Discussion

> "In the upper extremity, the prosthesis meets its greatest challenge. Here the lost function can only be imitated. . . . We must fit the prosthesis not only to the patient's limb but to his whole personality."
>
> (Kessler, 1947, p. 5)

Motivation is the most important factor in the acceptance and use of the prosthesis. This is a complex issue, because the prosthesis is chosen just when the patient is most confused and vulnerable. The patient's desire for a prosthesis is strongest after surgery and may wane as time passes, particularly for those with unilateral amputations, since compensatory one-handed techniques are soon perfected. The patient with a bilateral amputation

needs function and is likely to accept and use the prostheses.

What defines a successful wearer? When the prosthesis is viewed as necessary or meaningful for any activity, such as leisure activities or for cosmesis, it has added to the quality of life and is therefore successful (Fraser, 1998; Wright & Hagen, 1995). A patient with a unilateral amputation may use the prosthesis for particular activities, such as for sports, and these interests can change with time. Two sets of prostheses are strongly recommended for the person with high-level bilateral amputations; this ensures that the patient will always have use of the prostheses should one set need repairs.

The end goal of a therapeutic program is to ensure the highest level of independence and competency in life roles that the patient views as meaningful. This does not always assume prosthetic use. It is, however, the team's responsibility to present the options to the patient.

Prosthetic Training Program

The minimal training time is 6 hours for persons with transradial amputation; 15 hours for transhumeral, shoulder disarticulation, and bilateral transradial amputations; and 20 hours for bilateral transhumeral amputations.

Initial Stage of Treatment

The initial stage of treatment can generally be covered in one or two therapy sessions. Box 46-3 has treatment guidelines for this stage.

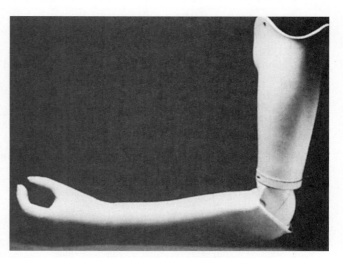

Figure 46-14 Utah arm with externally powered hand and elbow. Photo courtesy of Motion Control, Salt Lake City, UT.

BOX 46-3
PROCEDURES FOR PRACTICE

Treatment Guidelines for Initial Stage of Treatment

- Evaluate the prosthesis.
- Explain program goals to the patient.
- Describe the functions of each component; give the patient an illustration of the prosthesis with components labeled.

- Teach the patient to don and doff the prosthesis.
- Discuss the wearing schedule with the patient.
- Teach limb hygiene care.
- Teach care of the prosthesis.
- Begin controls training using the terminal device.

TABLE 46-2
Chart for Evaluating a Prosthesis

Activity	Yes	No	Comments
1. Does the prosthesis comply with the written prescription?			
2. Is the length of the prosthesis equal to the length of the sound arm? (Measure tip of TD to ground and compare to tip of thumb of sound hand to ground when the patient is standing. Compare elbow length for each side.)			
3. Are appearance and workmanship satisfactory? (Examine for smooth edges, smooth interior of socket, no loose rivets or screws, finished harness edges, satisfactory arm color.)			
4. Can the socket tolerate a downward pull of 50 lb without displacing more than 1 in?			
5. a. Is there pain or discomfort while the limb is in the socket? b. Does the limb show abrasions or discoloration when the prosthesis is removed?			
6. a. Does the housing cover the cable without restricting elbow flexion? b. Is the cable free of sharp bends?			
7. a. Is the axilla loop small enough to keep the figure 8 harness below the seventh cervical vertebra and slightly to the unamputated side? b. Is the axilla loop covered and comfortable? c. Are all straps of adequate length and in proper alignment?			
8. a. Does the triceps cuff fit firmly without gapping? b. Can the turntable be rotated manually with relative ease and remain in position?			
9. a. Do the TDs and wrist unit function smoothly? b. Is the glove covering for the hand satisfactory in color and fit? c. Does the TD have full opening, closing? d. Can the TD be fully opened and closed at the hip, at 90° of elbow flexion, and at the mouth?			
10. Can forearm rotation that is at least 50% of rotation without the prosthesis be achieved?			
11. Can elbow flexion that is only 10° less than flexion with prosthesis off be achieved?			
12. For transhumeral amputation: a. Can 90° of shoulder abduction and flexion and 30° of arm extension be achieved? b. Can the prosthetic elbow be flexed by flexing the humerus 45° or less?			

Adapted from Department of Prosthetics and Orthotics. (1986). *Upper limb prosthetics*, New York: New York University Medical Center, Postgraduate Medical School.

Evaluation of the Prosthesis

On the first visit the therapist checks out and evaluates the prosthesis before instituting training. The purpose of the evaluation is to determine (1) compliance with the prescription, (2) comfort of fit of the socket and harness, (3) satisfactory operation of all components, and (4) appearance (features) of the prosthesis and its parts. Table 46-2 has methods and standards for evaluation.

First Therapy Session

Generally, patients with unilateral amputations attend therapy on an outpatient schedule of 2 or 3 days a week; therefore, the first visit is a critical one. The aim from the outset is to minimize negative experiences to ensure acceptance and use of the prosthesis. In addition to evaluation of the prosthesis, the following must also be covered during the first visit: (1) donning and removing the prosthesis, (2) wearing schedule, (3) hygienic care of the residual limb if the patient did not receive preprosthetic care in that clinic.

Donning and Removing the Prosthesis

Donning and removing the prothesis can be achieved by one of two methods that simulate putting on a coat or pullover shirt. To use the coat method, the residual limb is inserted into the socket (Fig. 46-15), which is held in place with the intact hand, with the harness and axilla loop dangling behind the back. The intact arm reaches behind and slips into the axilla loop; a forward shrug of the shoulders positions the prosthesis in place. For the pullover method, the patient places the prosthesis in front of him or her and the intact arm is placed through the axilla loop while the residual limb is placed into the socket. Both limbs are raised to lift the prosthesis and harness over the head as the harness falls into place (Fig. 46-16). Initially, the prosthesis can be placed on a bed

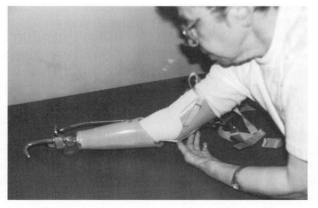

Figure 46-15 One method of donning a unilateral prosthesis.

or dresser to support it as the patient slips into the prosthesis.

Wearing Time

The patient must increase wearing time gradually to develop tolerance to the socket and harness. The initial wearing time may be 15 to 30 minutes. Each time the prosthesis is removed, the residual limb must be examined for excessive redness or irritation, and it must not be reapplied until any redness subsides. ***If redness does not disappear after approximately 20 minutes, this should be reported to the prosthetist for adjustment to the prosthesis.*** Otherwise, prosthetic wearing time can be increased in 30-minute increments until the prosthesis can be worn all day. The importance of gradually increasing the wearing time cannot be overemphasized, particularly for patients with decreased sensation and scar tissue.

Limb Hygiene

Because the residual limb is enclosed in a rigid socket where excessive perspiration can macerate the skin, it is important to instruct the patient to wash the limb daily with mild soap and lukewarm water and pat dry. The therapist can recommend that the patient wear a T-shirt or equivalent covering so that the harness system of a BP prosthesis is not in direct contact with the skin. This provides padding and absorbs perspiration. For the same reason, the patient is instructed to wear a sock over the residual limb. A roll-on silicone liner may be issued to those who perform heavy work; it provides secure suspension and minimizes piston action. However, this can cause excessive perspiration.

Care of Prosthesis

Mild soap and warm water are recommended to clean the interior of the socket. It can also be wiped with rubbing alcohol every several weeks. The patient must be cautioned about agents that may stain or damage gloves. The hook is more rugged, but care must be taken during work in areas where there is excessive dirt, grease, or water. The patient must be especially careful with externally powered components.

Intermediate Stage of Treatment

Training for Use of Body-Powered Prosthesis

The therapy program for the BP prothesis is addressed in two phases: (1) prosthetic controls training and (2) prosthetic functional use training.

Prosthetic Controls Training

Therapy for controls training begins with teaching the operation of each control, beginning with the TD

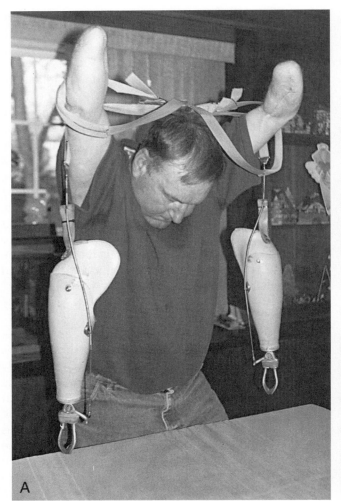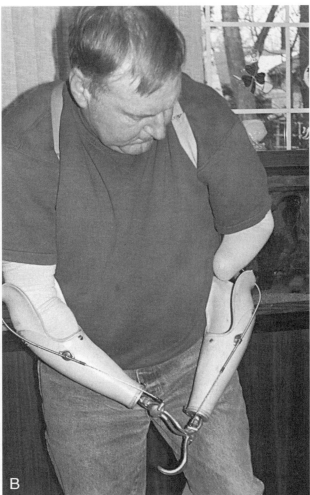

Figure 46-16 A. Donning bilateral harnesses overhead. **B.** Completing the process by inserting limbs into the sockets.

(Box 46-4). The therapist guides the patient to practice repetitive activation of each component. Transradial prostheses have a single control system that activates the TD by cable pull. Patients are instructed to activate the TD (Figs. 46-17 and 46-18) by using humeral flexion and scapular abduction (protraction). Transhumeral prostheses have a dual control system for the TD and elbow. The motions required to lock and unlock the elbow are a combination of humeral extension, abduction, and depression (Fig. 46-19). TD activation is achieved in the same manner as with the transradial controls except that the elbow must be locked. The patient with a transhumeral prosthesis may also have to learn to use the turntable to rotate the arm and possibly a shoulder joint to position the shoulder.

Practice in control drills requires coaching the patient in patterns of reach, grasp, and release for objects that vary in weight, size, texture, and configuration. Ordinarily, the sequence is from large, hard objects to small, fragile ones. These assortments are subject to the therapist's ingenuity and patient's interests. Initially, objects are placed on a tabletop for prehension practice, and then they are transported to various locations in the room. The therapist instructs the patient to determine the most natural and efficient position for the TD before grasping an item and to rotate it in the wrist unit. This is called prepositioning the TD.

Eventually the therapist instructs the patient to perform motion patterns in different planes, such as overhead, at tabletop, and at floor level. Overhead use is the most difficult because it is hindered by the harnessing system; it is particularly difficult, sometimes impossible, for persons with high amputations. The person with bilateral amputations has a harness system that is

BOX 46-4
PROCEDURES FOR PRACTICE

Controls Training for Body Powered Prostheses

Component	Movement	Intervention
Terminal device	Humeral flexion with scapular abduction (protraction) on side of amputation; bilateral scapular abduction for midline use of TD or when strength is limited.	Manually guide patient through motions. For transhumeral prostheses, keep elbow unit locked in 90° flexion; teach TD control first.
Wrist unit	Rotate TD to supination (fingers of hook up), midposition (fingers toward midline), or pronation (fingers down). For unilateral amputation patient uses sound hand to rotate TD. For bilateral amputation rotate TD against stationary object, between knees, or with contralateral TD.	Have patient analyze the task and determine the most efficient approach for grasp, avoiding excessive or awkward movements. Examples: TD in midposition for carrying a tray, in pronation for grasping small box from table.
Elbow unit	Depress arm while extending and abducting humerus to lock or unlock elbow mechanism.

Practice flexing and locking elbow in several planes. | Manually guide patient through motions. Begin with elbow unlocked. Patient listens for click as lock activates. Have patient exaggerate movements initially. Use a mirror.
Use humeral flexion to flex the elbow; go beyond desired height, since the arm will drop with gravity pull as patient is in process of locking the elbow unit. |
| Turntable | Rotate elbow turntable toward or away from body using sound hand. With bilateral amputations, push or pull against stationary object to rotate. | Teach patient to analyze task to determine need to use this component for more efficiency. |

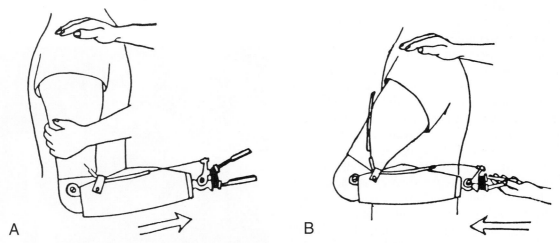

Figure 46-17 A. Teaching activation of VO TD. With elbow locked, therapist pulls the patient's upper arm forward to open TD. **B.** Teaching elbow lock and unlock. The therapist pushes the patient's arm back (*arrow*) into extension, abduction, and depression. It is brought back to the vertical plane between cycles. (Illustration by Gregory Celikyol.)

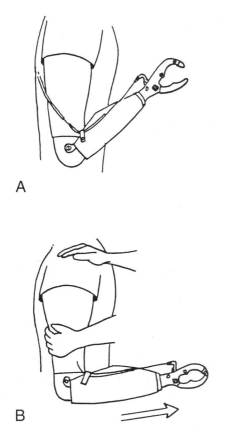

Figure 46-18 Activation of voluntary closing TD. **A.** the TD remains open at rest **B.** the TD closes with forward flexion. (Illustration by Gregory Celikyol.)

bilaterally attached; therefore, the patient must practice relaxing the musculature on the contralateral side while using one prosthesis.

Prosthetic Functional Use Training
Spontaneous, automatic skillful prosthetic use is a goal for functional use training. Another is completion of activities within a reasonable length of time while using minimal extraneous movement and energy expenditure. Figures 46-20 to 46-23 show functional tasks. The therapist encourages patients to analyze and see similarities among situations and reminds them of relevant principles. This prepares the patient to respond with a sense of control in unpredictable situations.

A person with a unilateral amputation can be expected to use the prosthesis primarily for sustained holding or for stabilization and to use it more slowly compared to the unaffected extremity. Table 46-3 suggests how some activities can be accomplished; Atkins and Meier (1989b) offer more comprehensive lists. An interesting study (Lake, 1997) revealed that individuals who received training surpassed those who did not in efficiency of use, skill, and spontaneity.

Several factors affect the degree of independence of the person with bilateral amputations, the major one being the level of amputation. Some adaptations may be necessary for those with high-level bilateral amputations. These may range from a simple buttonhook or dressing frame—a stand in which coat hooks are inserted to hold clothing—to high-tech solutions, such as electronic aids

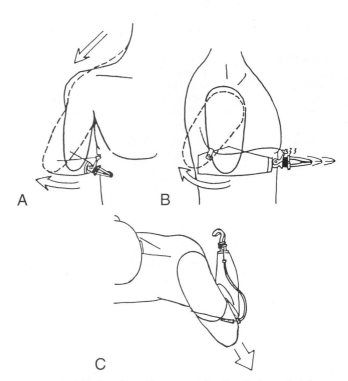

Figure 46-19 Motions (*arrows*) necessary for elbow lock or unlock for an above-elbow prosthesis. **A.** Abduction with depression. **B.** Extension. **C.** Combined movement pattern of extension, depression, and abduction. (Illustration by Gregory Celikyol.)

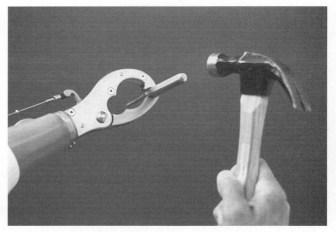

Figure 46-20 Use of the voluntary closing TRS Grip for bimanual task. Photo courtesy of TRS, Inc., Brooklyn, NY.

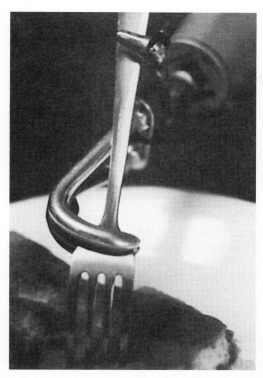

Figure 46-21 Grasping a fork using this method provides stability while the sound hand cuts the food.

for daily living (Lehneis & Dickey, 1992) and computers controlled by breath, voice, or mouthstick. The therapist is advised to encourage foot use when patients show potential and are agile. Persons who have developed this ability at an early age have a high degree of independence. Feet have the advantage of having sensibility, which serves them well in all activities and surpasses prosthetic use.

Myoelectrically Controlled Prostheses

Myoelectric prostheses are fast becoming standard choices and are frequently prescribed for transradial amputations. Figure 46-24 depicts a two-state system whereby two separate muscle groups are used to operate the TD. The intent is to choose muscles that physiologically closely correspond to the outcome motion and also produce strong electrical signals when contracted. Wrist flexors and extensors are commonly chosen to achieve grasp and opening of the TD. For transhumeral amputations, the common choices are the biceps and triceps. For higher-level amputations, as in shoulder disarticulation or forequarter amputations, the choices for control may be trapezius, latissimus, infraspinatus, or pectoralis muscles.

Most of the principles and treatment goals previously mentioned for BP prosthesis training apply to myoelectrically controlled prostheses. The therapy pro-

gram begins with evaluation of the prosthesis, with special emphasis on the control system (Spiegel, 1989). Factors to be addressed:

► Are the electrodes placed over the site offering the best muscle control potential?
► Is there good contact between the electrodes and the skin? (An imprint should be visible on the skin when the prosthesis is removed but should not be deep enough to cause irritation.)
► Can the patient open and close the hand in various planes?

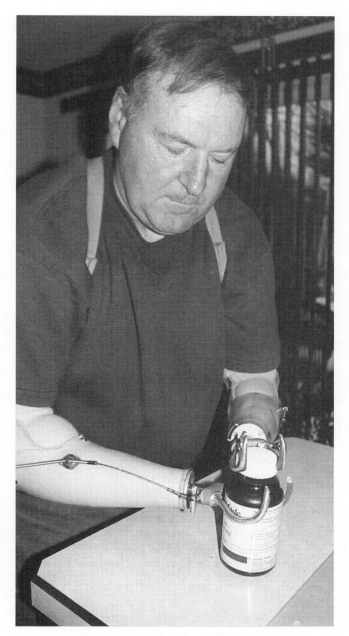

Figure 46-22 One way to open a jar using bilateral prostheses.

Case Example

MR. C.: TRANSRADIAL AMPUTATION

Patient Information

Mr. C., aged 53 years, sustained a crush injury of his dominant right arm in machinery at work that required a transradial (BE) amputation. He worked as a plant manager in a recycling plant. His responsibilities included supervising workers in the shop, but he was also required to adjust the machinery and do some lifting. He is married with two teenaged children and is the sole wage earner for the family.

Mr. C. received occupational therapy for preprosthetic training followed by prosthetic training using a body-powered prosthesis with interchangeable hook and hand. He chose to use the hand rather than the hook, as appearance was important to him. He developed exceptional dexterity in his remaining hand and has continued to improve writing skills. He had full day wearing tolerance and was independent in daily living skills but continued to have difficulty grasping objects above shoulder level and occasionally grasping items at floor level because of restrictions of the harnessing straps. Mr. C. has returned to work and resumed his position as plant manager and is working part time.

Reason for Referral to Occupational Therapy

Mr. C. has requested a myoelectrically controlled prosthesis with a hand. Approval was received from the insurance company and the patient was scheduled for occupational therapy to determine whether he is a candidate and to provide preprosthetic training if eligible. He was tested with the myotester and was able to achieve a sufficient although inconsistent level of muscle contraction of wrist flexors and extensors.

Occupational Therapy Problem List

- Inconsistency in maintaining strong muscle contractions
- Inconsistent isolation of muscle contractions
- Unable to grade (increase or decrease) muscle contractions at will

Occupational Therapy Goal List

- Achieve maximal muscle contraction of wrist flexors and extensors
- Maintain the level of contraction of the agonist at will while relaxing the antagonist muscle
- Control magnitude of contractions (grade contractions)

Treatment Plan

- Patient performs wrist flexion and extension with the sound hand and imitates the contractions using the residual limb.

- The patient views the myotester dial for feedback while practicing contractions.
- The patient controls opening and closing of the electronic hand, which is held by the therapist.

Mr. C. received 1-hour sessions three times a week for 2 weeks and achieved preprosthetic goals. He has received the permanent myoelectric prosthesis, which contains a supracondylar socket with no harness straps and a proportionally controlled electronic hand. Eight additional 2-hour therapy sessions have been approved. The patient wants to return to work full time and expressed anxiety with regard to resuming all his previous responsibilities.

Occupational Therapy Goal List II

- Patient will learn myoelectric control of the hand.
- Patient will use the prosthesis for IADL.
- Patient will use the prosthesis successfully at his work site.

Treatment Plan

- Instruct in donning and removing the prosthesis.
- Instruct in cleaning the socket and electrodes and battery charging.
- Practice maintaining grasp on objects.
- Simulate use of tools, lifting and placing items from floor to shelves at shoulder height.
- Practice graded control of pressure on objects.
- Arrange a job site visit.

Analysis of Reasoning

Mr. C. is already proficient in using the mechanical hand for life activities and for most tasks at work, so training was unnecessary to teach efficient grasp, since movement patterns of the mechanical and electric hands are identical. Therefore, myoelectric control training was the focus, with special emphasis on work-related tasks, the patient's prime goal.

CLINICAL REASONING
in OT Practice

Mr. C. is highly motivated to resume his previous work responsibilities; he feels confident with regard to performing desk skills but is fearful of lifting items that require bimanual grasp in various planes and in maintaining a firm grasp when adjusting machinery. How can the therapist design a program that will address these issues? What information is necessary to define the job requirements and how can they be obtained?

▶ Can the patient remove and replace the battery with ease?

The therapist should consult with the prosthetist for guidance with any concerns. Donning and removing the prosthesis may require collaboration with the prosthetist to determine the simplest method for the patient. Often, a slight twisting of the forearm when inserting the limb is helpful. Sometimes baby powder or a lubricant can be

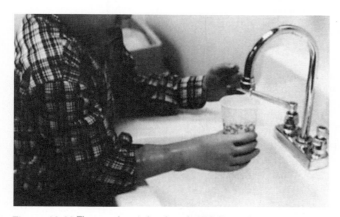

Figure 46-23 The myoelectric hand can hold delicate objects in bimanual activities.

used to ease donning, but these may inhibit electrode functioning.

Care of the socket requires daily cleansing with a damp cloth and mild soap to remove any residues of powder, lubricants, and perspiration. Other special concerns are care of the batteries, methods of charging the batteries, and operation of the on–off switch. Care of the glove was discussed earlier.

Controls and functional use training goals are similar to those for the BP prosthesis. This assumes that the patient has already received muscle site controls training during the preprosthetic period. When a myoelectric tester is used (a biofeedback unit can also be used), the goals are to isolate muscle contractions and increase muscle strength (see Chapter 25). If sustained grasp is required for an extended period, when one might inadvertently contract muscles that open the hand, a manual lock mechanism can be installed in the hand. This can be controlled by pushing it in with the remaining hand.

Final Stage of Treatment: IADLs

In the final stage, prosthetic functional use skills are further refined, and daily living activities that are more

---

TABLE 46-3
Suggested Approaches for Functional Activities: Unilateral Upper Limb Amputation

Task	Prosthesis	Sound Limb
Eating		
Cut food	Hold fork	Cut with knife
Butter bread	Stabilize bread	Spread toward body
Fill glass from faucet	Hold glass	Turn knob or lever
Carry tray	TD in midposition to hold	Hold in midposition
Peel fruit	Stabilize with TD	Peel
Dressing		
Don & doff shirt or blouse	Don: prosthesis in sleeve first; remove after sound arm	Don: sound arm last; remove sound arm first
Put clothing on hanger	Hold hanger	Place clothing on hanger
Buckle belt	Stabilize belt	Push belt through buckle
Tie bow	Stabilize lace	Manipulate & make loops
Button cuff on sound side	Use buttonhook, (or sew on button with elastic thread)	Hold cuff in place with fingertips while using buttonhook
Use zipper	Hold fabric with TD	Pull zipper
Desk skills		
Write	Stabilize paper	Write
Insert letter in envelope	Hold, stabilize envelope at end	Insert letter and seal
Use phone, dial, take notes	Hold receiver: TD or with chin & shoulder	Dial and write
Draw line with ruler; use paper clip	Stabilize ruler; hold paper	Draw line; apply clip
General skills		
Take bill from wallet	Hold wallet or stabilize on table	Manipulate wallet & remove bill
Wrap and unwrap package	Stabilize box and paper	Manipulate box, paper; tie
Thread needle	Hold needle	Thread needle

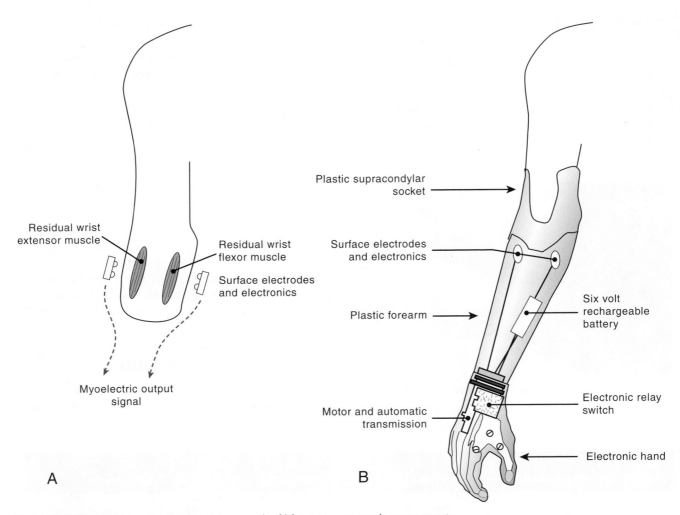

Figure 46-24 Myoelectric prosthesis, a two-state system in which two separate muscle groups operate the terminal device. **A.** 1. The muscle contracts and creates an electrical signal that can be measured in microvolts (1 millionth of a volt). 2. The EMG signal is detected by the surface electrode. 3. The EMG signal is processed by the electronics and transmitted to the electronic relay in the hand. **B.** 1. When the electronic relay receives an EMG signal from the wrist flexors, the circuit is complete and the electricity from the battery runs the motor to close the hand. 2. When the relay receives an EMG signal from the wrist extensors, the motor runs in the opposite direction to open the hand. (Illustration courtesy of Jack Hodgins, CPO, Kessler Institute for Rehabilitation, West Orange, NJ.)

demanding are introduced. Discharge planning should include exploration of vocational and recreational interests and driving and/or the use of public transportation. An adaptation for driving may require a simple knob or driving ring attached to the steering wheel. Foot controls can be installed for those with very high level bilateral amputations. The therapist can consult companies that do van conversions (see Chapter 31).

Visits to the community, home, school, and work are strongly advised. This brings the patient and therapist into the actual environment, away from simulated, static settings. Patients may be referred to a self-help group. These organizations vary in their goals, but most provide a forum wherein people can interact and share experi-

ences. Many groups provide ongoing educational programs on new prosthetic developments or on sports and recreational activities.

Sports and Recreation

Increasing numbers of individuals with amputations are pursuing recreational activities, and as a result, several customized prosthetic components are available for sports and recreational activities. Two comprehensive references, Radocy (1992) and Kegel (1992), discuss this topic. Figures 46-25 to 46-27 show modifications used to enable independence in sports activities. The Internet is a good source of information for this and related topics (see Resources).

Discharge Planning

At discharge, the team schedules a follow-up appointment for the clinic; this may be 1 to several months post discharge. The patient is encouraged to contact the prosthetist for repairs or maintenance as needed and to make an appointment for a clinic visit at any time. Patients' needs do not remain constant; as they resume their lives, they may want special modifications or different prostheses.

Partial Hand Amputations

As with any amputation, the surgeon performing a partial hand amputation attempts to preserve length with intact sensibility. At this level, retaining residual digits with adequate skin coverage and some degree of mobility and sensation is far superior to any prosthesis (Bunnell, 1990) and is the goal. The principles of preprosthetic

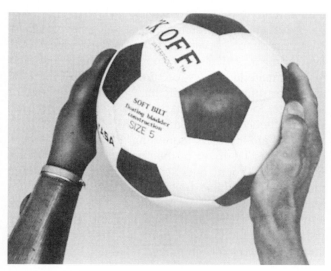

Figure 46-25 TRS Super Sport Passive Mitt, used for gross grasp. (Courtesy of Bob Rodocy, TRS, Inc., Boulder, CO.)

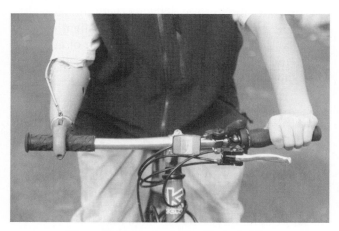

Figure 46-26 One-handed hand brake for bike.

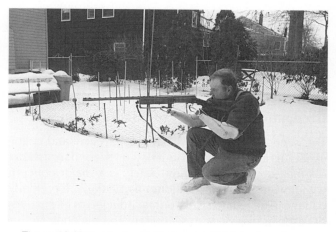

Figure 46-27 Modification of rifle for use with bilateral prostheses.

therapy (discussed earlier) apply to this level of amputation as well.

Some patients with a partial hand amputation want a prosthesis that closely replicates the look of the hand and provides dexterity as well. Although cosmetic hand coverings are truly artistic endeavors, once they fit over the residual hand, tactile sensation is lost, which limits function. For these reasons, it is fairly common for the glove to be discarded for a functional finger post.

Management of Lower Limb Amputations

The therapeutic program for persons with lower limb amputations requires collaboration between the physical therapist and occupational therapist. The physical therapist is responsible for skin care, limb wrapping, lower limb strengthening exercises, range of motion, and ambulation training. Training in some daily living activities may be shared, for example limb bandaging, bed mobility, and transfers. Critical care pathways can identify specific goals within a time frame for all professionals involved with patient care, ensuring maximum functional outcome (Esquenazi, 1996). The therapist can refer to a functional outcome guideline (Leonard & Meier, 1998) that lists specific daily living activities with expected outcomes for **transfemoral amputation** and **transtibial amputation** and to the *Locomotor Capabilities Index* (Gauthier-Gagnon, 1998) for an example of a questionnaire used to determine patients' perceived levels of independence in locomotor activities.

Often, functional conditioning groups are conducted by an occupational therapist. These are examples of topics included in such group sessions:

► Upper extremity strengthening exercises
► Safety precautions related to specific activities
► Energy conservation techniques

▶ Use of adaptive devices
▶ Review of dietary restriction when appropriate

Other staff may present topics in their areas of expertise, such as the dietitian on special diets.

Occupational Therapy Program Guidelines

The occupational therapist assesses physical and cognitive status and obtains information on secondary diagnoses that may affect function. Safety is a major concern with lower limb amputations, particularly for elderly patients. They may have a primary diagnosis of diabetes or vascular disease with secondary complicating factors that affect therapy, such as kidney disease, cardiovascular disease, chronic infection, respiratory disease, and arthritis. In the elderly, impaired vision and memory deficits may influence safe performance in activities of daily living. Energy expenditure 25 to 40% above normal can be expected for transtibial amputation, 68 to 100% above normal for transfemoral, more than 40% increase for bilateral transtibial, and 100% increase for bilateral transtibial–transfemoral amputation (Esquenazi, 1996).

The occupational therapist addresses activities of daily living in the following sequence: bed mobility; hygiene and grooming; dressing, including donning and removing the leg prosthesis; and wheelchair propulsion and management. Transfer skills are practiced with and without the prosthesis. Practice sessions include transfers to the bed, toilet, furniture, and car. The therapist teaches the family the transfer techniques when safety is a concern. The occupational therapist addresses mobility skills in the kitchen using a wheelchair and/or ambulating with the prosthesis, with or without a device. The therapist includes other IADL skills as appropriate, such as housecleaning and bed making. Home and community visits with the patient and a staff member may be indicated.

The therapist recommends home modifications and equipment to the patient and family. Equipment often includes transfer tub bench or seat and toilet safety arm rails. These rails fit around the toilet and provide a means of arm support that assists with lowering and coming to standing. The therapist makes the referral for driving assessment and training when appropriate. Installation of a left-foot accelerator bar and pedal is necessary for a person with a right-leg amputation. Hand controls can be installed for persons with bilateral leg amputations (see Chapter 31).

Emerging Trends in Prosthetics

Research and development of components for BP prostheses continue to receive attention: the Mica shoulder joint is one development. It can be locked in several positions, a feature previously unavailable (Jones & Davidson, 1996). Another development is a new design of humeral rotator for BP prosthesis that requires reduced effort to rotate (Ivko, 1999). A newly developed and promising cable of polyethylene is exceptionally strong and can withstand high abrasion (Jones & Davidson). In development is a VO BP prehensor with adjustable grip that can be controlled by rotating a stiff elastic band to obtain a range of 0.5 to 20 pounds grip (Frey, 1995). A prototype motorized arm from the United Kingdom (Edinburgh Modular Arm System) contains a motorized shoulder unit (see Resources). In the United States, a prototype hand allows for individual finger movement through tendon-activated pneumatic sensors in the forearm socket (Abboudi, 1999).

A surgical approach called osseointegration requires the implantation of a titanium peg fixed to the bone to which a finger or thumb prosthesis can be attached. This approach has also been used for lower limb amputations (Jones & Davidson, 1996).

Advances in lower limb prosthetics have also focused on use of graphite and carbon composites in the development of dynamic-response prosthetic feet. This resilient material allows for strong push-off of the foot, useful for running and jumping. New designs allow for additional foot movements, such as inversion and eversion and heel compression (Leonard & Meier, 1998).

What are the users requesting? Research and development must be driven by their needs. Atkins and Heard (1996) and Kyberd and Beard (1998) have identified these needs in their surveys. Here are some features identified for upper limb prostheses: better suspension and cable systems, additional wrist movement, more precision of pinch with more dexterity, coordinated motions of two joints, improved reliability for electronic hands.

As with research and development, the therapeutic program must be driven by the patient's needs. As the patient masters the basics of prosthetic control systems and practices their use in activities, with the therapist's guidance as facilitator or teacher, the patient chooses tasks that he or she values. The approach of analyzing tasks and problem solving serves the patient well throughout life.

Summary Review Questions

1. Why is the residual limb wrapped with elastic bandaging? How is it done?
2. What are the most common causes of acquired upper and lower limb amputations?

3. Which body movements are required for a patient with a transhumeral amputation to operate a conventional BP terminal device and elbow unit?
4. What are the positive and negative features of a hook? A hand?
5. Describe the differences between a VO and a VC terminal device.
6. What is myoelectric control?
7. What is the purpose of controls training and use training?
8. Why might a prosthesis be rejected?
9. What are the functional expectations for a person with a unilateral transhumeral amputation or a bilateral transhumeral amputation?
10. What is the role of the occupational therapist in the rehabilitation of the patient with lower extremity amputations?

Resources

Books and Pamphlets for Consumers and Professionals

Leavy, J. D. (1980) · *It Can Be Done: An Upper Extremity Amputee Training Handbook*, P. O. Box 515, Lake Almanon Peninsula, CA 96137.

Mooney, R. L. (1995) · *The Handbook*, Mutual Amputee Aid Foundation, P. O. Box 1200, Lomita, CA 90717-5200.

Sobolich, J. (1992) · *You're Not Alone*, 1017 NW 10, Oklahoma City, OK 73106.

Wilke, H. H. (1984) · *Using Everything You've Got!* Chicago: National Easter Seal Society.

Wilke, H. H. (1984) · *Reflections on Managing Disability*, Chicago: National Easter Seal Society.

Organizations

American Amputee Foundation, Inc. · P. O. Box 250218, Hillcrest Station, Little Rock, AK 72225. 501-666-2523.

American Orthotic and Prosthetic Association · 1650 King St., Suite 500, Alexandria, VA 22314.

Amputee Coalition of America · 6300 River Rd., Rosemont, IL 60018-4226.
www.amputee-coalition.org

Amputee Sports Association · 11705 Mercy Blvd., Savannah, GA 31406.

Web Sites on Topics Related to Limb Loss

Amputation: A Magazine for Persons With Amputations.
www.amputee-online.com/amputation

American Academy of Orthotics and Prosthetics.
www.oandp.org

Arm-Amp · Source of information and support for people with amputations.
www.amp-info.net/arm-amp.htm

International Children's Amputee Network.
www.amp-info.net/childamp.htm

Association for Children with Hand and Arm Deficiency.
http://www.reach.org.uk

Manufacturers and Distributors

Alternative Prosthetic Services · 159 Kings Drive, Southport, CT 06490. 203-256-9887. Manufactures silicone components, hand and arm anatomical coverings.

Edinburgh Modular Arm System.
http://www.reach.org.uk/spring99.htm
Developing a motorized shoulder unit.

Hosmer-Dorrance Corp. · 561 Division St., Campbell, CA 95008. 800-827-0070.
http://www.hosmer.com
Manufactures primarily BP components.

Liberty Mutual Research Center · 71 Frankland Rd., Hopkinton, MA 01748. 800-437-0024.
http://www.Libertytechnology.com
Manufactures electronic elbows, control systems, hands and gloves.

Motion Control, Inc. · 2401 South 1070 West, Suite B, Salt Lake City, UT 84119. 888-696-2767.
http://www.utaharm.com/
Manufactures the Utah electronic elbow and other electronic systems.

Otto Bock Orthopedic Industry · 300 Xenium Lane N., Minneapolis, MN 55441. 800-328-4058.
http://www.ottobock.com
Manufactures electronic hands and hooks; wrist, elbow, and other electronic systems; and BP components.

Ross Prosthetics · 17 Lynwood Rd., Scarsdale, NY 10583. 914-725-7785. Manufactures anatomical hand covers.

TRS, Inc. (Therapeutic Recreation Systems) · 2450 Central Ave., Unit D, Boulder, CO 80301-2844. 800-279-1865.
http://www.oandp.com/trs
Manufactures VC terminal devices and adaptations for sports activities and musical instruments.

References

Abboudi, R. L. (1999). A biomimetic controller for a multifinger prosthesis. *IEEE Transactions on Rehabilitation Engineering*, 7 (20), 121–129.

Atkins, D. J., & Heard, D. C. Y. (1996). Epidemiologic overview of individuals with upper-limb loss and their reported research priorities. *Journal of Prosthetics and Orthotics*, 8 (1), 2–11.

Atkins, D. J., & Meier, R. H. (1989a). Post-operative and pre-prosthetic therapy programs. In D. J. Atkins & R. H. Meier III (Eds.), *Comprehensive Management of the Upper-Limb Amputee* (pp. 11–15). New York: Springer-Verlag.

Atkins, D. J., & Meier, R. H. (1989b). Adult upper-limb prosthetic training. In D. J. Atkins & R. H. Meier III (Eds.), *Comprehensive Management of the Upper-Limb Amputee* (pp. 39–59). New York: Springer-Verlag.

Bunnell, S. (1990). The management of the non-functional hand: Reconstruction versus prosthesis. In J. M. Hunter, L. H. Schneider, E. J. Mackin, & A. D. Callahan (Eds.), *Rehabilitation of the Hand* (pp. 997–1017). St. Louis: Mosby.

Dise-Lewis, J. E. (1989). Psychological adaptation to limb loss. In D. J. Atkins & R. H. Meier III (Eds.), *Comprehensive Management of the Upper-Limb Amputee* (pp. 165–172). New York: Springer-Verlag.

Edelstein, J. E. (1992). Special consideration: Rehabilitation without prostheses: Functional skills training. In American Academy of Orthopaedic Surgeons, *Atlas of Limb Prosthetics: Surgical, Prosthetic and Rehabilitation Principles* (pp. 721–728). St. Louis: Mosby–Year Book.

Esquenazi, A. (1996). Rehabilitation in limb deficiency: 4. Limb Amputation. *Archives of Physical Medicine and Rehabilitation, 77,* S-18–S-28.

Flor, H., & Elbert, T. (1995). Phantom-limb pain as a perceptual correlate of cortical reorganization following arm amputation. *Nature, 8;* 375 (6531), 482–484.

Fraser, C. M. (1998). An evaluation of the use made of cosmetic and functional prostheses by unilateral upper limb amputees. *Prosthetics and Orthotics International, 22,* 216–223.

Frey, D. D. (1995). Voluntary-opening prehensors with adjustable grip force. *Journal of Prosthetics and Orthotics, 7* (4),124–131.

Friedmann, L. (1989). Functional skills in multiple limb anomalies. In D. J. Atkins & R. H. Meier III (Eds.), *Comprehensive Management of the Upper Limb Amputee* (pp. 150–164). New York: Springer-Verlag.

Fryer, C. M., & Michael, J. W. (1992). Body-powered components. In American Academy of Orthopaedic Surgeons, *Atlas of Limb Prosthetics: Surgical, Prosthetic and Rehabilitation Principles* (pp. 107–131). St. Louis: Mosby–Year Book.

Gauthier-Gagnon, C. (1998). *The locomotor capabilities index:* Content validity. *Journal of Rehabilitation Outcomes Measures, 2* (4), 40–46.

Geraghty, T. J., & Jones, L. E. (1996). Painful neuromata following upper limb amputation. *Prosthetics and Orthotics International, 20,* 176–181.

Heckathorne, C. W. (1992). Components for adult externally powered systems. In American Academy of Orthopaedic Surgeons, *Atlas of Limb Prosthetics: Surgical, Prosthetic and Rehabilitation Principles* (pp. 151-174). St. Louis: Mosby Year Book.

Heinze, A. (Producer). (1988). *Amputation, Rehabilitation and Prostheses* [videotape]. Washington: Universal Health Associates.

Ivko, J. J. (1999). Independence through humeral rotation in the conventional transhumeral prosthetic design. *Journal of Prosthetics and Orthotics, 11* (1), 297–322.

Jones, L. E., & Davidson, J. (1996). A review of the management of upper-limb amputees. *Critical Review in Physical and Rehabilitation Medicine, 8* (4), 297–322.

Kegel, B. (1992). Adaptations for sports and recreation. In American Academy of Orthopaedic Surgeons, *Atlas of Limb Prosthetics: Surgical, Prosthetic and Rehabilitation Principles* (pp. 623–654). St. Louis: Mosby–Year Book.

Kejlaa, G. H. (1993). Consumer concerns and the functional value of prostheses to upper limb amputees. *Prosthetics and Orthotics International, 17* (3), 157–163.

Kessler, H. H. (1947). *Cineplasty.* Springfield, IL: Charles C. Thomas.

Kessler, H. H. (1969). Extraordinary people seek an ordinary destiny. *Social Service Outlook* [Newsletter]. Trenton: New Jersey Department of Social Service.

Kyberd, P. J., & Beard, D. J. (1998). A survey of upper-limb prosthetic users in Oxfordshire. *Journal of Prosthetics and Orthotics, 10* (4), 85–91.

Lake, C., (1997). Effects of prosthetic training on upper-extremity prosthetic use. *Journal of Prosthetics and Orthotics, 9* (1), 3-9.

Lehneis, H. R., & Dickey, R. (1992). Fitting and training the bilateral upper limb amputee. In American Academy of Orthopaedic Surgeons, *Atlas of Limb Prosthetics: Surgical, Prosthetic and Rehabilitation Principles* (pp. 311–323). St. Louis: Mosby–Year Book.

Leonard, J. A., & Meier, R. H. (1998). Upper and lower extremity prosthetics. In J. DeLisa & B. M. Gans (Eds.), *Rehabilitation Medicine: Principles and Practice* (pp. 669–696). Philadelphia: Lippincott-Raven.

Liaw, M. Y. (1998). Central representation of phantom limb phenomenon in amputees studied with single photon emission computerized tomography. *American Journal of Physical Medicine and Rehabilitation, 77* (5), 368–375.

Maiorano, L. M., & Byron, P. M. (1990). Fabrication of an early-fit prosthesis. In J. M. Hunter, L. H. Schneider, E. J. Mackin, & A. D. Callahan (Eds.), *Rehabilitation of the Hand* (pp. 1048–1056). St. Louis: Mosby.

Malone, J. M., Fleming, L. L., & Robinson, J. (1984). Immediate, early, and late post-surgical management of upper-limb amputations. *Journal of Rehabilitation, 21,* 33–41.

Melzack, R. (1989). Phantom limbs, the self and the brain. *Journal of Canadian Psychology, 30,* 1–16.

Olivett, B. L. (1990). Adult amputee management and conventional prosthetic training. In J. M. Hunter, L. H. Schneider, E. J. Mackin, & A. D. Callahan (Eds.), *Rehabilitation of the Hand* (pp. 1057–1071). St. Louis: Mosby.

Pinzur, M. S., & Angelats, J. (1994). Functional outcome following traumatic upper limb amputation and prosthetic limb fitting. *Journal of Hand Surgery, 19A* (5), 836–839.

Radocy, B. (1992). Upper-limb prosthetic adaptations for sports and recreation. In American Academy of Orthopaedic Surgeons, *Atlas of Limb Prosthetics: Surgical, Prosthetic and Rehabilitation Principles* (pp. 325–344). St. Louis: Mosby–Year Book.

Schuch, C. M., & Pritham, C. H. (1994). International organization terminology: Application to prosthetics and orthotics. *Journal of Prosthetics and Orthotics, 6* (1), 29–33.

Sears, H. H., & Shaperman, J. (1998). Electric wrist rotation in proportional-controlled systems. *Journal of Prosthetics and Orthotics, 10* (4), 92–98.

Spiegel, S. R. (1989). Adult myoelectric upper-limb prosthetic training, In D. J. Atkins & R. H. Meier III (Eds.), *Comprehensive Management of the Upper Limb Amputee* (pp. 60–71). New York: Springer-Verlag.

Trombly, C. A. (1995). Theoretical foundation for practice. In C. A. Trombly (Ed.), *Occupational Therapy for Physical Dysfunction* (3rd ed., pp. 15–27). Baltimore: Williams & Wilkins.

Winchell, E. (1995). *Coping With Limb Loss.* Garden City Park, NY: Avery.

Wright, T. W., & Hagen, A. D. (1995). Prosthetic usage in major upper extremity amputations. *Journal of Hand Surgery, 20A* (4), 619–622.

47
Cardiac and Pulmonary Diseases

Nancy Huntley

LEARNING OBJECTIVES

After studying this chapter, the reader will be able to do the following:

1. Recognize the signs and symptoms of exercise and activity intolerance.
2. Identify the common cardiac diagnoses and their treatment in occupational therapy.
3. Understand various cardiac and pulmonary diagnostic studies and how these tests assist with treatment planning in occupational therapy.
4. Know the controllable risk factors for heart disease and ways to ameliorate their effect.
5. Be able to instruct patients with pulmonary disease in breathing techniques.
6. Know resources for further guidelines in cardiac and pulmonary rehabilitation.

*H*eart disease is the leading cause of death in the United States. Annually 41.4% of deaths in the United States are caused by coronary artery disease. Some 57 million, or 45% of Americans, are living with some form of the disease. About two-thirds of the people who survive a heart attack do not make a complete recovery. However, 88% of those under age 65 years return to their customary work (American Heart Association, 1998).

Pulmonary disease is also a significant cause of death in the United States. Chronic obstructive pulmonary disease (COPD) is the fourth leading killer of Americans (American Lung Association, 1995). Lung disease not only kills; it chronically and significantly alters the lives of those who have it. The incidence of lung disease has risen 17.5% in the past 10 years (American Lung Association, 1998).

The diagnosis of cardiac or pulmonary disease in a patient's medical history has implications for the occupational therapist's treatment plan. For instance, a patient may carry the primary diagnosis of a recent stroke. If that stroke occurred shortly after coronary artery bypass surgery, certain precautions should be taken to protect the patient's sternum. The therapist should also routinely measure the heart rate and blood pressure, both at rest and with activity, to determine the patient's cardiovascular

---

GLOSSARY

Angina pectoris—Temporary lack of blood flow to the myocardium that causes the sensation of chest pain, fullness, tightness, or pressure. The pain or discomfort from angina can be referred to the teeth, jaw, ear, or arm. Angina is relieved with nitroglycerin or rest.

Atherectomy—Procedure in which a catheter with a rotating blade cuts out the plaque in a coronary artery and suctions it out.

Athrogenic—Causing the development of plaque in an artery.

Atrial fibrillation—Rapid firing of cells in the atria of the heart with irregular response of the ventricles causing a fast irregular heart rhythm. With uncontrolled atrial fibrillation the patient often feels SOB and fatigue.

Cardiomyopathies—Diseases of heart muscle.

Cardioversion—Electrical shock delivered to the heart to stop a serious arrhythmia with the hope that the heart will restart in a normal sinus rhythm.

Congestive heart failure (CHF)—Condition in which the heart's pumping function is impaired for any of a number of reasons. This impairment results in the heart's inability to rid the body of excess fluid, which collects in the lungs and extremities.

Diaphoresis—Cold clammy sweat that comes on suddenly.

Hypoxemia—Insufficient oxygenation of the blood.

Myocardial infarction (MI)—Heart attack; death of heart muscle caused by lack of oxygen secondary to obstructed blood flow to the heart muscle.

Oxygen saturation (O_2 Sat)—Measurement of the amount of oxygen carried by the hemoglobin in the blood. Normal oxygen saturation is greater than or equal to 92%.

Sternotomy—Procedure used in open heart surgery in which the sternum is split in half to allow the surgeon access to the chest cavity. After surgery the sternum is wired together.

Tachypnea—Rapid shallow breathing

---

response to rehabilitation. Even though a clinician is working in neither cardiac nor pulmonary rehabilitation, heart disease or lung disease as a secondary diagnosis has direct implications for the treatment plan. The occupational therapist must therefore be aware of these disease processes and know how they influence treatment.

Heart Disease

Heart disease may be due to a blockage of the coronary arteries, diseases of the heart muscle, or structural anomalies of the heart.

Heart Attack

Heart attacks are the single leading cause of death in men and women in the United States (American Heart Association, 1998). A **myocardial infarction (MI)**, or heart attack, is death of the heart muscle caused by lack of blood flow due to obstruction of a coronary artery by plaque or spasm. The patient's clinical history, along with several diagnostic tests, is considered when diagnosing a heart attack. The patient may first have symptoms such as chest pain or pressure radiating to the teeth, jaw, ear, or arm. This may be accompanied by **diaphoresis**, shortness of breath (SOB), nausea, vomiting, and/or fatigue. The patient may present with one or more of these symptoms, and the severity and intensity

varies from person to person. An electrocardiogram (ECG) shows where the damage to the heart muscle occurred. Meanwhile, blood tests for certain structural proteins and cardiac enzymes confirm a heart attack and give an idea of the amount of damage done to the heart muscle.

If a person realizes he or she is having a heart attack and goes to the hospital immediately, a thrombolytic agent may be given to stop the damage to the heart muscle. Thrombolytics break up the clot in the coronary artery, restoring blood flow, but they must be given within 2 to 8 hours after the first symptoms start. The sooner the patient receives the thrombolytic, the more heart muscle can be saved. Patients treated with a thrombolytic within the first hour of onset of symptoms show the greatest benefit in terms of mortality. However, benefit from treatment with a thrombolytic is possible within the first 12 hours (Topol & Van de Werf, 1998).

The left ventricle is the main pump of the heart. It pumps the blood from the heart to the rest of the body. Since the left ventricle does more work, it has a higher oxygen requirement than the rest of the heart. It is the first area of the heart to suffer from any coronary artery perfusion deficiency. Blockage in the left main or left anterior descending artery of the heart—an anterior MI—damages the front of the left ventricle (Fig. 47-1). When the right coronary artery is involved—an inferior MI—the back and bottom of the left ventricle are damaged. The circumflex artery feeds the lateral wall of the heart, and blockage in it results in a lateral MI.

The heart muscle has three layers. A heart attack that affects all three layers is a transmural MI, also known as a Q-wave MI because of its identifying characteristic on the ECG. When damage occurs in one layer of the heart muscle, it is called a subendocardial MI, or non–Q-wave MI. Since transmural MIs cause more damage, they are more serious. Anterior transmural MIs are considered the most serious because of the large amount of muscle mass lost and the risk of complications (Topol & Van de Werf, 1998) (Box 47-1).

Open Heart Surgery

Open heart surgery usually entails a **sternotomy**, which allows the surgeon to work on the heart. There are several types of open-heart surgery.

Coronary artery bypass graft is the replacement of occluded coronary arteries with artery or vein grafts. These grafts are attached to the aorta and reconnected below the occlusion in the coronary artery. Sometimes the mammary artery, which comes directly off the aorta, is dissected from its original destination and used as a graft. Another arterial graft is the radial artery. Arteries are preferred as grafts because they stay patent longer than vein grafts. Vein grafts are usually harvested from the legs.

Valve replacement and/or repair may be necessary if disease or congenital malformation damages or destroys a heart valve. If the surgeon cannot repair the valve, it is replaced with a prosthetic, homograft (cadaver), or pigskin valve. If a prosthetic valve is used, patients must take thrombolytics for the rest of their lives. The thrombolytics prevent blood from clotting as it goes through the valve. Pigskin and homograft valves do not require thrombolytic therapy, and they usually last about

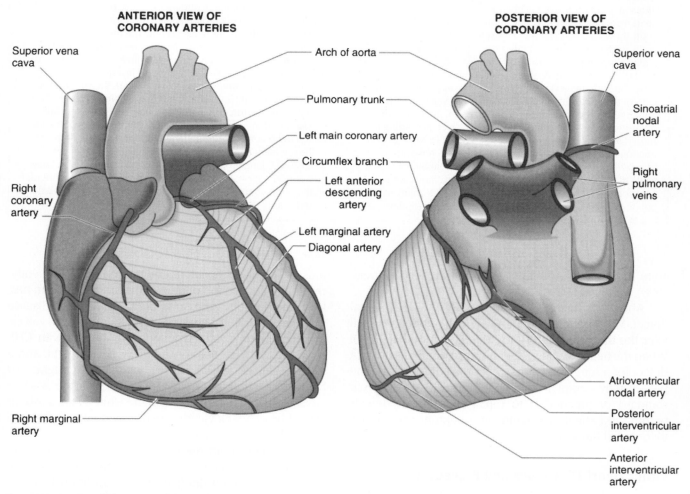

ANTERIOR VIEW OF CORONARY ARTERIES

- Superior vena cava
- Arch of aorta
- Pulmonary trunk
- Left main coronary artery
- Circumflex branch
- Left anterior descending artery
- Left marginal artery
- Diagonal artery
- Right coronary artery
- Right marginal artery

POSTERIOR VIEW OF CORONARY ARTERIES

- Superior vena cava
- Sinoatrial nodal artery
- Right pulmonary veins
- Atrioventricular nodal artery
- Posterior interventricular artery
- Anterior interventricular artery

Figure 47-1 Coronary arteries (anterior view). Location of damage to the heart depends on which coronary arteries are blocked. (Reprinted with permission from Willis, M. C. (1996). *Medical Terminology: The Language of Health Care* (p. 160). Baltimore: Williams & Wilkins.

BOX 47-1
Common Diagnostic Studies for Heart Disease

Blood tests are usually done for patients with probable symptoms of heart attack. The cells of the heart contain isoenzymes and structural proteins specific to that organ. Death of heart cells releases those isoenzymes and structural proteins into the bloodstream, where an increase in their levels can be measured. CPK MB is an isoenzyme that shows up in the blood within 3 to 5 hours after a heart attack (Gage & Radke, 1997). Myoglobin and troponin are two structural proteins whose levels rise with heart damage. Myoglobin levels start to rise within 1 hour of damage, allowing for early recognition of a heart attack. However, myoglobin is not specific to heart muscle. It can also rise with skeletal muscle damage, strenuous exercise, renal disease, open heart surgery and alcoholism, shock, and electrical defibrillation (Jairath, 1999). Troponin is specific to heart muscle. Troponin levels start rising after about 4 hours after an MI and stay elevated for up to 14 days, allowing detection of MI in patients who wait to seek treatment (Gage & Radke).

A stress echocardiogram is an exercise test usually conducted on a treadmill. Before the test starts, an ultrasound recording of the function of the heart at rest is taken. The patient is exercised to maximum capacity. After the exercise, another ultrasound recording of the heart is done to show how the heart responds to work. The results of the stress echocardiogram shows whether the heart muscle and valves work normally under pressure or whether some parts respond suboptimally. It is also possible to measure how much blood the heart ejects with each beat. A normal ejection fraction is above 60%. A person with an ejection fraction of 40 to 59% is mildly impaired. An ejection fraction below 40% is considered significant impairment. The lower the ejection fraction, the higher the risk of further events and complications. However, according to *Hurst's the Heart*, Volume 1, a person who has a low ejection fraction but can tolerate mild to moderate exercise has a better long-term outcome than those who cannot tolerate exercise well (Alexander et al., 1998).The ejection fraction does not always accurately reflect an individual patient's ability to work, but it is helpful as a starting point for making appropriate ex-

ercise and activity recommendations and precautions. A stress echocardiogram also reveals a person's maximum exercise capacity. Using 60 to 85% of the maximum heart rate attained during the stress test, the therapist can determine an appropriate level to start exercise and activity. Additionally, stress echocardiography is 85% accurate in predicting coronary ischemia (Fardy & Yanowitz,1995). When a stress test is given without the echo, the accuracy of predicting heart disease is reduced to 75%, but the patient's maximum exercise capacity and maximal heart rate with exercise will be known.

A thallium stress test is conducted with a 12-lead ECG as patients exercise to their maximum capacity on a treadmill. However, during this test patients are injected with thalium-210, a radioactive isotope, when the patient feels able to exercise for only 1 minute more. The patient is then placed under a scintillation camera, which can detect the radioactive isotope in the heart muscle. This isotope is readily picked up by healthy myocardium cells, more slowly by cells with poor perfusion, and not at all by infarcted myocardium. Thallium stays in the bloodstream for approximately 72 hours. Areas with restricted blood flow may eventually fill in with thallium, and these areas are said to have a reversible defect. Areas that do not fill in are infarcted, and the deficit is permanent (Padgitt & Kline-Rogers, 1997). Since this process may take several hours, the thallium test usually has an initial scan and then another scan 3 hours later (Padgitt & Kline-Rogers).

Coronary angiography is the definitive test in the diagnosis of coronary artery disease. A catheter is inserted into a blood vessel in the groin and wound into the heart, through which radiopaque dye is injected into the coronary blood vessels. The extent of the obstruction in any coronary blood vessel can be visualized. A blockage must be greater than 70 to 75% of the lumen to be considered significant. A lesion greater than 50% in the left main artery is considered equivalent to two-vessel disease. The length of any coronary artery lesions is also taken into consideration. In addition, heart valve function, ventricular wall motion abnormalities, and some heart defects can be detected (Fardy, Yanowitz, 1995).

---

10 to 15 years before they have to be replaced (Garcia, 1998).

About 7% of the population have an atrial septal defect. Many people are not aware of heart defects until after the third decade of life (Marelli & Moodie, 1998). When the heart has been attempting to compensate for a defect for a long time, it may become enlarged, and the patient may complain of fatigue and SOB. The current standard of practice is to repair these heart defects before the patient has significant symptoms or sustains myocardial damage.

Other Heart Diagnoses and Procedures

Congestive heart failure (CHF) describes the inability of the heart to function effectively as a pump. The heart muscle stretches beyond its ability to contract efficiently, resulting in collection of fluid in the lungs or extremities. CHF may result from any of a number of disease processes, such as multiple MIs, incompetent valves, cardiomyopathy, and hypertension. Patients with CHF have SOB, fatigue, possibly an increase in weight, and a dry, hacking cough. Often they complain of coughing or SOB while recumbent (Box 47-2). CHF is the leading cause of hospital admissions in the United States. About 20% of heart attack victims are disabled by CHF within 6 years (American Heart Association, 1998).

Cardiomyopathies are diseases of cardiac muscle. There are three main types of cardiomyopathy: dilated, hypertrophic, and restrictive. Dilated cardiomyopathy is the most common, comprising over 75% of cases. Some 75 specific diseases can cause dilated cardiomyopathy;

symptoms are an enlarged heart with decreased pumping capacity that usually results in congestive heart failure. Of those who are hospitalized for dilated cardiomyopathy, one-fourth will die within a year and half will die within 5 years unless they have a heart transplant (Wynne & Braunwald, 1998). However, some patients with cardiomyopathy for unknown reasons improve over time. An enlarged left ventricle and decreased heart function indicate a poorer prognosis (Wynne & Braunwald).

Angina pectoris is heart pain caused by a temporary inadequate supply of blood to the heart muscle. Angina may be described as pain, aching, tightness, or pressure. It is usually diffuse and located in the mid chest, but it may radiate to the teeth, ear, jaw, or arm. Angina typically comes on with activity and is relieved with rest. However, some people develop angina after a heavy meal or while resting. Nitroglycerin, taken by pill or spray under the tongue, usually relieves angina quickly. Angina is an indication of coronary artery disease, and it is fairly common to have angina after a heart attack. If the frequency or intensity of angina changes, the physician should be notified.

Percutaneous transluminal coronary angioplasty is used to improve the blood flow through an occluded artery and reduce the symptoms of angina. Angioplasty requires the insertion of a catheter into the coronary artery at the site of the occlusion. On the end of the catheter is a balloon that is inflated until the arterial walls at the point of the occlusion are pushed out to allow more blood flow through the area. Initially there is a 90% success rate with angioplasty, but approximately one-third to half of angioplasties close within 6 months, depending on how many vessels were opened. The more vessels opened with angioplasty, the higher the risk of closure (Fardy & Yanowitz, 1995). Sometimes a stent, which resembles a spring in a ballpoint pen, is used in conjunction with an angioplasty to hold the dilated area open. When a stent is used, the success of the procedure increases to about 85% (American College of Cardiology Expert Consensus Document, 1994). For patients whose lesions are too long or calcified to use the angioplasty balloon, another procedure, **atherectomy**, is available. In atherectomy, the catheter inserted into the coronary artery has a rotating blade that cuts out the plaque. As it cuts the plaque, suction pulls the plaque through a tube and out of the body. The long-term success of this procedure is comparable with that of angioplasty (Fardy & Yanowitz).

Cardiac Rehabilitation

Cardiac rehabilitation usually involves a multidisciplinary team. Doctors, nurses, occupational and physical therapists, exercise physiologists, dietitians, and social workers may all play a part in the patient's recovery. Dietitians and social workers perform their conventional role in treating the cardiac patient. However, none of the other health professionals are usually trained specifically to work in cardiac rehabilitation, and all need additional training. Geographical tradition and availability of staff seem to determine what role each health professional plays. Each discipline brings its own skills to rehabilitation of patients with heart disease, but official job expectations and responsibilities may essentially be the same. See Resources for information on key organizations in cardiac rehabilitation.

Occupational therapists are invaluable to the patient with heart disease. Therapists evaluate and analyze the patient's activities of daily living (ADL). The therapist can then assist patients in modifying activities, if necessary, so they can resume activities they previously enjoyed. The occupational therapist's expertise in rehabilitation and knowledge of comorbid diseases is extremely important for evaluating and adapting treatment for the needs of the individual patient. Patients who have undergone lifestyle changes and life-threatening diseases also benefit from occupational therapy intervention to help with psychosocial adjustment to their new situation.

Risk Factors for Heart Disease

One of the main goals of all phases of cardiac rehabilitation is primary and secondary prevention of heart disease. Primary intervention refers to efforts to prevent heart disease. Primary prevention efforts are usually limited to health fairs and lecture series, because health insurance does not cover the cost of primary prevention. Those costs are born either by a sponsor, such as a hospital, or by charging admission. Therefore, most of

---

BOX 47-2
Signs and Symptoms of Congestive Heart Failure

▸ Increase in weight of 2 to 5 pounds or more over several days
▸ Inability to sleep
▸ Persistent dry, hacking cough
▸ SOB with normal activity
▸ Swelling in ankles or feet
▸ Fatigue

Reprinted with permission from the American Occupational Therapy Association Inc. From Huntley, N. (1998). Reading the signs of heart disease. *OT Practice, 3* (6), 38–41.

the therapist's efforts are directed toward secondary prevention. Secondary prevention pertains to efforts made to stop or slow the progression of heart disease. Improving an individual's risk factor profile is the method used by therapists for secondary prevention of heart disease.

Ten risk factors increase one's risk of developing coronary artery disease. The three that are not controllable are age, family history, and gender. Risk of heart disease increases with age (Jairath, 1999). A first-degree relative, such as father, mother, or sibling, developing heart disease before age 50 increases one's risk. The highest risk of developing heart disease for both men and women occurs when another sibling has the disease. Indeed, studies suggest that a sibling with heart disease increases one's risk by three to four times that of a person without a sibling history of the disease (Jairath). Men are likely to develop heart disease an average of 10 years earlier than women, but as women approach menopause, they lose the protective effect of estrogen, and their risk of heart disease increases (American Heart Association, 1998). The risk of heart disease in women continues to rise after menopause until the 70s. Then their incidence of heart disease surpasses that of men (Jairath). So even though heart disease is commonly considered a man's problem, it is an equal opportunity killer. It remains the number one cause of death for both men and women (American Heart Association).

Controllable Risk Factors

The risk factors one can control are smoking, hyperlipidemia, hypertension, sedentary lifestyle, obesity, diabetes, and psychological stress. Smoking is a major modifiable risk factor in heart disease. People who smoke increase their risk of dying of heart disease by a factor of two to three. Smoking damages the endothelial lining of the coronary arteries, increasing their susceptibility to plaque formation. Nicotine causes vasoconstriction of the arteries and increases heart rate. Smoking makes the heart more susceptible to lethal ventricular arrhythmias and predisposes it to coronary artery spasm (Gordon, 1998). Carbon monoxide in cigarette smoke binds with hemoglobin faster than oxygen, resulting in less oxygen being distributed to the tissues. Nicotine also alters the metabolism of fats, increasing the levels of **athrogenic** low-density-lipoprotein (LDL) cholesterol and decreasing the levels of the heart-protective high-density-lipoprotein (HDL) cholesterol. Smoking causes the blood to coagulate more quickly and promotes thrombus formation (Jairath, 1999). Thus, smoking contributes to heart disease in multiple ways.

Hypercholesterolemia is a major risk factor among Americans. It has been demonstrated that a total choles-

terol level above 200 mg/dL, an LDL cholesterol above 130 mg/dL and an HDL cholesterol of less than 35 mg/dL significantly increase the risk of heart disease (Jairath, 1999). Just over half of American adults have cholesterol levels above 200 mg/dL (American Heart Association, 1998). Patients with known coronary artery disease should get their LDL cholesterol below 100 mg/dL. Cholesterol levels may be lowered through a low-fat diet, regular aerobic exercise, and weight loss. If these efforts are unsuccessful, the physician will probably prescribe a lipid-lowering drug. Some individuals inherit an inability to metabolize lipids normally. They have very high lipid levels in their blood because they manufacture their own cholesterol. These patients cannot lower their blood lipids sufficiently without medication. When they decrease their cholesterol level with the use of medication, they show decreased progression of coronary artery disease (Jairath).

Patients with hypertension have a progressive increase in both nonfatal and fatal cardiovascular disease because of high systolic and diastolic blood pressure (Gordon, 1998). The American Heart Association classifies blood pressures greater than 140/90 at rest as hypertensive. Hypertension damages the arterial walls and causes increased myocardial oxygen consumption because of the heart's need to do more work against high pressures. High blood pressure may be diagnosed after several elevated blood pressure readings. It is controlled by medication, weight loss, moderation in alcohol and sodium intake, and physical activity (Gordon).

Sedentary lifestyle is a risk factor for heart disease. The relative risk of a sedentary lifestyle for heart disease is comparable to the risk associated with smoking, hypercholesterolemia, and high blood pressure (American Heart Association, 1998). People who are physically inactive have twice the rate of heart disease as those who exercise regularly (Jairath, 1999). Regular physical exercise reduces blood pressure, lowers levels of atherogenic LDL cholesterol in the blood, raises the level of heart-protective HDL cholesterol, and increases insulin sensitivity and glucose tolerance (Gordon, 1998). The Center for Disease Control's *Behavioral Risk Factor Surveillance Study* defined adequate aerobic exercise as sustained physical activity 3 to 4 times per week for at least 30 minutes (American Heart Association). After an MI, patients who undergo aerobic exercise training have 20 to 30% fewer fatal myocardial infarctions than those who do not exercise (Gordon). Because of the effect of exercise on the heart, circulatory system, and other risk factors, aerobic exercise is an effective weapon against heart disease.

The precise role of obesity in coronary artery disease is difficult to determine, as it is closely associated with other risk factors, such as hypertension, diabetes, hyperlipidemia, and physical inactivity. Loss of even 5 to 10% of weight can improve these risk factors (Gordon, 1998). With every pound lost, the cholesterol level drops by 1 mg/dL (Jairath,1999). Blood pressure is also reduced with weight loss. Central or abdominal obesity is linked to increased risk of coronary artery disease (Lindsay, 1997).

Diabetes has long been recognized as a risk factor for heart disease. In fact, some form of heart or blood vessel disease kills two-thirds of people with diabetes (American Heart Association, 1998). Most people recognize that heart disease is a significant problem for people with insulin-dependent diabetes, but coronary artery disease is also the leading cause of death in those with non–insulin-dependent diabetes (Jairath, 1999). Women who have diabetes lose the protective effect of their hormones against heart disease, and their risk of coronary artery disease increases to seven times that of the general population (Jairath). It has been demonstrated that keeping blood sugar levels in tight control reduces macrovascular and microvascular disease in patients with type I diabetes, which reduces their risk of heart disease. Recent studies suggest that patients with type II diabetes also receive this benefit with tight blood sugar control (Jairath).

Stress is also considered to be a risk factor for heart disease, but its effect is difficult to quantify. What stresses one individual does not stress another. However, chronic stress impairs the cardiovascular system in several ways. Stress increases the heart rate, blood pressure, blood lipid levels, and blood clotting. Managing chronic stressors with relaxation techniques or through behavioral change in response to stress helps to minimize or eliminate the effect of stress on the body.

As part of secondary prevention, the therapist must direct considerable energy toward teaching the patient the significance of these risk factors and methods of ameliorating them. Education may take place in one-to-one sessions, such as with the patient while reviewing his or her home program, or with groups of patients before, during, or after exercise.

Phase I: Inpatient Cardiac Rehabilitation

The goals of inpatient cardiac rehabilitation are to prevent muscle loss during bed rest, monitor and assess the patients' ability to function, instruct patients in appropriate home activities, teach patients about their individual risk factors, and teach methods to lessen the risks.

Therapists treat each patient at least once a day and usually twice daily as soon as their medical status has stabilized, often within the first 24 to 48 hours after admission. Hospital stays for coronary events have declined significantly in the past 10 years. The average stay for both uncomplicated MI and for open heart surgery is 4 to 7 days.

The occupational therapist working in cardiac rehabilitation initiates therapy on a one-to-one basis so that the therapist can interview the patient regarding lifestyle and assess cardiovascular response to exercise. During exercise, physical measurements of heart rate, blood pressure, ECG response, and symptoms are noted. Occupational therapists working in cardiac rehabilitation need advanced training to read ECG's.

Patients who are stable are subsequently seen for group treatment. While programs vary in the type of exercise done, many begin with mild calisthenics for 2-minute bouts with a 1-minute rest. Initially the total time of the calisthenics is 4 to 8 minutes, depending on the patient's tolerance. As the patient progresses, the time doing calisthenics typically increases to 10 to 14 minutes. Programs may include other modalities, such as stair climbing, treadmill, bicycle ergometer, and/or hall walking. Regardless of the modality, each patient is started gradually (e.g., treadmill walking at 1 to 1.5 mph or less for about 3 minutes), and progression is based on the patient's tolerance. It is important to assess the patient's heart rate, blood pressure, ECG, and symptoms to establish the patient's tolerance for exercise (Box 47-3).

Clinical Pathways

A clinical pathway is a tool that describes a comprehensive program for a patient with a particular diagnosis, such as the MI pathway, the coronary artery bypass graft pathway, or the CHF pathway. The treatment plan for a patient with the diagnosis in question is delineated in a grid format. During each day of hospitalization, the grid lists the treatment the patient should receive. Areas included in a pathway are activities, rehabilitation, nutrition, interventions, education, treatments, psychosocial and spiritual considerations, and discharge planning. Each day, practitioners of the various disciplines record the care provided in checklist fashion. Deviations from the expected routine are recorded as variances in the progress record of the chart. Clinical pathways thus assist in evaluating outcomes and ensure a standard level of care (American Association of Cardiovascular and Pulmonary Rehabilitation [AACVPR], 1995).

Discharge Planning

Discharge planning begins early because of the short hospital stays. The cardiac occupational therapist provides information regarding the level of physical function the patient tolerates at discharge. The therapist also

BOX 47-3
PROCEDURES FOR PRACTICE

Assessing Patient's Tolerance for Exercise

Measuring Blood Pressure and Pulse

Blood Pressure (Jamieson et al., 1997)

▸ Wrap blood pressure cuff 1 to 1.5 inches above the antecubital space.
▸ The cuff should be wrapped smoothly and firmly around the arm.
▸ The bladder of the cuff should cover 80% of the arm circumference.
▸ Palpate the brachial pulse on the medial aspect of the arm.
▸ Place the stethoscope over the pulse.
▸ Close the valve on the inflation ball.
▸ Inflate the cuff 20 mm Hg greater than the point where you heard the pulse obliterated. Slowly open the valve on the inflation ball so the mercury or arrow drops at the rate of 2 to 3 mm a second.
▸ The first sound heard is the systolic pressure.
▸ Make note of that number.
▸ Continue to listen until the pulse starts to muffle and finally disappears.
▸ The point of disappearance is the diastolic pressure.
▸ Make a note of that number.
▸ Be sure to listen for 20 mm Hg longer to make sure you heard the exact last pulsation.
▸ Completely deflate the cuff and remove from the patient.

To be considered normal, blood pressure must be under 140/90 at rest. Systolic blood pressure should rise with exercise. The diastolic blood pressure should stay the same or drop slightly. The diastolic blood pressure while exercising should not be more than 10 mm Hg greater than resting. A patient who has a history of high blood pressure is likely to have an exaggerated blood pressure response with exercise.

Pulse

▸ Palpate the radial artery with the index and middle finger.
▸ Count the number of pulsations for 10 seconds.
▸ Multiply that number by 6 to determine the number of beats per minute (bpm).

▸ Notice whether the pulse is regular or irregular.
▸ Also note any skipped or early beats.

A normal heart rate range at rest is 60 to 100 bpm. However, someone who is very fit, such as a runner may have a heart rate in the 40s or 50s. After open heart surgery it is common for a patient to have a heart rate in the low 100s. In the first 2 weeks of convalescence, during exercise the heart rate should not increase more than 20 bpm above resting for a patient with an MI and about 30 bpm for a patient after surgery (ACSM, 1995). These are relative, not absolute, guidelines. It is fairly common for patients who have valve repair or replacement to develop a rapid heart rhythm called atrial fibrillation. This rhythm is usually controlled with medication or by **cardioversion. If the patient's heart rate is uncontrolled and is running 120 bpm or higher at rest, exercise is contraindicated.**

Signs and Symptoms of Exercise Intolerance

▸ Chest pain or pain referred to the teeth, jaw, ear, or arm
▸ Excessive fatigue
▸ Light-headedness or dizziness
▸ Nausea or vomiting
▸ SOB
▸ Unusual weight gain of 3 to 5 pounds in 1 to 3 days

A patient with chest pain or angina who has a prescription for nitroglycerin should try a nitroglycerin pill under the tongue. If the chest pain has not disappeared within 3 to 5 minutes, another nitroglycerin pill should be tried. Continue until a total of three nitroglycerin pills have been taken over a 15-minute period. If the chest pain persists, call 911. The doctor should be notified when the patient first has angina or if there are changes in the frequency or intensity of episodes of angina. Notify the physician if other symptoms of exercise intolerance persist after resting.

---

recommends further therapies and gives input on the need for home health care.

Home Programs

Each patient receives a home program before discharge. The type of program is individualized to the patient and his or her particular diagnosis. The general components of a home program are activity and exercise guidelines, work simplification, pacing, temperature precautions, social activity, sexuality, signs and symptoms of exercise intolerance, and/or a discussion of risk factors. Depending on the diagnosis, certain aspects of the home

program are emphasized or minimized. The information should be pertinent to the patient's lifestyle, including favorite activities, work, and/or hobbies, with suggestions for resuming these activities.

MI Home Program

The home program of a patient who has had an MI tends to highlight how to evaluate activity and exercise and determine the correct energy expenditure during recovery. Healing of the heart muscle takes about 4 to 8 weeks, depending on the amount of damage. Patients are usually asked to restrict their activities to 2 to 4 METs during this time (Box 47-4, Table 47-1). Pacing and work simplification may also be explained. This is especially important when the patient has had a significant amount of heart damage. (However, 88% of those under age 65 eventually return to work, according to the American Heart Association 1999 Statistical Update.) A walking or biking exercise schedule is given. Depression and sexuality are discussed because certain cardiac medications can play a significant role in mood, sexual function, and desire. Patients should be told that if there is a change in sexual ability or desire after their cardiac event, they should talk to their doctor to explore the role of any new medications in those changes. Sexual relations can be resumed when the patient is able to climb two flights of stairs without symptoms of intolerance (Texas Heart Institute, 1996).

Open-Heart Surgery Home Program

Patients who have had open-heart surgery receive more specific directions. They are in pain and under the influence of analgesics, which may affect retention of information. Patients are given information regarding what to expect during the healing process as well as what to do and what to avoid. They also receive information on stretches and mild exercises to assist in incisional pain management. Their sternum has been broken and is treated like any other broken bone. Surgical patients are to avoid lifting, pushing, and pulling, especially one-sided lifting or pulling, of objects weighing more than 10 pounds for 6 to 12 weeks. Therapists should recommend alternative ways of doing activities to avoid one-sided pulling. For example, it is desirable to use two hands to pull open a heavy door or to put one hand covered with an oven mitt on the bottom of a heavy coffee pot and the other hand on the handle. Patients who complain of feeling sternal shifting or clicking should try to avoid the activity that causes it and stop any upper extremity exercises. Usually the clicking goes away with a little care. Individual surgeons have their own views regarding the exact length of time

to avoid lifting and the amount of arm activity they will allow. Walking schedules per patient tolerance are also given. Patients are encouraged to express their affection. If they have sexual intercourse, they may wish to try positions that avoid strain on the sternum, such as side lying or sitting in a chair facing each other.

CHF Home Program

Many patients with CHF and/or cardiomyopathy have limited endurance. Their home program puts heavy emphasis on pacing and work simplification. It also includes a mild exercise program. Information regarding their diagnosis is given to help these patients understand that overexertion may put them back into heart failure. Signs and symptoms of CHF are included to alert the patient to signs of worsening medical status.

Angioplasty Home Program

Patients admitted solely for an angioplasty and stent or atherectomy are usually seen for home instruction. The goal is to teach risk factor recognition and awareness of ways to modify these risks. An aerobic exercise program positively affects most risk factors for heart disease. Therefore, a variety of ways to exercise are discussed, with the goal of finding one or several modes of aerobic exercise that may interest the patient. For example, if the patient chooses walking, options such as mall walking, treadmill, and video walking programs as well as outdoor walking are explored. Patients are taught how to start an exercise program and assess their physical response to exercise using the *Borg Rate of Perceived Exertion Scale* (*RPE*) (AACVPR, 1998) and heart rate monitoring, if appropriate. Again, the therapist reviews signs and symptoms of exercise intolerance. Stress reduction techniques may be covered, and other resources for stress reduction are given. If the patient is a smoker, willingness to quit is assessed. If the patient is in the planning or action phase of quitting, information regarding the effects of nicotine on the body is given, as well as assistance in planning how to beat the urge to smoke and resources for support groups. All information is written, so that the patient can refer to it later.

BOX 47-4
Approximate MET Values for Exercise and Activity

The MET is a unit of measure used to describe the amount of oxygen the body needs for a given activity (Armstrong, 1997). Extensive oxygen consumption tests have been done on a number of activities, and a small sampling of activities is included in Table 47-1. These values are approximate because they do not take into account environmental factors or skill. The more the body moves and has to work against resistance, the higher the MET level.

Phase II: Outpatient Cardiac Rehabilitation

Outpatient cardiac rehabilitation is a multifaceted program of ECG-monitored exercise and education for secondary prevention of heart disease. The goals for outpatient cardiac rehabilitation:

1. Continued medical surveillance and assessment of an individual's cardiovascular response to exercise
2. Limiting the physiological and psychological effects of heart disease

TABLE 47-1
Approximate Metabolic Values for Various Activities (Ainsworth et al., 1998)

1 to 2.5 METs

Home Activities	Leisure and Vocational Activities	Exercise and Sports
Sweeping floors	Power boating	Slow walking
Dusting	Fishing from boat	Playing catch with a baseball or
Straightening up	Pumping gas	football
Serving food	Typing, computer use	Horseback riding, walking
Table setting	Light office work, sitting	
Knitting, crocheting	Card playing, sitting	
Putting away groceries	Board games	
Making bed	Playing piano or organ	
Mowing lawn with a riding mower	Driving tractor	
Sexual activity	Sewing with a machine	
Dressing, undressing	Driving an auto or truck	
Sleeping	Sitting to study, read, or write	
Watching television	Casino gambling, standing	
Dishwashing	Standing quietly in line	
Changing lightbulbs		

2.6—4 METs

Home Activities	Leisure & Vocational Activities	Exercise & Sports
Child care, bathing and grooming	Pitching horseshoes	Very light stationary biking
Walk, run, play with children (moderate)	Home auto repair	Weight lifting, light to moderate
General housecleaning	Planting seedlings and shrubs	effort
Walking downstairs	Playing the drums	Stretching, yoga
Sweeping garage or sidewalk	Home wiring or plumbing	Golf using a cart
Raking lawn	Feeding small farm animals	Snowmobiling
Walking and carrying 15 lb	Standing to pack light to moderate boxes	Walking, moderate speed
	Bartending, standing	Water aerobics
	Walking and tidying yard	

4—6 METs

Home Activities	Leisure & Vocational Activities	Exercise & Sports
Major housecleaning, vigorous effort	Laying carpet or tile	General calisthenics, moderate
Moving furniture	Slow wood chopping	effort
Scrubbing floors on hands and knees	Farming, feeding cattle	Shooting hoops
Cleaning gutters	Outdoor carpentry	Golf, carrying clubs
Painting the outside of house	Carpentry, refinishing surfaces	Softball, fast or slow pitch
Painting and wallpapering inside of house	Hunting, general	Low-impact or dance aerobics
Weeding or cultivating	Road building, carrying heavy loads	Dodge ball, hopscotch
	Roofing	Bicycling, 10–11.9 mph

6–10 METs

Home Activities	Leisure & Vocational Activities	Exercise & Sports
Carrying groceries upstairs	Farming, bailing hay	High-impact aerobics
Moving household items in boxes	Concrete masonry	Running 10–12-min mile
Shoveling more than 16 lb/min (heavy)	Moving heavy objects, such as furniture	Basketball
Walking, standing with 50–74-lb load	Firefighter carrying hoses	Jumping rope
		Race walking
		Swimming laps, moderate pace
		Bicycling, < 12 mph

3. Stabilizing or reversing the progression of atherosclerosis
4. Maximizing psychosocial and vocational status

Patients usually start in outpatient cardiac rehabilitation 1 to 2 weeks after discharge from the hospital. The program runs 3 days a week for 4 to 8 weeks. It would be ideal if each patient had a stress test prior to starting rehabilitation so that the results could be used in developing an exercise prescription. However, many patients do not have a stress test until 6 weeks after an MI or percutaneous transluminal coronary angiography with stent and a year after a bypass. Often the therapist must take a careful history to determine risk stratification based on the patient's ejection fraction, hospital course, heart rate and blood pressure response, symptoms, and/or possible ECG changes with exercise. (Risk stratification refers to determination of the patient's risk of further cardiac events based on his or her medical history.)

After assessing the patient's risk stratification, the therapist must determine the appropriate exercise intensity. There are several ways to determine exercise intensity. The therapist could determine 50 to 85% of the patient's maximum age-adjusted heart rate (MAHR) (American College of Sports Medicine [ACSM], 1995). (Box 47-5). However, if the patient is taking a beta blocker, such as atenolol, metoprolol, or timolol, the heart rate response will be blunted, making the heart rate calculation inaccurate. Using the *Borg Scale of Perceived Exertion* is an additional way to measure the patient's tolerance of the exercise. The patient is usually asked to rate the intensity of exercise on the *Borg Scale* and try to keep it between 11 and 14 (AACVPR, 1995). The patient's cardiovascular response and symptoms assist in formulating the exercise prescription.

The exercise goal is usually equal to or greater than 5 METs (ACSM, 1995). However, the patient's heart function and previous vocational and leisure interests must be considered in determining the patient's exercise goal. The sedentary elderly and those who have low functional capacity can still benefit by increasing their maximum MET level. For example, a patient with CHF may have a functional capacity of 2.5 METs after a hospitalization. If the MET level increases to 3.5 to 4 METs, the patient will have significantly increased the number of activities or tasks he or she can do.

There are two primary methods of achieving exercise goals: continuous and discontinuous exercise. Continuous exercise works well for some. Others prefer short bouts of exercise on various pieces of equipment followed by a short rest of 1 to 2 minutes. With continuous exercise, increasing the total duration of the exercise to at least 20 to 40 minutes is the first goal. Later intensity is gradually increased. The advantages of continuous exercise are that you need less equipment and space and it more closely mimics what the patient will be doing at home. The disadvantages are that only certain muscle groups are targeted on one piece of equipment and the patient is exposed to just one form of aerobic exercise. In discontinuous exercise the amount of time a patient stays on a piece of equipment remains the same, but the intensity gradually increases. After finishing the allotted time on one piece of equipment, the patient switches to another ,and this process is repeated several times. The advantages of discontinuous exercise are that the patient is exposed to a variety of equipment, boredom is minimized, and multiple muscle groups are used. The disadvantages are that it takes a lot of space and equipment, it is sometimes hard to coordinate everybody shifting equipment at the same time, and it does not reflect what the patient will be doing for aerobic exercise at home. However, with either method of conditioning the patients achieve the same MET levels.

In outpatient cardiac rehabilitation a variety of exercise equipment may be used. Use of treadmills, bicycle ergometers, recumbent bikes, rowing machines, arm ergometers, and so on depends on the patient's preference and any orthopaedic problem. Weight training is usually started 4 to 6 weeks post event. Prior to weight training, patients must meet certain criteria regarding their exercise capacity, blood pressure control, and ejection fraction (ACSM, 1995).

Risk factor modification is a key focus of outpatient cardiac rehabilitation. Therapists help patients identify their own risk factors and choose which they would like to modify or eliminate. Risk factor education occurs in a variety of ways. Some centers have specific times on various days when health professionals lecture on a

---

BOX 47-5
PROCEDURES FOR PRACTICE

Determining the MAHR

- ▶ Take the number 220.
- ▶ Subtract the patient's age.
- ▶ This gives you that patient's MAHR.
- ▶ To get the patient's exercise heart rate range, multiply the MAHR by 50 to 85%.

For example, a 50-year-old's MAHR is 220 − 50 = 170. To determine the exercise heart rate, multiply 170 by 50% and 85%. A 50-year-old person's exercise heart rate range is 85 to 149 bpm.

MAHR, maximum age-adjusted heart rate.

particular topic. Other hospitals have short education sessions before, during, or after exercise sessions. The goal of educational sessions is to give patients the information they need to modify their risk factors.

Psychosocial issues of the patient who has heart disease must be evaluated. Depression post MI has been linked with poor prognosis and increased mortality (Taylor & Houston, 1998). Many centers use standardized questionnaires, such as the *Medical Outcomes Study Short Form* (SF-36) or *DUKE Health Profiles*, to determine depression (AACVPR, 1995). The results of testing will indicate whether the patient needs referral to a chaplain, social worker, or psychologist based on circumstance or preference.

Some patients have jobs that require heavy lifting. Feedback is given to the physician regarding their exercise capacity and cardiovascular response to aerobic exercise in cardiac rehabilitation. Following their outpatient cardiac rehabilitation program, they may also need a work-hardening program to ready them to return to work.

Phase III: Community-Based Cardiac Rehabilitation

Phase III is community-based cardiac rehabilitation with larger groups of patients and fewer staff members per participant. Phase III programs often take place in community centers, school gyms, or YMCAs. It may follow outpatient or phase II cardiac rehabilitation. However, a patient who is at low risk and has been active in the past may skip phase II and go directly to phase III. Only a small percentage of patients go to phase III after phase II, as it is generally not covered by insurance. Since reimbursement is difficult, it also means that these programs run on a very low budget and usually are lucky to break even.

A physician must refer a participant to phase III. Usually a stress test is required or the physician establishes heart rate guidelines. Trained personnel monitor blood pressure response and assist patients with monitoring their heart rate. ECG monitoring is typically limited to once per month. Goal setting for risk management continues, as does the education component. However, the education may be informal. Participants also enjoy the support and encouragement of others who have a common goal of reducing their risk of heart disease.

Chronic Obstructive Pulmonary Disease

COPD includes emphysema, bronchitis, and asthma (Ries et al., 1996). Emphysema is the progressive and irreversible destruction of the alveoli walls (Connors

et al., 1993). The walls of the alveoli have elastic fibers, and when these are destroyed the lung loses some of its elasticity, resulting in air trapping. This air trapping reduces the ability of the lung to shrink during exhalation, so the lung inhales less air with the next breath (MedicineNet, 1995). Chronic bronchitis is excessive sputum production and cough of at least 3 months' duration 2 years in a row (Connors et al.). Asthma describes an inflammatory process that causes the bronchial tubes to spasm, narrowing the airway. This inflammation also causes the bronchial tubes to increase their production of mucus. The result of these processes is that the patient has sudden SOB and may wheeze or cough (Reis et al., 1996). Patients with COPD have characteristics of all of these diseases (Box 47-6). COPD is a permanent and progressive condition (MedicineNet, 1999). Medications and good health habits can lessen the symptoms and maximize function.

The feeling of breathlessness called dyspnea is a key feature of COPD. Damage to the lung results in a flattening of the diaphragm due to hyperinflation. This flattening takes away the ability of the diaphragm to act effectively in assisting with expansion of the lungs during inspiration. To compensate for the lack of inspiratory pressure, patients with COPD tend to use their shoulder girdle muscles to expand their lungs, making it difficult

---

BOX 47-6
Pulmonary Function Tests

▶ Patients forcefully exhale as much air as possible into a spirometer. The amount of air exhaled in 1 second is called the forced expiratory volume (FEV_1). There are age-related norms for FEV_1, and there is an inverse relationship between the results of the FEV_1 and mortality (Peters, 1993).

▶ Arterial blood gases are drawn to determine the lungs' ability to oxygenate blood, remove carbon dioxide, and maintain the body's acid-base status. It is helpful to draw blood gases before and after exercise to see how well oxygenation is maintained during activity (Connors et al., 1993).

▶ A pulse oximeter is a noninvasive test to determine the amount of oxygen in the blood. A probe is wrapped around a fingertip. A light shines through the finger, and the amount of light reaching the other side indicates the amount of oxygen in the blood. Hemoglobin is red, and the more hemoglobin in the blood, the less light is able to penetrate the fingertip (MedicineNet, 1999). The oximeter occasionally gives a false reading. If the patient is anemic, wears nail polish, or has poor circulation, the pulse oximetry may be inaccurate. Often the oximetry machine also determines the patient's pulse. If the palpated pulse and the oximetry machine pulse match, **oxygen saturation (O_2 Sat)** is likely to be accurate.

Case Example

MRS. K.: OCCUPATIONAL THERAPY AFTER ANTERIOR MI AND CARDIOMYOPATHY

Patient Information

Mrs. K. is a married 32-year-old mother of a 3-year-old and a full time health worker. The day after the delivery of her second child, she suddenly developed a migraine headache. The headache became worse with any movement and was unrelieved with medication. Her condition continued to deteriorate over the next few days. The headache persisted, and she became extremely short of breath. She needed a rebreather mask with 10 L oxygen to maintain her oxygen saturation. Her heart rate ranged from 135 to 140. An echocardiogram revealed a left ventricular wall motion abnormality and an ejection fraction of 40%. The next day she was diagnosed as having an anterior wall MI. Several days later her pulmonary edema had resolved and she had a coronary angiogram. The angiogram showed normal coronary arteries but an ejection fraction of 25 to 30%. She was subsequently diagnosed as having cardiomyopathy.

A week after the delivery of her child and the start of her symptoms, Mrs. K. was referred to occupational therapy in cardiac rehabilitation. She was very weak, with poor tolerance for exercise and activity, and her balance was only fair when she walked. After several days of inpatient cardiac rehabilitation, her heart rate and blood pressure continued to increase significantly with mild exercise. However, at discharge she was able to do 8 minutes of calisthenics, 4.5 minutes of walking, and 12 stairs without difficulty. She was given a home program consisting of a calisthenics and walking schedule, home activity guideline, work simplification and pacing instructions, stress management techniques, and guidelines for resumption of sexual relations. When she left the hospital, Mrs. K.'s restrictions were to avoid lifting more than 10 pounds, which was close to the weight of her 3-week-old infant; to avoid stair climbing; and not to return to her job. Her limited endurance made her dependent on her husband and other relatives to maintain the house and care of the children. Mrs. K. was referred to home health occupational therapy services.

The home care occupational therapist saw Mrs. K. within 4 days of discharge. The therapist assessed Mrs. K.'s ability to do her own self-care and found her independent, but it took an hour and fatigued her. The occupational therapist observed that the patient could tolerate only 5 cardiac calisthenics done seated for 2 minutes each with a 1-minute rest between each exercise. Her walking was limited to 4.5 minutes. During her exercise and activity, Mrs. K.'s cardiovascular response was within normal limits. The therapist started discussion of energy-saving techniques with ADL and encouraged the patient to try standing while doing the exercise. Mrs. K. was noted to be deconditioned but highly motivated to improve.

Over the next month the occupational therapist saw the patient one to three times per week. Recommendations were

for a shower seat and hand-held shower nozzle to make showering less taxing. Continued guidance was given regarding the progression and cardiovascular monitoring of the patient's exercise and walking. There was further instruction in work simplification specific to time management and alternating heavy and lighter tasks throughout the day.

Mrs. K. felt significant stress over her diagnosis, financial concerns due to her inability to return to work, and her inability to care for her children and home. Her church provided volunteers around the clock to help with child care and homemaking. Although it was deeply appreciated, this too caused stress, because now there were always extra people around. Mrs. K. had had depression in the past and now confided in the therapist how overwhelmed she was with these stresses. The occupational therapist gave the patient written information on stress management techniques and practiced some relaxation exercises with her.

At the time of discharge from home health occupational therapy, the patient reported increased endurance. She was able to go up and down stairs, walk several blocks, and do 12 minutes of advanced cardiac calisthenics with a *Borg Scale* rating of perceived exertion of light, no cardiovascular symptoms and heart rate and blood pressure within normal limits. The occupational therapist recommended outpatient cardiac rehabilitation.

A week later Mrs. K. started outpatient cardiac rehabilitation. Mrs. K. still had volunteers around the clock in her home doing the majority of the housekeeping and child care. She arrived in the cardiac rehabilitation clinic in a wheelchair. She reported that she slept excessively and was exhausted with exercise. Her ejection fraction per echocardiogram was now at 50%. She was able to exercise for 20 minutes at a 2-MET level at her initial session without symptoms or abnormal cardiovascular response.

Outpatient Cardiac Rehabilitation Occupational Therapy Problem List

- ▶ Low physical capacity for work graded less than 3 METs
- ▶ Insufficient endurance to engage in previous work and leisure pursuits
- ▶ Depression over feelings of dependency and concern over cardiac diagnosis
- ▶ Dependence on volunteers for most IADL

Outpatient Cardiac Rehabilitation Occupational Therapy Goal List

- ▶ Learn normal physical response to exercise and activity through use of *Borg scale* and pulse monitoring.

▶ Gradually increase capacity for work through aerobic exercise and later strengthening exercises (2–5 METs).

▶ Gradually resume household tasks and leisure pursuits (1.5–5 METs).

▶ Learn to pace household activities.

▶ Learn work simplification concepts to maximize capabilities.

▶ Learn stress management techniques to cope with difficulties caused by illness.

▶ Learn methods to reduce risk factors for heart disease.

▶ Identify personal risk factors and ways to ameliorate their effects.

▶ Start regular aerobic exercise program.

Treatment Plan

Mrs. K. was seen three times per week for 6 weeks in outpatient cardiac rehabilitation. The treatment plan consisted of an exercise program designed to increase aerobic capacity and endurance plus brief educational sessions regarding risk factors for heart disease while the patients exercised. The occupational therapist also instructed the patient in appropriate activities for her aerobic capacity and included work simplification and energy conservation techniques. Stress management techniques and symptoms of depression were discussed with the patient. The goals for Mrs. K. were achieved.

Analysis of Reasoning

Mrs. K.'s physically weakened state made household chores difficult. As she regained physical strength through exercise, she could start resuming more of her usual activities and reduce her dependence on volunteers. Teaching Mrs. K. how to assess her own physical response to exercise and activity

gave her confidence that she was in control. Since Mrs. K. had difficulty with pacing, the therapist had her keep a diary of her day's routine. Later they reviewed it and the occupational therapist presented work simplification techniques and methods of pacing. The therapist assigned tasks within Mrs. K.'s current aerobic capacity to assist her in resuming her home responsibilities. Mrs. K. was also instructed in stress management techniques to help her deal with the stresses of her illness. Because she had a history of depression, the therapist reviewed with Mrs. K. the relation between depression and fatigue. The occupational therapist explored with her the possibility of seeking professional help and/or medication to deal with her depression. Additionally, Mrs. K. was instructed in the risk factors for heart disease. Her individual risk factors were identified, she was taught to ameliorate their effects. As part of her risk factor reduction, Mrs. K. initiated a walking program. The combination of exercise and education regarding heart disease and activity modification let Mrs. K. gradually resume her household and leisure activities. She planned to return to work within a month after discharge from the program.

CLINICAL REASONING
in OT Practice

Implications of a Diagnosis

Mrs. K. was initially diagnosed with anterior MI and later with cardiomyopathy. If a patient has had an MI, what symptoms or signs would you look for to determine whether he or she is tolerating an activity or exercise? How would those signs and symptoms be different if the patient has cardiomyopathy without MI?

---

to use those muscles in unsupported upper extremity activities (Scanlan et al., 1993).

Dyspnea, fatigue, cough, and sputum production are part of the disease process. The effort of breathing takes so much energy that often COPD patients find themselves without enough energy to do their daily tasks, from ADL to vocational and leisure endeavors. They are unable to increase their ventilation enough to meet physiological demands. Because of the unpleasant sensation of SOB, patients reduce their physical activities, resulting in muscle weakness and inability to use oxygen efficiently (Make & Glenn, 1996). Eating is made difficult by lack of air. Maintaining adequate nutrition is a problem for 40 to 60% of patients with COPD, and nutrition problems are a significant predictor of mortality (AACVPR, 1998). Many patients with COPD lose their appetite because of the excessive costs of their breathing efforts (AACVPR, 1998). Others use steroids to reduce

lung inflammation, and the resulting weight gain contributes to several problems. Weight gain exacerbates the problem of not having enough oxygen to metabolize food, and extra weight requires more oxygen to do any activity, including eating.

Depression is common with COPD. Between 51% and 74% of patients with COPD are depressed (AACVPR, 1998). As with any chronic disease process, the changes in lifestyle, the struggle to accomplish normal daily activities, the fear of extreme SOB, and feelings of hopelessness all contribute to depression.

Pulmonary Rehabilitation

The AACVPR sets standards of practice for pulmonary rehabilitation used by insurers and the Joint Commission on Accreditation of Healthcare Organizations. The AACVPR has published a book, *Guidelines for Pulmonary*

Rehabilitation Programs, to guide practice. It has also instituted a certification for pulmonary rehabilitation programs. A team of health professionals including doctors, respiratory therapists, dietitians, pharmacists, and occupational and physical therapists are ideally involved in the pulmonary rehabilitation program. As with other diagnostic categories the roles in reinforcing behaviors to enhance function may overlap. The goals of the occupational therapist in pulmonary rehabilitation (Scanlan et al., 1993; ACSM, 1998) are as follows:

▶ ADL evaluation and training to increase functional endurance
▶ Instruction and training in appropriate breathing techniques while doing ADL
▶ Evaluation and strengthening of the upper extremities
▶ Work simplification and energy conservation
▶ Evaluation of the need for adaptive equipment
▶ Assistance in adapting leisure activities
▶ Education in stress management and relaxation techniques

ADL Evaluation and Training

Patients with COPD often have limited ability to perform ADL because they have dyspnea. It is common to have significant muscle wasting from disuse. The therapist should note the patient's breathing pattern during the ADL evaluation. Many patients with COPD hold their breath, breathe shallowly and fast, or elevate their shoulders as they breathe. Oxygen saturation with activity should also be noted. If the patient's oxygen saturation falls below 90% during ADL, the use of oxygen with activity should be considered. If the patient does not have home oxygen, the physician should be informed of

the patient's low oxygen saturation. It should be noted that while **hypoxemia** is recognized at 90% oxygen saturation, Medicare does not pay for oxygen at home until the oxygen saturation is 88% or below (McInturff & O'Donohue, 1997). As part of the functional assessment, measurements of heart rate and blood pressure should also be taken.

Breathing Techniques

It is important to practice use of breathing techniques with ADL. After becoming familiar with diaphragmatic and pursed-lip breathing, the patient should use these breathing techniques while attempting tasks that previously caused them to be breathless. The pulse oximeter helps to reinforce the improvement in oxygen saturation with use of a breathing technique. Timing the breath with work is also helpful. For example, breathe out while pushing the vacuum cleaner and in while pulling the vacuum cleaner. Exhaling with the exertion of lifting is less taxing not only on the lungs but the cardiovascular system (Scanlan et al., 1993) (Box 47-7).

Upper Extremity Function

Muscle strength of the upper extremity must be evaluated. Since many pulmonary patients take steroids, their shoulder girdle, trunk, and hip muscles are usually weak (Scanlan et al., 1993). Patients with COPD commonly use the accessory muscles of the shoulder girdle to help them breathe, which makes it difficult for them to use these muscles in unsupported upper extremity activity. Upper extremity strengthening has been found to improve the quality of life by increasing the capacity to work and reducing the oxygen requirement of upper extremity activity (Reis et al., 1997).

BOX 47-7
PROCEDURES FOR PRACTICE
Breathing Techniques

Practice these techniques while sitting in a relaxed position, preferably with feet elevated.

After you have become proficient using these breathing methods at rest, try using them while doing pleasant activities such as reading or watching television. Next, try using one of these techniques while doing a difficult task, such as stair climbing (Garritan, 1996).

Pursed-Lip Breathing
▶ Breathe in through your nose
▶ Exhale slowly with lips pursed (as if to kiss your aunt)
▶ Take twice as much time to exhale as to inhale

Diaphragmatic Breathing
▶ Place your hand on your abdomen.
▶ As you inhale through your nose, try to feel your abdomen push out as your lungs fill with oxygen.
▶ Next, feel your abdomen go down as you slowly breathe out through pursed lips.
▶ Continue to repeat this process until you become comfortable doing it.
▶ Stop the diaphragmatic breathing if you become light-headed or fatigued.

Case Example

MR. L.: OCCUPATIONAL THERAPY FOR COPD

Patient Information

Mr. L. is a 73-year-old widower with a history of COPD. He has been hospitalized for lung surgery for cancer. Mr. L. lives alone in a one-story house. The entrance to his house has three steps with railings. His house is air-conditioned. He has a car and has been driving. He has a cordless phone and knows 911. Patient's neighbors have been helpful with snow removal, but Mr. L. has been doing all of the lawn care until recently. In the hospital he needs 2 L oxygen to achieve an oxygen saturation of 95% but has never needed oxygen at home. He has inhalers and prednisone to maintain airways. He has never received therapy for COPD management beyond this medical approach.

Reason for Referral to Occupational Therapy

Mr. L. was hospitalized for a month and was referred to occupational therapy for evaluation and treatment to optimize self-management abilities. He was seen by occupational therapy for 14 visits during his hospital stay.

Assessment Findings

During the assessment, Mr. L. was alert and oriented. He was also cooperative and motivated to learn new techniques for managing his COPD, though was noticeably anxious. His sensory systems were intact, but he was mildly hard of hearing. He did not need eyeglasses for reading. Mr. L. was independent in his ADL, such as dressing, feeding, sink hygiene, grooming, and showering in the tub. However, he became SOB easily and required extra time to complete these tasks. He had never received any adaptive equipment to use for his ADL. Mr. L. was independent in such tasks as shopping and cooking, preparing a lot of TV dinners. He also took care of his own finances, household tasks, laundry, and home maintenance. Because of his increased SOB, he planned to get help with most of these activities after discharge from the hospital.

Formal evaluation revealed that active range of motion and strength were within normal limits. He had fair endurance for activity, tolerating 3 minutes 18 seconds of activity before needing a rest. He stated that he would often get SOB in groups, especially if the participants were noisy or loud. Mr. L. was independent in supine to sit and sit to stand, and he walked long distances behind a wheelchair so he could use the oxygen attached to the chair.

Occupational Therapy Problem List

► Lack of knowledge of COPD breathing and energy conservation techniques
► Decreased endurance for ADL
► SOB even at rest

Occupational Therapy Goal List

► Will complete COPD educational program to learn how to manage his disease
► Will be able to list 10 energy-saving techniques he could use in his daily life to decrease SOB in 3 weeks
► Will tolerate 5 minutes of continuous upper extremity activity without needing a rest to increase ease of ADL performance before discharge
► Will purchase recommended adaptive equipment
► Will successfully use relaxation techniques that control anxiety and allow him to participate in group activities before discharge

Treatment Plan

The COPD treatment plan consisted of an education program, including a four-part pulmonary self care video series and a folder of print materials. Next he practiced the diaphragmatic and pursed-lip breathing he learned in the videos. He was instructed in energy conservation and work simplification, and the need for adaptive equipment was evaluated. In addition, Mr. L. engaged in graded activities in occupational therapy to increase his endurance.

Analysis of Reasoning

After learning about COPD, Mr. L. would be better able to understand the triggers for his SOB and how diaphragmatic and pursed-lip breathing could minimize his breathlessness. Learning energy-saving techniques helped him maximize his energy capacity. The therapist and patient also found benefit from use of a shower chair, hand-held shower hose, dressing stick, long-handled shoehorn, a pistol-grip reacher, Velcro straps on his shoes, and a sock aid to assist Mr. L. in completing his ADL while minimizing SOB. Mr. L. increased his endurance through use of a Theraband exercise program, which enabled him to tolerate 5 minutes of upper extremity activity without needing a rest. Finally pursed-lip and diaphragmatic breathing provided him with a coping measure to use when he was anxious because of breathlessness.

Mr. L. accomplished all of his goals through the educational and exercise program in occupational therapy. He kept his oxygen saturation above 90%, so he was discharged without supplemental oxygen. In addition, he received Meals on Wheels and assistance with housework and lawn care, which allowed him to remain in his own home.

CLINICAL REASONING
in OT Practice

Maximizing COPD Patients' Capabilities

As part of his occupational therapy goals, Mr. L. was supposed to list 10 work simplification and/or energy saving techniques he could use. If you were the therapist working with this patient, what 10 work simplification or energy-saving techniques do you think might be beneficial?

It is easy to measure improvement in upper extremity strength with the arm ergometer, but the best method of strengthening the upper body has not been determined (Reis et al., 1997). Use of free weights, Theraband, or other upper body strengthening techniques appear to be of equal value. Several studies have shown improvement in functional status when leg training is added (Reis et al.).

Work Simplification and Energy Conservation

Since their work capacity is significantly reduced, patients with COPD benefit from instruction in work simplification and energy conservation. Bathing is a particularly strenuous activity because the hot, humid air makes breathing difficult. Therapists encourage patients to use the ventilation fan or leave the door open while bathing to keep the humidity down. Using a chair in the shower and using a thick terry robe after showering instead of toweling off help to reduce energy expenditure. Unsupported upper extremity activity fatigues patients with COPD. It is important to teach these patients to support their arms during upper extremity activities, such as hair combing and shaving. Sometimes a machine, such as an electric toothbrush, is helpful. They can also accomplish more if they do relatively strenuous activities after they use the inhaler and are feeling better (Romanik, 1994).

Not all patients with COPD need adaptive equipment. However, as the disease progresses, some adaptive equipment is useful. Since bending over to tie shoes or put on pants may cause significant SOB, elastic shoelaces, long-handled shoehorn, or a reacher to assist with putting on slacks may be helpful.

Promoting Self-Enhancement Roles

Having COPD tends to isolate the person. Just completing daily necessities takes so much energy that there is little or none left for leisure activities. Many patients fear extreme SOB in front of others or are embarrassed to use oxygen. The occupational therapist can help patients evaluate previously enjoyed activities and see if those activities can be adapted to fit their health status. Informing patients of programs or activities available in their community is also helpful. Sometimes a helper or companion may make an activity more feasible.

Stress Management

The feeling of being unable to get enough air is frightening. Patients with COPD often feel panic with breathlessness. Teaching patients to cope with extreme SOB can lessen their fear. Leaning forward and resting their arms on the table releases the diaphragm and makes breathing easier. Using pursed-lip and diaphragmatic breathing helps to slow the pace of breathing so that the patient is not breathing so shallowly and rapidly. A stress management technique, such as visualization, may help patients calm themselves by mentally transporting them out of the stressful situation. It is important to practice these options prior to needing them. Having a well-practiced plan of action for the panic associated with breathlessness gives patients confidence in their ability to control the situation.

Heart disease and pulmonary disease, as the first and fourth leading causes of death, respectively, pose major health problems. As either a primary or secondary diagnosis, both heart disease and COPD require specialized attention in planning occupational therapy. If a patient has a history of heart disease or COPD, the occupational therapy practitioner must assess the patient's cardiovascular response to activity or exercise. Precautions for the patient's cardiac or pulmonary problem must be incorporated into the treatment program.

Summary Review Questions

1. A person is admitted to the hospital with an acute MI and is given thrombolytics to reverse clot formation in his coronary arteries, but the thrombolytics

cause a cerebral bleed. In evaluating and treating for stroke related deficits, what physiological parameters should the therapist take to measure the workload on the patient's heart? What factors might increase these parameters?

2. What cardiac symptoms might a patient who has a previous heart history exhibit if he or she were not tolerating the treatment you prescribed for a current shoulder injury?

3. What symptoms would a person going into CHF exhibit?

4. In reviewing a patient's medical record after hip replacement surgery what cardiac diagnoses might impinge on your treatment? What cardiac diagnostic tests might provide information to help you make decisions about the severity of their heart disease?

5. Describe in detail the differences between a home program for a patient with an MI, a coronary artery bypass graft and an angioplasty. How would you customize the program for the individual?

6. Describe the different ways of conditioning an outpatient in cardiac rehabilitation? What are the advantages and disadvantages of each method?

7. List the risk factors for heart disease. What methods might an occupational therapist use to decrease patients' risk for coronary artery disease?

8. Develop a treatment plan for a patient with COPD who is having problems with SOB while doing their ADL.

9. Describe pursed-lip and diaphragmatic breathing. How would you teach it to a patient with COPD?

10. If you were the only occupational therapist in a small rural hospital, where could you find information pertaining to the treatment of the patient with cardiac or pulmonary disease?

Acknowledgments

Thanks to Margie Swanson, OTR, geriatric specialist from the Veterans Affairs Medical Center, Minneapolis, for submitting the case study on the patient with COPD.

Resources

Two organizations dominate the administration and policies of cardiac rehabilitation. The AACVPR published *Guidelines for Cardiac Rehabilitation and Secondary Prevention Programs*. Government agencies and third-party payers use this publication to determine appropriate cardiac rehabilitation policies and procedures. The American College of Sports Medicine (ACSM) has several nationally recognized certifications for health professionals who wish to work in cardiac rehabilitation. Both organizations offer continuing education courses in cardiac rehabilitation, and together they shape the practice of cardiac rehabilitation.

AACVPR · 7611 Elmwood Ave., Suite 201, Middleton, WI 53562. 608-831-6989.
aacvprtmdhq.com
www.aacvpr.org
ACSM National Center · 401 West Michigan St., Indianapolis, IN 46202-3233. 317-637-9200.
E-mail: crt2acsm@acsm.org
www.acsm.org

References

Ainsworth, B., Haskell, W., Leon, A., Jacobs Jr., D., Montoye, H., Sallis, J., & Paffenbarger R. Jr., (1998). Compendium of physical activities: Classification of energy costs of human physical activities. In J. Roitman (Ed.), *ACSM'S Resource Manual for Exercise Testing and Prescription* (pp. 657–665). Baltimore: Williams & Wilkins.

Alexander, R. W., Pratt, C. M., & Roberts. R. (1998). Diagnosis and management of patients with acute myocardial infarction. In R. W. Alexander, R. Schlant, & V. Fuster (Eds.) *Hurst's the heart* (p. 1407). New York: McGraw-Hill.

American Association of Cardiovascular and Pulmonary Rehabilitation [AACVPR] (1995). *Guidelines for Cardiac Rehabilitation Programs and Secondary Prevention Programs*. Champaign, IL: Human Kinetics.

American Association of Cardiovascular and Pulmonary Rehabilitation [AACVPR] (1998). *Guidelines for Pulmonary Rehabilitation Programs*. Champaign, IL: Human Kinetics.

American College of Cardiology Expert Consensus Document (1994, September). Coronaryartery stents. *Journal of American College of Cardiology, 28*, 782–793.

American College of Sports Medicine (1995). *ACSM'S Guidelines for Exercise Testing and Prescription*. Media, PA: Williams & Wilkins.

American College of Sports Medicine (1998). *Guidelines for Pulmonary Rehabilitation Programs*. Champaign, IL: Human Kinetics.

American Heart Association (1998). *1999 Heart and Stroke Statistical Update*. Dallas: Author.

American Lung Association (1995). *Fact Sheet*. New York: Author.

American Lung Association (1998). *Lung Disease in Minorities*. Retrieved April 15, 1999, from http://w.w.w.lungusa.org/pub/minority/copd.htm.

Armstrong, G. (1997). Lifestyle management: Exercise. In G. M. Lindsay & A. Gaw (Eds.), *Coronary Artery Disease Prevention* (p. 158). New York: Churchill Livingstone.

Connors, G. L., Hilling, L, & Morris, K. (1993). Assessment of the pulmonary rehabilitation candidate. In J. E. Hodgkin. G. L. Connors, & C. W. Bell (Eds.), *Pulmonary Rehabilitation Guidelines to Success* (pp. 64–66). Philadelphia: Lippincott.

Fardy, P. S., & Yanowitz, F. G. (1995). *Cardiac Rehabilitation, Adult Fitness and Exercise Testing*. Baltimore: Williams & Wilkins.

Gage, R. C., & Radke, J. (1997). Laboratory tests. In S.VanRiper & J. VanRiper (Eds.), *Cardiac Diagnostic Tests: A Guide for Nurses* (pp. 113–114). Philadelphia: Lippincott-Raven.

Garcia, M. (1998). Prosthetic valve disease. In E. J. Topol (Ed.). *Textbook for Cardiovascular Medicine* (p. 584). Philadelphia: Lippincott-Raven.

Garritan, S. (1996). Physical therapy interventions for persons with chronic obstructive pulmonary disease. In J. Bach (Ed.), *Pulmonary Rehabilitation the Obstructive and Paralytic Conditions* (p. 95). Philadelphia: Hanley & Balfus.

Gordon, N. F. (1998). Conceptual basis for coronary artery disease risk factor assessment. In J. Roitman, (Ed.), *ACSM'S Resource Manual for Guidelines for Exercise Testing and Prescription* (pp. 3–8). Baltimore: William & Wilkins.

Jamieson, E. M., McCall, J. M., Blythe, R., & Whyte, L. (1997). *Clinical Nursing Practices.* New York: Churchill Livingstone.

Jairath, N. (1999). *Coronary Heart Disease and Risk Factor Management.* Philadelphia: Saunders.

Lindsay G. M. (1997). Risk factor assessment. In G. M. Lindsay & A. Gaw (Eds.), *Coronary Heart Disease Prevention* (pp. 22–23). New York: Churchill Livingstone.

Make, B., & Glenn, K. (1996). Outcomes of pulmonary rehabilitation. In J. Bach (Ed.) *Pulmonary Rehabilitation: The Obstructive and Paralytic Conditions* (p. 196). Philadelphia: Hanley & Belfus.

Marelli, A. J., & Moodie, D. (1998). Adult congenital heart disease. In E. J. Topol (Ed.), *Textbook for Cardiovascular Medicine* (p. 775), Philadelphia: Lippincott-Raven.

McInturff, S., & O'Donohue, W. (1997). Respiratory care in the home, alternate sites. In G. G. Burton, J. E. Hodgkin, & J. J. Ward, (Eds.) *Respiratory Care: a Guide to Clinical Practice* (p. 898). Philadelphia: Lippincott.

MedicineNet (1999). *Chronic Obstructive Pulmonary Disease (COPD) a.k.a. Chronic Obstructive Lung Disease (COLD).* Retrieved March 19, 1999 from http://w.w.w.medicinenet.com/S. . ./asp?li=MNI&d=193&cu=16583&w=1&ArticleKey=197.

Padgitt, E., & Kline-Rogers, E. (1997) Nuclear medicine studies and positron emission tomography. In S. VanRiper & J. VanRiper, (Eds.), *Cardiac Diagnostic Tests: A Guide for Nurses* (pp. 179–180). Philadelphia: Saunders.

Peters, J. (1993). Preventive care in pulmonary rehabilitation. In J. E.

Hodgkins, G. I. Connors, & C. W. Bell, (Eds.), *Respiratory Care: A Guide to Clinical Practice* (p. 103). Philadelphia: Lippincott.

Reis, A., Carlin, B., Carrieri-Kohlman, V., Casaburi, R., Celli, B., Emery, C., Hodgkin, J., Mahler, D., Make, B., & Skolnick, J. (1997). Pulmonary rehabilitation: Joint ACCP/AACVPR evidenced-based guidelines. *Journal of Cardiopulmonary Rehabilitation, 17,* 378–379.

Reis, A. L., Moser K. M., Bullock P. J., Limberg T. M., Myers, R., Sassi-Dambron, D. E., & Sheldon, J. B. (1996). *Shortness of Breath: A Guide to Better Living and Breathing.* St. Louis: Mosby.

Romanik, K. (1994). *Around the Clock with C.O.P.D.* Minneapolis: American Lung Association.

Scanlan, M., Kishbaugh, L., & Horne, D. (1993). Life management skills in pulmonary rehabilitation. In J. E. Hodgkin, G. L. Connors, & C. W. Bell (Eds.) *Pulmonary Rehabilitation Guidelines to Success* (pp. 251–258). Philadelphia: Lippincott.

Taylor, C. B., & Houston, N. M. (1998). Psychopathology. In J. Roitman (Ed.), *ACSM'S Resource Manual for Exercise Testing and Prescription* (p. 537*).* Baltimore: Williams & Wilkins.

Texas Heart Institute (1996). *Heart Owner's Handbook.* New York: Wiley.

Topol, E., &Van de Werf, F. (1998). Acute myocardial infarction early diagnosis and management. In E. J. Topol (Ed.), *Textbook of Cardiovascular Medicine* (pp. 410–411). Philadelphia: Lippincott-Raven.

Wynne, J., & Baunwald, E. (1998). The cardiomyopathies and myocarditis. In E. J. Topol (Ed.), *Textbook of Cardiovascular Medicine* (Vol. 2, p .408). Philadelphia: Lippincott-Raven.

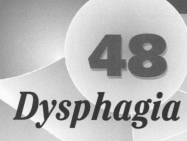

48
Dysphagia

Wendy Avery-Smith

LEARNING OBJECTIVES

After studying this chapter, the reader will be able to do the following:

1. Discuss normal swallowing.
2. Identify types of dysphagia and their presentation.
3. Describe how to perform a clinical dysphagia assessment.
4. Employ basic compensatory and rehabilitative strategies to treat dysphagia.
5. Describe instrumental evaluation procedures for dysphagia.

*D*ysphagia, or difficulty with any stage of swallowing, interferes with functional independence for many recipients of occupational therapy services: 33% of acute-care hospital inpatients (Groher & Bukatman, 1986), 32% of rehabilitation hospital inpatients (Cherney, 1994), and 59% of nursing home residents (Siebens et al., 1986) may be dysphagic. Dysphagia care is a rapidly evolving science and a relatively new treatment area for health care practitioners. Safe swallowing is a critical and life-supporting capacity that is addressed by occupational therapists in many environments, including acute care and psychiatric hospitals, rehabilitation centers, outpatient clinics, nursing homes, and schools.

Occupational therapists assist patients with dysphagia in rehabilitation of abilities that affect swallowing, including self-feeding, cognition, perception, sensory and motor skills, and postural control. In some settings, occupational therapists serve as the primary swallowing therapist (Avery-Smith, 1998); in other settings, speech–language pathologists do so. In many facilities, dysphagia care is provided by a designated dysphagia team that may include the disciplines of speech–language pathology, physical and respiratory therapy, nursing, physiatry, radiology, and gastroenterology.

Because of the prevalence of dysphagia, basic knowledge of swallowing disorders and their treatment is important for occupational therapists. This chapter introduces the entry-level skills required for the evaluation and treatment of dysphagia in adults. Independent treatment of the dysphagia patient

---

GLOSSARY

Aspiration—Entrance of food or secretions into the larynx below the level of the vocal cords.

Bolus—Food or liquid in the mouth.

Deglutition—The act of swallowing.

Direct therapy—Therapeutic techniques involving ingestion of food or liquids.

Dysphagia—Difficulty with any stage of swallowing.

Eating—Ingestion of food and liquid, including the preoral, oral preparatory, oral, pharyngeal, and esophageal stages.

Feeding—Taking or giving nourishment.

Indirect therapy—Therapy addressing the prerequisite capacities associated with swallowing without ingestion of food or liquid.

Instrumental evaluation—Use of technological tools to assess aspects of swallowing.

Laryngeal penetration—Entrance of food or secretions into the larynx above the level of the vocal cords.

NPO (nil per os)—Latin, *nothing by mouth*: no food or medication to be administered orally.

Swallowing—Ingestion of nourishment, beginning with introduction of food into the mouth and ending with reception of food into the stomach; includes the preoral, oral preparatory, oral, pharyngeal and esophageal stages.

Videofluoroscopy—Recording on videotape of moving radiographic images of structure and physiology; in this case, of swallowing.

---

requires advanced knowledge and skills on the part of the occupational therapy clinician. The American Occupational Therapy Association (2000) delineates entry-level and advanced-level skills in dysphagia care for occupational therapists and assistants. Further information about dysphagia can be acquired by seeking basic and advanced learning opportunities, researching new developments, attending workshops and conferences, and receiving mentoring.

Normal Swallowing

Deglutition is a complex process involving both volitional and nonvolitional behaviors. The cranial nerves execute the sensory and motor processes that constitute swallowing. Cortically mediated factors, including appetite, attitude, attention span, appreciation of food, and body position influence swallowing and must be considered in evaluation and treatment. Oral, pharyngeal, and esophageal structures involved in swallowing are shown in Figure 48-1.

The stages of swallowing include the preoral, oral preparatory, oral, pharyngeal, and esophageal stages (Box 48-1). The preoral, oral preparatory and oral stages are voluntary. The length of the oral preparatory stage varies considerably with the type of bolus (Hiiemae et al., 1996) and age (Logemann, 1998). Oral transit time, the length of time to accomplish the oral stage, is normally 1 to 1.5 seconds (Tracy et al., 1989). The pharyngeal stage is involuntary, although volitional

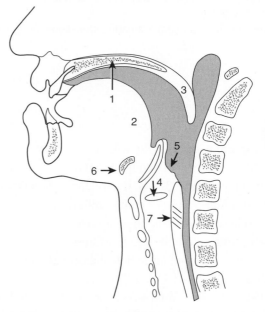

Figure 48-1 The oral, pharyngeal, and esophageal structures involved in swallowing. 1. The hard palate. 2. The base of the tongue. 3. The soft palate and uvula. 4. The vocal cords. 5. The laryngeal vestibule. 6. The hyoid bone. 7. The upper esophageal sphincter. Adapted with permission from Groher, M. E. (1997). *Dysphagia: Diagnosis and Management* (3rd ed). Boston: Butterworth-Heinemann.

movements can alter it. Normal pharyngeal transit time is 1 second (Tracy et al., 1989). While the patient's position may affect the esophageal stage because of gravity, this stage is involuntary.

Impaired Swallowing

Many disease processes cause dysphagia, including those that affect the central nervous system, peripheral nervous system, motor end plate, muscles, and other anatomical structures. Trauma may affect anatomy and physiology, resulting in dysphagia. Dysphagia can lead to dehydration (Musson et al., 1990), malnutrition (Finestone et al., 1995), and pulmonary complications due to aspiration, including aspiration pneumonia (Schmidt et al., 1994), airway obstruction (Eckberg & Feinberg, 1992), adult respiratory distress syndrome (Garber et al., 1996), and death (Schmidt et al., 1994). The limited ability to participate in social and cultural activities because of chronic dysphagia can profoundly affect an individual.

Types of Dysphagia

Dysphagia occurs in three types: paralytic, pseudobulbar, and mechanical. Paralytic dysphagia results from lower motor neuron involvement that causes weakness and sensory impairment of oral and pharyngeal structures, including weakness or absence of the swallowing reflex. Pseudobulbar dysphagia results from upper motor neuron involvement, causing hypotonicity or hypertonicity of oral and pharyngeal structures and a slow or poorly coordinated swallowing reflex. Paralytic and pseudobulbar dysphagia are neurological dysphagias. Mechanical dysphagia is caused by loss of oral, pharyngeal, or esophageal structures, weakness and/or sensory deficits due to trauma or surgery. Secondary disorders in addition to the primary cause of a particular type of dysphagia may complicate the presentation. Pulmonary diagnoses and their treatment also pose special challenges (Box 48-2).

Clinical Dysphagia Presentation for Various Diagnostic Groups

The following review of the literature provides an overview of the typical clinical dysphagia presentation for diagnoses frequently encountered by occupational therapists.

Alzheimer's Disease: Pseudobulbar Dysphagia

Patients with Alzheimer's disease demonstrate decreased attention span and apraxia for swallowing and self-feeding. They demonstrate slowed oral and pharyngeal responses and a need for physical and verbal cues to self-feed (Priefer & Robbins, 1997). Patients with moderate to severe Alzheimer's are prone to aspiration (Horner et al., 1994).

Brain Injury: Pseudobulbar, Paralytic Dysphagia

Type and severity of dysphagia in brain injury depends on the cause of the injury and location and size of brain lesions. Behavioral and cognitive problems that affect self-feeding and swallowing are often present. There may be abnormal pathological reflexes affecting oral and pharyngeal control (Logemann et al., 1994). In the oral stage there may be increased or reduced muscle tone causing decreased mouth opening, decreased lip closure, drooling, decreased tongue control, and pocketing of the bolus in the cheek (Logemann et al.;

BOX 48-1
The Stages of Swallowing

Preoral Stage
The food is visually and olfactorily appreciated. This stimulates salivation, and there are preparatory movements of the mouth to ready the oral cavity to receive and mobilize the food or liquid. Spontaneous upper extremity movements occur as the person reaches for and grasps the utensil, cup or finger food, and brings it to the mouth.

Oral Preparatory Stage
The food is received and contained by the mouth. It is then formed into a **bolus** of food and mixed with saliva. Pureed or liquid boluses require little mastication and may briefly be held centrally in the mouth by the tongue and cheek musculature. If solid, the food may have to be bitten off to be contained in the mouth. The bolus is chewed in a rotary motion by the molars and is moved between the left and right molars. The buccal muscles contract to prevent food from pocketing between the cheeks and the teeth. Once masticated or formed, the bolus is brought to the center of the tongue.

Oral Stage
As the cheek and tongue muscles retain the bolus centrally in the mouth, the tongue squeezes it against the hard palate, moving it posteriorly to the level of the faucial arches.

Pharyngeal Stage
The soft palate elevates to close off the nasopharynx. The larynx elevates and retracts, minimizing the size of the laryngeal vestibule (its opening), as the epiglottis tips to cover the vestibule. Breathing stops, which reduces the possibility of **aspiration** or **laryngeal penetration** of food or liquid. The vocal cords close. Simultaneously, the pharyngeal constrictor muscles sequentially contract to propel the bolus through the pharynx. The elevation of the larynx causes the upper esophageal sphincter (UES) to relax, allowing the bolus to pass through it.

Esophageal Stage
The UES returns to its normal tonic state and the bolus is transported through the esophagus via esophageal peristalsis and gravity. The lower esophageal sphincter relaxes, allowing the bolus to pass through into the stomach.

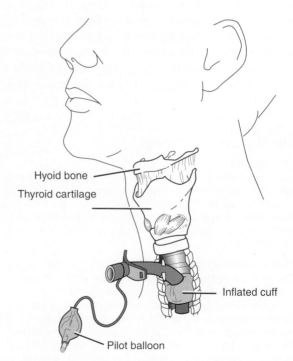

BOX 48-2
SAFETY BOX

Pulmonary Concerns

As the respiratory and swallowing mechanisms share anatomy and physiology, respiratory problems may contribute to dysphagia and vice versa.

► **Secretion management**—The patient's airway must be clear of excessive secretions. Intermittent suctioning through the nose or tracheostomy may be needed to clear the airway. The swallowing therapist should work closely with nursing and respiratory staff to assess whether airway protection and the ability to maintain oxygenation are adequate. Personnel should be available to suction the airway as necessary.

► **Tracheostomy**—A tracheostomy tube reroutes breathing through a stoma in the neck. Tracheostomy tubes may be temporary or permanent and are used to keep the airway open (Fig. 48-2). Tracheostomies provide easy access for suctioning or ventilator use but can cause or exacerbate dysphagia. They cause reduced smell and taste sensation, as the patient is not breathing through the nose. Tracheostomy reduces the ability to clear the upper airway if laryngeal penetration occurs. It increases the risk of aspiration due to pooling in the pharynx, delays trigger of the swallow reflex (Devita & Spierer-Rundback, 1990), decreases duration of vocal cord closure (Shaker et al., 1995), and reduces laryngeal movement.

► **Mechanical Ventilators**—Ventilators are machines that assist patients to breathe if they cannot do so on their own. Positive pressure ventilators may be used temporarily to assist a patient through an acute illness, or chronically, for a patient with a long-term respiratory deficit. Positive pressure ventilators deliver breaths to patients through a tube in the nose or mouth or through a tracheostomy. Patients who use a ventilator to breathe via a tracheostomy may be able to eat by mouth. Breathing and swallowing alternate (Logemann, 1998). A well-coordinated swallow is needed to interpose the swallow between inhalation and exhalation. Patients who have had mechanical ventilation for more than a week have been shown to have multiple swallowing deficits once the ventilator is removed (Tolep et al., 1996). Patients who are ventilator dependent via tracheostomy are prone to aspiration during eating (Elpern et al., 1994).

(pseudobulbar dysphagia) display mild oral transit delays and some delay in pharyngeal trigger and laryngeal elevation (Lazarus, 1995). The pharyngeal stage lasts longer, and there may be penetration of the larynx and aspiration (Robbins et al., 1993). There may be neglect or denial of swallowing problems. Patients with left hemispheric stroke (pseudobulbar dysphagia) display delays in initiating the oral stage and in triggering the pharyngeal stage (Lazarus). The pharyngeal stage takes longer (Robbins et al.). There may be apraxia for eating and swallowing. Patients with subcortical stroke (paralytic dysphagia) demonstrate mild oral transit delays and a delay in triggering the swallow. There is general weakness of pharyngeal swallow, as seen in reduced laryngeal elevation, reduced tongue base retraction, and unilateral pharyngeal weakness (Horner et al., 1991; Robbins et al.). There may also be reduced upper esophageal sphincter (UES) opening (Horner et al. 1991).

Developmental Disabilities: Pseudobulbar, Paralytic Dysphagia

Cerebral palsy (CP) and mental retardation, together or in isolation, may present a variety of eating and swallowing deficits. In a population with both diagnoses, Rogers et al. (1994) noted deficits of bolus formation and transit, delayed swallow reflex, pharyngeal dysmotility, esopha-

Figure 48-2 A tracheostomy tube. Tubes come in different sizes, and may come with or without the cuff as pictured. The pilot balloon is used to inflate the cuff with a syringe, and indicates relative inflation of the cuff. The inflated cuff prevents food or secretions from falling further into the airway. Adapted with permission from: Logemann, J. A. (1998). *Evaluation and Treatment of Swallowing Disorders* (2nd ed.). Austin, TX: Pro-Ed.

Mackay et al., 1999). In the pharyngeal stage, delayed pharyngeal swallow trigger, nasal regurgitation, decreased base of tongue movement and decreased laryngeal elevation with resulting pharyngeal residue may be seen (Logemann et al.). Overall mealtime is longer (Mackay, et al.).

Cerebrovascular Accident: Pseudobulbar Paralytic

Pharyngeal and laryngeal sensory deficits occur in right and left hemispheric as well as subcortical strokes (Aviv et al., 1996). Patients with right hemispheric stroke

geal disease, and aspiration. The following may also be observed in the CP population: abnormal oral reflexes, oral hyposensitivity or hypersensitivity, pharyngeal stage delay, decreased laryngeal elevation, and aspiration (Logemann, 1998). Poor postural, head, neck, and limb control can affect swallowing.

Head and Neck Cancer: Mechanical Dysphagia

Swallowing problems with head and neck cancer vary with tumor type, size, and location, as these determine how extensive surgery, radiation therapy, and chemotherapy must be. In general, the more extensive the surgery, the worse the postoperative swallowing function. In oral cancer, bolus control and containment problems result from surgery to the lip (McConnel & O'Connor, 1994). Resection of tumor from the floor of the mouth causes difficulty with bolus control, reduced laryngeal elevation, and its accompanying reduction in UES opening (McConnel & O'Connor). Glossectomy, or removal of some or all of the tongue, causes difficult or absent bolus mobilization; a resection of the tongue base limits the elevation needed to initiate the pharyngeal swallow (McConnel & O'Connor). Unilateral laryngeal cancer may require a vertical laryngectomy or hemilaryngectomy; this may cause reduced vocal cord closure, reduced posterior tongue movement, and reduced UES opening (McConnell & O'Connor). A supraglottic laryngectomy is done if the tumor is above the level of the glottis; this surgery reduces glottic closure, laryngeal elevation, and opening of the UES (McConnell & O'Connor). Extensive cancer of the larynx necessitates a total laryngectomy, which separates the foodway and airway tracts and creates a permanent anatomical tracheostomy. While aspiration is no longer a threat, there is no laryngeal elevation, hence there is a reduced movement and force of the UES (McConnell & O'Connor). Adjunctive radiation therapy causes edema in areas adjacent to the radiation field, fibrosis, and reduced salivary flow, causing dry mouth or xerostomia. Radiation therapy combined with chemotherapy without surgery can reduce tongue base movement, laryngeal elevation, and pharyngeal range of motion and speed (Lazarus et al., 1996). Radiation therapy combined with surgery can cause longer oral transit time, increased pharyngeal residue, and reduced UES opening (Pauloski et al., 1998).

Multiple Sclerosis: Pseudobulbar, Paralytic Dysphagia

Dysphagia symptoms vary with location of plaques in the central and peripheral nervous systems. Weakness of the oral structures and the neck muscles may be seen (Thomas & Wiles, 1999), as may delayed pharyngeal swallow and weakness of pharyngeal contractions (Logemann, 1998).

Parkinson's Disease: Pseudobulbar Dysphagia

Impulsiveness and poor judgment can affect swallowing (Leopold & Kagel, 1996). Jaw rigidity, abnormal head and neck posture, impaired coordination of tongue movements and mastication, and difficulty with coordination of upper extremity movements for self-feeding are seen (Leopold & Kagel, 1996). There may be oral residue, poor oral bolus manipulation, residue in the pharynx, delayed laryngeal elevation and delayed oral and pharyngeal transit times (Nagaya et al., 1998). Impaired pharyngeal motility and aspiration may be seen (Leopold & Kagel, 1997).

Psychiatric Disorders: Pseudobulbar Dysphagia

Tardive dyskinesia caused by long-term use of neuroleptic agents causes dystonia of the tongue and larynx and hyperkinesis of the face, jaw, tongue, and UES (Groher, 1997; Sokoloff & Pavlakovic, 1997). There can be choking due to eating too quickly (Fioretti et al., 1997).

Dysphagia Assessment

A dysphagia assessment involves two components, a clinical assessment and an instrumental evaluation.

Clinical Assessment

Clinical assessment of dysphagia must be thorough, with examination of all areas relevant to swallowing. It is best done using a reliable and valid tool (Avery-Smith et al., 1997). A reliable and valid tool allows for accurate assessment and reassessment by different test administrators, and ensures that each test item provides accurate assessment of performance components. Figure 48-3 illustrates use of a chartable form to document evaluation results.

History, Nutrition, and Respiratory Considerations

The clinician reviews the patient's medical and surgical history, with special attention to any diagnoses and procedures that are relevant to dysphagia. The patient and caregiver also provide information about any history of swallowing disorders. Specific signs and symptoms and modifications in behaviors relevant to mealtime are noted, as are changes in food intake and weight loss. The current nutritional sources are recorded, including the length of time the patient has been **NPO**, or not eating by mouth, if applicable. The therapist also documents any cultural and religious dietary preferences and practices. Information regarding respiratory status is gathered from the hospital chart and staff, especially any tracheostomy and/or mechanical ventilation and the level of independence with secretion management.

Text continued on p. 1100.

DYSPHAGIA
Evaluation Protocol
RECORD FORM

Client name: *Doe, John*   DOB: *1/1/20*   Age: *80*   Date: *1/1/00*

Physician: *Dr. Physician*   Location: *bedside*   Type of service: *neuro*

Type of eval ☑ Initial ☐ Re-eval   Assistive or postural devices used: *wheelchair*

Diagnosis: Ⓛ CVA, Ⓡ *hemi*   Date of onset: *12/25/99* Reason for referral: *s/s dysphagia*

Last oral feeding: *breakfast*   Clinician/Title: *Wendy Avery-Smith, OTR*

HISTORY AND OBSERVATIONS

Feeding History

Normal preexisting function?   ☑ No   ☐ Yes

   When did change occur? Describe change.

   Coughing with all textures, p̄ CVA

Has consistency of food changed?   ☐ No   ☑ Yes

   When, and how did client compensate? *MD ordered*
   Level I Aspiration Prevention Diet

Has food intake changed?   ☐ No   ☑ Yes

   When, and how? *Reduced, p̄ CVA*

Weight loss?   ☑ No   ☐ Yes

   Number of lbs: _____ When? _____

   Other changes: _____

Nutritional Status

Nutritional Route:

   ☐ NPO   ☑ PO

Alternative feeding method used:

   ☐ NGT ☐ PEG ☐ TPN ☑ Other: *IV for fluids*

Current diet:

   ☐ Regular   ☑ Other: *Level I, Aspiration*
   Prevention

Special dietary requirements:

   ☐ No concentrated sweets ☐ Low salt ☐ Kosher

   ☐ Other: _____ *none*

Respiratory Status

Auscultation of pooling?   ☑ No   ☐ Yes

Suctioning required?   ☑ No   ☐ Yes

   Frequency: _____ Route: _____

Tracheostomy?   ☑ No   ☐ Yes

   Type: ☐ Cuffed   ☐ Cuffless

      ☐ Fenestrated   Size: _____

   Position of cuff:

   ☐ Fully inflated ☐ Partially inflated ☐ Deflated

Comments: _____

_____

Ventilator? ☑ No ☐ Yes ☐ Cannot be removed

   Weaning parameters: _____

Receiving chest physical therapy? ☑ No ☐ Yes

   Type of treatment: _____

Comments: _____

_____

General Status

Alertness:

   ☑ No deficit ☐ Partial deficit ☐ Moderate/Severe deficit

Follows directions:

   ☑ verbal   ☐ gesture

   ☑ 3-step   ☐ 2-step   ☐ 1-step   ☐ Unable

If client responds to fewer than 3-step directions, note reason

for difficulty: _____

_____

> *If the client has difficulty with two- or three-step directions,*
> *see Alternative Administration Protocol section of the manual*
> *for information about continuing the evaluation.*

Recognizes swallowing problems:

   ☑ Good insight ☐ Partial insight ☐ No insight

> *Record the appropriate rating of this item after observing*
> *client's performance during the Feeding Trial portion of*
> *the evaluation.*

Perceptual/Cognitive observations:

   ☑ No deficit ☐ Partial deficit ☐ Severe deficit

Comments: _____

_____

Physical Status

Assistance needed to attain and maintain position:

   ☑ Independent   ☐ Minimal/Moderate assistance

   ☐ Maximal assistance

   Comments: _____

_____

Head and neck control

   Range of motion: ☐ Normal ☑ Impaired

   Manual muscle testing   ☐ Normal ☑ Impaired

   ☐ Nonfunctional for eating

> *If head and neck control is nonfunctional for eating, stop the*
> *evaluation and refer to the Manual for additional information.*

Upper-extremity control

   for self-feeding: ☐ Normal ☑ Impaired

   ☐ Nonfunctional

> *Record rating for upper-extremity control during the feeding trial.*

Comments: *↓ tone R side of neck; needs*
cues to keep head erect; decreased
R UE tone for utensil manipulation

1

Figure 48-3 A completed evaluation for the case example from the *Dysphagia Evaluation Protocol*. (Copyright 1997 by Therapy Skill Builders, a Harcourt Health Sciences Company. Reproduced by permission. All rights reserved.)

(continued)

CLINICAL EVALUATION OF SWALLOWING

Observations

☐ Drooling	☐ Tongue or lip biting
☑ Excessive oral secretions	☐ Tongue thrust
☐ Dry mouth	☐ Oral-motor apraxia
☑ Poor oral hygiene	☐ Excessive coughing (more than twice)
☐ Residual food in the oral cavity	☐ Hoarse or wet voice
☐ Food remnants on the lips	☐ Frequent clearing of throat
☐ Dentures	☑ Other observations: *Dentition intact*

Oral Control

	Tone		ROM		Strength		Sensation		Comments
	Intact	Impaired	Intact	Impaired	Intact	Impaired	Intact	Impaired	
Lips		↓ R		✓		✓	✓		
Cheeks		↓ R		✓		✓	✓		
Jaw	✓		✓		✓		✓		
Tongue		↓ R		✓		✓	✓		

Primitive and Abnormal Reflexes

Jaw jerk	☑ Absent	☐ Present
Rooting	☑ Absent	☐ Present
Sucking	☑ Absent	☐ Present
Bite	☑ Absent	☐ Present

Pharyngeal Control

	Normal	Impaired	Absent	Comments
Soft palate function		✓		
Gag reflex		✓		
Vocal quality			✓	*Unable to phonate 2° vocal cord weakness*
Volitional cough		✓		

2

Figure 48-3 *(Continued).*

FEEDING TRIAL

Appetite/Willingness to Participate

☑ Positive

☐ Neutral

☐ Negative

Consistencies Used: (Description)

☑ Moist, cohesive _Applesauce, pudding_

☐ Soft, chewable _____

☐ Thick liquid _____

☐ Thin liquid _____

☐ Crunchy, chewable _____

Special Tools and Techniques: _Hand over hand guiding to self-feed c̄ (R) hand, use (L) hand to maintain lip closure and massage (R) cheek to prevent pocketing of food in cheek_

Ability to Swallow Without Food Bolus: ☐ Normal   ☑ Impaired   ☐ Absent

Oral Stage

	Normal	Impaired	Absent	Comments
Bolus containment in oral cavity		✓		
Bolus formation		✓		
Bolus propulsion		✓		
Mastication				_not tested_

Pharyngeal Stage

Laryngeal elevation   ☑ Normal   ☐ Impaired   ☐ Absent

Voice quality after swallow   ☐ Normal   ☐ Impaired   ☑ Absent _(was not present pre-swallow)_

Auscultation:

   Audibility of upper esophageal sphincter: ☐ No   ☑ Yes

   Pooling   ☑ No   ☐ Yes

   Comments: _Delay in trigger of pharyngeal swallow response._

Repetitive swallows   ☐ No   ☑ Yes   Number of swallows: _1_

Cough reflex   ☑ No   ☐ Yes

   ☐ Before swallow   ☐ During swallow   ☐ After swallow

Other Observations:

O₂ saturation level remained at 96% before, during and immediately after feeding trial

During the feeding trial, record the patient's recognition of swallowing problems and upper extremity control for self-feeding.

Comments:

Pt is aware of inability to swallow fluids and chewable solids. He required hand over hand assistance to load spoon and bring to mouth. Able to hold a plastic cup with two hands, and bring to mouth.

3

Figure 48-3 *(Continued).*

IMPRESSIONS

Summary

This 80 yo gentleman is s/p CVA c̄ Ⓡ hemiplegia and aphasia. He shows reduced oral tone and control in the Ⓡ tongue and cheek. He is managing soft, formed boluses with extra time for oral manipulation and a slowed swallow response. No pooling or coughing was noted after swallowing. There were no clinical signs of laryngeal penetration or aspiration.

Functional Level (Physical and verbal assistance needed for positioning, hand-to-mouth movements, and swallowing):

Pt was able to self-feed c̄ hand over hand guidance to use utensil, but was able to use cup Ⓘ c̄ 2 hands. He needed supervision to transfer to the wheelchair to eat and verbal cues to prepare his tray to eat.

Intermittent supervision at meals and snacks, as well as assistance to self-feed c̄ Ⓡ hand is recommended.

Recommendations/Plan:

☐ NPO (No food by mouth)

☐ Nutrition consultation: _____

☑ Videofluoroscopy *To assess laryngeal protection c̄ fluids.*

☐ Prefeeding program

☑ Special positioning, Adaptive equipment: *Seated to eat*

☑ Mealtime supervision ☐ Constant ☑ Intermittent ☐ Set-up

☑ Diet recommendation: *Continue c̄ Level I, Aspiration Prevention*

☑ Other: *Short-term goals:*
  ① Advance diet to Level II, including cooked fruit and pasta.
  ② Tolerate soft chewables without s/s aspiration
  ③ Ⓘ use of techniques to maintain lip closure and prevent food pocketing
  ④ Ⓘ vocal cord adduction exercises
  ⑤ Modified Ⓘ self-feeding c̄ equipment and adapted tech.

Figure 48-3 (*Continued*).

Assessment of Cognitive, Perceptual, and Physical Abilities

Important cognitive and perceptual considerations include the level of alertness and arousal, orientation, ability to attend to a feeding session or meal, ability to follow multi-step commands, and any visual deficits or neglect. The clinician notes the patient's insight into his or her dysphagia and observes head, neck, trunk, and

BOX 48-3
SAFETY BOX

Precautions for the Therapist and Patient

The swallowing therapist stays close to the patient during eating and is exposed to oral secretions and respirations. Likewise, the patient is exposed to pathogens on the therapist's clothing and hands and in the therapist's respiratory tract. Universal precautions should be used. The use of gloves is mandatory anytime the therapist touches the face or inside the oral cavity.

Dysphagia patients are prone to difficulty with airway obstruction and aspiration during eating. For the safety of the patient, the swallowing therapist should be trained in suctioning of the airway, the Heimlich maneuver, and cardiopulmonary resuscitation.

Signs and Symptoms of Potential or Actual Aspiration

While laryngeal penetration or aspiration may be silent, occurring without overt warning signs and symptoms, the following indicate that it may occur or be occurring. If observed during a dysphagia evaluation, these signs or symptoms can indicate that a feeding trial should not be initiated or should be discontinued. Specific items of concern (Avery-Smith et al., 1997):

1. The patient cannot remain awake for the clinical evaluation.
2. The oral and/or pharyngeal sensation and motion assessment reveal poor ability to manipulate and contain the bolus.
3. The bolus remains in the mouth, and the patient cannot initiate or complete the oral preparatory stage within a reasonable time.
4. There is excessive coughing or choking before, during, or after swallowing.
5. There is no swallow response once the oral stage is completed.
6. There is a change in voice quality, often wet, or no voice, after swallowing.
7. Severe pooling or wetness is heard on auscultation or by the naked ear; secretions are poorly managed.
8. Silent aspiration is suggested by a change in the patient's color, and/or respiratory rate, increased congestion on auscultation of the chest, and/or a reduction in oxygen level in the blood as recorded by pulse oximetry.

BOX 48-4
PROCEDURES FOR PRACTICE

Preparation for Eating

Prior to the feeding trial portion of an evaluation and snacks or meals, measures must be taken to optimize the patient's swallowing performance. As these strategies do not involve ingestion of food, they are **indirect therapy** techniques.

1. Provide a quiet environment to encourage concentration.
2. Position the patient upright in a chair to minimize the risk of aspiration. The feet should be supported and the arms free for self-feeding. Patients with pseudobulbar dysphagia may need special attention to positioning before eating and special positioning devices; they may need assistance to maintain head and neck alignment and facilitation to stimulate oral and pharyngeal motions prior to and during eating (Fig. 48-4).
3. Complete oral hygiene activities before the trial, as this stimulates sensation and range of motion in oral structures.
4. Present a simplified visual array of food and utensils for the patient with visual neglect and/or other visual deficits. Anchors, colorful cues to call attention to the side of the plate, are helpful for patients with neglect.
5. Present appetizing, culture-specific foods, utensils, and tableware.
6. Provide adaptive equipment and/or use hand-over-hand guiding to facilitate self-feeding.
7. Provide simple explanations and one-step verbal directions if necessary.
8. If the patient eats too quickly or is confused by multiple food choices, present one food at a time.
9. Use small-bowled utensils and verbal or manual assistance to load just a teaspoon-sized bolus. Pinch the straw to limit the amount of liquid consumed or use a covered cup with a small opening.

limb control and endurance for being out of bed at mealtimes. The ability to self-position and self-feed and need for or use of adaptive eating equipment are assessed.

Assessment of Oral and Pharyngeal Abilities

Once direct physical assessment begins, the clinician must observe universal precautions to prevent exposure to pathogens for both the clinician and the patient (Box 48-3). Clinicians begin by assessing oral and pharyngeal control, including tone, range of motion, strength, and sensation of the lips, tongue, jaw, and cheeks and any abnormal oral reflexes. To assess pharyngeal control, the clinician observes soft palate movement, gag reflex, vocal quality and volitional cough. A stethoscope may be used to listen for pooling of fluid above the level of the vocal cords, as pooled liquids resonate during breathing. The clinician rates the patient's hunger and level of enthusiasm for a snack or meal.

The Feeding Trial

Interventions that maximize performance must be initiated before the feeding trial begins (Box 48-4). The safest food textures are chosen for the trial. Easy-to-manage foods and thick fluids are attempted first, especially if the patient has been NPO and/or has a diagnosis or clinical picture that suggests a high risk of aspiration. During the oral stage, the clinician observes bolus containment, formation, propulsion, and mastication. During the pharyngeal stage, the clinician assesses laryngeal elevation, voice quality after swallow, repetitive swallows, and cough reflex. The clinician should observe for signs and symptoms of laryngeal penetration or aspiration, especially during the first feeding trial (Box 48-3). The evaluation concludes with a summary, recommendations, and a plan (Avery-Smith et al., 1992).

Specific techniques are helpful during the feeding trial. Auscultation of the swallow with a stethoscope (Fig. 48-5) can reveal the efficiency and safety of the oral and pharyngeal stages (Zenner et al., 1995). Gentle palpation of the neck (Fig. 48-6) during the swallow reveals symmetry, strength, and speed of oral pharyngeal movement and may be done simultaneous to auscultation. Use of a pulse oximeter, a noninvasive monitoring device that measures the patient's oxygen saturation in the bloodstream, may be effective in assessing whether aspiration or respiratory difficulties are occurring (Sherman et al., 1999). Normal oxygen saturation

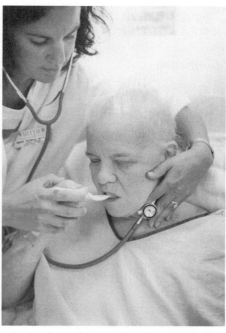

Figure 48-5 Auscultation of the swallow using a stethoscope. The therapist may be able to facilitate head position and guide self-feeding while listening to the sounds of the swallow.

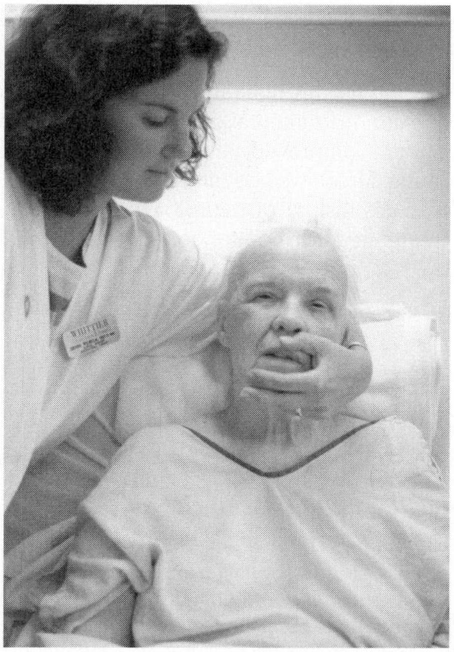

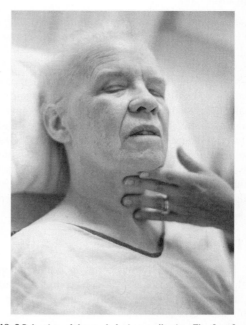

Figure 48-6 Palpation of the neck during swallowing. The first finger is under the chin; The second finger is at the base of the tongue; the third finger is over the thyroid cartilage; the fourth finger is at the base of the throat. A very light touch should be used so as not to inhibit motion.

Figure 48-4 Using the half-nelson position to assist with head and neck control. The therapist can also assist with jaw, cheek, and lip control at the same time.

Case Example

MR. D.: DYSPHAGIA EVALUATION AND TREATMENT FOR A PATIENT WITH LEFT CEREBROVASCULAR ACCIDENT

Patient information

Mr. D. is an 86-year-old man whose medical history includes hypertension, coronary artery disease, peptic ulcer disease, and transient ischemic attacks with aphasia. He was admitted to the hospital with aphasia and right upper extremity weakness. A computed tomography scan was positive for cerebral atrophy consistent with his age and for left hemispheric CVA. A dysphagia evaluation was done in the acute care setting, using the *Dysphagia Evaluation Protocol* (see Resources). The evaluation (Fig. 48-3) revealed that he had hypotonicity and reduced control of his lips, cheek, and tongue on the right side. Decreased airway protection skills were evidenced by his inability to phonate because of vocal cord weakness, inability to cough volitionally, and reduced laryngeal elevation during swallowing. He was not aphasic. Mr. D. was able to swallow beginning-level dysphagia diet foods, including soft, moist textures, such as pudding and applesauce, with mild food spillage out of the mouth due to poor lip control, delayed formation and propulsion of the bolus, and delayed initiation of the swallow. He had difficulty grasping utensils and cups because of hypotonicity of his dominant right hand.

Recommendations

Mr. D. was seen daily for occupational therapy during a week as an inpatient. Constant supervision at mealtime was recommended, and all meals and snacks took place with him upright in the chair. Occupational therapy intervention addressed exercises to enhance tone and control of oral motor skills, laryngeal exercises to strengthen his vocal cords and improve laryngeal elevation, and facilitation of tone and movement in his hypotonic right upper extremity to improve self-feeding skills. The patient and caregiver were informed of the nature of his dysphagia, exercises, and mealtime procedures and precautions. Long-term goals included tolerating a regular diet consisting of a variety of solid and liquid textures and self-feeding with his right arm without adapted equipment or techniques.

Short-Term Goals

- ▶ Mr. D. will tolerate a more advanced dysphagia diet, adding soft chewables such as cooked fruit and soft pasta.
- ▶ Mr. D. will tolerate these textures without clinical signs of aspiration (Box 48-3).
- ▶ Mr. D. will be independent in vocal cord adduction exercises.
- ▶ Mr. D. will support the right side of the lower lip and massage the right cheek during the oral preparatory stage to prevent food spillage and pocketing in the right cheek.

- ▶ Mr. D. will feed himself with his right hand with built-up utensils and an adapted cup while weight bearing on his right elbow.

Mr. D. achieved the short-term goals within a week and was able to add soft chewables and honey-thick fluids to his diet. He and his caregiver were taught to thicken fluids with commercial thickeners at home. As his vocal cord strength returned, his volitional cough became stronger, and he gradually became able to speak in a loud whisper; laryngeal strengthening exercises continued. Mr. D. was able to discontinue use of external lip control strategies as oral motor control returned. He continued use of built-up utensils and weight bearing at the elbow while self-feeding.

Revised Goals

Within a week Mr. D. was discharged from the hospital to home in the company of his full-time caregiver. He continued with outpatient occupational therapy for 4 more weeks. During that time the following long-term goals were accomplished:

- ▶ Mr. D. will tolerate dry cut-up chewable solids and thin liquids without signs or symptoms of aspiration.
- ▶ Mr. D. will eat independently with his right upper extremity without the use of adaptive equipment and without compensatory movements.

Mr. D. could use his right arm in dominant fashion for all other basic and instrumental activities of daily living. His laryngeal strength improved, and he could speak at almost normal volume. Mr. D. was comfortable at this point eating in public. Given his history of neurological events, he and his caregiver continued to monitor for signs and symptoms of aspiration.

CLINICAL REASONING
in OT Practice

Dysphagia Evaluation and Treatment for Stroke Patients

Mr. D., with a left-sided brain lesion, demonstrated impaired oral bolus control due to reduced muscle tone of the oral structures, reduced laryngeal elevation during the swallow, and weakness of the vocal cords as evidenced by the inability to phonate. How would his symptoms be different if he had a right-sided brain lesion? How would his treatment be different?

in the bloodstream falls between 93 and 98%; a level below 92% after swallowing suggests aspiration. If the patient can self-feed, palpation and auscultation may be done simultaneously. If the patient needs help to self-feed, auscultation and guiding with hand-to-mouth efforts may be done simultaneously.

Recommendations and Plan

Once the clinical evaluation is complete, recommendations and a plan are formulated. As seen in Figure 48-3, recommendations may include whether eating by mouth is advisable; whether an instrumental evaluation is advised; whether a nutritional consultation with a dietitian is needed; recommended diet type; mealtime positioning and supervision; adaptive equipment; and type and amount of assistance. Evaluation of the patient is ongoing, and with additional information from clinical observations, instrumental evaluations, and input from other dysphagia team members, the treatment plan and goals change.

Instrumental Evaluation

Clinical assessment goes hand in hand with instrumental evaluation, which uses imaging and diagnostic studies to provide critical information about the unseen parts of the oral, pharyngeal, and esophageal stages of swallowing. Various types of instrumental evaluations for dysphagia are discussed in Box 48-5. These evaluations are usually performed by physicians, often together with a swallowing therapist. Aspiration of food or fluid may be silent (Linden et al., 1993). Imaging studies such as **videofluoroscopy** are needed to identify aspiration (Splaingard et al., 1988). These studies also provide information about the quality of the swallow and the efficacy of compensatory therapy techniques used during swallowing.

Dysphagia Treatment

One consideration in treatment is remedial versus compensatory goals. Remedial treatment focuses on restoring a normal level of swallowing function. Potential for partial or full recovery is anticipated when goals are remedial. Compensatory treatment circumvents a problem with the use of alternative strategies and techniques. Use of these techniques implies either that full recovery is not anticipated or that these techniques are necessary for a safe, functional swallow prior to recovery of normal swallowing. Table 48-1 discusses

---

BOX 48-5
Instrumental Evaluation of Swallowing

Instrumental evaluation uses technology, including the following:

Electromyography
Electrodes are placed either into the muscle via a small needle, or on the skin over a muscle, to record contractions of the muscle. Surface electrodes have been used to assess aspects of oral bolus management in neurological dysphagia patients and pharyngeal, laryngeal, and esophageal activity (Ertekin et al., 1996, 1998).

Fiberoptic Endoscopic Swallowing Study
A fiberoptic laryngoscope, a narrow flexible tube with a small camera on its tip, is introduced through the nose into the nasopharynx, where structures including the palate, pharynx, and larynx are viewed for assessment of anatomy and movement. Food is administered in different consistencies to observe posterior oral and pharyngeal function and airway protection during eating.

Manometry
A catheter with transducers to measure pressure is introduced into the esophagus. The force, timing, and sequence of the esophageal contractions are measured.

Scintigraphy
A radioactive isotope is mixed with food. As the bolus is swallowed, a gamma camera tracks the radioactive particles. This test measures the speed of bolus transit and can accurately measure the amount of bolus that is aspirated.

Ultrasonography
An ultrasound transducer held under the chin produces images of oral and pharyngeal stages of swallow, revealing the mobility of structures and boluses swallowed.

Videofluoroscopy
The patient is seated between a movable camera and a fluorescent screen. Radiographic images of oral, pharyngeal, and esophageal structures are delivered to a television screen from the camera as barium-impregnated fluids and foods are swallowed. The images are recorded on videotape. Figure 48-7 illustrates a videofluoroscopic image of the oral, pharyngeal, and upper esophageal structures. Swallowing pathology and the effectiveness of compensatory swallowing techniques and positions can be observed. The patient may be positioned in a lateral and/or anteroposterior position to view structure and function from both perspectives. Videofluoroscopies are often repeated to assess progress. A swallowing therapist is usually present to ensure that the test reproduces compensatory maneuvers and food textures being used and to ensure that it mimics real eating as accurately as possible. In some instances, the swallowing therapist may perform the videofluoroscopy. Therapists assisting with or performing videofluoroscopies must be expert swallowing clinicians; they must be fully trained in use of the equipment and procedures used in videofluoroscopy.

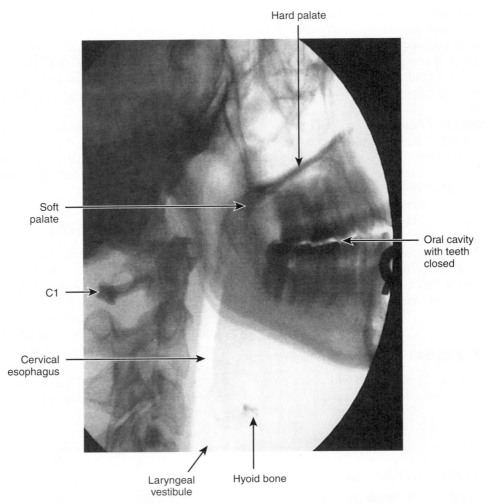

Hard palate

Soft palate

Oral cavity with teeth closed

C1

Cervical esophagus

Laryngeal vestibule

Hyoid bone

Figure 48-7 A videofluoroscopic image of the oral, pharyngeal, and esophageal structures. Videoprint image courtesy of Bette Pomerleau, MS, SLP, and Ray Autiello LPN, RT, of Universal Mobile Services, Haverhill, MA.

compensatory and remedial interventions for specific swallowing deficits. Compensatory swallowing maneuvers and their indications are discussed in Box 48-6. Goals may be remedial, then change to compensatory once a plateau in function is reached.

Another consideration is the type of therapeutic techniques used. Indirect therapy addresses the prerequisite abilities or the capacity to swallow without ingestion of food or liquid. Patients who are at high risk for aspiration often begin with indirect therapy only. Indirect therapy can include range of motion, strengthening, and coordination exercises for weak or hypotonic oral and pharyngeal musculature; strengthening of pharyngeal and laryngeal structures; techniques to reduce or stimulate sensitivity of oral musculature; and techniques to improve the pharyngeal swallowing response. Indirect therapy also involves manipulating the environment to optimize behaviors that affect swallowing (Box 48-4). **Direct therapy** rehabilitates prerequisite abilities or the

capacity to swallow during therapeutic snacks or meals. This entails exercises and/or the use of compensatory swallowing maneuvers that include ingestion of food. Indirect therapy may continue once direct therapy has begun. An individualized treatment plan usually includes a selection of direct and indirect techniques. The complexity of a treatment plan depends on the ability of the patient and/or caregiver to process complex information. Treatment techniques, especially in the pharyngeal stage, where the effect of techniques are unseen, should be evaluated by videofluoroscopy or fiberoptic endoscopy to assess their efficacy.

Progression of Diet With Swallowing Therapy

As indirect therapy begins, a patient may receive all nutrition, hydration, and medication via a nonoral source, such as intravenous or gastrostomy tube feedings. As the patient recovers the ability to swallow

TABLE 48-1
Compensatory and Remedial Interventions for Specific Problems

Patient problem	Compensatory intervention	Remedial intervention
Swallowing apraxia	Provide a natural mealtime setting; enhance self-feeding skills to facilitate oral skills. Provide a variety of boluses to stimulate oral movements (Logemann, 1998).	
Weakness of cheeks, lips	Provide soft solids and thick fluids for easy oral manipulation; place food at back and stronger side of mouth; tilt head toward stronger side; massage cheek to prevent pocketing; hold lips closed; inspect mouth after meals to check for residue.	Use tapping, vibration, and quick stretch to stimulate movement; provide range of motion and stretching exercises progressing to resistive sucking and blowing exercises.
Abnormal oral reflexes	Avoid stimuli that provoke rooting, bite, tongue thrust, sucking, and hyperactive gag. Elicit movements antagonistic to undesirable reflex; for example, encourage mouth opening to weaken bite reflex. Seat patient with body well supported to minimize proximal extensor tone, which can provoke abnormal distal movements and reflexes.	
Facial, intraoral hypersensitivity		Provide systematic desensitization to face and intraoral area. If sensory defensiveness affects whole body, a program of sensory diet, graded sensory stimulation to body, should precede stimulation to oral area, followed by careful introduction of food. Use systematic desensitization with guided imagery to reduce muscle tone and anxiety regarding eating and mouth (Brown et al., 1992).
Oral hyposensitivity	Place bolus on more sensitive areas of mouth; use warmer or colder bolus and flavorful food to stimulate sensation (Logemann, 1998). Use heavy or viscous boluses.	Sensory diet providing heightened tactile and proprioceptive input to intraoral structures may stimulate sensation and movement before and during a meal or snack.
Reduced lingual control	Introduce diet requiring little oral manipulation, including soft solids and thick fluids; use posterior and/or lateral placement of food on stronger side; inspect mouth for residue after meals.	Introduce active and passive tongue range of motion exercises, activities; provide quick stretch to tongue with tongue depressor or gloved fingers; provide articulation exercises.
Slow oral transit time	Use cold boluses to hasten oral transit time; take care in case they melt into a difficult-to-manage liquid. Sour boluses, such as those infused with lemon juice, can speed oral manipulation (Logemann et al., 1995).	
Delayed swallow	Use a sour bolus to reduce swallow delay (Logemann et al., 1995). Try chin tuck to enhance airway protection; increase bolus volume and viscosity to reduce pharyngeal delay time (Bisch et al., 1994).	Try thermal-tactile stimulation: stroke anterior faucial arches with iced laryngeal mirror (Fig. 48-8); hastens initiation and overall speed of swallow immediately after application (Rosenbek et al., 1996).
Reduced laryngeal elevation	Use Mendelson maneuver to prolong laryngeal elevation or chin tuck to elevate larynx; use supraglottic or super supraglottic swallow to clear or minimize any material in airway (Logemann, 1998).	
Reduced laryngeal closure	Use supraglottic or super supraglottic swallow to enhance airway protection (Logemann, 1998) or chin tuck to elevate and close off larynx.	Introduce vocal cord adduction exercises (Logemann, 1998).
Tracheostomy	Occlusion of tracheostomy tube minimizes aspiration, improves swallow biomechanics (Logemann et al., 1998); use of one-way speaking valve can decrease frequency of aspiration (Dettelbach et al., 1995). Chin tuck may be useful.	

The swallowing therapist typically has to try several interventions, preferably with the assistance of videofluoroscopy, to assess which techniques work most effectively. Clinicians should work under the guidance of an experienced therapist when using a technique that is new to them.

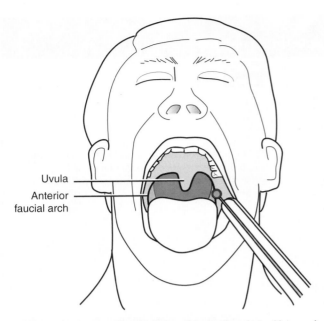

Uvula
Anterior
faucial arch

Figure 48-8 Thermal-tactile stimulation of the swallow. An iced laryngeal mirror is used to stroke the faucial arches to elicit or improve strength of the swallowing reflex. Adapted with permission from: Logemann, J. A. (1998). *Evaluation and Treatment of Swallowing Disorders* (2nd ed.). Austin, TX: Pro-Ed.

without laryngeal penetration or aspiration, direct therapy with the clinician present begins during snacks and progresses to meals. As improvement continues and the patient learns compensatory techniques, he or she may progress to eating under the supervision of nursing personnel and trained significant others, then progress to eating independently. Calorie counts are initiated by the dietitian to assess the adequacy of oral intake. Once food intake improves and calories are consistently sufficient, nonoral feeding sources may be used only for hydration and/or medication. Finally, as the patient improves and fluids and medications are safely ingested by mouth, the use of nonoral feeding sources can be discontinued. Diet textures are upgraded as skills develop. Depending on the diagnosis and potential for recovery, patients may level off at any point in the described progression.

Dysphagia Diets

Dysphagia diets are designed to provide stepwise gradation of food and fluid textures that are matched to the patient's improving oral and pharyngeal skills. Groher (1987) found that a diet of mechanical soft foods that form a cohesive bolus and thickened fluids significantly

---

BOX 48-6
PROCEDURES FOR PRACTICE

Compensatory Swallowing Maneuvers: Their Purpose and Execution

These techniques are ways to use volitional movement to improve the quality of the pharyngeal swallow. As most of them are complex, they require a good attention span and the ability to follow complex directions on the part of the patient.

Maneuver	Purpose	Execution
Chin tuck	Moves base of tongue back; narrows opening to larynx, protecting airway; helps protect airway when larynx is low and swallow is delayed (Ohmae et al., 1996; Welch et al., 1993).	Tuck chin down toward chest while swallowing.
Effortful swallow	Helps to elevate base of tongue (Pouderoux & Kahrilas, 1995).	Squeeze hard with throat muscles while swallowing.
Mendelsohn maneuver	Prolongs opening of UES when larynx is low (Logemann, 1998).	Push tongue into roof of mouth; try to keep Adam's apple up while swallowing.
Neck rotation	Closes weaker side of pharynx; uses stronger intact musculature in cases of unilateral weakness of pharynx and/or vocal folds (Logemann et al., 1989).	Turn head to the weaker side while swallowing.
Supraglottic swallow	Compensates for weak vocal cord closure, reduces penetration of food into larynx during swallow by closing vocal cords (Ohmae et al., 1996).	Swallow while holding breath; then cough. Volitional cough after swallow helps to ensure that anything in airway returns to pharynx to be reswallowed.
Super supraglottic swallow	Reduces penetration of food into larynx during swallow by narrowing opening to airway (Ohmae et al., 1996).	Hold breath and bear down; maintain breath-hold, keep bearing down while swallowing; cough after swallowing.

reduced the incidence of aspiration in a group of patients with pseudobulbar dysphagia, compared with pureed food and thin fluids. Most dysphagia diets follow this progression:

1. Thick purees, such as pudding and applesauce
2. Very soft moist chewables, such as soft cooked vegetables, fruits, and soft pastas
3. Drier chewables, such as cookies and breads
4. Foods requiring biting, firmer chewables such as meats, and mixed textures like cereals and milk, pills and water

The progression of fluids advances thus:

1. No fluids at all
2. Honey-thick fluids
3. Nectar-thick fluids
4. Thin, flavored fluids
5. Water

Fluids are easily thickened with commercial thickeners, which can be mixed with hot or cold beverages.

Patient and Caregiver Training

While the occupational therapist alone may carry out aspects of treatment, the plan for treatment also includes education of the patient, nursing staff, and caregivers. The patient and family should understand the cause of and prognosis for the patient's dysphagia and the importance of direct and indirect strategies to be carried out at home. It may be helpful to have the patient view the videofluoroscopy or fiberoptic endoscopy to clarify his or her condition and the benefits of compensatory techniques. Mealtime positioning, adaptive equipment, and the type and amount of assistance must be taught to caregivers. Meal preparation practice and community outings can reinforce diet modifications, enhance patient and family education in various settings, and motivate the patient.

Efficacy of Dysphagia Treatment

Numerous studies cite the efficacy of dysphagia treatment in both acute and chronic populations with a variety of diagnostic cohorts. Odderson et al. (1995) found that early management of dysphagia in the acute care setting prevents incidents of aspiration and is cost-effective. Dysphagia intervention has been shown to be effective for patients with traumatic brain injury (Shurr et al., 1999), acute neurogenic dysphagia (Bartolome et al., 1997), chronic dysphagia following brainstem lesions (Huckabee & Cannito, 1999), head and neck cancer (Dejonckere & Hordijk, 1998), and for the pro-

foundly mentally retarded CP population (Helfrich-Miller et al., 1986). Examples of proven therapeutic techniques to manage dysphagia are presented earlier in the chapter.

As the emphasis on evidence-based medicine and rehabilitation advances, clinicians must keep abreast of new knowledge. Useful resources on dysphagia care for both beginning and advanced level swallowing therapists are noted under Resources. I encourage the reader to explore further learning and expertise in dysphagia care. In many facilities, problem-oriented rehabilitation team goals are supplanting discipline-specific goals to target improvement of specific abilities that pose barriers to discharge, creating a need for occupational therapists versed in dysphagia management. Also, early discharge from acute care and rehabilitation hospitals and minimized staffing in skilled nursing facilities create situations in which competence in dysphagia intervention has become a mandatory skill for occupational therapy practitioners. Occupational therapists, with their background in the many abilities and capacities that influence eating and swallowing, make logical primary swallowing therapists.

Summary Review Questions

1. What are the stages of swallowing, and what events occur during each stage? Which stage or stages are most amenable to therapeutic intervention, and why?
2. What is aspiration, and what are its warning signs and symptoms?
3. Outline the three types of dysphagia; compare the specific dysphagia symptoms of selected diagnoses with the typical manifestations of the appropriate category: paralytic, pseudobulbar, and mechanical dysphagia.
4. Which components of a thorough dysphagia evaluation are most accurately completed with a patient who can follow multiple-step commands? How would you alter bedside evaluation for patients with various cognitive and perceptual deficits?
5. What are the instrumental evaluations for dysphagia, and how does the information that each provides assist in dysphagia rehabilitation?
6. What recommendations should a dysphagia evaluation provide?
7. Define compensatory and remedial and direct and indirect dysphagia treatments and provide examples of each for specific diagnoses.

Acknowledgments

I thank my husband, Scott R. Smith, for his invaluable assistance with the writing of this chapter, and Denise Jules Wilhelm, OTR, for her assistance with photographs used in this chapter. Thanks also to Bette Pomerleau, MS, SLP, and Ray Autiello, LPN, RT, of Universal Mobile Services in Haverhill, Massachusetts, for their assistance with the videofluoroscopic image reproduced in this chapter.

Resources

American Dietetic Association · *Practice Guidelines for Dysphagia*. Book on dysphagia screening and diets, patient education, and discharge planning. The ADA's Task Force on Dietetics in Physical Medicine and Rehabilitation is developing a publication on a national dysphagia diet to standardize dysphagia diets throughout the U. S. 800-877-1600. http://www.eatright.org

Dysphagia Resource Center
Dysphagia.com
Web site provides information and links on anatomy and physiology pertinent to dysphagia, organizations, print materials, case studies, research information, and funding. Information for clinicians and lay persons.

Dysphagia Evaluation Protocol · Assessment of dysphagia in adults developed by occupational therapists and tested for reliability and validity. Chartable record form and easy-to-use flip book format. Therapy Skill Builders. 800-211-8378.

Dysphagia Research Society · Houston, TX.
http://www.uiuc.edu/drs/

Dysphagia · Official journal of the Dysphagia Research Society. Springer-Verlag. 713-965-0566.
http://www.springer.de/
Peer-reviewed journal devoted to publication of scholarly articles about dysphagia. Abstracts and subscription information available on line. Subscription information by telephone.

References

American Occupational Therapy Association (2000). Specialized knowledge and skills for eating and feeding in occupational therapy practice. *American Journal of Occupational Therapy, 54*, 629–640.

Avery-Smith, W. (1998). An occupational therapist-coordinated dysphagia program. *OT Practice, 3*, 20–23.

Avery-Smith, W., Rosen, A. B., & Dellarosa, D. (1992). Clinical assessment of dysphagia in adults. *Occupational Therapy Practice, 3*, 51–58.

Avery-Smith, W., Rosen, A. B., & Dellarosa, D. (1997). *Dysphagia Evaluation Protocol*. San Antonio, TX: Therapy Skill Builders.

Aviv, J. E., Martin, J. H., Sacco, R. L., Zagar, D., Diamond, B., Keen, M. S., & Blitzer, A. B. (1996). Supraglottic and pharyngeal sensory abnormalities in stroke patients with dysphagia. *Annals of Otology, Rhinology and Laryngology, 105*, 92–97.

Bartolome, M., Prosiegal, M., & Yassouridis, A. (1997). Long-term functional outcome in patients with neurogenic dysphagia. *Neurorehabilitation, 9*, 195–204.

Bisch, E. M., Logemann, J. A., Rademaker, A. A. W., Kahrilas, P. J., & Lazarus, C. L. (1994). Pharyngeal effects of bolus volume, viscosity, and temperature in patients with dysphagia resulting from neurologic impairment and in normal subjects. *Journal of Speech and Hearing Research, 37*, 1041–1059.

Brown, G. E., Nordloh, S., & Donowitz, A. J. (1992). Systematic desensitization of oral hypersensitivity in a patient with a closed head injury. *Dysphagia, 7*, 138–141.

Cherney, L. R. (1994). Dysphagia in adults with neurologic disorders: An overview. In: L. R. Cherney (Ed.), *Clinical Management of Dysphagia in Adults and Children*. Gaithersburg, MD: Aspen.

Dejonckere, P. H., & Hordijk, G. K. (1998) Prognostic factors for swallowing after treatment of head and neck cancer. *Clinical Otolaryngology, 23*, 218–223.

Dettelbach, M. A., Gross, R. D., Mahlmann, J., & Eibling, D. E. (1995). Effect of the Passy-Muir valve on aspiration in patients with tracheostomy. *Head and Neck, 17*, 297–302.

Devita, M. A., & Spierer-Rundback, L. (1990). Swallowing disorders in patients with prolonged orotracheal intubation or tracheostomy tubes. *Critical Care Medicine, 18*, 1328–1330.

Eckberg, O., & Feinberg, M. (1992). Clinical and demographic data in 75 patients with near-fatal choking episodes. *Dysphagia, 7*, 205–208.

Elpern, E. H., Scott, M. G., Petro, L., & Ries, M. H. (1994). Pulmonary aspiration in mechanically ventilated patients with tracheostomies. *Chest, 105*, 563–566.

Ertekin, C., Aydogdu, I., & Yuceyar, N., (1996). Piecemeal deglutition and dysphagia limit in normal subjects and in patients with swallowing disorders. *Journal of Neurology and Neurosurgery, 61*, 491–496.

Ertekin, C., Aydogdu, I., Yuceyar, N., Tarlaci, S., Kiylioglu, N., Pehlivan, M., & Celebi, G. (1998). Electrodiagnostic methods for neurogenic dysphagia. *Electroencephalography and Clinical Neurophysiology, 109*, 331–340.

Finestone, H. M., Greene-Finestone, L. S., Wilson, E. S., & Teasell, R. W. (1995). Malnutrition in stroke patients on the rehabilitation service and at followup: Prevalence and predictors. *Archives of Physical Medicine and Rehabilitation, 76*, 310–316.

Fioretti, A., Giacotto, L., & Melega, V. (1997). Choking incidents among psychiatric patients: Retrospective analysis of thirty-one cases from the west Bologna psychiatric wards. *Canadian Journal of Psychiatry, 42*, 515–520.

Garber, B. G., Hebert, P. C., Yelle, J. D., Hodder, R. V., & McGowan, J. (1996). Adult respiratory distress syndrome: A systemic overview of incidence and risk factors. *Critical Care Medicine, 24*, 555–556.

Groher, M. E. (1987). Bolus management and aspiration pneumonia in patients with pseudobulbar dysphagia. *Dysphagia, 1*, 215–216.

Groher, M. E. (1997). *Dysphagia: Diagnosis and Management* (3rd ed). Boston: Butterworth-Heinemann.

Groher, M. E., & Bukatman, R. (1986). Prevalence of dysphagia in two teaching hospitals. *Dysphagia, 1*, 3–5.

Helfrich-Miller, K. R., Rector, K. L., & Straka, J. A. (1986). Dysphagia: Its treatment in the profoundly retarded patient with cerebral palsy. *Archives of Physical Medicine and Rehabilitation, 67*, 520–525.

Hiiemae, K., Heath, M. R., Heath, G., Kazazoglu, E., Murrary, J., Snapper, D., & Hamblett, K. (1996). Natural bites, food consistency and feeding behaviour in man. *Archives of Oral Biology, 41*, 175–189.

Horner, J., Alberts, M. J., Dawson, D. V., & Cook, G. M. (1994). Swallowing in Alzheimer's disease. *Alzheimer Disease and Associated Disorders, 8*, 177–189.

Horner, J., Buoyer, F. G., Alberts, M. J., & Helms, M. J. (1991). Dysphagia following brainstem stroke. *Archives of Neurology, 48*, 1170–1173.

Huckabee, M. L., & Cannito, M. P. Outcomes of swallowing rehabilitation in chronic brainstem dysphagia: A retrospective evaluation. *Dysphagia, 14*, 93–109.

Lazarus, C. L. (1995). Conference notes from *Dysphagia Symposium: Management of Swallowing Disorders in the Medical Setting*. North Shore Medical Center, Salem, MA.

Lazarus, C. L., Logemann, J. A., Pauloski, B. R., Colangelo, L. A., Kahrilas, P. J., Mittal, B. B., & Pierce, M. (1996). Swallowing disorders in head and neck cancer patients treated with radiotherapy and adjuvant chemotherapy. *Laryngoscope, 106*, 1157–1166.

Leopold, N. A., & Kagel, M. C. (1996). Prepharyngeal dysphagia in Parkinson's disease. *Dysphagia, 11*, 14–22.

Leopold, N. A., & Kagel, M. C. (1997). Pharyngo-esophageal dysphagia in Parkinson's disease. *Dysphagia, 12*, 11–20.

Linden, P., Kuhlemeier, K. V., & Patterson, C. (1993). The probability of correctly predicting subglottic penetration from clinical observations. *Dysphagia, 8*, 170–179.

Logemann, J. A. (1998). *Evaluation and Treatment of Swallowing Disorders*. Austin: Pro-Ed.

Logemann, J. A., Pepe, J., Mackay, L. E. (1994). Disorders of nutrition and swallowing: Intervention strategies in the trauma center. *Journal of Head Trauma Rehabilitation, 9*, 43–56.

Logemann, J. A., Kahrilas, P. J., Kobara, M., & Vakil, N. B. (1989). The benefit of head rotation on pharyngoesophageal dysphagia. *Archives of Physical Medicine and Rehabilitation, 70*, 767–771.

Logemann, J. A., Pauloski, B. R., & Colangelo, L. (1998). Light digital occlusion of the tracheostomy tube: A pilot study of effects on aspiration and biomechanics of the swallow. *Head and Neck, 20*, 52–57.

Logemann, J. A., Pauloski, B. R., Colangelo, L., Lazarus, C., & Fujui, M. (1995). Effects of sour bolus on oropharyngeal swallowing measures in patients with neurogenic dysphagia. *Journal of Speech and Hearing Research, 38*, 556–563.

Mackay, L. E., Morgan, A. S., & Bernstein, B. A. (1999). Swallowing disorders in severe brain injury: Risk factors affecting return to oral intake. *Archives of Physical Medicine and Rehabilitation, 80*, 365–371.

McConnel, F. M. S., & O'Connor, A. (1994). Dysphagia secondary to head and neck cancer surgery. *Acta Oto-Rhino-Laryngologica Belgica, 48*, 165–170.

Musson, N. D., Kincaid, J., Ryan, P., Glussman, B., Varone, L., Gamarra, N., Wilson, R., Reefe, W., & Silverman, M. (1990). Nature, nurture, nutrition: Interdisciplinary programs to address the prevention of malnutrition and dehydration. *Dysphagia, 5*, 96–101.

Nagaya, M., Kachi, T., Yamada, T., & Igata, A. (1998). Videofluorographic study of swallowing in Parkinson's disease. *Dysphagia, 13*, 95–100.

Odderson, I. R., Keaton, J. C., & McKenna, B. S. (1995). Swallow management in patients on an acute stroke pathway: Quality is cost effective. *Archives of Physical Medicine and Rehabilitation, 76*, 1130–1133.

Ohmae, Y., Logemann, J. A., Kaiser, P., Hanson, D. G., & Kahrilas, P. J. (1996). Effects of two breath-holding maneuvers on oropharyngeal swallow. *Annals of Otology, Rhinology, & Laryngology, 105*, 123–131.

Pauloski, B. R., Rademaker, A. W., Logemann, J. A., & Colangelo, L. A. (1998). Speech and swallowing in irradiated and nonirradiated postsurgical oral cancer patients. *Otolaryngology—Head and Neck Surgery, 118*, 616–614.

Pouderoux, P., & Kahrilas, P. J. (1995). Deglutitive tongue force modulation by volition, volume, and viscosity in humans. *Gastroenterology, 108*, 1418–1426.

Priefer, B. A., & Robbins, J. (1997). Eating changes in mild-stage Alzheimer's disease: A pilot study. *Dysphagia, 12*, 212–221.

Robbins, J., Levine, R. L., Maser, A., Rosenbek, J. C., & Kempster, G. B. (1993). Swallowing after unilateral stroke of the cerebral cortex. *Archives of Physical Medicine and Rehabilitation, 74*, 1295–1300.

Rogers, B., Stratton, P., Msall, M., Andres, M., Champlain, M. K., Koerner, P., & Piazza, J. (1994). Long-term morbidity and management strategies of tracheal aspiration in adults with severe developmental disabilities. *American Journal of Mental Retardation, 98*, 490–498.

Rosenbek, J. C., Roecher, E. B., Wood, J. L., & Robbins, J. (1996). Thermal application reduces the duration of stage transition in dysphagia after stroke. *Dysphagia, 11*, 225–233.

Schmidt, J., Holas, M., Halvorson, K., & Reding, M. (1994). Videofluoroscopic evidence of aspiration predicts pneumonia and death but not dehydration following stroke. *Dysphagia, 9*, 7–11.

Shaker, R., Milbrath, M., Ren, J., Campbell, B., Toohill, R., & Hogan, W. (1995). Deglutitive aspiration in patients with tracheostomy: Effect of tracheostomy on the duration of vocal cord closure. *Gastroenterology, 108*, 1357–1360.

Sherman, B., Nisenboum, J. M., Jesberger, B. L., Morrow, C. A., Jesberger, J. A. (1999). Assessment of dysphagia with the use of pulse oximetry. *Dysphagia, 14*, 152–156.

Shurr, M. J., Ebner, K. A., Maser, A. L., Sperling, K. B., Helgerson, R. B., & Harms, B. (1999). Formal swallowing evaluation and therapy after traumatic brain injury improves dysphagia outcomes. *Journal of Trauma, 46*, 817–821.

Siebens, H., Trupe, E., & Siebens A. A. (1986). Correlates and consequences of eating dependency in institutionalized elderly. *Journal of the American Geriatrics Society 34*, 192–198.

Sokoloff, L. G., & Pavlakovic, R. (1997). Neuroleptic-induced dysphagia. *Dysphagia, 12*, 177–179.

Splaingard, M. L., Hutchins, B., Sulton, L. D., Chaudhuri, G. (1988). Aspiration in rehabilitation patients: Videofluoroscopy vs. bedside clinical assessment. *Archives of Physical Medicine and Rehabilitation, 69*, 637–640.

Thomas, F. J., & Wiles, C. M. (1999). Dysphagia and nutritional status in multiple sclerosis. *Neurology, 246*, 677–682.

Tolep, K., Getch, C. L., & Criner, G. J. (1996). Swallowing dysfunction in patients receiving prolonged mechanical ventilation. *Chest, 109*, 167–172.

Tracy, J., Logemann, J., Kahrilas, P., Jacob, P., Kobara, M., & Krugler, C. (1989). Preliminary observations on the effects of age on oropharyngeal deglutition. *Dysphagia, 4*, 90–94.

Welch, M. V., Logemann, J. A., Rademaker, A. W., & Kahrilas, P. J. (1993). Changes in pharyngeal dimensions effected by chin tuck. *Archives of Physical Medicine and Rehabilitation, 74*, 178–181.

Zenner, P. M., Losinski, D. S., & Mills, R. H. (1995). Using cervical auscultation in the clinical dysphagia examination in long term care. *Dysphagia, 10*, 27–31.

Index

Page numbers followed by an "f" denote figures; those followed by a "t" denote tables.

Radio frequency (RF)
assistive technology control technologies, 393
definition, 390
Raimiste's phenomenon, in Brunnstrom Movement Therapy approach, 546
Rancho Los Amigos Levels of Cognitive Functioning Scale, in traumatic brain injury (TBI) assessment, 860–861t
Random access memory (RAM), computer, definition, 402f
Random practice, 495
definition, 482, 630
in learning, 632
in Occupational Therapy Task-Oriented Approach, 495
Range of motion
active (*See* Active range of motion)
in activity analysis, 264
in amputations, 1050
assessment of, 387f, 397–398
in burn injuries, 1033
compensatory strategies, 635f, 643–647
basic activities of daily living, 643–646
bathing, 645–646
dressing, 644–645, 645f
gardening, 646
grooming, 643–644
instrumental activities of daily living, 646–647
opening containers, 646
sexual activity, 646–647
shopping, 646
telephoning, 646
toileting, 644
in fractures assessment, 913–914
in hand therapy assessment, 932
measurement, 48–82
case example, 50–51
elbow, flexion-extension, 62, 62f
forearm
pronation, 64, 64f
supination, 63, 63f
goniometer use, 49, 51, 51f
interpretation of results, 81
recording, 52, 53f
reliability, 49, 51–52
shoulder
abduction, 56, 56f
extension, 55, 55f
external rotation, 60, 60f, 61, 61f
flexion, 54, 54f
horizontal abduction, 57, 57f
horizontal adduction, 58, 58f
internal rotation, 59, 59f, 61, 61f
thumb
abduction, 73, 73f
carpometacarpal extension, 70, 70f

carpometacarpal flexion, 69, 69f
interphalangeal flexion and extension, 72, 72f
metacarpophalangeal flexion and extension, 71, 71f
opposition, 73, 73f
upper extremity, 54–80
wrist
extension, 66, 66f
flexion, 65, 65f
radial deviation, 68, 68f
ulnar deviation, 67, 67f
passive (*See* Passive range of motion)
in rheumatoid arthritis, 1005, 1011
treatment methods, 468–470, 471–472
positioning, 469
stretch
active, 471
passive, 472
Rao Cognitive Screen for MS, for multiple sclerosis assessment, 891
Rapid Estimate of Adult Literacy in Medicine (REALM), assessment of literacy, 218f–219f
Rapport (*See* Therapeutic rapport)
Ratings of perceived exertion (RPE), 133–134
Reaching
body mechanics for, 923
treatment, 513, 515, 517t
Readily Achievable Checklist, physical environment assessment, 249
Reading, compensatory strategies
muscle weakness, 640–641
visual impairment, 656
Reasonable accommodation
accessibility and, 237–238, 788
definition, 236, 784
Reasoning, 201
clinical (*See also* Clinical Reasoning), 445
as cognitive capacity, 201
conditional, 217
defined, 198
Rebif, for multiple sclerosis, 889
Recent memory, 200f
Reconstructive surgery, in burn injuries, 1037–1039
Recreation (*See also* Leisure)
definition, 746
in leisure, 746
Rectus femoris muscle, strength testing, 125, 125f
Reeducation
muscle, 567–568, 567f
sensory (*See* Sensory reeducation)
Referred pain
definition, 422
physical agent modalities for, 424
Reflex-hierarchical model, of motor control, 140–142, 140f
knowledge of results (KR), 141
long-term memory, 140–141

motivation, 140
program development, 141
program execution, 141
Reflex hyperexcitability, definition, 577
Reflex-inhibiting pattern (RIP), 525, 531–532, 532f
definition, 522
Reflex model, of motor control, 138–139
Reflexes
brain stem, 546f, 547
tonic, 545
Rehabilitation
definition, 18
development of occupational therapy and, 23–24
Rehabilitation Accreditation Commission (CARF)
definition, 444
documentation and, 446
Rehabilitation Act of 1973, 785
Rehabilitative approach, in Occupational Functioning Model, 13–14
Reintegration to Normal Living Index (RNL), 35
Relaxation response, definition, 762
Reliability, 49, 51–52, 240
Box and Block Test, 934–935
computation of, 933, 933f
definition, 32, 48, 49, 168, 236
Minnesota Rate of Manipulation test, 933
of measurement, 33
sensory, 168, 170–171
Purdue Pegboard Test, 935–936
TEMPA, 937
Remedial therapy, 452–453, 611–613, 611t
for cognition, 611–613, 611t
effectiveness of, 612–613
graded cognitive exercises, 611–612
effectiveness of, 612–613
graded cognitive exercises, 611–612
Remote memory, 200f
Repetition maximum (RM), in muscle strengthening, 473
Repetitive strain injury (*See* Tendinitis)
Residential community reintegration programs, for traumatic brain injury, 875
Residential neurobehavioral programs, for traumatic brain injury, 875
Respiration, 1082
in chronic obstructive pulmonary disease, 1083, 1085t
in spinal cord injury, 969
Resting splint
case example, 341, 343f
construction, 360f–362f
wrist, 341, 343f
Retribution, definition, 762
Retrieval
definition, 284
in learning, 284